Watson's
Clinical Nursing and Related Sciences

Senior Commissioning Editor: Ninette Premdas
Project Manager: Andrew Palfreyman
Design Direction: Erik Bigland
Illustrations Manager: Merlyn Harvey
Illustrator: Antbits

Watson's
Clinical Nursing and Related Sciences

Seventh edition

Edited by

Mike Walsh PhD BA PGCE RGN DipN A&ECert
Reader in Nursing, St Martin's College, Carlisle, UK

Alison Crumbie RGN DipAppScN BSc MSN NP
PGCE DoctorateNSc
Nurse Practitioner, Windermere and Bowness Medical Practice, Cumbria, UK

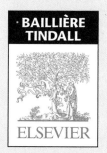

BAILLIÈRE TINDALL

ELSEVIER

Edinburgh London New York Oxford Philadelphia St Louis Sydney Toronto 2007

BAILLIÈRE
TINDALL
ELSEVIER

First edition 1972
Second edition 1979
Third edition 1987
Fourth edition 1992
Fifth edition 1997
Sixth edition 2002
Seventh edition 2007

ISBN: 978 0 7020 2825 0
IE ISBN: 978 0 7020 2826 7

British Library Cataloguing in Publication Data
A catalogue record for this book is available from the British Library

Library of Congress Cataloging in Publication Data
A catalog record for this book is available from the Library of Congress

Note
Knowledge and best practice in this field are constantly changing. As new research and
experience broaden our knowledge, changes in practice, treatment and drug therapy may
become necessary or appropriate. Readers are advised to check the most current
information provided (i) on procedures featured or (ii) by the manufacturer of each
product to be administered, to verify the recommended dose or formula, the method and
duration of administration, and contraindications. It is the responsibility of the
practitioner, relying on their own experience and knowledge of the patient, to make
diagnoses, to determine dosages and the best treatment for each individual patient, and to
take all appropriate safety precautions. To the fullest extent of the law, neither the
Publisher nor the Editors assume any liability for any injury and/or damage to persons or
property arising out of or related to any use of the material contained in this book.

The Publisher

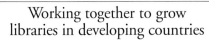

Working together to grow
libraries in developing countries

www.elsevier.com | www.bookaid.org | www.sabre.org

ELSEVIER   BOOK AID International   Sabre Foundation

  your source for books,
journals and multimedia
in the health sciences

www.elsevierhealth.com

The
publisher's
policy is to use
**paper manufactured
from sustainable forests**

Printed in China

Contents

Contributors

Margaret Abbott RGN BA(Hons) PGCE NDN CertCPT
(Chapter 7)
Senior Lecturer, Department of Nursing and Midwifery, St Martins College, Lancaster, UK

Mark Edward Collier BA(Hons) RN ONC RCNT RNT V3000
(Chapter 25)
Lead Nurse Consultant – Tissue Viability, United Lincolnshire Hospitals NHS Trust, c/o Pilgrim Hospital, Boston, Lincolnshire, UK

Alison Crumbie RGN DipAppScN BSc MSN NP PGCE DoctorateNSc
(Chapters 1, 3 ,4, 5, 12, 15, 19)
Nurse Practitioner, Windermere and Bowness Medical Practice, Cumbria, UK

Wendy Fairhurst-Winstanley BA(Hons) RGN, PGCE, MScClinicalNursing
(Chapters 13, 18)
Nurse Practitioner/Partner, Marus Bridge Practice, Wigan, UK

Lesley Kyle BA MSc RCN Nurse Practitioner Award DN SCM RGN
(Chapter 23)
Nurse Practitioner/Nurse Partner, Esk Valley General Practice, Canonbie, UK

Helen L. Leathard BSc PhD FBPharmacolS MA
(Chapter 6)
Professor of Healing Science and Pharmacology, Faculty of Health and Social Care; Director of St Martin's College Graduate School, St Martin's College, Lancaster, UK

Sue Lee RGN BA(Hons) MSc ENB 998 &100 FETC
(Chapters 16, 17)
Associate Head of Department of Nursing Studies, St Martin's College, Lancaster, UK

Claire Mavin MSc BSc (Hons) PGCE RGN ENB 148
(Chapter 20)
Practice Development Sister, Institute of Neurological Sciences, Southern General Hospital, Glasgow, UK

Miriam K. Rowswell MSc BSc(Hons) RGN DipN OncCert
(Chapter 11)
Macmillan Lead Nurse – Cancer Services, Portsmouth Hospitals NHS Trust, Portsmouth, UK

Susan Skinner MAEd BA SRN SCM ENB 904 RCNT DipNurseEd
(Chapter 10)
Senior Lecturer, Neonatal Health, Anglia Ruskin University, Chelmsford, UK

Veronica Thomas PhD BSc RGN DipN PGDipCouns PGDipCBT Cpsychol
(Chapter 8)
Consultant Health Psychologist, Department of Haematology, Guy's and St Thomas' NHS Foundation Trust, London; Senior Lecturer, Department of Psychology, Institute of Psychiatry, King's College London University, London, UK

Mike Walsh PhD RGN BA(Hons) DipN(London) A&Ecert(Oxford) PGCE
(Chapters 1, 2, 9, 19, 21, 22, 24, 26)
Reader in Nursing, St Martin's College, Lancaster, UK

Audrey Yandle MSc BA PGCEA RN
(Chapter 14)
Lecturer, Florence Nightingale School of Nursing & Midwifery, King's College, London, UK

Preface

Welcome to this new edition of what has been for many years a standard nursing textbook for pre registration nurses. If you look at the last edition, you will notice a new name has appeared on the cover of this book. Alison Crumbie, a very experienced nurse practitioner, has joined me in co-editing this 7th edition. Since the 6th edition many things have changed in health care and therefore Alison's involvement is an important step in the development of this book. Let me explain further.

Health care in many countries is moving increasingly towards a primary care focus and Alison's role as a nurse practitioner in primary care ensures she brings precisely that perspective to this book. Nurses are expanding their role in many directions including enhanced health assessment. Alison brings her nurse practitioner expertise to bear on this crucial aspect of nursing and between us we have pushed the realm of nursing assessment beyond what you would normally find in a conventional pre-registration textbook. A further key development has been that of non-medical prescribing and we have brought our collective expertise to bear on this exciting area of practice.

No preface would be complete without looking at the impact of technology on health and we have reflected this by our development of extra learning resources associated with this book, which are accessible on the Elsevier Evolve Website. Go there and you will find myself narrating power point summaries and extra diagrams which underpin the basic anatomy and physiology needed to support this book. Add to that a mix of case studies contributed by Alison, and you will have plenty of supplementary material which takes the traditional printed page into new territory.

As a result we feel this book will not only equip you with the knowledge you need but also get you used to a new way of thinking about patient care that is going to be increasingly important for the future. You need to think primary care, you need to think assessment and you need to think decision making. Above all, you need to realise the implications of the increased levels of accountability and autonomy for you as a registered nurse. May you enjoy your nursing career as much as I have.

Mike Walsh
Cumbria
2007

Getting the best from *Evolve* and this book

When you buy a copy of this book you gain access to the Elsevier *Evolve* website containing a series of case studies and narrated PowerPoint presentations as an extra learning resource. The PowerPoint presentations summarise the basic anatomy and physiology of the main body systems and will help to underpin your nursing studies. If you are not familiar with narrated PowerPoint, you may find the following advice useful.

Check your computer has PowerPoint software (it should as part of a standard Microsoft package), a sound card, which is activated and a speaker (s). Check also that the volume control is turned up. This may sound very basic but we have taught students who complained narrated PowerPoint didn't work and the problem has been traced to each of these simple mistakes.

We suggest you print out the slides contained in each presentation as follows:

1. Go to the print option then in 'Print what:' click the drop down box then highlight 'Handouts' as your choice
2. Go to 'Color/grayscale' and click the drop down box, highlight 'Pure Black and White'
3. Then click 'OK' to print out the PowerPoint slides as a student handout.

Now you can start the PowerPoint presentation and listen to the narration explaining the basic anatomy and physiology. Listening and reading at the same time is difficult which is why it should help to print out the basic text and then concentrate on listening to the narration.

There are diagrams in the presentation, and you can print out the full size diagrams if you want. These narrated PowerPoints are not a substitute for a good anatomy and physiology textbook, but they provide a rapidly accessible summary of what you need to know for the main body systems. The systems covered are:

- Cardiovascular
- Respiratory
- Endocrine
- Gastrointestinal
- Neurological
- Integumentary
- Renal
- Musculoskeletal
- Haematological
- Immune

You will also find case studies linked to each narrated PowerPoint presentation. They should help to relate the material within each chapter to the information presented in the narrated PowerPoint. The case studies bring the anatomy, physiology and pathophysiology to life. Reflective questions at the end of each case study help to explore everyday issues that are faced by patients and nurses in the world of clinical practice. You may want to think about the case studies and consider how they relate to experiences you have with patients and their families as you work through your nurse training.

We hope these additional materials will help you to get the most from the seventh edition of *Watson's Clinical Nursing* and make the crucial link between the written text and your clinical practice.

Mike Walsh
Alison Crumbie

Context of care

INTRODUCTION

Nothing in life can ever be divorced from its context if it is to be fully understood and nursing is no exception. For a complete understanding of how to care for a patient recovering from pneumonia or injury, it is essential to look at the professional context within which the nurse is attempting to work, as well as at the family and wider social environment. Direct nursing care therefore depends upon a wide-ranging set of factors, which are explored in this first section of the book. It is essential that nurses know nursing and understand why nursing exists, for the benefit of patients above all else. A professional sense of self identity is crucial if nursing is to avoid merely being a collection of odd jobs that nobody else wants. At the core of that identity is the primacy of the patient.

Clinical care also depends heavily upon therapeutic communication, which is a two-way process. The word 'therapeutic' is crucial as this denotes communication as part of treatment and care. Effective communication will prevent many mishaps and improve patient outcomes. 'Effective' means that the patient not only fully understands what is being said and done, but also has a part in that action and in the decision-making process. This means in turn that you as the nurse need to be a good listener and culturally aware. Hear what the patient is telling you and be sensitive also to the non-verbal channels of communication.

Section one of this book helps set the scene for what follows but will also allow you to make better sense of later chapters when you have read them. You are encouraged to revisit these early chapters later in your education and reflect upon their content in the light of your experience. Remember that at all times you owe it to your patient to deliver safe and effective care and that means you are obliged to follow your professional code of conduct. Increasingly this requires you to familiarize yourself with evidence-based practice (EBP) in order that you can justify your care. This is the essence of accountability and if the EBP language is a bit daunting at times, take a look at Appendix 2.

The nature of nursing

Mike Walsh and Alison Crumbie

INTRODUCTION

Large textbooks of this nature frequently start with an introductory overview of the big issues facing nursing today and a summary of the content that follows in the next thousand-odd pages. This one does not. Instead we want to start with a real person's story, a story that is not unusual for patients of her age and encapsulates many of the problems and issues that you will have to learn to deal with as a qualified nurse in the years ahead. Let us introduce you to Pat (see Case Study 1.1) and ask you to reflect upon her story as you read the rest of this introductory chapter.

CASE Pat's Story

Pat was born in the 1920s at the height (or depth?) of the Great Depression. She had a brother and a sister, her father having survived the horrors of World War I as an army sergeant, wounded and invalided out of the carnage at the Battle of the Somme in 1916. She grew up in a strict authoritarian family background that was always poor, her father finding work whenever he could. She left school at 14 with no qualifications and went to work in a shop. During World War II she met her husband to be and worked in the munitions industry, suddenly finding herself employed as a draftswoman as there were insufficient skilled men to meet the demands of making Spitfire engines. She also experienced the horror of being buried alive in an air-raid shelter that took a direct hit during a heavy German bombing raid. Today we would understand the mental distress that followed this event and which dogged her for the rest of her life as post-traumatic stress disorder and Pat would have counseling to help her recover. In those days you were just glad to have survived and had to get on with things as best you could.

After the war Pat went back to working in a soap factory as de-mobbed men reclaimed their old jobs. She married Bernard and had one child, working part time as a cleaner thereafter. In the early 1960s the family was re-housed from a slum with no electricity or bathroom to a council estate. It was never a happy family, with their son enduring a psychologically and occasionally physically abusive childhood as endless arguments between parents raged around him.

Things deteriorated further. Both Pat's parents developed **type 2 diabetes**, her father had a stroke, developed gangrene in his foot, had his leg amputated and then developed gangrene in his other foot and died a miserable death in great pain. Her marriage fell apart when she was in her 40s, and after much argument her husband left home for another woman. Pat became depressed, began drinking heavily and took a series of overdoses, usually of the benzodiazepines that her general practitioner was supplying on an endless series of repeat prescriptions without actually seeing her. Pat had become drug dependent as well as alcohol dependent. She suffered from episodes of abstinence syndrome when she could not get enough alcohol and in one such episode attacked her son (now aged 21) with a bread knife attempting to kill him, such was the extent of her hallucinations. She lost the tenancy of the council house and moved to a small one-bedroom flat. Admission to a large psychiatric hospital followed to detoxify and then to attempt to treat her anxiety and depression. Her son moved away and did not come back for many years. Pat spent most of the next few years in one of two large psychiatric hospitals before finally being discharged to a 'half-way house', aged nearly 60. She was no longer drinking and had finally given up smoking, but had become very institutionalized. Subsequently she was discharged from care into a small council flat. Shortly afterwards, her brother died, aged 60, as a result of renal failure and multiple other complications secondary to type 2 diabetes, which he had also developed.

Pat now became very reclusive, refusing to leave the flat or see a doctor or any other healthcare professional. She had put on a great deal of weight during her lengthy stays in the two mental hospitals. Despite becoming increasingly disabled with osteoarthritis and having a strong family history of type 2 diabetes, she put on further weight after discharge. She dealt with the problems of her **obesity** and high risk for type 2 diabetes by denial. She had never divorced her husband (he was Catholic) and he still visited her weekly to get shopping and do odd jobs for her. Her son, who lived away from the area, now began visiting whenever he could and helped with shopping and odd jobs. The home help who came in twice a week was Pat's only other contact with the outside world. Her son noticed a strong odour on one visit and, despite her protestations, lifted back the bedclothes to find a gangrenous infected foot. Admission to hospital failed to save the leg and it was amputated as the diagnosis of type 2 diabetes was confirmed.

A short while after being discharged to a nursing home Pat was readmitted with a gangrenous ulcer on the heel of her remaining foot, caused by the foot being elevated on a footstool for long periods without any pressure relief. The other leg was amputated as, in addition, she was critically ill with septicaemia and heart failure. She was discharged to another nursing home where she was reasonably happy for a further 2 years, but then this home closed down and Pat was transferred to a third home. By now her husband had died after suffering a succession of strokes. In this final nursing home she became very disoriented and confused; she had lost her sight as a result of cataract formation and received little stimulation from the environment. Finally, aged 78, Pat was admitted to hospital for the last time where she died from bronchopneumonia. Her sister died shortly afterwards suffering from type 2 diabetes.

And what of her son? He survived a miserable and abusive childhood which he coped with by denial and obliterating it from conscious memory. Psychological problems followed him around but it was only after both his parents had died that he could begin to work through all the buried psychological trauma of his childhood. A long and painful spell of counseling was necessary before he could lay those ghosts to rest and get on with the rest of his life. So far he has not developed type 2 diabetes, exercises regularly, and follows a healthy lifestyle quite different from his parents.

What can we learn from this true story? Understanding health is clearly a great deal more than the physical process of disease. Social and psychological factors played a large part in shaping Pat's life. Her illness and care needs can be understood only in the context of the great social events that shaped the twentieth century and the lives of today's older people. How did her father's experiences in World War I and the Depression of the 1920s impact upon her upbringing? What were the long-term consequences for her mental health of her own wartime experiences? Psychological factors are also paramount in this story: witness Pat's denial of her type 2 diabetes and the catastrophic results that had. Yet some aspects of disease and health are beyond our control, as shown by the strong family trait of type 2 diabetes that dogged Pat and her family. Social isolation was a major factor in her later years whilst lack of stimulation in her last nursing home contributed to her final confusional state. Pat experienced nursing care in large psychiatric institutions, accident and emergency departments, acute hospital wards and nursing homes at various stages of her life. She was never an easy patient and presented a complex challenge whenever she came into contact with the caring system. Perhaps the nursing staff in the mental hospitals could have prevented Pat becoming so obese. Care in the community could have prevented many of her problems after discharge, but only if she had been a willing and cooperative partner in her care, which she was not. A small pressure sore, which could have been prevented, set in motion a chain of events that led to the loss of her remaining leg. These are examples of how effective nursing care improves quality of life and prevents illness.

Pat is the sort of patient you will encounter: a real person with multiple interrelated problems that have physical, social and psychological origins. Nursing can make a huge difference in caring for people like Pat and that is the challenge you face in your career. This book will help you rise to that challenge and help all the Pats you will encounter in the years ahead.

THE NURSE AND THE HEALTHCARE SYSTEM

There have been many changes in nursing over the past decades. Perhaps two of the most significant have been the rise of accountability and health as key concepts in nursing. Nurses have always been responsible for the care they delivered but that is not the same as being accountable. The traditional model that we largely worked with was the biomedical model with its focus on illness, not health. As Pat's story illustrates, this approach misses out a great deal that is essential to care for people who, in the majority of cases, will not be cured of their illness, only helped to live with it. This crucial shift in emphasis has led to nurses being seen as *accountable healthcare practitioners*, with a consequent growth in autonomy that is redefining our relationship with both patients and the medical profession. We need to explore how nurses fit into the healthcare system if we are to understand the implications of increased levels of autonomy and a greater focus on health.

There are various agencies that directly or indirectly control and affect your everyday nursing practice. This will become increasingly apparent to you as you progress in nursing and become more aware of the context within which you operate. The key agencies can be summarized as:

- the higher education institution where you are educated
- the patient and his or her family

- the community
- registered nurses and other healthcare professionals
- employers and managers who run the healthcare system
- the statutory bodies that regulate nursing.

As a student you are responsible to these agencies but when you qualify you will become fully accountable to them (except of course to your university). Accountability means simply being able to give an account of why you did what you did, when you did it. This is very different from responsibility, which is concerned with following instructions and guidelines conscientiously, rather than acting as you see fit and then being able to justify your actions. Accountability therefore involves making decisions for yourself that you can justify. For a registered nurse to be accountable, therefore, she or he must have the necessary authority and autonomy to make decisions and act upon them, and also the necessary knowledge to make the right decisions. Full accountability comes only with registration, but even as a student you are always responsible for your actions. Initially you are likely to be most aware of your teachers and the college environment but, as you start to gain practical experience, patients, their families and staff involved in direct care will become foremost in your concerns. As your career develops, never forget that the patient is always the most important person to whom you are accountable. The patient is also a member of the wider community and increasingly becoming aware of his or her rights.

The staff involved in giving care, such as your mentor on the ward or in the health centre, are in turn accountable to those who manage the service at local, regional and national level. We are also accountable to our colleagues in other professions such as medicine. Health service managers are in their turn accountable to the elected government of the day. But there is another major force involved in controlling practice. In the UK, it is the Nursing and Midwifery Council or NMC for short. This statutory body is responsible for the regulation of nursing and you can call yourself a registered nurse only if the NMC has you on its live register.

Ultimately, in the UK, there are three main mechanisms for holding you accountable as a registered nurse:

1 The NMC holds registered nurses to account via the Code of Professional Conduct.
2 The patient holds the nurse and the National Health Service to account via the civil law, which permits the patient to sue for damages should things go wrong.
3 The employer holds the nurse to account via a contract of employment, which is also enforceable by law.

In addition, no nurse or health professional is above the law, either criminal or civil, and, as we have seen in the infamous cases of nurse Beverly Allitt and Dr Harold Shipman in the UK, nurses and doctors can be convicted of murder.

Whatever country you work in, from the day you qualify, you will find yourself pulled three different ways by these competing forces of accountability: to the patient, to the national statutory body that regulates nursing and to your employer. The consequences of this tension for nursing have been explored in some depth by Walsh (2000). While it certainly presents complex problems, accountability also leads to real opportunities as increasing levels of autonomy in practice and better educational opportunities flow logically from the basic principle of accountability. This can, however, lead to potential conflict with other professional groups.

CHANGE AND THE HEALTHCARE SERVICES

Changes in the delivery of healthcare services have been in response to three major social trends in the second half of the twentieth century: the explosion in scientific knowledge, the escalating costs of health services and the changing needs of the healthcare consumer population. These trends give rise to complex issues that involve economic, political, social, cultural, educational and ethical considerations.

Scientific discoveries in medicine, notably advanced medical technology, have influenced the delivery of healthcare services and nursing practice. Advances in medical technology permit intense monitoring of and interventions into human biological processes on a scale hitherto unimagined. Life and death decisions may be made on the basis of nurses' interpretations of information from high-technology equipment. These advances have led to increasing specialization within nursing, in both hospital and community settings.

Advances in computer technology, as part of the explosion in scientific knowledge, have influenced the delivery of health care. Computers have automated and consolidated information and increased the speed and efficiency of information processing. Nurses in a variety of healthcare settings are using computers to enter, store and retrieve patient information, check nursing and medical orders, and request services for their patients from other sectors of the healthcare system as diverse as pharmaceutical and social services.

Genetic engineering developments have brought in their wake very complex ethical problems and nurses have increasingly to be aware of the need to offer patients opportunities to talk through these issues in a supportive environment. Counseling skills are increasingly becoming part of the nurse's repertoire and the next chapter will explore this further.

A second trend, the rising cost of restoration to health through acute care hospitalization, in competition with other public needs and wants and in the face of finite resources, has provoked a search for alternative healthcare delivery strategies and sites. Health promotion and health maintenance through public education and community-based programmes have become widespread. Nurses have played a significant role in providing these alternatives and have been given the lead role in the NHS Direct 24-hour telephone health advice service and NHS walk-in centres in the UK. In addition, increased attention has been given to threats to human health emanating from personal lifestyles, pollution of the environment and poor socioeconomic circumstances.

The Conservative government in the UK was responsible for a marked reduction in the number of hospital beds during the 1990s and a reduction in student nurse numbers. This has belatedly been recognized as a major mistake and the Labour government that took office in 1997, after an initial period of hesitation, finally started to commit the necessary resources to reverse these trends. In the run up to the 2001 election, pre-election promises from the Conservatives signalled an intention to match Labour's expenditure on the NHS. Since the election, Labour seem to have raised the stakes and pledged even higher levels of expenditure on the NHS in a bid to bring UK health expenditure up to the EU average. However, as the government are finding out to their discomfort, it takes many years to have an impact upon an organization as large as the NHS. Things have been further complicated by major arguments in government about the extent to which private healthcare providers should be involved in the NHS, whilst despite record expenditure, many NHS Trusts struggled with serious overspending on their budgets in 2006. New and very expensive treatments for cancer are making major competing demands upon resources leading to agonizing choices between, for example, treating a limited number of cancer patients or spending the money on larger numbers of people with less newsworthy health problems such as mental illness or those associated with just growing old. In the short to medium term, therefore, serious pressure on resources will remain the norm. This means finding new, smarter and more effective ways of working; this will involve challenging many traditional professional boundaries.

The care in the community policy means that elderly patients are seen as belonging in private nursing homes or being supported at home by the local social services department rather than cared for by the NHS (see Ch. 3). A major new initiative is the provision of intermediate care for older people in order to avoid acute hospital beds becoming blocked by patients whose acute medical problems have been largely resolved, but whose discharge is not possible because of predominantly social and psychological problems. Rapid response teams have also been set up in a bid to keep older people out of the hospital system. A similar community philosophy has been applied to caring for those with a learning disability or mental health problems. If such initiatives are seen purely as a cost-cutting opportunity, however, there is a danger that vulnerable groups will suffer. Community care is not necessarily cheaper and will achieve results only if the patient is a cooperative partner (reflect on Pat's story). Criticism of the care in the community policy relates to underfunding of its implementation rather than to the policy itself. It is not a means of saving money in a way that, perhaps, day-care surgery is.

A third trend, the changing needs of the healthcare consumer population, stems from changing patterns of mortality and morbidity, coupled with consumers' increased participation in their own healthcare decisions. The proportion of the population that is elderly is increasing, as is the incidence of long-term illness. The older segment of the UK population is increasingly including people from ethnic minority backgrounds born in the Indian subcontinent or the Caribbean, for whom culturally sensitive care is required. Meanwhile social disruption in other parts of the world has produced a significant number of refugees and asylum seekers who do not speak English. Their health needs must be met as must the needs of people from eastern Europe who under European Union legislation are free to seek work in the UK.

Longitudinal studies show a pattern of decreasing mortality and increasing incidence of morbidity (illness) in middle-aged and older people. Previously, acute infectious diseases were the greatest threat to health; today, chronic disabling diseases, from infancy to old age, represent our major health problems. However, as this book is being written, there is great concern that a new pandemic of flu could possibly pose a major and global health threat (the H5N1 version of avian flu). Long-term and disabling diseases are attributed to detrimental social, environmental and lifestyle factors, which are much more difficult to control than infections. Chronic illness represents a broad spectrum of diseases. Some are life-threatening, such as **heart disease**, **cancer**, **acquired immune deficiency syndrome (AIDS)** and **stroke**, while others are more physically or cognitively debilitating, such as **diabetes** (as shown by Pat's story) or **Alzheimer's disease**.

Consumers' involvement in their own health care changed considerably in the latter half of the twentieth century. In the 1970s, the women's movement and other activist groups began to assert their rights in health care. Today, consumers are much more knowledgeable about health problems and interventions. More consumers want to participate actively in their health care; they seek information to make informed decisions. The formerly dependent, acquiescent patient may now prefer to be an active partner with the healthcare team members.

Nurses have responded to the changing needs of patients by focusing less on the medical emphasis of disease cure and more on the holism of patient health promotion, maintenance and restoration. Thus, the role of the nurse incorporates that of adviser, counselor and collaborator. Nurses work in partnership with patients. Nurses increasingly provide information for patients, assisting them to examine their own values, beliefs and goals, and helping them to evaluate and choose from available courses of action.

THE FOCUS OF NURSING

Nursing is recognized as an emerging profession with a unique perspective on people, environment and health. It is the application of nursing knowledge to the promotion, maintenance and restoration of health for the individual and family as they experience stressful events, which may include death and bereavement. In recent years, nursing has derived its focus not from the medical model, with its emphasis on the treatment and cure of pathological problems, but from the relationships between people, the environment and health outlined in the holistic philosophy that underpins the nursing model of care.

It is noteworthy that, from the time of Florence Nightingale, nursing has described as its focus the health of human beings. What have changed over time are the skills, scope and settings of nursing practice. Nurses maintain that care is at the core of nursing practice, but we should remember that nurses do not have a monopoly on care. Any doctor or physiotherapist would state that they care for their patients as well. The key is to understand what we mean by that little four-letter word 'care'.

This has been discussed extensively by Walsh (2000) and he concludes that, while it is axiomatic that nursing is about caring, there is uncomfortable evidence to question the commitment of some nurses to caring, especially for other nurses. The literature may be summarized by saying that caring is:

- a one-to-one interpersonal reaction. You have to recognize the person in the patient and in yourself, to really care
- context dependent – the environment is crucial in the delivery of care
- about being involved and having things matter rather than performing a series of tasks in a cold, detached manner
- taking into account the person's emotional and psychological needs together with the social circumstances in which he or she lives
- about seeing things from the patient's point of view
- universal in nature: to be cared for is a fundamental human right. It is a moral imperative that the nurse discharges equally for all people.

You should reflect upon this analysis at various stages of your education. Memorable incidents occur to all nurses in their training and you will be no exception. These critical incidents can be either positive or negative but will still be valuable learning experiences if you reflect upon them critically with this view of caring in mind.

CONCEPTS CENTRAL TO NURSING

During your education in nursing you will come across a number of nurse theorists who have explored the concepts that are central to nursing (Orem 1985, Peplau 1952, Rogers 1970, 1980, 1987, Roper et al 1980). Central to all theories of nursing are the concepts of the patient, the environment, health and nursing.

The patient

The patient is the recipient of nursing care and fundamentally must always be seen as a person. The patient is viewed in the context of being both a human being and being unique, with a particular make-up, experiences and responses. The person has a distinct identity, in addition to being a member of a family and community, and is in constant interaction with the environment. Interactions and responses are influenced by sociocultural background, lifestyle, values, capabilities, interests, past experiences and the patterns of behaviour laid down as a result of those experiences. These factors contribute to the uniqueness of the person, who should be regarded as having worth, dignity and the right to pursue health, happiness, love, security, purpose and freedom. The nurse considers the individual holistically by focusing the nurse–patient encounter on the total person and not merely the component parts.

The patient should always be informed about his or her health status, make informed decisions compatible with personal beliefs and values, and actively participate (as far as possible) in the care process. All people have essential basic human needs; nursing intervention may be indicated when the individual cannot independently satisfy these needs. Basic biological needs include the intake of oxygen, fluids and food, the elimination of wastes, rest, sleep, activity and maintenance of body temperature within a definite range. Significant psychosocial needs of each person include: a sense of security, the maintenance of an identity as an individual, acceptance, a sense of being wanted and belonging, the opportunity for socializing, independence (and at times dependence and interdependence), freedom to make decisions, and opportunities to develop and use innate potential. He or she should have interests and goals and the opportunity to feel self-respect, in addition to feeling useful and having a sense of achievement.

Environment

The relationship between the individual and the environment is dynamic and influences both health and lifestyle. Within the context of nursing, the internal environment comprises everything within the skin and mucous membranes of the body. It encompasses all structural and physiological aspects of the human body and may be modified by psychological and sociocultural experiences. The external environment includes physical surroundings, patterns of relationships and interactions with family and society, outside resources, and the ways in which the individual has contact with a healthcare delivery system.

Nursing is directed towards managing the way in which the patient interacts with the environment, promoting health, preventing disease and delivering care in illness. Specific strategies and actions enabling the nurse to direct or manage the patient–environment interaction vary according to the individual, the environment and the health problem.

Health

The meaning of health is a matter of considerable controversy (see p. 14). Some nurses see health as a state, others as a process. Most recognize health as a goal to be attained and maintained. How health is perceived by the individual is influenced by cultural and educational background and by past experiences. An individual's health is measured against some yardstick or set of standards. The standard used may be absolute; for example, it may be the presence or absence of disease, or the ability or inability to function as a contributing, independent member of society. Other measurements may be relative and give greater consideration to subjective components such as the sense of well-being and quality of life but, overall, health remains an illusive concept to try to measure absolutely.

Besides the physiological and functional aspects of health, nursing is also concerned with subjective factors contributing to the quality of life and the opportunity the individual has to realize potential. Effects of the internal environment on functioning, well-being and lifestyle are readily apparent. The effects of unfavourable external environmental factors significant to health, such as polluted air, water, noise and adverse living conditions, are complex and more difficult to identify and change. Other factors related to lifestyle, such as the amount of physical exercise a person takes, dietary and smoking habits, levels of **stress** and relationships with others, can also affect health and perception of health.

Nursing

Nursing takes place within the context of the nurse–patient relationship, which is characterized as a professional or therapeutic relationship. This differs from a social relationship in that it is collaborative and is directed towards meeting the patient's goals. It may be time limited and take place within a structured and designated setting, such as a health centre or hospital. People often have preconceived ideas about the nurse as well as about how they themselves should behave as patients. Clarification of these perceptions may be necessary before an effective rapport can develop. The professional purpose of the relationship gives direction to the role assumed by the nurse and to the way in which the nurse applies nursing knowledge and skills. The nurse brings to the relationship respect for the person's uniqueness and integrity, and an appreciation of the patient's right to participate in or receive care. The patient, as an active participant, brings certain abilities and values, as well as a background of culture, education, experiences and needs, with the right to demonstrate and apply these in decisions and in the care process. Mutual acceptance is fundamental to the effectiveness of the nurse–patient relationship.

As the nurse develops empathy with the patient and strives to earn trust and confidence, the patient should develop trust and confidence in the nurse. With each encounter, the nurse's role is mutually agreed upon by the nurse and patient. A sincere interest and willingness to help may be demonstrated by the nurse being non-judgmental, accepting the patient, demonstrating thoughtfulness, anticipating needs, showing concern and, most importantly, by being ready to listen and answer questions. You have to care for the patient as they are, not as you would like them to be. Recognition of identity by addressing the patient by name, respect for personal preferences and the demonstration of flexibility, contribute to a satisfactory relationship. Appreciation of the family's concerns and each member's need for an interpretation of what is happening fosters trust and confidence. Expressing and sharing information with the family may prove therapeutic for them as well as the patient.

During the total nurse–patient relationship, the nurse's responsibilities include that of being the advocate. When acting on behalf of the patient, attempts are made to assess the situation carefully from the patient's point of view, rather than simply deciding what is 'good for' the patient on the basis of past nursing experience. As advocate, the nurse should provide information to assist the patient and/or the family to make informed decisions about the individual's health care (e.g. about a procedure, a form of therapy or a change in circumstances). Confidentiality must be respected; it is an important factor in establishing and maintaining good nurse–patient relationships. When information must be shared with other members of the healthcare team, the patient should be advised of the reasons and the advantages of communicating it to others.

The nurse–patient relationship lies at the heart of nursing and it is not surprising, therefore, to find that the NMC, the regulatory body for nursing, makes this the cornerstone of its *Code of Professional Practice* (NMC 2004). This document is binding upon all nurses and sets out guiding principles for ethical and safe practice with regard to issues such as advocacy and confidentiality. You should have been issued with a copy of the code when you commenced your nurse education and are well advised to revisit the document at regular intervals. Always remember that it tells you first and foremost to safeguard the interest of individual patients and that you will always be held accountable for your actions as a registered nurse.

Rapid changes taking place in practice mean that you will find nurses in situations where in the past they did not practise. New therapeutic skills and techniques (e.g. prescribing), radical changes in clinical practice (e.g. day-care surgery), shortages of junior medical staff and increasing demand for health care in the community are only some examples. The principle of accountability within the *Code of Professional Practice* (NMC 2004) together with recent government policy (DoH 1999a, 2000, 2002), underpin all such new developments. These documents take the concept of accountability and uses it to show how nurses may expand and develop their roles into new areas, provided they remember that they will always be held accountable for what they do.

An exciting new development in the recent past has been the growth of the *nurse practitioner* role. The concept was developed in the USA and has several key distinguishing features. The nurse practitioner sees patients with an undifferentiated diagnosis, utilizing both nursing and medical assessment skills to arrive at a diagnosis before either initiating treatment or referring on as appropriate. The nurse practitioner, therefore, can carry out physical examinations, take a medical history and utilize clinical decision-making skills to operate on the boundaries of nursing and medicine. She or he brings together the best of both nursing and medicine to deliver high-quality health care to the patient. There is a high degree of autonomy involved and the nurse may work in a primary care environment such as a health centre or in an acute hospital (e.g. A&E department) providing a health service that is complementary to, but different from, the conventional medical consultation. Nurse practitioners may develop clinical specialist roles in areas such as diabetes or ophthalmology. Alternatively they may work with specialist client groups, such as sex workers or refugees, who are often on the fringes of society.

It became apparent that the nurse practitioner role had become established in the UK when in April 2000 the *British Medical Journal* and the *Nursing Times* ran simultaneous feature issues of their journals which were focused on the changing roles of nurses and doctors and particularly on the evaluation of nurse practitioner practice. These two influential journals thus marked a significant moment for healthcare delivery in the UK. Nurse practitioners have gradually become established in general practice over the last two decades. The Cumberlege report on community nursing can be seen to have provided the groundwork for such developments by stating that 'the principle should be adopted of introducing the nurse practitioner into primary health care' (DoH 1986, p. 32). In 1991 the National Health Service Executive Management published *Junior Doctors: the New Deal* which paved the way for the reduction in junior doctors' hours (National Health Service Executive 1991). With junior doctors being less available and fewer recruits entering general practice a need was developing for nurses to advance their roles and to take on some of the work that had previously been the domain of doctors. This has been recognized more recently in a government document *Making a Difference: Strengthening the Nursing, Midwifery and Health Visiting Contribution to Health and Health Care* (DoH 1999a). In addition to the supportive policy emanating from the UK government, the British Medical Association has also recognized the contribution of nurses by stating that a nurse practitioner could be the first point of contact for most patients in primary care (BMA 2002). In the light of such support, nurse practitioners have been gradually expanding their roles and have been moving into areas of practice that would have previously been seen as the domain of medicine.

Examples now exist of nurse practitioners taking on triage roles (Reveley 1999), running minor illness clinics (Marsh and Dawes 1995), accepting same-day clinic appointments (Kinnersley et al 2000, Venning et al 2000) and operating open access clinics (Stilwell et al 1987, Salisbury and Tettersell 1988). The nurse–patient interaction, however, remains governed by the holistic philosophy outlined earlier; the nurse is at all times working as a nurse, remains bound by the NMC *Code of Professional Practice*, and is accountable for everything that he or she does. As this book goes to press, we are awaiting government approval for an NMC proposal to open a new part of the nursing register for advanced nurse practitioners. If this goes ahead it will set the seal upon many years campaigning for this important recognition of advanced nursing practice.

A very important part of the Code of Conduct reminds nurses that all patients are equal and all deserve equally high standards of care. The nurse must not be judgmental about patients and has no right to refuse to give care. As the NMC points out, the law does not confer upon the nurse any right of conscientious objection to participation in treatment; the nurse should consider any strongly held beliefs when applying for posts in the first place. Nurses cannot refuse to care for a patient without simultaneously breaching the NMC *Code of Professional Practice* and their contract of employment, whilst placing themselves at risk of a civil lawsuit for negligence.

Within different nurse–patient relationships, the nurse may find theories from other disciplines very useful in describing, explaining, making predictions about, or controlling the events that occasion the relationship. For example, the nurse may derive insights from knowledge of the psychological and physiological changes associated with ageing to assist the elderly patient; alternatively, learning theory may assist the nurse in patient teaching. Depending upon the context, theories from other disciplines have considerable relevance to nursing as descriptions, explanations and/or predictors of the relationships between patient, environment and health, and as the basis for rational nursing actions. It is, however, nursing's unique perspective that directs us to select from among the theories of other disciplines those that are useful in each nurse–patient relationship.

The growth of evidence-based practice also requires nurses to base their practice upon firm evidence. There are three sources of evidence for practice, and research is only one of them. The other two key areas are patient preferences and the practitioner's own experience of what works best. Accountable nursing practice, therefore, means that the nurse must be able to discuss the evidence base upon which practice is based. Following orders is not a valid evidence base and does not constitute accountable practice. Doing something because we have always done it or because 'Sister likes it that way' is not a sufficient foundation for professional practice and leads to ritualistic, unthinking nursing that may be positively harmful to the patient.

THE DELIVERY OF NURSING CARE

Nursing care has to be based upon the individual needs of each patient, planned with the involvement of the patient and then evaluated for its effectiveness. Consistency of care and good communication are also essential. Nursing developed the *nursing process* as a means of achieving these goals. Ford and Walsh (1994) and Walsh (1998) have, amongst others, critiqued this concept in depth. Increasingly the traditional nursing care plan derived from the nursing process is being replaced by the critical pathway, which heralds a less cumbersome, more quality-oriented approach. These two methods of planning care will now be considered

THE NURSING PROCESS

The nursing process was developed as a tool for teaching care planning and was then implemented across the whole of nursing, but unfortunately with little research to support such a major step. The result has been much criticism and a sense amongst many nurses that it is all too time consuming. It involves a series of stages that begins with assessing the patient, identifying problems, setting goals, implementing care to achieve those goals and finally evaluating the effectiveness of care given. That sounds reasonable until it is realized that this all has to be written down, in detail, for each individual patient. The writing down of copious notes, by hand, to cover each of these stages is both tedious and extremely time consuming. It leads to a great deal of documentation, which nurses feel they have not got the time for.

THE CRITICAL PATHWAY

The critical pathway is an alternative to the traditional nursing process care plan and is based upon the realization that, for most patients with the same condition, the same stages in care should be reached at the same time. Patient outcomes and the care to be delivered to achieve these goals can be pre-planned by the multidisciplinary care team as standards whose achievement can be measured. These are then written down as a pathway the patient will follow and the patient is assigned, if suitable, to that pathway upon admission. The result is a multidisciplinary document that all the care team can use which sets out what the patient should achieve on each day. In very acute areas shorter timescales can be used, based on hours or even minutes. The pathway requires only charting by exception. In other words, the nurse (or other health professional) writes in the document only when something is different from the pre-planned care; otherwise it is merely a matter of signing to say that the care was delivered and the goal achieved as per the pathway.

The pathway consists of sections based on key areas of activity such as discharge planning, investigations, pain control, wound care, mobility, personal hygiene and medical interventions. The targets for each day are set in advance for each of these sections of patient care. This document is a powerful quality assurance tool as it may be readily audited to see whether care is deviating from that which has been set as the desired standard. A consistent pattern of deviation may emerge suggesting there is a particular problem such as a delay in obtaining lab results or discharge medication. This can then be rectified. Patients should also be given their own version of the pathway. This keeps patients and families informed of what is happening, when and why.

PRIMARY AND TEAM NURSING

The nursing process and critical pathways are ways of planning and documenting care. It still remains to organize the delivery of that care. Traditionally this was done on a task basis with the nurse in charge delegating to each nurse a group of tasks to perform for all the patients. This was known as task allocation and, while it may seem an efficient way to operate, there are major problems. Patients cease to exist as whole individuals and become broken down into tasks: the holistic philosophy that distinguishes nursing from the reductionist medical scientific model is lost. Communication is very difficult and some things do not get done, whilst others may be done twice. A crucial point is the lack of accountability for any individual nurse in such a system.

Alternative methods of organizing care delivery grew out of a general dissatisfaction with this fragmented approach, and they became known as *team nursing* or *primary nursing*. In team nursing, as its name suggests, a team of nurses is responsible for care delivered to a group of patients. The team has an experienced registered nurse as its leader and patients are assigned to a team for their care. This system can work in both primary care and hospital settings. A variation on this approach, often encountered in hospitals, is patient allocation which involves patients being allocated to teams on a shift by shift basis. As the shifts change, so do the members of the teams. It is still possible for fragmented, task-centred care to occur within such a team nursing approach, but care should become more holistic as nurses and patients are able to build up more of a relationship.

The primary nursing approach was commonly understood to involve one nurse being held accountable for all care delivered to a patient 24 hours a day. She or he admits the patients, plans all care, delivers much of it while on duty, and is also responsible for discharge planning. When the primary nurse is off duty, an associate nurse carries on with care according to the primary nurse's plan. This is a simplified account but covers the main elements described by Manthey (1980), who is credited with being the first nurse fully to develop and advocate this way of nursing. The fragmentation and task focus of traditional nursing is replaced by accountable professional care with the advantages of continuity and the opportunity to develop a good nurse–patient relationship. This is particularly important for the hospital nurse given the ever-shorter inpatient stays that characterize the rapidly changing healthcare system.

As care moves towards a more multidisciplinary focus and the government is keen to develop completely new professional caring roles such as the surgical practitioner, such a 'nursing-centred' approach may increasingly find itself unsustainable. The critical pathway model encourages multidisciplinary working as a replacement for the traditional primary nursing approach.

PATIENT CARE PLANNING

Whether a primary nursing or team nursing approach is used, patient care still has to be planned. The logical place to begin, therefore, is with patient assessment, as this always comes first.

Assessment

Assessment underpins the traditional care planning approach of the nursing process or the newer critical pathway technique. All good nursing care starts with assessment, which is a continuous process of collecting data about the patient's responses, health status, strengths and concerns. Information should be both current and historical, reflecting biological, psychological and social functioning, as well as environmental and lifestyle factors that may affect health. The patient is the primary source of data, but a variety of data sources should be used, such as the family, health records and other health professionals. A good assessment includes subjective data such as the patient's own story, their view of what is wrong and a carefully structured interview which asks questions designed to elicit information about the person's health status. Direct observation of the patient is essential, together with objective measurement of appropriate physical parameters such as vital signs, height and weight, pulse oximetry, peak flows, capillary blood glucose, urine testing, etc. Increasingly, nurse practitioners are learning medical physical examination techniques such as auscultation, and combining these findings with a structured medical history to carry assessment to a new level, integrating medical and nursing skills to carry out an in-depth holistic assessment. This approach is essential if the nurse is acting as the first point of contact in seeing patients with undifferentiated diagnoses. If evidence from countries such as Australia and the USA is any guide, these skills may soon become part of normal pre-registration education rather than the preserve of advanced post-registration courses. At the end of the assessment, it is important to confirm or validate any data and impressions with the patient. This ensures that messages conveyed by the patient are being received and interpreted accurately by the nurse.

Problem identification

Problem identification must have the patient as a focus; a correctly stated patient problem is the starting point for effective, individualized nursing care. Data obtained in the assessment need to be sorted into categories and compared with accepted norms, as defined by sciences such as anatomy, physiology or psychology, in order that actual or potential health problems may be discovered. It is also essential to seek the patient's point of view, as the patient may not agree with the nurse that a behaviour constitutes a problem; for example, the patient may see smoking as beneficial because it is perceived as reducing stress. The patient may cope with problems simply by denying they exist. Where possible, the likely cause of a problem should also be identified as this helps to focus intervention into appropriate areas.

Goal setting

Goal setting (planning) occurs when the patient and nurse identify activities to prevent, reduce or correct the patient's problems. The steps in planning are to:

- set priorities among the identified problems
- establish patient goals and outcome criteria
- identify intervention strategies
- weigh alternative actions and predict outcomes
- determine nursing interventions
- write the nursing care plan.

Once patient problems (actual and potential) have been identified, priorities are set to provide direction for nursing interventions. Knowledge, experience and, in some critical situations, intuition are applied in setting priorities. If the situation is life-threatening, airway, breathing and circulation (ABC) assume priority. In many situations, priority setting involves patient and family participation to prevent conflicts arising and to enhance active cooperation in care activities.

There is no one tool or framework available that assists in making decisions on priorities of care in all situations. Emergency and life-threatening circumstances readily dictate priorities for intervention; other situations may require different considerations. Nurses have often used Maslow's hierarchy of needs framework to assist in the ranking of patient problems (Maslow 1954). Maslow's hierarchy presents an ordered classification of human needs, and is based on motivation theory, implying that the patient contributes to the decision about priorities. Physiological needs (for oxygen, water, food) are ranked as the most immediate priorities, followed by safety and security, love and belonging, self-esteem and self-actualization. Communicating the reasons for priorities helps in establishing mutual goals: failure to consider what is important to the patient may create conflict and delay in achieving health goals.

Goals and objectives describe the patient's expected outcomes and may be the focus of multiprofessional effort rather than just the preserve of nursing. Each goal is derived from the identification of patient problems and the goals are directed towards the promotion, maintenance and restoration of health, the alleviation of suffering and the giving of support to the dying. Goals may be either short- or long-term statements, should be relevant to the identified problem and within the patient's capabilities and limitations. Short-term goals may be discrete steps leading to achievement of a specific long-term goal and should always reflect mutual planning with the patient. An important feature of a patient goal is that it must be measurable, otherwise how will we know whether the patient has achieved it? A 'fluid intake of 3 litres per day' represents a measurable goal which also contains a statement of the time limit (24 hours) on goal achievement, whereas a statement such as 'increase fluid intake' is too vague to be measurable as a goal and has no concept of time attached to it. Goals should therefore be stated in terms of observable behaviour and should also be realistic. Goals that are unrealistic will only discourage both patient and nurse, and are a waste of time.

Intervention strategies are selected with the patient from alternatives. They are considered in the light of anticipated effectiveness in achieving outcomes, the benefits and risks involved, and the availability of resources, including people, equipment, time, finances and facilities.

The care plan should contain written statements describing the nursing interventions required to help the patient achieve the various goals outlined in the plan. They should be stated in concise, specific terms, and in the sequence in which they are to occur. They may include strategies for the promotion, maintenance or restoration of health, or for peaceful dying. The nursing interventions support the medical regimen of care and should be kept current, revised, and describe alternative plans, as necessary.

When problems are identified by the nurse that are outside the realm of nursing, a referral may be made to the appropriate member of the healthcare team. Similarly, when problems are identified that are beyond the expertise of one particular nurse, referrals may be made to other qualified nursing colleagues. These may be clinical nurse specialists, nurses practising in a special care area or specialty, or community nurses. Collaboration, cooperation and sharing of knowledge and skills provide quality and continuity of care. Medical orders and the plans developed by other healthcare workers should be integrated with the planned nursing actions to develop an overall schedule for patient care.

The critical pathway approach uses goal setting in the same way to identify desired patient outcomes. The key differences are that they are group outcomes for all patients with a common condition (e.g. myocardial infarction or undergoing breast surgery for cancer) and are placed on a timeline, giving specific deadlines by when they are normally to be achieved for all patients.

Implementation

Implementation is the performance of nursing interventions described in the nursing care plan. The scope of nursing actions include the following:

- supportive measures designed to assist with activities the patient is unable to perform and to reinforce adaptive coping mechanisms
- therapeutic measures such as breathing exercises or a dressing change

- continuous data collection and monitoring of the patient's health status
- health promotion and health maintenance activities such as teaching
- coordination of care by other members of the healthcare team
- reporting, recording and consultation.

Evaluation

Evaluation encompasses comparing the patient's health status with the goals and objectives of health care, and determining progress toward goal achievement. Evaluation is a continuous process that occurs during ongoing assessment and implementation of nursing care. When behaviour indicates that goals have been achieved, the nurse and patient either move to the next level of expectation or the relationship is terminated. If the goals are not achieved, the nurse may explore the reasons for this by questioning. For example: Were the goals realistic? Were they stated in measurable terms? Were the actions inappropriate, or did the patient's situation alter? Goals are then re-examined, modified if necessary, and priorities are re-established in relation to the patient's level of achievement and/or change in health status.

If a critical pathway is in use, the nurse or other health professional, if appropriate, will be responsible for initiating action when a goal is not achieved. Continual monitoring of outcome achievement is a powerful quality assurance tool as significant patterns may emerge showing that patients frequently fail to achieve certain goals. This, in turn, may either indicate that the goals are unrealistic or highlight a problem in the care delivery system.

DOCUMENTATION

The patient's health record can be used as a legal document. The nurse is accountable for ensuring that information recorded in the notes is accurate, clear, concise, factual and complete. Data collection, identification of patient problems, plan of care, interventions and results of the interventions, and evaluation of the outcome criteria are recorded. Under the UK legal system, a patient may bring a case for negligence up to 3 years after the event. The nursing staff will only have their documentation to rely on in such an instance; you are very unlikely to even remember the patient, let alone the details of their care, over 2 years later.

All members of the healthcare team should share the patient's record. Increasingly care teams are developing multidisciplinary documentation which places all the different professions' records in a single document. This greatly improves communication between different members of the care team. If the patient has a chronic condition that is managed largely in the community but still requires occasional admissions either for acute exacerbations or respite care, the patient record can be held by the patient. Some health staff find this a rather radical suggestion but it is increasingly gaining acceptance. If involving patients as partners in care is to be meaningful, why not let them look after their own notes? It means staff know exactly what community care has been given before admission, and vice versa upon discharge. It thus becomes a means of providing information about the patient's condition and the health professionals' care plans, and contributes to continuity of care. Accurate and comprehensive written documentation facilitates collaboration and cooperation among members of the various healthcare professions to ensure optimal use of resources on the patient's behalf. The record is a confidential document; it is available only to those participating in the care by permission of the patient and employer.

NURSING ETHICS

The moral premise of nursing practice is founded in the nurse–patient encounter, embodied in the concept of caring. Nursing practice and hence caring are underpinned by an ethical approach that in the UK is embodied in the NMC Code of Professional Conduct (NMC 2004). Nurses have become increasingly aware of ethics in recent years; indeed, Robertson (1996) studied a team of doctors and nurses who worked together in a gerontological psychiatric setting and concluded that ethical theory can usefully illuminate the moral considerations present in the everyday provision of health care. As nurses become more accountable and autonomous they are increasingly finding themselves caught in very uncomfortable positions, juggling a conflict of accountability between the patient on the one hand and powerful NHS managers and doctors on the other. Lindseth et al (1994), for example, explored ethically difficult care episodes and the reflections of physicians and nurses upon those episodes; Kelly (1991) found numerous examples of value conflict in her study of the values of nursing undergraduates and Varcoe et al (2004) found tensions and conflicts in values in their study of ethical practice in nursing. Nurses do not make ethical decisions in a vacuum. As Holm (1997) points out, they are influenced by society at large, the environment in which they live and the healthcare system and institution within which they work. Nurses and other professionals are caught between personal, clinical and bureaucratic/legal tensions leading to many potential ethical dilemmas. However, Holm (1997) argues that these may be grouped together under broad headings such as truth telling, termination of treatment and the role of families in decision-making, for which ethical guidelines and policies may be developed in advance. This should result in staff sharing their perspective and arriving at a common ethical position. This approach denies the power of medicine and pre-eminence of *medical* ethics in favour of a more egalitarian *healthcare* ethics.

Nursing ethics rest on caring as the moral basis for both the social role of nursing as a profession, and for nursing practice. It is also underpinned by fundamental ethical principles derived from analytical philosophy (Benjamin and Curtis 1992). This ethic is governed by an appeal to principles of moral conduct. These principles of moral conduct, sometimes expressed as moral duties, include:

- *Autonomy* – the obligation to respect the personal choices another person makes
- *Beneficence* – the obligation to do good
- *Fidelity* – the obligation to keep one's word
- *Justice* – the equitable distribution of risks and benefits among people
- *Non-maleficence* – the obligation to do no harm
- *Veracity* – the obligation to tell the truth.

The principles of moral conduct have been derived from several different world views of human relationships. The world views articulate rights and obligations in human encounters through principles of moral conduct. One world view, *teleology*, argues that the goodness of an act is determined by its consequences. It further argues that the collective good takes precedence over the good of the individual: the greatest good and least harm to the greatest numbers. In contrast, a second world view, *deontology*, argues that the goodness of an act is independent of its consequences and is determined by its conformity to obligations that arise from the fact of being human. It further argues that the good of the individual takes precedence over the collective good, based on the premise that no one be treated as a means to the ends of another.

Conduct based upon any one of the principles, and not in conflict with any other principle, is morally right conduct. However, when two or more moral courses of conduct come into conflict, we have an ethical dilemma.

Nursing ethics wrestles with problems that arise when alternative courses of conduct, each moral in itself, come into conflict in a particular situation. An example in nursing practice of conflicts between alternative courses of moral conduct is the conflict between beneficence and autonomy. For example, consider the person who refuses nursing care that would greatly benefit his or her health (such as Pat). If the nurse respects the person's autonomy, the obligation to do good and do no harm may be difficult to achieve and Pat's health status may be harmed. If the nurse coerces the individual into receiving nursing care, or fails to elicit consent for nursing care, the nurse violates the autonomy of the person, and possibly the law, as such an act may be construed as common assault, for which a patient may sue to obtain damages. The nurse may have to choose one over the other as a basis for the course of action.

An alternative ethical dilemma often occurs over the issue of how much information to give a patient. Nurses have traditionally identified themselves in the role of patient advocate, although authors such as Porter (1988) have questioned the validity of this assertion. A key element of nursing involves giving information in order that a patient may make informed decisions about treatment and care. The NMC Code of Professional Conduct (2004) requires nurses to be truthful with patients. In some circumstances a patient's family may ask the nurse not to inform the patient of his or her diagnosis. This can, on occasion, happen in situations where the diagnosis is one of cancer. The family often seem to believe that they are protecting the patient by shielding them from the knowledge of their condition. The nurse may therefore be placed in the position of having to choose between lying to the patient when asked 'What is wrong with me?' or telling the truth and contradicting the family in the process. There are no easy answers, except to say that nurses must be able to support their actions with sound rationales (such as the NMC Code of Conduct), which is the essence of being an accountable practitioner. In cases of difficulty, the nurse would also derive great benefit from membership of a professional organization such as the Royal College of Nursing.

It is possible to read texts on ethics that present detailed analytical frameworks for various situations based on the principles of moral conduct outlined above. Debates in class over what to do in various situations are a good way of rehearsing the arguments and learning about the complexities of modern health care. However, when difficult ethical situations occur in practice, nurses usually have little time and are under a great deal of pressure to make a decision that they may not agree with. Under such circumstances the niceties of analytical philosophy and moral frameworks are just academic exercises. The nurse needs safe and simple solutions that will avoid harm to the patient and protect the individual nurse. Pragmatic advice is that, if in doubt, adhere to the Code of Conduct at all times with its fundamental principle that the patient's interests are paramount: tell the truth, seek an opinion from a senior colleague and do not be rushed or 'bounced' into anything. Above all, remember that *you* are accountable for *your* actions; following doctors' orders is not a defence. Document immediately what you did and why (remember that accountability is about justifying your actions). A final piece of advice is to belong to a professional organization and, if you feel morally compromised, involve it at the earliest opportunity.

THE NURSE AS A PROMOTER OF HEALTH

It will be helpful to begin by defining what is meant by health and two other much-used terms: health promotion and health education. Many different definitions of each are found in the literature. It is important to realize that there is no one 'right' definition, but the definitions chosen will give you a basis for understanding the other concepts presented. Some historical perspectives will also be discussed.

HEALTH

It is important when thinking of health not to see it just in *biological terms*, as health also has important social and psychological dimensions. Many theories of health differ principally on how much weight they attach to these three components. A more philosophical view of health sees it as empowering people to fulfill their potential (Seedhouse 1986). This presents the nurse with a very challenging and rewarding perspective on nursing as our job is to help people achieve their maximum personal development. Health is therefore a very dynamic and positive concept that is all about the growth and development of both the individual and the society in which they live (Ewles and Simnett 1999). The biomedical or Western scientific model of health has been summarized by Naidoo and Wills (2000) as having the following characteristics:

- *Biomedical* – it is associated with living organisms
- *Reductionist* – disease and health may be understood by breaking down the body into smaller and smaller units from systems to cells
- *Mechanistic* – the body is conceptualized as functioning like a machine
- *Allopathic* – opposing forces of health defeat the threat of disease (e.g. medication or surgery).

In reviewing this approach to health, Naidoo and Wills (2000) point out that improvements in living conditions since the mid-1800s probably had far more to do with improving health than specific biomedical interventions. These authors cite interesting statistics concerning death rates from infectious disease such as tuberculosis (TB). In 1838 the death rate from TB was approximately 4000 per million in England and Wales. By the time the causative organism had been discovered in 1882, the mortality rate from TB had already more than halved to 1750 per million. When effective chemotherapy to treat TB became available in the late 1940s the figure had dropped to 650 per million and by 1960 had fallen to 250 per million. Only a small proportion of the reduction in death rate from its 1838 levels (approximately 10%) can therefore be assigned to the introduction of effective drugs and the BCG vaccination programme. Gough et al (1994) point out that medical dominance led to the NHS becoming a disease- and hospital-focused service rather than a true health service. Despite these criticisms, the biomedical model remains the dominant approach to health care in the UK and there is a great deal of evidence to support its validity. Much of your work as a nurse will take place within the context of the biomedical model; however, we have to ask whether it is the whole story.

There are alternatives to the biomedical model of health. The *social–positivist* approach applies the methods of the natural sciences to social enquiry in order to identify the causes of health and illness, while *interactionist* explanations concentrate on the meanings that people give to the experiences of health and illness. Finally, there is the *structuralist* approach, which sees health in terms of how power and authority are distributed in the broader context of society; the effects of capitalism, class structure and the power of

men over women are examples of how this view seeks to explain health.

We know that there is a significant social component to health by considering the Black Report (Davidson and Townsend 1982). This was commissioned by the Labour government in the UK in the late 1970s and was ready for publication as the new Conservative government came to power in 1979. It found little favour with Prime Minister Thatcher but was published in paperback in 1982 and widely discussed. As a major study of the health of the UK, the Black Report proved very embarrassing for the government of the day. It pointed out that health and mortality were closely linked to social class and wealth. The investigators showed that, for a whole range of medical conditions, *mortality* (death rate) and *morbidity* (reported illness) were lowest amongst the wealthiest and highest amongst the poorest. Much research has followed in the 25 years since the Black Report was published, but the findings remain the same: your life expectancy and health are heavily influenced by where you are in society. Authors such as Bywaters and McLeod (1996) claim that there is substantial evidence to show that social inequalities continue to undermine health and, what is worse, during the 1990s the gap between the better off and the poorest in our society steadily widened. Research into health inequalities demonstrates that, while the biomedical model of health has much validity, it is only part of the story. Health cannot be seen in purely scientific reductionist terms, divorced from sociological and environmental factors.

An alternative perspective on health is provided by the interactionist model, which suggests that health can look very different when it is examined either from the individual's or the professional's view. This is an issue that can be usefully illustrated by exploring the differences in meaning between illness and disease. Illness can be viewed as a human experience and refers to the perceptions of the patient and family and their responses to the symptoms and suffering caused by the disease process. Disease on the other hand refers to a problem that can be viewed from the medical perspective and can be defined by alterations in the structure and function of the body. Helman (1994) writes of illness as something that you go to the doctor with, whereas disease is something you have when you leave the surgery. Each person is aware of their own symptoms and attaches their own meanings to these; this subjective experience is the illness. However, the medical profession has objective models of disease that when applied to the person's complaints (illness) give it a label which is the disease. There is often a mismatch between the severity of a symptom as perceived by the individual when compared with the clinician's view. What may seem trivial to the person may be important to the nurse or doctor, and vice versa.

A further example of the potentially conflicting views of patients and members of the healthcare community involves patients who live with chronic conditions. Patients may live with a particular condition (e.g. hypothyroidism)

and yet consider themselves to be perfectly healthy. If the condition is managed adequately with appropriate replacement therapy, the intrusion of the disease into the patient's daily life may be minimal. For other patients with more intrusive conditions (e.g. type 1 diabetes) the perception of poor health may be ever present and patients may consider themselves to be unwell. In these examples the body may be described as losing its silence (Bleeker and Mulderij 1992, Morse et al 1994) describe the person with a chronic condition as having a body in disease. Ultimately it is not the condition that determines whether the patient is living with illness, rather it is a complex interaction between the individual and the condition, and each person will respond in a unique and individualized way.

As an illustration of the many personal views of health (interactionist models) that people have, the work of Stainton-Rogers (1991) is very illuminating. Her research was carried out in the UK and her sample was biased towards professional people. She found the following personal accounts of health, some of which have already been encountered:

1 The *'body as machine'* account sees illness as natural and real, and as something that can be dealt with only by modern biomedical science.
2 The *'body under siege'* account views the body as under attack from outside forces such as stress and difficult relationships, which act through the mind to affect the way the body works, in addition to biological agents such as bacteria.
3 The *'inequality of access'* account supports modern medicine but sees health as threatened by poverty and lack of access to health care.
4 A *'cultural critique'* views exploitation and oppression within modern society as determining health.
5 A *'health promotion'* account recognizes the adoption of a healthy lifestyle and the responsibility of the individual in achieving health.
6 The *'robust individualism'* account is concerned with doing whatever the person wishes and attaches little importance to health as long as freedom of choice is present.
7 The *'God's power'* account sees health as in the hands of a deity; the person therefore needs to follow religious teachings to achieve God's care.
8 The *'willpower'* account places the person in complete control of their own health and stresses the need to use 'will' to maintain health.

Setting aside criticism about the representativeness of the sample chosen by Stainton-Rogers, this work is important to you as a future registered nurse. It shows that people have a whole range of views about health and you need to explore these views with each patient before any meaningful care or health education work can take place. The strength of this work is the way it shows such a wide variation in personal perspectives. A person who subscribes to the 'robust individualism' account is much less likely to pay

attention to messages about health than somebody who identifies with the 'health promotion' account.

An additional factor in understanding health is the variability introduced by different cultures. The increasing globalization of the world means that any one country is likely to have significant numbers of people from other countries, cultures and religious backgrounds who will all have different perspectives on health. Research that might shed light upon this phenomenon is rather sparse in the UK. Smaje (1995) was very critical of the lack of rigorous data gathering that could provide evidence about the health of people from minority ethnic groups. What little evidence there is suggests that people in the UK who were born abroad tended to have better health than the population in their native countries but had worse mortality statistics than UK-born citizens. Of all the ethnic groups in the UK, those born in Ireland had the worst mortality statistics.

There is a complex interplay of genetic, cultural and environmental factors at work in explaining the health records of minority ethnic populations. This is illustrated by the example of diabetes, where mortality statistics for England and Wales show that the standardized mortality rate due to type 2 diabetes for men aged 20–69 years who were born in the Indian subcontinent or the Caribbean is three times higher than that for the general population. However, the incidence of type 2 diabetes is also increasing amongst the native UK population (as it is in the USA and elsewhere) because of dietary and life-style changes. This is what Helman (1994) describes as the 'malnutrition of the West' meaning eating larger amounts of 'junk' food of low nutritional value.

In the introduction to this section it was stated that there are many different definitions of health, and perhaps it is best to conclude with the views of the World Health Organization (WHO). In 1958, the WHO reported that 'health is a state of complete physical, mental, and social well-being, not merely the absence of disease and infirmity' (WHO 1958, p. 459). This definition was an acknowledgement that health is more than non-disease, but it has been criticized for proposing an ideal, rather than a measurable goal for which strategies for achievement can be devised. It has since been altered to present health not as a 'state' but as a 'resource':

Health is the extent to which an individual or group is able, on the one hand, to realize aspirations and satisfy needs and, on the other hand, to change or cope with the environment. Health is seen as a resource for everyday life, not the objective of living, it is a positive concept emphasizing social and personal resources as well as physical capacities.

(WHO 1986)

Although regarded as an improvement on the earlier definition, this has not increased its measurability and, as Gough et al (1994) point out, this is one of the main problems surrounding health debates. If it is not possible to agree what health actually is, how can we agree measures of health and therefore know when it is improving or getting worse?

This introduction to health has shown there are many definitions of health ranging from those of learned academics in medicine and the social sciences through to the everyday personal understandings that we all carry around with us. It is these latter definitions that you will have to work with as a nurse, trying to set them within the wider academic and clinical framework of health as you care for, and discuss health, with each patient.

HEALTH EDUCATION AND HEALTH PROMOTION: THE DEBATE

It will not surprise you that, given the difficulties surrounding the definition of health, there is little agreement about what constitutes health promotion and how this differs from health education. Naidoo and Wills (2000) give an excellent account of the debates that have taken place around this topic and you are referred to their text for a full account.

A commonsense definition of health education sees it as teaching individuals about steps they can take to enhance their health (e.g. exercise) and avoid disease (e.g. use of a condom during sex). The relationship of this activity to health promotion was described by Tones (1993) in terms of a simple formula:

$$\text{Health Promotion} = \text{Health Education} \times \text{Healthy Public Policy}$$

In this view, health education is seen as empowerment which, when combined with a health-oriented public policy, leads to the promotion of health. Nurses have a key role in this process as they can make a major contribution to individual empowerment. Tones (1992) has argued that health education has three main strands:

1 Critical consciousness raising – creating an empowered population that can exert pressure on governments for change.
2 Convincing a wide range of occupational groups that they have a role in health. Examples might be teachers, local authority housing staff, the transport industry, those responsible for planning economic growth and development.
3 Direct and individual patient-focused health education such as teaching a person newly diagnosed with diabetes about managing their diet and insulin regimen.

Nurses have traditionally been involved only in the third of these options, but are beginning now to realize that they should get involved in the other areas (see Box 1.1).

Early public health strategies were related to the eradication of illness and prevention of communicable disease (see Box 1.2). Although disease prevention and health protection are still important activities, there is a danger that health

Box 1.1   A nurse practitioner-led farmers' health service

Farmers are a group who face serious health problems due to the hazardous and arduous nature of their work. Their health needs have not always been met by a health service designed for a predominantly urban population. Since the mid-1990s British agriculture has been gripped by its most serious crisis for 60 years causing a dramatic increase in mental health problems and farm suicides on top of the serious physical health problems farmers and their families face. A nurse-led project in the southern part of the English Lake District and adjacent Pennines has started providing a unique health service to individual farmers by means of a mobile clinic visiting auction marts. The nurses regularly attend farming meetings to discuss issues ranging from first aid to stress management. The project has also become involved with agricultural organizations, working to raise consciousness about risks such as mental health and organophosphate poisoning. It is working with the Health and Safety Executive as well as farmers to bring about change in accident prevention work. The project is also lobbying NHS providers to make their services more appropriate for the farming community and to increase knowledge amongst health professionals about farming problems. The nurses have shown their solidarity with the farmers by joining them on protest marches. All three of Tones' modes of health education are being addressed by this project.

Box 1.2   The three levels of prevention

- *Primary* – activities to decrease the probability of illness and to protect against illness; includes both risk avoidance and risk reduction

- *Secondary* – activities for early diagnosis and early intervention to reduce the duration and severity of illness

- *Tertiary* – rehabilitation, coping with disability or chronic disease.

promotion will remain a very limited concept if we do not look further afield than the actions outlined in Box 1.2. Naidoo and Wills (2000) observe that a disease prevention perspective does not look beyond readily identified risk factors to the real origins of ill-health such as poverty and social breakdown. This approach may define health education as merely information giving by health experts and measure success in terms of the extent to which clients follow the advice given. In the UK, The 1999 Department of Health publication *Our Healthier Nation* (DoH 1999b) can be criticized from this point of view. What is missing is a willingness to work with people to help them make informed choices for themselves (empowerment), as simply telling people what to do is an ineffective health education strategy. Other models for health promotion include the social model aimed at influencing key decision makers, and the community model aimed at achieving collective action in pursuit of health. The community model brings more than just health professionals into the field of health promotion as teachers, welfare workers, workplace managers and social workers, for example, could all be involved. These models are discussed further in the next section.

Nevertheless, as Delaney (1994) observes, health education is inseparably linked to health protection and disease prevention measures. This is characterized by the WHO, which see health promotion as an umbrella concept pulling together various aspects of health and involving public policy. This clearly makes it the business of national governments. Delaney, however, discerns amongst the WHO's general statements on health promotion two specific elements: attention to *individual lifestyle* and *living conditions*.

In the UK, health promotion has been linked to health policy for some time. Various government publications since the 1970s have carried the message that many health problems are the product of lifestyles and therefore the individual is responsible for preventing much illness. That is the message from the government at policy level and the government has the power to legislate accordingly (e.g. banning smoking in public places, car seatbelt legislation).

This latter point is crucial because, as the Black Report and much subsequent work (Whitehead 1988) has shown, social constraints are very real. Advice about a healthy diet is meaningless if the person cannot afford it. The devastating psychological effects upon an individual of redundancy and unemployment may drown out completely any health education messages. The political or economic refugee with little or no English is in no position to act upon health education messages. How many healthy options (joining an exercise group or getting support from friends to stop smoking) exist for a socially disadvantaged single woman who is the head of the household with three young children to care for? Nurses need to be sensitive here to the dangers of what is known as 'victim blaming'. This occurs where society places a double burden upon the sick: it creates the conditions that lead to health problems then establishes a model of health care that makes the individual responsible for their own sickness, and even stigmatizes them for it.

MODELS OF HEALTH PROMOTION

There are various approaches to health promotion, and Naidoo and Wills (2000) offer an excellent discussion of these models. They summarize them as follows:

1 *The medical or preventive approach*. This method seeks to increase medical interventions that will prevent ill-health. It is medically led, makes use of epidemiological methods and screening techniques, and works on the principle that the prevention or early detection of disease

is much cheaper than treating the established disease later. The success of vaccination programmes in eliminating diseases such as smallpox and polio are testimony to the power of this approach. However, access for disadvantaged groups remains a problem.

2 *Behaviour change*. Government publicity campaigns aimed at persuading people to change their behaviour are examples of this approach. This is expert-led and targeted at the individual.

3 *The educational approach*. This method does not directly set out to persuade people to change behaviour but rather to provide knowledge and information in the hope that the person will subsequently modify their behaviour as a result of their own choice. Both the educational and behaviour change approaches suffer from disadvantages as human health behaviour is far more complex than they acknowledge and the individual may not have the resources necessary to make individual lifestyle changes, even if they wanted to.

4 *Empowerment*. This is a bottom-up approach which involves facilitating people, either as individuals or in communities, to decide for themselves what health-promoting activity they wish to participate in and to proceed to act for themselves. The current government have acknowledged the importance of empowering individuals and patients in such publications as *The Expert Patient* (DoH 2001) and *Choosing Health Making Health Choices Easier* (DoH 2004).

5 *Social change*. This radical approach aims to change the physical, social and economic environment as a means of achieving healthier lives for people.

The nurse may be involved in any of these approaches, whether working as a practice nurse giving vaccinations, running a well woman clinic or putting up posters in the A&E waiting room. However, as Delaney (1994) has observed, nurses have tended to view health promotion as being about preventing specific diseases or promoting general good health rather than getting involved in the more contentious political and 'conditions of living' arena. At an organizational level, bodies such as the Royal College of Nursing do lobby government departments, often in conjunction with the medical Royal Colleges, on a range of health issues. Some individual nurses are also becoming involved in health promotion by empowerment. They are, for example, working with high levels of autonomy in community centres in certain deprived urban areas of the UK, following a precedent set by nurse practitioners in the USA 40 years ago. One of the defining principles of nurse practitioner practice today is the desire to enable patients to care for their own health. Nurses in the UK have moved into the nurse practitioner role to meet the needs of underserved populations (Smith 1992), to enhance the capacity of general practice in areas of poor GP recruitment (Kenny 1997) and to deliver innovative healthcare services to populations with specific needs (Walsh and Howkins 2002). Delaney's

observation is still valid in general terms, however, and it remains to be seen whether nurses will become more aware of the importance of political power as a key health-promoting factor. It now remains to move to the one-to-one level in which the nurse engages in health education.

HEALTH EDUCATION AND PATIENT TEACHING

Patient education is an important function of nursing practice. As we have already seen, it can be about raising people's awareness about an issue, working on key groups of decision makers or working with the individual client. Ewles and Simnett (1999) fill in some detail by stressing that this process involves the whole person throughout their entire life, regardless of how ill or well that person may be at any one time. They see health education as helping people to help themselves, either individually, in families or in larger communities, by using a wide range of teaching techniques to achieve goals that often involve changing behaviours, attitudes and social circumstances. In the past, nurses have tended to teach patients within a disease-oriented framework rather than from a health perspective. Focusing only on the disease is a narrow and blinkered approach that ignores a wide range of social and psychological factors and is also very limited in its goals. As Seedhouse (1986) reminds us, a major theme in health education tends to be the prevention of illness rather than the creation of wellness. In his view, health is the foundation for all human achievement; this gives a much deeper significance and meaning to health education. Patient education is an interactive process whereby learning, which may subsequently be used to influence behaviour, takes place. This leads to a more humanistic view of patient education in which the nurse and patient share responsibility for learning.

Autonomy is the key to patient-centred education. In education that is medically centred, notions of compliance and a paternalistic viewpoint tend to dominate. Freire (1985) pointed out that real education must entail emancipation; that is, liberating people to make their own decisions on their own terms. Historically, however, nurses and other professionals have hesitated to allow patients the control that they need to make their own choices and decisions. At times this reluctance has stemmed from our maternalistic or paternalistic view of patients. Hospitals and other healthcare agencies have also created organizational barriers that prevent the patient from having the freedom to make decisions about health.

If we accept the validity of the patient-centred approach to health education, what are its goals? Box 1.3 shows a more structured approach to individual health education and is derived from standards set by the US Joint Commissioning Authority for Health Organizations (JCAHO).

These standards emphasize the empowering nature of health education and the need to involve family members in

---

Box 1.3 Goals for patient education

The nurse should focus on:

- assisting the patient and family in their understanding of the nature of their health problems and the treatment options available to them

- involving the patient and family in the decision-making process

- developing the skills and coping strategies needed for self-care

- encouraging a healthy lifestyle

- ensuring that patients and families are involved in continuing, long-term care

---

the process, recognizing that clients do not exist in a vacuum, but have to be seen in their social context. As we have already seen, though, promoting a healthy lifestyle is possible only if the patient has access to the necessary resources.

Seedhouse (1986) commented that the meaning of health cannot be understood from a dictionary, nor is it enough to say that health is desirable and then leave the issue at that: action is needed. In his view, health education has two main broad aims: (1) to ensure that people have a good standard of general education and (2) to develop people's powers of intellectual conception so that they can maximize the information with which they are presented. This is an enabling point of view consistent with the JCAHO standards outlined in Box 1.3. It is about giving people the tools with which to tackle their own health problems; health education is definitely not about indoctrination and propaganda.

Every patient has the right to seek information and participate in the educational plan. Simply providing information about health matters is a waste of time. The purpose of education is to encourage patients to use knowledge to modify behaviour and perform activities that will result in improved health status. The role of the nurse, therefore, is to plan learning experiences with the patient, as a component of total care, so that adults share responsibility for health. Ideally, the outcome of learning is that the patient is able to make rational decisions with respect to health, participate effectively in self-care and adjust to the realities of the lifestyle changes that are required. However, various environmental factors can seriously hinder the patient's ability to change lifestyle.

PRACTISING HEALTH EDUCATION: AN EXAMPLE

A prime example of the importance of health education is provided by AIDS where, in the absence of any known cure or immunization programme, the main defence against the disease is education. Nurses are one of the key groups that can carry out the educational function in a wide range of situations and, in view of the importance of the issue of health education and AIDS, this is worth exploring in some detail.

There are two critical goals in the global management of **HIV** infection:

- Intervention needs to be focused on the prevention of transmission of the virus into healthy individuals
- Intervention must be focused on appropriate and humane care of individuals affected by the virus. Self-care for the person is critically important.

Despite the agreed wisdom that prevention of the spread of human immunodeficiency virus (HIV) is so important, the evidence worldwide is not encouraging as the number of new cases continues to climb remorselessly. This trend led Lifson (1994) to speculate that, with regard to preventing HIV infection, we have all lost our way and now face a growing crisis. He suggested there are five key principles involved in meeting the threat:

1 We must emphasize the viral nature of the disease and the fact that progression towards serious illness begins with infection; therefore AIDS prevention means HIV prevention.

2 The highest priority must be given to preventing the sexual transmission of HIV and other sexually transmitted diseases that facilitate its spread. This means shifting public attention away from the occasional unfortunate healthcare worker who is infected or from speculation about a protective vaccination to the reality that HIV is spread most readily by unprotected sex.

3 The problem of HIV spread amongst drug users must be tackled irrespective of political concerns or other niceties. This should include safer sex messages.

4 Prevention programmes must be planned and carried out that are sensitive to local needs.

5 Strong leadership is needed at national and international level to ensure that HIV is tackled as the major public health threat that it is.

Health education forms the core of the first four principles, whereas the final point relates more to health promotion (see Tones' formula on p. 16). The nurse is in the front line of this campaign whether talking to a patient and family about the risks of blood transfusion before routine surgery, working as a school nurse with adolescents or in a family planning clinic.

Prevention of HIV infection is everyone's responsibility. Abstaining from or minimizing the degree of risky behaviour is an important deterrent in decreasing transmission of the virus. It is crucial that information is provided in a culturally acceptable manner and in a language that is easily understood. Previously, the weight of responsibility has fallen on individuals infected with HIV to practise safer sexual practices or to inform sexual partners of their HIV status. However, self-protection is equally the responsibility of a non-infected partner. Sexual relationships require individual responsibility. For individuals to be motivated to adopt a new behaviour they must perceive a certain degree of risk or vulnerability. One of the problems of preventive education is that repression and denial are often used to minimize the degree of threat to the person. Therefore, individuals do not adopt safer behaviours because they deny they are at risk.

The nurse can teach the importance of using safer sexual practices; however, it is often difficult to motivate people to change practice. It is usually more effective to focus teaching around both partners. An atmosphere that feels safe needs to be created so that individuals feel comfortable discussing intimate behaviours. Safer sexual practices need to be incorporated so that they are pleasurable and in keeping with the individual's cultural and moral values. The individual needs to understand that safer sex is used because the person wants to stay healthy, not because their partner is suspect. Attention needs to be given not only to the mechanics of sexual behaviour but also to areas of maintaining intimacy and closeness.

The key message is that unprotected sex constitutes the highest risk behaviour, in particular:

- male to male via penetrative anal intercourse
- male to female via penetrative anal or vaginal intercourse.

Transmission from an infected passive male to an active male or from an infected female to a male is less likely as the concentration of infectious particles is lower in vaginal or anal secretions than in semen. Intercourse during menstruation greatly increases the risk of infection. Oral sex carries less of a risk of infection, but it is still possible. The risk for a receptive male having oral sex with an infected male partner is approximately one-sixth that of having receptive anal sex, but is still very real. An infected woman can infect a man via oral sex, although there is no conclusive evidence that 'French kissing' has caused HIV transmission. Other factors that increase the risk of infection are if the man is uncircumcized, has multiple sexual partners, there is trauma or bleeding during sexual activity, and if other sexually transmitted diseases are present.

In addition to information on safer sexual practices, the nurse also needs to provide information on the use of condoms and lubricants. Obstacles to incorporating behaviour change may include knowledge deficits, fear, lack of skill, lack of social support or inadequate resources to purchase products such as condoms. The nurse can be of vital importance in helping individuals learn how to negotiate a sexual relationship. In particular, it may be difficult to get a sexual partner to use condoms. Many people are unsure how to initiate this discussion. Among men, a variety of reasons have been cited for the underutilization of condoms, including lack of ready access, failure to plan for sexual intercourse, the use of alcohol and drugs prior to sex, beliefs that condoms impair sexual pleasure, and the belief that condoms are unnatural or immoral. These same questions have not been asked of women. With particular groups of clients, it may be useful to role-play prospective situations to try to minimize these barriers (Table 1.1). When men and women are empowered with information and negotiating skill, they are less likely to place themselves in risky situations. The management of HIV and AIDS demonstrates the complexity associated with health education relating to particular illnesses and disease. The nurse must not only focus on the

Table 1.1 Talking about condom use – suggestions for role play

He says	She says
I haven't had sex with anyone for ages so I must be clean.	But you could be infected with something and not know it – I think I'm clean as well, but I don't know for sure.
It doesn't feel the same; it takes the fun out of it.	Yes I know that, but think of the fun we can have putting it on.
Condoms smell.	Let's try some of the scented ones, especially if they have different flavours as well – do you know my favourite flavour?
All that fiddling around may make me lose the urge.	So we make it part of the fun before we get down to some serious bonking!
If I mess around putting one on I'll lose my erection.	If I help you put it on, you won't, I promise!
You know I love you too much to risk giving you something nasty.	And I love you too but I want to protect ourselves and our thing together – often people don't find out they're infected for years after.
It may burst or come off anyway so what's the point of spoiling the fun?	I'll help you put it on so it won't come off and the chances of it bursting are very remote and even if it did, we would be no worse off than not using one.

individual patient's social situation and personal beliefs but must also be aware of the national and international dimensions of the condition and the enormity of the economic and human impact on a global scale.

EXPECTATIONS FOR PATIENT EDUCATION

Patients are becoming better consumers of health care. They are better informed and they want to know more. Because of the consumer movement and greater media attention to healthcare issues, patients are aware of their rights and are more demanding about receiving information on their condition and treatment. Many want to be involved in decision making regarding their care and treatment.

Patient education has become part of total, comprehensive patient care. To provide quality care, all of the patient's needs must be addressed, including the need to know about health education, disease prevention and health promotion. Factors such as shorter hospital stays, reduced convalescent facilities and higher incidence of chronic illness mean that more patients are being cared for at home by family carers. Family carers cannot be expected to care for ailing relatives without learning the necessary skills.

The nurse is the health professional in most contact with a patient and has a broad overview of the patient's health status; this would appear to make the nurse the ideal person to engage in health education work. While authors such as Black and Hawks (2005) see education as an essential part of the nurse's role, pressure of time tends to mean that patient teaching suffers as a result. Nurses have to work hard to establish the validity of patient teaching as an essential part of caring. They still have to justify longer consultation times with patients in primary care settings or setting time aside on busy wards in order to engage in patient teaching.

Giving nurses more accountability for individual patient care may also facilitate patient education, although there is a range of factors, mentioned above, that is seen as interfering with the nurse's educative role. One key factor that is missing from the discussion, however, is whether the patient is able to respond to education to make appropriate lifestyle changes. The limitations imposed upon people by poverty, culture and environmental factors have already been mentioned, while the advertizing industry spends huge sums of money persuading people to smoke, eat unhealthy food and drink more alcohol than is good for them. There is, therefore, a powerful critique of the individualist account of health that also needs to be considered. Dines (1994), in discussing the limitations imposed upon individuals, cautions against being too fatalistic. Although there are powerful forces at work in people's lives over which they have little control, individuals still retain some autonomy, and to target health education work the nurse needs to find those areas where people retain a larger degree of control. In Dines' view health education is a constrained activity as a result of such social forces, but nevertheless is worthwhile as positive results may be obtained in limited areas.

Despite such strong historical evidence that patient education can be effective, the introduction of new education programmes should be monitored for effectiveness. Health education consumes scarce resources (such as nursing time) and the evidence must be gathered to show that it is a cost-effective use of those resources.

In summary, it is clear that there are expectations placed on nurses to teach. Quality assurance standards, professional standards and a focus on risk management emphasize the nurse's role in patient education. Nurses perceive that patient education is an important component of total patient care, yet are faced with external constraints that limit their ability to teach effectively. These constraints include time restrictions, unrealistic expectations of managers, patients who are too acutely ill to learn, and workload factors. With greater expectations on the part of patients who want to learn and demand to know, the challenge is for nurses realistically to meet these expectations.

Compliance and concordance

Much time, effort and expense is devoted to patient education by health professionals. Patient education, if viewed as a total process, can be a key component in enabling patients to act on the recommendations of the health professionals. However, patients cannot carry out a treatment or recommendation that they do not understand or *do not accept*. Refer back to Pat's story, which introduced this chapter, to see the importance of this observation. The degree to which patients follow recommendations is usually called *compliance* or *patient adherence*.

Compliance can be viewed as coercive obedience and for this reason the Royal Pharmaceutical Society of Great Britain launched a paper in 1997 entitled 'From compliance to concordance: towards shared goals in medicine taking' (Marinker 1997). Concordance is defined as:

> *… a new approach to the prescribing and taking of medicines. It is an agreement reached after negotiation between a patient and a health care professional that respects the beliefs and wishes of the patient in determining whether, when and how medicines are to be taken. Although reciprocal, this is an alliance in which the health care professionals recognise the primacy of the patient's decisions about taking the recommended medications …'*
>
> (Concordance Co-ordinating Group 2000)

Concordance is not a substitute for the word compliance; there are subtle differences in the approach taken when concordance with medical regimens is the focus. Concordance requires the agreement of two parties; it cannot be imposed. If concordance is being used as a framework for the development of treatment plans, the patient will be encouraged to express concerns about the treatment and will be involved in decision-making about their medications. If concordance is successful some patients will decide not to take their medication and the outcome may not be what the healthcare professional thinks is in the best interests of the patient (Dickinson et al 1999). It is important to accept this situation and review the goals of treatment which may differ with each individual patient. In this sense, concordance is part of the helping relationship between the health professionals and patient; it is the outcome of nurse–patient communication and interaction.

Increased attention to the area of concordance has been generated because of the impact of compliance or non-compliance on health outcomes. Rankin and Stallings (1996) cite extensive evidence to show that a high percentage of patients do not follow the recommendations of health professionals. It has been estimated that the rates of non-compliance with prescribed medications are 50% (Haynes et al 2006) and others have found that the number of patients who do not take their medications as prescribed ranges from 10% to 94%. Non-compliance is therefore costly; it wastes medical and human resources, and may have serious consequences for the patients and their families or significant others.

Non-compliance can take many forms: failure to keep scheduled appointments, to take medications as directed, to follow recommended dietary or lifestyle change, or to follow recommended preventive health practices. Factors that may contribute to non-compliance include financial problems (inability to pay for expensive prescriptions), inconvenience (such as taking medications during working hours), religious beliefs, denial of illness, lack of family or other support, feelings of fear or shame, and feelings of helplessness or lack of control. All of these factors can impact on the patient's decision not to follow suggestions or recommendations regarding health.

The Health Belief Model is useful in helping nurses to understand the important factors in developing concordance with patients. This model theorizes that the likelihood of patient compliance varies with:

- the patient's perception of susceptibility to the disease
- the prediction of the impact of the illness on the patient's life
- the patient's perception of barriers to taking recommended action
- the patient's perception of the benefits of taking the action (Naidoo and Wills 2000).

It suggests that people carry out cost–benefit analyses in which they assess the threat and cost of illness compared to the possible benefits of seeking medical help and also the costs (in the broadest sense) of obtaining that help. The fundamental question becomes 'Is it worth it?' If the answer is 'yes', then the person is likely to seek help and to co-operate with treatment; if the answer is 'no', then he or she either will not seek help or, if they do, will not follow advice and treatment requirements. Walsh (1995) has found, for example, that this model explains much patient behaviour in attending A&E departments. This should be seen as only one amongst several factors at work in determining patient behaviour. However, the model gives the nurse some important insights into health education activity as the client has

first to perceive that there is a threat to themselves, and second that the potential advantages (benefits) outweigh the disadvantages (costs) in taking therapeutic action. Those who think that only gay men and drug users contract HIV will not use a condom whilst having heterosexual sex, as infection cannot happen to them. Teenage smokers cannot really imagine what it is like to be 45 years old, so they are unlikely to perceive the long-term risks of smoking as something that will affect them, however serious they may be.

It is important for nurses to understand that all individuals are influenced by their beliefs and values (attitudes) about their health or illness. Nurses are also influenced by their own beliefs and values. At times, the individual's values and the nurse's beliefs may be very different. For effective teaching to occur, the nurse has to base the educational plan on the individual's perception of what is important and achievable because beliefs are strong motivators of human behaviour.

Yet another factor influencing education is the rapport and relationship established between the nurse and patient. In the next chapter we will explore this further as we discuss the area of therapeutic communication.

Contracting

Contracting with patients has been shown to be effective in achieving cooperation. The purpose of a contract is to promote the patient's active participation in health care by assisting the patient to identify and accomplish specific goals. Contracting helps to facilitate the patient's self-esteem, as well as promoting a trusting relationship.

Contracting promotes the patient's autonomy, involvement and responsibility for health. The patient exercises the right to self-determination and ability to solve problems. Furthermore, when nurses use contracting as a strategy, they are demonstrating belief in the dignity and worth of the patient.

The steps used in developing a contract are outlined in Box 1.4.

When helping patients to adjust to major lifestyle changes, the nurse can use contracting as a method to achieve co-operation. Contracting breaks down what might be overwhelming change into small incremental steps. The patient who feels in control of what can be accomplished will be more likely to achieve the desired objective.

Box 1.4 Steps in developing a contract
1 Identification of the priority health concerns or needs of the patient
2 The setting of *mutual* goals
3 Writing the contract
4 Implementation of the task or activities agreed upon
5 Evaluation of the outcomes of the contract

INFLUENCE OF CULTURE ON PATIENT EDUCATION

Culture determines many of the beliefs and values held by individuals; it therefore has a strong influence on health behaviour. Conflicts can arise when the nurse and patient hold different beliefs and values about what constitutes appropriate health behaviour.

Assessment of the beliefs, values and practices of the patient is vital to tailoring educational interventions (Helman 1994). The patient should be assessed as an individual, so that cultural preferences come out naturally, rather than being forced into a preconceived ethnic stereotype. For example, to teach about therapeutic changes in diet, the nurse must determine the patient's preferred and current diet, and the meaning of food in the patient's life.

The nurse needs to elicit the patient's views on the illness experience. For example, in some cultures it may be undesirable for a man to be bathed by a woman, and to put the patient in this situation would jeopardize his self-esteem. Conflicts in perspectives should be acknowledged openly and clarified. The nurse cannot enforce a teaching plan that contradicts the patient's beliefs. The patient's plan may not be the nurse's first choice but it may be more acceptable than the patient rejecting all interventions.

When English is the patient's second language, it is important for the nurse to speak slowly, use simple sentence structure, avoid medical or technical jargon, provide sequential steps in teaching, and not assume that the patient understands. Even if English is the first language, jargon and abbreviations should be avoided. The nurse should also consider the educational level of the patient and, without being patronizing, speak in terms that are appropriate and readily understood by the individual.

HELPING PATIENTS CHANGE

Individual health education involves the client making significant lifestyle changes. Nurses have increasingly turned to the work of Prochaska and DiClemente (1986) on change as providing useful insights into how people may be helped to change their behaviour. These authors propose that change does not happen in one 'big bang' but rather involves the person working through a series of stages in a cyclical process. The model may be summarized as described below.

Stage 1: Precontemplation

Here the person has not become aware of any health problem and is unaware of the existence of a health risk or the need for change. Consider Graham Smith, a 50-year-old bus driver who smokes 20 cigarettes a day, takes no exercise, eats a diet high in fats and processed food, weighs 12 kg more than he should for his height, and is regularly in the local pub consuming substantial quantities of beer. He sees no reason to change his lifestyle until …

Stage 2: Contemplation

Individuals are now aware of the benefits of change but have not actually decided to make any changes. They may be seeking help to make the decision to change, but so far have not decided to do anything about it. Some people never progress beyond this stage. Graham Smith has entered the contemplation stage as a result of a 'healthy heart' initiative by the bus company's occupational health nurse. She set up an exhibition in the canteen one lunch time and gave Graham a 'cardiac MOT', as she called it. It took only 10 minutes but made him aware that he really was overweight, unhealthy and had several risk factors for serious cardiac problems including raised blood pressure. He began thinking about these facts and talking to his wife. A few days later, and coincidentally, his brother was admitted to hospital, seriously ill after a heart attack. This led on to …

Stage 3: Preparing to change

At this stage the person now sees that there is a real threat and that the advantages of changing their lifestyle outweigh the costs (remember the Health Belief Model). They also perceive that change is possible and feel ready to change, although they may need support to do so. His brother's heart attack came as a great shock to Graham, especially as his brother was 2 years younger than he was. Graham realized he should be thinking in terms of another 25–30 years of active life, yet here was his closest living relation (his father died from a heart attack 12 years ago) seriously ill in hospital with something that he had been warned only that week could happen to him. As he talked with his wife she showed him some photographs from a few years ago of a much slimmer Graham turning out for the pub football team; he also considered how much money he could save by giving up smoking, just like his mate Roy had at work. 'If Roy can, I can', he concluded. It was time for action.

Stage 4: Making the change

In order to start the change process people need to make clear decisions about what they are trying to achieve and how they will do this. Key features of making a successful change are clear goals, realistic plans, support, and some kind of reward for achieving those goals. Graham got his support from his wife (who did not smoke) and from the occupational health nurse who he went to see to discuss his health. He agreed with her to give up smoking completely, a realistic programme of exercise, starting with a brisk 20-minute walk three times a week, and took home a dietary advice sheet to consider with his wife. The nurse also provided him with advice about foods to avoid at the works canteen and listed the healthier options she had just succeeded in getting the company to put on the menu (an example of health education by organizational campaigning). He also made an appointment to see his GP to discuss his blood pressure problem, reassured by the occupational health nurse that the practice nurse would also be very supportive. Having made the change, Graham realized that the hardest part was sticking at it or, in other words …

Stage 5: Maintenance

Sustaining the new behaviour pattern, moving to a healthier lifestyle and staying there is the hardest part of all, as reversion or relapse may easily occur. This puts the person back to one of the earlier stages. Few people, in fact, go through all these stages in an orderly way; relapse is common, but eventually each person will have moved through each stage. So it was with Graham as he found his first attempt at giving up smoking failed after only a week. However, reassurance from the practice nurse that this does happen and does not make him a failure led to a second successful attempt. Six months later, Graham had acquired a lively Border Terrier, which needed walking three times a day, had lost 5 kg in weight, been tobacco free for 4 months, had reduced his beer intake by a third and was feeling much better with a healthier diet.

The stages of change model outlined above depends fundamentally upon client motivation for success and this must be the focus of the nurse's efforts when working with any individual. The more involved the client is in planning the changes that are to be made, the more motivated he or she will be and therefore the more likely the nurse is to be successful in promoting healthy lifestyle changes for the client. Social support networks are very important in maintaining changes once begun. The nurse must be aware of the existence of the precontemplative stage because, if the patient is in this stage, there is little chance of achieving success. Change will occur only when the client is aware of the need for change and is willing to make the effort to do so; change must therefore come from within rather than be imposed from outside by an authoritarian or paternalistic approach. Change is more likely to be maintained if it becomes part of the person's everyday routine, such as walking the dog, rather than something that involves a special effort. We also have to be realistic in understanding how much change and uncertainty a person can cope with at any one time (Naidoo and Wills 2000). If the person is going through a very turbulent period in their life such as a divorce or struggling with the effects of redundancy, or they are living in a chaotic poverty-stricken environment, it may be unrealistic to expect significant health-related changes to occur in their lifestyle.

In working through the stages of change model with a client, the nurse should pay particular attention to the following:

1 *Attitudes to health and customs.* The patient's attitude towards health, and the degree of belief that it is possible to be in control of your own health, will influence learning. Religious and cultural beliefs influence eating habits, lifestyle and receptiveness to health care and prescribed therapy. This information is also useful to the nurse who is helping the patient to make decisions about care.
2 *Past experience of illness.* Information about past health history should be collected, including how the person coped with illness and what changes in health habits and lifestyle resulted.
3 *Physical condition.* The patient's general feeling of well-being or illness influences the capacity and readiness to learn. The ability to carry out activities of daily living and to manage tasks and procedures necessary for self-care should be assessed. **Vision**, **hearing**, **touch**, manual dexterity and mobility all need assessment because they are important to physical functioning.
4 *Emotional state.* Emotions affect an individual's readiness to learn and to respond to teaching. In illness, and when there is a permanent loss of function, patients may progress through stages of adaptation or grieving. These stages include denial, anger and resentment, recognition and acknowledgement of the problem. When recognition and acknowledgement occur the patient begins to participate in decision-making.
5 *Intellectual ability.* As well as willingness and desire to learn, the patient's ability to understand the condition and solve related problems will contribute to effective learning. The length of the individual's attention span, basic knowledge and fluency in the language being used should be kept in mind when considering comprehension and learning. This is particularly important if an interpreter is being used, especially when the interpreter might be a young child acting for his or her mother.
6 *Support system.* The response of family and friends to the situation can play an important part in the patient's education. If supportive, it facilitates learning and provides reinforcement for positive changes in behaviour.
7 *Barriers to learning.* Individual deterrents to learning include sensory deficits, decreased ability to comprehend, lack of orientation to time, place and person, decreased manual dexterity and loss of physical mobility. Learning is also inhibited by lack of motivation. Severe anxiety can interfere with learning, so that worries about lack of social and financial support and resources may inhibit effective patient education. If the language or form of words used by those teaching is unfamiliar or too technical (or perhaps too patronizing), that can also act as a barrier to understanding.

It is important early in the process to establish what the learning needs of the person are. A learning need is the educational gap between the present and the desired or required level of competence. It is mutually identified by the nurse and the patient from the analyses of the data collected and the needs expressed by the patient. The identification of learning needs should include a description of what the patient should know or be able to do and the factors influencing this.

Identifying educational needs and setting priorities requires assessing the patient's and family's present knowledge, how they see the patient's present level of functioning and what the desired level of competence may be. It is important to know whether they are able to look at the long-term implications or are able to focus only on what is happening today. This sort of assessment must be a continuous process, as changes occur once the patient has achieved the initial goals, coped with the impact of illness and begun to accept the changes in lifestyle.

Once learning needs have been identified, the nurse works with the patient to establish goals for learning, to determine priorities for teaching content and to select methods of teaching. Learning goals are usually divided into *short-term goals*, for immediate learning needs, and *long-term objectives*, for defining the eventual expected outcomes. The knowledge or skill to be achieved is defined, and the expected level or degree to which it will be met is stated. The final component of objective setting is defining the time in which the desired change is expected to occur. Behavioural objectives are worded in simple, basic terms that are clear to the patient and to all members of the healthcare team. They break learning tasks into small, sequential steps that can be tackled independently before the total goal is achieved.

The teaching plan must be written and placed in the patient's record. Without a written plan, other members of the healthcare team cannot actively participate in the teaching process. The plan must also be shared with the patient so that he or she can actively work towards achieving results.

Using a patient with **diabetes** as an example, behavioural objectives for the patient might be to:

- *state* the action of insulin
- *demonstrate* the technique of self-injecting with an insulin pen
- *talk about* feelings related to self-injection with insulin.

Teaching content must be accurately expressed in terms and language understandable to the patient and family, and adapted to age, cognitive ability, education and culture. The amount of time necessary and opportunities for questions, correction and repetition should be given consideration when planning teaching programmes.

Practical procedures should be broken down into a logical sequence of steps. First, the procedure should be demonstrated as a whole so that the patient is provided with an overview; then each step should be shown slowly and in detail. Time and opportunity should be allowed for practising the technique as soon as possible after the demonstration. The nurse should be aware that, in teaching any body of information, the first and last parts are recalled best; therefore, the most important points should come first and last. Repetition and receptiveness to questions reinforces learning.

Evaluation of the teaching programme and the patient's learning should be continuous. Revisions are made as indicated, and in some instances are made on the spot if the patient is not responding positively to the planned strategy. Outcomes of teaching are assessed: what effect the teaching has had, whether the objectives have been met, and whether the patient has acquired the knowledge and skills needed. Role playing or simulation may be used to assess changes in the patient's behavioural responses and in the ability to apply knowledge to real-life situations. The patient must also be an active participant in the ongoing and final evaluation of the educational plan. Observation and feedback are the primary ways in which the nurse determines whether (behavioural) change has occurred.

The process outlined above provides a framework for health education. It has not, however, referred to the many possible moral dilemmas that may be thrown up in day-to-day practice. Clarke (1993) has discussed health education with regard to the basic ethical principles of respecting the autonomy of the individual, acting to benefit the person (*beneficence*), not harming the individual (*non-maleficence*) and finally giving people what they deserve (*justice*). As she observes, health education involves choices and, if the wrong choices are made, a great deal of harm can follow; therefore the nurse must always be able to defend his or her actions ethically.

Health screening is an example chosen by Clarke, especially with regard to **cervical screening**. It is intended to be beneficial to the patient and to do no harm. But consider the stresses involved in the procedure and afterwards waiting for the results. Suppose that the woman is recalled for another smear or a mistake is made? The Health Belief Model would predict that, if the fears and anxieties generated by the procedure were too great, they might outweigh the possible advantages, leading to women failing to attend for screening at all.

It was issues such as these that led Foxwell and Alder (1993) to investigate whether a simple 10-minute nurse teaching package before screening could reduce anxiety levels. A large sample of 187 consecutive women (who were well educated and from a predominantly middle-class background) were allocated at random to either a control group that experienced the standard procedure or an experimental group that was given an additional nurse teaching presentation about the procedure. Anxiety levels after the smear were significantly reduced in the experimental group compared with the control group, suggesting that patient teaching in this case reduced anxiety. The researchers predict that this effect would be more pronounced in women who were less well educated or well informed, although this remains to be tested.

Encouraging women to attend for screening therefore generates anxiety, despite our principle of beneficence, but this study suggests these adverse effects may be minimized by further health education and information giving. This is consistent with Clarke's argument that the tension between beneficence and non-maleficence shown by this example can best be resolved by the nurse engaging the patient in full and open discussion about such procedures. This is what is meant by informed consent: the patient consents but only after being given all the information. Debate still continues about how much information is required for consent to be fully 'informed'. The current UK position seems to be that it is as much as the doctor thinks the patient needs to know. The furore created in 2001 by the scandal of organ removal at autopsy without parental consent, which was highlighted by the practices at Alder Hey Children's Hospital, has brought the issue of informed consent again to the fore. The medical profession's traditional view can be criticized as paternalistic and in need of a significant shift towards a more open approach.

Health education and promotion work continually throw up these dilemmas and you may find that the basic ethical principles that underpin nursing sometimes appear to contradict one another. Ultimately, the answer lies in open communication between nurse and patient, respecting the wishes of the patient at all times. Health education is set to become an increasingly important part of the nurse's role, particularly as nursing develops its community profile in response to the future shift in health care out of hospital. However, the limitations of what can be achieved, as pointed out by Dines (1994), should be borne in mind.

SUMMARY

The practice of nursing is dynamic and evolving, shaping and being shaped by the context within which nursing practice takes place. Changes in the healthcare delivery system have influenced the scope, skills and settings for the practice of nursing.

Nursing is growing slowly in self-confidence and is developing increased levels of autonomy. Nurse theorists have provided perspectives unique to nursing that emphasize the knowledge, research, ethics and practice of the profession. These perspectives provide a framework for applying knowledge from other disciplines to the practice of nursing, delineating the nurse–patient relationship and giving individualized, planned patient care. The nursing process is one method used by nurses to provide a systematic framework for nursing care, although alternative, more efficient, approaches, such as critical pathways have now been introduced. Accountability for care is a constant theme whatever method of care planning and documentation is used. All nursing care must rest on a sound ethical basis. Nursing ethics is premised upon principles of moral conduct, which include autonomy, beneficence, fidelity, justice, non-maleficence and veracity. The NMC provides guidelines for the ethical practice of nursing in its Code of Professional Conduct.

The following chapters provide the reader with the introductory knowledge, rationale and nursing perspective for the practice of nursing. Excellence depends upon the nurse applying this knowledge to clinical practice. During your nursing career you will work alongside a vast array of individual patients, their families and their communities. Each of these interactions will be unique. We hope that this text will provide you with the knowledge to address the needs of the patients you work with and also the flexibility to remain aware of the personal and particular perspective of each individual, their family and friends.

REFERENCES

Benjamin M, Curtis J (1992) Ethics in nursing, 3rd edn. Oxford: Oxford University Press.

Black J, Hawks J (2005) Medical surgical nursing, 7th edn. Edinburgh: Elsevier Saunders.

Bleeker H, Mulderij K (1992) The experience of motor disability. Phenomenology and Pedagogy 10, 1-18. Cited in: Price B (1996) Illness Careers: the chronic illness experience Journal of Advanced Nursing 24: 275–279.

British Medical Association (2002) The future healthcare workforce. BMA. Online. Available: http://www.bma.org.uk/ ap.nsf/Content/The+Future+Healthcare+Workforce 1 Dec 2004.

Bywaters P, McLeod K (1996) Working for equality in health. London: Routledge.

Clarke J (1993) Ethical issues in health education. British Journal of Nursing 2(10): 533–538.

Concordance Co-ordinating Group (2000) What do we mean by concordance? http://www.concordance.org/ Dec 2000.

Davidson N, Townsend P (1982) Inequalities in health. London: Penguin.

Delaney F (1994) Nursing and health promotion; conceptual concerns. Journal of Advanced Nursing 20: 828–835.

Department of Health (1986) Neighbourhood nursing – a focus for care. A report of the community nursing review. London: HMSO.

Department of Health (1999a) Making a difference: strengthening the nursing, midwifery and health visiting contribution to health and health care. London: HMSO.

Department of Health (1999b) Saving lives: our healthier nation. London: HMSO.

Department of Health (2000) The NHS plan. London: Department of Health.

Department of Health (2001) The Expert patient: a new approach to chronic disease management for the 21st century. London: HMSO.

Department of Health (2002) Liberating the talents: helping primary care trusts and nurses to deliver the NHS plan. London: Department of Health.

Department of Health (2004) Choosing health making health choices easier. London: HMSO.

Dickinson D, Wilkie P, Harris M (1999) Taking medicines: concordance not compliance. British Medical Journal 319: 787.

Dines A (1994) What changes in health behaviour might nurses logically expect from their health education work? Journal of Advanced Nursing 20: 219–226.

Ewles L, Simnett I (1999) Promoting health. A practical guide. London: Baillière Tindall.

Ford P, Walsh M (1994) New rituals for old; nursing through the looking glass. Oxford: Butterworth-Heinemann.

Foxwell M, Alder E (1993) More information equates with less anxiety. Professional Nurse October: 32–36.

Freire P (1985) The politics of education, culture power and liberation. New York: Macmillan.

Gough P, Maslin-Prothero S, Masterson A (1994) Nursing and social policy. Oxford: Butterworth-Heinemann.

Haynes R, Hassan N, Hasanah C (2006) Identification of psychosocial factors of non-compliance of hypertensive patients. Journal of Human Hypertension 20: 23–29.

Helman C (1994) Culture, health and illness, 3rd edn. Oxford: Butterworth-Heinemann.

Holm S (1997) Ethical problems in clinical practice. Manchester: Manchester University Press.

Kelly B (1991) The professional values of English nursing undergraduates. Journal of Advanced Nursing, 16: 867–872.

Kenny C (1997) Fighter pilots. Nursing Standard 93(45): 14–15.

Kinnersley P, Anderson E, Parry K et al (2000) Randomised controlled trial of nurse practitioner versus general practitioner care for patients requesting 'same day' consultations in primary care. British Medical Journal 320(7241): 1043–1048.

Lifson A (1994) Preventing HIV; have we lost our way? Lancet 343: 1306–1308.

Lindseth A, Marhaug V, Norberg A et al (1994) Registered nurses' and physicians' reflections on their narratives about ethically difficult care episodes. Journal of Advanced Nursing 20: 245–250.

Manthey M (1980) The practice of primary nursing. Oxford: Blackwell.

Marinker M (ed) (1997) From compliance to concordance: achieving shared goals in medicine taking. London: Royal Pharmaceutical Society.

Marsh GN, Dawes ML (1995) Establishing a minor illness nurse in a busy general practice. British Medical Journal 310(6982): 778–780.

Maslow A (1954) Motivation and personality. New York: Harper & Row.

Morse J, Borttorff J, Hutchinson S (1994) The phenomenology of comfort. Journal of Advanced Nursing 20: 189–195.

Naidoo J, Wills J (2000) Health promotion, 2nd edn. London: Baillière Tindall.

National Health Service Executive (1991) Junior doctors: the new deal. London: National Health Service Executive Management.

Nursing and Midwifery Council (2004) The NMC code of professional conduct: standards for conduct, performance and ethics. London: NMC.

Orem D E (1985) Nursing: concepts of practice, 3rd edn. New York: McGraw-Hill Book Company.

Peplau HE (1952) Interpersonal relations in nursing. A conceptual frame of reference for psychodynamic nursing. New York: GP Putnam's.

Porter S (1988) Siding with the system. Nursing Times 84(14): 30–31.

Prochaska J, DiClemente C (1986) Towards a comprehensive model of change. In: Miller WR, Heather N, eds. Treating addictive behaviours: processes of change. New York: Plenum.

Rankin S, Stallings K (1996) Patient education; issues, principles and practices. Philadelphia: JB Lippincott.

Reveley S (1999) The role of the triage nurse practitioner in general medical practice: an analysis of the role. Journal of Advanced Nursing 28(3): 584–591.

Robertson D W (1996) Ethical theory, ethnography, and differences between doctors and nurses in approaches to patient care. Journal of Medical Ethics 22(5): 292–299.

Rogers M (1970) An introduction to the theoretical basis of nursing. FA Davis: Philadelphia.

Rogers M (1980) Nursing: a science of unitary man. In: Riehl JP, Roy C, eds. Conceptual models for nursing practice, 2nd edn. New York: Appleton Century Crofts.

Rogers M (1987) Rogers's science of unitary human beings. In: Parse RR (ed) Nursing science. Major paradigms, theories and critiques. Philadelphia: WB Saunders Company, p 138–149.

Roper N, Logan W, Tierney A (1980) The elements of nursing. Edinburgh: Churchill Livingstone.

Salisbury C J, Tettersell M J (1988) Comparison of the work of a nurse practitioner with that of a general practitioner. Journal of the Royal College of General Practice 38(312): 314–316.

Seedhouse D (1986) Health: the foundation for achievement. London: Wiley.

Smaje C (1995) Health: race and ethnicity. London: King's Fund.

Smith S (1992) The rise of the nurse practitioner. Community Outlook, November/December, p 16–17.

Stainton-Rogers W (1991) Explaining health and illness. London: Harvester Wheatsheaf.

Stilwell B, Greenfield S, Drury M et al (1987) A nurse practitioner in general practice: working style and pattern of consultations. Journal of the Royal College of General Practice 37(297): 154–157.

Tones K (1992) Health education; politics and practice. Geelong, Australia: Deakin University Press.

Tones K (1993) Theory of health promotion; implications for nursing. In: Wilson-Barnett J, Clark J, eds. Research in health promotion and nursing. London: Macmillan.

Varcoe C, Doane G, Pauly B et al (2004) Ethical practice in nursing: working the in-betweens. Journal of Advanced Nursing 45(3): 316–325.

Venning P, Durie A, Roland M et al (2000) Randomised controlled trial comparing cost effectiveness of general practitioners and nurse practitioners in primary care. British Medical Journal 320(7241): 1048–1053.

Walsh M (1995) The health belief model and use of A&E services by the general public. Journal of Advanced Nursing 22: 694–699.

Walsh M (1998) Models and critical pathways in clinical nursing. London: Baillière Tindall.

Walsh M (2000) Nursing frontiers; accountability and the boundaries of care. Oxford: Butterworth-Heinemann.

Walsh M, Howkins D (2002) Lessons from a farmers' health service. Nursing Standard 16(16): 33–40.

Whitehead M (1988) The health divide. London: Penguin.

World Health Organization (1958) The first 10 years of the WHO. Geneva: WHO.

World Health Organization (1986) Ottawa Charter for Health Promotion. Ottawa: WHO.

Therapeutic communication and nursing practice

Mike Walsh

INTRODUCTION

In chapter 1 we saw that the nurse–patient relationship lay at the heart of nursing care whether the nurse was in the active role of caregiver or in a more supportive or educational role. Any relationship depends upon good communication if it is to work properly and in this chapter we will be looking at the key elements that go to make up effective communication. The chapter will seek to apply these principles in three major areas of nursing activity: assessment, patient teaching and offering psychological support. The management of patients with long-term illness, a crucial area for nursing, draws heavily upon these three aspects of communication skills. The most difficult practice area of all is perhaps giving patients bad news and supporting bereaved relatives. As these are such difficult topics they have been given chapters of their own (see Chs 00 and 00); however, the general principles covered in this chapter underpin these chapters in particular, as well as the rest of the book.

THE IMPORTANCE OF COMMUNICATION

It is essential to be clear about what we mean by caring if we are to see the real importance of communication. Caring used to be seen as getting the work done, performing a series of tasks, carrying out sister's or doctor's instructions. That was largely the case when I started my nursing career back in the 1970s. If caring is defined purely in terms of physical tasks, communication with the patient becomes of less importance. This is particularly true if the patient adopts a passive attitude of 'nurse/doctor knows best' and allows staff to carry out procedures in an unquestioning way. Patients were expected to be compliant with therapy and nurses were advised not to get involved with patients. We were to remain at a distance so that we could concentrate on the tasks in hand without feelings getting in the way.

We have moved on since then. The word 'care' has come to take on new meanings in the nursing literature. By the 1990s Sadler (1997) was writing of care as being about mutual interaction with a person and Wilde (1997) stressed the connected nature of care. Care is a deliberate and intentional process that depends upon a relationship being established and maintained between nurse and patient, not a collection of jobs to be performed in a shift.

Writers such as Chase (2004) have emphasised that in order to care for a person, we have to try to understand the complex web of interrelationships and interdependencies that involve that person. We cannot surgically remove the person from that network and treat his/her pathophysiological problem in isolation then drop him back in there (discharge) and hope all will be well. That isolationist or reductionist approach will often lead to unsatisfactory results.

A major new idea that has gained widespread acceptance in the scientific community in the last 20 years is that of complexity theory. The basic principles may be summed up by saying that we have to recognize that various parts of a system can interact with each other to produce an outcome (known as an emergent property) that was not obvious by just considering the bits alone. The likelihood of this happening is greatly increased in the presence of positive feedback and sensitive dependence upon initial conditions. This idea is summed up by the familiar phrase 'the whole is greater than the sum of the parts'.

Let me give you an example. In September 2005 in the UK rumours began to spread of an impending petrol shortage due to a combination of planned protest action against fuel tax by hauliers and the damage caused by Hurricane Katrina to the US petroleum industry. People are very sensitive to petrol shortages as the car is the only way to travel around in many parts of the UK (sensitive dependence upon initial conditions). Some people began going to petrol stations to fill up their cars (and spare containers) even though they had plenty in their tanks. This resulted in queues at the petrol pumps. Drivers going past saw the queues and thought that there really was a problem so they joined the queues to buy extra petrol, making the queues longer. Other motorists saw the lengthening queues and joined in (positive feedback). The dramatic surge in demand meant that petrol stations ran out of petrol, sending panicking motorists on journeys of many miles looking for petrol, which caused more shortages. The result was several days of chaos and a real shortage when there was absolutely no reason for one, all caused by sensitive dependence upon initial conditions and positive feedback. An objective analysis of the components of the system would have shown petrol stocks at their normal levels, no action being taken to disrupt supplies and no reason for a sudden increase in mileage by motorists, the components therefore could not have predicted the crisis that ensued. However, the process of interaction in a dynamic system with positive feedback produced a completely unexpected result (an emergent property): a fuel crisis!

The point of this story is to get you to think of human health in terms of interactions between things in the presence of positive feedback, i.e. complexity. Normally our body operates multiple systems of *negative* feedback to dampen down changes and continually fine tune and adjust our metabolism to produce homeostasis. However, when positive feedback acting on sensitive initial conditions creeps in, things have a habit of going badly wrong. The development of chronic renal failure (p. 615) involves a set of circumstances whose interactions cause renal cells to die. The more renal cells die, the fewer normal functioning cells are left, however, the work they have to undertake on behalf of the whole body remains the same so each cell is working harder at the same time as it is being affected by a spreading disease process. This leads to more cell death which further overworks the survivors so they more readily succumb, and so the process feeds back on itself as runaway positive feedback, leading to total destruction of the kidneys and end-stage renal failure which will be ultimately fatal without a kidney transplant. This is an example of complexity: interacting systems with positive feedback. Let us consider another example. Adolescents think it is cool to smoke – they get enhanced prestige from the behaviour which makes them feel good; this means they smoke more which makes them feel better (psychologically speaking); however, the addictive properties of nicotine take over, rewarding the behaviour with a pleasant sensation, which results in a major health problem. Pathologists are increasingly beginning to understand significant areas of pathology in these terms, such as how infection spreads through populations or how daily blood sugar levels vary in diabetic patients. As Wilson and Holt (2001) explain, illness arises from dynamic interaction within and between biological and psychosocial systems rather than the failure of a single component. The key to it all is dynamic interrelationships and positive feedback and that is where we began this analysis of caring. Communication is clearly critical to these two processes.

Communication is therefore an essential prerequisite for connection and the building of a therapeutic relationship with the patient and their family. This relationship may last a long time for, as we shall see in Chapter 5 on long-term illness, an increasing proportion of patients receive nursing care from the same team for the same problem over periods of many years. Communication is essential if the meaning and context of the patient's needs are to be understood; this is what Chase (2004) calls 'engaged knowing'. Trying to understand the situation from the patient's perspective is known as empathy and while this is a valuable insight for the nurse, it is not always easy to achieve.

We need to recognize that caring means different things to different people in different situations. This is a challenge to the nursing quality of empathy as it means the nurse must ask whether she or he can *really* appreciate what it is like to be 82 years old and have suffered a fractured hip. Good communication is therefore essential to understand the patient's individual perspective on their health status and strive for empathy (see p. 37).

Nurses are present in the caring situation and so may use that presence as a therapeutic tool, and do so creatively. By the very act of being there, you change the situation and make it different for the patient. You cannot be in the presence of the patient without communicating, even if you do not speak. Non-verbal communications such as the expression on your face or body posture will speak volumes. Caring is therefore multidimensional work as you have to draw upon the social sciences as well as the biological sciences to practise nursing care. Communication is of course a constant theme running through the social sciences and essential if you are to connect with the patient and begin to explore the psychological, social, ethical and spiritual dimensions of that person's needs.

Communication is a two-way street; the nurse and patient have to understand each other. Chase (2004) observes that nurses are not primarily concerned with the disease but rather with the person who is experiencing an illness. It is essential we get the balance right and do not lose sight of the medical dimension of the patient's condition, but also that we never forget that this is a real person and not another case of osteoarthritis. The crucial point is that by being open and honest (an authentic relationship) with patients, they are more likely to be similarly open and honest with us, which is essential if we are to achieve any degree of insight into their problems and to empathise with their experience.

BARRIERS TO EFFECTIVE COMMUNICATION

One of the biggest historical barriers to communication has already been referred to: the way nurses were encouraged to distance themselves from patients, as 'getting involved' was seen as detrimental to carrying out tasks. It is still possible to see nurses rapidly changing the subject if they feel uncomfortable, or resorting to bland reassurances such as 'It will be OK' or 'We do hundreds of these operations every year'. The patient's take on this might be 'How do you *know* it will be OK?' or 'You may do hundreds of operations on other people, but this is *my* operation!'. Patients who are gay or lesbian may find that sexuality is completely missing from their care as nurses avoid all mention of a partner. To care is to connect and that cannot happen across a distant void.

The problem of distancing leads into the problem of avoiding disclosure as the nurse worries that exploring an area might be too personal, too painful or do more harm than good. In the past, medicine has been criticized for this patriarchal approach of knowing what is best for the patient and telling only what the doctor thinks the patient should know. However, times are changing and medicine now places great emphasis on communication within a consultation and emphasises the need to build a relationship with a patient before collecting both subjective and objective data and then moving on to *agree* a management plan (Gask and Underwood 2003). The patient is the only person able to decide where they wish a conversation to go, and questions must be answered honestly rather than avoided along with attempts made to change the topic on to safer ground. Patient care can be an emotional minefield but nobody ever said nursing was easy. Feelings such as anger, fear or despair may not be far away. You need to be aware of this at all times and tread carefully – although this is no reason for not treading at all!

Once expressed, a patient's feelings do need to be explored, not ignored. Feelings may not be immediately expressed, however, and you also have to recognize the meaning of silence. A patient's silence can be quite intimidating and you may feel like breaking in with some small talk. This is a mistake as the reason for the silence may be that what the patient is thinking of is so painful and difficult that they are desperately struggling to bring themselves to verbalize these deep feelings. The silent listener who remains engaged and attentive is the compassionate listener (Seidal et al 2003) and eventually the patient may start to express themselves. Look for clues such as trembling hands, a reddening face and eyes filling with tears, which are telling you that something is too painful to talk about. Be prepared to give the patient a tissue and to say something like 'That's OK, I can see you are feeling really bad about this …' and to allow the patient the emotional release of the tears that will follow. As a student you also need to recognize when you might be getting out of your depth with a patient. It is not an admission of defeat or failure to ask a registered nurse to take over or to refer a patient's questions to a registered nurse because you do not know the answer. Neither is it an admission of defeat to find yourself getting emotional as well; self awareness is a valuable tool for the nurse and you cannot deny your own emotions and life experiences.

Getting into sensitive areas with patients is not easy. Price (2004) suggests one approach which he calls 'laddering' and this is based on the observation that patients generally find questions about events and activities easiest to answer and least threatening. He suggests starting there and moving up to the next 'rung' which involves meaning and knowledge. These are areas patients find less easy to deal with. Here we ask about the meaning of symptoms to patients or their knowledge of a disease such as diabetes. Finally we move to the hardest 'rung' of all which involves feelings, beliefs, attitudes and values. Here we might explore how the patient sees themselves now and what she/he thinks the future holds for them. Price's argument is that we move progressively into more sensitive areas, only after developing a trusting relationship built on less sensitive, more factual areas. Only then can we intrude into the patient's inner world therapeutically.

Dealing with a distressed patient needs even more skill than normal. However, you must recognize that communicating effectively with even the most open, stable and cooperative patient needs skill. Lack of communication skills can therefore be a major barrier. Each individual who becomes a nurse is different and so brings a unique mix of skills and life experience to nursing. Lucky is the nurse who is a born natural communicator. Most of us have to learn communication as a set of skills that we can deploy in different situations and, by reflecting on what worked and what did not as we go along, steadily improve our communication skills.

Communication is a two-way process, and however good you may be, this is only half the story. Patients may not be particularly good at expressing themselves for a range of reasons, such as linguistic skills (even if English is their first language), cultural beliefs or previous life experience. A significant proportion of the population does not have English as a first language, and in some circumstances the services of a translator are required. This can be very difficult, especially if the translator is a child and the patient is the mother, as she may not wish to share intimate details with her 10-year-old son and a complete stranger.

The two-way nature of communication means that you have to be aware of the fact that the patient's perceptions may be very different from your own, especially in relation to health. Lay beliefs about health may be very different from yours and the patient may be lacking in the technical language we take for granted. Seidal et al (2003) cite the clinical pearl of a patient who presented to a nurse practitioner (NP) complaining of 'low blood, high blood, bad blood and thin blood' all at once. It took some considerable time and skill (and superb communication skills I suspect) to establish that this patient thought he was anaemic (low blood), hypertensive (high blood), suffering from syphillis (bad blood) and had been overtreated with anti-coagulants (thin blood).

The patient may have a very different agenda for the consultation than you have. It is essential that you find out at the beginning exactly what is the patient's purpose, perceptions and levels of knowledge about their health. This can save a great deal of frustration and misunderstanding later. Consider the real case of a traveller who presented with his wife to an NP in UK primary care, announcing he had cancer of the rectum. The NP took a comprehensive health history which did not contain one single possible hint of bowel cancer and proceeded to undertake a full physical exam with the same nil result. Upon being reassured that there was absolutely no indication of the possibility of bowel cancer being present the man became extremely angry and proceeded to vent his anger on his wife (who had fading bruising around one eye) and left the surgery still shouting at her as they strode off into the flatlands of the Fen country. As a stand-up comic might say 'What was all that about?' The man probably had another agenda but the NP never had a chance to explore this.

The old adage that 'first impressions count' has been borne out by much experimental research in the field of social psychology. Humans tend to make perceptual short-cuts and place people in stereotypical categories based upon an initial first impression (see below). Again this works both ways. You, as a nurse, need to beware of falling into the perceptual trap when you meet a patient for the first time. You must look beyond the clothes and appearance to get to know the person within the patient. By the same token, how you appear to the patient on first meeting is equally important.

We quickly move from our first impressions concerning a person's appearance and behaviour to make inferences about their personality. Your patients are doing this about you whilst you are doing this about them! We therefore need to have some insights into what is going on in order that we can be more self-aware and try to avoid making errors; however, we will never be totally objective, but we should try our best and at least be aware of how bias might be creeping in. According to Taylor et al (2000) the key factors in the way we process and make sense of our impressions are:

1 *Evaluation*. This boils down to simply liking or disliking the other person and we naturally form a like or dislike very early in an interaction. Patients, however, have to be worked with and helped as they are, whether we like them or not, rather than how we would like them to be.

2 *Positivity bias*. Humans tend to want to see the best in people and often form a more positive first impression than perhaps they should. It is postulated that this is because we need to feel good about things and so like to rate others positively.

3 *Negativity bias*. Given that our 'default setting' is to be positive about strangers, when we notice something negative it tends to stand out much more and make a disproportionate impact. This can easily bias a history as one negative factor can be the focus of attention and other positive things are down-played. The patient may be a single parent receiving benefit payments, but she may also have a very supportive extended family, a resilient

personality and her child may be attending an excellent nursery which is also very supportive.

4 *Emotional information bias*. Overt emotional behaviour (e.g. sadness or happiness) is a potent source of bias. We tend to let this dominate and not see the whole person. Your assessment could become fixed on the person's low mood, which although it could be important and perhaps very important, should not blind you to looking at the whole health picture. The 30-year-old woman may appear sad, but you still need to check her diet and bowel function; the 16-year-old may appear happy but you still need to check how things are at school.

5 *Imputing meaning*. We are always trying to give meaning to what we learn about a person. As a consultation proceeds and new pieces of information are elicited, we tend to interpret the information in light of the impression we have already formed.
Example. You see a newly registered patient at the practice for the first time and begin to realise that he is fixed in his thinking and does not readily change his mind or actions; in short he is stubborn. If we already know this person has type 2 diabetes mellitus, a body mass index (BMI) of 32, smokes a packet of cigarettes per day and refuses to change his lifestyle despite 3 years of effort by the rest of the practice team, our impression is negative and we may conclude he is a stubborn, uncooperative patient. The same person could present as someone who does not suffer from type 2 diabetes mellitus, BMI 22, does not smoke, but who is feeling stressed and tired because he has been leading the campaign to keep the local community hospital open and refuses to take no for an answer from all the various tiers of authority in the NHS. He is still stubborn and uncooperative but we may interpret his stubbornness quite differently now!

6 *Imputing consistency:* This is about the halo effect. If we have initially evaluated a person positively or negatively, we tend to make other inferences about the person that are consistent with that initial judgment.

7 *Schemas:* These are mental short cuts or 'organized structural sets of cognitions' based on the little we know about the person and a series of examples drawn from previous life experience. These are mental pigeon-holes and we tend to stick the person rapidly into one of these standard pigeon-holes and assign a whole host of attributes to them accordingly. This can lead to a negative or positive judgment. This of course leads to the formation of stereotypes and blinds us to the individual.

Ethnic stereotyping, as we saw above, leads to assumptions being made about ethnic groups. The fact that a person belongs to a particular ethnic or religious group does not allow you to make assumptions about what they might eat, their views on privacy or who may treat them. All patients must be treated as individuals and your interaction with them will probably get off on the wrong foot if you start with a series of assumptions made based upon a stereotypical view of the ethnic or religious group to which they belong.

One final point concerning barriers to communication concerns the point of communication. If the aim is to discover information (assessment), then effective communication with the patient will not have occurred if effective communication with other colleagues does not follow. Whatever you may discover about the patient is wasted if it is not passed on to other members of the care team in clear and concisely written note form as well as verbally. The reverse is also true: effective communication with the patient for teaching or support purposes can occur only if you have the correct information to pass on.

The environment in which communication occurs can have a major influence on effectiveness and therefore constitutes a major barrier. Walsh (2006) expands upon this observation to point out that lack of privacy, the layout of furniture in a room, the distance between you and the patient (too far or too close), the mood or feeling in a room (stark and clinical or soft and relaxed), whether the area is quiet or noisy are all factors that can interfere with communication. There are also interpersonal factors that affect the environment and hence communication. Excessive formality on the part of the nurse together with emphasis upon status and position will inhibit communication by the patient. Sitting behind the barrier of a desk with the patient on the other side is an example of how a combination of furniture, room layout and status can interfere with communication. Brusqueness, hurrying the patient and lack of eye contact only make things worse.

In summary, therefore, the main barriers to communication are:

- distancing from the patient associated with lack of involvement
- fear of where a conversation may go and a desire to stay on safe ground
- lack of awareness of communication skills
- patient difficulties in communicating with you
- perceptions and first impressions of people
- stereotyping and making assumptions about people
- environmental factors
- interpersonal factors surrounding role and status.

Whether you are assessing the patient, engaging in teaching, or offering support and help with difficult decisions, these factors must be taken into account. Failure to do so leads to what Riley (2000) calls non-therapeutic communication. There is a range of communication techniques that, consciously or unconsciously, are used to maintain distance from a patient or to control the direction of a conversation in order that uncomfortable areas (for the nurse) are avoided. Riley (2000) has produced a comprehensive list of such techniques to avoid (Table 2.1) and we will consider some of the main ones below.

A truism in communication work is that it is not so much the message sent that counts as the message received. In other words, listening skills are crucial, particularly active listening (see p. 36). The converse of this statement is that a failure to listen properly to the patient will inhibit therapeutic communication as you will not receive the message that the patient is trying to send you. This may occur because of distractions in the immediate environment – hence the importance of environmental factors in preventing effective communication. However, there may be factors within

Table 2.1   Non-therapeutic communication – mistakes to avoid

Mistake	Result
Failing to listen	Do not receive message from patient
Failure to probe	Inadequate data collection
Parroting	Irritates patient who comes to doubt your competence
Being judgemental	Suggests you have a right that you do not: the right to judge the patient. Prevents establishment of good relationship with patient
Bland reassurance	Negates patient's fears, feels not taken seriously
Refusing to discuss topics	Patient feels personally rejected
Defensive attitude	Patient feels staff will stick together rather than listen to his or her complaint
Giving advice or instructions	Contradicts patient as partner in care
Stereotyping	Makes patient feel devalued as an individual
Changing topics	Tells patient that the nurse is in charge and sets the agenda rather than discuss topics the patient wants to talk about
Patronizing	Insults and devalues patient

Adapted from Riley (2000).

yourself that interfere with listening. Your mind may be on something else, such as worrying about home or social matters, thinking about the next job you have to complete, concern about another patient or getting that essay completed by the deadline. Whatever the distraction, if you are not giving 100% of your attention to what the patient is trying to tell you, you will not be able to obtain a good health history and carry out a full patient assessment.

To engage with a patient who is distressed and in need of psychological support, you have to focus completely on what she or he is telling you. Any apparent disinterest on your part will be quickly picked up by the patient and the therapeutic element in the dialogue will evaporate. If you are teaching a patient, it is important to check that they have learnt what you have taught them and to provide opportunities for them to question you. Another important truism is that it is not what is taught that matters, but what is learnt. You can assess what has been learnt only by listening to the patient's questions and asking questions of your own to check understanding. It all comes back to good listening.

A potential pitfall at the start of an interview is jumping to conclusions. This relates to making assumptions and stereotyping people. If you make a decision very early on about a patient's health problems or needs, you will tend to foreclose other options. Consequently you may not actually hear the messages that are being given to you as you try to interpret the patient's statements in the light of your initial judgement. You may be totally focused on what the patient is saying, but still not listening as you manipulate their words to fit your judgement or hypothesis about the problem as you see it. It is very important to maintain an open mind if you are to maintain 'open ears' and really listen to the patient's story.

A major assessment problem is failure to probe, resulting in superficial, inaccurate or confusing data. If the nurse is worried about where the interview may lead, then the result is likely to be that questions are vague, lacking in depth or even omitted altogether. There is a cultural dimension to this problem. The British are notoriously reserved, whereas other societies (e.g. North America) are much more open. A Caucasian British nurse may feel very uncomfortable trying to assess the health needs of an Asian woman and therefore conduct a very superficial interview. Areas such as feelings, emotions and sexual practices are frequently omitted from assessments even though they are directly related to the patient's health problems. Sometimes the patient gives a hint in an answer that there is a problem without initially telling the full story. The nurse who is listening carefully will detect that hint and further gentle probing can lead to the patient opening up a whole area of their life that has remained hidden until now and that can shed light on apparently unrelated health problems. Obviously the nurse needs to ask such questions gently, unhurriedly and explain the reasons for asking, giving the patient the opportunity to decline to answer. Getting the balance right between asking sensitively about difficult areas and appearing intrusive or inquisitorial comes with experience and critical reflection upon your performance.

Adherence to rigid assessment schedules will lead to inadequate assessment. A standardized interview will tend to produce standardized data, not a holistic picture of the individual patient. An assessment framework is certainly very useful to ensure all the main areas are covered for all patients. However, you must be prepared to ask questions that are not on the schedule to arrive at a full assessment of the patient's health history. Obvious physical clues that need investigating may present themselves, such as signs of bruising which may indicate domestic violence. The patient may reply that they do not sleep very well in response to a question about sleeping habits. You must follow that up and explore further in order to discover why they do not sleep very well. This may be a clue to severe anxiety, a depressive illness, or frequent visits to the toilet to micturate due to an enlarged prostate or difficulty breathing whilst lying flat caused by heart failure, to name but four of many possible reasons.

We have already stated that patient teaching requires the nurse to check how much the patient has learnt. This requires not only effective listening but also effective questioning to ensure there are no misunderstandings. The patient who is upset and in need of psychological support will benefit also from a gentle probing approach which invites the patient to go as far as they feel comfortable in disclosing their problems.

Allied to a failure to probe the area being assessed is a tendency to change topics if the nurse is uncomfortable with the direction the interview is taking or if she or he wishes to explore other areas that the nurse considers of more interest. This gives the message to the patient that the nurse is not interested in what the patient has to say and may lead to important information being missed. There are times, however, when time is short and there are patients who have a tendency to ramble away from the topics that you do need to assess. The skill of therapeutic communication lies in gently guiding the patient into the key areas that you want to talk about without abruptly cutting across the patient's flow of conversation. It is also helpful to promise to come back later and continue the conversation. Such promises must be kept!

A lack of awareness of communication skills can be as bad as incompetent application of such skills. A good example of this is the skill of reflecting (see p. 36); unfortunately, in unskilled hands this sometimes becomes more like parroting as the nurse continually repeats the patient's words back to them. This can be interpreted by the patient as meaning that the nurse is not really listening to what they are saying. It can also be very annoying to the patient. Either way, parroting the patient's own words back to them will interfere with effective therapeutic communication.

Jumping to conclusions has already been mentioned as a serious problem. As nurses, we have to be aware of our own human weaknesses and the tendency to be influenced by first impressions and stereotypes (p. 31). Where this really becomes a problem is if it is linked to being judgemental about patients. Nurses do not have the right to sit in judgement on patients, approving or disapproving of their actions. It is very difficult to engage with a patient who you know has committed a serious crime such as rape. Your religious beliefs may make you very uncomfortable about nursing a woman having a termination of pregnancy. The patient brought to the A&E department with a drug overdose may be regarded as the author of his or her own misfortunes. However, you need to remember that your NMC Code of Professional Conduct forbids such judgemental attitudes, which will obviously interfere with your ability to communicate effectively with the patient. However difficult it may be, judgement has to be suspended and patients treated equally with unconditional regard. Negative attitudes towards the patient will adversely affect both communication and care, which – ultimately – is the purpose of nursing.

The question of making judgments about patients links to the whole area of inferring causality. A basic human characteristic is to try and understand any event in terms of what caused it or, in other words, to infer causality. The event in question could be a presentation in clinic or the actual illness itself. This area of social psychology is known as attribution theory and there are some important insights to be gained from a brief consideration of its key principles.

The most fundamental attribution we make is whether a behaviour stems from something within the person (internal attribution) or the situation/context within which they are located (external attribution). A human characteristic is to err on the side of internal attribution and neglect the possible role of context (Taylor et al 2000). This is such a consistent and major flaw in our perception of the world that it is referred to as the fundamental attribution error. The implication is that whenever a patient presents with a health problem (a behaviour) we are programmed to explain it in terms of something within the person (internal attribution) rather than consider external factors. Consider the issue of substance misuse discussed in Chapter 26; there is a tendency to expect people to deal with their own substance misuse problems themselves as the cause is assumed to lie within themselves. I am not arguing against personal responsibility for one's own actions, but merely pointing out that there are a range of external factors which could also explain the substance misuse problem. These include childhood experiences, peer group pressures, ready availability and aggressive advertising campaigns. Ignoring these external factors will mean it is unlikely that the substance misuse can be effectively treated. We therefore have to be aware of our natural, fundamental attribution bias when taking a health history or trying to help a patient with health education. Self awareness on the nurse's part is the key.

Another obstacle to therapeutic communication comes in the form of patronizing the patient. This clearly sends the message that the nurse is superior to the patient and may creep in unintentionally as the nurse tries to make the situa-tion less formal. A clumsy use of humour may inadvertently have the same effect. First names should be used only when the patient has been asked for permission to do so. Terms such as 'dear', 'chuck' and 'love' should be avoided, particularly when caring for older people, as they are extremely patronizing. Patient teaching should be carried out at the correct intellectual level for the patient, which should therefore have been determined beforehand. Clearly the approach required in dealing with a retired university lecturer is different from that needed with a builder's labourer. Children will frequently be encountered in the A&E department or primary care settings and, once again, you should ascertain their intellectual level of functioning and developmental stage before engaging them in conversation, even if their parents are present. Children hate being patronized just as much as anybody else.

A statement commonly read in care plans and student essays is that 'The patient will be reassured'. The word reassurance is much used and abused. In many cases it is inappropriate. A moment's reflection will suggest that a few words to the effect 'It will be OK' will have little impact upon a patient facing a life-threatening illness or surgery as they have multiple complex fears and anxieties to deal with. Reassurance like this can be little more than a meaningless platitude which might insult the patient's intelligence. The patient will probably think 'How do you know?', although rarely bother to say so. Dismissing the patient's fears with such a bland reassurance negates the patient's feelings and can make them feel trivialized. Alternatively it can convey a message of not caring – almost dismissing the patient's worries as not important.

Stereotyped responses can have the same effect as bland reassurances. A typical nursing comment at the end of an assessment is 'Everything will be OK and we will have you home inside 3 days'. At best, the patient is likely to be unimpressed by this comment and it may have exactly the opposite effect from that which was intended. If something does not quite go according to plan and there are complications, your credibility will be the first casualty, closely followed by the patient's trust in anything they are told. By the same token, if a patient is anxious about their care and needs time to talk through their anxieties, they should be given that time and not quickly dismissed with bland reassurances that prevent the conversation getting into difficult areas. You have to be honest and realistic with patients when discussing progress; if you do not know the answer to a question, be honest enough to say so. Rather than hazard a guess or give vague reassurance, contact a trained member of staff or a doctor and ask them to talk to the patient.

It is only a short step from avoiding real discussion by giving bland reassurance to refusing to discuss topics with patients altogether. Such a rejection makes therapeutic communication impossible as the patient may feel that not only has their question been rejected, but so have they. When the patient asks what the chances are of something going seriously wrong with their operation, the answer should not be 'We do not discuss things like that, Mr Smith', as the author once heard a nurse reply. Refusing to discuss an area of concern with a patient is as negligent and unprofessional as refusing to give a patient an injection to relieve pain. The basic principle remains that, if you do not know the answer or feel the topic lies beyond your area of expertise, you are obliged to find someone who *can* deal with the subject.

A potential problem surrounding role and status issues arises when staff become defensive in response to questions and challenges. The principle of informed consent requires patient knowledge and good communication rather than an obsession with compliance. Patients know how to search the internet for medical information and may attend clinic with an armful of printed downloads concerning their condition. This is to be welcomed as it shows the patient is interested in their condition and is likely to be better informed as a result (although the websites visited should be checked as there is a great deal of complete rubbish available over the internet as well as good reliable sources).

A good starting point for a discussion on informed consent is the NMC Code of Professional Conduct (2004) which states that all patients have a right to information about their condition and reminds nurses that they must be both sensitive to patient needs and respectful of the wishes of those who refuse information or who cannot receive information about their condition. The Code points out the patient's autonomy means they have the right to decide whether to undergo any treatment even if refusal may result in harm or death to themselves or an unborn fetus (unless a court orders to the contrary). For consent to be informed it must be given freely and without coercion. There is controversy, however, on how much information a patient should be given before consent is *informed* consent. The Code does state that we assess the patient's ability to understand what is told to them, and the context in which it is told. That is true, but it still avoids the question of exactly 'what' the patient should be told. Should we tell the patient every known possible risk of a treatment or only those which *we consider* more likely or sufficient for the patient to make a decision? The latter course of action is pragmatic but potentially patronizing and disempowering as we are making decisions *for* the patient and not *with* the patient. In a thorough review of this topic, Cable (2003) concluded that from a nursing perspective, patients should be *fully* informed about interventions and told in such a way that they can understand the risks and benefits; however, we cannot speak for the medical profession. The logical deduction from this statement is that nurses not only must be effective communicators but they must also understand issues of risk, probability and mathematical concepts such as the difference between statistical and clinical significance. In short they need to understand the mathematics that underpin evidence-based practice, yet this is an area missing from the

nursing curriculum which seems to be a weakness. The law permits patients who think they have not been fully informed of the risks and benefits of a treatment to bring legal action for damages. Perhaps in considering whether you should tell patients something as part of the process of gaining their consent, you might reflect on how it would look in court a few months later if you were called upon to justify *not* telling the patient of a known risk or side-effect?

It is possible that staff still feel threatened when care is questioned and, rather than engaging in a meaningful discussion to explain what is happening and why, go on the defensive. Defensive responses negate the patient's right to express opinions and say what is on their mind. They can lead to suspicions of a cover-up and the opinion that the staff are withholding the truth. Differences in social status can be exaggerated by defensiveness, leading to more antagonism. Sometimes you can explain things repeatedly in as reasonable a way as possible and the patient just will not listen, usually indicating that a more deep-seated problem is present. However, in many cases, unnecessary friction and poor communication can be avoided if staff accept that patients are entitled to question and challenge the care they receive. This is about putting the rhetoric of 'patients as partners in care' into practice and treating them accordingly. This means giving them equal status and not responding defensively to their questions and criticisms.

Involving patients as partners in care does not mean telling them what they should do as this negates the contribution of the patient. It is tempting to give advice and lapse into informal everyday conversation with phrases such as 'If I were you I would …' or 'What you really should do is …'. This is the common approach frequently overheard when two people are talking on the bus or in a pub. It might be common conversation, but it is not therapeutic communication. This is being directive, not valuing the patient's contribution and always invites the rejoinder 'But you aren't me!' or 'It's OK for you to say that but …'. A therapeutic approach needs to discover the patient's view of his or her problems first and then perhaps put forward the correct health promotion message or therapeutic interventions that would be required, but in a non-directive way. This can be followed up with the simple question 'How do you feel about that?' or 'Have you considered this?' The scene is then set for a discussion and negotiation in which you are fully aware of the patient's knowledge about the topic and his or her feelings about the problem. The patient is then a fully involved, active partner rather than a passive recipient of nursing or medical advice and instruction.

This section has summarized some of the communication pitfalls and mistakes to be avoided. It now remains to move on and look at more positive aspects and the kind of skills that will facilitate therapeutic communication. These are all skills that can be learnt and must be practised if you are to achieve effective communication with patients and members of staff also.

SKILLS FOR EFFECTIVE COMMUNICATION

STARTING THE INTERACTION

Every conversation has a beginning and, as first impressions are so important in human communication, you must make a good start to the interview. That means you must explain who you are and what the purpose of the interview is. It is easy for hospital patients to become confused as they see so many different people in a day. The move away from traditional nursing uniforms is to be welcomed for all manner of practical reasons, but it may leave the patient unsure who this person in a top and trousers actually is. Small print on badges is often difficult to read, so there is no substitute for a full introduction of yourself.

If you are carrying out a health assessment interview it is important to explain that you are asking questions to try to obtain a whole picture of the person's health. The patient who is coming in for surgery on their knee may be very puzzled as to why you are asking about their diet, smoking and drinking habits, sleep patterns and whether their parents are still alive. Do avoid asking unnecessary questions such as age, date of birth and address as these are available on the patient's notes or admission form. Patients find it irritating to be asked the same questions six times on the same day by six different people.

A health education session should always start with you finding out how much the patient knows already. It is necessary to explain at the beginning that you will be asking a few questions to ascertain the patient's knowledge and views about the problem. This allows the patient to understand why these questions are being asked, which in turn is more likely to result in meaningful, helpful answers.

The patient may be reluctant to begin talking and at first remain silent. This should suggest to you that the person is very anxious and unsure. Gentle prompting such as just stating their name in a questioning way (Mr Wilson …?) and pausing may be needed to elicit an initial response, rather than repeating the initial question.

Non-verbal aspects of communication are very important at the beginning of an interview and throughout. They will be addressed below.

ASKING QUESTIONS

Questions are basically open or closed. An open question might be 'How can we help you today?' or 'What brings you to the surgery this afternoon?'. The response is entirely the patient's; there is no right or wrong answer nor is there a limited choice of responses. Open questions can elicit information about patient knowledge or feelings such as 'Let's recap. What can you tell me about the two different types of inhaler that you use for your asthma?' or 'How do you feel about things since getting home from hospital?'. These sorts of question allow patients to say what they want to say and

are an essential characteristic of a genuine therapeutic partnership with patients.

The closed question is characterized by a limited choice of responses (frequently yes or no) or a simple factual answer (How many days is it since those stitches were put in?). They are useful for gaining factual information and when there is a sense of urgency, such as in an emergency situation (Is this patient a known diabetic?). However, they are very limiting and do not allow patients to express their feelings. Consider a patient who has just been admitted to a surgical ward. If you begin your assessment with 'Do you know why you have been admitted today?' you will discover little. However, 'Can you tell me why you think you have been admitted to hospital today?' will start to gain an understanding of the patient's perceptions and can easily be followed up with further questions.

Another example of a closed question is to ask whether the patient is in pain. All this will obtain is a yes/no response, which is of limited value. A closed question could still be used, but one that will gain far more information such as asking the patient to rate their pain on a scale of 0–5. Perhaps a better approach would be to ask how the patient is feeling as this opens up other possible responses such as anxious or worried as well as in pain. You could then focus on pain assessment with some closed questions to elicit how severe the pain is, but should use open questions to discover *where* the pain is and what the *character* of the pain is. A closed question such as 'Is the pain in your left side?' may obtain a 'yes' answer but fail to discover a highly significant finding that it is also radiating into the patient's groin, as there is no opportunity for the patient to state this. 'Tell me where the pain is … Can you show me?' is a far more useful line to follow. A trap that the unwary may fall into, in trying to avoid a closed question, is to ask 'Is the pain in your left side?'. This is a leading question as it is suggesting the answer to the patient who may agree in order not to appear difficult. Similar questions might be 'I am sure you are happy to be going home today?' or 'Is your pain a lot better since we changed your medication?'. At all times, be careful to avoid suggesting the answer when asking questions.

ACTIVE LISTENING

This involves attending skills in which, by both verbal and non-verbal cues, you indicate to the speaker that you are receptive and paying attention to what she or he is saying. This means it is a dynamic process as you convey to the original speaker that you have heard and understood what the speaker is saying. Active listening involves integrating non-verbal cues from the speaker and the tone of his or her voice with the actual words the person is saying. It is about listening to the person's voice and not to a stereotype that you may carry around of that *type* of person. It is possible, for example, that the tone of voice and body language do not match the content of the speech, indicating deep-seated problems that need careful exploration.

The work of Egan (1986) has been drawn upon extensively by nurses as the basis for active listening. He suggests that the following key non-verbal skills make a simple but essential framework for effectively demonstrating to the patient that you are listening to what he or she is saying:

S sit squarely to your patient in order that you may engage them fully
O adopt an open posture that is welcoming and receptive
L lean slightly forward suggesting attention and interest
E maintain good eye contact, which again shows interest
R show a relaxed approach.

You do not have to sit square on to the patient, leaning forward at all times for the entire interview. This is unnatural and will probably give you backache and prove unnerving for the patient. Move around in a relaxed way but keep returning to this position for important parts of the patient's story to show maximum interest and encouragement. Sitting with your arms and legs folded gives a 'closed' message to the patient. The relaxed open posture is encouraging and facilitates patient expression.

The SOLER skills need to be practised so that they come naturally to you. If you are concentrating on getting these things right during an interview you will not be listening to the patient! They should be practised until they are second nature. Video recordings of interviews, whether real or simulated with other students, are a very effective way of learning these skills via direct feedback. A word of caution is necessary, however, as if these techniques are used incorrectly they can actually be intimidating or even provocative. You can get *too close* to the patient and inappropriate eye contact becomes *staring* at the person and construed as provocative.

There are other important non-verbal aspects of the interview that will enhance its therapeutic value:

1 Avoid having a barrier such as a desk, bed or trolley between you and the patient.
2 Sit with your chair at an angle to the patient. This allows you to engage the patient fully by sitting square on but without being confrontational.
3 Ensure your chair is at the same level as that of the patient, emphasizing the sense of equality.
4 Do not sit with your back to the light (e.g. a window). This means the patient cannot see your facial expressions clearly and, if the light is bright, may be squinting into the light in a way that can be disconcerting.
5 Ensure privacy and quiet whilst carrying out the interview.
6 Consider carefully the delicate issue of touch. British society is not a very 'touchy feely' society, so touching the patient can be inappropriate and unwelcome. There are some circumstances when the offer of an arm to help

somebody to their feet is very welcome. A hand laid gently on a patient's arm or a soft touch on the shoulder when they are struggling with painful emotions can be a very effective piece of nursing when done at the right time with the right patient. Knowing when to do this is about experience and expertise, and the expert nurse knows intuitively when to do this. As a student, watch, listen and learn.

Just as your body posture will encourage patients to tell their story, verbal prompts and rewards will have the same effect by demonstrating your interest and appreciation of the fact that they have chosen to share what can be very painful feelings with you. Prompts include 'Go on …' or 'And then …'. Another useful technique is to turn the end of a statement into a question and put this back to the patient. For example, the patient may say 'I felt so angry at what she said', to which you reply: 'What she said...?' This demonstrates careful attention and interest on your part and encourages the patient to expand upon what could be difficult emotional experience.

One final skill is the skill of silence. Do not dominate the conversation as the interaction is for the patient's benefit. Sometimes a carefully placed silence can encourage patients to carry on with their story, especially if followed by a slight prompt such as 'Yes …' or 'And then …'. There are times when silence is all that is required. Here you are using your presence as a therapeutic tool. Being with a patient so they are not alone at a time of great distress, or even at the ultimate end of life, is an act of immense nursing care. It merely requires presence. Do not be afraid if you can think of nothing to say; just being there is enough. Such occasions arise frequently in A&E or critical care nursing, for example when a bereaved relative is alone in the relative's room, perhaps waiting for family members to arrive, numbed by the awful truth of the death of their loved one. Your presence, alone with that person, is high-quality nursing care. Words may be of little importance in such a situation.

The skills of active listening described in this section are important in assessment and teaching, but particularly so in working with a patient who is very distressed or upset and in need of psychological support.

EMPATHY

Empathy involves attempting to understand the experience and feelings of others as they experience them or, in other words, putting yourself in the other person's shoes and trying to understand how things appear to them. We have already seen on page 29 that this is not as simple as it sounds, especially when there are large differences of age or culture between the nurse and the patient. It is also important to retain your own sense of objectivity and not become lost in the patient's subjective reality with resultant clouding of your judgment. We all possess the potential for some degree of empathy and the older we are the more we are likely to possess it as a result of life experience. Student nurses may have to work on what they start out with and develop it into a valuable tool to aid communication.

It is essential, however, to signal to patients that you are trying to see things from their point of view to make maximum use of this technique. Consider the following example from Jarvis (2004).

You are called over to the bedside of a 55-year-old man who says in a sarcastic tone: 'This is just great. Here I am running my own company and telling people what to do all day and now I have to ask you for every little thing, including going for a pee.'

A response such as:

- 'I can see that's difficult, one day having so much control and now feeling totally dependent on others ...' is empathic and helpful.

On the other hand:

- 'Oh don't worry, you'll soon be out of here, back at work and telling everybody what to do in no time' is unhelpful, probably irritating or even annoying as it shows you do not understand what he is feeling and it is possibly untrue!

Empathy should also make you aware that perhaps patients are only half expressing themselves. A woman may be telling you that she is terrified of a simple operation to remove a benign lump from her breast because of her fear of needles and pain and also because her neighbour's sister actually woke up in the middle of her operation because she was not given enough anaesthetic. Pause to think and put yourself in her position: is there something else she is not telling you because it is too frightening to talk about? Empathy might suggest the woman is actually afraid she might have breast cancer, even though the lump is a benign cyst.

Seidal et al (2003) suggest the following are the kind of open-ended questions that can show empathy:

- How are you feeling today?
- What do you think is causing your symptoms?
- How are you feeling about your illness?
- How are you coping with your illness?
- How would you like me to address you?

Empathy allows you to use two other important skills, *reflection* and *rewording*. If you are in tune with the patient you will be able to pick up on certain feelings and emotions that can be explored further. Reflecting the patient's feelings can be achieved by rewording what they are saying and putting this back to the patient in your own words. To do this you have to use active listening skills to be aware of the tone of the person's voice and their non-verbal cues as well as what they are saying. The woman sitting in front of you with tears in her eyes and who is fiddling with her hands in an agitated way and yet who says 'I am OK', clearly is not

OK. This distress can be gently reflected back to the patient: 'Mmmm ... are you sure? How are things at home?'.

Rewording can be used on the content of speech to clarify meaning. The woman who says 'I told my husband to go to hell!' might be helped by the nurse saying 'You were really angry with him' as this allows her to clarify her feelings and signals that the nurse is on her wavelength. She may well press on to explain why she was so angry without you even having to ask why.

A useful way of reflecting feelings that involves rewording is the formula 'I think I hear what you are saying. It sounds to me like ... Am I correct?'. This should be used sparingly, however, as the patient will become irritated by continual rewording and reflecting as they feel they are going round in circles and getting nowhere. It may also encourage the person to wallow in destructive or distressing emotions without moving forward to deal with those feelings constructively.

Egan (1986) offers the following useful tips in the use of empathy:

- Pause before you speak and think carefully. Do not rush into glib statements
- Keep your responses short as it is the patient who should be doing most of the talking
- Recognize the emotional tone of the patient through your active listening skills and pitch your responses accordingly.

Finally, it is important to not confuse empathy with sympathy. Identifying too closely with the patient may cloud your judgement. This is especially true if the patient is the same age as yourself (see above).

HANDLING EMOTION

In the course of the interview, especially if offering support to a distressed patient, a range of emotions may be unleashed that you have to handle. These can include anger, guilt, denial and fear. This is particularly likely when talking to the relatives of a person who has just died or who is critically ill (see Ch. 4 for a discussion of bereavement and breaking bad news).

Anger may arise from several factors such as the need to blame something or somebody for a serious illness such as cancer or a stroke that has apparently come out of the blue. The patient may complain bitterly that life is not fair. The patient may be angry because of delays in treatment or cancellations, none of which are your fault but you happen to be the person on whom the patient vents their anger. If the anger is dismissed or denied and you become defensive, this is very unproductive and will probably lead to an escalation of anger that could spill over into abusive behaviour and even violence. Responding to anger with anger will only lead to an even quicker escalation and confrontation.

A more effective approach is clearly needed which has to start by acknowledging the anger expressed by patients as a real expression of their feelings. It is essential to show that you are taking their complaint seriously and then to find out exactly what the nature of the complaint is. Only by finding out what is the root cause of the anger is it possible to move forward and resolve the potential conflict. Keeping a cool head and not reacting to harsh words is not easy but it is essential if you are to defuse the situation. Patients must be allowed to have their say and ventilate their feelings as part of the defusing process. In many circumstances the anger has resulted from a lack of communication or information compounding a sense of frustration, injustice or fear. Good listening skills and defusing techniques will usually calm such situations.

However, there may sometimes be a difficult dilemma if the outburst takes place in front of very sick patients or young children in the A&E department. You need to manoeuvre the person away from such an environment, but also beware of becoming isolated from the rest of the staff for your own safety. Remain visible to others and do not become penned into a corner or side room with the aggressor between you and the exit route.

When dealing with an angry person the 'SOLER' framework needs modification. You need to place distance between yourself and the person and be out of arm's reach. This is for your own safety because, if the person suddenly lashes out at you, it gives you a chance to take avoiding or blocking action. Increasing distance from the person and not leaning towards them at a time like this is also less confrontational. The best posture is with your weight slightly on your back foot and your body placed slightly oblique to the person. This gives you the best position to defend yourself if you are attacked. Eyeball to eyeball contact can be very provocative if you are handling an aggressive person: keep your gaze at about the level of the first shirt button, as this is less threatening but shows you are paying attention. If the person is under the influence of drugs or alcohol, then you are much less likely to succeed in resolving the situation; such individuals are best dealt with quickly by security and/or the police.

Guilt is not so easy to resolve as anger. It tends to be something that has accumulated over many years, sometimes quite irrationally. The best that can be done with guilt in the short term is to be aware that it may be there and could explain otherwise inexplicable behaviour. Patients can be facilitated to expand upon their feelings and talk about their guilt as part of a supportive relationship. This is particularly important in the management of long-term illness where the nurse builds up a relationship with the patient possibly over several years. Their guilt is as much a part of them as their diabetes or asthma. Guilty feelings surface particularly after bereavement and have to be worked through as part of grieving (see p. 63).

Denial is a means of coping with events by simply pretending they are not happening. I remember a woman in her sixties presenting to my A&E department protesting all the way in that she did not need to see any doctors. She had a massive fungating malignancy of the breast that was grossly contaminated and highly odorous. I can still see the look of amazement on the face of the female student who had undressed her. 'How on earth could she have pretended that there was nothing wrong?', she asked me. Denial was of course the answer.

It can be very frustrating when patients resort to such an ineffective coping mechanism. It may be the young adult who denies their **diabetes** or **epilepsy**, ignores medication and advice about lifestyle, and continues to present as a regular emergency admission, or the middle-aged man who denies that he has had a **myocardial infarct** and continues as before. Complete denial presents a brick wall to therapeutic intervention. However, we should not become judgemental and must treat the patient as an adult who is making his or her own decisions about their life. Maintaining communication and contact at least holds out the hope that at some stage in the future the person will come to see things differently and reach out for help as they begin to accept the truth of their situation. Therapeutic communication means that a bridge to that person can be built eventually which will do some good, even though it may be late in life and after much harm to their health. The patient who is terminally ill and yet in denial has to be handled with great sensitivity. Eventually reality will intrude and nursing must be there for that person when this occurs.

Anxiety and fear are very common human emotions. In fact they are essential for survival. However, they can become distressing and debilitating especially when bottled up inside. Cultural and social norms play a major part in the expression of such emotions, with men in northern European society often feeling unable to admit fear and anxiety. Therapeutic communication is about giving the person the room and space to admit to such feelings. It allows you to discover the focus that lies at the root of fear. Sometimes this can be dealt with directly by clearing up misunderstandings, which will alleviate fear. Sometimes the person just feels better for talking about things and realizing that they are not the only person with this problem. On other occasions patients can be encouraged and facilitated to discuss their problems with relevant family members, perhaps including referral for skilled counselling. When fear and anxiety become totally debilitating and/or irrational, specialist mental health professionals need to be involved.

THE UNPOPULAR PATIENT

Unfortunately some patients, despite all our professional ideals to the contrary, become labelled as 'difficult' or 'manipulative'. In short they are unpopular. Significant amounts of research have been carried out on this phenomenon and Riley (2000) summarizes the following characteristics of 'the unpopular patient' by saying they are a person who:

- argues, complains and fails to cooperate
- states that they do not like being in hospital and want to go home

- states that they are suffering more than nurses believe
- suffer from conditions that should be treated elsewhere such as another ward or by their GP (it is not the patient's 'fault' they are on your ward, yours was the only bed available that day)
- require more time and attention than the nurses believe they should have
- have complex diagnoses with difficult illness pathways involving various complications over a long time period, especially if the nurse knows little about the condition
- are considered to be of low social value and moral worth
- are stigmatized by virtue of sexual orientation, race, religion, etc.
- have an 'own fault' diagnosis such as a drug overdose or alcoholism.

Many of these factors are easily linked to an internal attribution so the discussion (p. 00) about fundamental attribution error is particularly pertinent. You should reflect upon this list as you work your way through your education. How many patients can you identify towards whom the nursing and medical staff have a strongly negative attitude, and how many of these characteristics are present? Pause for a moment and check this list against Table 2.1 to see how many items involve the nurse using *non-therapeutic* communication techniques such as being judgemental, using stereotypes or rejecting. The problem of the unpopular patient in health care can be greatly reduced by the use of therapeutic communication, avoiding preconceptions and treating the person as a person, not as a patient with a reputation.

SUMMARY

This chapter has been a brief introduction to key aspects of communication, which has to be effective if it is to be thera- peutic. Therapeutic communication is as important as any other skill you will learn in your career – and probably more important than most. However, it needs practice and can always be improved upon. Critical reflection is one particu- larly effective technique that will assist you in developing this aspect of your nursing. If knowing what to do is the science of nursing and knowing how and when to do it is the art, then therapeutic communication is the essential underpinning of both the science and art of nursing.

REFERENCES

Cable S (2003) Informed consent. Nursing Standard 18(12): 47–53.

Chase S (2004) Clinical judgment and communication in nurse practitioner practice. Philadelphia: F.A. Davis.

Egan G (1986) The skilled helper. Monterey, California: Brooks/Cole.

Gask L, Usherwood T (2003) The consultation. In: Mayou R, Sharpe M, Carson A, eds. ABC of Psychological Medicine. London: British Medical Journal.

Jarvis C (2004) Physical examination and health assessment. St Louis: Saunders.

Nursing and Midwifery Council (2004) The NMC code of professional conduct: standards for conduct, performance and ethics. London: NMC.

Price B (2004) Conducting sensitive patient interviews. Nursing Standard 18(38): 45–52.

Riley J (2000) Communication in nursing, 4th edn. St Louis: Mosby.

Sadler J (1997) Defining professional nurse caring; a triangulation study. International Journal of Human Caring 1(3): 12–21.

Seidal H, Ball J, Dains J et al (2003) Mosby's guide to physical examination. St Louis: Mosby.

Taylor S, Peplau L, Sears D (2000) Social psychology, 10th edn. New Jersey: Prentice Hall.

Walsh M (2006) Nurse practitioners, clinical skills and professional issues. Edinburgh: Butterworth Heinemann Elsevier.

Wilson T, Holt T (2001) Conplexity and clinical care. BMJ 323: 685–688.

CRITICAL INCIDENT

Conversation overheard on a surgical ward one day involving a medical student clerking a 70-year-old man:

Student: Do you smoke?

Patient: Yes.

Student: How many?

Patient: About 20 a day.

Student: You know that is very bad for you?

Patient: Don't be daft, a fag in the morning makes me cough and clears my chest. Smoking relaxes me and makes me clear my chest with a good cough, so don't go giving me any of your medical lectures!

Student: But the cigarettes are making you cough because they are harming your chest.

Patient: But a good cough is good for me!

The medical student pursued this circular argument with the patient for a further 10 minutes, becoming increasingly frustrated and irate while the patient became increasingly annoyed. The rest of the clerking was finally concluded in a very strained atmosphere and the patient's first afternoon on the ward had got off to a bad start.

Reflection

Reflect upon the communication technique used by the medical student and how he failed to appreciate the patient's point of view. How might you have approached this patient and discussed his smoking?

See Appendix 2 for guidelines on reflection.

3

Ageing and health

Alison Crumbie

INTRODUCTION

This chapter focuses on older people. In your work as a nurse you are more likely to come into contact with older people than any other group. In the UK, it is this group who are more likely to experience poor levels of health than the rest of the population (Office of Population Censuses and Surveys (OPCS) 2006); they will attend casualty or outpatients departments more frequently and when they are admitted they will have longer hospital stays than the rest of the adult population (Office of National Statistics 2004). This chapter will explore the context of care for older people located within and influenced by current policy. An overview of the common theoretical perspectives on ageing will provide a variety of standpoints from which to view the older person. The importance of assessment will be highlighted as a mode of accessing nursing and in recognition of advancing roles in gerontological nursing and the role of nurses in prescribing medications, normal variations in the physical examination of older people will be addressed alongside variations in the pharmacokinetics and pharmacodynamics. Throughout, discussion will be linked to a critical care pathway in which the experiences of Mr Jacob Brown are followed through a potential healthcare experience. The chapter concludes with a consideration of the context of care in relation to the ongoing development of nursing expertise in the specialty of gerontology.

DEMOGRAPHY

There is a folk-saying that 'everyone wishes to live a good long life, but no one wishes for old age' and another that 'getting old is no fun but the alternative is not attractive either!'. These two folk-sayings demonstrate the way in which we automatically associate old age with ill-health,

disability, increasing vulnerability and greater dependency upon others.

Ageing takes place within a global village where the boundaries between nations and continents are blurring different lifestyles and cultures. The key challenges for the future include:

- the older population is increasing in absolute terms and as a percentage of the total population
- the fastest growing segment is the 'oldest old' – 80 years plus
- there is a declining birth rate
- people are deferring child rearing.

In 2003 there were 20 million people aged over 50 years in Great Britain (OPCS 2005a) and in 2001, 8100 people were estimated to be 100 and over (House of Commons Hansard 2003). The trends in Great Britain have shown that the population is becoming older and that the composition of the ageing population is changing. In 1951, 1.6% of the 50 years and over population were aged 85 and over, in 2003 5.5% of the 50 years and over population were aged 85 and over and in 2031 it is projected that 7.9% of the 50 years and over population will be aged 85 and over (OPCS 2005a). Women are expected to live longer than men with a life expectancy at birth being 76 years for men and 81 years for women (WHO 2004). This compares with life expectancy for men and women in China which is 70 and 74 years respectively, in India which is 61 and 63 years, in Spain which is 77 and 83 years, in the USA which is 75 and 80 years and in South Africa which is 47 and 49 years (WHO 2004). The UK currently compares favourably with many other countries but If we reflect back a century, then we see that of boys born in 1881 only half reached 55 years and a mere 20% survived to 75 years. Girls fared slightly better, with 40% dying before the age of 55 years; many of these deaths occurred in infancy. Only one-third of the girls survived to 75 years (Grundy 1994). Such dramatic statistics herald a survival revolution, achieved largely through reduced infant mortality and the near eradication of infectious diseases such as tuberculosis. These demographics have some important implications for the provision of healthcare services.

Whilst women have a longer life expectancy than men they also report more years in poor health. Simply getting older increases the possibility of living with long-term illness and in 2001 three-quarters of the population of women and two-thirds of the population of men aged 85 years and over reported disability or long-term illness (OPCS 2005b). In 2003, 20% of those aged 65–74 years had consulted with an NHS GP, this compares with 14% in 1972. Of the people aged 50 and over, one-fifth had attended an outpatients' department or casualty in the preceding 3 months and one-tenth had stayed in hospital in the preceding 12 months (OPCS 2005c).

Birth rates have always been the most important influence on the size and composition of the population. The relative size of the older age groups is due mainly to falls in the birth rate, which result in fewer children and younger people. However, in the UK, where the birth rate has been low for some time (Murphy and Grundy 2003), changes in death rates at older ages are having a stronger effect on age composition. The combination of previous fertility patterns and improvements in life expectancy have resulted in increasing numbers and proportions of older people aged 85 years and over (OPCS 2005d).

The statistics show that older people, in particular the very old, make up an increasingly large segment of our population. Whilst this should be a cause for celebration, it is more frequently seen as a cause for concern. Certainly it is considered to pose a major challenge to society. Most people are aware of the fears regarding the rising cost of health and social care, but there is less understanding of changing family patterns, such as the rise of divorce, the increase in the number of single parents and those living outside any form of partnership (Haskey 1995). How these factors will affect the capacity of younger generations to support the old is still not yet fully understood (Murphy and Grundy 2003). Given that the most important source of practical and emotional support for older people currently is from their spouse, partner or family (OPCS 2005d), the trend for living alone has the potential to influence future patterns of care. Interestingly though, Murphy and Grundy (2003) have predicted that there will be a higher proportion of older people in the UK who have a surviving child in the next quarter of a century than there ever has been before. This is due to the changing trends in fertility and child bearing. The world of work is also changing, with older workers becoming an increasingly significant group. Over 1 in 4 workers will be aged over 60 by the year 2020, compared with 1 in 5 in 1990. This is viewed as a positive development, with more people using a variety of skills and talents into later life (Phillipson 1997). A number of companies in the UK, have policies of positively seeking the employment of older people, who they see as offering many skills to the consumer. These sorts of initiative, along with a rise in the traditional retirement age, could encourage older people to retrain and remain in active employment for longer, if this is their choice (Moore et al 1994). This may affect the capacity for some people to take up informal caring roles, which presently support many older people. Today, it is estimated that about 3 million people aged 50 years and over in England and Wales are involved in unpaid caring activities (OPCS 2005d).

In addition to family configurations and future employment trends, health will be influenced by the way in which we live. Our geographical distance from one another and the houses we occupy, in town or countryside, will affect our access to one another and to health services. The conditions of the houses people live in are important, as is the ability to get about. Living in a balanced community, where a mixture of types of people, in terms of age, class, income and household are represented, is considered to work to everyone's advantage (Russel 1999).

So, in summary, whilst there are clear reasons for celebrating our ageing society there remain some valid reasons for concern, most commonly the cost of health and welfare services for older people.

CONTEMPORARY POLICY CONTEXT

CURRENT HEALTH AND SOCIAL CARE PROVISION

Current provision of services for older people originated in divisions of welfare that go back to the nineteenth century. They reflect the gradual extension of public sector activity and its changing historical role in relation to the individual, the workplace and the voluntary sector (Jones 1994). Healthcare policies will continue to be heavily influenced by the economic and political context in which they operate.

Community care in the UK was fully introduced in 1993 (DoH 1990), with the intention of reducing the emphasis on institutional care and promoting home-based approaches, supported by health and social services. In the vast majority of cases, older people living at home will depend largely upon their own resources, their partner, family, friends and neighbours to meet their daily living needs. Directly relevant to these needs has been the policy focus on enabling people where possible to remain in their own homes, an objective that research has shown undoubtedly matches what older people themselves prefer (Audit Commission 2000, Tinker 1984).

In the UK, practical support for carers by service providers is advocated in several policies, such as the Carers Recognition and Services Act (Department of Health/Social Services Inspectorate 1995) and Caring about Carers (Department of Health 1999a). There has been recognition that the UK's 6 million carers save the tax payer approximately £33.9 billion each year (Neno 2004). But concerns have been expressed that the balance of care has shifted away from state provision towards the community, resulting in stress upon the carers of some vulnerable older people (Evandrou 1992).

In recent years in the UK older people's needs have been the focus of national policy, with the Royal Commission's report on long-term care (Royal Commission 1999), the establishment of national care standards (DoH 1999b), the formation of local eligibility criteria (DoH 1995), challenges to the equity of these criteria (DoH 1999c, Royal College of Nursing (RCN) 2000a), proposals for the enhancement of partnerships between health and social services (DoH 1998) and assessment (Ford and McCormack 1999, RCN 1997a,b). In addition The NHS Plan (DoH 2000a) highlighted the delays in hospital discharge for older people and this led to the development of the Singal Assessment Process (SAP) (Evans and Means 2005). Currently in the UK, nursing is free at the point of delivery for all older people except those who live in nursing homes, where means testing occurs. The National Plan (DoH 2000a) proposed a change to the funding of long-term care, with entitlement to nursing care as a 'free' component. This highlights the importance of assessment and the difficulty of differentiating between nursing and personal care (Royal Commission 1999); the differentiation of nursing care and personal care could become the new 'grey' area, replacing the previous health and social care debate (Loux et al 2000). The National Plan (DoH 2000a) and the UK government's response to the Royal Commission's 1999 recommendations for long-term care do not define nursing care, other than to indicate that registered nurses will assess the need for nursing care. To establish a broader understanding of nursing as more than a series of tasks (RCN 1997b), nurses working with older people will need to articulate the ways in which the presence of a registered nurse provides a constant overview or supervision of the care provided. Registered nurses will also provide actual care, while they also monitor, direct, manage and supervise care (RCN 1997a).

The NHS National Plan (DoH 2000a) requires an NHS-registered nurse to establish a component of the older person's care which is nursing. The hope is that these nurses will assess in a way that reflects a clear view of the complex ways in which a nurse contributes to the care and support of an older person – in essence, with a broad view of nursing that looks beyond tasks and hopefully prevents the new grey area of confusion in relation to the boundaries of nursing and personal care from developing.

In many instances older people will require input from both health and social services, which is best provided in an integrated way. The recommendations of the Royal Commission identified lack of integration as a problem and promoted good practice examples of partnership between health and social services providers. Current UK government policy seeks to encourage such partnerships (DoH 1998). The development of integrated services for older people has gained much support (e.g. Henwood 1999).

Primary care is currently seen as the leading partner in determining healthcare provision, which seeks to increase the decentralization of services, bringing them closer to the older person, perhaps in the form of primary care centres (Warner et al 1999). Services might be provided in more inventive ways, the National NHS Beds Inquiry (DoH 2000b) explores options which include making better use of nursing homes in the independent sector, through the provision of intermediate care facilities, for example. The National Plan aims to expand intermediate care services (DoH 2000a); this acknowledgement of the need for services for older people that afford additional time for recovery and access to appropriate expertise (Audit Commission 2000) holds promise for expansion in the primary and independent care sectors. However, all services must be mindful of the potential for ageism within the NHS (Age Concern 2000), especially if older people are seen as users of specific services, instead of accessing all services equally.

EMERGING TRENDS

Future services will be influenced both by policy and a variety of other factors. Heath (2006) states that a shift towards preventive care and community-based services has become evident in recent policy. The *National Service Framework for Long Term Conditions* (DoH 2005) and *Our health our care our say: a new direction for community services* (DoH 2006) are examples of this shift in England. In Scotland the move towards preventive health is reflected in *Delivering for health* (Scottish Executive 2005) and in Northern Ireland the new primary care strategy (Department of Health, Social Services and Personal Safety 2005) focuses on elderly people. The National Assembly for Wales also has a strategy for older people and the intention across the UK is that most health care will be delivered at home and in the community wherever possible (Heath 2006).

In addition to policy shifts, services for older people can be influenced by perceptions of old age. The media has a significant impact upon such perceptions through exposure to images on the television, film, radio and journals, and in newspapers. Many representations of older people in the media are less than positive; they are caricatured as a cohesive whole, wrinkled and frail, or they are infantilized. Hockey and James (1993) explore a variety of media reports, which form analogies between old age and childhood, or treat the example of fit and vital old age as the remarkable exception. As older people's individuality and vitality receives a fair hearing, health professionals can draw attention to positive models of ageing.

The independence and inclusion of older people is becoming more commonplace (Help the Aged 1997). The focus for health and social care professionals is being drawn toward user consultation. Users are articulate in expressing their viewpoint and the need to listen to what older people want from services is something that should not be ignored

(NHS Executive 2000) and, indeed, should influence policy. The ideal is not the disenfranchisement of any group, but the empowerment of all age groups within society (Warner et al 1999).

Standards of care services are becoming highly formalized, both in the independent sector, with the introduction of national required standards (DoH 1999b), and within the National Health Service, with the formation of the National Institute for Health and Clinical Excellence (NICE). NICE was established to give new coherence and prominence to information about clinical costs and effectiveness. In addition the National Service Framework (NSF) for older people (DoH 2001a) establishes standards for use within the NHS. The NSF is a complex framework with eight standards, under the four themes of:

- respecting the individual
- intermediate care
- providing evidence-based specialist care
- promoting an active healthy life.

The NSF seeks to guide service and practice development in the care and support of older people, these developments will be measured by the use of performance indicators and predetermined milestones for each standard. The setting of standards may in part respond to the findings of bodies such as the Health Advisory Service (2000), whose inquiry into the care of older people on acute care wards in general hospitals resulted in the following recommendations:

- increased user consultation in relation to all aspects of their care from older people
- the challenging of negative views about old age, from patients, their relatives and staff – particularly the belief that prospects for recovery are gloomy
- for the poor image and profile of older people to be tackled at every level of the health and social care system
- that the crucial role of the ward manager in creating a supportive culture of care should be developed and promoted
- better education for staff working with older people, in all settings.

Neno (2005) points out that multidisciplinary teamwork is required to ensure the success of high-quality care for older people. A number of models of care were outlined by the DoH (2001b) in order to deliver intermediate care and these included:

- rapid response
- hospital at home
- residential rehabilitation
- supported discharge
- day rehabilitation.

Each of these models of practice have a part to play in service delivery and a truly integrated service should include all of the models to ensure the needs of specific individuals are met in a timely and appropriate manner. The future for older people and the nurses who work with them has the potential to be challenging and rewarding, as we all adapt to the policy changes and move into a system that could create new partnerships across organizational boundaries and, more importantly, with older people themselves.

MEETING MR JACOB BROWN

Making sense of all the issues that could relate to the health and social well-being of an older person can be challenging. As a focus for the rest of this chapter, Jacob Brown is introduced. First you meet him as ageism would define him. In this first scenario (Case 3.1) Jacob is receiving informal caring and is encouraged to stay in his home, in keeping with the community care act (DoH 1990). In the second scenario (Case 3.2) Jacob's situation is described as it might be with the new policy developments and in a society without ageism.

The second of Mr Brown's scenarios is tracked as he travels on a critical pathway through service provision. Later Mr Brown is met again in relation to assessment.

CASE **Mr Jacob Brown: scenario 1**

Mr Brown lives alone. He can't do much for himself, and his nephew, who lives in the next village, is tired of going to drop off his dinner, only to find the next day that he hasn't eaten it. Mr Brown used to be a factory storeman for a large firm, but he retired 10 years ago and does nothing now. He used to fish but has given it up, the river being a couple of miles off, and he doesn't drive now – his nephew said a man his age would be a danger behind the wheel, so the car was sold.

Jacob lost his wife many years ago from cancer and they had no children. He has lots of nieces and nephews, because he has a brother and two sisters who have been married more than once. He sees them only at Christmas because they live all over, but they telephone now and then.

He fell last year and gave himself a fright. He went to the hospital and stayed in for 2 days; since then he has lost weight and still gets giddy when he gets up sometimes. He asked the doctor about getting a bit of help but wasn't eligible to go into the nursing home because the local criteria did not measure his needs as nursing. Jacob used to work with Bill Taylor, who lives in a residential home, but Jacob has never been there; it might be awful – you do hear things.

These days Jacob gets the paper delivered and reads that while it's light, to save on the electricity. Then he has a cup of soup and just waits for Colin, his nephew, to call. Nice lad, but he tends to be busy ferrying his two children about, so doesn't stay long. Sometimes Jacob feels miserable; the house is too big, and one day is like the next. He thinks he probably isn't good company.

In this first scenario, Jacob is seen from an ageist viewpoint:

- His ability to work beyond traditional retirement age is not acknowledged

- His skills are not utilized for the benefit of his family or local community
- He receives informal care from his nephew, which is not formally acknowledged
- He cannot maintain his lifestyle and relationships because he is viewed as unable to drive owing to his age
- Screening has not been carried out to alert his general practitioner to his dizzy spells, and Jacob has not accessed expert practitioners with specialist knowledge in gerontology
- Assessment has been carried out in light of local eligibility criteria, which does not view Jacob's needs as nursing
- Residential care is viewed as dependent living, in an institutional setting

Jacob has not been valued as an individual.

CASE **Mr Jacob Brown: scenario 2**

Mr Brown lives alone. He drives a Morris Minor, which he has had for years. On the advice of his nephew, Colin, he has a check-up from the practice nurse once a year, just to be sure he is still safe, but he's pleased to be getting around independently as he is quite a busy chap. He likes to fish at the weekend with an old work colleague, Bill Taylor. He collects Bill from the residential home where he lives and they usually go back to Bill's for a drink and a bit of a meal. If he ever needed to, Jacob thinks he would try to get a room there – you have a small bed-sit and it's all self-catering, which is lovely.

Jacob decided to move last winter after he had a nasty fall; the place was too big for him and he was keeping the lights off to keep the bills down. Looking back, that fall had been a godsend in a funny way. He ended up with a black eye, but no broken bones. The hospital assessed him and a nurse came along; she explained she was part of a team, which had a doctor and social workers in it. As a result of his assessment, they found out that Jacob had high blood pressure, and he now takes something for that so doesn't get dizzy.

The assessment helped him to think about living alone in that huge house – empty since his wife's death 30 years ago – and he decided to move nearer to his nephew. He got a first floor flat near the pub, where he's a regular feature, running the pub quiz and having his tea if he's feeling lazy. Jacob also gives Colin's children lifts here and there in return for the odd Sunday lunch at their house. Jacob is pleased to have his health, because some don't.

In this second scenario, Jacob exists in a positive framework which values older people for their ability to contribute to society:

- His skills are utilized and he remains an active member of his community
- He is able to spend time with his nephew's children, in a positive role

- His health problems have been identified and preventive measures put in place
- Jacob maintains his individuality and lifestyle choices
- His future decisions will be made in collaboration with professionals
- Residential care is viewed as communal living in a supportive environment.

Such a positive scenario demands a society in which equity and justice are central and in which individuals' ability to choose and take their own path in life is not hampered by stereotypes of old age. In the current context, however, issues of inequity for older people exist; the next section explores this in more detail.

ISSUES OF EQUITY

Equity is defined in *The Oxford Dictionary* as 'fairness, the application of principles of justice'. This definition suggests that everyone should have an equal voice and value in society. The question of equity for older people in health and social care has received increasing attention in recent years, largely as a result of the debate about rationing and prioritization (Grimley Evans 1997, Williams 1997). This chapter focuses on rationing as an extreme example of inequity. Rationing is defined as 'a fixed allowance, to limit or share out'.

Rationing by age polarizes perspectives. For example, Williams (1997, p. 820) cautions against the 'vain pursuit of immortality', claiming that we have reached a point at which no one must die, until everything possible has been done for them. Henwood (1999) agrees, and suggests ways in which a dignified death can be achieved; however, she also reminds us that this is a separate argument from the one that supports rationing in relation to age. For example, Grimley Evans (1997, p. 883) counters Williams' argument, stating that it is unethical to 'use age as a criterion for depriving people of health care from which they could benefit'.

There is evidence that rationing of health care does take place, for instance in end-stage renal disease (Mallick 1994) and coronary care (Dudley and Burns 1992). These findings also reflect the ageism associated with pharmaceutical and clinical research. Half of all malignancies occur in people over 70 years of age, yet people of this age are excluded from clinical trials of cancer treatment. The rationing debate is part of the wider debate about equity in health care, as the Acheson Report (Acheson 1998, p. xiii) observed:

Although average mortality has fallen over the past 50 years, unacceptable inequalities in health persist. For many measures of health inequalities have either remained the same or have widened in recent decades.

The main barriers to equity for older people are structural and attitudinal: *structural* in terms of age-segregated services and access difficulties, and *attitudinal* in terms of prejudicial ageist attitudes. Attitude refers to a person's favourable or unfavourable evaluation of an object (Yurick et al 1988).

Structural barriers to equity for older people occur as a result of the way in which services are organized within the NHS. Speed of recovery is emphasized, and older people who require time to improve and reach their maximum potential are disadvantaged. This system encourages increased dependence and loss of role and ability for older people, with a resulting resource implication (Audit Commission 2000). Structural barriers often re-enforce attitudinal barriers to equity. Older people are treated as a burden for taking up a hospital bed, labeled negatively as 'bed blockers' to be discharged quicker and sicker, making their potential for read-mission more likely (Audit Commission 1997, Yates 1998).

The attitudes of some care providers towards older people have been considered by gerontologists to have a major influence on the kind of care provided and on the self-image of the older person. A recent report from Age Concern (2000) presented evidence that the NHS discriminates against older people. Many accounts from older people themselves have described the way in which they felt healthcare personnel stereotyped them; the following comment was typical of others in the report (Age Concern 2000, p. 14):

Elderly people have the feeling that they are expendable. People are waiting for them to die. We have excellent maternity services, and services for children, psychiatry and drug abuse. Action this and action that! Action for the elderly should be equally good or better. After a long life, it is no less than we deserve. We want to feel loved and valued as we approach the end, not just fit for the scrap heap.

As can be seen, older people do not see themselves as passive recipients of care. However, the old, and particularly those aged over 75 years, are portrayed as a burden on society and a drain on our nation's resources (Birch et al 1999). This group of people is considered to be non-productive and therefore a burden to economically active younger people (Jeffreys 1989). As Stokes (1992) has identified, people are unwilling to accept the reality of ageing as it is commonly associated with physical and mental decline. Today's society is youth oriented: concepts such as energy, creativeness and beauty are valued and considered the sole prerogative of youth.

One solution could be to foster interactions between older and younger members of society, thereby developing a tolerance for the differences between generations and mutual concern. Voluntary organizations that promote foster grandparenting and schemes in schools that enable older people to assist in the classroom as teachers' aides might encourage this. Old age holds out promises as well as challenges. More contact with older people may help younger people to look beyond the caricature of decrepitude and dependency, instead seeing lifestyles that are free from the anxieties of childcare and the pressure of full-time work.

When negative beliefs are held about older people they often result in a paternalistic welfarization of the old. This view reinforces the beliefs that older people, and particu-larly the very old, are dependent and require help from the state in order to function (Johnson 1997). Whilst this sort of attitude is being challenged (Birch et al 1999), there is still a belief that an increase in the numbers of older people will pose a crisis in our society. Inevitably, health and social care professionals, as members of society, are affected by such stereotypes.

As a result of these attitudes, older people are often treated as passive consumers of health and social services (Ford 1989, Heath 1993). For example, most older people who sustain a **stroke** will require some form of rehabilitation to ensure that they regain maximum independence. This may take the form of being taught how to regain sitting balance, a technique that is essential in order to regain any degree of mobility. This is a skilled activity. Yet if health and social care workers have not been taught the principles of re-enable-ment, if older people are discharged before they have made a complete recovery, and if rehabilitation services are not available in the community, then that older person will never reach his or her potential and may even deteriorate further (RCN 1997b).

When we see people as a homogeneous group, we over-look their individual strengths and capabilities. This is as true of older people as it would be of any other group (Ford and McCormack 2000). It is worth noting that there are several generations of older people, all of whom will have had different life experiences. Within each generation there are many individuals, all different from one another. Such concepts of individuality and personal differences are not new, and if incorporated into professional practice result in rewarding practice which locates our interactions between the older person and practitioner in a person-centred way. Such person-centred approaches aim to reduce the deper-sonalization of older people in care settings, where images of dependency, someone to be moved and fed, abound (Ford and McCormack 2000). Person-centred assessment helps the process of really seeing the person to begin with (RCN 2000b); we will address assessment in some depth later.

Nurses working with older people aim to provide good quality care, but they also know that the reality of achieving this rarely sits comfortably alongside frameworks of patients' rights which focus on the ideal – an ideal not always met within systems and buildings that do not afford the level of choices or comfort a person might experience in their own home. Barriers to equity have been discussed, which occur through structures and systems. Nurses have to operate within these structures and may not be able to effect substantial change in them. However, by concentrating on overcoming attitudinal barriers to equity, nurses can effect a change; the concepts of respect, partnership and interdependence are often more helpful than strict adherence to principles of autonomy (British Medical Association/RCN 1995). These concepts build upon knowledge of biological and physiological perspectives of normal ageing, which are examined next.

NORMAL AGEING

The study of **ageing** is a multidisciplinary enterprise. Each discipline and profession brings its own theoretical perspectives and methods. In this chapter it is possible only to introduce the reader to some of these theories; further reading will be recommended at the end of the chapter.

Biological, psychological and sociological theories of ageing tend to focus on different aspects of the ageing process and do not necessarily contradict one another. They make different assumptions and use concepts in different ways, posing different questions and explanations along the way. Perspectives, then, are different. This does not make them right or wrong.

BIOLOGICAL AND PHYSIOLOGICAL PERSPECTIVES

While it is important to distinguish between the changes in an older adult resulting from disease or injury, exactly how we age is not yet clear. However, there are some inconclusive theories. Kyriazis (1994) claims that the theories converge into two main camps:

1 Ageing is caused by factors that damage our body, including radiation, toxic byproducts of the metabolism, random everyday damage and the genes that promote ageing.
2 The damage is not repaired properly; this may be because of a lack of metabolic energy, hormone deficiencies, lack of genetic support, failure of the immune system, and so on.

There is a lack of precise information on normal ageing processes. Much of the research has been cross-sectional (comparing average results of a group of older people with a younger group), so that the differences found in these studies between age groups may have been due, not to age, but to the effects of environment, diet or activities interacting with the groups at different points in time. In some instances it would seem that performance actually increases with age. It has been found that exercise, diet, not smoking and practicing intelligence tests have produced changes in the level of fitness, heart reserve, blood pressure, memory and reaction time of some older adults (Fries 1989).

The existing knowledge related to changes with age can serve as general guidelines for care which are aimed at preserving and prolonging function. New knowledge may alter these conceptions of old age. Most older people function well at rest but their functional capacity may be altered under conditions of stress, such as illness, surgery, trauma, physical exercise and emotional stress, which may exceed the body's threshold of physiological reserves resulting in an inability to maintain homeostasis. Older people are also more likely to develop complications and to take longer to recover than younger individuals. Physiological changes may not occur until well after 70 years of age. The older person may continue to engage in all the activities of middle age with perhaps a modification of the pace of life. Table 3.1 displays physical and functional changes that occur with ageing along with key nursing implications. Later in this chapter we will review the impact of these changes on the expected findings during physical examination.

Ageing **skin** is generally characterized by diminishing function and reserve capacity. Local sensation of heat, pressure and painful stimuli may be less acute. **Wound healing** is slower, and nail and hair growth declines.

Adult **bone loss** (osteoporosis) begins to take place in both sexes around the age of 40 years and is thought to be related to diet, physical activity, hormonal changes and possibly ribonucleic acid (RNA) activity.

The **neurological system** reacts more slowly with increasing age due to vision changes, decreased numbers of axons in the nerves and synapse changes resulting in slow nerve conduction. This may result in slower reflexes, decreased pain sensation and more time being required for problem solving.

There are obviously changes to the special **senses**, of which sight and hearing are the most commonly affected. Communication involves the use of symbols and motor articulation or speech. With ageing, simple reaction time is decreased and learning occurs at a less rapid rate; normal ageing, however, does not account for speech difficulties. This is more likely to be attributed to teeth alignment or breath control. Atrophy of vocal cords affecting pitch may alter speech, but generally it remains functional. There is a decreased sense of taste and smell for some individuals.

In the **cardiopulmonary system**, cardiac output drops due to fibrosis and sclerosis in the endocardium, left ventricular wall thickening and increased fat infiltration in the right atrium and ventricle. The **heart rate** slows with age and cardiovascular stress response is less efficient in the older adult. A decrease in fluids affects the removal of dust and mucus through coughing and sneezing; this predisposes the person to bronchopneumonia. Additionally there is less pulmonary elasticity and capillary action decreases, which leads to less efficiency and contributes to bacterial growth.

The **gastrointestinal system** has such a large reserve capacity that decreases in normal function can occur with little effect on physiological processes. Periodontal disease becomes the major cause of tooth loss and there is less salivary activity. The gag reflex is weaker and the cardiac sphincter more relaxed; this predisposes the older person to aspiration difficulties. Less gastric acid and weaker musculature leads to a need for smaller and more frequent amounts of food. Decreased intestinal peristalsis and duller nerve sensations can cause a missed signal for defaecation.

Degeneration of the **renal system** for some leads to a slowing of filtration functions. Bladder capacity decreases from about 500 to 250 mL, resulting in frequency and nocturia. For some, bladder emptying is more difficult because of a weakening of the muscles; this can lead to urine

Table 3.1 Physical and functional changes related to ageing

Changes	Nursing implications
Skin	
Decreased elasticity	Attention to skin care, nail care, position changes and hygiene
Dryness, scaling of skin	Insulatory effect of clothing
Wound healing retarded; increased vascular fragility	Avoiding exposure to sun and heat
Nails thicken, become brittle and yellow	
Thinning of hair, loss of pigmentation	
Sweat glands atrophy	
Musculoskeletal	
Decreased subcutaneous tissue, muscle mass and strength	Accident prevention and rest
Bone demineralization	Exercise programme
Joints stiffen, lose flexibility	Weight control
	Aids to movement
	Diet high in calcium, vitamin D and protein
Neurological	
Slowed reaction, especially to multiple stimuli (neurone loss)	Slower pacing of activities
Decreased temperature regulation and pain perception	Monitor trauma or illness carefully
Increased time for problem solving	Assess sudden confusional states
Decreased overall sleep time and REM sleep	5–7 hours of night sleep may be sufficient
Sense of balance declines	
Special senses	
Diminished visual activity (presbyopia); increased sensitivity to glare and difficulty adjusting to darkness	Regular vision and hearing tests
Decreased depth perception	Avoid night driving, glare
Diminished hearing activity (presbycousis)	Home safety (lighting, furniture)
Diminished colour perception (especially blue and green)	Communication techniques (auditory, visual and tactile)
Decreased sense of taste and smell	Use of yellows, oranges against contrasting backgrounds
	Use of spices/herbs and low calorie foods
	Smoke detectors
Cardiopulmonary	
Less able to increase heart rate and cardiac output with activity	Regular blood pressure readings
Blood vessels less elastic	Posture, breathing and walking exercise
Venous return less efficient	Avoid prolonged immobility; early ambulation
Peripheral oedema and pooling may occur, especially with immobility	Avoid irritants
Pulmonary elasticity and ciliary action decrease, leading to less efficient gas exchange and slowed cough reflex	Limit salt intake
	Pacing activities
	Attention to prolonged infections
	Vaccinations (pneumococcal and influenza)
Gastrointestinal (including dentition)	
Diminished saliva, digestive juices, and decreased nutrient absorption	Regular diet low in fat and calories, high in fibre and fluids
Delayed oesophageal and gastric emptying	Small, frequent servings more readily digested
Reduced muscle tone and decreased peristalsis	Discourage long-term laxative and other non-prescription drugs
Decreased blood flow to liver lessens drug detoxication	Accessible toilet facilities
Decreased taste buds	Community resources for help with meals
Teeth more brittle, some reabsorption of gum tissue	Dental and oral hygiene
	Regular dental examinations
Genitourinary (including reproductive)	
Decreased blood flow to kidneys	Encourage hydration
Bladder capacity diminishes; reduced glomerular filtration	Minimum daily 1500–2000 mL of fluid
Decrease in bladder size and sphincter control may result in incomplete emptying	Accessible toilet and hygiene facilities
	Avoid constipation

Continued

Table 3.1 *cont'd*	
Changes	**Nursing implications**
Enlarged prostate, reduced testosterone, slowed erection	Recognize drug toxicity
Atrophy and decreased lubrication of female genital tract; reduced oestrogen	Continence promotion
	Adaptation of sexual practices
Endocrine	
Decreased testosterone	Maintain normal weight
Glucose tolerance deteriorates	Limit use of fat and sugar
Temperature regulation less efficient	

Modified from Gioiella and Bevil (1985) and Taylor et al (1989).

retention. Tissue changes associated with oestrogen deficiency in women result in relaxed pelvic floor muscles. In men, prostate enlargement and atrophy of periurethral structures can occur. These changes may lead to uninhibited bladder contractions (stress incontinence and dribbling).

Age-related changes to the **reproductive system** do not prevent sexual function or alter libido. Research to date has tended to concentrate on three areas: sexual performance or behaviour; changes in sexual responses with age; and sexual problems or dysfunction. It often omits consideration of older people. This research has tended to be male and heterosexually oriented, and pays little attention to the experiences or feelings of older people. Older people who do not have an active sex life are likely to be lacking a partner or fear the attitudes of society. This is particularly difficult if they share a sexual relationship with a partner of the same sex.

A loss of **mental function** is not a normal part of the ageing process. There is, however, less capacity for adaptation, especially in stressful or unfamiliar settings, and if the older person has impaired senses. Older people experience a decreased ability to respond to multiple or complex stimuli, so they tend to respond to the stimuli of greatest intensity. If all stimuli are of low intensity then the person may well become disinterested. This is of particular importance for those who live alone or who are residing in a home or hospital.

Older people's need for personal expression and mental health support is apparent, with an estimated 750 000 people in the UK with some form of dementia and one in five people over the age of 80 suffering from the condition (Alzheimer's Society 2006). Essink-Bot et al (2002) found similar prevalence rates for dementia across six European countries. These sorts of statistics can lead us to lump old people into a homogeneous group, but this could not be further from the truth. Older people continue to learn and problem-solve. Intellectual performance is stable but response time is slower. This results in slower absorption, processing and response to information and environmental cues. Memory is generally stable except where distractions or time pressure is present. There is no reliable data relating to dementia in developing countries because methods of detection need to be culturally sensitive and as yet many cultures do not have the relevant tools for diagnosis (WHO 1998).

PSYCHOLOGICAL PERSPECTIVES

Age-related psychological changes may be associated with internal stressors, such as changes in memory, sleep patterns, hearing and vision, and gastrointestinal metabolism. These and other factors may lead the older adult to feel isolated, frustrated, bored or apathetic. External stressors such as retirement, loss of a partner or friends, and diminished resources can all contribute to a loss of self-worth and independent functioning. Developmental theories seek to explain the diverse growth processes that occur with ageing.

Erikson's theory of development

Erickson's theory or 'eight stages of life' is perhaps the most well-known example (Erikson 1964). Erikson is considered one of the precursors of what is known as lifespan developmental psychology (Sugarman 1986). The emphasis on integrity of the lifespan is Erikson's lasting contribution, and one that is vital to the understanding of old age (Bond and Coleman 1994). In order to understand people in late life it is necessary to see them in the context of their whole life history with the challenges of life that may or may not have been resolved at earlier stages. Clearly such an approach has several implications, namely that older people are individuals and as such will vary according to their histories. Such courses of development are likely to diverge as we age, and therefore it is likely that we become even more individual as ageing takes place.

It is likely that development occurs on a number of different fronts. Bond and Coleman (1994) point out that there is no reason to think that intellectual, physical and social development all follow the same pathway.

A third characteristic of the lifespan approach is that the reciprocal influences between the environment and the individual are recognized. This was emphasized by Erikson, who stressed the interdependence of the generations, with the old needing the young and the young needing the old. Such a model of ageing may be too idealistic: the nature of modern society makes it difficult for someone to achieve such positive qualities. Erikson does not offer a well-worked-out theory of adjustment in later life (Bond and Coleman 1994), but he points to key elements that have to be taken into account in any consideration of ageing. He raises the special issues of adjustment which older people must face.

SOCIOLOGICAL PERSPECTIVES

One starting point in analyzing the conditions of older people in society is the influence exerted by sociological theory. As the numbers of older people have increased, they have become more 'visible' and as such have become the subject of much discussion and study. From these studies various theories have emerged about ageing which frequently reflect society's perception and treatment of our older citizens.

Socially constructed life course

Concern with old age in our time has tended to focus attention on this stage of life in isolation from the entire life course. Without denying the unique rewards and challenges of this period of life, it is important to interpret it as part of the life course, and with historical context. Hockey and James (1993) contend that the recognition of old age in the twentieth century is part of a larger historical process involving the emergence of new stages of life and their societal recognition.

Disengagement theory

Disengagement theory is generally defined as a triple withdrawal: a loss of roles, a contraction of contact, and a decline in the commitment to norms and values. The theory arose from research in the USA, which was conducted on older people (Cummings and Henry 1961). The theory proposes that, independent of poor health or poverty, ageing involves a gradual decline that inevitably results in a withdrawal from interaction between individuals and society. At the same time disengagement theory suggests that society prepares older people to play fewer active roles, with the result that the ageing person slowly and inevitably withdraws, experiencing deterioration in both the quality and quantity of relationships. However, most of the evidence is ambiguous and little attention has been paid to individual variations. A further difficulty is the implicit value judgment that disengagement is a good thing for society and the individual. Blau (1973, p. 152), an American sociologist, has argued that:

> The disengagement theory deserves to be publicly attacked because it can so easily be used by the non-old, who constitute the 'normals' in society, to avoid confronting and dealing with the issue of the olds' marginality and rolelessness in American society.

Role and activity theory

Harris (1990) suggests that the major role losses associated with old age come with retirement, loss of a partner and institutionalization. Role and activity theory, developed in the 1950s and 1960s, claims that individuals play a variety of roles throughout their lives which offer them social development leading to status and identity.

This view was combined with a sense of concern about older people's abilities to use leisure, leading to the development of activity theory. This is an extension of role theory and emphasizes the importance of maintaining a range of activities. This has led to the development of pre-retirement courses and a variety of studies on the meaning of work and retirement.

Continuity theory

Developed by Atchley (1980), this theory proposes that adaptation to ageing can proceed in several directions depending on the individual's past life. Personality and adjustment to stress remain stable over the lifespan. This theory has gained support as it accounts for factors in other theories and considers individual variation.

Exchange theory

Disengagement, role and activity theories all focus on discontinuity from one phase of life to another. Exchange theory focuses on discontinuity in terms of a loss of power. Markides and Cooper (1987) argue that, implicit within this theory, is the importance of reciprocity: the ability to return favours or rewards so that the bargaining position of social relationships is maintained. The theory is based on the assumption that much social interaction may be reduced to rewards and cost. The concept of reciprocity in relationships and society in general is basic to survival, and for Ebersole and Hess (1990) the ability of older people to survive is dependent on their ability to 'barter in the market place of human relationships' in an environment of 'generational equity'. In other words, unequal patterns of exchange create dependency. Interdependence is based on concepts of time, equity, caring and sharing; in old age an increasing amount of dependency may occur. It is therefore important to maintain a strong position of reciprocity in order to avoid the erosion of self-esteem.

Essentially this is a theory about power and status, and is therefore particularly useful for nurses as it suggests that steps to correct loss of power in older people may be an important element in any therapeutic regimen. It is clearly relevant, particularly in rehabilitation and longer-term care, in which nurses are key providers. This theory relates directly to interdependence, the opportunity for giving as well as receiving.

Political economy theory

Fennell et al (1988) suggested that in the UK and the USA the process of ageing needs to be viewed in the context of advanced capitalist societies, because the way in which resources are allocated is central to the status and experience of older people. Social gerontology has become highly political, linking the political economy to a moral economy approach which questions how ideas of fairness and human values influence policy. Taking this view one can see the importance for nurses to maintain links to national policies, so that they can influence decisions that impact on older people as they are developed.

Political economy theory focuses on the structural changes and processes that affect older people. Many themes have been developed, in particular through the works of Townsend (1979, 1981), Estes (1979) and Phillipson and Walker (1986). The theory was first developed after the public spending crisis of the mid-1970s, which led to cuts in public expenditure. Much of the money had previously been targeted at older people; they subsequently were viewed as an economic burden and the subject for political attack. Political economy theory is actually a study of the interactions between government, the economy and those groups of people who may be defined socially as 'the poor' or 'the old'. Older people came to be viewed as an intolerable burden on Western economies, with demographic changes seen as causing intolerable pressure on public spending.

In this theory, it is argued that dependency in old age is not the inevitable outcome of ageing but rather the result of social structuring. The state plays a large part in this in that it determines the events of later life that create dependence, poverty or isolation (Townsend 1981). Little attention has been paid previously to the structural relationship between older people and the rest of society and the differential impact of social and economical institutions upon older people. Implicit within this theory is that ageing is a social rather than a biologically created status.

At the start of this section it was pointed out that no one theory provides all the answers, and no single theory is right or wrong. Rather they serve to guide thinking and in this way encourage nurses to explore the relationships between theory, policy and practice. A particular challenge for nurses is the development of their relationship with older people, from a basis of genuine mutual respect and valuing or reciprocity, where each gains from the other. A key factor in this relationship will be the assessment undertaken by the nurse but which, in fact, is likely to be a two-way process in which the older person will also be assessing the nurse – albeit less overtly. In this way the nurse–user relationship should seek to establish equality, with both parties bringing skills and information that are different but of equal standing.

ASSESSMENT

Assessment is a complex activity, requiring skill in its execution (Ford and McCormack 1999, Heath 2000, Lewis et al 1999). It is a multidisciplinary process which can initiate person-centred care (Ford and McCormack 2000, Kitwood 1997, RCN 2000a). The methods used to engage older people in the assessment process will call upon story telling and the use of biography (RCN 2000b, Schofield 1994) and as nurses advance their roles in work with older people, assessment will also involve aspects of physical examination and medical history taking. The specific focus of an individual's assessment will be guided by the presenting needs and concerns. Here, we will firstly consider the tools of nursing assessment before moving on to the physical examination; however, in reality the older person's more

pressing need may be a medical examination before other issues can be given thorough consideration.

A tool may be used to guide the assessment, whilst the practitioner remains mindful of the need always to record the individual person's personal and particular perspective. Consequently the selection of any tool intended to provide a framework for assessment should consider the following questions (Wills and Ford 2001):

- Does the tool facilitate a holistic view of the individual, which considers individual needs, wants and aspirations?
- Does the tool account for ethnicity and cultural context?
- Does the tool utilize biography as an essential component of assessment?
- Does the tool call for skilled application?
- Is the tool valid and reliable?
- Can the tool be completed in a reasonable time frame: does it have a practical application within the resources that exist?
- Does the tool have a common language?
- Does the tool indicate the level of input needed, i.e. personal or nursing care?
- Does the tool account for changes over time, lending itself to the fact that assessment is a continuous process?
- Does the tool maintain a focus on the individual with room for the older person's own involvement, as opposed to the professional's needs?
- Is the tool part of the multidisciplinary assessment?

Facilitation of the assessment process for older people includes the ability to respond to any sensory needs (e.g. poor auditory or visual ability) and to monitor and respond to changes as they occur (e.g. fatigue or breathlessness) (Heath 2000). Assessment provides information that is critical to the development of a plan of action that can enhance personal health status, decrease the potential for or the severity of chronic conditions, and assist the individual in gaining control over health through self-care (RCN 1997a, 2000c). In recent years the focus on assessment has intensified (Loux et al 2000) as it is the gateway to continuing care and re-enablement services for many older people. The political climate, with its emphasis on eligibility criteria and the funding of nursing care, has highlighted the importance of assessment for several reasons.

The shortcomings of current approaches to assessment have been widely reported:

1 Assessment does not have an unambiguous meaning (Ford and McCormack 1999).
2 Assessment may have an underlying fiscal drive (Royal Commission on Long Term Care for the Elderly 1999).
3 Assessments are disparate, with many different practitioners, organizations and health authorities using a variety of different tools, which cannot easily be compared with one another (Lewis et al 1999, Stewart et al 1999).
4 Assessments are of varying quality (Stewart et al 1999).

5 Assessments may be undertaken by practitioners without the appropriate expertise to carry them out (Ford and McCormack 1999).

6 Assessments may use formats that lose the older person's biography and individuality, thereby losing some of the richness and detail that makes the assessment a true representation of the older person (Ford and McCormack 1999, Royal Commission on Long Term Care for the Elderly 1999, RCN 2000b).

There is considerable debate over which tools are best, and whether or not there should be a move towards greater standardization of assessment tools (Ford and McCormack 1999). The development of an integrated service provision, which delivers a comprehensive service to older people, is achievable through the adoption of a standardized approach to assessment. It has been advocated that there is a need to distinguish between standardized assessments and a standardized approach to assessment (RCN 2000d). The use of one standardized assessment tool and one protocol to assess all older people may overlook the individuality of the older person. However, a standardized approach to assessment adopts a common approach to assessment through specific domains that may make use of standardized tools. Such an approach should utilize assessment tools that foster a re-enablement approach. For example, the RCN assessment tool (Ford and McCormack 1999, RCN 1997a) for nursing older people has been developed by expert gerontological nurses to identify the areas where nursing is needed and provide evidence for the prescribed level of registered nurse intervention. The assessment tool aims to promote a re-enablement model of care, which maximizes the potential of the individual by building upon the abilities needed to achieve those things they consider to be important to them (RCN 1997b).

When selecting a tool to guide the assessment process the nurse needs to consider the importance of the individual's biography, with the emphasis on the older person's potential to achieve desired, realistic health choices. This maximizing of potential is one of the aims of the assessment: to determine the person's needs, wants and aspirations, and to plan healthcare interventions in accordance with these and in partnership with the older person. Assessment for older people often involves members of the multidisciplinary team, which means that all the healthcare and social services professionals should be mindful of the need to maximize the sharing of information and the avoidance of duplication.

The initiation of the nursing assessment marks the beginning of a relationship between the nurse and older person. The interview that follows requires skill in establishing trust and confidence. A considerable amount of time is required to undertake a comprehensive health assessment. It requires specific skills of the nurse such as the ability to listen patiently, to allow for pauses, to ask questions that are not often asked, to obtain information from all the available sources and to recognize normalities of late

life that would be abnormal in those who are younger. The quality and speed of the assessment is an art that is born of both experience and a genuine valuing of older people in this way.

Maximizing the potential of the older person through the process of assessment, the RCN (1997b, 2000b) calls for the skilled nurse to focus on independence and ability, as opposed to dependence. The rehabilitation of older people is not a short-term intervention usually associated with acute hospitals, but a process with potential in continuing care settings (Nocon and Baldwin 1998, RCN 2000c). The RCN views this extension of the traditional view of rehabilitation (Warren 1981) as re-enablement, helping people to adapt to changes in their life circumstances. It is a shared activity between the person affected, other people close to them and multiprofessional teams. It means recognizing that older people are experts on themselves and that professionals provide expertise in their own field. Re-enablement must have a therapeutic value for the person concerned, with the ultimate aim of maximizing their social well-being. It is not time limited with set outcomes, but may cover the lifespan of the individual; its goals are person-centred, selected and set in partnership with the older person (RCN 1997a,b).

Such a philosophy promotes assessment that accesses various models of care and that could take place in a variety of settings: the older person's home, the community hospital, the nursing or residential home, or acute hospital. The family and others close to the older person may naturally have key involvement, which poses a challenge in the balancing of different perspectives. Re-enablement ways of working also offer the community in which the older person lives (whether in their own home or in more formal care) the opportunity to be involved.

Many nurses are now expanding their roles to include physical examination and history taking. This can provide an extra dimension to the assessment of older people and is particularly valuable in the work of modern matrons, intermediate care support teams, rapid response teams, nurse practitioners in casualty settings, nurse practitioners in general practice and gerontological nurse specialists. In all of these roles, a physical examination carried out by the nurse can help to prevent unnecessary trips to see the GP; or the examination can help to identify and diagnose problems sooner, leading to timely intervention and ultimately less distress for the elderly person and their family. Nurses working with older people do need to be aware that there may be variations from the normal expected findings on physical examination but that these findings are completely normal for the older population. A summary of these findings follows, which has been adapted from *Mosby's Guide to Physical Examination* (Seidel et al 1999).

Ear, nose and throat

Hearing tends to deteriorate after about the age of 50. Due to deposition of bone cells the stapes may become fixed to the tympanic membrane; there may be sensorineural deficit and due to a reduction in the activity of sebaceous glands the cerumen may become dry and more likely to block the external ear canal. Cartilage formation continues in the ears and nose, making the pinna of the ear more prominent. Loss of teeth can lead to changes in the appetite and difficulty with chewing. The teeth often appear longer as the gums retract.

Eyes

The major change in ageing is the development of presbyopia (problems with near vision). This occurs as the lens becomes more rigid and the ciliary muscles of the iris become weaker. The lens gradually becomes more dense as fibres continue to be laid down and are gradually compressed in the central region causing loss of clarity and ultimately the formation of cataracts.

Head and neck

With ageing it is not uncommon for the thyroid gland to become more fibrotic and to feel nodular and enlarged on palpation. Caution should be exercised when asking the patient to go through range of motion movements with the head as the increased likelihood of arthritic changes in the neck can cause pain and neural damage with excessive movement. The older person's face may provide a number of clues about his or her health status. Many years of smoking will alter an older person's face as will many years of breathlessness which results in obvious vertical lines around the lips as the person with chronic obstructive pulmonary disease has used pursed lipped breathing to control their respirations.

Skin, hair and nails

The changes of old age are particularly noticeable in the skin, hair and nails. The skin loses its elasticity, subcutaneous tissue decreases, the epidermis thins and flattens and sebaceous and sweat gland activity decreases. The result is dry, parchment-like skin which tends to be thin, wrinkled and dry. The person looks more angular as bony prominences become more obvious, making them more prone to developing pressure areas and more prone to skin damage in general. The lack of elasticity in the skin can result in 'tenting' when testing for turgor, therefore do not rely on this finding as a test for hydration status.

There are several lesions that can be found on the skin of normal health older people and these include: cherry angiomas, seborrheic keratoses (or warts), cutaneous tags, hyperkeratotic horns, senile letigines (often referred to as 'age spots' or 'liver spots') and sebaceous hyperplasia. It remains important to be alert to the signs of malignant disease of the skin and therefore to approach each lesion with caution and suspicion.

Melanocyte function decreases resulting in the graying of hair, and axillary and pubic hair production declines. Hair loss on the trunk and extremities is common. Hair loss may also result from peripheral vascular disease and it is therefore important to remain alert to this possibility when assessing the older person. Nail growth slows and toenails,

in particular, tend to become thicker, ridged and more prone to breaking.

Chest and lungs

Chest expansion in the older adult is often decreased as the muscles of respiration become weaker and calcification of the rib articulations interfere with respiratory movement. This may result in them using accessory muscles to aid breathing and you may therefore find them obviously using the sternocleidomastoid muscles or their abdominal muscles with each breath. In some older people the dorsal curve of the thoracic spine becomes pronounced (kyphosis) and the lumbar curve flattens. This alters the diameter of the chest. An older person may tire quickly during examination of the chest and they may find repeated deep inspirations quite demanding. Therefore, even for a perfectly well older person, the pace of the examination needs to be slowed and their physical comfort should be considered at all times.

Cardiovascular system

Due to the increased anteroposterior diameter of the chest (as described above) the apical beat may be difficult to locate. The range of normal heart rate for older people is 40 beats per minute to 100 beats per minute. A rate below 60 beats per minute should be investigated further but may still turn out to be normal for that individual. Ectopic beats are not uncommon and once again, can be a normal finding. These findings should be considered within the context of the rest of the physical examination and any concern regarding the rate and rhythm of the heart should be followed up with an ECG and further investigations.

Loss of elasticity in the blood vessels results in an increase in systolic pressure. This makes the older person more prone to hypertension. In addition the more superficial vessels are more likely to appear tortuous and distended and the dorsalis pedis and posterior tibial pulses can be more difficult to find.

Breasts

The appearance of the breasts in post-menopausal women changes due to the reduction in hormones. The breasts become pendulous, flattened and elongated and the nipples become flatter and smaller. On palpation the breast tissue feels finer and granular and less glandular. Post-menopausal women should be encouraged to continue to be breast aware as cancer of the breast occurs more frequently in older women than it does in the younger population.

Female genitalia

The skin of the labia undergoes the same changes as skin elsewhere and therefore it may appear drier; the labia may appear flatter and the clitoris may appear smaller than it does in the younger woman. The introitus may narrow and therefore you may need to use a small speculum for the vaginal examination. In some women (particularly those who are multiparous) the introitus may gape and the vaginal walls may roll out towards the opening. The vagina may be narrower and shorter and the cervix may also be smaller and appear paler than the cervix of a younger woman. Older women are prone to atrophic vaginitis as their level of oestrogen falls. It is therefore important to observe for this and to look for bleeding, infection, inflammation and tenderness, all of which may be the uncomfortable signs of the ageing process, but also all of which should be taken seriously, investigated and treated accordingly.

Male genitalia

The ejaculatory volume may actually increase with age although the viability of the sperm may decrease and the chances of conception may be reduced. The scrotum becomes more pendulous, erection may develop more slowly and the sensation of orgasm may be less intense.

Gastrointestinal system

Palpation of the abdomen in the older adult may be easier than in a younger person as the abdominal musculature becomes thinner and the contents of the abdomen become more palpable. The contour of the abdomen becomes more rounded as muscle tone is reduced and there are often fatty deposits in the abdominal cavity even though there is loss of fatty tissue in the extremities. There is decreased intestinal motility with ageing and therefore intestinal disorders are common in older people. It may be possible to palpate soft stool in the region of the sigmoid colon and there may be increased tympany with percussion over gaseous or bloated areas. Older people may exhibit atypical pain symptoms as a normal part of the ageing process and therefore complaints of pain may be completely absent. Therefore physical examination findings should take into account other elements of the related history. The incidence of gastrointestinal cancer increases with age and therefore you must be alert to symptoms such as nausea, weight loss, anorexia, haematemesis, malena, and changes in the frequency and consistency of the stool.

Anus rectum and prostate

In some older people the sphincter tone of the anus is decreased resulting in faecal incontinence. Older men are highly likely to have an enlarged prostate which should feel smooth, rubbery and symmetrical.

Musculoskeletal system

Joint and muscle agility have tremendous extremes in the older population. There is a reduction in muscle mass which may be exacerbated through disuse and the joints may become less supple. You may notice that the person walks with their arms held slightly away from the body to aid balance and the posture may change with a kyphosis of the thoracic vertebrae and flexion at the hips.

Neurological system

The older person tends to have decreased sensations of smell, taste, vision and hearing. Their proprioception declines and therefore their gait becomes unsteady. Tactile sensation and vibratory sensation are reduced and so it is not uncommon for older people to need stronger stimuli to detect a sensation. The reflexes tend to be less brisk and the lower extremities tend to be affected first. Fine motor coordination tends to be diminished and a benign tremor is common.

Mental function

There is a decline in synthesis and metabolism of neurotransmitters in older age and at times of stress the metabolism may be inadequate to respond; this may result in an increased risk of delirium with acute illnesses. Some problem-solving skills may deteriorate with age but this can be related to lack of use. Some people report that their recall of distant memories improves with age, although short-term memory and the ability to reason abstractly and spatially may all deteriorate.

In summary there are a number of changes which are a completely normal part of the ageing process and such findings can be expected during the physical examination of the older adult. Nonetheless, it is essential to remember that the finding may be normal for an older person but it may be abnormal for this particular individual. Always think of the differential diagnosis and put the findings into the context of the patient history and presenting problems. The incidence of disease and illness increases with increasing age and therefore you need to be alert to all possibilities at all times. An additional confounding factor to consider during examination of the older person is the medication they are taking. Polypharmacy in the older adult is not uncommon and the affects of the medications plus the interactions between drugs can have profound affects on the patient's physical and mental functioning.

Pharmacology in older people

As people get older they are likely to have developed various illnesses and are more likely to be living with long-term conditions. It is therefore not uncommon to find people over the age of 65 taking more than four medications to manage their hypertension or diabetes or to prevent further heart attacks or strokes. As the number of medications increase so does the potential for error. Equally as the number of medications increase so does the potential for drug interactions and adverse reactions (Grahame-Smith and Aronson 2002).

It is important to consider the pharmaceutical factors which may contribute to problems with medications. Old people might have problems swallowing large tablets, or they may have difficulty drinking an adequate quantity of fluid to make sure the tablet lands in the stomach. Pharmacokinetics in older people also contribute to the difficulty with drug treatments as renal excretion falls with age, metabolism of particular drugs may be reduced and distribution of the drug throughout a body which has altered in composition of fats and water changes; this results in elderly people tending to be more sensitive to particular drugs (e.g. ACE inhibitors) and hence the starting doses must be lower than they are with the younger adult population.

Pharmacodynamic factors affecting the older person include altered sensitivity to particular drugs because of the altered sensitivity of the pharmacological receptors. In some cases they may be more sensitive to the effects of certain drugs (e.g. digoxin) and less sensitive to others (e.g. salbutamol) because the sensitivity of the receptors is decreased (Grahame-Smith and Aronson 2002). There are also all sorts of practical problems associated with medications for older people such as physically getting the prescription from the chemist, being able to remove the child-safe tops on medication bottles, not being able to read labels properly because of the size of the writing, the list is endless. Suffice to say, the use of medication with older people is associated with a set of particular problems related to the ageing process. In our work with older adults we need to be aware of these problems so that we can monitor them and ensure that they receive their treatment in as safe and effective manner as possible.

ASSESSMENT, PHYSICAL EXAMINATION AND JACOB BROWN

Let us return to Jacob Brown, to explore how some of the principles that relate to assessment might apply to him (see Case 3.3).

CASE Assessment and Jacob Brown

Unexpectedly one night Jacob awoke, breathless and uncomfortable. When he tried to get out of bed he felt weak. He didn't want to bother the doctor, so he stayed in bed waiting for his nephew, Colin, to pop in, as he usually did. Jacob had forgotten that Colin and the family had gone away for a long weekend. By Sunday, he was very poorly, in pain, had a sore bottom and **swollen legs**, and hadn't eaten since Thursday night, although he had sipped squash. He managed to look for help and appeared, dishevelled and seemingly incontinent of urine, in the pub next door. The landlord called an ambulance, which took Jacob to casualty. Jacob wasn't making much sense at that point. He was muddling up his words and saying that he needed to get back to work and check that the building was secure.

After being assessed in casualty Jacob was transferred to the medical assessment unit. Here, the nurse practitioner took a history and assessed Jacob initially by observing him, carrying out a full examination of his cardiovascular system, respiratory system, mental ability, urinary system and gastrointestinal system. The nurse then ordered a series of tests including blood tests for electrolytes, full blood count, liver function test and erythrocyte sedimentation test, a urine test for leucocytes, nitrites, blood, glucose and culture and sensitivity and a chest X-ray to assess for pulmonary oedema, signs of infection or other underlying lung disease. The nurse practitioner explained everything that was happening to Jacob and arranged for Colin to be informed. The nurse also discussed Jacob with medical colleagues and, realizing that he would need a number of treatments, arranged for admission to the ward.

It can be seen how Jacob's usual independent self may be lost, as his present physical condition and confusional state take precedent in the A&E department. It is important that his physical condition is treated, so that he is hydrated, and the cause of his breathlessness and discomfort discovered, but it is also important that the nurse assesses Jacob's previous lifestyle, ability and needs, so that the goals of his recovery may be matched to his desire for independence. In Box 3.1 we consider which elements of Jacob's needs might be included in an assessment, as he is admitted to hospital.

A PROFESSION EQUIPPED TO SUPPORT AND WORK WITH OLDER PEOPLE

In the discussion about assessment it becomes apparent that the professionals working with older people need to be knowledgeable doers (Benner 1984). In the UK, Reports from the UKCC (1997) on the continuing care of older people and from Age Concern (1998) regarding training and qualifications for work with older people recommend a concentrated effort to formalize and expand the qualifications of those working with this group. Heath and Ford (1999) have explored this further, describing their vision for a gerontological nurse specialist, a band of expert, skilled and knowledgeable gerontological nurses who transcend care boundaries, moving in and out of the care location anticipating and responding to need. Such nurses could be employed in any setting; what will matter is that they are able to practise at an advanced level in an autonomous way. These practitioners would continue to promote the use of evidence in the planning and implementation of practice.

Ford and McCormack (1998) do not believe that older people have more or fewer needs depending on whether

---

Box 3.1 Elements of Jacob's assessment and biography (adapted from Johns 1991)

- How does Jacob deal with his admission, discomfort and distress? How can his individual reaction be supported?

- What physical needs does Jacob have (breathlessness, nutrition and hydration, skin integrity)?

- What medications is Jacob taking and what medications will he need subsequently?

- What were Jacob's previous abilities and how do they match with his present abilities?

- Which people support and interact with Jacob when he is at home? How might they be a part of his recovery?

- How can Jacob be helped and supported by the nurses and the rest of the multidisciplinary team?

- How does Jacob view the future for himself and others in his life?

they are in an acute ward, a nursing home or in their own home, and do not believe that a nurse needs more or less knowledge and skills to work in an acute ward, nursing home or the community. The establishment of gerontological nurse specialist roles, as case managers or coordinators of care services, is an achievable option for the future (RCN/BGS 2001). If a total systems approach to services for older people is to be adopted, then roles such as these, which transcend existing organizational boundaries, would appear to be essential. It seems unlikely that we will ever achieve a state where organizational boundaries do not exist; therefore, establishing roles that help older people to cross the boundaries safely and securely seems an important way forward. Some gerontological nurse specialist posts have recently been initiated in line with such a policy. How could such roles impact on the care of Jacob Brown? (See Case Study 3.4.)

CASE Jacob Brown and the gerontological nurse specialist: scenario 4

Whilst on the re-enablement ward for older people, Jacob met Natalie Smith, the gerontological nurse specialist, again. He knew her from the last time he had been in the hospital after his fall. She remembered him and was sorry to find him in hospital again. She knew he had moved to the flat last year, as she had visited his home. She explained to Jacob and Colin, his nephew, that Jacob had a chest infection and some heart failure. The doctor had talked to him already, so there had been time for him to think of some questions. The nurse spent lots of time talking about medication and looking after himself. She helped him plan his discharge with the nurses on the ward. Jacob had given himself and Colin a scare, so he decided to stay in the residential home until he had fully recovered, and then go home.

Natalie Smith has arranged for Bill Taylor to come in and visit him from the home today. She just popped in there to talk to the staff about Jacob's needs and sorted it out. Jacob still feels a bit washed out but he's on the road to recovery, so seeing Bill will be nice.

The post of gerontological nurse specialist, as it has been described (Ford and McCormack 1998, Heath and Ford 1999), would take a broad view of the older person's needs. This view would promote health and wellness, discussed below.

HEALTH PROMOTION AND WELLNESS

Kalache et al (1988) argue that the development of priorities and practices for health promotion for a nation are dependent upon the prevailing economic and cultural conditions. There are some fundamental requirements for the health of any individual, such as income, shelter and food. These need to form the basic foundation. Without them, they argue, improvement in health is merely an abstraction.

Complementary requisites are: information and knowledge about health factors, skills to promote health, supportive environments that enhance health, and the opportunity for healthier choices.

It has been suggested that healthy lifestyles for older people should encompass 'self responsibility for health, nutrition, exercise, **stress** management, interpersonal relationships/support, spiritual growth and self actualization, accident and injury prevention, safe/moderate use of medications and alcohol, smoking avoidance, self-care regimes for chronic illnesses and accessing preventative health services (Burnard and Phillipson 1991, p. 320). Balanced against this view, however, is the reality of poor housing, low income and an extensive range of social difficulties that many older people face.

The importance of health promotion is reflected by the development of Health Action Zones and Health Improvement Programmes (RCN 2000e), which aim to improve the health of communities. A whole-systems approach is suggested; this has the potential to enhance the care that is already taking place, and plan future partnerships that make the most of the available skills and resources. Joint training for all disciplines, across agencies, could raise awareness for many practitioners about the potential for joint working and the sharing of case notes and information, offering opportunities to build relationships and knowledge about one another's services, with the potential benefit of more fluid referrals between agencies for older people. Working in this way could reduce the number of practitioners an older person sees, thereby avoiding duplication of effort, whilst building more meaningful relationships for the older person.

A total population approach to the organization of services for older people recognizes that those in care homes or in receipt of long-term care services are a part of the healthcare population. Currently, people in care homes do not account for a natural component of that population, other than in considerations of medical support to care homes. A total population approach would utilize Health Improvement Plans as the basis for decision-making and would recognize the care needs of older people in care homes as part of that population. Resources would be allocated according to care need, rather than location of care delivery, using the total population approach. This reinforces the need for a standard approach to assessment. This changing focus on healthy communities aims to keep older people healthier for longer.

The postponement of chronic illness is something in which we all have interest. Fit and healthy older people not only enjoy a better individual quality of life, but have the resources to continue to participate in society.

Screening and health promotion for older people has been brought to the fore by UK government publications. The White Paper on community care (DoH 1989) lists the promotion of healthy lifestyles through education and effective health surveillance and screening as its first priority for older people and for those with a disability. Screening should be based on guidelines (RCN 1990). The RCN (1990, p. 2) chose to define screening and assessment as follows:

Screening can be defined as the process of identifying unrecognised disease or illness by application of tests, examinations and other procedures. Screening tests differentiate between apparently well people who may have a problem from those who do not. Screening is a component of the assessment process and is not in itself a means of assisting individuals to improve and maintain their health.

Health assessments give an opportunity to do more than just identify problems. Other forms of preventive activity (both medical and social) can take place.

Health assessments provide nurses with opportunities for health promotion in general and can include subjects such as exercise, smoking, prevention of accidents, preservation of autonomy, social contact and self-care. Information can also be given regarding services and resources available in the locality.

A number of preventive practices have been found to yield important benefits for older people, and have been summarized well by Gambert and Gupta (1989). Health education programmes are shifting from a focus on disease-specific conditions and individual responsibility to developing comprehensive health promotion programmes. Such programmes are aimed at the prevention of illness and injury, and the understanding of the determinants of health, such as socioenvironmental factors. More research studies, particularly longitudinal ones that evaluate the effectiveness of various programmes, are required.

Older people who wish to manage their own health may choose to do this through the use of complementary therapies. Many of the complementary therapies involve touch, and offer the older person 30–45 minutes per session in which they can discuss their health needs as they receive treatment. This may be one of the potential advantages of these therapies, although they are not currently widely available as part of NHS provision and therefore a cost may sometimes be attached to such an option. Studies are emerging that support the use of complementary therapies, such as aromatherapy, reflexology and Reiki (a form of hands-on healing) in NHS and other care settings (Brett 1999, Hudson 1996, Taylor 1995). More research is required to see how older people might benefit from these therapies in a variety of settings and situations.

For the nurse involved in health screening programmes that include people aged over 75, certain criteria must be met to ensure competence. In order to carry out such screening the nurses should therefore:

- understand the normal ageing process
- have knowledge of the social and health resources available to older people within the locality
- understand the principles of anticipatory care
- demonstrate an ability to put anticipatory care needs into practice

- recognize the need for and understand the principles of re-enablement
- undertake effective assessment procedures, particularly the assessment of ability and disability
- understand the purpose of a health check
- recognize and utilize the opportunities for health promotion
- be able to apply knowledge and expertise relating to the medical, nursing and social needs associated with old age
- have the skills pertaining to visiting older people at home, including effective communication skills
- demonstrate positive values and beliefs about older people and their needs.

The value of screening programmes for older people continues to be a subject of considerable contention (McGarry and Arthur 1999). If health checks and health promotion can help older people to achieve greater independence, then whatever the controversy regarding the 'medical' benefits of health promotion, there is likely to be a greater recognition of the rights of older people to access health screening and assessments. A case can be made for the value of paying more attention to older people's health by arguing for the broadening of the model of screening to incorporate a true health promotion approach. Nurses are in a key position to do this and as such have the potential to help older people remain active and independent for as long as possible and thereby lessen the crisis-driven, reactive, short-term approach to our ageing population.

SUMMARY

In this chapter the demographic picture has been examined in relation to older people; this has been related to current policy with an exploration of possible future care provision. Mr Jacob Brown provided an insight into issues of equity for older people, as he travelled on a care pathway that highlighted the importance of assessment and concluded with his discharge into the care of an expert nurse. Normal ageing was reviewed from a biological, physiological, psychological and sociological perspective, and the need to maintain health promotion and wellness as perspectives in the support of older people was discussed. Innovative new ways of working with older people were explored, and the gerontological nurse role was introduced.

As illustrated, ageing is a process of continued development and adaptation. It is now recognized that those who survive beyond 65 years are a highly diversified group, most of whom remain well and function independently until only a short time before death. Stereotypes about older people persist and frequently lead to efforts that prevent older people from reaching their full potential. Fortunately there is a growing body of knowledge about ageing, which is challenging such negative stereotypes. This increased social awareness and greater participation by older people themselves has helped to improve equity and access to services.

However, for the momentum to be maintained, it is necessary for older people to use their 'vote' judiciously. Health and social care professionals should endeavour to work in partnership with older people. This will assist the process of information exchange which, in turn, should empower the older individual. There is nothing disloyal about giving older patients the facts, as with the facts they can act on their own behalf.

The future for nurses working with older people is bright, as some of the most well-known innovations in nursing have been developed in services for older people (Heath and Schofield 1999). Nurses working with older people will continue to require a range of advanced and complex skills and knowledge, but these must be shared with colleagues as services for older people are increasingly provided within the community. The potential exists for the gerontological nurse specialist role to expand our knowledge about the creative ways we might develop further partnerships with older people. Policy developments look set to change the frameworks in which we support and care for older people. There is an increasing and exciting future for nurses who choose to learn the special skills that are required to work with older people.

ACKNOWLEDGEMENT

The author would like to acknowledge the work of Pauline Ford in her original work on this chapter in the previous two editions of *Watson's Clinical Nursing and Related Science*; much of her original work remains as does the work of Tina Wills.

REFERENCES

Acheson D (1998) Independent inquiry into inequalities in health. London: DoH.

Age Concern (1998) Training and qualifications for work with older people. London: Age Concern.

Age Concern (2000) Turning your back on us older people and the NHS. London: Age Concern.

Alzheimer's Society (2006) Facts about dementia. Online. Available: http://www.alzheimers.org.uk/ Facts_about_dementia/Statistics/index.htm 26 Jan 2006.

Atchley R (1980) Social forces in later life. Belmont, CA: Wadsworth.

Audit Commission (1997) The coming of age. Improving care services for older people. London: Audit Commission.

Audit Commission (2000) The way to go home: rehabilitation and remedial services for older people. London: Audit Commission.

Benner P (1984) From novice to expert. New York: Addison Wesley.

Birch R, Hancock R, LeGrys D et al (1999) Paying for age in the 21st century. The millennium papers. London: Age Concern.

Blau Z (1973) Old age in a changing society. New York: New Viewpoints.

Bond J, Coleman P (1994) Introduction to social gerontology, 2nd edn. London: Sage.

Brett H (1999) Aromatherapy in the care of older people. Nursing Times 95(33): 5–6.

British Medical Association/Royal College of Nursing (1995) The older person: consent to care. London: BMA/RCN.

Burnard M, Phillipson C (1991) Self care and health in old age. In: Redfern S, ed. Nursing elderly people, pp. 316–327. Edinburgh: Churchill Livingstone.

Cummings E, Henry W (1961) Growing old. New York: Basic Books.

Department of Health (1989) Caring for community care in the next decade and beyond, Cmnd 849. London: HMSO.

Department of Health (1990) NHS and Community Care Act. London: HMSO.

Department of Health (1995) NHS responsibilities for meeting continuing healthcare needs. HSG(95)8. London: HMSO.

Department of Health (1998) Partnership in action (new opportunities in joint working between health and social services). London: HMSO.

Department of Health (1999a) Caring about Carers. London: HMSO.

Department of Health (1999b) Fit for the future? National required standards for residential and nursing homes for older people. Consultation document. Modernising social services. London: HMSO.

Department of Health (1999c) HSC 1999/180 EX parte Coughlan; follow up action. London: HMSO.

Department of Health (2000a) The NHS plan. A plan for investment. A plan for reform. London: The Stationery Office.

Department of Health (2000b) Shaping the future of the NHS; long term planning for hospitals and related services. Consultation document on the findings of the National Beds Inquiry. London: Department of Health.

Department of Health (2001a) National service framework for older people. Modern standards and service models. London: HMSO.

Department of Health (2001b) Intermediate care. HSC 2001/01: LAC. London: HMSO

Department of Health (2005) National service framework for long term conditions. London: HMSO.

Department of Health (2006) Our health our care our say: a new direction for community services. London: HMSO.

Department of Health/Social Services Inspectorate (1995) Carer's Recognition and Services Act. London: HMSO.

Department of Health, Social Services and Personal Safety (2005) A healthier future: a twenty year vision for health and wellbeing in Northern Ireland 2005–2025. Belfast: Department of Health, Social Services and Personal Safety.

Dudley N, Burns E (1992) The influence of age on policies for admission and thrombolysis in coronary care units in the UK. Age and Ageing 21: 95–98.

Ebersole P, Hess P (1990) Towards healthy ageing, 3rd edn. St Louis: CV Mosby.

Erikson E (1964) Child and society. New York: Norton.

Essink-Bot M, Pereira J, Packer C et al (2002) Cross-national comparability of burden of disease estimates: the European disability weights project. Bulletin of the World Health Organization 80(8): 644–652.

Estes C (1979) The ageing enterprise. San Francisco: Jossy Bass.

Evandrou M (1992) Changing the invisibility of carers; mapping informal care nationally. In: Laczko F, Victors C, eds. Social policy and older people. Aldershot, UK: Avebury, p 142–158.

Evans S, Means R (2005) Single assessment for older people: new dawn or continued confusion? Nursing Older People 17(2): 16–19.

Fennell G, Phillipson C, Eves H (1988) The sociology of old age. Milton Keynes: Open University Press.

Ford P (1989) Reactions to Griffiths (implications for care of the elderly). Nursing Standard 29: 19–20.

Ford P, McCormack B (1998) Gerontological nurses specialist conference paper. Third European Nursing Older People Conference, Harrogate, UK, 1998. Ludlow: Lang & Bussion.

Ford P, McCormack B (1999) Determining older people's need for registered nursing and continuing health care: the contribution of the Royal College of Nursing's assessment tool. Journal of Clinical Nursing 8: 731–742.

Ford P, McCormack B (2000) Keeping the person in the centre of nursing. Nursing Standard 14(46): 40–44.

Fries J (1989) Ageing well: a guide for successful seniors. Reading: Addison Wesley.

Gambert S, Gupta K (1989) Preventive care: what it's worth in geriatrics. Geriatrics 44: 61.

Gioiella EC, Bevil CW (1985) Nursing care of the aging client: promoting healthy adaptation. Norwalk CT: Appleton Century Crofts.

Grahame-Smith DG, Aronson JK (2002) Oxford textbook of clinical pharmacology and drug therapy. Oxford: Oxford University Press.

Grimley Evans J (1997) Rationing health care by age. The case against. British Medical Journal 314: 822–825.

Grundy E (1994) Live old, live well. MRC News 64: 22.

Harris D (1990) Sociology of ageing, 2nd edn. New York: Harper & Row.

Haskey J (1995) Trends in marriage and cohabitation: the decline in marriage and the changing patterns of living in partnerships. Population Trends 80: 5–15.

Health Advisory Service (2000) Not because they are old; an independent inquiry into the care of older people on acute wards in general hospitals. London: HAS.

Heath H (1993) Ageism: spell out the facts. Elderly Care 5(3): 34.

Heath H (2000) Assessing older people. Elderly Care 11(10): 27.

Heath H (2006) Older people in primary care. Primary Health Care 16(3): 18–20.

Heath H, Ford P (1999) The development of nursing with older people. In: Heath H, Schofield I, eds. Healthy ageing; nursing older people. London: Mosby, p 516–517.

Heath H, Schofield I, eds (1999) Healthy ageing; nursing older people. London: Mosby.

Help the Aged (1997) A life worth living. The independence and inclusion of older people. London: Help the Aged.

Henwood M (1999) The future health and care of older people: the best is yet to come. The millennium papers. Debate of the age. London: Age Concern.

Hockey J, James A (1993) Growing up and growing old. Ageing and dependency in the life course. London: Sage.

House of Commons Hansard (2003) Written answers 3 March col841W Crown Copyright

Hudson R (1996) The value of lavender for rest and activity in the elderly patient. Complementary Therapies in Medicine 4: 52–57.

Jeffreys M (1989) Growing old in the twentieth century. London: Routledge.

Johnson M (1997) The meaning of older age. In: Norman I, Redfern S, eds. Mental health care for elderly people. Edinburgh: Churchill Livingstone, p 308–314.

Jones H (1994) Health and society in twentieth century Britain. London: Longman.

Kalache A, Warnes A, Hunter D (1988) Promoting health among elderly people: a statement from a working group. London: King Edward's Hospital Fund for London.

Kitwood T (1997) Dementia reconsidered – the person comes first. Buckingham: Open University Press.

Kyriazis M (1994) Age and reason; theory of ageing, ageing mechanisms. Nursing Times 90(18): 60–62.

Lewis H, Wistow G, Arbott S et al (1999) Continuing health care; the local development of policies and eligibility criteria. Health and Social Care in the Community 7(6): 455–463.

Loux A, Kerrison S, Pollock AM (2000) Long term care; social care or health care? (editorial) British Medical Journal 320: 5–6.

Mallick N (1994) End stage renal failure. In: Tunbridge M, ed. Rationing in health care in medicine. London: Royal College of Physicians, p 14–20.

Markides K, Cooper C (1987) Ageing and ethnicity. California: Sage.

McGarry J, Arthur A (1999) Can over-75 health checks identify unmet need? Nursing Standard 13(33): 37–42.

Moore J, Tilson B, Whitting G (1994) An international overview of employment policies and practices towards older workers. Research series no. 29. London: Department of Employment.

Murphy M, Grundy E (2003) Mothers with children living and children with living mothers: the role of fertility and mortality in the period 1911–2050. Online. Available: http://www.statistics.gov.uk/articles/population_trends/fertility mortality_pt112.pdf 26 Jan 2006.

Neno R (2004) Spouse caregivers and the support they receive: a literature review. Nursing Older People 16(5): 14–15.

Neno R (2005) Intermediate care: policy rhetoric or an effective strategy? A review of the literature. Nursing Older People 17(3): 16–19.

NHS Executive (2000) Advocacy: a code of practice. Mental Health Task Force User Group. London: DoH.

Nocon A, Baldwin S (1998) Trends in the rehabilitation policy. A review of the literature. London: King's Fund.

Office of National Statistics (2004) General household survey trends in self reported sickness by sex and age. National Statistics Crown Copyright

Office of Population Censuses and Surveys (2005a) Ageing. Online. Available: http://www.statistics.gov.uk/ 17 March 2006.

Office of Population Censuses and Surveys (2005b) Health and well being. Online. Available: http://www.statistics.gov.uk/ 17 March 2006.

Office of Population Censuses and Surveys (2005c) Health and social care. Online. Available: http://www.statistics.gov.uk/ 17 March 2006.

Office of Population Censuses and Surveys (2005d) Health and social care. Online. Available: http://www.statistics.gov.uk/ 17 March 2006.

Office of Population Censuses and Surveys (2006) Health status higher social groups report best health. Online. Available: http://www.statistics.gov.uk/CCI/nugget.asp?ID=916&Pos=1&C olRank=2&Rank=320 25 Jan 2006.

Phillipson C (1997) Employment and training: planning for 2020 and beyond. In: Erandou M, ed. Baby boomers ageing in the 21st century. London: Age Concern, p 41–42.

Phillipson C, Walker A (1986) Ageing and social policy, a critical assessment. London: Gower.

Royal College of Nursing (1990) Guidelines for assessment of elderly people. London: RCN.

Royal College of Nursing (1997a) Assessment tool for nursing older people. London: RCN.

Royal College of Nursing (1997b) Nursing homes, nursing values. London: RCN.

Royal College of Nursing (2000a) Rationing by stealth. A review of the legality of health authorities' continuing care policies in England and Wales. London: RCN.

Royal College of Nursing (2000b) Nursing assessment with older people: a person centred approach. Oxford: RCN Institute.

Royal College of Nursing (2000c) Rehabilitating older people. The role of the nurse. London: RCN.

Royal College of Nursing (2000d) Internal briefing paper prepared by P Ford and B McCormack. London: RCN.

Royal College of Nursing (2000e) Internal paper. Recommendations for NHS modernisation plan, with regard to the needs of older people. Gerontological nursing programme. London: RCN.

Royal College of Nursing and the British Geriatrics Society (2001) Older people's specialist nurse, a joint statement by the RCN and BGS. London: BGS/RCN.

Royal Commission on Long Term Care for the Elderly (1999) With respect to old age. London: HMSO.

Russel L (1999) The future of the built environment. The millennium papers. Debate of the age. London: Age Concern.

Schofield I (1994) An historical approach to care. Elderly Care 6(6): 14–15.

Scottish Executive (2005) Delivering for Health. Edinburgh: Scottish Executive

Seidel HM, Ball JW, Dains JE et al (1999) Mosby's Guide to Physical Examination, 3rd edn. St Louis: Mosby.

Stewart K, Challis D, Carpenter I et al (1999) Assessment approaches for older people receiving social care; content and coverage. International Journal of Geriatric Psychiatry 14: 147–156.

Stokes G (1992) On being old; the psychology of later life. London: Falmer Press.

Sugarman L (1986) Life span development: concepts, theories and interventions. London: Methuen.

Taylor A (1995) Back in touch. Nursing Times 91(26): 18.

Taylor C, Lillis C, Lemone P (1989) The fundamentals of nursing: the art and science of nursing care. Philadelphia: JB Lippincott.

Tinker A (1984) The elderly in modern society. London: Longman Press.

Townsend P (1979) Poverty in the United Kingdom: a survey of household resources and standards of living. Harmondsworth, UK: Penguin.

Townsend P (1981) The structured dependency of the elderly: creation of social policy in the twentieth century. Ageing and Society 1: 5.

UKCC (1997) The continuing care of older people. UKCC Policy Paper 1. London: UKCC.

Wales Assembly Government (2003) Strategy for older people in Wales. Cardiff: Wales Assembly Government.

Warren MD (1981) The need for rehabilitation. In: Mattingley S, ed. Rehabilitation today in Great Britain, 2nd edn. London: Update Books.

Warner M, Longley M, Gould E (1999) Healthcare futures 2010. Welsh Institute for Health and Social Care. London: UKCC.

Williams A (1997) Rationing health care by age, the case for it. British Medical Journal 314: 820–822.

Wills T, Ford P (2001) Assessing older people – contemporary issues for nursing. Nursing Older People 12(9): 16–20.

WHO 1998

World Health Organization (2004) Health core indicators. Online. Available: http://www.who.int/whosis/core/core_select_process.cfm 27 Jul 2006.

Yates A (1998) Social responsibility; an issue of age. In: Marr J, Kershaw B, eds. Caring for older people. Developing specialist practice. London: Arnold, p 222–234.

Yurick A, Spier B, Ebert N (1988) The aged person and the nursing process, 3rd edn. Norwalk, CT: Appleton & Lange.

FURTHER READING

For further information about the sociological changes that have occurred and have impacted on older people, including the older person's voice:

Evandrou M, ed. (1997) Baby boomers, ageing in the 21st century. London: Age Concern.

Johnson J, Slater R, eds (1993) Ageing and later life. London: Sage.

Phillipson C (1998) Reconstructing old age. New agendas in social theory and practice. London: Sage.

For recent policy developments for older people:

Department of Health (2001) National service framework for older people. Modern standards and service models. London: HMSO.

For an extensive background to person-centred ways of working with and assessing older people:

Heath H, Schofield I (1999) Healthy ageing, nursing older people. London: Mosby.

Royal College of Nursing (2000) Nursing assessment with older people: a person centred approach. Oxford: RCN Institute.

Wills T, Ford P (2001) Assessing older people – contemporary issues for nursing. Nursing Older People 12(9): 16–20.

For further information about normal ageing:

Audit Commission (1999) Forget me not: mental health services for older people. London: Audit Commission.

Bond J, Coleman P (1994) Introduction to social gerontology, 2nd edn. London: Sage.

Cummings E, Henry W (1961) Growing old. New York: Basic Books.

Ebersole P, Hess P (1990) Towards healthy ageing, 3rd edn. St Louis: CV Mosby.

Erikson E (1964) Child and society. New York: Norton.

Estes C (1979) The ageing enterprise. San Francisco, CA: Jossy Bass.

Fennell G, Phillipson C, Evers H (1988) The sociology of old age. Milton Keynes: Open University Press.

Hockey J, James A (1993) Growing up and growing old. Ageing and dependency in the life course. London: Sage.

Kyriazis M (1994) Age and reason, theory of ageing, ageing mechanisms. Nursing Times 90(18): 60–62.

Markides K, Cooper C (1987) Ageing and ethnicity. Thousand Oaks, CA: Sage.

Phillipson C, Walker A (1986) Ageing and social policy, a critical assessment. London: Gower.

Sugarman L (1986) Life span development, concepts, theories and interventions. London: Methuen.

Townsend P (1979) Poverty in the United Kingdom, a survey of household resources and standards of living. Harmondsworth: Penguin.

Townsend P (1981) The structured dependency of the elderly: creation of social policy in the twentieth century. Ageing and Society 1: 5.

Williams R, Tibbitts C, Donahue W, eds (1963) Processes of ageing. New York: Atherton.

USEFUL WEBSITES

Age Concern
http://www.ageconcern.org.uk/
Help the Aged
http://www.helptheaged.org.uk/default.htm
The Practitioner Network on Ageing
http://www.pnoa.co.uk

Death, grief and loss

Alison Crumbie

INTRODUCTION

… dying involves more than a body becoming dead. Dying is a psychological and social phenomenon as much as a physical one. It involves the relationships and behaviours of others toward the dying person as a dying person. It is like an intricate dance in which friends, associates, caregivers and dying persons learn to play their parts.

(Cassell 2004. p. 257)

In your work as a nurse you will have the privilege of being intimately involved with people at some of the most important moments of their lives. The act of dying is one of those moments and yet it is commonplace in our society to hide from death; we do not talk about it openly and those people who do share their thoughts about it (often older people) are thought of as being morbid. Nurses encounter death and dying repeatedly and because of this, people often look to us to know how to act and respond at these times. The skilled actions of nurses in these situations is often a product of past experiences and familiarity with the normality of this intensely emotional and painful event. Now, as the educational opportunities relating to care of dying people grow, nurses' actions are also based on knowledge of the grieving process for the dying person and his or her significant others, and an understanding of death and loss. This chapter aims to provide you with an introduction to some of the major theories relating to grieving, death and loss and will also invite you to consider your own responses to the grieving process.

The experience of loss, and the grieving that is associated with it, can be experienced in a number of situations which include not only death and dying but also: the loss of a limb, the loss of one's sight, the loss of a job and the status that goes with it, the loss of a driving licence and all that that

symbolizes. The expression of grief is a universal response by which people adapt to a significant loss – the loss of something that was theirs, a valued possession that had special meaning. The most traumatic loss is that of a significant person (i.e. a person with whom an individual has had an important relationship, one that had special meaning) through death, separation, divorce or distance.

Grief can also result from loss of a pet – through disappearance, separation or death – and loss of objects due to burglary or fire. Objects can be replaced but the feelings attached to them cannot. Objects have sentimental value because they are associated with a particular moment in time. People can experience loss when they move house too – the loss of leaving a place that is familiar and the scene of special memories. Another kind of loss is that associated with human development and life's milestones. This can include loss of opportunity to be a mother or, in older people, loss of strength or physical well-being.

Previous experiences of loss may provide people with the ability to cope with a new loss. This means that what is a loss to one person may not be a loss to another. Emotional and physical well-being also gives people greater resources to handle losses. Nurses meet people who have varied emotional and physical resources for handling their loss and varying levels of social support. Family attitudes to loss, and different cultural, ethnic and religious backgrounds, will influence the way people deal with loss or death. A number of issues may all interfere with what is regarded as the 'normal' grieving process and this might result in a person experiencing an abnormal or a pathological response to loss.

Although most people would view loss through death as the most significant loss, this chapter looks at all areas of loss and grief. Nurses spend a lot of time helping clients come to terms with many different losses and at these times it is important and valuable to have a sound knowledge base from which to provide support for the grieving person and their significant others.

Philosophers and scientists have attempted to understand and even control death. Indeed, Western medicine could be construed as being solely focused on the preservation of life and the denial of death. We create heroes out of the celebrities who cheat death and survive cancer against all the odds and, with the exception of the hospice movement and some critical care units, we rarely embrace death as an important process that can be skillfully managed. Unfortunately, even today, patients and their families are left to get on with the dying process with little support from healthcare professionals. It has been reported that approximately 50% of people who contacted a regional bereavement support group did so because they had feelings of anxiety and anger relating to the care they received from hospital staff at the time of the death (Wiseman 1992). Anxiety and anger are emotions that are completely normal in the grieving process; nonetheless, the fact that the source of those reactions in Wiseman's study were healthcare personnel, including nurses, is a concern. We need to learn more about the grieving process so that we can provide patients and their families with the most appropriate and skillful support possible at their time of need. And at that time we need to be sensitive, flexible and self aware so that we can be alert to signs of abnormal grieving, remain alert to situations which might lead to potential problems in the future and be in touch with our own emotions so that we might seek help if we ourselves are experiencing difficulty.

The fact that everyone must face their own death as well as the death of others not only creates anxiety but also gives meaning to life. A person's thoughts about death will affect the way he or she lives. These thoughts can be threatening, painful or inspirational and give deeper meaning to a relationship. It is essential that you, as a nurse, examine your own thoughts and feelings on these difficult issues in order to help others cope with them. This chapter confronts you with some of the more painful and difficult areas of life. If you are to be an effective nurse it is important that you explore these uncomfortable thoughts and continue to work on them throughout your career.

Loss, separation and dying are very personal, individual experiences. This chapter offers some guidelines for sharing with, understanding and caring for people who are encountering these experiences. As a nurse you may feel you are intruding into someone's most private moments, but the very nature of your work means it is almost impossible to avoid such intimacy. The understanding you gain from working through the issues of loss and grief will help you to value and respect the individual needs and beliefs of your patients, as well as giving you an insight into what you can actually do to help.

Working as we do in the area of health care, we are frequently in close contact with people who face or experience loss. Occasionally we will become involved with someone who does not even know the patient but suddenly becomes involved in the patient's life; for example, the driver who fatally injures someone or the pedestrian who witnesses an horrific accident. In these examples nurses will be dealing with distress that is acute and immediate and in other settings (e.g. the community) the problems of grieving and loss may be less obvious and more insidious. In either setting the skills of the nurse need to be adapted to the particular needs of the individual and this requires knowledge, understanding and sensitivity.

As we look at death, grief and loss, and its effects upon individuals, some of the losses will be actual losses, others will involve the threat of a loss and all the ensuing fear associated with major life transitions. This is termed 'anticipatory grieving' and we will explore this later in the chapter.

Much of our time as nurses will be spent caring for people who are physically ill. Studies have demonstrated how death, grief and loss produce many physical symptoms (Stuart and Laraia 1998) because of all the associated anxiety. Therefore, it is important, when we take a patient's history of important life events, to identify episodes of death, grief and loss which are part of any evaluation of what may be contributing factors to the illness. Dysfunctional grieving may be a major contributing factor. Parkes (1996) showed that people who are bereaved are twice as likely to become ill as the rest of the population.

Experience of loss and normal grieving are universal and are accompanied by psychological and physical reactions. Normal grieving is the process by which we adapt to loss (Worden 1993), and it is important that we help individuals to grieve as this will be the means by which the pain of the loss is healed. The experience of loss applies to something or someone that was owned in some way, and which was valuable or meaningful. We will consider some of the theories on the process and stages of grief, how anticipatory grief may occur before the actual loss, and how dysfunctional grieving can result in serious psychological distress or illness.

NORMAL GRIEVING

Normal grief is also known as uncomplicated grief. It describes a range of feelings and behaviours commonly seen and experienced after a loss. Worden (1993) states that one way of conceptualizing normal grieving behaviour is the frequency with which that behaviour is found among a bereaved population. The more a behaviour or feeling is observed, the more it is defined as normal.

Freud (1917) described how the normal grieving process is triggered by a significant loss, and that it is a process to be expected. He went on to say that a person experiencing normal grieving loses the capacity to give attention to others, to engage in a meaningful attachment whilst the pain of the loss is consuming them. The loss takes away the ability to focus on normal everyday activities. Even as long ago as 1917, when Freud began writing about this, he indicated that it would be a period of 1–3 years before a satisfactory resolution of the difficulty would be achieved.

Another early attempt to look at normal grief reactions was the work of Eric Lindemann. He wrote his classic paper after extensive work with the relatives of victims of the Coconut Grove night club fire in which 500 people lost their lives (Lindemann 1944). From Lindemann's observations of 101 people, he described repetitive patterns in the characteristics of acute grief. These are listed in Box 4.1.

Lindemann's much-quoted study has some limitations. Parkes (1972) criticized the lack of information in Lindemann's work about how much time elapsed between the death and the interview. Despite this criticism, much of the behaviour and many of the feelings outlined by Lindemann are apparent in interactions with patients in everyday practice. Kent and McDowell (2004) brought together a number of the major works on grieving and created a list of the many and varied psychological, physical and behavioural manifestations of grief (Box 4.2). It is clear that Kent and McDowell's more recent work is congruent with Lindemann's work and

that the observations made in 1944 still have a resonance with the grief reaction today.

Bowlby (1980) described normal grieving as resulting from the loss of others, of part of self or of objects. Box 4.3 shows his description of the three phases of response to loss. In the first phase, expression of anger, denial, shock and disbelief will be underlined by periods of yearning or longing for the deceased. Crying, searching to recover the loss, and appeals for help may run alongside sleep disturbances and changes in appetite. The second phase of disorganization is described as being driven by despair and depression. This will often result in social isolation because of the withdrawal and/or regression, with psychomotor retardation. The third phase, reorganization, describes a disengagement from the attachment, a development of new interests and attachments, and a restructuring of lifestyle. This should return the individual to a level of functioning experienced before the loss, although life will be different.

Kubler-Ross (1969) described five stages of grief in the dying patient (Box 4.4), and also suggested that this process is also experienced in those close to the dying patient. The first stage is denial and this is said to offer an opportunity to deal with the shock and disbelief in the short term, whilst organizing more effective defensive strategies. The use of denial has often been viewed negatively, but Davidhizar and Newman-Eiger (1998) emphasize that nurses need to appreciate the importance of denial. They indicate that it may be the only psychologically safe way of coping with the unimaginable. Some factors reduce the need for denials; for example, how much time remains to ground the eventual death in reality, and the way the information is given, will influence the extent to which individuals remain with the denial. The second stage is anger and this may well be expressed in some form of protest: 'Why me?' 'Why now?'.

Box 4.1   Lindemann's characteristics of the bereaved

- Somatic or bodily distress
- Preoccupation with the image of the deceased
- Guilt relating to the deceased
- Hostile reactions
- Inability to function as before the loss
- Developing traits of the deceased in their own behaviour

Box 4.2   Manifestations of grief

Psychological reactions	Physical reactions
Anger	Anorexia
Anxiety	Change in weight
Apathy	Chest pain
Denial	Fatigue
Depression	Gastrointestinal disorders
Disbelief	Hair loss
Emotional lability	Headache
Guilt	Immunodeficiency
Hallucinations of the deceased's presence (visual or auditory)	Trouble initiating and …maintaining sleep
Helplessness	**Behavioural reactions**
Impaired concentration	Agitation
Irritability	Crying
Lowered self esteem	Fatigue
Numbness	Social withdrawal
Sadness	
Searching for the deceased	

(Kent and McDowell 2004 with permission)

Box 4.3   Bowlby's three phases of response to loss

1 Protest

2 Disorganization

3 Reorganization.

Box 4.4   Kubler-Ross's five stages of grief in the dying patient

1 Denial and isolation

2 Anger

3 Bargaining

4 Depression

5 Acceptance

Resentment and expressions about injustice may quickly be verbalized, and may be projected on to others – perhaps the nurses. Nurses may find this difficult to tolerate, and may take it personally.

The bargaining stage is said to be about trying to postpone the death. Some kind of agreement or deadline will be offered, to prevent or postpone the inevitable. In the depression stage the inevitable can no longer be denied or displaced elsewhere. The reality is recognized, producing some apparent sadness and a resignation that the course of events cannot be prevented. At this time you may witness withdrawal, silence and perhaps helplessness. This is said to be part of the anticipatory grief process in the preparation for the death. Finally, in acceptance, energy to prevent the inevitable death is no longer needed. Contemplation of the death, and giving up the struggle, should indicate that the individual is more relaxed or, as often described, peaceful. This stage is thought to make the pain less acute, as emotional distress is thought to exacerbate the intensity of pain (Dossey 1994). The five-stage model of grief was developed from Kubler-Ross' work with dying patients and it has been used as a means of understanding the ways in which people cope with dying (Dunne 2004). It should not be seen as a linear model or a recipe that each person experiencing grief with have to follow, rather it should be viewed as a dynamic process with individuals moving back and forth through the stages, sometimes possibly missing a stage altogether. The model has its use in providing a framework to aid understanding and to help people realize that what they are experiencing is normal and to be expected.

Kubler-Ross (1969), Bowlby (1980), Lindemann (1944) and Freud (1917) have all contributed to the idea that there is a normality to the grieving process. There are a number of manifestations which are common and reasonable responses to loss and there are identifiable phases and stages that a person may move through. Parkes (1996) also made a major contribution to the study of grief by identifying the determinants that influence the whole grieving process (Box 4.5). These six determinants or predictors of grief are the circumstances surrounding a death that will influence the outcome or resolution; they identify the difficulties that people may need to address so they can begin to process the grief.

Box 4.5   Parkes' six determinants of grief

- Mode of death
- Nature of the attachment
- Who was the person?
- Historical antecedents
- Personality variables
- Social variables

MODE OF DEATH

If the death was from an illness, even if it was sudden, it is likely to cause fewer problems than traumatic death. In many instances death from an illness allows the patient and their family to plan ahead and to have addressed a number of difficulties before the event of the death. In contrast, death by injury can be sudden and unexpected, it may cause physical damage to the body, and is more likely to be perceived as an injustice by the family. In traumatic death most people will ask whether the deceased suffered or knew anything about the process or act of dying. Much time and effort will be needed to explore the issues around this.

Death by road traffic accident, or accident at work or at home, can cause anger and a sense of injustice far greater than natural sudden death. Things are even worse when monetary compensation is an issue: this usually always falls short in that it somehow devalues the deceased. The verdict of the coroner's court or the finding of a Fatal Accident Enquiry is often discussed at length, as is the question of whether the deceased is entirely blameless in relation to his or her own death. If the deceased was not to blame, some thing or some person is usually felt to be responsible. The area of responsibility may be even wider: if a person or organization was not to blame then the whole of society may be blamed. In some extremes, civilization or humankind is blamed and the bereaved person may isolate him or herself from society, resulting in an even greater sense of loss.

The place where the death occurred becomes an integral part of the grief. Was the deceased on home ground, or in a strange place? The pain can be exacerbated if she or he was far away from home and alone during death. The fact that many families are now scattered throughout the world presents an added dimension to grief. This is particularly difficult if friends and neighbours of the remaining family did not know the deceased. The nurses, friends and neighbours may be at a disadvantage in having no sense of who the person was and it can therefore reduce their ability to understand and empathize.

One mode of death that produces some tremendous difficulties is suicide. The process of grieving becomes very complicated both emotionally and intellectually. The bereaved are not only sorting out their own loss but speculating about how the victim might have emerged from the difficulty had she or he remained alive. They may come up with actions that may have prevented the suicide, and this holds the potential for profound feelings of guilt.

NATURE OF THE ATTACHMENT

The grieving person will have had a unique and complex relationship with the person who is deceased. The nature of their relationship, in addition to the mode of death, will have an impact on the grieving process. The strengths of the relationship, and the security or aspects of safety gained from the relationship, are useful areas to explore. One feeling that may occur in crisis involving death is ambivalence, and this can give rise to heartache and soul searching. The difficulty lies in the strong sense that this feeling is inappropriate in grief and the grieving person needs to be given time to express their concerns and guilt relating to this reaction.

WHO WAS THE PERSON?

Who the deceased was in relation to the client must be ascertained. The deceased's position in the hierarchy of the family is not necessarily a clue to the enormity of the loss, and we must not make assumptions. Families are made up of an enormously complex web of relationships. You might find yourself comforting the lover of the deceased who was unknown to the rest of the family; you might find yourself making assumptions about the relationship between husband and wife when in fact they had been estranged for many years, or you might find yourself supporting the same sex partner of the deceased who had never been accepted by the rest of the family. The important lesson here is not to make any assumptions, allow the grieving person to express their feelings and concerns, and let them tell you their story so that you might start to appreciate and understand their loss.

HISTORICAL ANTECEDENTS

A previous life crisis, particularly a sudden death, will present as a major factor in coping. If I have experienced a previous life crisis with a good or reasonable outcome, then in theory this should help me. I will have programmed into my head something that identifies difficulty but removes or diminishes some fear about the outcome. This may be useful, provided I can get in touch with the previous experience. However, if the previous outcome was one of pain and suffering, the present problems are compounded. Previously unresolved loss, or failure to confront loss, may result in its re-emergence, causing difficulty for the helper in establishing the focus of the loss.

Other recent life changes, crisis or recent depressive illness will result in more difficulty in handling the loss. Energy and resources used up in tackling these will have left the person drained or depleted of resources.

PERSONALITY VARIABLES

Positive coping with the immediate grief does not guarantee a lack of long-term problems. Someone who has a personality that allows self-actualization, a feeling of some control over one's own life, and sees problems as a challenge seems to be most likely to recover. Raphael (1984) writes that, although no specific risk factors have been demonstrated, certain personal characteristics may carry a risk of poor outcome. These include ambivalence and dependent or clinging relationships. Earlier personal experience of grief, especially childhood loss of parents, contributes to vulnerability. The key factors influencing outcome appear to be personality in combination with the pre-existing relationship of dependence.

SOCIAL VARIABLES

Some loss alienates and isolates, whereas other loss produces gain. There is a shifting of relationships and the bereaved person may welcome this change or, conversely, may mourn the loss of connections with people who relied on the presence of the now deceased person.

Some religions and cultures will support the bereaved, showering them with offers of help. People who are grieving are known to lose their appetite and subsequently lose weight and therefore people surrounding the bereaved person often bring gifts of food and offer their support in making sure the person is eating adequately (Neuberger 2004). In the UK there are diverse examples of community response to death; clear confrontation of it or avoidance may be apparent. Whilst members of a religious community are assumed to be a help and support in sudden death, the bereaved may feel otherwise. The grieving person may wish to be left alone and may not welcome the intrusion of the well-meaning religious community; others may welcome the distraction and may appreciate the opportunity to talk about the deceased, however painful that might be.

Wright (1996) highlights how the six determinants (Box 4.5) will give some indication of who is likely to need some help and support through the whole process of grief. Very early in the process (even before the death has occurred) major negative determinants may indicate who is at risk from dysfunctional grieving.

ANTICIPATORY GRIEVING

Lindemann (1944) first used the term 'anticipatory grief' when he described the reactions of relatives who were in the armed forces. The relatives had gone through a grieving process because their loved ones were in situations where they were highly likely to lose their lives. When they returned from their time on the front line, the families had often already gone through the grieving process and, in some cases, had even achieved a sense of resolution causing enormous difficulty for the subsequent relationship on their return. Anticipatory grieving is said to combine the beginning and the actual process of grieving, and takes place when anticipating a significant loss before the loss actually takes place. This significant loss can refer to the potential death of a significant person who is facing a terminal illness, or the potential loss of a body part where some surgery is to take place. One's own impending death, or moving away from one's permanent place, can fall into this category of grieving (Clayton et al 1973). People experiencing anticipatory grief exhibit similar feelings and behaviour as those found in normal grieving. There is great value in being alert to anticipatory grief as it provides an opportunity for intervention and support from the nurse (Kubler-Ross 1969). The use of Parkes' (1996) determinants of grief can assist in identifying the potential for abnormal or dysfunctional grieving, allowing the nurse to work with the patient

and his or her family to avoid unnecessary suffering and pain in the long term.

Anticipatory grieving is difficult to define clearly (Dunne 2004), nonetheless a number of studies have explored this phenomenon and have concluded that: the period immediately before death allows adaptation to begin (Costello 1999) and that there are common dimensions among people who are anticipating the death of a loved one, such as anger, despair, anxiety and distress (Chapman and Pepler 1998). The hospice movement has acknowledged this process and has worked to minimize the suffering of the patient and the significant others by addressing their specific needs at the time leading up to death. Neuberger (2004) states that those who are dying or are about to be bereaved need reassurance, and need to understand that what they are experiencing, albeit horribly painful, is an entirely normal human process. Nurses have an enormously important role to play at this time in people's lives and with skillful judgment and sensitive actions and words they can anticipate problems and relieve some of the suffering of those experiencing death.

LIFE TRANSITIONS WITH A CAPACITY FOR GRIEF

Other life changes or transitions can result in a loss, and may even result in a life crisis (Caplan 1964). The work of crisis intervention is underpinned by Caplan's theories and studies, which acknowledge Erikson's 1950 model of developmental (maturational) and situational (accidental) crisis (Box 4.6).

Caplan described developmental crisis as transitional periods in personality development, characterized by disturbances in affective and cognitive functioning. A sudden unexpected threat to, or loss of, basic resources or life goals constitutes a situational crisis. Situational crises can lead to intensive periods of psychological, behavioural and physical disarray. Caplan observed that situational crises are often new to the client and that their usual coping methods do not work.

Some crises may be compounded by fitting into both categories. A 20-year-old woman, for example, may suffer the death of her husband in a road traffic accident within a month of her marriage. We cannot treat her loss, and the emotionally painful experience of the loss, without discussing the distress of this happening within a month of her marriage.

Whilst this example identifies clearly the two types of crisis, others may not be so easily identified. We need to be aware of where the client is on the developmental scale (life's milestones) in order to appreciate fully the implications of a sudden death. Placing a client's experience of loss on his life milestone graph (Box 4.7), noting the stage she or he is now at or may be heading towards or leaving, is a useful exercise. Further discussion with clients about their perception of their life situation may alter assumptions we have made about them.

Some situational crises, such as redundancy, divorce or separation, produce a loss of status and security. Again, if these are marked along the line of life's developmental crises, their overwhelming nature may be perceived. Caplan (1964) says that even individuals with relatively stable personalities can change in unexpected ways during such a crisis.

The change needed to deal with crisis may have positive aspects, highlighting the opportunities that crisis can bring. On the other hand, the crisis can result in an increased inability to cope, and lead to feelings of chaos and disorder. This leads to the view that a crisis is a transitional period offering the individual an opportunity for growth or increasing their vulnerability.

Time is another aspect to consider. A crisis cannot be tolerated for a long period because it involves intense feelings of distress and disorder which have the capacity to damage. Nurses not only have to respond quickly but also frequent and lengthy periods of care will be necessary to prevent damage and restore equilibrium. Caplan (1964) viewed crisis intervention as a major part of preventive psychiatry. He believed that individuals could be supported and offered the right conditions to deal effectively with crisis, thereby preventing mental disorder. This chapter aims to explore mechanisms for helping the patient and others use the process of grief to deal with the loss in the long term. Crisis intervention

Box 4.6 Erikson's model of developmental and situational crises	
Situational	**Developmental**
(accidental)	(maturational)
Sudden illness	Birth
Accident	Puberty and adolescence
Redundancy	Courtship
Loss of income	Marriage
Loss of status	Pregnancy
Loss of security	Menopause
Divorce or separation	Death

Box 4.7 Examples of life's milestones

- Birth
- Puberty
- Adolescence
- Courtship
- Marriage
- Pregnancy
- Children leaving home
- Midlife crisis
- Retirement
- Death

helps them to begin this process, and offers the nurse a framework to use in assisting them.

Rogers and Reich (1988) recognized the importance of reassuring and affirming a person's feelings – from the moment of impact through ongoing support – in healing the grief. The crisis model shown in Figure 4.1 provides a useful framework for intervention, identifying three routes to explore when dealing with the crisis of sudden death.

SUDDEN DEATH

When a death is sudden, it can be difficult to ground the event in reality because it was unexpected and therefore there has been no preparation for it. At this time the three factors identified in the crisis model (perception of the event, external resources and internal resources) become even more important in helping the bereaved to deal with the loss.

PERCEPTION OF THE EVENT

It is important to explore if the bereaved person understands what has happened. A realistic appraisal of the event and what led up to the death is valuable in helping the client to ground the death in reality. Information will help this process as well as checking the client's understanding of what happened. The opportunity to see or be with the deceased will further confirm the client's perception of the reality. This can be a challenge when the deceased's body is disfigured through injury but it seems, on the whole, that relatives value the opportunity to view the body and often the sight is less horrific than they anticipated.

EXTERNAL RESOURCES

The external resources available to help the client cope with this event are the second factor to work with. The disordered activity resulting from the impact of the event often makes it difficult for the client to think logically about sources of strength, comfort and support, and may actually prevent the client accessing them. The first resources to explore are usually family and friends, or other people close to or on intimate terms with the client. The person in crisis knows his or her need of them, but the disarray and distress produce fear that they will not be reached. This may be expressed clearly as: 'Please help me find my brother. He will help me, he will know what to do'. This expectation of the help to be received may well be unrealistic initially, but as time progresses – and this will help – more order will

replace disorder. The external resources may also include other disciplines, caring agencies and organizations or self-help groups. It is important to be aware of local resources and the types of help available.

INNER RESOURCES

The client may be able to access inner resources in coping with the crisis, and should be helped to realize strengths and vulnerabilities. The overwhelming feeling at a time of crisis is that any forward movement is impossible; the client is rendered impotent and this increases distress. The fear produced by being immobilized is tremendously powerful; it can make one feel totally weak or lead to panic. Acknowledging inner strengths and feelings can result in activity and forward movement, enhancing potency or effectiveness. This feels positive and suggests some advance towards management of the problem. It is important for clients' self-esteem that they can ask 'What can I do about this?' and begin to look at answers and alternatives for themselves.

If we can help the client to look at and work positively with these three aspects of coping with a stressful event – perception of the event, external resources and inner resources – a crisis may be averted. Perception of the event will have strong negative content if there is denial of the meaning or the reality of the situation. Negative responses will also arise if external resources are poor or not available. The client's inability to access strengths, resources or insights within him or herself will make exploration of the third area a non-productive exercise. One or two negative responses in these areas are likely to lead to a life crisis if the client's position remains unchanged.

THE FOUR PHASES OF CRISIS

There are four recognized phases of crisis (Fig. 4.2), although individuals do not necessarily experience all phases. Using the three routes of coping as described earlier to can enable the client to leave the process of crisis (i.e. begin to manage it) before reaching the final, severe stage. However, this is not a magic formula. In sudden death there is no quick answer but we can help clients to *begin* the process of managing their feelings of chaos and disorder.

STATUS

A sudden death can instantly or more insidiously damage a person's position or standing in society that governs the respect or rights people receive. Their status may give them a role or place, somewhere they belong. If this is suddenly removed it leaves them vulnerable or seeking a new status:

● 'Where do I stand now?'
● 'Does this relate to what I thought I had?'
● 'This is like starting over again.'

Some people describe having to make a completely new start or an about-turn after a crisis. Image and status can be

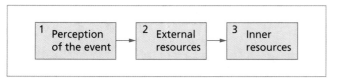

Figure 4.1   Three routes to explore when attempting to cope with a crisis.

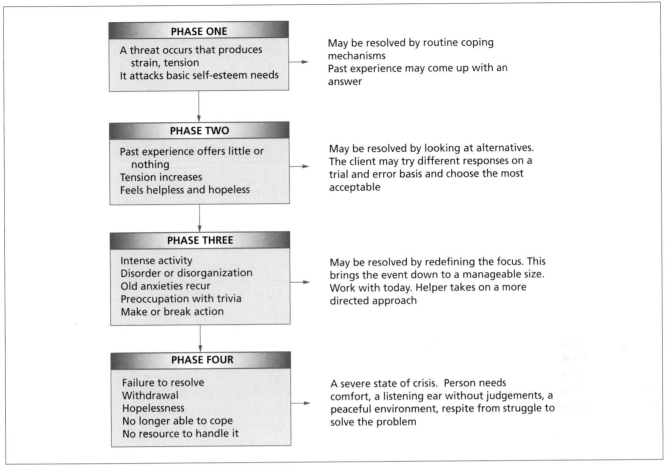

Figure 4.2   The phases of crisis.

closely bound together. We have discussed how a client's place along life's milestones graph may indicate a developmental crisis; it may also highlight a threat to a client's status. For example, a shift towards retirement, or a mother's children growing up and leaving home, or the end of a woman's sexually reproductive period, indicates a new role and a change in status. If you look at a sudden death using the phases of crisis in Figure 4.2, you will see that it cannot be resolved immediately, so work needs to be done in each phase of crisis. Much of this work with a sudden death will be the concern of A&E departments and critical care units, but there will be occasions when it has to be addressed on a ward, or in someone's home or other community setting.

One of the difficult elements of a sudden death is that this emergency is imposed upon clients suddenly, leading to disempowerment and loss of autonomy. Most therapeutic relationships result from clients asking for help for themselves: people are usually in a position to make the decision to ask for help or are referred for help with their agreement. However, in the case of sudden death the element of choice is absent and this alters the whole nature of the relationship. Family or loved ones are thrust into the position of being helpless, disempowered and needing immediate help (Wright 1999). Not only is this death difficult to grieve

because of the number of negative determinants, but it can also result in post-traumatic stress disorder (Ornstein 1998).

The resulting disempowerment may mean that the nurse has to be more assertive in providing people with the conditions they need to move into the process we call grief, because many people will experience chaos and disorder in all the dimensions of their person (Box 4.8).

The theories discussed earlier suggest the need for some action on the part of the helper and indeed they demonstrate that the response should be clearly proactive. As we walk that line of acknowledging the unique needs of the individual, and recognizing their autonomy and choice, we may be prevented from being more proactive. If we are proactive in providing certain conditions at the time of death and suggesting that it would be helpful to do this or that, we could be accused of being prescriptive. An example is viewing the body.

VIEWING THE BODY

In Wright's (1996) study on this subject, relatives who saw the body after the death spoke about the definite value of contact with the deceased. Viewing the body is especially

Box 4.8	The five dimensions of the person
Physical	Nausea, blurring of vision, tachycardia, weakness in legs, faint, restlessness, dry mouth and more
Emotional	A whole range of emotion can be experienced over a short timespan, for example numbness, intense sadness, helplessness, anger, frustration and occasionally rage
Cognitive	Unable to receive, retain or process information. Inability to access familiar information such as a well-known telephone number
Social	May be surrounded by family and friends and feel totally alone. Unable to perceive anything as a resource
Spiritual	Loss of faith or belief. Intense distress at loss of belief in their life and in their vision for self. Too many questions and no answers. Perplexity, confusion, loss of purpose

valued by relatives not present at the point of death. The chance to say 'I am sorry I was not with you' and to affirm the death was described as providing comfort. The place where the body was viewed was also commented on.

Wright's (1996) study revealed that it is important to see the deceased where they died. This may be a resuscitation room or a treatment room. Some relatives viewed the body again later, in the chapel next to the hospital mortuary, but said they were most comforted by seeing the person where they had died. This seems to take the bereaved person closer to the event, which they have a strong need to feel part of. There was not one negative response to viewing the body. When a phone-in on sudden death on local radio was conducted by Wright and Ashdown, most of the problems concerned the absence of a body. One woman rang to say her son was lost overboard at sea 20 years ago and she still expected him to walk through the door. Wives of pilots missing in the war talked of their difficulty at not having a body to see in order to confirm death (Wright 2002).

The debate about bringing the bodies of the dead from the Falklands War back to Britain highlighted the focus on the deceased's body. More recently, the need to retrieve bodies after fishing boat incidents has been discussed. Raphael (1986) in her experiences with bereavement, and particularly disaster, points out that not being able to see the body contributes to later difficulties. Whilst Cathcart (1988) noted that the relatives' reluctance to see the body should be respected, she went on to say that they should be encouraged to view, and that photographs should be kept.

Currently an assertive response to viewing the body is being adopted. The previous response to the question 'Should I see the body?' was often a passive one: 'If you want to' or 'It is your decision'. There is value in saying: 'Yes, I think you should'. We can make it the most natural thing to do: 'I am sure you would want to see him, even if it's only to say goodbye'.

It is unusual to hear of someone regretting seeing the deceased. More regrets and difficulties arise from not seeing the body, and later it is, of course, too late. The risk of regret seems worth taking when a beneficial outcome is most likely. A study by Jones and Buttery (1981) of relatives of sudden death victims who spent time with the body in the emergency department also concluded that the viewing process was helpful. Most people stated that the whole episode seemed like a fantasy or bad dream, and that the viewing made it a reality. Reality, whilst painful, is more manageable than fantasy. Several people in Wright's study who did not see the deceased had difficulties with fantasies about how the body looked (Wright 1996). Fantasies can be intrusive and are less controllable, whilst reality is preferable and frees you from bizarre and distressing images.

People state that it is helpful to have things explained before viewing the body, for example if someone looks blue after death. In cases of head and facial injuries one might assume it is wiser to prevent someone from seeing the body. This is not so – as long as people are told what to expect before viewing the body. If necessary, the injuries can be covered, and it need not prevent them holding the deceased's hand. Being with the deceased is certainly a major issue and affirms that the time and effort spent with relatives and the deceased is tremendously valuable. There seems little doubt that it helps to begin the process of grief.

ADVOCACY

Advocacy is seen as an integral part of practical nursing (Seedhouse 2000). An advocate speaks on behalf of some other person (or persons) as he or she perceives the person's interests. A nurse advocates for a patient if he or she is convinced that to do so is a health priority. Another interesting thought from Seedhouse (2000) is that a thorough ethical analysis is in order, to ensure that advocacy for this patient will not unreasonably compromise the health of others.

Some clients need to have an advocate at the time of death of their loved one. In Wright's study there was overwhelming evidence that younger women need an advocate at the time of a death. Many examples were given of male relatives and friends answering on behalf of younger bereaved women and making major decisions for them. These women later complained that the staff should not have allowed this to happen. We know how each dimension of the person is disempowered, yet we still wait to see how things progress, perhaps waiting for them to decide what they need to do. A death is a very personal, intimate time for individuals and families. Many nurses express the anxiety that they feel like an intruder encroaching on a private family moment. If we leave it to the families, this assumes they will know what to do and know the responses that facilitate good grief. Skillful intervention from nurses at these times of crisis in people's lives can assist in relieving subsequent suffering and help to prevent regrets when the time has passed for the bereaved person to reasonably view the body.

ABSENT AT THE TIME OF DEATH

Because most sudden deaths require vigorous attempts to resuscitate the patient, relatives are often not present at the time of death. Many will not be present at the hospital, and others will be kept waiting in a different room. When death is confirmed, the majority of relatives will ask whether the person suffered, whether they would have known what was happening, and whether they had said anything. Some people can place the focus more precisely on the issue most important to them and say: 'Did he ask or say anything about me?'.

Strong ambivalence is expressed at not being present at the time of death – a great need to have been there and an equally great need to run in the opposite direction. When this ambivalence has settled, many will regret or feel guilt at not having been present.

Nurses can give clear information and should not avoid answering questions. Often they will be confirming that the patient was unconscious and had no awareness of what was happening. At other times the nurse will be informing them that strong analgesic drugs were given to deal with the pain. Supplementary information about the nature of these drugs is helpful and can alleviate further distress. We may say, for example, 'The drug was a powerful narcotic, like morphine'. Most people have heard of morphine and understand its useful properties.

Despite all these reassurances, issues such as why they did not get to the person on time, and their helplessness in trying to facilitate this, can become prolonged difficulties for the people who are left behind. Because of the value for most people of being present at the time of death, we must not forget waiting relatives when attempts at resuscitation have failed. Some patients will continue to have a heartbeat for a short time after attempts have ceased. The relatives can be brought to the patient to spend a short time with them before they die.

The separation of family from patient has been identified as causing difficulty and often disruptive aggression in hospitals (Wright 1993). Work in a UK hospital explored whether relatives should be present while resuscitation was taking place (Doyle et al 1995). It was found that relatives might wish to be with family members who may be dying, even though resuscitation efforts are being made. Seventy people who participated in the study were taken to the resuscitation room, accompanied by a member of staff who explained what was happening. None of the participants interfered with the resuscitation efforts.

This demonstrates a need for a much greater input from staff involved at the impact of a sudden death. This will result in spending much longer periods with the relatives, and in staff training and support. This will enable people to re-emerge from this difficult, traumatic and distressing life crisis and ultimately to avoid the potential for dysfunctional grieving once they have departed from the confines of the hospital setting.

Caring for the suddenly bereaved will test all our skills of communication with people in crisis. Communication is the vehicle by which nurses establish a therapeutic relationship with clients; it involves passing on information and exchanging thoughts and feelings. This exchange influences the behaviour of others: communication is critical to the successful outcome of all nursing interventions (Stuart and Laraia 1998). Working with the immediate care of the suddenly bereaved will demand major resources of communication from the nurse, and studies highlight how the nurse can, as a result, suffer from post-traumatic stress disorder (Chandler 1993). This is particularly a problem when breaking bad news.

BREAKING BAD NEWS

You may not have any control about where the bad news is given. It will certainly make a difference if you are in the patient's home as opposed to a hospital corridor, so if we can influence the conditions in which the bad news is given this will help with a difficult task. A quiet place where people are not walking through, without telephones and other disturbances, will help. Frequently the person breaking the bad news feels they have done it badly.

Communication is a dynamic, complex, continuous exchange: it is quite common to feel ineffective and at a loss as to which direction to follow (British Medical Association 1992). A study of the parents of critically ill children (Farrell and Frost 1992) found that, although the information they received was distressing and traumatic, there was an overwhelming need to know that it was correct and honest. Euphemisms for death should be avoided: words such as 'dead' or 'died' are unequivocal. Phrases such as 'She has passed away', 'We have lost him', 'She has just gone' are open to misinterpretation.

As discussed earlier, when perception of the event is distorted or there is a possibility of denial, we must ground the event in reality. The bearer of bad news may feel they have inflicted pain on the recipient by honest, direct information. Whilst the loss is the real focus of the event, there is a need for clear, understandable information. In a situation that is outside the realms of understanding there is a need to introduce some order and remove some of the perplexity.

Honest, direct information about the death and the sequence of events, from people who do not skirt around the issues, is valued by the clients. This role involves painful confrontation and the recipient may show some cognitive disarray as a result. This leads on to the second component useful in the management of a crisis: finding some external resources.

HELP TO FIND IMMEDIATE RESOURCES

Some extremely simple tasks become difficult or complicated at times of crisis. Information usually familiar to people can become difficult to locate. Family, friends or significant others, although geographically near, may seem far away. Those who are far away will cause the helplessness and frustration to intensify. For example, people familiar with telephone directories will ask you to find someone's number, because they cannot understand its sequence. It is not at all uncommon for people not to be able to use the telephone or dial a number. Which persons are significant in their lives, and how you can arrange for them to join you, is an important issue. It often requires painstaking discussion to elicit where these people are.

In a large and busy hospital, it is important that relatives and friends are able to ask for a named member of staff on arrival. To arrive distressed and find that reception staff do not know who you are puts both staff and relatives in a difficult position. It also suggests that this most significant of events is not being given priority.

Prior to the arrival of others, some relatives will negotiate with the nurse as to who should give the bad news. It is important that the relatives impart the information to new arrivals, and nurses must encourage this, however reluctant the relatives may be.

THE ARRIVAL OF OTHER RELATIVES AND FRIENDS

The arrival of other relatives and friends will produce some intense distress and a feeling for the nurse of beginning it all again. The events leading to the death will be reviewed, perhaps more than once. The nurse may use this opportunity to evaluate how the person who was at the hospital from the start perceives and relates to the event. Allowing people to relate the events to those who join them will again confront them and allow them an opportunity to review the death.

When the story is repeated, other things may well be clarified. Other family and friends arriving may give further opportunity to spend time with the deceased. This is often a time when all the pain and anguish becomes apparent. The family may need to be alone together, but do not assume that this is what they want. Check first.

There are a number of very practical actions a nurse can take when working with people who are suddenly bereaved. Kent and McDowell (2004) developed a summary of the principles of best practice in these situations and this can be found in Box 4.9. Simple actions such as using paper bags specifically designed for the purpose of returning a patient's belonging to their relatives is so much better than using hospital bin bags. Allowing significant relatives to participate in the last offices can also have an enormously beneficial

effect in helping them to come to terms with the reality of the event and providing them with the opportunity to do one last caring thing for their loved one.

LOSS

Working with loss is a major part of a nurse's day and many of the losses will have a tremendous impact on people's lives. Box 4.10 lists several examples of loss associated with healthcare issues – but the list is endless.

Some losses are associated with our image, our sexuality and our status. Our image is our view of ourselves: as we grow and walk about, this image becomes well established; it becomes very important during adolescence. Young people receive messages from others and from the media about how they should look and what others will value when they see them. Many people will think that a person's body is the most important expression of who they are as an individual. At vulnerable times, like the years of growing into adulthood, we are strongly influenced by messages about our appearance from our peer group, some of whom will express values about others according to looks, body, clothes and style. These early messages are exploited by the media and advertisers, who suggest ways to achieve and maintain our attractiveness.

The ideal body image and the way you see your own body image become associated with your idea of your physical appearance. Your awareness of your own body image has important emotional consequences.

Your body image is open to change. Its shape, size, how it is structured and how it functions may alter. This can happen slowly and may not be obvious, or it may be sudden and dramatic. Your hair may gradually turn grey and lines appear on your face; you may be aware of this or choose to deny it. Some people make these changes part of their view of themselves; others deny them and then experience a sudden feeling of crisis or loss at the change. Some people undergo cosmetic surgery with high hopes that the results will change their lives. However, it is not always possible for the result of surgery to meet people's expectations, as the example about Mrs Patel shows (see Case 4.1).

CASE Mrs Patel was 50 years old and worked as a buyer of fashionable clothes for a large department store. She had to make predictions about future trends in fashion and take risks when calculating the volume of certain clothes she bought. Mrs Patel had always felt that her personal appearance (her body image) was very important to her overall performance and ability. She became preoccupied with the lines on her face, and when some of her fashion predictions were wrongly timed she began to worry that she was losing her ability and judgment. She told herself she was getting old and that she was no longer functioning efficiently.

Mrs Patel decided she needed to have cosmetic surgery to alter her image. She was sure that after surgery she would return to her former self and once again experience the energy and skill she had known when she was younger. What Mrs Patel failed to see was that the real problem was not her wrinkles but the fact she was out of touch with current trends. She had lost some of her former contacts with whom she could discuss forthcoming changes in the market, and was miscalculating the moment when new styles and ideas emerged.

Because Mrs Patel's expectations of the outcome of the surgery were wrong, when the change in her image failed to have the expected result in her life, she blamed it on poor-quality surgery. Soon she was involved in a long-standing dispute with the doctors, nurses and health authority.

How people think about the effects of an illness depends on how they cope with change. Changes in physical appearance, or in people's body image, result in changes in other areas of their lives too. Change involves leaving behind things that are familiar and accepted parts of our existence.

Box 4.9   Principles of best practice when caring for those who are suddenly bereaved in an acute care setting

Contacting relatives or friends
Communicate by telephone
Speak to the most significant relative or friend, state own name and position held
Give the name of the hospital and the patient's full name
Convey the severity of the situation
Check understanding

Arrival of relatives or friends
Allocate one support nurse to the family or friends
Meet them on arrival
Take relatives or friends to an appropriately furnished private sitting room

Resuscitation
Inform relatives or friends of the situation, assure them that every effort is being made to save the patient
Provide an honest update every 10–15 minutes (support nurse)
Encourage relatives or next of kin to witness resuscitations if they wish

Informing relatives or friends of the death
Inform relatives or friends promptly of the death, using clear unambiguous language
Express care and concern, support bereaved relatives and friends whatever their reaction
Allow time to talk, listen and answer questions

Viewing the body
Present the deceased person to look as peaceful as possible
Encourage relatives or friends to see, touch and talk to the deceased person
Allow time alone with the body
Allow relatives or friends to participate in last offices
Provide the opportunity to see the place of death

The deceased person's belongings
Fold clothing, place in a specially designed container, avoid plastic clothing bags
Explain soiled or cut clothes, place a note with the clothing stating the same

Concluding procedures
Accommodate cultural or religious rituals
Discuss organ or tissue donation
Inform relatives and friends about the post-mortem
Provide information on arranging a funeral, registering a death and bereavement support groups
Retain photograph or lock of hair

Follow-up
Provide a hospital contact number and name of support nurse or doctor
Provide follow-up care in the week following the death by telephone or written note

(Kent and McDowell 2004 with kind permission)

Box 4.10   Some losses associated with health care

- Mastectomy
- Alzheimer's disease
- Chronic obstructive disease
- Diabetes
- Amputation of a limb
- Miscarriage
- Hysterectomy
- Prostatectomy
- Stroke

Box 4.11   Patterns of behaviour that may follow body change

- Passivity
- Denial
- Reassurance
- Isolation
- Hostility

- make people feel vulnerable and ill at ease with themselves, and produce grief.

Body image is closely associated with feelings, inner beliefs and personal goals: our own ideas of our strengths and weaknesses are the result of the way we see our image. A change in a small area of a person's body, whether internal or external, can take on great significance.

Work on patients with chronic leg ulcers (Bland 1999) reveals how, along with the body breaking down, there is a breaking down of relationships with others. New, long-term relationships with healthcare professionals have to be forged, and care taken not to offend these experts. The care and management is often undertaken by district nurses and this contact may last years. This study explores the reality of living with a body that can no longer be relied upon and the enormity and significance of that loss. It is not necessarily useful that people insist the client/patient concerned is still the same and that it is all perfectly acceptable. This person is not the same: they feel different and may look different and have had to make the change between who they were and who they are now.

Responses such as 'It could be worse' are well meaning but take away from the painful consequences of the change. Clients need someone to validate their reactions and fears, someone who will not try to dilute or dismiss them.

It would be easy to say that image is not important and that people value other aspects of a person much more. People say that other characteristics such as loyalty, self-determination and creativity are more important, but in practice they often place more importance on image and appearance. The advertising industry exploits this fact.

Altered body image may:

- threaten a person's status
- change a familiar and long-accepted part of a person
- weaken people's security by raising issues of whether they possess or have lost control of what they assumed would always be theirs
- suddenly become difficult to cope with after a long period of gradual change

RESPONDING TO ALTERED BODY IMAGE

It can be useful for a client to express concern and anxiety about body image. It is a way of exploring the possible effects of the change with another person. This outward expression of inner concerns is both necessary and healthy for many clients. The nurse can use the occasion to reassure the client that she or he continues to recognize the client as a person. Certain patterns of behaviour may follow body change, including those in Box 4.11.

PASSIVITY

If the client is passive she or he appears withdrawn and listless, simply accepting the care that is offered. Lowered morale and reduced self-esteem can lead to this sadness and withdrawal, which may result in the person not wanting to be involved in his or her own care. Demotivation and apathy will follow.

DENIAL

The client may show denial by refusing to touch or look at an altered part of the body, such as a colostomy, operation scar or damaged tissue. If the client has a limb amputated or a breast removed, he or she may deny its absence. For the nurse, it can be very distressing when the client resists any attempts to return attention to the loss or change. The nurse then feels that by trying to do this she or he is inflicting pain and distress on the client, and worries that this may strain their relationship.

REASSURANCE

The client may seek constant attention from the nurse and from his or her own family. In order to gain reassurance concerning their acceptability the client may make dismissive remarks such as 'Nobody every really fancied me anyway'.

Paying the client a compliment can have a powerful effect on these occasions because it indicates that appearance or image does not take away from the attractiveness of the complete person.

ISOLATION

The client's isolation may be self-imposed because she or he feels unacceptable. Avoidance may be used as strategy to prevent rejection. If the client says that he or she is less acceptable to family and friends, it is easy for the nurse quickly to deny it and say it is all imagination. However, the client may have sensed the family's response correctly: it is not unusual for family members or friends to reject a client because of body changes. They make remarks like: 'He is not the person he was' or 'It has altered his personality'. This could be true, but it could be that they themselves are unable to cope with the physical changes they see in the client. Their attitude both to the physical changes and to the changes in the client's emotional state may be the reasons for their rejection.

HOSTILITY

Feelings of hostility and anger emerge frequently when clients feel strongly about their altered or damaged body image. Their protests may be intended for someone else but may be directed at the nurse because she or he is there. If the client feels that some other person is responsible, but cannot express anger towards them, she or he may become rebellious or provocative towards the nurse.

Any of these changes in behaviour may occur after a sudden death as well as after the loss of a limb or organ or a change in appearance. The loss of some organs also results in the loss of masculinity or femininity. These losses can result in as much grief as death does.

Feelings of separation and loss associated with illness or injury remind us that we are not totally in control. We become attached to and familiar with ourselves, and feel sad if we 'lose' parts of ourselves. The bonds we develop with what is familiar, for example self and others, are threatened. If the bond is broken or continues to be threatened, we feel acute anxiety.

PHASES OF LOSS

Bowlby (1973) described the loss of self (or part of self) and the loss of objects as being in three phases (Box 4.12). Bowlby's theory is task oriented, that is, the phases he describes are demonstrated by the things people are involved in at the various stages of grief. For example, in the first phase people wander around looking for the lost one or for signs that the person may still be available; in the third phase people learn new skills. Bowlby suggests that we can recognize which phase a person is going through by looking at the purpose of the tasks they are carrying out.

Box 4.12	Bowlby's three phases of loss
Protest	Characterized by the feelings of anger, disbelief, shock and yearning (great longing). The person focuses on thoughts of loss by crying, searching consciously (or unconsciously) to recover the loss and by making appeals for help. Sleep, digestion and appetite may be disturbed during this stage
Disorganization	This stage is indicated by despair, depression, withdrawal, social isolation and a slowing down of physical activities. There may also be obvious signs of regression – return to an earlier, more primitive, form of behaviour
Reorganization	The person breaks away from the attachment, developing new interests and attachments. Return to a level of functioning similar to that experienced before the loss

SUMMARY

You may feel that the work discussed in this chapter involves only sadness, misery and pain, but loss and grief are part of everyday life and no one can avoid the strong feelings that surround them. You may also think you would prefer not to work with clients in such distressing situations because you find it too upsetting or difficult. Yet nurses who do tackle the issues of loss and grief find the work very rewarding. They gain great insight into the nature of relationships and the ways in which people view life and give it meaning. Many nurses find that the challenge of working with loss and grief contributes to their own personal growth. They develop a clear understanding of some of the difficult issues of life and gradually feel more comfortable with them. Caring for those experiencing loss, grief and separation can make an obvious difference to people's lives, be a positive experience and make a useful and meaningful contribution to care. Sensitive and skillful nursing interventions directed towards people who are experiencing dying and grieving can enhance the lives of all concerned. It is the ultimate and final act of caring for the dying person and can have lasting effects for the people who survive. There is no universal way of providing help; each situation will be unique and special. All we can do is be guided by the principles of practice based on the theories of grieving and loss to act in the best ways we can to support and care for people who are dying or bereaved. It is a privilege to share these significant milestones of life with people, and it is not wrong to find that you actually enjoy the work. Whatever the challenges, the uniqueness of each event will make it an experience to value.

CRITICAL INCIDENT

You are accompanying a district nurse from the local health centre whilst on your community placement as a student. The district nurse is asked to visit Mary, a 70-year-old woman who is giving her GP some concern. Mary has visited the surgery regularly with numerous minor ailments over the past year. Prior to this she rarely visited her GP. The only other significant detail is that her husband died the previous year, but as it is now a year ago she is coping with that.

On entering Mary's house you introduce yourselves, and Mary appears flustered and panicky that you have arrived. She apologizes for this but says she is just preparing a meal and if you do not mind following her she will have to complete what she was doing. You all go into the kitchen and she continues chopping up carrots, puts them in a pan of water, puts the pan on the stove and turns on the gas. Mary notices you looking at a picture of an elderly man on the kitchen dresser. She walks over, picks it up and clutches it to her chest. You then have to remind her that she has not lit the gas. She is embarrassed about this and explains that she cannot concentrate very well. You notice her husband's coat hanging behind the door and two places already set at the table. The district nurse remarks how very difficult it must have been since her husband died and how the doctors were concerned about how unwell she had been recently.

Mary looks at the district nurse and at you for what seems like a long time, before saying how he just loved organizing things and that she never had to lift a finger. If they were going on holiday, every detail was decided upon by him – it was organized meticulously. She smiled and remarked how she never had to do a thing. Her friends had said they would not like that, but she said it suited her fine. She stands and ponders this.

Then, as if startled, she apologizes for not sitting you down and offering you some tea, and leads you to the sitting room. Here are more pictures of them in faraway exotic places such as India, and one of them on a kind of bobsleigh in the Canadian Rockies.

The district nurse says how she must miss him, and tears immediately well up in Mary's eyes. She apologizes and says she must not get upset, as it was now beginning to annoy people: two friends had remarked recently that she was living in the past and needed to get on with her life. She then remarks how she must be getting on people's nerves as they are visiting her less frequently, and how she is not expecting anyone to visit until the weekend (it is now Tuesday). The district nurse suggests various opportunities for Mary to socialize; she says she does not want to seem ungrateful for the suggestion but at her time of life she will not change now. She always got what she wanted from just the two of them. 'He did not like me mixing with others', she remarks, 'He says they may ask too many questions'.

You then say you are not aware of all the circumstances of his death. Mary immediately launches into all the detail. She was baking and had forgotten to get the sultanas; she apologized for this saying how it was her fault, she had not put them on his shopping list. He always did the shopping as he liked to control the money. She said she would run down to the corner shop and get some, but he was adamant that she would not. It was dusk and, as he had said to her before, 'You are too trusting, and I have told you before about talking to anyone'. He insisted he would go to the shop but then complained bitterly and became quite angry, saying how she was becoming more and more stupid and forgetful.

Mary becomes more subdued at this stage, and tearful. She says she hated it when he was angry with her and she knows it was all her fault. After half an hour she suddenly became aware that he had not returned – he should have been back after 15 minutes but she had forgotten this as she became engrossed in something on TV. She had heard the ambulance sirens but thought nothing of it. When the woman from the shop hammered on Mary's door she was frightened by the urgency of it. The woman explained that two young boys were playing football outside the shop and the ball had hit him; when they laughed he became angry and then suddenly collapsed. When Mary had arrived at the hospital she was too late.

Mary pauses then and looks away. 'He had already gone, you see, I was too late. He never got to the shop and I have not had the heart to bake since then.' When the hospital staff heard her only sister lived 200 miles away, they got her a taxi home. Eventually, the next day she thought it was, her sister arrived and took over, made all the arrangements and that was it. She agrees she is eating all right, not always sleeping very well and not very well organized. She laughs and tells you her sister said she would have to get her act together – she was her own worst enemy. Mary says she makes a point of walking down to the shops just to get out, and remarks that it is difficult to get excited about cooking for herself. She agrees the district nurse can visit her again, and if she is getting very upset or unwell she will contact her.

Reflection

From your knowledge of the grief process and negative determinants, what information did you gain that would indicate Mary is having problems with her grief process?

REFERENCES

Bland M (1999) Living with chronic leg ulcers. In: Madjar I, Walton JA, eds. Nursing and the experience of illness. London: Routledge, p 36–57.

British Medical Association (1992) A stressful shift. BMA Board of Health Science and Education teaching package. London: BMA.

Bowlby J (1973) Separation. London: Penguin.

Bowlby J (1980) Attachment and loss: loss, sadness and depression. Vol. 3. New York: Basic Books.

Caplan G (1964) Principles of preventative psychiatry. New York: Basic Books.

Cassell E (2004) The nature of suffering and the goals of medicine, 2nd edn. Oxford: Oxford University Press.

Cathcart F (1988) Seeing the body after death. British Medical Journal 297: 997–998.

Chandler E (1993) Can post traumatic stress disorder be prevented? Journal of Accident and Emergency Nursing 1: 87–91.

Chapman K, Pepler C (1998) Coping, hope and anticipatory grief in family members in palliative home care. Cancer Nursing 21(4): 226–234.

Clayton PPJ, Halikas JA, Maurice WL (1973) Anticipatory grief and widowhood. British Journal of Psychiatry 122: 47–51.

Costello J (1999) Anticipatory grief: coping with impending death of a partner. International Journal of Palliative Nursing 5(5): 223–231.

Davidhizar R, Newman-Eiger J (1998) Patients' use of denial. Nursing Standard 12(43): 34–36.

Dossey L (1994) Healing words. New York: Harper Collins.

Doyle CJ, Post H, Burney RE et al (1995) Family participation during resuscitation – an option. Annals of Emergency Medicine 16(6): 673–675.

Dunne K (2004) Grief and its manifestations Nursing Standard 14(45): 45–51.

Erikson EH (1950) Childhood and society. New York: WW Norton.

Farrell MF, Frost C (1992) The most important needs of parents in critically ill children. Journal of Intensive Care and Critical Care Nursing 8(3): 104–106.

Freud S (1917) Mourning and melancholia. Cited in: Stachy J, Freud A, eds (1964) The complete works of Sigmund Freud. London: Hogarth Press.

Jones WH, Buttery M (1981) Sudden death: survivors' perceptions of their emergency department experience. Journal of Emergency Nursing 7: 1.

Kent H, McDowell J (2004) Sudden bereavement in acute settings. Nursing Standard 19(6): 38–42.

Kubler-Ross E (1969) On death and dying. New York: Macmillan.

Lindemann E (1944) Symptomatology and management of acute grief. American Journal of Psychiatry 101: 141–148.

Neuberger J (2004) Dying well: a guide to enabling a good death, 2nd edn. Oxford, San Francisco: Radcliffe Publishing.

Ornstein R (1998) Approach to the patient following a traumatic event. In: Stern T, Herman J, Slavin P, eds. The MGH guide to psychiatry in ordinary care. New York: McGraw-Hill, pp. 327–334.

Parkes CM (1972) Studies of grief in adult life, 1st edn. London: Tavistock.

Parkes CM (1996) Bereavement: studies of grief in adult life, 3rd edn. London: Routledge.

Raphael B (1984) The anatomy of bereavement – a handbook for caring professions. London: Hutchinson.

Raphael B (1986) When disaster strikes. London: Hutchinson.

Rogers MP, Reich P (1988) On the health consequences of bereavement. New England Journal of Medicine 319(8): 510–511.

Seedhouse D (2000) Practical nursing philosophy: the universal ethical code. Chichester, UK: John Wiley.

Stuart G, Laraia M (1998) Pocket guide to psychiatric nursing, 4th edn. St Louis: Mosby.

Wiseman C (1992) Bereavement care in an acute ward. Nursing Times 88(20): 34–35.

Worden JW (1993) Grief counselling and grief therapy, 2nd edn. London: Routledge.

Wright B (1993) Caring in crisis, 2nd edn. Edinburgh: Churchill Livingstone.

Wright B (1996) Sudden death – a research base for practice. Edinburgh: Churchill Livingstone.

Wright B (1999) Autonomy and disempowerment at the time of a sudden death. Journal of Accident and Emergency Nursing 17(3): 154–157.

Wright B (2002) Death grief and loss in: Watson's clinical nursing and related science, 6th edn. Walsh M, pp.59–74. London: Ballière Tindall.

FURTHER READING

Aguilera DC (1997) Crisis intervention: theory and methodology. St Louis: Mosby.

Practical methods for dealing with situational and maturational crisis. Offers an explanation as to why people behave as they do around the more acute loss.

Bowlby J (1978) Separation. Harmondsworth: Penguin.

Bowlby J (1981) Attachment. Harmondsworth: Penguin.

Bowlby J (1981) Loss. Harmondsworth: Penguin.

This classic trilogy and much acclaimed work examines ways in which young children and families respond to loss. Gives a perspective on the background to the grief process.

Kubler-Ross E (1970) On death and dying. London: Tavistock.

Particularly helpful at exploring the dying process for the patient and family.

Neuberger J (2004) Dying well: a guide to enabling a good death, 2nd edn. Radcliffe Oxon

A useful resource with practical advice and explanations for people working with dying patients.

Parkes CM (1986) Bereavement: studies of grief in adult life. London: Routledge.

Long recognized as the most authoritative work of its kind.

Walker T (1999) Bereavement – the culture of grief. Milton Keynes: Open University Press.

This book looks at the social positions of the bereaved and how people find themselves caught between the living and the dead. It offers some sociological insights into this most personal of human situations.

Wright B (1996) Sudden death – a research base for practice. Edinburgh: Churchill Livingstone.

Looks at the death from the point of view of the bereaved and examines the long-term implications.

Primary health care and working with patients with long-term conditions

Alison Crumbie

INTRODUCTION

Over the last few decades there has been a marked shift in healthcare provision from secondary to primary care in the UK. The government's plans for modernizing the National Health Service (NHS) have placed primary care centre stage (DoH 2001). The emphasis on primary health care has resulted in a vast increase in the number of nurses working in community settings and there is therefore a need for nurses to understand how health care is delivered outside the hospital. Simultaneously there continues to be a rise in the number of people who live with long-term health problems. The prevalence of diabetes alone looks set to rise from 1.8 million people in the UK to 2.7 million by 2030 and globally the rise is expected to jump from a staggering 171 million to 366 million by the year 2030 (WHO 2005). It is estimated that over 17 million people in the UK live with a long-term condition (Metcalfe 2005). The prevalence of many of the long-term conditions is increasing partly because people are living longer with long-term conditions and also partly because people are living longer generally.

It is in this climate that you will find yourself working as a nurse. This has relevance for all areas of nursing. Nurses working in hospital settings will be working with patients who have long-term chronic conditions, and liaison with colleagues in the community setting will be vitally import-ant to ensure effective discharge planning. Nurses working in the community will find that they are now expected to perform aspects of care that were previously available only in the hospital setting. The purpose of this chapter is to consider the concept of primary health care and the impact of this approach to health care on our work with people who live with long-term conditions.

WHAT IS PRIMARY HEALTH CARE?

In recent years we have heard a great deal of rhetoric in the media over the primary-care-led National Health Service. 'Primary-care' would appear to be a simple term and there is an assumption that we all have a shared understanding of what it means. However, there has been much debate over the definition of primary care. In 1978 the World Health Organization (WHO) stimulated an international reorientation of healthcare services towards primary health care, and at that time provided a comprehensive definition of primary care. The WHO (1978) definition of primary care is:

> *... essential health care based on practical, scientifically sound and socially acceptable methods and technology, made universally available to individuals and families in the community through their full participation and at a cost that the*

community and country can afford to maintain at every stage of their development in the spirit of self-reliance and self-determination.

This is a rather complex and broad definition, and further on in the document, primary care is described as 'the first level of contact of individuals, the family and the community with the national health system, bringing health care as close as possible to where people live and work'. Cook (1999) suggests that this second description of primary care is more useful to nurses who work in the UK. There are, however, other perspectives that can enrich our understanding of this complex concept.

PRIMARY CARE AS AN APPROACH, ACTIVITIES, LEVEL OF CARE OR A PHILOSOPHY

PRIMARY CARE AS AN APPROACH

Macdonald (1992) describes primary health care as an approach to the planning and delivery of health services. The primary healthcare approach encompasses comprehensive healthcare systems which include cure, prevention, health promotion and rehabilitation, with the people who receive the care as equal partners in the process (Blackie 1998). This approach also emphasizes the importance of including primary healthcare professionals in the commissioning of services. An example of this is the introduction of primary care groups (PCGs) and primary care trusts (PCTs) in England. The PCGs and PCTs consist of a group of healthcare professionals and lay people who make decisions about the provision of healthcare services for their population. The NHS plan in the UK (DoH 2000a) is a further example of the primary care approach to the delivery of health services. The plan states that patients are the most important people in the health service, and a variety of measures has been suggested to help empower and respect patients. These include the provision of more information for patients and greater patient choice. We can see the results of this approach to healthcare provision in services such as NHS Direct and walk-in centres.

PRIMARY CARE ACTIVITIES

Primary care activities include, for example, community dentistry and pharmacy, community nursing, childhood immunization programmes and general practitioner (GP) services. It would not matter where these activities took place; primary care in this example would be defined by the activity rather than the approach or location. It would be possible, then, for a child to receive **immunizations** at the GP surgery or at their school. GP services can be delivered as an out-of-hours service from a base at the local hospital or by the GP travelling to a patient's home. In each of these examples the service that is delivered to the patients is a primary care service, even though the locations may vary enormously.

LEVEL OF CARE

The level of care refers to the idea of the 'first contact' with health services. A patient may present to the GP surgery as a first point of contact, but they may also present to a minor injuries unit, a pharmacy or make a phone call to the NHS Direct 24-hour telephone helpline. Each of these presentations would be an example of a first point of contact, and would therefore represent primary care. This perspective demonstrates that care provided by a rapid response team in the community setting would not be primary care. The patient would first have accessed health services by contacting a healthcare professional who would then have referred the person on to the rapid response team. The team would then deliver healthcare services to the patient in his or her home, such as the administration of intravenous fluids, monitor the patient and hopefully prevent admission to hospital. In this example the nursing activity would have taken place in the community, but it does not qualify as primary care because the first point of contact was with another healthcare professional.

A PHILOSOPHY OF CARE

A fundamental feature of the philosophy of primary care is the notion that health is a basic human right. The philosophy of primary care is further defined by Vuori (1986), who states that a country can claim to practise primary care only if its entire healthcare system is characterized by an acceptance of the broad definition of health, social justice and equality, self-responsibility and international solidarity. It is clear from this definition that the active participation of people using health services is placed at the heart of the philosophy of primary care.

It is clear that there is a variety of approaches to understanding the concept of primary care. We can think of it as an approach, a group of activities, a level of care or a philosophy of care. It is evidently not defined by the place in which the activity occurs, although there is an underlying theme that primary health care involves moving service provision closer to the patient. In 1996 the Department of Health (DoH) identified the principles of good primary care in the document *Primary Care: Delivering the Future* (DoH 1996). These are summarized in Box 5.1. It can be seen that these principles reflect the definitions of primary care discussed above, identifying the importance of focusing on the needs of the local population. There is also an emphasis on the healthcare professionals' responsibility to be knowledgeable about the patients they are working with and the conditions that present in primary care.

POLICY AND PRIMARY CARE

The founding principles of the UK National Health Service have served to provide the basis for the delivery of primary care in the UK over the past 50 years. On 5 July 1948 the

---

Box 5.1 Principles of good primary care

Quality

- Professionals should be knowledgeable about the conditions that are present in primary care and skilled in their treatment and in contributing to their prevention.

- Professionals should be knowledgeable about the people to whom they are offering services.

- Services should be coordinated with professionals aware of each other's contributions, with interprofessional working and with no service gaps.

- Premises and facilities should be of good standard and fit for their purposes, and equipment should be up to date, well maintained and safe to use.

Fairness

- Services should not vary widely in range or quality in different parts of the country.

- Primary care should receive an appropriate share of overall NHS resources.

Accessibility

- Services should be reasonably accessible when clinically needed.

- Necessary services should be accessible to people regardless of age, sex, ethnicity, disability or health status.

Responsiveness

- Services should reflect the needs and preferences of the individuals using them.

- Services should reflect the health demographic and social needs of the area they serve.

Efficiency

- Primary care services should be based on evidence of clinical effectiveness.

- Primary care resources should be used efficiently.

From Department of Health (1996)

NHS was launched on the principles of equity and universality; the service would be comprehensive, funded by the state and managed by a consensus of professionals. In the early days there was a focus on hospitals as the source of administrative power. As there was concern over the use of resources, the administrative power was moved away from the hospitals to regional, area and district authorities. In the early 1980s there was an attempt to reduce bureaucracy by abolishing area health authorities; however, criticism of the inefficiency and unresponsiveness of the system continued. Towards the end of the 1980s three White Papers were released: *Promoting Better Health* (DoH 1987), *Caring for People* (DoH 1989a) and *Working for Patients* (DoH 1989b). This provided the basis for some major reforms in the health service, with a particular shift towards primary care. The NHS and Community Care Act in 1990, provided the statutory basis for the changes outlined in the White Papers. This resulted in radical reform of the health service, with the introduction of the internal market, the development of NHS trusts, GP fundholding and a new GP contract (DoH 2003).

In 1997 the White Paper *The New NHS: Modern, Dependable* (DoH 1997) was published in England. This heralded the end of the internal market with plans to set up PCGs and ultimately PCTs. Typically the PCGs served a population of 100 000 patients and one of their functions was identified as the development of primary care. They were also charged with working closely with social services and with taking responsibility for commissioning services for the local community. The PCGs rapidly progressed to PCTs and, as a result of *Shifting the Balance of Power in the NHS* (DoH 2001), health authorities were abolished in April 2002 and were replaced by a small number of strategic health authorities (SHA). The SHAs are responsible for managing the performance of the PCTs. This shift of power towards primary care resulted in the claim that 75% of the entire budget of the NHS for England is now devolved to local, primary-care-based organizations (Glendinning and Dowling 2003). A diagram representing the current organizational structure of the new NHS in England can be found in Figure 5.1. As devolution had taken place during this time, Wales, Scotland and Northern Ireland put forward their own proposals for a reconfiguration of health services, and information about the organizational structure of primary care can be found on the Welsh Office web site for Wales (http://www.wales.gov.uk), The Scottish Office web site for Scotland (http://www.scottishsecretary.gov.uk) and the Northern Ireland Executive web site for Northern Ireland (http://www.nics.gov.uk).

The organizational structure of primary care outlined above reflects a major move away from centrally controlled health

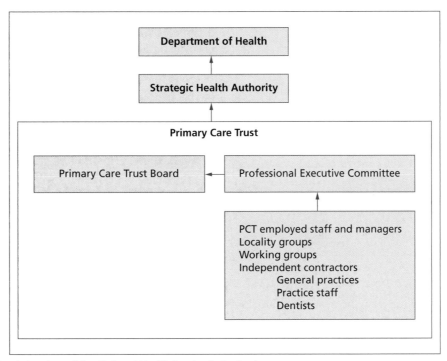

Figure 5.1 Organizational structure of the National Health Service in England.

service provision to locally led initiatives, with power for commissioning services moving closer to the patient. In July 2000 the NHS Executive in England published the NHS plan (DoH 2000a), and this is a further example of the general shift towards a primary-care-led health service. There is evidence of the national plan operating from the perspective of a primary care approach, focusing on primary care activities, addressing the level of care and operating within a philosophy of primary care. The primary care approach to health services is evidenced in recommendations for improvements in curative procedures, prevention of disease, promotion of health and rehabilitation. For example, the national plan suggests that ambulance paramedics be trained to provide thrombolysis for patients who are experiencing myocardial infarction; this is estimated to save up to 3000 lives per year and should protect patients against the potential damage to their heart. There is a variety of approaches to prevention of disease, one of which is the fact that the NHS breast screening programme has been extended to include women aged 65–70 years, resulting in 400 000 more women having mammography each year. Health promotion is being implemented through a commitment to smoking cessation across the country, and rehabilitation is addressed through the promotion of independence in old age through active recovery and rehabilitation services.

There is also evidence of the plan focusing on the activities of primary care such as community pharmacy and GP services, and there is a pledge to increase the number of walk-in centres across the country. The level of care is addressed through the issue of speed of access to services. The plan guarantees that patients will have access to a primary care professional within

24 hours and to a primary care doctor within 48 hours. The plan addresses equity of access to services and closer liaison between social services and health service management. It could therefore be suggested that a philosophy of primary care underpins the English NHS plan, creating an exciting climate for the work of primary care nurses.

THE NURSE'S ROLE IN PRIMARY HEALTH CARE

Primary care represents the context in which community nursing is delivered. There are a number of roles in the community that can be identified as areas of specialist practice for nurses. There are also many nurses who work as generic community nurses and do not have a specialist qualification. The most recognized areas of specialist practice are listed in Box 5.2. There is a great deal of overlap between these specialist areas and it is therefore difficult to identify tight definitions of each role; instead, some broad comments can be made about the type of work carried out by nurses in each of these roles.

District nurses tend to deliver nursing care to people in their own homes. To carry out this work, the district nurse needs to have a whole range of technical nursing skills to manage effectively patients who are increasingly being discharged early from hospital. District nurses also need to have case management skills so that they can organize the delivery of nursing care. The district nursing team needs to be able to liaise effectively with people in the hospital setting to assist with discharge planning, and with social

Box 5.2   Specialist nurses in the community

- District nurses
- Practice nurses
- Community mental health nurses
- Community learning disabilities nurses
- Community children's nurses
- School nurses
- Occupational health nurses
- Public health nursing/health visiting.
- Community matrons (England)

services to help coordinate a team of people to care for people in their home setting.

Practice nurses have traditionally been employed directly by GPs to work in general practice surgeries. Practice nurses cover a whole range of healthcare activities in the surgery including travel health, cervical cytology, women's health clinics, immunizations, **diabetic** and respiratory clinics, venepuncture, coronary heart disease clinics and many more. The role of the practice nurse has developed differently in different surgeries according to the skills of the nurse and the needs of the local population. Some practice nurses have extended their work to include minor injuries clinics and telephone triage, and others visit people in their homes to deliver their specialist skills to those who could not otherwise access their services. This is an example of the way in which the role of a district nurse and a practice nurse might overlap and provides an illustration of the value of working together as an integrated team where the boundaries between roles are flexible.

Community mental health nurses are known in many parts of the UK as community psychiatric nurses. Mental health nurses may be based in a surgery or community clinic and many develop a specialty in a particular area of care, such as working with children or the elderly. Preparation for this role begins with the mental health branch following the common foundation programme of pre-registration education.

Community learning disabilities nurses work in the community setting to support people with learning disabilities in their homes. The learning disabilities nurse will have particular skills in the assessment, planning and implementation of specialist clinical nursing for individuals who have a learning disability. This may include the management of critical events such as challenging or violent behaviour. The aim of learning disabilities nurses is to maximize the clients' potential for independent living and to minimize the effects of their disability. This may involve working with families, carers and other agencies, such as social services, speech therapists and other members of the multidisciplinary team.

Like community mental health nurses, community learning disabilities nurses begin their educational preparation in pre-registration courses by choosing the learning disabilities branch following the common foundation programme.

Community children's nurses assist children to stay in their own homes as long as possible, thereby avoiding admission to hospital whenever possible. Some children's nurses have become extremely specialized, focusing on childhood oncology or **cystic fibrosis**, for example, and different models of practice operate in different areas of the country. In some areas, community children's nurses operate an 'outreach' service where the nurses are based in the hospital and visit children at home when they are in need of their specialist skills; in other areas the nurses offer an 'in-reach' service where community-based children's nurses maintain some responsibility for children when they are in the hospital. Again, nurses who wish to specialize in this area of community nursing will choose the child branch of the common foundation programme.

School nurses are responsible for the health-related needs of children at school. The school nurse is involved in health screening, health surveillance and therapeutic techniques to maintain the health of children, adolescents and the family. The nurse working in a school may act as the first point of contact for children in the school setting and will therefore need a whole range of skills associated with children's nursing, including the identification of child protection issues and methods of minimizing risk. Like all the specialist community roles, school nurses will be involved in the health education of children, and many school nurses get involved in health fares for children and after-school activities. Some school nurses have extended their role to include the provision of clinics away from the school setting after school hours, to allow children to consult with them away from the watchful eyes of their peers. This can help to reduce embarrassment and meet the needs of children who would not have otherwise approached the healthcare system for support. This is yet another example of the fluid boundaries in the primary healthcare setting.

Occupational health nurses are specialists in the provision of services to people in their work settings. This group of nurses can be involved in a whole variety of activities including the management of clinical emergencies, the assessment of people who feel unwell at work, health promotion activities and carrying out health checks for people in the workplace. Occupational health nurses also have a responsibility to interpret and apply health and safety legislation and approved codes of practice with regard for the environment, well-being and protection of those who work and the wider community.

Public health nursing/health visiting is concerned with health promotion and the prevention of ill-health (Blackie 1998). In 1977 the Council for the Education and Training of Health Visitors (CETHV 1977) set out the principles of health visiting; these include the search for health needs, stimulation of the awareness of health needs, influence on policies affecting health, and the facilitation of health-enhancing activities. A quarter of a century later, these four principles remain important and relevant. The NMC definition of Specialist Community Public Health nursing is that it: 'aims to reduce health inequalities by working with individuals, families, and communities promoting health, preventing ill health and in the protection of health. The emphasis is on partnership working that cuts across disciplinary, professional and organisational boundaries that impact on organised social and political policy to influence the determinants of health and promote the health of whole populations' (NMC 2005). In practice, health visitors work in a variety of settings in the community including health centres, surgeries, community halls and hostels. The health-visiting role can lead to work with travelling families and other populations that tend to have difficulty accessing mainstream healthcare services.

The *community matron* is a new clinical role for nurses in England. This role was first described in the *NHS Improvement Plan* (DoH 2004) and its focus is to meet the needs of patients who require high intensity healthcare services. Community matrons are highly skilled nurses who act as case managers for particularly vulnerable patients. They are able to make referrals, order investigations and arrange admissions for patients (DoH 2005). They will usually be supplementary and independent prescribers and they will become a trusted key contact for the patient and the patient's family (Metcalfe 2005).

There are many other nurses who work in the community and form part of the primary healthcare team. There are nurses who work as continence advisers, who may be based in the hospital setting but 'reach out' into the community, and others who work in the community and 'reach in' to the hospital. There are family planning nurses, sexual health nurses, respiratory specialist nurses, diabetes specialist nurses and many more. There are also new ways of operating in primary care such as NHS Direct, where the patient's first point of contact with the healthcare service (and often the only point of contact) is with a nurse at the end of a telephone line. The nurse on the telephone may not be one of the community nurses, but instead will be a nurse with specialist training in telephone consultations using a computer programme to guide decision-making and the provision of advice.

In recognition of the overlap between nurses in the various specialist roles in the community setting and the need for each group to understand the role of others in the team, the educational preparation for community specialists has been based on a shared core curriculum with additional specialist competencies for each of the specialist areas. One of the aims of this educational approach is to enhance the possibility of nurses in the community working as an integrated team. As previously mentioned there are a variety of other nurses working in primary care including sexual health nurses, continence advisers, stoma nurses and others. Healthcare professionals in primary care will also interact with nurses from specialty areas in secondary care such as

respiratory health, **diabetes**, **rheumatology** and dermatology and it could be suggested that this group of practitioners should also be included in the team. The following section will focus on teamwork in primary care.

THE PRIMARY HEALTHCARE TEAM

The provision of primary health care is a complex and massive task. The Department of Health (DoH 1997, 2000b, 2005) has identified the need to develop the roles of healthcare professionals working in the primary care team in recognition of the fact that nurses, doctors, pharmacists and other healthcare professionals all have a great deal to offer patients, and their potential should therefore be realized. It is no longer possible for one healthcare professional to deliver all the care required by a particular population, and so it is necessary to work in teams. Working in a team can be a challenge, although it also has several potential benefits. The benefits of teamwork include the following (Blackie 1998, Pritchard and Pritchard 1994):

● Care given by a group is greater than the sum of its parts
● Team members are better supported and have increased job satisfaction
● Rare skills can be made more available to patients
● Prevention and curative work can be better coordinated
● Team members can learn from one another
● The patient receives more efficient care when ill.

Membership of the primary healthcare team is an issue that is frequently debated. Some suggest that the team should be defined by the provision of day-to-day clinical care and therefore the team members would include the health visitor, district nurse, practice nurse and GP (Blackie 1998). Others have suggested that the team is defined by the GP and the members of staff employed by the GP, which would therefore include receptionists, practice managers, and the practice nurse, and in many cases exclude the district nurse and health visitor. Bryar and Bytheway (1996) found that there seemed to be a multiplicity of teams working together to provide primary care services. They found that the team would come together to meet the needs of different sections of the population. One team might develop around the provision of services to people with diabetes and another might emerge in relation to screening for cervical cancer. It could be suggested that a particular healthcare professional's inclusion in the primary healthcare team is determined by the needs of the patient, so you can see that the primary healthcare team is not a fixed entity: rather it is a dynamic system that has the patient at its core.

Pritchard and Pritchard (1994) state that a team can be described as intrinsic, functional or full. The intrinsic team has the patient at its core as an active participant in care. Other members of the intrinsic team will then be determined by the needs of the patient so that, in the example of a patient with **hypertension**, the team might include the patient, the practice nurse and the GP. If this particular patient had a **stroke**, membership of the intrinsic team might change to include the patient's carer, district nurse, social worker, occupational therapist and physiotherapist (see Fig. 5.2).

A functional team is defined by its purpose. An example of a functional team might be the group of people who come together to provide maternity services or healthcare services for people with diabetes. It might be suggested that the patient or the group of patients should still remain firmly at the core of the functional team as this provides the purpose for the team's existence.

On some occasions, the full team needs to gather, perhaps to make decisions related to major issues such as altering the health centre's times of opening, changing the way referrals are made between team members, or developing new protocols for the provision of health services by the team. Clearly, the full team would involve many more people than the intrinsic team; however, there are times when it is essential to include as many people as possible to make sure that the team continues to operate smoothly and that communication between team members remains effective.

Another important issue to consider here is how the team carries out its work. Teamwork can be described as multidisciplinary or interdisciplinary (integrated). The approach taken has an impact upon the healthcare professionals in the team and – more importantly – the patient's experience.

MULTIDISCIPLINARY TEAMWORK

The multidisciplinary team is the model most commonly used in primary healthcare teams. Multidisciplinary teamwork can be defined as a group of professionals providing their own expertise regardless of the techniques used by other team members. The patient in this example is perceived as a series of 'problems' to be solved. If a 75-year-old man was dying at home after surgery for gastric cancer, the district nurse might attend the patient to deal with his **wound**, the Macmillan nurse might attend to address his pain control needs and the social worker might attend to provide advice on benefits and support. An advantage of this approach is that team members tend to have a fairly clear idea of their own and others' role in the work of caring for a particular patient: roles are clearly demarcated and overlap between roles is minimized. The disadvantage is that the patient becomes split into a series of parts and some of his needs may therefore be missed. He may, for example, be experiencing depression but because there is no mental health nurse included in the team this particular problem may be overlooked and the patient may have to struggle with his problem without assistance.

INTERDISCIPLINARY TEAMWORK

Interdisciplinary or integrated teamwork delivers coordinated, non-hierarchical, holistic care involving the patient

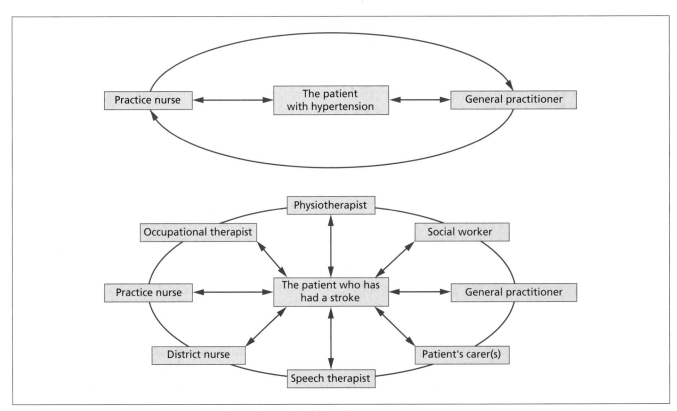

Figure 5.2 The intrinsic team changes according to the needs of the patient.

and family (Blackie 1998). The interdisciplinary team is focused explicitly on the patient's needs and is involved in formal, structured meetings to plan goals. If we consider the example outlined above, the team involved in the provision of care for this 75-year-old man would meet and aim to identify his needs and how best to meet them. The provision of care would then be determined by the needs of the patient, not by the make-up of the team that happened to be visiting him.

A further example might be the team's approach to the provision of care for people with **diabetes**. The team would need to meet regularly to plan a unified approach to patient education in relation to dietary advice, for example, and the ongoing monitoring of people with diabetes; some overlap of role would be expected and a unified approach would be developed. The advantage of this approach is that the patient is treated more holistically and is more likely to be able to see the value of the service provided.

A difficulty with the interdisciplinary approach is that roles between professionals can become blurred and this can cause some problems in the team as people become less clear of their own purpose within the team. A great deal of teamwork skill is required to overcome this problem. If all team members can manage to live with the lack of clear boundaries between their roles, working in a model such as this can be extremely satisfying for everyone, including the patient. All members of the primary healthcare team have an important role to play in working with people who have long-term conditions, and in this area, more than most, it is vital that the team is integrated and works together effectively.

LONG-TERM CONDITIONS

As a nurse working in the primary healthcare setting you will have an important role in working with people who live with long-term conditions or chronic illness. The nurse working in general practice, for example, may run clinics aimed at the management and monitoring of a variety of conditions. Practice nurses run clinics for people with **asthma**, diabetes, **coronary heart disease**, **hypertension** and **epilepsy**, for instance. District nurses will frequently be working in the home with people who have any one of these conditions, and health visitors work with families with children who live with a long-term condition such as asthma, eczema or epilepsy. Long-term conditions cannot be cured (Thomas 2005) and patients who live with these conditions often have complex needs requiring sensitive and highly skilled nursing care.

Working with people who live with chronic illness is described by Funk et al (1993) as being at the heart of nursing. So, what is chronic illness and how does it differ from a condition or disease? Often these words are used interchangeably and yet there are important, although subtle, differences between the three. Illness refers to the human experience and to the perceptions of the patient and family and their responses to the symptoms and suffering caused by the disease process. Disease, on the other hand, refers to a problem that can be viewed from the medical perspective and can be defined by alterations in the structure and function of the body. A condition is a state of being and as such it describes the whole experience of a person who lives with chronic illness.

Chronic disease management, then, refers to the activities carried out in the primary care setting with patients who live with diseases such as diabetes, hypertension, epilepsy and asthma. The patient's disease is managed with the help of the healthcare professional through annual monitoring for the signs of neuropathy in the feet in diabetes, or of **blood pressure** recordings in the hypertensive patient, for example. The role of nursing, however, goes way beyond the assessment of feet and the recording of blood pressures. Because we work with people who live with these diseases, we need to consider their experience of the illness. Our nursing assessment includes a review of their understanding of the condition, how they are managing with their medications, and what involvement their family has in the process. There are many roles that a nurse can assume when working with a patient who has a chronic illness; these are explored later in this chapter.

Having considered what we mean by the terms condition, illness and disease, we now need to develop an understanding of the term 'chronicity'. Curtin and Lubkin (1998) state that it is extremely difficult to define chronicity. Many authors have attempted to capture the essence of this concept, some with simple and brief definitions and others with lengthy and complex explanations. Several of these definitions will be explored here to provide a variety of perspectives on the term 'chronic'; you may find one that you feel relates well to the people with whom you work, or two or three that capture the essence of chronic illness from your own perspective.

Kelly and Field (1996) point out that chronic illness results in the physical reality of 'bad' bodies. The body changes in chronic illness and can be seen as letting the person down. Bleeker and Mulderij (1992) speak of the body losing its silence, and Morse et al (1994) describe a body in dis-ease. These are simple but effective comments on the experience of living with a chronic illness. The patient becomes acutely aware of his or her body. People who are without chronic illness do not experience this. The constant monitoring required in type 1 diabetes means that the patient becomes acutely aware of responses to certain foods, exercise, and simple colds and infections. People who do not have a chronic condition usually live alongside their bodies with little awareness of daily fluctuations in response to the stressors placed upon them. Clearly, chronicity involves a heightened awareness of the physical self which permeates the whole being.

Cameron and Gregor (1987) argue that chronic illness is a lived experience that involves a permanent deviation from the norm caused by unalterable pathological changes. The problem with this definition is that it labels people who have chronic illness as being abnormal. Certainly one of the important aspects of defining chronicity is the notion of permanence. Chronic conditions are not curable and this has an enormous impact upon our approach to working with people who live with chronicity. An important point to note is that most people live with rather than die from a chronic condition (Verbrugge and Jette 1994).

Several authors have offered more complex definitions of chronicity. Lyons et al (1995) state that a chronic illness is not a singular event, rather it signifies a set of complex processes that develop and endure over time. This links with the trajectory model of chronic illness outlined by Corbin and Strauss (1992), who refer to the journey of chronic illness as a trajectory, a course that varies over time and can be divided into subphases. The course of the chronic illness can be shaped and managed, and this is where we can have an impact upon the patient's experience of their disease. Funk et al (1993, p. 3) quote the 1956 definition of chronic illness by the Commission on Chronic Illness as 'being caused by pathological changes in the body that are non-reversible, permanent or leave residual disability; they may be characterised by periods of recurrence and remission and they generally require extended periods of supervision, observation, care and rehabilitation'. Curtin and Lubkin (1998, p. 6) offer a further definition of chronic illness as 'the irreversible presence, accumulation, or latency of disease states or impairments that involve the total human environment for supportive care and self-care, maintenance of function and prevention of further disability'.

It is valuable for us to develop our understanding of what it is like to live with a chronic illness because it will assist in our nursing assessment of the patient. Two important themes that seem to run through the various definitions of chronicity are the idea of the condition being permanent and that it alters the patient's awareness of his or her body. There is also a sense of *living with* the condition and being on a journey. This helps to put our interventions with patients into perspective and, as we now move on to consider the management of patients with chronic illnesses in primary care, you might want to consider how your actions could have an impact upon the patients' lived experience of their condition.

WORKING WITH PATIENTS WHO LIVE WITH A LONG-TERM CONDITION IN PRIMARY CARE

There is no doubt that a structured approach to working with people who live with a chronic condition will enhance the standard of care (DoH 2000). The structure needs to span the primary healthcare/hospital divide and should be flexible enough always to have at its centre the individual patient. The following discussion will outline the elements of a structured approach to care of the person with a long-term condition in primary health care and will go on to

consider the nursing skills that you can utilize with this specific group of patients.

SETTING UP A REGISTER

A starting point for working with patients who have long-term conditions is the development of a register of patients who have specific chronic conditions. If you work in a general practice, the patient population can be scanned to identify each individual who has a particular condition. If you are a health visitor attached to several practices, you can search your own caseload of children, for example, and identify how many of them have certain conditions. If the practice nurse finds that there are 40 patients with diabetes mellitus in her practice population when the total population is 2000, the prevalence of diabetes in that practice would be 2%. This is an important finding because we know that the national prevalence of diabetes mellitus in the UK is 3%; it can be as high as 10% in people over the age of 75 years and as much as 16% in the 40 to 65-year-old Asian population. If your practice seems to have a low prevalence of diabetes, it is worthwhile considering whether there are undiagnosed patients in the practice and therefore whether it is worth developing a screening programme to find the missing patients. Many practices now have well-developed registers for all their patients who live with long-term conditions such as heart disease, asthma and diabetes. Some registers will be less well developed because the presence of the condition may be less immediately obvious, for example osteoporosis or chronic obstructive airways disease.

The example of a practice profile in Table 5.1 demonstrates the interesting information that can be elicited when a register is compiled. The information shown was gathered after a search for patients with **chronic obstructive airways disease** had taken place at the surgery. The healthcare team used various approaches to identify patients who had chronic obstructive airways disease. A computer search was carried out to identify all the patients who were using inhalers and from this group of patients, those who had straightforward asthma were excluded. The healthcare team also had a working knowledge of who in their care had respiratory illness, and so this knowledge was used to identify further patients on the register. Eventually the numbers shown were presented as the practice register of people with chronic obstructive airways disease.

A list such as this, then, raises some important questions. We know that the national prevalence of chronic obstructive airways disease in the UK is 1.4% and yet the practice information shows a prevalence of 0.9%. This may be because this particular population does not have many risk factors for chronic obstructive airways disease and therefore the prevalence is low; it may also be because the patients with chronic obstructive airways disease have not been fully identified in the practice. It is also interesting to note that there is a higher prevalence of chronic obstructive airways disease in the male population when compared to the female

Table 5.1 Chronic obstructive pulmonary disease register

	Males	Females
Age group (years)		
0–44	0	0
45–54	2	0
55–64	2	1
65–74	4	9
75–84	10	2
85–89	2	0
>90	0	0
Total males	20	
Total females	13	
Total both sexes	33 (0.9%)	

population. Armed with such information the practice can now start to target high-risk patients for a series of health checks including spirometry and assessment of smoking status as there may be a number of patients in the practice with undiagnosed chronic obstructive pulmonary disease.

The register of people with a particular condition is not only valuable for identifying undiagnosed patients who, in the case of diabetes, might benefit greatly from early diagnosis and treatment, but is also useful for structuring and evaluating a programme of care. The programme of care will depend upon the nature of the condition. For people with **asthma**, for example, the patients may be recalled for an assessment in the asthma clinic on an annual basis, or for people who suffer with mental health problems a review of their records might take place at regular intervals to ensure that appropriate investigations have taken place for blood levels such as lithium and that a person has been identified as the main healthcare worker responsible for their care.

This information has become even more important with the development of national standards such as the National Service Frameworks (NSFs) for England and Wales. The NSFs outline national standards and, once a register of people with a particular condition has been created, an assessment can be made as to the level of care they are receiving. For example, the NSF for **coronary heart disease** states that 'general practitioners and primary healthcare teams should identify all people with established cardiovascular disease and offer them comprehensive advice and appropriate treatment to reduce their risks' (DoH 2000b, p. 4). Clearly it is important for the primary healthcare team to identify how many people have clinical evidence of occlusive arterial disease in the practice population and then to identify who these people are so that their treatment and the advice they

have received can be measured against the agreed national standards.

CALL/RECALL SYSTEMS

To manage the register of people effectively, a call/recall system should be developed. This can involve any member of the primary healthcare team; the important thing is that someone is identified as the person responsible for the system and that all members of the team involved in the care of people in a particular group feed back into the system. In the area of asthma, for example, the practice might have its own register of people who live with asthma. The health visitor might also know who in his or her caseload has been diagnosed with asthma, and the school nurse might have a similar register. The school nurse might also notice a child who seems to be short of breath in the playground and will refer potential new cases of asthma to the general practice.

The important issue is that someone in the team is reviewing the people with asthma at least annually. If the school nurse carries out the review, that information needs to be shared with the practice and the health visitor, and similarly, if the practice carries out the review, the fact that a review has taken place needs to be shared with the rest of the team. In some situations patients may be reviewed in secondary care. People with **rheumatoid arthritis**, for example, are often managed by specialist nurses and/or hospital consultants, and this information needs to be fed back to the general practice. It is important that the whole healthcare team communicates, and that for each condition someone is identified as the person responsible for maintaining the call/recall system.

People with the following types of chronic condition could benefit from a register and a call/recall system:

- thyroid disorders
- diabetes mellitus
- asthma
- chronic obstructive pulmonary disease
- epilepsy
- rheumatoid arthritis
- severe mental health problems
- coronary heart disease
- hypertension
- cerebrovascular disease.

EVALUATING THE PROGRAMME OF CARE

Once the register and the call/recall systems have been set up, you can readily evaluate your programme of care for a particular group of people by carrying out an audit. Indeed, if you are planning to introduce a new approach to clinical practice in your area it is valuable to carry out an audit before you implement the change. In this way you can identify areas of weakness before changes are made and you will be able to use the audit to evaluate how effective your intervention has been.

The main reason for carrying out an audit is to improve patient care. The patient should always be placed at the centre of the cycle of audit so that we do not lose sight of the reasons for carrying out this activity. Carrying out an audit can also help to educate everyone involved in the process; it can enhance teamwork and help people to understand one another's roles in more depth. Audit involves several steps, which are summarized as a cycle in Figure 5.3.

Assess need and choose a topic

The first step is to identify an area of clinical practice that needs to be evaluated through audit. You can make this choice in several ways. The subject area may come to you when a patient mentions something to you in practice. For example, a patient might comment that it seems to be a long time since he had his blood pressure checked. You look back in the notes and find that it is over 18 months since the last recorded **blood pressure** reading. This patient has a history of **cardiovascular disease** and during this consultation you find that his blood pressure is 160/95 mmHg. You are aware that the NSF for **coronary heart disease** (DoH 2000b) recommends that people with established cardiovascular disease should receive advice and treatment to maintain blood pressure below 140/85 mmHg, and you therefore become concerned that your primary healthcare team might be falling short of the national standards for health care.

Alternatively, you may identify an area for evaluation by reading about standards of health care in journals or in the publications from the national organizations. You may note that Diabetes UK recommends that all people who live with diabetes in the UK should expect to have their vision checked by an appropriately qualified healthcare professional at least once a year. You may then start to ask yourself whether your practice meets this standard; you can carry out an audit to check whether you meet this standard. These are examples of the ways in which you can implement evidence-based practice in the clinical setting.

Select the audit team

There is great value in approaching an audit from a team perspective. Various members of the team will have different suggestions to offer regarding the appropriate standards to use, the methods of collecting information, and methods for improving performance once the data have been collected. Audit can be as easy as pressing a button on a computer or it may require a trawl through many sets of patients' notes. This can be very time consuming and it may require several members of the audit team to assist with the retrieval of information. Involving the team also has the added benefit of raising the profile of whatever the subject area is and raising general awareness of the issue in the team.

Decide on criteria

A criterion is an item of care or some other aspect of clinical practice that we can use to assess quality. Each criterion should be recorded in a statement. The NSFs have helped to provide clear statements that serve as criteria for audit; for example, the coronary heart disease NSF (DoH 2000b) states that all people with clinical evidence of occlusive arterial disease should have advice and treatment to maintain their **blood pressure** below 140/85 mmHg. This is

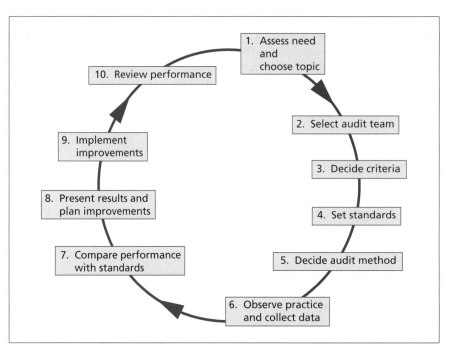

Figure 5.3 Audit cycle.

supported by the British Hypertension Society guidelines on the management of hypertension (Williams et al 2004). Your primary healthcare team could identify this as the criterion and record the statement that all people with clinical evidence of occlusive arterial disease should have their most recent blood pressure recorded as 140/85 mmHg or below.

Set standards

Once the criteria have been identified, the standards need to be agreed by the team. A standard is a statement of the proportion of occasions or patients that must fulfil the criteria. For example, in the example of blood pressure recordings in people with coronary heart disease the team might agree that the target should be set at 80%. The NSF states that the blood pressure target of 140/85 mmHg is challenging and it will not be possible to achieve this for every patient. Whilst it is acceptable, then, to set a standard that is less than 100%, practitioners should not be satisfied with any blood pressure recording over 150/90 mmHg. So the standards for the audit in this example might be recorded as '80% of the patients who are identified as having clinical evidence of occlusive arterial disease should have their most recent blood pressure recorded as 140/85 mmHg or below' and '100% of the patients who are identified as having clinical evidence of occlusive arterial disease should have their most recent blood pressure recorded as 150/90 mmHg or below'.

Decide on the audit method

Clearly the method of carrying out the audit will depend upon the subject area and the criterion chosen. In the example of blood pressure recordings and the group of patients with occlusive arterial disease, a computer search could be carried out to find all the people who have blood pressure recordings that fall within the acceptable range. If the audit had been focused upon the safe transport of specimens to the laboratory, the criterion might have been that all specimens should be securely placed in a sealed bag for transport to the laboratory, the standard set might have been 100% and then the audit method might involve a review of the specimens before they are handed to the person who will transport them to the laboratory. Each specimen could be checked for the way it had been packaged for transport and whether the bag had been sealed appropriately.

Observe practice and collect data

The team needs to decide for how long they are going to collect data and/or how many data they need to acquire in order to obtain an accurate reflection of what is actually happening in practice. In computerized systems it is quite straightforward to audit all the patients on the system, and therefore our example of blood pressure recordings and **cardiovascular disease** could be carried out on the whole practice population. However, when the audit is focused on something that is not readily available on the computer, the team may need to decide to look at a sample of the overall

population to gain a general impression of the standard of practice in that particular area. The question is how many instances of a particular practice does one need to observe in order to gain an accurate picture of the whole? This decision can be made by calculating the number of occurrences of the criterion, and then collecting data on the size of the sample required. In the example of the specimens for transport, the team might find that 2000 samples are sent to the laboratory annually. The team may decide to sample 10% of the specimens and would therefore need to collect data on the next 200 samples sent to the lab. It is clear that the larger the sample the more valid your results will be. You may therefore decide to sample 80% of people with diabetes when you are carrying out an audit of diabetes care, thus enhancing the validity of the results of your audit.

When you are collecting data you might also want to consider the time of year you carry out your audit. If, for example, you were looking at the use of **bronchodilators** in people with **asthma**, you might find that during the winter months there is a rise in the use of relief inhalers in this population, and again during times of high pollen counts the rate of inhaler use might increase. In a situation like this you may benefit from conducting an audit that runs over a whole year by taking the fourth week in every month to collect your data. It is important to be continually aware of threats to the accuracy of your audit. The results of your audit will inform your subsequent practice and therefore it is essential to make sure that the information you produce is accurate.

Compare performance with standards

Once the data have been collected, you are in a position to determine how close you are to the standards that you set yourself. If you find that only 50% of the people in the coronary heart disease group have a blood pressure of 140/85 mmHg or below, then you can start to search for reasons why this is so. If you find that 90% of the target group has a blood pressure in the desired range, you can be pleased that the team's performance measures up to the agreed standards; however, the cycle does not stop there.

Present results and plan improvements

An important part of the audit cycle is dissemination of your findings to other members of the team. You may choose to present the results in a report or to share your results at a meeting. Whatever the results, the team needs to be aware of them in order to analyse the findings and either seek to maintain the standard or work out a plan for improvement. If the results of your audit into blood pressure readings found that only 50% of the population had a **blood pressure** in the agreed range, the team could be invited to suggest reasons for this. It may be that people with cardiovascular disease are not systematically reviewed every 12 months, or it may be that the cardiovascular disease clinic is being held at inappropriate times for the people it is seeking to attract. It may be that not all healthcare professionals in the team were aware of the guidelines for the management of blood pressure in this particular group and were therefore not considering this group for rigorous treatment of hypertension. Whatever the reasons identified in an area such as this, it is most likely that there will be several approaches to improving care. These need to be identified by the team, agreed upon and a plan of action should be documented.

If you found that you exceeded the standard and that 90% of the target population had a blood pressure recording in the agreed zone, you might ask yourself whether this could be improved even further and adjust the standard to 95% on the next audit occasion. You might also try to identify areas of good practice that have allowed your team to reach such a good standard. This can then be shared with other primary healthcare teams, and your findings can be disseminated with a wider group so that others may learn from your good practice.

Implement improvements

The team then needs to decide how the plans are to be implemented. You may have identified the need for more flexible surgery times or the need for different members of the team to become involved in this area of practice. For example, the primary healthcare team may have thought that the GP had sole responsibility for the maintenance of blood pressure in the group of people with cardiovascular disease, when in fact your audit identified that several housebound people had blood pressures exceeding the target and these people were being visited regularly by the district nursing team. An improvement that could be implemented might be that the district nurses assess the patients' blood pressure when they visit them at home and that they record this reading in the practice notes and speak with the rest of the primary healthcare team if the recording exceeds the acceptable limit.

Review performance

Once you have implemented the planned changes you will need to revisit the audit to see whether you have really made a difference in practice. You might carry out the same audit and compare your findings with the previous audit, or you might focus on one area of practice that was highlighted as problematic in the first audit. The cycle of audit is continuous as we strive for more effective and efficient ways of working.

THE NURSE'S ROLE IN WORKING WITH PATIENTS WHO LIVE WITH A CHRONIC CONDITION

In addition to developing registers of people with chronic conditions, managing call/recall systems and ensuring that the existing provision meets agreed standards of care, there are many aspects of the nursing role that can have an impact upon the patients' experience of their condition. When you consider the uncertainty, stigma, grief, management of

treatment regimens and alteration in family relations that are characteristic of life with a chronic illness, you can see that your role as a nurse can have an enormous impact upon the patient in a variety of ways.

It is sad to note, however, that nurses do not appear to value working with patients whose conditions are not curable (Metcalfe 2005). Instead we seem to prefer to work with patients who will recover fully from their disease, and our actions with people who have a long-term condition are focused as though the patient was suffering from an acute episode of illness. Gibson and Kenrick (1998) studied a group of people who had peripheral **vascular disease** and found that the patients tended to think of the revascularization surgical approaches used as being curative and the medical team did nothing to refute this belief. In fact, the patients' vascular disease was not being cured, it was simply being managed temporarily, and therefore the patients needed to receive an approach to care that acknowledged the chronicity of their condition. Gibson and Kenrick (1998) concluded that this particular group of patients suffered from the inappropriate application of therapeutic approaches designed for use in acute episodes. It is possible that this is an example of the healthcare professionals' desire to work with people who have acute episodes of care rather than people who live with chronic conditions. As the numbers of people who live with chronic illness increase, it is possible that work in this area of practice will be recognized as a specialty in its own right. As this happens we will begin to appreciate that different approaches are required with this group of patients and nursing skills will be identified as being especially appropriate.

In your role as a nurse in primary care you have a great deal to offer a person who lives with a long-term condition. The ability to communicate effectively and to be able to listen to the patient's concerns can have a huge impact upon the patient and his or her family. When we make a nursing assessment of the patient with a long-term condition we need to consider the individual patient and alter our approach accordingly. It is important to remember that the patient has the most important role to play, as people who live with long-term conditions do most of the work associated with managing the illness themselves. There are, however, many roles we can take on in this situation; the exact nature of our role will be determined by the patient's individual needs at the time and the projected needs for the future. There is no doubt that we need to be clinically skilled in the area of disease management for that particular patient. When working with people who have continence problems, for example, there is no substitute for an in-depth knowledge of the management of continence and the clinical application of this knowledge. In addition to the specialist knowledge required it will also be important to be able to work effectively with patients who have general needs such as the acquisition of new knowledge and skills. One of the important roles we can play in this instance is the role of educator.

THE NURSE AS EDUCATOR

When a person is first diagnosed with a chronic condition they are likely to have many questions about their condition. People with diabetes might ask whether the condition is going to shorten their life, or people with asthma might want to know whether this will stop them playing sport. It is important that you discover the patient's beliefs and values, and what the most pressing questions are for him or her. An example of the particular and personal concerns of a patient who has been diagnosed with diabetes mellitus can be found in the critical incident at the end of this chapter. If you do not address the immediate questions, the patient will not be able to internalize any of the important self-care messages you might want to pass on, and the rest of the educative role becomes meaningless.

Bopp and Lubkin (1998) suggest that the teaching–learning process involves four phases: assessment, planning, implementation and evaluation (Fig. 5.4). The assessment process involves an analysis of the patient's readiness to learn. The critical incident provides an example of a patient who was not particularly ready to learn. You should also assess the patient's current knowledge about the condition, some of which might be inaccurate or based on experiences of friends or family. In working with patients who have a chronic condition it is also important to assess the family's desire to learn and the patient's willingness to include them in the process.

Planning the educational process involves deciding with the patient where and how the teaching will take place. At this point goals should be established and a period of review and evaluation can be determined.

The implementation stage of the process includes the actual act of teaching. This might take a variety of forms including one-to-one teaching in the home setting, self-directed learning through the use of the internet or other resources such as videos, leaflets, tapes or books, group sessions with local support groups, or informal learning through networks of family and friends.

After the implementation stage, evaluation of the educative process should take place. The patient and nurse can consider what the goals were at the outset and evaluate whether learning has occurred. This is part of the feedback loop and, if learning has not occurred, this information can form part of a further assessment before planning ongoing education. If learning has occurred, new goals can be set and the education can move on to different areas of interest.

When you are working with patients to educate them about their condition and its management, it is essential to remember that you are working with an individual and not a 'diabetic', an 'asthmatic' or an 'epileptic'. No two people with diabetes will be the same and part of your assessment at the outset must include an appreciation of the individual characteristics of the patient. It is particularly important to take note of the patient's culture, age, readiness to learn, language ability, reading ability and motivation to learn. The patient may also be experiencing physical barriers to learning, such as pain, decreased mobility, lack of energy, breathlessness or nausea. In this state of discomfort the patient will be limited to focusing on meeting immediate basic physical needs: he or she may, at this point, be less concerned about the potential long-term complications of the condition.

Bopp and Lubkin (1998) state that a patient might also experience emotional obstacles to learning. Patients may be in denial of the condition; they may be angry, depressed or withdrawn. Denial is one method of coping with a condition, particularly in the early days of diagnosis, and it is therefore important to acknowledge this and to work with the patient to accept the condition so that learning might take place at a later time. A summary of the potential barriers to learning is given in Box 5.3.

THE NURSE AS CHANGE AGENT

The diagnosis of a chronic illness results in the patient and his or her family members having to prepare to make changes in their lives. Corbin and Strauss (1992) developed

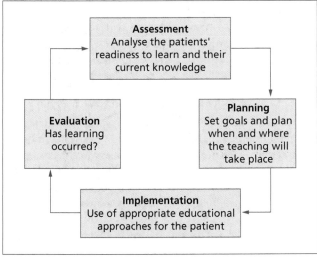

Figure 5.4 Teaching and learning process.

Box 5.3	Barriers to learning	
Physical	**Patient**	**Emotional characteristics**
Pain	Age	Denial
Shortness of breath	Culture	Anger
	Language ability	Depression
Poor vision	Reading ability	Anxiety
Poor mobility	Motivation to learn	Withdrawal
Poor hearing		
Nausea		
Lack of energy		

the trajectory model of chronic illness, which suggests that a person who has a chronic illness is on a journey that will present the patient with a variety of challenges along the way. In the same way that we identified barriers to education, Dixon (1998) points out that there may be barriers to change. Resistance to change is a most important problem that needs to be recognized in order for us to work effectively with the patient. People tend to resist change in order to maintain the status quo in their lives, and this can cause problems when change is forced upon a patient due to the nature of his or her disease. New and Couillard (1981) identified five reasons why individuals might resist change: threatened self-interest, inaccurate perceptions, objective disagreement, psychological reactance and low tolerance for change.

THREATENED SELF-INTEREST

If patients weigh up the cost of change and decide that it threatens their personal interests, they may become reluctant to make the change. An example of this might be when you work with a patient who has a respiratory problem, such as chronic obstructive **pulmonary disease**, and you are advising the patient to stop **smoking**. The patient considers how stopping smoking would affect his or her social life and the joy of sharing a cigarette with friends at the pub. The positive feelings associated with smoking could far outweigh the argument that shortness of breath is going to deteriorate over time if the patient does not stop smoking. In this case you would need to act in your role as change agent to point out as many benefits as possible for engaging in smoking cessation and try to eliminate the costs associated with stopping smoking, for example pointing out that the patient can still socialize with friends without using a cigarette as the focus.

INACCURATE PERCEPTIONS

If a patient has an inaccurate belief about a particular change it is less likely that the change will take place. For example, if a woman who has experienced a heart attack has a perception that exercising will put a strain on her heart and therefore do it some harm, she may avoid **exercise** and remain at home in the safety of her own surroundings. In this example you would have to work with the patient to find out what her perceptions and beliefs are. Once you had determined what she understood about heart disease and the effects of exercise, you could then begin to offer her some education and support to alter her perceptions of exercise and heart disease.

OBJECTIVE DISAGREEMENT

In some situations a patient might have accurate information that is in disagreement with the information you have in your role as nurse. It might be that the patient has alternative information to your own and you will need to explore this to determine whether the patient's approach is not going to cause any problems. An example of this might be the Buteyko breathing exercises that some patients with **asthma** use instead of salbutamol inhalers. This approach has been used in countries such as Russia and the information relating to it has been publicized in the UK. However, research into Buteyko breathing exercises is ongoing in this country to date, and you might find that you do not have the evidence to be able to support or discourage the patient in the use of this alternative approach. In a situation such as this you might need to share with the patient the best available evidence and be prepared to support the patient if a decision to use the breathing exercises is made.

PSYCHOLOGICAL REACTANCE

This describes the tendency of people to engage in behaviours that have been identified as problematic. For example, if you suggest to a young man with type 1 diabetes that drinking eight pints of beer at the weekend is going to create difficulties with **blood glucose** control, he might begin to think of this activity as even more desirable than he had previously. You might find that he has repeated episodes of hypoglycaemia due to the alcohol consumption followed by hyperglycaemia owing to the rebound effect following a hypoglycaemic episode. Often in situations involving psychological reactance, patients are unable to articulate why they are engaging in these risky behaviours, and this makes your task even more difficult because rational explanation will not help to persuade patients to alter their actions. It is important in examples such as this to continue to try to understand the patient's perspective and what his or her particular values and beliefs are concerning this behaviour. Continually encouraging the patient and reinforcing the messages you have been giving regarding the diabetes will gradually help to improve the chances of making a change in the patient's behaviour.

LOW TOLERANCE FOR CHANGE

Some people have more difficulty in dealing with change than others. A patient who has low self-confidence, poor self-esteem and a poor sense of self-efficacy may feel unable to engage in the change. An example of this might be a patient who completely understands the value of exercise in reducing the risks associated with hypertension; she or he is fully able to engage in exercise but seems resistant to making the change. This might result from low self-esteem and a low tolerance for uncertainty. In this case you can encourage the patient and support them at every opportunity and, when small changes are made, praise them for what they have achieved and gradually aim to enhance their self-respect and sense of self-reliance.

In addition to the five areas listed above, Dixon (1998) points out that *alienation* is another important reason why a person might be resistant to change. This refers to the

alienation between the patient and the nurse. There may be a huge gap between the client's experiential knowledge of a condition and the nurse's technical knowledge, so that the two are alienated from each other. This may result in conflict as the patient and the nurse do not understand one another. Factors that might lead to a situation of alienation include cultural, age or gender differences. You might find yourself encouraging a man to stop smoking when he has four great aunts in their nineties who have all smoked 20 cigarettes a day since they were 16. His personal experience will have provided strong messages that far outweigh the risks you might be discussing with him and therefore he will be reluctant to engage in changing his behaviour. Once again, you need to spend time understanding the patient's values and beliefs to help contextualize your messages.

SUMMARY

A recurring theme in working with patients who have chronic illnesses is the need to understand the perspectives of the patient and, on many occasions, the patient's family.

Without this, our messages are meaningless and we are unlikely to be successful in helping the patient adapt to the challenges associated with their particular condition. Assess the patient thoroughly before engaging in your nursing interventions and allow the patient time to talk to express worries and concerns. Ultimately the patient has the information you need to do your job effectively; if you provide the opportunity for open communication and develop a shared understanding, your chances of success will be increased. Nurses working in the primary healthcare setting have a great deal to offer patients who live with chronic illness, both in clinical skills and approaches to managing change and providing education.

REFERENCES

Blackie C (1998) Community healthcare nursing. Edinburgh: Churchill Livingstone.

Bleeker H, Mulderij K (1992) The experience of motor disability. Phenomenology and Pedagogy 10: 1–8. Cited in: Price B (1996) Illness careers: the chronic illness experience. Journal of Advanced Nursing 24: 275–279.

CRITICAL INCIDENT

A week after I had arranged for a series of blood and urine tests, I met with Mr A to discuss the results. The blood tests had confirmed our suspicions that he had type 2 diabetes mellitus. I asked him whether he knew what diabetes was; he said he knew very little and did not know anyone who had the disease. I explained what was happening and began to discuss the first line of management, which is to follow the general healthy-eating guidelines. I asked him to describe his usual pattern of eating and then I began to explain in detail the approach to dietary management. I was also aware that I needed to explain to him that he should have his eyes checked, feet assessed, a follow-up for determination of his blood sugar levels in 3 months' time, a referral to a dietician and careful monitoring of his blood pressure and cholesterol levels.

It was clear, though, that Mr A was distracted. After explaining the first steps of dietary management I asked him whether there was anything that was bothering him about the diagnosis. After a short silence he asked me: 'What does this mean? Am I going to die?'. We discussed his fears and concerns, and I returned to the explanation of diabetes and the importance of monitoring and treating raised blood glucose levels and blood pressure readings. I talked about the risks of complications and emphasized all that he could do to prevent their development. The consultation ended there with a plan to meet again in 2 weeks' time to see how he was managing with his dietary changes. My plan was to review some of the areas we had discussed during this consultation and to introduce some of the topics we had not covered on this first encounter.

Reflections

I felt that this consultation was fairly straightforward. The diagnosis of diabetes was expected and I felt competent to explain this to Mr A. I was aware that it is possible to overload patients with information when they are first given the diagnosis of diabetes and I was therefore attentive to the cues Mr A was giving off. I was quite taken aback by his question 'Am I going to die?' and, knowing the statistics on the mortality rates for people with diabetes, I felt lost for an immediate answer to his question. It would have been easy to say 'Of course not!', but I did not want to reassure him falsely. I was struck by the enormity of the question and realized that there was no way he could listen to what I was saying until we had discussed his fears and concerns regarding the impact of diabetes on his life.

Questions for reflection

- How might you break the news of the diagnosis of diabetes to a patient?
- What questions could you use to learn more about the patient's concerns?
- What support mechanisms are available to Mr A?
- What would be your plan for follow-up?
- Which members of the interdisciplinary team might you include in Mr A's care?
- Identify examples of communication skills that would be helpful in addressing Mr A's needs.

Bopp A, Lubkin I (1998) Teaching. In: Lubkin I, ed. Chronic illness impact and interventions, 4th edn. Sudbury, UK: Jones and Bartlett, p 343–361.

Bryar R, Bytheway B (1996) Changing primary health care. Oxford: Blackwell Science.

Cameron K, Gregor F (1987) Chronic illness and compliance. Journal of Advanced Nursing 12: 671–676.

Cook R (1999) A nurse's survival guide to primary care. Edinburgh: Churchill Livingstone.

Corbin JM, Strauss A (1992) A nursing model for chronic illness management based upon the trajectory framework. In: Woog P, ed. The chronic illness trajectory framework. New York: Springer, p 29–38.

Council for the Education and Training of Health Visitors (1977) An investigation into the principles of health visiting. London: CETHV. Cited in: Blackie C (1998) Community health care nursing. Edinburgh: Churchill Livingstone.

Curtin M, Lubkin I (1998) What is chronicity? In: Lubkin I, ed. Chronic illness impact and interventions, 4th edn. Sudbury, UK: Jones and Bartlett, p 3–25.

Department of Health (1987) Promoting better health. London: HMSO.

Department of Health (1989a) Caring for people. London: HMSO.

Department of Health (1989b) Working for patients. London: HMSO.

Department of Health (1996) Primary care: delivering the future. London: HMSO.

Department of Health (1997) The new NHS: modern, dependable. London: HMSO.

Department of Health (2000a) The NHS plan. A plan for investment, a plan for reform. London: HMSO. Online. Available: http://www.nhs.uk/nhs plan

Department of Health (2000b) Coronary heart disease national service framework. London: DoH.

Department of Health (2001) Shifting the balance of power in the NHS: Securing delivery. London: HMSO.

Department of Health (2003) Investing in general practice. The new GMS contract. London: HMSO.

Department of Health (2004) The NHS improvement plan: putting people at the heart of public services. London: HMSO.

Department of Health (2005) Supporting people with long-term conditions: liberating the talents of nurses who care for people with long-term conditions. London: HMSO.

Dixon E (1998) Change agent. In: Lubkin I, ed. Chronic illness: impact and interventions, 4th edn. Sudbury, UK: Jones and Bartlett.

Funk S, Tornquist M, Champagne MT, Wiese R, eds (1993) Key aspects of caring for the chronically ill. New York: Springer.

Gibson J, Kenrick M (1998) Pain and powerlessness: the experience of living with peripheral vascular disease. Journal of Advanced Nursing 27: 737–745.

Glendinning C, Dowling B (2003) Introduction: 'modernising the NHS'. In: Dowling B, Glendinning C. The new primary care. modern, dependable, successful? Berkshire: Open University Press, p 3-20.

Kelly MP, Field D (1996) Medical sociology, chronic illness and the body. Sociology of Health and Illness 18: 241–257.

Lyons RF, Sullivan MJL, Ritvo PG et al (1995) Relationships in chronic illness and disability. Thousand Oaks, CA: Sage.

Macdonald J (1992) Primary health care: medicine in its place. London: Earthscan.

Metcalfe, J (2005) The management of patients with long-term conditions. Nursing Standard 19(45): 53–60

Morse J, Borttorff J, Hutchinson S (1994) The phenomenology of comfort. Journal of Advanced Nursing 20: 189–195.

New JR, Couillard NA (1981) Guidelines for introducing change. In: Hein EC, Nicholson MJ, eds. Contemporary leadership behaviour: selected readings, 2nd edn. Boston: Little Brown. Cited in: Lubkin I (1998) Chronic illness impact and interventions, 4th edn. Sudbury, UK: Jones and Bartlett.

Nursing and Midwifery Council (2005) Specialist community public health nursing. Online. Available: http://www.nmc-uk.org/ (n40go255h0t4a4esdcgvvjet)/aSection.aspx?SectionID=29 28 Oct 2005.

Pritchard P, Pritchard J (1994) Teamwork for primary and shared care, 2nd edn. Oxford: Oxford Medical Publications.

Thomas, S (2005) Supporting people with long-term conditions. Primary Health Care 15(1): 13–14.

Verbrugge LM, Jette AM (1994) The disablement process. Social Science and Medicine 38(1): 1–14.

Vuori H (1986) Health for all, primary health care and general practitioners (keynote address), WONCA, 1986. Cited in: Cook R (1999) A nurse's survival guide to primary care. Edinburgh: Churchill Livingstone.

Williams B, Poulter NR, Brown MJ et al (2004) The BHS guidelines working party. British Hypertension Society guidelines for hypertension management, 2004 - BHS IV: summary. British Medical Journal 328: 634–640.

World Health Organization (1978) Report of the international conference on primary health care, Alma Ata, USSR. Geneva: WHO. Cited in: Cook R (1999) A nurse's survival guide to primary care. Edinburgh: Churchill Livingstone.

World Health Organization (2005) Diabetes programme. Country and regional data. Online. Available: http://www.who.int/ diabetes/facts/world_figures/en/ 28 Oct 2005.

FURTHER READING

Blackie C (1998) Community healthcare nursing. Edinburgh: Churchill Livingstone.

This book explores the meaning of primary health care, describes the NHS reforms and explains the organization of community care. It is a useful text for community nurses and student nurses as it addresses the core knowledge for nurses who work in the community setting.

Cook R (1999) A nurse's survival guide to primary care. Edinburgh: Churchill Livingstone.

This is a pocket-sized guide to primary healthcare nursing which addresses a range of issues of relevance to both student nurses and qualified staff. The book covers major policy issues, key principles of clinical care, information relating to the range of agencies operating in primary care, and valuable insights into health promotion and public health.

Crumbie A, Lawrence J (2001) Living with chronic illness. A practitioner's guide. Oxford: Butterworth Heinemann.

This book aims to equip the healthcare practitioner with the necessary knowledge and skills to manage the impact of chronicity on patients' lives. Section one is focused on developing an understanding of what it is like to live with a chronic condition and the ways in which healthcare professionals can enhance sensitivity to patients. Section two focuses on

specific chronic diseases, providing an overview of the epidemiology, pathophysiology, assessment and treatment options for the patient with that particular condition.

Lubkin I (1998) Chronic illness – impact and interventions, 4th edn. Sudbury, UK: Jones and Bartlett.

This text covers a wide range of issues that influence clients and families who are living with chronic illness. Sociological, psychological, ethical, organizational and financial aspects of chronicity are dealt with in depth. A case study approach is used to add relevance to the clinical environment and to illustrate ways in which healthcare professionals can contribute to the care of people who live with chronic illness.

Lyons RF, Sullivan MJL, Ritvo PG et al (1995) Relationships in chronic illness and disability. Thousand Oaks, CA: Sage.

This book provides a series of valuable papers focused on the dynamics of relationships of people who live with chronic illness. The impact of chronic illness on interpersonal relationships is explored and interventions such as relationship-focused coping are examined.

Key clinical principles

INTRODUCTION

Specific medical diagnostic labels become attached to patients as they make their way through the complex and increasingly specialised world of modern health care. However, several problems are common to many patients regardless of whether they are under the care of a general practitioner, orthopaedic surgeon or cardiologist. This section will address these broad themes of pain management, principles of pharmacology and infection control.

The ability to transfer and adapt skills from one clinical environment to another is an essential characteristic of high-quality nursing care. The clinical themes outlined in this section will run through the rest of the book when specific conditions are discussed in a broadly systematic way. You will therefore find it useful to refer back to this section to reflect upon both your clinical experience and to expand the more detailed content of subsequent chapters. You should also remember that the principles discussed in these chapters apply with just as much validity in primary care settings as they do in the acute hospital.

Principles of pharmacology

Helen L. Leathard

INTRODUCTION

Pharmacology is the study of *drugs*. A comprehensive definition of drugs is that they are chemicals that can influence the functioning of the body or its constituent tissues. In this sense hormones and neurotransmitters are included along with substances that we would normally think of as drugs, i.e. those that are foreign to the body and are produced by different organisms or by chemical synthesis. A medicine is a drug formulated for medical use, and many drugs are used in medicines. Some other substances that are classed as drugs are used recreationally or misused, some are used in the investigation of physiological processes, and others are toxins found in the environment. In this chapter, however, we will concentrate on the basic principles of those aspects of pharmacology that are relevant to nursing.

The term *pharmacotherapy* is often used to refer to the therapeutic use of medicines in the treatment of patients who are acutely ill, and the prophylactic use of drugs to reduce the frequency of recurrence and/or the severity of symptoms in chronic relapsing conditions such as asthma, peptic ulcer and inflammatory bowel disease. The term pharmacotherapy is also used to refer to hormonal contraception and **menopausal** hormone therapies used by healthy people; but not recreational or abusive taking of drugs. The pharmacological principles discussed in this chapter apply equally well to all drugs, regardless of the purpose for which they are used.

The sequence in which we will cover the pharmacological content is unconventional but appropriate to the requirements for nursing practice. First, we consider how active drugs are administered and reach their intended site or sites of action. Second, we explore quite simply the various ways in which drugs can cause their actions and effects in the body and, third, we discuss ways in which the actions and effects of drugs are terminated by inactivation and elimination from the body. Specificity and selectivity of drug action are key features of the effectiveness and safety profile of any medicine. Adverse and unwanted effects of individual agents and the problem of drug interactions in people taking more than one medicine are, therefore, examined in separate sections. First of all let us look at the relationship of pharmacology to nursing practice.

PHARMACOLOGY AND NURSING PRACTICE

The administration of medicines has, for a long time, been an important part of registered nurses' practice that requires thought and the exercise of professional judgement (NMC 2002). Key roles can be grouped in three clusters:

- *Appropriate administration*: confirming the correctness of the prescription and judging the suitability of administration at the scheduled time
- *Patient support*: reinforcing positive effects of treatment and enhancing patients' and their carers' understanding of prescribed medication, so minimizing the risk of misuse of medicines
- *Evaluation of treatment*: helping assess the effectiveness of medication and recognition of adverse effects or interactions in individual patients.

More recently in the UK, *group protocols* (Box 6.1) for the supply and administration of medicines and, for appropriately qualified nurses, prescribing from a Nurse Prescribers' Formulary (since 1998) and an Extended Nurse Prescribers' Formulary (since 2001) have been introduced (DoH 2005). Sound understanding of relevant pharmacology is required to underpin these aspects of professional practice. With the exception of those specifically entitled to prescribe, nurses

Box 6.1 Group protocol

This is a specific written instruction for the supply or administration of named medicines in an identified clinical situation. It is drawn up locally by doctors, pharmacists and other appropriate professionals, and approved by the employer, advised by the relevant professional advisory committees. It applies to groups of patients or other service users who may not be individually identified before presentation for treatment.

(Data from Crown 1999, Department of Health 2005, p. 79)

Box 6.2 Gaining knowledge about pharmacology

Ives et al (1996) studied the actual and self-rated pharmacology knowledge of first year registered, graduate nurses in Victoria, Australia, using a postal questionnaire. The findings demonstrated that there was a very wide range of extent of knowledge of pharmacology as assessed by multiple choice questions (test scores ranged from 16% to 92%), with respondents who had participated in a graduate-year programme attaining higher test scores than those who had not. The means by which their pharmacology education had been delivered varied considerably and respondents valued their practical, clinical experience more highly than theory sessions as a means of gaining knowledge, emphasizing the importance of relating theory to practice.

Their ability to assess this is, however, questionable because self-rating of their knowledge correlated with their test scores only in relation to therapeutic effects. They overestimated their knowledge of drug administration and legal aspects by considerable margins and somewhat overestimated their knowledge of adverse effects, but underestimated their knowledge in relation to client education. These findings can, therefore, be interpreted as demonstrating that clinical experience reinforces learning of those topics that are subject to discussion and critical appraisal in the workplace. Experience has less impact, however, on topics where competence is assumed but is less subject to scrutiny by colleagues or clients.

may only supply and administer under a group protocol or administer according to a medical prescription.

Pharmacology education requirements differ between groups of nurses, and people's requirements will depend partly upon their current employment and partly upon their career ambitions. In this short chapter I aim to provide an account of the basic principles of what I like to refer to as 'nursing pharmacology' – those aspects that are relevant to nursing practice. This is analogous to, but not identical with, clinical pharmacology – a medical specialty involving the application of pharmacology for individual patients consequent upon diagnosis, and integrated within care plans that include other therapies; or clinical investigations of new drugs as potential medicines. The application of these basic principles in nursing will be illustrated in Section 3 of this book, where particular types of medicines are included as aspects of the care provided for various groups of patients.

To provide good patient support in relation to medicines, nurses require sound and comprehensive knowledge of the actions and effects of all medicines being taken by patients in their care. They also need to know about common, clinically significant, interactions between drugs, and the reasons for which the medicines are used. Integral to this is broad familiarity with the durations of courses of treatment (for the foreseeable future, fixed-duration course or as required), dose frequency and what to do when one or more doses is or are missed. Such broad knowledge needs to be based upon secure understanding of the principles of *pharmacokinetics* (how bodies handle drugs) and *pharmacodynamics* (how drugs act upon bodies). Although retention of detailed information on a wide range of drugs is not feasible, nurses might reasonably have comprehensive understanding of medicines that are commonly encountered in their particular practice and the ability to look up appropriate information about others.

Some sound and relevant research demonstrates clearly that more pharmacology education correlates with better knowledge (Box 6.2) and clinical practice (Box 6.3). This work has been followed up by Grandell-Niemi et al (2005) who have shown that pharmacological skills continue to increase in post-registration clinical practice and have argued

Box 6.3 Applying knowledge in clinical practice

Jordan and Hughes (1998) have published a very substantial study of the impact on nursing practice of a part-time post-registration diploma in nursing in Wales, which included 100 taught hours of applied physiology that clearly included pharmacology. Examples taken from 'academic diaries' kept by their subjects for 6 months (recording instances of the course affecting working practices), together with findings from questionnaires and interviews, demonstrated that most students were applying their new knowledge in practice. Their participation in interprofessional discussions and team decisions increased, as did their ability to understand, assess and question medical decisions. It was evident that the quality of their caring for patients improved.

that this increase is necessary for safe and effective administration of medicines. Allied with this is the finding of Banning (2005) that nurse prescribers have varying degrees of understanding of research and evidence-based practice. She argued, therefore, that their education needs to include work on randomized controlled trials and more naturalistic studies of the effectiveness of medicines. In recognition of these professional requirements, in this chapter I aim to provide the basic information that can underpin the development of the pharmacological expertise that is necessary for safe and effective medicines-related practice.

The *British National Formulary* (BNF, see Further reading), or its equivalent outside the UK, is a widely available, standard source of information about currently available medicines. It is a reference book for prescribers and includes the use of many specialist technical terms without explaining their meaning. Medical education engenders ready familiarity with and good understanding of this clinical pharmacological language. Nurses, too, are increasingly using the BNF as a reference book, so this chapter will provide clear explanations of the requisite specialist terminology.

The limited familiarity of most nurses with chemistry can be a great cause of anxiety in their approach to the study of pharmacology, and yet it is unrealistic to argue the case for extensive study of this subject as a prerequisite to a career in nursing. In this chapter the principles of pharmacology will be discussed as simply as possible from the chemical point of view. The chapter on **chemistry** in Montague et al (2005) provides appropriate background information.

CLASSIFICATION AND NAMING OF MEDICINES

Medicines are known by a mixture of therapeutic, pharmacological and chemical classifications. None is perfect and various combinations are in common usage. The BNF uses primarily a therapeutic classification, but many drugs appear in multiple sections. Pharmacological classifications are really helpful because they serve as concise reminders of mechanisms of action and this can act as a key to recall of actions and effects. The chemical classifications are the most difficult for those without extensive understanding of organic chemistry, and chemical names tend to be used as labels without full understanding of their meaning. In practice, what is needed is familiarity with all the classifications in common usage, such as: opioid analgesics, non-steroidal anti-inflammatory drugs or benzodiazepine anxiolytics.

It is also important to remember the difference between *drugs* and *medicines*, as explained on p. 00. The distinction between *non-proprietary (generic or approved) names* of medicines (which specify the active ingredients, and are the names under which medicines appear in the BNF) and *proprietary (brand or trade) names* (which specify a particular pharmaceutical company's product) is also important. A useful indication of the status of a medicine's name is that non-proprietary names are treated as common nouns and have a capital initial letter only where they start a sentence. Brand names are treated as proper nouns and always have a capital initial letter and often some indication that the name is a registered trademark. For example, paracetamol is a non-proprietary (generic, British approved) name, whereas

Panadol® is one particular company's brand of paracetamol. Generically named drug combinations have their name prefixed by 'co-' (combination), which draws attention to the complex nature of the medicine. Thus, co-codamol 8/500 and co-codamol 30/500 are generic names for combinations of 8 or 30 mg codeine respectively with paracetamol (500 mg). Proprietary products with the lower codeine content are available over the counter (OTC) either by the generic name, co-codamol, or as Panadeine®, Paracodol® or Parake®, whereas those with the higher codeine content are prescription-only medicines (POMs) and are marketed by different pharmaceutical companies as Kapake®, Solpadol® and Tylex®.

An individual drug may be marketed in a variety of formulations and doses under a range of brand names. Continuing the above example, paracetamol oral suspension 120 mg per 5 mL (Paediatric Mixture) is marketed by this generic name or as Cupanol® Paediatric, sugar-free; Disprol® Paediatric, sugar-free; Panadol,® sugar-free; Calpol® Paediatric or Calpol® Paediatric, sugar-free. Conversely, a single brand-named medicine may contain multiple active drug ingredients, any one of which may be a source of adverse effects or interactions. Typical contents of 'cold and flu remedies' are paracetamol (antipyretic analgesic), pholcodine (antitussive, mild analgesic) and pseudoephedrine (nasal decongestant) with the addition of a sedative antihistamine for night-time use or caffeine for daytime alertness.

ADMINISTRATION, ABSORPTION AND DISTRIBUTION OF MEDICINES, AND BIOAVAILABILITY

The essentials of nursing practice in relation to the administration of medicines are summarized in Box 6.4. In the present chapter we will cover the pharmacological principles that enable understanding and make links between the practice of administration of medicines and the theory of how the active drugs reach their sites of action. Separate sections are devoted to administration for local action and administration for systemic action. There is an additional short section on drug access to the central nervous system because of its distinctive features and clinical significance.

Box 6.4 Administration of medicines

The administration of a medicine involves giving:

- the correct dose
- to the correct patient
- in the correct formulation
- by the correct route
- at appropriate time intervals.

BASIC PRINCIPLES: FACTORS INFLUENCING DRUG MOVEMENT

The pharmacological principles are founded in physiology because, as we shall see, drug molecules enter (or are prevented from entering) the body or specific body compartments in just the same way as other molecules. A sound understanding of the properties of cell surface membranes and the functioning of various epithelia, gastrointestinal and circulatory systems, blood and the blood–brain barrier is an essential prerequisite. Relevant information can be found in textbooks such as Montague et al (2005).

Types of cells and tissues through which drug molecules might need to pass include:

- **epithelia**, such as the gastrointestinal mucosa or the skin
- **vascular endothelium**, which is more or less permeable in different tissues, being quite readily permeable in the **gastrointestinal** mucosa and liver, but nearly impermeable in the **central nervous system** - contributing to the **blood–brain barrier**
- **connective tissues**, especially areolar tissues and the blood.

Drug molecules move down concentration gradients from higher to lower concentrations, generally by simple diffusion. In principle they can pass through or between cells, but in practice the passage of molecules between cells (the intercellular route) is rare or constitutes only a very small proportion of drug movement. Exceptions occur in the immature gastrointestinal mucosa of infants or where **capillary permeability** is enhanced by an inflammatory reaction.

Most commonly the movement of drug molecules into and within the body depends upon their ability to cross **cell membranes**. This is determined by the phospholipid bilayer structure of the cell surface membranes and by the chemistry of the drug molecules. As noted above, we are familiar with cell membrane structure and functioning from studying the physiology of cells, so here we need to consider the properties of drug molecules that influence their ability to cross the cell membranes. The two most important factors are *size* and *solubility*.

Size

Small molecules with suitable solubility properties can cross membranes much more readily than larger molecules of similar solubility. Molecules with very low molecular masses, such as water (H_2O = 18), oxygen (O_2 = 32) or nitric oxide, which is the active molecule released from nitrovasodilator drugs (NO = 30), move freely across biological membranes. In contrast, molecules with a mass of around 1000 or greater do not, regardless of their solubility properties. Specific biochemical transporters or mechanisms such as **endocytosis** and **exocytosis** are required to move these large molecules into and out of cells. Endocytosis involves the plasma membrane of the cell forming a vesicle that engulfs the molecule and transports it into the cell, while exocytosis involves vesicles moving molecules out of a cell by fusing with the plasma membrane then opening outwards to release the molecules on the outside of the cell.

Solubility

Between these extremes of size, it is the solubility of drug molecules in water and lipid at pHs encountered in the body that determines their ability to diffuse across cell membranes. Hydrophilic (water attracting, water soluble) molecules dissolve readily in intracellular and extracellular fluids but are unable to cross cell membranes unless they also have lipophilic (lipid attracting, lipid soluble) properties that enable them to dissolve in the lipid of the cell membranes. Equally, hydrophobic (water repelling, lipophilic) molecules dissolve readily in cell membrane lipid but are unable to dissolve in and move through the aqueous intracellular and extracellular body fluids unless they also have hydrophilic properties.

Drug molecules, like many natural hormones and neurotransmitters, combine these properties. Without going into chemical detail, this is achieved by them being relatively small molecules with a covalently bonded core consisting of atoms held together by sharing electrons. This arrangement confers lipophilic properties on the molecule. Attached to this core are various 'functional' groups that confer various degrees of water solubility. This combination of chemical properties enables most clinically used drug molecules to access the systemic circulation when administered by various routes, although the ability to cross membranes varies considerably between drug molecules, influencing their ability to penetrate into the central nervous system (CNS) and their susceptibility to metabolism and excretion. In some cases chemical 'anchors' are attached to active drug molecules to restrict their freedom of movement. For example, propionate additions help retain inhaled corticosteroids within the respiratory tract, and decanoate, palmitate or enantate additions retain antipsychotic and contraceptive agents, respectively, within oily intramuscular depots.

Blood flow

The rate of **blood flow** through various tissues, and the possible influences upon this of ageing and some diseases, can have a marked influence on drug absorption from subcutaneous and intramuscular injection sites, from applications to the skin and from the gastrointestinal tract. Vigorous exercise, for example, by increasing cutaneous blood flow, can increase the rate of absorption of insulin from subcutaneous sites, raising the blood level of the hormone and possibly leading to **hypoglycaemia**. In contrast, many elderly people who are ill and in pain have very poor cutaneous blood flow. Transdermal absorption of the analgesic fentanyl from patches can be impaired by this, leading to inadequate analgesia. Similarly, migraine is known to reduce gastrointestinal mucosal blood flow and this then impairs the absorption and, therefore, the effectiveness of migraine medication taken orally.

ADMINISTRATION FOR LOCAL ACTION

One way of achieving selectivity in the action of a drug is to administer the medicine locally to its desired site of action on or in:

- eyes
- ears
- nose
- respiratory system
- mouth and throat
- gastrointestinal system
- urinary system
- uterus or vagina
- skin and/or scalp
- cerebrospinal fluid
- other locations.

The main advantage of local application is that it is possible to achieve a pharmacologically active concentration of the drug at its intended site of action without causing unwanted or adverse effects by raising concentrations elsewhere in the body. For example, chemicals that are quite toxic can be used to kill parasites such as head lice, scabies or intestinal worms without poisoning the person needing the treatment. Similarly, corticosteroid drugs can be taken quite safely by the inhalation route for the treatment of asthma. The risk of harmful side-effects such as adrenal suppression, immuno-suppression and an increased risk of osteoporosis, which could occur with systemic administration for extended time periods, can be avoided in this way.

In the sections that follow we will consider the pharmacological principles relating to local actions in the respiratory and gastrointestinal systems, and on the skin. These principles can then be applied by the reader to the localization of drug action elsewhere.

Respiratory system

There are two main aspects to achieving local action within the **respiratory system** for treatment of conditions such as **asthma** where the available drugs could produce marked or even severe unwanted effects if given systemically. One of these is to get the active agent to its site of action on the bronchial mucosa and smooth muscle, and the other is to prevent it from being removed too quickly by the pulmonary circulation. To enable the drug to reach the bronchial mucosa it needs to be inhaled as strongly as possible. *Metered dose inhalers* (MDIs) are delivery devices that help with this, but their use does need to be coordinated carefully with the timing of inhalation if an effective proportion of the active medication is to reach the bronchus rather than simply be deposited in the mouth, swallowed and inactivated. The need for skill in coordinating inhalation and MDI usage is reduced by use of *spacer devices* (used with MDIs) and *nebulizers*, but these have the disadvantage that they are cumbersome.

Diffusion of drugs from the respiratory system into the pulmonary circulation can be disadvantageous for two distinct reasons. One is loss of medication from its desired site of action resulting in reduced duration of action, which makes it necessary to give the medicine more frequently. Reduced intensity can also be compensated for by increasing the dose. The other is the risk of adverse effects on other tissues if the active agent is not sufficiently diluted in the blood to render it inactive. Acute palpitations from use of β_2-adrenoceptor stimulants (e.g. salbutamol) and long-term adverse effects of corticosteroids in asthma sufferers are problems the pharmaceutical companies have succeeded in reducing considerably. One key to success has been the use of molecules with structures that restrict their ability to diffuse across cell membranes, such as beclometasone dipropionate. Another solution has been to devise molecules, such as fluticasone propionate, that are very rapidly inactivated by the liver so that they do not persist in the general circulation. This also solves the problem of safe disposal of any fraction that is swallowed and absorbed from the gastrointestinal tract.

Gastrointestinal system

Although many medicines that are taken orally and swallowed are intended to reach the general circulation by being absorbed from the **gastrointestinal tract**, various ulcer-healing agents, laxatives and anthelmintics, among others, are taken orally for local action within the gut. The gut has evolved to absorb a wide range of molecular types for nutrition, so drugs that are retained within the tract or absorbed to a minimal extent are characteristically large or strongly hydrophilic (with poor lipid solubility), or both. Those taken for action in the stomach or duodenum are at risk of being flushed away very quickly by digestive secretions so they need to be administered in some way that helps them to coat and bind to the mucosal surface. Thick liquid formulations are efficacious.

With medications taken for their action within the colon there is likely to be a delay of at least 4–6 hours before they produce any effect, and this needs to be borne in mind when choosing suitable times for their administration. Lactulose and senna, for example, are relatively inert in the upper gastrointestinal tract and their effectiveness depends upon the release of active products by the action of colonic bacteria. This is why at least 6–8 hours usually elapses before the urge to defaecate is stimulated, and why these agents should be administered either at bedtime or early morning but not late afternoon or evening. The need for these drugs to be activated by colonic bacterial action explains why their effectiveness can be impaired by a course of antibacterial drug therapy.

Skin and scalp

The same factors that influence the passage of drugs across cell membranes also influence the rate and extent of their penetration into and through the **skin**, although the skin is thicker and a more effective waterproof barrier. Because of this, water-based treatments for skin parasites pose minimal risks of systemic toxicity, and they can be removed by washing (or bathing) after the specified treatment period.

Treatments for inflammatory skin conditions such as eczema and psoriasis are generally applied as creams or oily lotions because these are partly absorbed into the epidermis and remain at their sites of action for reasonable periods without being rubbed off on to clothing. When they are removed by hand washing, they need to be reapplied. Corticosteroids and other lipid-soluble skin treatments tend to diffuse into the local blood vessels and thence into the systemic circulation. The risk of pharmacologically active concentrations being reached elsewhere in the body is minimal so long as recommended doses are adhered to.

ADMINISTRATION FOR SYSTEMIC ACTION

Systemic action is a widely used shorthand phrase to denote the potential access of drug molecules to all organs and tissues that are nourished directly from the circulatory system. It excludes the CNS, which is protected to a large extent from bloodborne chemicals by the blood–brain barrier. Routes of administration for systemic action are generally subdivided into *enteral* and *parenteral*. Other specialist routes are beyond the scope of this chapter. There are differences of opinion between various authorities as to which group some routes belong to. The classification below is that of Bennett and Brown (2003). Enteral routes include:

- oral
- buccal
- sublingual
- rectal.

Parenteral (not enteral) routes include:

- intravenous
- intramuscular
- subcutaneous
- transdermal.

Oral administration

Oral administration refers to medicine being swallowed and absorbed from the gastrointestinal tract (mainly the small intestine). It is the most widely used route of administration for both prescribed and OTC medicines. Its greatest advantages lie in its familiarity, convenience and acceptability to most people and its suitability for most drugs. There is often a choice between solid (tablets, capsules, caplets) and liquid (syrup, elixir) formulations to suit people of differing ages and with differing abilities to swallow solids. *Sustained-release formulations* of some medicines are also available (Box 6.5).

The challenges to reaching effective blood concentrations by this route lie in the body's defence mechanisms against ingested foreign materials and the **digestive processes**. Nausea and vomiting are common reflex responses to the ingestion of foreign substances and serve to protect against poisoning. Because of this, the first few days of treatment with a wide range of medicines can cause nausea, with or without vomiting, in susceptible individuals, but normally subsides with continued usage.

Box 6.5   Sustained-release formulations

Desirable frequencies of administration for orally administered drugs are between one and three times a day, whereas many medicines, when given in safe dosages, have durations of action of only a few hours. Sustained-release formulations that retain part of a relatively large dose of a drug within the gastrointestinal tract for several hours enable twice-daily administration of medicines. These help patients who need to take one or more medicines over extended periods to accommodate these within a relatively normal lifestyle. Excessive dose frequency can impact negatively on a patient's ability to adhere to their treatment even when *concordance* (agreement on treatment) has been achieved during a consultation.

Gastric acid provides a powerful defence against ingested bacteria but inactivates some drugs, such as benzylpenicillin, which would be ineffective if administered by the oral route. Similarly, digestive enzymes are essential for our ability to absorb nutrients from proteins, carbohydrates and lipids, but these will also break down and inactivate protein, carbohydrate and lipid medicines, such as insulin, heparin and natural prostaglandins, which cannot, therefore, be administered orally.

Once absorbed across the intestinal mucosa into the bloodstream, the drug molecules are carried by the **portal venous system** to the **liver**, where varying proportions of the ingested dose are subject to metabolic transformations, as discussed in the section on inactivation, metabolism and elimination (see p. 108). From an evolutionary perspective these are detoxification reactions through which the liver provides protection from foreign substances. Only after surviving into the hepatic vein do orally administered drugs become available for systemic action. The terms *first-pass metabolism* or *first-pass effect* are used to refer to the inactivation of orally administered drugs before they reach the systemic circulation.

The proportion reaching the systemic circulation is quantified as the *oral bioavailability*. It is expressed as a percentage of the dose given. For some drugs there is considerable interpatient variation in the factors that affect their oral bioavailability, either genetically determined (such as differences in liver enzymes) or influenced by disease. This can necessitate careful *titration* (adjustment according to effect) of doses to achieve the best balance between beneficial and adverse effects in individual patients. Once orally administered drugs reach the systemic circulation, the rate at which they reach their sites of action will depend on the blood flow to target areas and upon their ability to cross the vascular endothelium and any other tissue barriers.

If drugs are taken orally on a fairly empty stomach their action can commence in as little as 15–20 minutes, although it will continue to increase for at least 1–2 hours. The absorption of drugs can be delayed and extended significantly if medicines are taken on a full stomach. Some medicines, such as oral flucloxacillin, need to be taken on an empty stomach to ensure full effectiveness, whereas others such as the non-steroidal anti-inflammatory drugs are best taken with food to minimize the risk of dyspepsia.

Buccal or sublingual administration

These terms refer to medications being retained in the mouth or under the tongue for local effect or to enable their rapid absorption directly into the bloodstream without being subject to first-pass metabolism. It is the second of these that concerns us here. Glyceryl trinitrate is a commonly encountered example of a drug administered in this way. It is available as tablets or aerosol spray (which can be sprayed into a patient's mouth by a carer if necessary) for rapid relief of anginal symptoms.

Rectal administration

This route of administration seems to be much less popular in the UK than in continental Europe, for sociocultural reasons rather than pharmacological ones. It provides a non-invasive route for quite rapid absorption of drugs into the bloodstream for patients who are unable to take oral medication due to vomiting, migraine or inability to swallow. A proportion of the rectal venous drainage, which varies between individuals, is independent of the hepatic portal system. This contributes to quite variable blood levels of drugs that are subject to substantial first-pass metabolism, with attendant risks of ineffectiveness and toxicity. A further disadvantage of this route for regular medication is the risk of causing local inflammation.

Intravenous administration

Medicines that are given intravenously reach the systemic circulation immediately and without any loss due to metabolism or barriers to diffusion. *Injection* or *continuous infusion* can be used, depending on the duration of action required. This route can be used for volumes that are too large for subcutaneous or intramuscular injection, but care needs to be taken to ensure that large doses of potentially cardiotoxic agents are given slowly enough to allow for adequate dilution in the blood before they reach the heart. Sterile precautions are required to avoid risk of infection at the site of injection.

Intramuscular administration

The intramuscular route of administration carries lower risks of cardiotoxicity and systemic infection than the intravenous route and yet can provide rapid onset of drug action because of the good blood flow through commonly used gluteal muscles or those of the upper arm. For example, it is used for opioid analgesics, antiemetics and antimicrobial drugs when rapid and reliable action is desirable. Because of the scarcity of pain-sensitive nerves in skeletal muscle, mildly irritant drugs can be given by this route. Also, volumes somewhat larger than are suitable for subcutaneous injec-

tion may be used. The intramuscular route is unsuitable for self-administration because of its inherent risks, although some patients, such as those with Addison's disease, may be taught to give their own intramuscular injections in emergency situations.

In addition to providing for rapid onset of action, the intramuscular route can provide for prolonged drug action through the use of depot injections. The active drug molecules or their formulations (or both) are modified to ensure very slow release of active molecules into the systemic circulation. Some antipsychotic drugs and contraceptive progestogens can be given at fortnightly or longer intervals. One disadvantage is that drugs given in this way cannot be removed if adverse reactions occur.

Subcutaneous administration

Small volumes of non-irritant formulations can be injected or infused just under the skin to achieve quite rapid systemic effects. The rate of onset of action is influenced by local blood flow, and exercise can alter the rate of absorption into the circulation. This is the least invasive route available for protein- and carbohydrate-based drugs such as insulin and heparins, and is considered suitable for self-administration by people who have received appropriate training. The duration of action, and therefore the frequency of injections, depends on the form and vehicle in which the active agent is injected. This route is commonly used for insulins and for patient-controlled analgesia.

Transdermal administration

The **skin** forms a relatively impermeable barrier to many drugs, but lipophilic molecules can penetrate the skin in suitable conditions. Transdermal administration, from *patches* (adherent occlusive dressings), which release the active drug over extended time periods, is increasingly being introduced as a means of achieving relatively constant blood levels and avoiding first-pass metabolism of susceptible drugs without requiring infusions. It is used for analgesia, antiemetics or menopausal hormone therapy, and as an alternative to sublingual administration for glyceryl trinitrate.

BIOAVAILABILITY

The idea of oral bioavailability was introduced above. Bioavailability is also used to describe the proportion of drug given by any route that reaches the systemic circulation, and by this definition intravenous administration achieves 100% bioavailability. The concentration of drug at its sites of action in the tissues is, however, not necessarily the same as its plasma concentration because of *plasma protein binding*. Plasma protein binding reduces availability of drugs at their sites of action because molecules are not free to diffuse out of the bloodstream to target tissues while they are attached to plasma proteins. Their duration of action is, however, increased by this means because the drugs are also unavailable for hepatic metabolism or renal excretion.

Competition for plasma protein binding sites between different drugs and between drugs and natural hormones can cause adverse effects, as discussed below. In patients taking warfarin (or warfarin plus regular low-dose aspirin), intermittent use of aspirin in analgesic doses causes varying degrees of *displacement* of the anticoagulant from a large plasma protein-bound reservoir, increasing the concentration of free warfarin and leading to risks of bleeding episodes.

Drug access to the central nervous system

The **CNS** is quite effectively protected from blood-borne chemicals by the **blood–brain barrier**. This is formed by close apposition of vascular endothelial cells, by the high proportion of lipid (as myelin) in the brain and by selective filtration of blood solutes by the choroid plexus during the formation of cerebrospinal fluid. The ability of drugs to penetrate the blood–brain barrier and influence CNS functioning is dependent on them being strongly lipophilic. Drugs produced for actions in the CNS are either lipophilic (e.g. morphine) or they are selectively transported into the cerebrospinal fluid (e.g. levodopa).

Many drugs that are weakly or moderately lipophilic can diffuse into the bloodstream from the small intestine and reach peripheral sites of action but are relatively too hydrophilic to access the CNS in pharmacologically active concentrations. Modest differences in ability to penetrate into the CNS can have quite marked effects on the adverse effect profiles of otherwise similar drugs used for their peripheral actions. Instructive pairs to contrast in this way are propranolol with atenolol and cimetidine with ranitidine.

HOW DRUGS ACT

Most drugs work by activating or blocking receptors or by inhibiting enzymes that either synthesize or inactivate biological mediators. Therefore, the understanding of pharmacodynamics depends upon understanding of drug–receptor and drug–enzyme interactions, and recognition that many receptors are, or are closely linked to, enzymes. Drug–receptor and drug–enzyme interactions largely determine the quantitative relationships between concentration of drug and its pharmacological effect, and are responsible for selectivity of drug action. For the remainder of this chapter the phrase drug–receptor interaction will be used to imply drug–enzyme interaction also, because characteristics of drug interactions with both types of site are closely similar. A few drugs act independently of either of these mechanisms, and these, together with *placebo effects*, are explored in brief sections below. Some key pharmacological and related terms are defined and explained in Box 6.6.

QUALITATIVE ASPECTS OF DRUG–RECEPTOR INTERACTIONS

Most drugs that are used as medicines interact reversibly with receptors or enzymes, so that the degree of their action is related to the concentration of the drug in the circulation. For those drugs that have irreversible interactions with receptors or enzymes, their duration of action depends upon the rate of synthesis of new receptor or enzyme proteins, and this varies from tissue to tissue. Similarly, the effects of

---

Box 6.6 Pharmacological and related terms

Receptors are defined as those parts of a cell with which a drug or biological mediator interacts in order to produce its effect. They have evolved to mediate the actions of hormones and neurotransmitters but serve also as targets for drug action.

Enzymes, or enzyme systems, are biological catalysts that promote biochemical reactions in the body without being altered by them.

Agonist is a technical word used to describe a drug that interacts with a receptor to activate (or stimulate) it and thus produce a direct effect.

An *antagonist* is a drug that interacts with a receptor or adjacent site to interfere with the activation of the receptor by a biological mediator or other drug. It produces its effect indirectly by reducing or preventing an ongoing process as a result of *antagonizing* (inhibiting) the action of a natural hormone or neurotransmitter, or another drug.

Enzyme inhibitors also work indirectly because they increase or decrease the concentration of biological mediator available for action by inhibiting their destruction or formation respectively.

For each drug, a *therapeutic index* can be calculated from toxic and therapeutically effective doses. Where the toxic dose is only a little higher than the effective dose, the index is low. For drugs, such as digoxin, with a low therapeutic index there is limited scope for increasing the dose to obtain an increased effect without causing adverse effects.

The terms *toxicity* or *toxic dose* are not rigidly defined but tend to be used in relation to adverse effects that are serious or life-threatening rather than unpleasant or inconvenient.

For some drugs (notably tricyclic antidepressants) there is a *therapeutic window* of concentrations below and above which the drug is ineffective. The reasons for this are not well established, but *receptor desensitization* (*downregulation* or *internalization*) by high drug concentrations has been postulated.

Similar mechanisms may underlie the development of *drug tolerance*, a phenomenon that occurs with opioids, benzodiazepines and glyceryl trinitrate, for example, involving progressive loss of sensitivity to the drug and requiring progressively increasing doses to maintain the desired therapeutic effect.

those drugs that act genomically (affecting genes in the cell nucleus) to stimulate the formation of new tissues or enzymes outlast the duration of the drug in the circulation.

The mechanism of action of many drugs involves interaction with receptors or active sites of enzymes, either by mimicking the action of a physiological mediator (agonist) or by blocking it (antagonist). An analogy is provided by reference to locks and keys. Two similar but not identical keys can be inserted into the same lock, but only one will activate the mechanism (agonist), while the other (antagonist) fails to activate the mechanism and prevents access of the correct key to the activating mechanism (see Box 6.7). The selectivity or specificity of drugs for particular receptors, and whether they act as agonists or antagonists, is related to the properties of *functional groups* on covalently bonded molecular cores, and also to the molecular size.

Cell membrane receptors are complex proteins within the cell membrane. There is a number of families and superfamilies of receptor structures, such as those that regulate

ion channel opening or those that are linked to intracellular G proteins and thereby regulate intracellular enzyme activities. The duration of binding of a drug to a receptor can be very short (milliseconds) when only hydrogen bonding is involved, or may be virtually permanent when covalent bonds are formed. Covalently bound drugs are rarely encountered in therapeutics because their long action tends to make dosage adjustment very difficult.

The binding sites of the receptor protein that are responsible for interactions with biological mediators or drugs have chemical properties that are specific for a single molecule or a small number of closely similar molecules. A single biological mediator or drug can have different types or subtypes of receptors in various tissues (see adrenaline (epinephrine)-related examples in Box 6.8). As in this example, letters of the Greek alphabet are sometimes used to differentiate main receptor types, followed by subscript numbers to distinguish between subtypes. Alternatively, capital initial letters of the naturally occurring receptor activator are used (e.g. H for histamine receptors, B for bradykinin receptors, 5-HT for 5-hydroxytryptamine receptors), with subscript numbers, sometimes followed by subscript letters, indicating receptor type and subtype respectively (e.g. 5-HT_{1A}).

QUANTITATIVE ASPECTS OF DRUG–RECEPTOR INTERACTIONS

The magnitude of response of a tissue or organ depends upon the number or proportion of receptors activated by an agonist. Receptor activation, and usually the consequent response, has been found empirically to be related to the logarithm (base 10) of the drug concentration by a sigmoid curve (Fig. 6.1) with an approximately straight-line section

---

Box 6.7 Fundamental concept of drug–receptor interactions

Agonist + Receptor → Active drug–receptor complex

→ RESPONSE

Antagonist + Receptor → Inactive drug–receptor complex

→ NO RESPONSE

A receptor that is occupied by an antagonist cannot be activated by an agonist.

Box 6.8 Adrenaline (epinephrine)-related examples of receptor subtype specificity

Adrenaline (epinephrine) acts as an agonist at α_1, α_2, β_1, β_2, β_3 receptors.
Noradrenaline (norepinephrine) acts as an agonist at α_1, α_2, β_1, β_3 receptors.
Some drug examples related to adrenaline (epinephrine) and noradrenaline (norepinephrine) (adrenoceptor agonists and antagonists) are:

Receptor	Drug	Clinical use
α_1	Agonist: phenylephrine	Nasal decongestant[b]
	Antagonist: prazosin	Antihypertensive[b]
α_2	Agonist: clonidine	Antihypertensive[b]
	Antagonist[a]	
β_1 and β_2	Agonist: isoprenaline	Bronchodilator[b]
	Antagonist: propranolol	Antihypertensive[b]
β_1	Agonist: dobutamine	Cardiac stimulant
	Antagonist: atenolol	Antihypertensive[b]
β_2	Agonist: salbutamol	Bronchodilator[b]
	Antagonist[a]	
β_3	Agonist[a]	(lipolysis)

[a]There is currently no clinically used drug of this type; experimental tools exist.
[b]Only one important effect is listed although these substances have many actions.

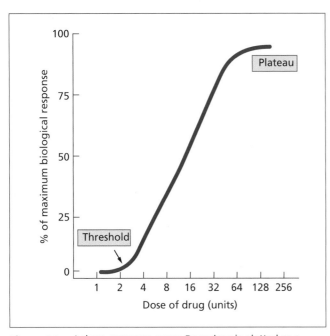

Figure 6.1 A dose–response curve. Drug dose is plotted as a logarithmic scale. The threshold is the dose of drug required to produce a measurable response. The plateau is the area of the curve where increasing the dose has no further measurable therapeutic effect. From Clark et al (2000), with permission.

between 20–25% and 75–80% of the maximum response (Neal 2002). The logarithmic relationship between concentration and response is the reason why drug doses are generally altered by doubling or halving, rather than arithmetic step increments of, say, 1 mg at a time. Ideally, therapeutic doses should give rise to free drug concentrations (in blood, interstitial fluid, cerebrospinal fluid) that are around the middle of this concentration–response curve. Owing to biological variation, low doses will be ineffective in a proportion of people and high doses may be toxic in some people. In clinical practice the range of doses recommended for adults is often quite narrow despite the wide range of variation in sizes of people, but there are different formulations and dose recommendations for infants and children aged under 12 years. For any drug with a low therapeutic index, such as cancer chemotherapeutic agents, the doses for adults can be calculated in proportion to body weight or body mass index.

DRUG ACTIONS THAT ARE INDEPENDENT OF RECEPTOR OR ENZYME INTERACTIONS

Gastric antacids and dietary fibre are widely used examples of the few types of drug that do not interact with specific receptors.

Gastric antacids, such as sodium bicarbonate, magnesium hydroxide and calcium carbonate, neutralize gastric acid by reacting with it to produce non-irritant chloride salts (e.g. sodium chloride, magnesium chloride, calcium chloride). The

quantity of acid neutralized depends upon the dose, and the action effectively ends when the drug leaves the stomach.

Dietary fibre is not absorbed from the gastrointestinal tract, and retains water with it by osmotic forces as it passes along in the lumen. Thus it increases the intraluminal bulk and stimulates increased peristalsis. Fermentation of the fibre by colonic bacteria increases the number of osmotically active particles (and carbon dioxide and water) in this organ, and thus enhances the stimulant effect here.

PLACEBO EFFECTS

Randomized controlled clinical trials generally show that about 30% of the population respond to inert 'treatments' (placebos) as if they had received effective medication, and also suffer side-effects. Such placebo responses are not well understood but they show us that psychological factors such as expectation of recovery, being cared for by healthcare professionals and others, or perhaps just being encouraged to rest can contribute to the diminution of symptoms. It would be unethical to treat people with placebos when effective treatments were available, but it is equally important to appreciate that placebo effects probably contribute something to the effectiveness of all pharmacological treatments. There is fuller and illuminating discussion of placebo effects in the clinical pharmacology textbooks of Grahame-Smith and Aronson (2002) and Bennett and Brown (2003).

INACTIVATION, METABOLISM AND ELIMINATION

The rate at which a drug is inactivated (or activated) by metabolism or eliminated from the body is a major factor in determining its duration of action. This, in turn, determines the range of possible frequencies of its administration to provide a continuous therapeutic effect. Because metabolic rate in general and renal clearance, and hepatic functioning in particular, can be influenced by age and disease, we can understand the need for caution in particular patient groups (paediatric, elderly, those with renal or hepatic impairment). Medicines administered too frequently to people who cannot inactivate or eliminate them rapidly enough can cause adverse effects as drugs accumulate in blood and tissues.

In this section we will look first at the elimination of drugs (focusing on renal clearance, which is quantitatively the most important for the majority of systemic drugs), and then at the metabolic inactivation of drugs and their conversion into molecules suitable for excretion in urine or bile. Finally, we will cover briefly some other facets of drug metabolism that are clinically important, and explain some widely used terms.

ELIMINATION

The concentration of drug in the circulation represents not only the concentration available to act but also the concentration available for metabolism and excretion. Because of the potential impact of organ-specific disease on duration of drug action and potential toxicity, it is important to be aware of the major sites of elimination of each drug:

- the kidneys and *urinary excretion*
- excretion via the liver into *bile*, and then *faeces* or *enterohepatic circulation* (see Box 6.13, p. 110)
- exhalation.

There are diverse other means of eliminating locally administered medicines:

- washing the skin, or loss on to clothing
- *mucociliary clearance* from the bronchial tree
- tears from the eyes
- saliva from the mouth
- digestive and mucous secretions, and faecal elimination, clear the gastrointestinal tract
- mucous secretions and urine clear the urinary and genital tracts.

Urinary elimination of drugs or drug metabolites

The **kidneys** treat drug molecules and drug-derived molecules (metabolites) in just the same way as they handle other blood-borne solutes, being subject to:

- glomerular filtration
- concentration as the urine is concentrated, leading to
- various degrees of reabsorption by passive diffusion
- active tubular secretion or absorption.

All molecules of up to about 20 000 in molecular mass are filtered through the *fenestrated capillaries* of the glomerulus into the renal tubular fluid. Apart from large protein or glycoprotein drugs, such as insulin and heparin, and those drug molecules that are bound to plasma proteins, molecules of drugs and their metabolites are generally filtered in this way. As the tubular fluid is gradually concentrated, so too are the drug molecules, creating a concentration gradient for them between tubular fluid and the blood. Molecules that are sufficiently lipophilic to cross the membranes of the tubular epithelial cells and capillary walls will then tend to diffuse back into the blood at a rate that is proportional to the concentration gradient, and little if any will be excreted in the urine. More hydrophilic molecules, however, will tend to remain in the tubular fluid and be excreted in the urine.

The rate of elimination of drugs in the urine is, therefore, determined largely by their extent of plasma protein binding and lipid solubility, with both of these factors tending to reduce the rate of excretion and prolong the duration of action. Highly lipid-soluble drugs can be eliminated in the urine only after they have been converted into more hydrophilic molecules by hepatic metabolism.

One other factor that influences the rate of urinary excretion of a few drugs is active tubular secretion. Benzylpenicillin, for example, is secreted into the urine by the epithelial cells of the renal tubules, and would have a very short duration of action unless injected in large doses, as a depot injection, or administered with probenecid, which inhibits tubular secretion.

DRUG METABOLISM FOR INACTIVATION AND EXCRETION

Drug molecules are rendered inactive and prepared for excretion in various tissues (Box 6.9). Hepatic metabolism is quantitatively the most important for the vast majority of drugs.

Hepatic metabolism generally yields compounds that are less lipophilic and more hydrophilic than the parent compound. The metabolic processes detoxify ingested poisons and inactivate many medicines, although a few drugs are activated (see Boxes 6.10 and 6.11). The hydrophilic metabolites are more readily excreted in urine or bile than lipophilic parent compounds.

Box 6.9 Drug metabolism

Sites of drug metabolism:

- liver – hepatocytes

- gut – mucosal cells

- lungs – epithelial and endothelial cells

- kidney – epithelial and endothelial cells

- blood and circulation – endothelial cells, blood platelets, plasma enzymes.

Those sites in contact with the external environment are specialized to deal with foreign molecules, whereas those in contact solely with body tissues are specialized to regulate endogenous substrates, but also metabolize drugs that resemble the natural substrates.

Very few experimental studies have attempted to distinguish whether parenchymal cells or vascular endothelial cells are responsible for their metabolic capabilities in tissues, such as lungs and kidneys, with an abundance of blood capillaries.

Box 6.10 Active metabolites

Some drugs have pharmacologically active hepatic metabolites, produced by *phase 1 reactions* (see Box 6.12). The active metabolites can contribute to effect and extend the duration of action of the medicine that contains such drugs. Illustrative examples are:

Active drug	Active metabolite
amitriptyline	nortriptyline
codeine	morphine
diazepam	oxazepam

Two distinct categories of chemical reactions involved in drug metabolism are commonly referred to as *phase 1* (Box 6.12) and *phase 2* (Box 6.13) reactions. These may occur independently or sequentially, depending on the available functional groups of a particular drug. The combined effect of inactivation and elimination determines the duration of action or effect of a drug in the body and this, in turn, influences the frequency of administration. The half-life of a drug (Box 6.14) is a useful indicator of the rate of its inactivation and elimination, and is used by clinical pharmacologists as a guide to frequency of administration (Fig. 6.2). The duration of therapeutic effect of a medicine can, however,

Box 6.11 Pro-drugs

Some drugs depend on metabolism to produce pharmacologically active molecules from inactive molecules at various sites following oral administration of inactive substances. Illustrative examples are:

Pro-drug	Site(s) of conversion	Active drug
cyclophosphamide	liver	4-keto-cyclophosphamide
enalapril	liver	enalaprilat
levodopa	dopaminergic nerves[a]	dopamine
sulfasalazine	colonic bacteria	5-aminosalicylic acid

[a]Conversion of levodopa to dopamine by dopa-decarboxylase in the sympathetic nervous system is inhibited by peripheral decarboxylase inhibitors that are unable to cross the blood–brain barrier.

Box 6.12 Phase 1 reactions

These reactions cause an increase in water solubility by oxidation[a], hydroxylation[a], dealkylation[a] or deamination[a] of the drug (or by various combinations of these). Many drugs, such as paracetamol, have several different metabolites.
Many phase 1 reactions are catalysed by the microsomal, *mixed-function oxidase* system, but not all oxidation reactions involve this system, for example:

- *monoamine oxidases* (in neurones and blood platelets as well as liver) inactivate many biogenic monoamines and related drugs, such as dobutamine and isoprenaline

- ethanol is metabolized by a soluble *cytosolic enzyme*, alcohol dehydrogenase.

[a]These chemical terms refer to addition of oxygen, addition of hydroxyl groups, removal of alkyl groups and removal of amine groups respectively, all of which increase the hydrophilicity (water solubility) of the molecules. For further information about these and other chemical groups that are of biological importance, see Montague et al (2005, ch. 1.2).
As the science of pharmacogenomics develops these mixed function oxidase enzymes are increasingly being referred to in textbooks as CYP enzyme types, such as CYP3A4 or CYP2D6, because **cy**tochrome **P**$_{450}$ is involved in their functioning (Bennett and Brown 2003).

Box 6.13 Phase 2 reactions

These reactions involve the conjugation (joining) of drugs, or their metabolites from phase 1 reactions, to highly water-soluble entities such as sulfate, glucuronyl or acetyl groups which are available from the circulation or other hepatic metabolic processes. Morphine, for example, is converted to various conjugates.

The resulting conjugates can then be excreted in urine (which often contains a mixture of several metabolites) or bile. Conjugates excreted in bile may undergo deconjugation by enzymes when they reach the small intestine or pass out in the faeces. Those undergoing deconjugation may be reabsorbed into the circulation, and have their action prolonged through this process, referred to as **enterohepatic circulation**. Ethinylestradiol, the oestrogen in many oral contraceptives, has its action prolonged in this way.

Box 6.14 Half-life of drugs

The half-life ($t_{1/2}$) of a drug is the time it takes for the plasma concentration of the drug to fall by half. The concentrations of most drugs (alcohol is a notable exception) fall exponentially regardless of the size of the dose taken within the therapeutic range (see Fig. 6.2). This means that the half-life is the same irrespective of the starting concentration, and its value can be reported as a constant characteristic of that drug.

Half-life is normally measured in human volunteers at a very early stage in clinical trials, by frequent monitoring of plasma levels following a single intravenous injection.

As mentioned above, although the half-life of a drug (in minutes, hours or days) is one useful parameter of the duration of action of a drug, it is not the only factor that determines possible frequency of administration.

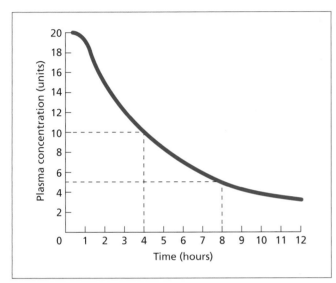

Figure 6.2 Drug half-life curve. In this example the drug has a half-life of 4 hours: at 4 hours the concentration has halved, and at 8 hours the concentration is half of what it was at 4 hours, etc. From Clark et al (2000), with permission.

also be altered by varying the dose (usually, the larger the dose, the longer its action) within limits determined by its effectiveness and safety.

ENZYME INDUCTION AND ENZYME INHIBITION

Certain drugs (including barbiturates, carbamazepine, ethanol, phenytoin, rifampicin and St John's Wort), components of foodstuffs and environmental toxins can stimulate an increase in the synthesis of mixed-function oxidase enzymes in the liver and consequently the activity of this enzyme system. The result of *enzyme induction* is an increase in the rate of metabolism and reduction in concentration and/or duration of action of any drug or endogenous substrate. This can lead to serious drug–drug interactions (see below) and/or ineffective concentrations of drugs or hormones. For example, the effectiveness of oral contraceptives is impaired in this way by various antibacterial, antiepileptic and antifungal drugs or by regular consumption of ethanol.

For many drug groups, inhibition of specific enzymes (angiotensin-converting enzyme, cholinesterases, cyclo-oxygenases) is the mechanism of their therapeutic effect, and this has been referred to above. Some drugs, however, inhibit the hepatic mixed-function oxidase system and thus prolong and/or increase their own actions and those of other drugs or endogenous substrates. Cimetidine, for example, has been found to cause clinically significant adverse effects by enhancing the actions of various antiarrhythmic, anticoagulant and antiepileptic drugs in this way.

UNWANTED AND ADVERSE EFFECTS OF MEDICINES

Nurses are well placed to help patients work out whether various signs or symptoms might be adverse effects of their medication, and whether they are mild or transient (unwanted) effects or sufficiently adverse to be a cause for concern. Anything serious or persistent, or any uncertainty, needs to be referred to the patient's doctor or other prescriber, and may merit reporting to the Medicines Control Agency and the Committee on Safety of Medicines through the yellow card system. Morrison-Griffiths et al (1998) have presented a very clear outline of this system in relation to nursing.

Unwanted and adverse effects can be part of the pharmacological activity profile of a drug, or arise from pharmacokinetic interactions with other substances being taken at the same time. The principles relating to these have been outlined above. These pharmacologically based adverse effects are generally dose related and can often be eased by reducing the dose of the medication, although some are so serious that it is essential to stop the medication immediately. Other adverse effects can be the result of immunological reactions to drugs or *haptens*. A hapten is an immunogen formed when a small molecule is attached to a larger carrier molecule. Haptens can be formed in the body from drugs or their metabolites binding covalently to tissue or plasma protein molecules. Penicillin may sometimes have this effect. Hapten formation can result in serious allergic reactions to medicines that are not dose related and are sometimes referred to as idiosyncratic or bizarre.

The reader is referred to the BNF (or its equivalent) as a readily available source of detailed information on possible side-effects, cautions and contraindications for medicines.

INTERACTIONS BETWEEN DRUGS WHEN USED TOGETHER

Interactions between drugs can be pharmacodynamic or pharmacokinetic in origin. *Pharmacodynamic* interactions arise when drugs enhance or, more commonly, inhibit the actions of one another at the receptor level, and are predictable from the pharmacological profiles of the drugs. *Pharmacokinetic* interactions arise when drugs interfere with the absorption, distribution, metabolism or excretion of one another. Some examples are given above, and numerous possible drug–drug interactions are listed in an appendix to the BNF, including many that are not usually of clinical significance. Nurses will be familiar with interactions that are relatively common within their area of practice, but it is not possible to memorize all possibilities.

There is a particular risk of drug–drug interactions when patients are on multiple drug therapies. If such people develop unexpected signs or symptoms, the possibility that these might have their basis in a drug–drug interaction should always be considered, and the possible interactions of all of their treatments should be checked.

DRUG DISCOVERY, DEVELOPMENT AND EVALUATION

'They test new drugs don't they?' In a chapter under this quizzical title Freeman (1991) asserted that many people who prescribe or administer medicines have little understanding of the preclinical and clinical stages of the production of a new medicine. I am, therefore, including this section because I believe it is important that nurses should have some understanding of how medicines are discovered and tested. In fact, the introduction of a new medicine is underpinned by more rigorous regulation than is applied to any other therapy. Such rigorous appraisal is not applied to food additives, diverse complementary therapies, surgical techniques or, indeed, other orthodox therapies.

An understanding of the principles of drug discovery, development and clinical evaluation enables people to have justified confidence in the effectiveness and safety of medicines, and an appreciation of why animal studies are an essential part of this process. This contentious issue has been debated by Blake and Collins (1999). Blake, who has Friedrich's ataxia, an incurable genetic disease that affects the CNS, argued cogently for the need for medical research that includes carefully regulated and monitored experiments on animals. Collins provided a contrasting, emotive argument that not all adverse effects of drugs are detected by animal experiments and, therefore, their use is unjustified. Such debates will undoubtedly continue.

Currently, pharmacological studies on animals almost invariably precede trials in humans. Clinical trials then proceed in four main phases:

1 *Phase 1*: safety and dose-ranging studies in healthy volunteers to establish the profile of actions and effects, half-life, and patterns of inactivation and elimination.
2 *Phase 2*: small-scale, pilot studies in patients with the disease(s) to be treated. These are 'open' trials in which both doctors and patients know the type and dose of the medication being tested. These can produce large placebo effects, at least in the short term, if the healthcare staff conducting the trials are very enthusiastic about the new treatment. Their main purpose is to discover whether or not the new treatment is effective in the illness(es) for which it was designed, and to establish what doses are effective in patients.
3 *Phase 3*: randomized controlled trials in groups of patients, in which new treatments are compared as objectively as possible with either placebo or currently available medicines, or both. Both effectiveness and safety (adverse effects) are measured and documented as accurately as possible. It is rightly regarded as unethical to use placebo controls in life-threatening or serious conditions for which there are treatments available.
4 *Phase 4*: post-marketing surveillance, in which recently licensed medicines are monitored as they are introduced to a wider population than the carefully selected groups used in phases 2 and 3. It is only at this stage that rare adverse effects are detected.

An understanding of these stages and the principles of design of clinical trials will enable nurses to evaluate claims of effectiveness and safety based on publications in journals or appearing in promotional literature. Specific information on clinical trials is provided in many textbooks of clinical pharmacology, such as that of Bennett and Brown (2003), and authors such as Sackett et al (1997) have produced more general guidance on interpretation of research findings to underpin evidence-based practice.

SUMMARY

This chapter commenced with definitions of pharmacology and pharmacotherapy, followed by some consideration of the aspects of pharmacology that are particularly relevant to nursing practice. The ways in which medicines are classified on the basis of their clinical applications, pharmacological properties or chemical nature, and various combinations of these, were discussed. This led into an illustrated explanation of generic and brand naming of medicines.

The administration of medicines is an important part of nursing practice, so pharmacological principles relating to this have been covered in some detail, with a 'chemistry free' account of drug inactivation, metabolism and elimination, emphasizing how these influence the duration of drug action and therefore the necessary frequency of administration.

The topic of 'how drugs act' has been treated quite briefly, as have the subjects of drug discovery, development and evaluation, because detailed coverage of these is beyond the scope of a single chapter, although awareness of them is important. Nurses can play crucial roles in the observation and identification of adverse drug reactions and interactions, and the principal mechanisms by which these can be caused by pharmacotherapy are explained.

The chapter also includes definitions and brief explanations of many of the specialist clinical pharmacological terms used in the BNF to enable readers to use this valuable, readily available, reference book.

REFERENCES

Banning M (2005). Issues in clinical nursing: conceptions of evidence, evidence-based medicine, evidence-based practice and their use in nursing: independent nurse prescribers' views . Journal of Clinical Nursing, 14(4): 411–417.

Bennett PN, Brown MJ (2003) Clinical pharmacology, 9th edn. New York: Churchill Livingstone.

Blake A, Collins B (1999) Animal testing: for and against. Nursing Times 95(8): 32–33.

Clark J, Queener S, Burke V (2000) Pharmacologic basis of nursing practice, 6th edn. St Louis: CV Mosby.

Crown J (1999) Review of prescribing, supply and administration of medicines. Final Report. London: Department of Health

Department of Health (2005) Online. Available: http://www.dh.gov.uk/PolicyAndGuidance/ MedicinesPharmacyAndIndustry/Prescriptions/NursingPrescribing

Freeman J (1991) They test new drugs don't they? In: Glaxo Group Research, eds. Drug safety – a shared responsibility. Edinburgh: Churchill Livingstone, p 13–26.

Grahame-Smith DG, Aronson JK (2002) Oxford textbook of clinical pharmacology and drug therapy, 3rd edn. Oxford: Oxford University Press.

Grandell-Niemi H, Hupli M, Leino-Kilpi H et al (2005). Issues in clinical nursing: Finnish nurses' and nursing students' pharmacological skills. Journal of Clinical Nursing 14(6): 685–694.

Ives G, Hodge K, Bullock S et al (1996) First year RNs' actual and self-rated pharmacology knowledge. Australian Journal of Advanced Nursing 14(1): 13–18.

Jordan S, Hughes D (1998) Using bioscience knowledge in nursing actions, interactions and reactions. Journal of Advanced Nursing 27: 1060–1068.

Montague SE, Watson R, Herbert R (2005) Physiology for nursing practice, 3rd edn. London: Ballière Tindall.

Morrison-Griffiths S, Pirmohamed M, Walley T (1998) Reporting of adverse drug reactions: practice in the UK. Nursing Times 94(10): 52–54.

Neal MJ (2002) Medical pharmacology at a glance, 4th edn. Oxford: Blackwell Science.

Nursing and Midwifery Council (2002) Guidelines for the administration of medicines. London: Nursing & Midwifery Council. Online. Available: http://www.nmc-uk.org/ (4eer2y55dwjqndqiot4fe555)/aArticleSearch.aspx?SearchText= administration%20of%20medicines

Sackett DL, Richardson WS, Rosenberg W et al (1997) Evidence-based medicine. New York: Churchill Livingstone.

FURTHER READING

Bennett PN, Brown MJ (2003) Clinical pharmacology, 9th edn. New York: Churchill Livingstone.

This is one of many good clinical pharmacology books produced in the UK, and relating closely to the BNF. It is highly readable and, while it has much less content than 'Goodman and Gilman', it is largely evidence based, with annotated references provided as footnotes on individual pages and a fairly extensive guide to further reading at the end of each chapter.

British Medical Association/Royal Pharmaceutical Society British National Formulary. London: BMA/RPS.

The BNF is published every 6 months (March and September). It contains four main sections: (1) guidance on prescribing; (2) emergency treatment of poisoning; (3) notes on drugs and preparations; and (4) appendices and indexes. The concise and current synopses of available medicines, which constitute the majority of the formulary, are written in the professional language of clinical pharmacologists. It is the hope of the author that those who have read the present chapter on Principles of Pharmacology will be able to understand this very convenient and informative reference work.

Department of Health (2005) Online. Available: http://www.dh.gov.uk/PolicyAndGuidance/ MedicinesPharmacyAndIndustry/Prescriptions/NursingPrescribing

The website above is useful for keeping up to date on prescribing and other policy matters that relate to pharmacology and nursing.

Downie G, Mackenzie J, Williams A (2003) Pharmacology and drug management for nurses, 3rd edn. Edinburgh: Churchill Livingstone.

This is a very sound basic textbook that presents quite a simple account of pharmacology and medicines management in a way that is related to nursing. Summaries of relevant physiology, immunology and pathophysiology are provided to explain how drugs work. As befits a basic textbook, there are some references to original research but no analysis of it. Useful further reading or reference lists are provided at the end of each chapter.

Hardman JE, Limbird LE (eds), (2001) Goodman & Gilman's the pharmacological basis of therapeutics, 10th edn. New York: McGraw-Hill.

This substantial book contains a huge quantity of information, presented in a readable, scholarly style. The content is research based and critical/analytical where appropriate, with references to seminal, empirical research and careful selection of review articles. Although it originates in the USA, the book is intended for an international readership, and the fact that it is based on the United States Pharmacopoeia *causes few difficulties.*

Luker K, Wolfson D, eds (1998) Medicines management for clinical nurses. Oxford: Blackwell Scientific.

This is not a pharmacology textbook. Produced following Karen Luker's involvement in the evaluation of nurse prescribing, this book is really a manual of a wide range of related professional issues for those who are or are intending to become prescribers, and is very useful in that context. It is a multiauthor book, and the quality of evidence base, levels of referencing and extent of further reading lists varies between chapters.

Montague SE, Watson R, Herbert R (2005) Physiology for nursing practice, 3rd edn. London: Ballière Tindall.

Of the many anatomy and physiology textbooks currently available for students of the healthcare professions, this one has the advantage of being specifically focused on nursing. A significant advantage of this text over many 'functional anatomy' physiology books is that the physiology provided by Montague et al contains sufficient biochemistry and chemistry to underpin 'nursing pharmacology' also.

Neal MJ (2002) Medical pharmacology at a glance, 4th edn. Oxford: Blackwell Science.

This attractive, slim volume provides clear, concise summaries of all of the main aspects of basic pharmacology that are relevant to medical practice. Each topic is covered on a double-page spread, starting with a very clear diagrammatic representation of the system involved. Its disadvantage for students of nursing is that it presupposes familiarity with quite advanced chemistry (a good 'A' level grade is required for entry to medical school). Inevitably in such a condensed presentation, the style is descriptive and assertive, rather than evidence based, and the list of further reading is limited.

Nursing and Midwifery Council (2002) Guidelines for the administration of medicines. London: Nursing & Midwifery Council. Online. Available: http://www.nmc-uk.org/ (4eer2y55dwjqndqiot4fe555)/aArticleSearch.aspx?SearchText= administration%20of%20medicines

This website is useful for keeping up to date with regulations relating to the administration of medicines.

7 Non-medical prescribing

Margaret Abbott

HISTORICAL REVIEW OF NON-MEDICAL PRESCRIBING IN THE UK

Nurses were the first healthcare profession apart from doctors, dentists and vets to acquire prescribing powers in the UK. However, UK policy has moved on rapidly so that it is now better to talk about non-medical prescribing rather than nurse-prescribing. Historically, the fight for prescriptive authority for British nurses began as far back as 1978, when the Association of Nursing Practice of the Royal College of Nursing identified the problems district nurses encountered when acquiring dressings for their patients (Jones 1999). It also has to be recognized that in North America, nurses and in particular nurse practitioners, have enjoyed prescriptive authority for many years. The exact nature of their authority is, however, determined on a state by state (USA) or province by province (Canada) basis.

A key milestone to acquiring prescriptive authority was marked by the report *Neighbourhood Nursing – A Focus for Care* (DoH 1986) which became known as the Cumberlege Report after its author Baroness Cumberlege. Amongst other things, this highlighted the plight of terminally ill patients whose pain management was impaired as community staff had to contact GPs to authorize a change in medication. A Department of Health (DoH) advisory group chaired by Dr June Crown reviewed the recommendations of the Cumberlege Report and published their findings in the Crown Report in 1989 (DoH 1989). This report recommended that suitably qualified community nurses, i.e. those holding a District Nurse (DN) or Health Visiting (HV) qualification should be allowed to prescribe from a limited Nurse Prescriber's Formulary (NPF). The Crown Report also recommended that nurses should be able to supply medicines within group protocols and that dosage and timing could also be altered within patient specific protocols.

In spite of the above recommendations it was not legally possible for nurses to prescribe without a change in the legislation. The Medicines Act 1968 governs all aspects of the licensing, supply, storage and administration of drugs along with the Misuse of Drugs Act 1971. This act is now almost 40 years old and UK health care today has changed dramatically since this act was passed.

Primary legislation was therefore necessary to allow nurses to prescribe and this was achieved with the Medicinal Products: Prescription by Nurses, etc., Act 1992 (Humphries and Green 2002). Although it was then legal for nurses to prescribe, an amendment to the Pharmaceutical Services Regulations 1994 was required to allow pharmacists to dispense nurse's prescriptions (Gibson 2001). Once primary legislation is in place, government departments can make legal changes relatively quickly by the introduction of Statutory Instruments. Although the relevant government department makes the change, they have to be authorized by central government. This is known as delegated legislation (Elliott and Quinn 2000).

To understand the development of non-medical prescribing it is necessary to have an appreciation of how the UK government agenda is set out for the development of health care. Non-medical prescribing should be seen therefore in the wider context of government policy. The White Paper *Primary Care: Delivering the Future* (DoH 1996) set the agenda and the key aims were:

- extending the professional's role (including the national roll-out of DN/HV prescribing)
- reviewing the supply and administration of medicines
- the expansion of the community pharmacist's role, to incorporate reviewing patient medication regimens
- enhancing collaboration between primary and secondary care.

By 2000 the UK had a new government in the shape of New Labour which set out its health care vision in *The NHS Plan* (DoH 2000). This included the Chief Nursing Officer's 10 key roles, one of which was prescribing medication. To help deliver the plan, and therefore make the nurse prescribing aspect happen, the government in 2002 published *Liberating the Talents* (DoH 2002a) which stressed:

- high national standards and clear accountability
- devolution of power and resources to the front line to give health professionals who deliver care the freedom to innovate
- increased flexibility between services and between staff to cut across outdated organizational and professional barriers
- a greater diversity of service providers, and choice for consumers.

Although *Liberating the Talents* was directed at primary care in England, this framework could be applied to secondary care and the other UK countries also. The three core functions of nurses, midwives and health visitors were identified as:

- first contact/acute assessment, diagnosis, care, treatment and referral
- continuing care, rehabilitation, chronic disease management and delivering the national service frameworks
- public health/health protection and promotion programmes that improve health and reduce inequalities (DoH 2002a).

A moment's reflection on these three core functions makes it apparent that in order to achieve these goals, nurses (and others) had to have extensive prescriptive authority. Effective treatment and chronic disease management can only be achieved if the practitioner has the authority to prescribe autonomously from an extensive formulary, unlike the very restricted formulary that was made available to the minority of nurses who had prescriptive authority at this time.

Mental Health was not to be left behind and *Improving Mental Health Services by Extending the Role of Nurses in Prescribing and Supplying Medication: Good Practice Guide* was published jointly by the National Prescribing Centre, the National Institute for Mental Health in England and the Department of Health in 2005.

THE STORY IN SCOTLAND, WALES AND NORTHERN IRELAND

Scotland, Wales and Northern Ireland in the UK have generally followed the principles established by the UK government and the UK nursing regulatory body (NMC). However, devolution has given the Scottish Parliament and the Welsh Assembly powers of their own over health care whilst in Northern Ireland different arrangements have also applied. We therefore need to note the following.

SCOTLAND

The necessary legislation which allowed DN/HV prescribing from a narrow nursing formulary was introduced in 1996 before devolution and there are now 3000 such prescribers in Scotland (NHSS 2005). In May 2001 Scottish ministers announced an extension of prescribing and with it the introduction of supplementary prescribing similar to that in England. Since 2002 prescriptive authority has been extended to all first level registered nurses who have completed an appropriate higher education qualification in prescribing. However, they may only prescribe from the nurse prescriber's extended formulary or basic formulary, as in England. Proposals now being discussed will extend prescriptive authority to a much wider range of drugs and allow pharmacists the same privileges.

WALES

Nurse prescribing has followed a similar history to England and Scotland but lagged slightly behind. So whilst England and Scotland announced a review of nurses' prescriptive authority that included the option of independent prescribing from the whole BNF (except controlled drugs) in 2005, it was January 2006 before a similar announcement, including pharmacists, was made in Wales (BBC 2006). All political parties and the BMA in Wales have supported the move. As the announcement was made, the *Western Mail* reported only 200 nurses and pharmacists in Wales with supplementary prescribing privileges only and none with independent prescribing authority (icwales 2006).

NORTHERN IRELAND

The situation in Northern Ireland has been hampered by uncertainty over the fate of the Northern Ireland Assembly due to political difficulties. However, plans were announced in 2005 that do suggest a real expansion will take place with both the universities (University of Ulster and Queen's University Belfast) putting out a joint press release on November 11 2005, welcoming government proposals to extend non-medical prescribing in Northern Ireland in line with other parts of the UK (Ulster.ac.2005).

THE GROWTH AND DEVELOPMENT OF NON-MEDICAL PRESCRIBING

What happened next involved a journey into some arcane jargon and rather clumsy phraseology that could only have been thought up by civil servants. The reader will have to live with some of the language which is not easy to follow but each phrase has a specific meaning in law, so we must be precise even if it as the expense of brevity!

The first steps which granted a nurse prescriptive authority, involved undertaking a Nursing and Midwifery Council

(NMC) approved course (code V100) and initially only district nurses (DNs) and health visitors (HVs) were allowed to do this and prescribe from their own limited formulary.

In 2001 it was announced that nurse prescribing was to be extended to allow more nurses to prescribe a wider variety of medicines for patients in the four categories of minor ailments, minor illness, health promotion and palliative care (DoH 2002b). They could, for example, prescribe from a list of approximately 150 prescription only medicines (PoM). This became known as extended nurse prescribing. Since then the limits have been gradually removed so the four distinct categories have been abandoned and the English Department of Health is regularly updating the lists of medications that 'extended nurse prescribers' can access.

At the same time, the government also announced plans for supplementary prescribing:

Supplementary prescribing is a voluntary prescribing partnership between an independent prescriber (doctor) and a supplementary prescriber (SP) to implement a patient specific Clinical Management Plan (CMP) with the patients agreement.

(DoH 2002c)

Supplementary prescribing is relevant for those healthcare professionals who are responsible for the continuing care of patients, i.e. monitoring a chronic condition and issuing repeat prescriptions following initial assessment and diagnosis by the independent prescriber. The aim is that the independent prescriber (initially assumed to be a doctor) will discuss the treatment with the supplementary prescriber and patient and all parties agree to the clinical management plan. Initially nurses could have supplementary prescriptive authority from the whole BNF with the exception of controlled drugs; however, in 2005 the restriction on controlled drugs was lifted and supplementary prescribers can now use the whole of the BNF. However, their prescriptions cannot stray from agreed clinical management plan. Supplementary prescribing is now seen as of great benefit to patients as practitioners can adjust existing medication regimens without continually having to refer back to the doctor or the nurse who prescribed the drugs by virtue of his/her authority as an 'extended formulary nurse prescriber'. The NMC approved course which gave the nurse extended and supplementary prescriptive authority was coded as V300 and access was no longer restricted to DNs and HVs only.

In 2003 supplementary prescribing for pharmacists was introduced. This enabled pharmacists to prescribe for patients with long-term conditions under a clinical management plan. Currently pharmacists can only prescribe as supplementary prescribers. Further developments came with the announcement of supplementary prescribing for allied health professionals (AHPs) in 2004. This includes, podiatrists, physiotherapists, radiographers and optomotrists. Health care is moving towards a more multidisciplinary approach, at least in the area of prescribing medication, and when tomorrow's registered nurses (RNs) are furthering their education in the field of prescribing, they will be sharing in classes with a range of disciplines. This has obvious potential advantages because, as we all have to work together for patient care, we might as well learn together. However, staff will be coming from different backgrounds with different levels of knowledge and different perspectives on care. This looks set to present some interesting challenges as it is essential for consistent care, that all staff achieve the same level of competence in prescribing.

The Drug Tariff is a useful resource and contains a plethora of information. It is compiled by the Prescription Pricing Authority (PPA) and published monthly on behalf of the DoH. Although many non-medical prescribers see this as a community pharmacist's handbook as it contains the basic price of drugs, it is an essential reference guide for those prescribers who wish to ensure that the patient receives the correct stoma/continence appliance, or urinary catheter by writing the code number on the prescription. A prescriber only has to note the 13 pages of urinary catheters to realize how useful this book can be to the continuity of patient care.

The Drug Tariff lists wound management dressings by type, brand name, wound contact size and where relevant, the size of the border. It is permissible for dressings to be prescribed by brand rather than generically, to ensure continuity of care. The price of each individual dressing is also listed which enables the prescriber to compare the prices of the various products. It must be noted that when prescribing dressings and bandages, the quantity required must be stated as the number of individual dressings, not the number of boxes. Initially many district nurses were met at the patient's house with one dressing when they expected to find one box that might contain five or ten. Many trusts have prepared a local formulary to which the non-medical prescriber is expected to follow. In addition to this the drug tariff contains such information as who is exempt from prescription charges, pre-payment certificates and lists drugs and other substances not to be prescribed under the NHS pharmaceutical services.

SEVEN PRINCIPLES OF GOOD PRESCRIBING

The National Prescribing Centre (NPC) devised the prescribing pyramid and this is helpful to all prescribers. The philosophy behind it is to contemplate each of the seven steps of the 'pyramid' before moving on to the next stage (NPC 1999).

STEP 1: CONSIDER THE PATIENT

Nurses are relatively new to the idea of diagnosis, having traditionally worked with the concept of nursing models of assessment. However, the development of the Nurse Practitioner (NP) role in the UK has changed all this. As this book is being written, the NMC are proposing to open up a new part of the register for Advanced Nurse Practitioners

(ANPs) and part of their remit will include diagnosis. The ANP is required to combine a nursing assessment with a physical exam and medical history to arrive at a decision over what may be wrong with the patient (Walsh 2006). This may be aided by ordering investigations such as bloods, pathology or radiographs. The ANP then has the authority to decide what is wrong and may initiate treatment which could include drug therapy. Alternatively she or he may refer to a medical practitioner for their expert opinion and possible therapeutic interventions. The nurse therefore starts the prescriptive process with the patient and their symptoms.

A structured medical history will obviously explore the symptoms the patient is experiencing but must include ascertaining what, if anything, the patient has done to relieve their symptoms. There must be a detailed account of all medications the patient is taking, including over the counter (OTC) and complementary medications and recreational substances (legal and illegal). Drug–drug interactions may occur and can only be avoided if the practitioner knows exactly what other substances the patient is taking. An important check in the assessment stage is to establish *who* the medicine is for, as a prescription should never be issued for a third party who is not actually present.

It is necessary to establish not only the presenting condition, but to also consider the patient's beliefs and lifestyle. These factors may impact not only on the prescriber's decision about the treatment, but also the likelihood of the patient actually taking the prescribed medication.

STEP 2: CONSIDER THE APPROPRIATE PRESCRIPTIVE STRATEGY

By no means all patients require prescriptions. Practitioners are accountable for their prescribing budgets and should consider carefully whether the patient will be helped in a cost-effective way by a prescription. It is therefore important to consider the alternative options available to treat the patient, such as advice or health education backed up by a patient information leaflet.

A key part of your assessment should be checking whether the patient has had the complaint before and if so, how they treated it. This can guide your decision-making. Additionally, patients may have medications from previous episodes at home in the medicine cupboard. This is a good opportunity to suggest the patient check the expiry date and give some education concerning the risks of accidental (or deliberate) drug overdose which are increased if there are large quantities of drugs being kept under such circumstances.

In considering a prescribing strategy, the practitioner must remember they are always liable for their actions and are required by the NMC to always operate within their scope of competence. Referral to another health professional may therefore be more appropriate, especially if the required medication is not included in the practitioner's formulary. We always have to stay within the law as well as our NMC Code of Professional Conduct.

STEP 3: CONSIDER THE CHOICE OF PRODUCT

Prescribing decisions should be evidence based and guidelines are very helpful in this regard. Access to the internet and intranet facilitates the use of guidelines while practitioners visiting patients in their homes should avail themselves of paper versions as appropriate. A current BNF is obviously an essential tool for prescribing.

To help with the choice of product the NPC (1999) suggest another mnemonic EASE:

E how Effective is the product?
A how Appropriate for this patient?
S how Safe is it?
E is the prescription cost Effective?

Good guidelines should inform the practitioner how effective the treatment is for the target condition and she or he must also consider how appropriate the medication is for that *individual* patient. Guidelines are only guides that will work for most patients most of the time, not all patients every time, so there is room for individual judgment, providing the practitioner can justify a deviation from the guideline. That justification is the essence of being an accountable practitioner. Individual patient factors must be considered alongside known contraindications, side-effects, interactions, and recommendations concerning dose, route and timing of drug administration.

In considering the safety of a drug, the practitioner needs to be aware of any previous adverse drug reactions (ADRs) experienced by the patient. If any ADR is experienced after a newly licensed drug, the practitioner *must* report it to the Committee on Safety of Medicines. A serious reaction in a well-established drug should also be reported. Reporting takes place through the yellow card system, which is explained at the back of a BNF and non-medical prescribers can now complete these cards. Information relating to ADRs can be found near the front of a current BNF. Reactions to medical devices are reported to the Medicines and Healthcare products Regulatory Agency (MHRA).

A decision about the choice of product cannot be made without considering the cost effectiveness. Local guidelines usually advise the use of cost-effective preparations and when writing the prescription, prescribers are advised to use the non proprietary (generic) name for medication, i.e. paracetamol not Panadol, although in some cases the brand name may be dispensed if the item is prescribed using the non-proprietary name (BNF 2006). There are some exceptions to this guidance, for example, the proprietary name is often used in prescriptions for antiepileptic treatment.

STEP 4: NEGOTIATE A CONTRACT AND ACHIEVE CONCORDANCE WITH THE PATIENT

Health care is now a partnership between the professional and the patient. Patients tend to be more knowledgeable about their conditions and the treatment options available than in previous years. The internet has played a major role in improving patients' levels of knowledge and understanding which in turn should ensure they get maximum benefit from their medication. The Association of the British Pharmaceutical Industry and the Ask About Medicine not-for-profit organization have produced a useful guide *Health and Medicines Information Guide and Directory* which is available on the internet (AAM 2005, ABPI 2005).

Patients need to understand:

- what is wrong with them
- how the medication will help
- how to take the medication, i.e. dose, timing, length of time to take the medication
- other healthy lifestyle measures that will assist, e.g. exercise
- side-effects to look out for
- indications that the medication is or is not working
- possible interactions with other medications
- when to return to see the practitioner for review.

With this level of understanding patients are more likely to be cooperative. They can also supply the practitioner with important and relevant information which will act as feedback concerning how effective the medication is. This will inform future prescribing decisions. This level of cooperation and partnership is the essence of concordance as opposed to the older term of compliance which just meant the patient did what they were told.

All of the information should be given in a manner that will enable the patient to make an informed decision without being manipulated in any way by the practitioner. Time spent in discussing the medication will be well spent if it results in patient concordance, which in turn is more likely to produce a favourable result. The consultation is therefore crucial to a good partnership with the patient (Weiss and Britten 2003).

There will always be those patients who do not wish to enter into this partnership for whatever reason and this wish must be respected. Factors such as the patient's beliefs about the medication and the influences of culture and religion must be considered. However, stereotypes must be avoided and each patient treated as an individual.

The general public are becoming more aware of the developing problem of antimicrobial resistance and its linkage with over-prescribing. Despite this, there will always be the patient who demands antimicrobials for a minor condition such as a simple sore throat, which is probably viral in origin anyway. The practitioner needs tact and diplomacy to explain why antimicrobials have not been prescribed. As in all professional matters the practitioner is accountable for their actions and must be able to justify them at all times.

The final element for successful concordance is that the patient is supported in the taking of their medication. Medicines Partnership (2005) divides this into four sections:

1 Medication is reviewed regularly with patients. It is becoming common for community pharmacists to take on this role and it would be beneficial for any pre-registration student to spend some of their time during their community placement with the community pharmacist reviewing patient medication. One of the advantages of the medication review is the opportunity to ask patients if they still require medication that is on repeat prescription. Patients may tick all of the items on the repeat request, regardless of whether they need them or not. This could be very wasteful. More than £100 million of unused medicines are returned to pharmacies each year (DoH 2000b).

2 Practitioners should use every opportunity to discuss medicines and medicine taking with patients. The patient with a long-term condition may be an 'expert patient' and know exactly how the medication affects them. If the patient has not taken the medication as prescribed it is important to ask them why. Patients need to know their opinions are valued. In discussing medication with patients you need to be knowledgeable, not only about the medication you prescribe, but also how they may interact with medication prescribed by other healthcare professionals. Diet and supplements can also interact with medication and therefore you must be aware of the possibility of these interactions. If a patient reports that the medication has not been effective, then you need to investigate why.

3 The practical problems of taking medication must be considered, from the form of the medication to the packaging, frequency of dose, and any issues surrounding access to a pharmacy for dispensing. Pharmacists are required to dispense medication in suitable containers. Medicines are now dispensed in child-proof containers which sometimes prove problematic for patients with impaired manual dexterity. Medication will not be effective if the patient cannot remove it from the bottle and she or he will therefore require a container she or he can open. It is also possible for the pharmacist to dispense the medication in 'dosette' boxes, which are useful for patients who have difficulty remembering when they have to take medication.

Care must be taken with regards to the form of medication when prescribing. Not all patients can swallow large tablets or find soluble alternatives palatable, particularly if they are complaining of nausea. For those patients who have difficulty getting to the surgery to collect the prescription, many pharmacies now offer a free service collecting the prescription from the surgery, dispensing it and then delivering the medication to the patient's house.

4 The last area that we are going to look at is information sharing, both with the patient and other healthcare professionals. Record keeping is of paramount importance and will be discussed later. The importance of keeping all staff informed about patient care cannot be over-emphasized. With more healthcare professionals involved in the prescribing process there is more potential for

confusion and the prescription of medications that may interact with others. The records also allow the patient's view of medication to be widely shared with different staff. Copies of the care plan are given to the patient, as well as being stored with the medical notes. This will enable the patient to look at it and make a note of any questions they might have before the next consultation. The care plan can also be useful for patients with long-term conditions to take on holiday in case they need to access medical care whilst they are away.

STEP 5: REVIEWING THE PATIENT

The practitioner must inform the patient if and when they need to return for review. For acute conditions the patient should be told approximately when they may expect to notice an improvement in their condition, and who to contact if that does not happen or if the condition becomes worse. For those patients suffering from long-term conditions, a month's supply of medication is the usual practice. This may have financial implications for patients who pay for prescriptions. Patients should be informed about pre-payment certificates which in some cases will be more cost effective for them. For oral contraceptives the prescriber will usually give 12 months' supply. Medication diaries are useful for monitoring the effectiveness of treatment.

STEP 6: RECORD KEEPING

Record keeping has always been an integral part of health care, but with increasing numbers of practitioners becoming involved with prescribing, accurate record keeping is becoming even more important. One of the purposes of record keeping is to improve communication (NMC 2005).

Good communication requires accurate record keeping of what has been prescribed (generic name), when, by whom (signatures must be legible) and why (including details of differential diagnosis). Records should also include the dosage of current medication, previous medication and any known allergies or previous adverse drug reactions. Other substances such as OTC medicines, herbal remedies and recreational drugs should be noted as they are an essential part of all patient assessment anyway.

There are local policies to determine the time span for notifying doctors of a prescription issued by a non-medical prescriber; however, it is good practice to record your prescribing as soon as possible and within 24 hours on a weekday and within 48/72 hours at weekends and bank holidays.

One of the UK areas in which nurse prescribing has become increasingly common is the Walk in Centre (WIC). In these, nurses see patients for an initial contact, frequently out of hours and often without any access to medical records. This is particularly common in patients who are not registered with a GP, or at venues such as holiday resorts and airports. The nurse must make a professional decision on the facts presented to him/her and ultimately make

accurate, contemporaneous records to be forwarded to the patient's GP and any other relevant healthcare professionals. Equally, nurses in A&E are involved in prescribing, and they also do not always have access to patient's medical records. There should be systems in place to inform GPs and other healthcare professionals of the treatment given.

It is important to record what the patient has told you even if it is a negative response to a question. Healthcare records are legal documents and should be afforded an appropriate level of care and accuracy. Dimond (2002) reminds us that 'Any document requested by the court becomes a legal document'. It is often the records that prove to be the healthcare professional's downfall in a court of law (Swage 2000). Cases of medical negligence may not come to court until many years have elapsed since the original incident. The practitioner will only have the records written at the time to fall back on as their defence as human memory will not suffice. Medical records should be written therefore, always bearing in mind that one day they may be required by a court of law and may constitute your best defence against litigation or accusations of unprofessional conduct. Nurses must follow the NMC 'Guidelines for Records and Record Keeping' (NMC 2005) and ensure accurate, factual and clear notes are kept of any consult. It is also important to document advice that has been given to the patient but avoid common mistakes such as illegible handwriting, meaningless phrases and unprofessional comments such as 'sweet old lady' (Dimond 2002).

Abbreviations should be avoided as they can lead to confusion and mistakes, especially as the same abbreviations can have different meanings to different people. For example, BP to a pharmacist could mean British Pharmacopaeia rather than blood pressure and medicines TTA (to take away) would puzzle any teacher who was the patient as they may wonder what their care had to do with the Teacher Training Agency.

The same rules for record keeping apply to prescription writing. There is a list of accepted abbreviations in the back of the BNF and an accompanying statement advising that directions should be written in full English. The pragmatic, time-saving approach is usually to use abbreviations, however these should be from an approved list. Jargon and abbreviations that are not understood may not only sow the seeds of confusion but destroy any notion of the patient as a partner in care. See Chapter 2 for a review of the importance of communication in therapy.

Open questions permit the patient to express their personal experience of a problem and they are an important part of assessing the patient (Sully and Dallas 2005). To ask the question 'Are you taking any paracetamol?' may not be sufficient. The patient may not know that many OTC remedies contain paracetamol, therefore a question phrased as 'Can you tell me what other medication you are taking at the moment or have taken today?' will elicit more information. In some instances it may be necessary to explain to the patient why you are asking the question, particularly if you ask if they have taken any herbal remedies or illegal substances, as they may not want to divulge this information. By explaining that herbal and illegal substances may interact with conventional medicines you will tell the patient why you need to know and be more likely to get an honest answer.

A common error in prescription writing is the instruction 'as directed'. Unless this is for a medication that is taken as required it can cause a lot of confusion. When a prescription is dispensed the instructions on the label will be copied from the prescription, therefore the prescription must state clearly the dose, timing and route of administration if the medicine is to be properly labelled. Records must also state exactly what was prescribed with the same level of detail.

The person who has written the prescription should be the person to sign the records, or enter data on to the computer. Where clerical staff type up records, it is the responsibility of the qualified professional to countersign any records. You should apply the same principles to computerized records as written records. It is becoming increasingly common for healthcare professionals to share records and this system will enhance patient care in non-medical prescribing, if the records are unambiguous, accurate, contemporaneous and legible. Records are audited on a regular basis to identify any areas of risk and training needs of staff.

STEP 7: REFLECTING ON YOUR PRESCRIBING

Audits are a regular occurrence in professional practice, and are used not only to monitor financial costs, but to provide information about current practice. Clinical guidelines, for example, cannot only be of value to practitioners, they can also be subject to regular audit (Pollock 2004). Every time a prescription is issued the practitioner is spending public money and is accountable for that expenditure. In secondary care the budget holder will have a statement of the medicines budget. As non-medical prescribing is still relatively new to secondary care, systems for monitoring practice are still being implemented. In primary care, prescribing has been monitored by the Prescription Analysis and Cost Trends (PACT) data for many years. This information is prepared monthly by the Prescription Pricing Authority (PPA) and distributed to all prescribers in the community.

Reflection on practice is of value in all areas, not just in learning to be an effective and safe prescriber. A brief review of reflection may be found in Chapter 1 and these principles should be applied to prescribing, especially with critical incidents in mind.

ACCOUNTABILITY

You are personally accountable for your practice. This means that you are answerable for your actions and omissions, regardless of advice or directions of another professional.

(NMC 2004, p.4)

In other words the buck stops with you! Accountability means simply being able to give an account of your actions and being able to justify them. Following doctor's orders is not the justification of an accountable practitioner. Citing evidence and explaining your decision-making process is, however, being accountable. This might, for example, be a situation where you have declined a request for antimicrobials in a patient with a minor sore throat that is probably viral in origin. It could even be a situation where you have not followed a guideline because of some individual factor in that patient. As long as you can justify the decision, you are being an accountable practitioner. Accountability of course depends upon having the necessary knowledge to base your decisions on (note this excludes intuition) and also the authority to implement them (i.e. prescriptive authority). This also means you must not overstep the mark in terms of what you are legally or professionally allowed to prescribe.

As a registered nurse who can prescribe, the practitioner is therefore held accountable for:

- assessment and diagnosis
- deciding whether to prescribe and if so what to prescribe, its dosage, route and frequency, taking into account possible interactions and side-effects
- negotiation with the patient to effect informed consent and also to give advice about storage of medicines, disposal of unused medicines and an agreed review date
- ensuring records are correctly written up, the prescription is correctly written and there is effective communication with other staff.

The registered nurse who delegates work, such as the administration of medicines, is accountable for ensuring that the task is carried out satisfactorily (Tilley and Watson 2004). You are therefore accountable for ensuring that the person who will administer the medication is capable of doing so, whether it is the patient or their carer (family member or paid carer). In some instances such as the management of asthma, teaching the patient to use their inhaler is just as important as the diagnosis and prescription. Patient education obviously includes the correct timing and method of administration as in some cases the patient may return complaining the treatment has not worked when in fact the problem is one of inappropriate administration.

SUMMARY

This chapter has given a brief overview of non-medical prescribing from its inception to the present day. Undoubtedly by the time this book is published even more changes will have taken place. Future practitioners who aspire to prescriptive authority will need a knowledge of physiology, pathology, health assessment, pharmacology and decision-making substantially beyond that covered in pre-registration nursing education today. You must therefore be prepared to further your education in these fields in line at least with the new minimum standards being discussed by the NMC as this book goes to print in 2006. Ideally, you may wish to go beyond that minimum standard to achieve the new level of practice that is being introduced by the NMC; the advanced nurse practitioner. There will probably continue to be heated debate about non-medical prescribing with some sections of the medical profession having major reservations. However, the passage of time and experience will resolve the issue and we have to ensure a favourable outcome for patients by adopting a responsible attitude to our new found prescriptive authority.

REFERENCES

Ask About Medicine (AAM) (2005) Health and medicines information guide and directory. Online. Available: http://www.askaboutmedicines.org 23 Jan 2006.

Association of the British Pharmaceutical Industry (ABPI) (2005) Health and medicines information guide and directory. Online. Available: http://www.abpi.org.uk 23 Jan 2006.

BBC (2006) BBC news. Online. Available: http://www.news.bbc.co.uk/1/hi/wales4627564.stm

British Medical Association, Royal Pharmaceutical Society of Great Britain 2005 BNF (2006) British National Formulary. London: British Medical Association, Royal Pharmaceutical Society of Great Britain.

Department of Health (DoH) (1986) Neighbourhood nursing – a focus for care. A report of the community nursing review. London: HMSO.

Department of Health (DoH) (1989) Report to the advisory group on nurse prescribing (The Crown report). London: HMSO.

Department of Health (DoH) (1996) Primary care: delivering the future. London: DoH.

Department of Health (DoH) (2000) Pharmacy in the future implementing the NHS plan. London: DoH.

Department of Health (DoH) (2002a) Liberating the talents London: DoH.

Department of Health (DoH) (2002b) Extending independent nurse prescribing within the NHS. London: DoH.

Department of Health (DoH) (2002c) Supplementary prescribing. London: DoH.

Dimond B (2002) Legal aspects of nursing, 3rd edn. Harlow: Pearson Education.

Elliott C, Quinn F (2000) English legal system, 3rd edn. Harlow: Pearson Education.

Gibson B (2001) Legal and professional accountability for nurse prescribing. In: Courtney M. Current issues in nurse prescribing. London: Greenwich Medical Media.

Humphries J, Green J (eds) (200) Nurse prescribing 2nd edn. Basingstoke: Palgrave.

Icwales (2006) Online. Available: http://www.icwales. icnetwork.co.uk/women/o80403health

Jones M (ed.) (1999) Nurse prescribing politics to practice. London: Harcourt.

Medicines Partnership (2005) From compliance to concordance. London: Medicines Partnership.

National Prescribing Centre (NPC) (1999) Principles of good prescribing. Liverpool: NPC:

NHSS (2005) Extended independent nurse prescribing within National Health Service Scotland. Edinburgh: NHSS.

Nursing and Midwifery Council (NMC) (2004) The NMC code of professional conduct: standards for conduct, performance and ethics. London: NMC.

Nursing and Midwifery Council (NMC) (2005) Guidelines for records and record keeping. London: NMC.

Pollock L (2004) Accountability and clinical governance in nursing: a managers perspective. In: Tilley S, Watson R, eds. Accountability in Nursing and Midwifery 2nd edn. Oxford: Blackwell Science.

Sully P, Dallas J (2005) Essential communication skills for nursing. Edinburgh: Elsevier Mosby.

Swage T (2000) Clinical governance in health care practice. Oxford: Butterworth-Heinemann.

Tilley S, Watson R (2004) Accountability in nursing and midwifery, 2nd edn. Oxford: Blackwell Science.

Ulster.ac (2005) Online. Available: http://www.ulster.ac.uk/news/releases2005/1927.html

Walsh M (2006) Nurse practitioners; clinical skills and professional issues, 2nd edn. Oxford: Butterworth Heinemann.

Weiss M, Britten N (2003) What is concordance? The Pharmaceutical Journal 271: 493.

The management of pain

Veronica Thomas

INTRODUCTION

Before focusing on pain control it is necessary to consider the phenomenon of pain generally. If pain relief strategies are to be effective, they must integrate the knowledge of the physiological pain experience and response, pharmacology, and the personal or psychological experience of the patient. These elements are introduced in this chapter because they are basic to the control and management of all types of pain.

PAIN PATHWAYS

We now know that **pain** is mediated by free, unspecialized nerve endings. These nerve endings are present in the dermis and epidermis, and with their afferent fibres they form integral parts of single neurones, the bodies of which are situated in the posterior root ganglia associated with the spinal cord. The **receptors** are specialized for dealing with different types of noxious stimuli. The thermoreceptors respond only to heating and cooling, while some nociceptors are responsive to mechanical injury. Polymodal receptors are responsive to mechanical injury, noxious heat and chemical irritation.

It is now well established that there are two types of pathway for the conduction of pain from these nociceptors. First, there are medium-diameter nerve axons called A-delta (A-d) fibres. These are myelinated and consequently conduct nerve impulses very quickly. Sharp, pricking pain sensations are conducted via these fibres to the brain in less than 0.1 s. The other type of fibre is known as a C fibre; this is narrower than the A-d type and not myelinated. As a result, conduction is much slower (1 s or more) and aching, throbbing pain sensations tend to be conducted. A painful stimulus may therefore be felt twice: an immediate sharp pain and then a duller, aching pain developing seconds later.

The afferent nerve pathways that conduct pain and other sensations away from nerve endings in the various tissues have ultimately to deliver their messages to the sensory areas of the cortex. This usually happens via a relay system involving three neurones (first, second and third order) which connect at their respective synapses. Pain impulses are conducted to the brain via the following system of neurones:

1 First-order neurone, which connects the receptor in body tissue to the spinal cord. The actual cell body of the first-order neurone is located at the posterior root ganglion and its axon synapses with the …
2 Second-order neurone, whose cell body is located in the posterior grey horn of the spinal cord. The axon of this cell crosses to the opposite side of the spinal cord and passes upwards in the spinothalamic tract. This has two components: the lateral or anterior tract. The axon terminates in the thalamus.
3 The third-order neurone, which conducts pain impulses from the thalamus to the cortex.

The information contained in the spinothalamic tract consists of rather diffuse pain and heat sensations. Associated with the spinothalamic tract is the spinoreticular tract. These ascending sensory nerve fibres are found in the anterior segment of the spinal cord and relay messages to the reticular formation of the brainstem. This part of the system is crucial for consciousness and awareness. Another key group of ascending nerve fibres is the dorsal column medial lemniscal pathway, which carries very precise information to the brain about touch and limb movement.

Various naturally occurring substances have been shown to play a major role in pain transmission. Substance P is a neurotransmitter found in unmyelinated fibres, and bradykinin, serotonin, histamine and prostaglandin E either excite or sensitize nociceptors.

COMPONENTS OF PAIN

Pain can be regarded as having three components: the sensory–discriminative, the motivational–affective and the cognitive–evaluative.

Sensory–discriminative

This component of pain allows the injury to be identified in time and space, and its exact extent to be determined. In addition to transmission of nociceptive stimuli, this component requires large-fibre transmission of touch and other sensory stimuli to enable the source, site and severity of the pain to be identified.

Motivational–affective

This component produces somatic (bodily) and autonomic activity, which result in various protective processes such as movement away from pain, immobilization of damaged tissue or preparation for flight. No spatial or temporal information is involved at this stage. The neural areas of the reticular formation and the limbic system are involved in the motivational–affective features of pain.

Cognitive–evaluative

This is a complex component in which response to the painful stimulus is influenced by cultural values, anxiety, attention and many other factors. These activities, which involve cortical processes, may affect the sensory–discriminative and motivational–affective dimensions. Arousal in situations of extreme danger may block the sensory–discriminative and motivational–affective components of pain. Suggestion and placebo may modulate the motivational–affective component and leave the sensory–discriminative component relatively undisturbed (Melzack and Dennis 1978).

THE GATE CONTROL THEORY OF PAIN

Our current understanding of pain is based upon the **gate control theory** of Melzack and Wall (1965) and incorporates the three components mentioned above. The basic idea is that within the substantia gelatinosa of the dorsal horn of the spinal cord there is a gating mechanism, which controls the **transmission** of information to the brain. As a result large-diameter A-β fibres from touch and pressure receptors can inhibit the conduction of impulses through the smaller-diameter fibres that connect pain receptors with the cerebral cortex (A-δ and C fibres). Nerve impulses from the A-β fibres are preferentially conducted to the cerebral cortex, closing the gate on pain impulses in the smaller-diameter fibres. Pain impulses have to reach a certain threshold intensity to force open the gate and be conducted via the spinothalamic tract to the cerebral cortex and also to reach the reticular formation via the spinoreticular tract (Fig. 8.1).

The theory also proposes that descending fibres from the brain synapsing in the dorsal horn areas can modify the transmission of incoming pain signals. This opens up the possibility that psychological factors may play a major part in the perception of pain. Cerebral function can also be linked to physiological processes that reduce pain perception. One mechanism for doing this is secretion of chemicals that occur naturally within the body called **endorphins** and **enkephalins**, which are thought of as naturally occurring opioids. This takes place in response to stimulation from the effect of the neurotransmitter, substance P. Acupuncture is thought to stimulate the release of enkephalins, explaining its analgesic effects, whereas the placebo effect may be due to psychogenic release of endorphins. The placebo effect refers to the phenomenon whereby a patient reports a reduction in pain even though the medication that has been given has no analgesic properties.

The gate control theory also sheds light on **phantom limb pain**. Here, the patient experiences disturbingly real sensations and pain from a limb that has been amputated. This may continue for many years after amputation. Destruction of the large-diameter nerve fibres that normally input to the spinal cord from the lost limb means that their overriding effect on the surviving smaller-diameter fibres is lost, and therefore these fibres are much more sensitive than normal – hence the increased perception of pain. The brain may also interpret the input it receives from proximal surviving sensory nerves as if the impulses were coming from the distal portion of the nerve in the limb that is no longer there. An alternative proposal is that the brain actually constructs its own virtual reality model of the body based upon neural networks within the brain. If this is true, then the loss of a real part of the body will not affect the way we perceive ourselves as this is based upon the virtual model constructed by the still intact neural networks in the brain.

A related phenomenon is that of **referred pain** in which the brain interprets pain as coming from a different part of the body to where the painful stimulus actually arises. A classic example is myocardial pain, which is often described as being in the left arm or jaw. What is happening here is that the damaged area and the area where the pain is perceived are both served by the same part of the spinal cord, and synapses between pain fibres from the two regions occur. The sensory nerve input from the left arm enters the spinal cord at levels T1–T5, the same levels as those from the myocardium. Synapses between the neurones that receive pain from the skin in the left arm and those neurones receiving visceral (myocardial) pain result in a shared ascending pathway to the brain. Pain impulses from the myocardium can then be perceived as coming from the left arm and the pain is said to be referred to the left arm.

PSYCHOSOCIAL FACTORS IN THE EXPERIENCE OF PAIN

Melzack and Wall (1988) argue that **pain perception** cannot be described simply in terms of stimulus intensity, and draw our attention to the complex interplay between physiological and psychological factors. In this chapter, I will

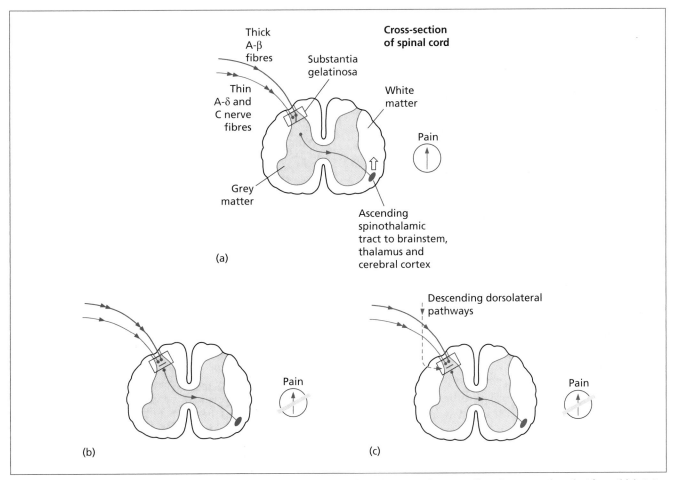

Figure 8.1 The gate control theory of pain transmission. (a) When input from the A-δ and C nerve fibres is greater than that from thick A-β fibres, the gate is open and pain is felt. (b) When input from A-δ and C nerve fibres is less than that from thick A-β fibres, the gate closes and pain is not felt. (c) The influence of the cerebral cortex via descending dorsolateral pathways closes the gate by the release of neuromodulators (e.g. endogenous opiates), neurotransmission and chemical mediators. Pain is not felt or is substantially reduced. Adapted from Davis (1993).

explore some of the psychological and social factors that contribute to accounting for this highly individual experience. I will look at the role of gender, age, culture and emotional states in explaining individual differences in the response to pain. An awareness of the pertinence of psychosocial factors in the experience and expression of pain is very useful to healthcare professionals because it provides them with potential insights and explanations for understanding individual reactions and behaviour to pain.

GENDER DIFFERENCES

The role of gender in an individual's response to pain has received considerable attention in the literature but the findings have not been unequivocal. In some research it seems that women report more pain or required more analgesic medication than men (Bond 1979, Taenzer et al 1986), whereas others have found the reverse pattern. Both of these findings contrast to other studies where no significant difference between males and females has been established (Khun et al 1990, Streltzer and Wade 1981).

In more recent times, a review of the literature on gender in pain experience by Unruh et al (1996), reveal that in most studies women report more severe pain levels more frequently and for longer duration than men. According to Unruh and colleagues, women are more likely to experience moderate and severe pain from menstruation and childbirth and increased risk of disability. Despite this fact Unruh and colleagues have argued that women are more likely to be given purely psychological explanations for their pain (Unruh et al 1996). There is therefore no research evidence to support a consistent pattern of pain appreciation related to sex.

AGE DIFFERENCES

The literature addressing the influence of age on pain experience is also not straightforward and the discussion takes account of pain experience at both ends of the developmental cycle. Not a great deal is known about the epidemiology of pain in children (Anand and Hickey 1987, Eland 1985), and Llewellyn (1997) has argued that the reason is attributable to the fact that children's pain has little social

KEY CLINICAL PRINCIPLES

impact. This is because the costs cannot be calculated in terms of lost work-days and benefits claimed. Consequently the incentive to investigate the extent of the problem has hitherto been small (Goodman and McGrath 1991). More recent research has revealed that up to 25% of children and adolescents report persistent or recurrent pain (Perguin et al 2000). Whilst a smaller proportion presents repeatedly with extensive pain associated distress and disability to multiple healthcare providers (Perguin et al 2001).

When considering the adult's pain experience some researchers have found that ageing is associated with enhanced analgesia, indicating that the elderly can obtain effective relief for longer periods with smaller doses of opioid analgesics than younger people (Belville et al 1971, Berkowitz et al 1975, Burns et al 1989, Taenzer et al 1986) and younger patients express greater dissatisfaction with pain relief (Donovan 1983). The picture is further complicated by the differences in the amount of pain reported by different age groups. Older people may systematically under-report the amount of pain they perceive. On the one hand, Miller and Shuter (1984) found that patients aged over 40 years reported more pain than those of a younger age group, whereas Khun et al (1990) found no relation between the amount of reported pain and age.

Cognitive impairment in the elderly is frequently attributed to the effects of opiates and they are often discontinued as a consequence. Interestingly, it is now recognized that pain itself causes cognitive impairment and effective pain relief is the remedy (Lorenz et al 1997).

ETHNIC DIFFERENCES

It is apparent from empirical studies and observations that pain experience cannot be fully explained without reference to cultural and ethnic differences. Culture seems to influence the expressiveness rather than the sensory experience itself (Melzack and Wall 1988). Cultural norms determining when and where to express pain are learnt at an early age (Peck 1986). Seminal research on cultural differences in pain has, over the years, revealed that people from Latin origins are typically more expressive and are inclined to dramatize pain expression with excessive vocalization and posturing (Lipton and Marbach 1984). People of Scandinavian origin tend to be more stoical and are on the whole less expressive about pain (Chapman 1984). Black English people of African/Caribbean ethnicity have been found to report more pain than the white Anglo-British population (Woodrow et al 1972), but other evidence (Thomas and Rose 1991) has indicated that the white population is better able to tolerate pain than those born in the UK whose parents originated from the Indian subcontinent. Other studies have failed to find differences between 'Old Americans', southern US blacks, Irish, Italian and Jewish subjects in the amount of reported pain (Flannery et al 1987). Lipton and Marbach (1984) have argued that the relationship between pain experience and ethnicity may be subtler than customarily thought, and that

it may be only possible to describe certain responses as more or less characteristic of one group relative to another.

A related issue is the effects of culture on language, which in turn influences how pain is reported. For example, a study of 50 Arabic speaking hospitalized patients revealed that nurses who spoke the same mother tongue as the patients were more accurate at assessing their pain than nurses who spoke a different language (Harrison et al 1996). This issue of culture and language will be discussed further in the section on pain assessment.

EMOTIONAL STATES IN THE EXPERIENCE OF PAIN

The influence of various emotional states on pain experience has been the subject of much research.

Neuroticism

Neuroticism refers to emotional stability, and studies that have used Eysenck's Personality Inventory (EPI) or Questionnaire (EPQ) to measure preoperative neuroticism have tended to find a significant positive relationship between high levels of neuroticism before surgery and pain experience after surgery in both men and women. This positive relationship between pain experience and neuroticism has also been observed by others (Thomas et al 1990, 1995).

Anxiety and pain

The association between anxiety and pain is well known. Anxiety has been distinguished as:

- *state anxiety* – a transitory emotional state that varies in intensity and fluctuates over time and is associated with threatening anticipatory circumstances
- *trait anxiety* – a stable personality disposition that is said to predict state anxiety, i.e. it predisposes people to react in a highly anxious manner in stressful situations (Spielberger 1966).

It is well known that people awaiting surgery become extremely anxious and Spielberger (1973) has shown that anxiety trait remained stable in surgical patients before and after surgery, but those patients with high trait anxiety scores reacted in a highly anxious manner just before the operation. In other words, patients with an anxious predisposition (trait anxiety) become acutely anxious in threatening situations. Numerous studies have shown that both state and trait anxiety are positively correlated with the degree of pain experienced in acute and chronic pain settings (Lim et al 1983, Seers 1997, Taenzer et al 1986, Thomas 1991, Thomas et al 1995).

In the context of acute surgical pain, a research report identified state anxiety as an important variable in the post-operative pain experience (Leinonen and Leino-Kilpi 1999). In a recent study, involving 87 women undergoing gynaecological surgery, Carr et al (2005) found that preoperative anxiety was highly predictive of long-term post-operative anxiety for as long as 4 days after surgery which was also positively correlated to pain experience over the same time period.

Fear is related to anxiety states and some people choose to minimize the expression of pain because they are frightened. One group is the needle-phobic patients who under-report pain because they are fearful of needles and injections. Victims of needle phobia are at high risk of morbidity and death because they have a tendency to avoid health care at all costs. The use of sedatives, local anaesthetic cream such as EMLA (Frayling et al 1990) or skin coolant (Eland 1981) before injections or venepuncture is helpful in reducing pain. However, such measures are not helpful in removing the phobia because it is the sight of the needle that produces distress; psychological interventions in the form of cognitive behaviour therapy (see p. 133) provide effective solutions for people who have needle phobia (Trijsburg et al 1992). Another group of people who experience fear in relation to pain are those who suffer with chronic long-term pain. When patients suffer with chronic pain they tend to avoid or limit activity to prevent discomfort on movement. Vlaeyen et al (1995) propose that avoidance arising from the innate drive to reduce discomfort and thoughts/beliefs that activity will produce pain and suffering leads to a vicious cycle characterized by decreased self efficacy, fear and further avoidance and subsequent disability.

Overall it does appear that anxiety and fear as emotional states have important roles to play in the perception of pain and therefore there is some value in attempting to reduce pain and distress by directly addressing anxiety in the pre-operative and post-operative situations.

Depression and pain

The threat of pain and its experience can lead to low mood and negative affect (Eccleston 2001). Depression has been found to be a common feature of chronic pain, and is characterized by feelings of hopelessness, withdrawal, lethargy and feelings of worthlessness (Eccleston et al 2003, Romano and Turner 1985, Tyrer 1992, Tyrer et al 1989). Anger is frequently associated with depression and Eccleston (2001) suggests that when patients have chronic pain, anger is a means by which people attempt to gain self-control or to enhance their self-esteem. Classically, depression has been studied only in the context of chronic pain but recent evidence suggests that depression also has an important role in the experience of acute pain (Carr et al 2005, Gillies et al 1999, Taezner 1986). In the post-operative period, Gillies et al (1999) studied the depression-pain relationship in 351 adolescents undergoing elective surgery and found that pre-operative depression scores had risen from 4% to 29% after surgery with depressed patients being more likely to experience severe pain post-operatively. Similarly, Carr et al (2005) examined the role of depression over time on surgical pain experience among 85 women undergoing gynaecological surgery. Using the hospital anxiety and depression scale (HADS) they assessed the patients pre-operatively and then on days 2, 4 and 10 post-operatively, and found depression to have increased significantly by day 4.

When people experience the prolonged stress of unrelieved pain and feel that nothing they do helps, they may stop striving to achieve goals and come to believe that they have no control over events in their lives. In other words they develop a sense of helplessness.

Helplessness and controllability

Learned helplessness (inability to effect change in spite of repeated efforts) is a major component of depression (Beck 1976). The psychological state of uncontrollability or helplessness is therefore a key feature of anxiety, depression and pain. There is an abundance of human and animal studies that supports the link between perceived control, anxiety, and painful or aversive events (Mandler 1972, Miller et al 1989).

Patients who live with chronic pain typically perceive that they have a lack of control, which may be related to their unsuccessful attempts to control their pain. Psychological techniques aimed at enhancing personal control and reducing the sense of helplessness are a basic feature of an effective approach to pain control (Jensen and Karoly 1991, Wells 1994).

THE ROLE OF MEANING

People attach meaning to their pain, and evidence suggests that such meaning may influence the ways individuals tolerate pain. The meanings associated with pain and suffering may dramatically affect the intensity and quality of the individual experience of pain. An early example of the powerful effect of meaning was described by Henry Beecher in 1956 (Beecher 1956). He made comparisons between seriously wounded soldiers (during World War II) and civilians in an American hospital during peace-time and observed that, in spite of their extensive wounds, the soldiers reported significantly less pain than the civilians and required less analgesic medication. Beecher suggested that the relief at finding themselves alive and removed from the line of fire was significant. For the soldiers their wounds marked release from life-threatening trauma, but for the civilians the hospitalization marked the start of personal disaster and disruption in their lives.

In a study involving 148 hospital inpatients, Copp (1974) assessed personal meanings of pain. The results showed that more than half saw pain as a challenge, something to fight and conquer, to promote self-searching and increasing understanding of others, and a quarter saw pain as weakness or punishment. These socio-cultural meanings influence attitudes towards pain and also have an impact on the patient's subsequent behaviour.

Fordham and Dunn (1994) have argued that the search for and the attribution of meaning is not only necessary for response but provides a way of coping with pain. Like pain, cancer has special meanings for people. It is commonly perceived to be uncontrollable and unpredictable, linked closely to extreme pain, suffering and death. Cassell (1982) provides an example of a patient who reported that when she believed the pain in her leg was sciatica she was able to control it with small doses of codeine. However, when she discovered that it was due to the spread of malignant disease, much greater amounts of medication were required for relief. This example introduces the notion of the effects of pain when it is perceived as a threat to well-being. In another study Daut and Cleeland (1982) found that the impairment of normal activities and life enjoyment was greatest in patients who believed their pain to be caused by cancer, intermediate for those attributing pain to cancer treatment, and lowest for those who did not believe cancer was causing the pain. Pain then can be perceived as a threat and in research to explore the impact of this perception, Crombez et al (1998) found that threatened patients experienced greater disruption on task performance than non-threatened patients.

Other research has considered the ways in which pain appraisals relate to coping. Eccleston and Crombez (1999) found that fear of pain produced catastrophic thinking, less engagement in cognitive distraction and reduced pain tolerance; Unruh et al (1999) reported similar results. More recently, Jackson et al (2005) found that healthy adult volunteers in a threatened situation experienced a reduction in pain tolerance, cognitive coping strategies and used more catastrophizing than those in control conditions.

Whether the pain is **acute** or **chronic**, it is closely related to the meaning the patient attaches to the pain and hence how they will cope with it. The pain of childbirth is severe and acute but the woman knows it is self-limiting. That is very different to the chronic pain of an advanced cancer, a disease that the person knows will probably lead to their death. Post-operative pain is again severe and acute, but the patient knows that eventually it should resolve. Contrast that with the chronic pain of osteoarthritis, which the patient knows will not go away and is caused by disease that, while not life threatening, is progressive and disabling. Psychological factors therefore play a major role in the patient's perception of pain. Many patients adapt to chronic pain and just live with it as part of their everyday routine. They still feel the pain, but they do not show it in the same way that a person shows acute sudden pain.

ASSESSMENT AND EVALUATION OF ACUTE PAIN

The efficacy of pain management strategies can be assessed and improved only if some form of measurement is made. Many studies have shown that lack of assessment (Paice et al 1991) or inadequate pain assessment (Larue et al 1997, Sloan et al 1996) are major causes of poor pain control.

Objective **assessment** techniques have relied upon the assessment of biochemical indices such as changes in plasma concentrations of hormones, but these tend to be inaccurate, expensive and not applicable in clinical practice (Mitchell and Smith 1989). However, simple respiratory function tests may be a useful indicator of pain severity after abdominal and thoracic surgery (Chapman 1989) and posture, restlessness and facial expression can all be observed and are part of the behavioural aspects of acute pain. Although an experienced observer may be able to use these indicators to make a rough assessment of the degree of pain suffered by the patient, absence of the behavioural or physiological signs of pain does not necessarily mean that the patient is not experiencing pain.

It is widely accepted that the amount of suffering can only be assessed accurately by the patient themselves (McCaffrey and Beebe 1989. McCaffrey and Pasero 1999).

According to McCaffrey and Pasero (1999) nurses avoid asking patients about their pain because it may reveal a pain problem that they do not know how to relieve. Additionally our conscious and unconscious biases and misconceptions can, on some occasions, get in the way of us asking patients about their pain.

In recent years some advances have been made in the clinical measurement and evaluation of pain. A huge area of research has been devoted to the development of assessment tools, which are aimed at enhancing the person's verbal expression of their suffering so that they can convey their subjective experience. Meinhart and McCaffrey (1983) have argued that comprehensive assessment of pain should include the following information:

- location
- quality
- pattern
- intensity
- factors that increase the pain
- verbal statements about the pain (this should include asking the patient about his or her usual manner of expressing pain)
- non-verbal expression
- associated symptoms.

A useful tool for analysing pain as a symptom is the PQRST tool described by Walsh (2005). This tool can be used to analyse the nature of any symptom such as a cough or stiff knee joint and is particularly useful for the analysis of pain. The letters PQRST give the following framework to the assessment:

P Provocation/Palliation – What brings on the pain? What relieves the pain?

Q Quality – What does the pain feel like? Stabbing? Dull ache? Sharp? Throbbing?

R Region/Radiation – Where do you feel the pain? Does it radiate anywhere?

S Severity – A simple approach is simply to ask the patient to rate the pain from 0 to 10, where 0 means no pain at all and 10 the most severe pain imaginable. This should be assessed at rest and when moving, if appropriate. See below for other pain severity rating scales.

T Time – How long have you had the pain? Does it vary through the day?

Pain is an intensely personal experience and no nurse can ever really know the patient's pain experience. Pain represents the limits of empathy in many cases. Unfortunately there are still many misconceptions concerning pain, and they are summarized in Box 8.1.

UNIDIMENSIONAL RATING SCALES

There are a number of rating scales that are commonly used to measure pain, and these have been described as simple and reproducible. They enable the patient to express the severity of pain in a way that is quantifiable. They vary according to the nature and number of anchor points supplied, numbers, words or the presentation of visual analogue lines, and are available in a variety of languages (McCaffrey and Pasero 1999). *Visual analogue scales* (VASs) consist of a straight line with numerical, verbal or pictorial anchors with the ends representing the extreme limits of pain.

Verbal rating scales (VRSs) consist of a sequence of words corresponding to escalating pain. The more words in the scale, the more sensitive it is; however, it has been found that the patient is less likely to choose the same word on different occasions even if the pain is the same.

Visual analogue scales

The VAS consists of a straight line, usually 10 cm long, with the ends representing the extreme limits of pain (McCaffrey

Box 8.1 Misconceptions about assessment of patients who indicate they have pain	
Misconception	Correction
1. The health team is the authority about the existence and nature of the patient's pain sensation	The person with pain is the only authority about the existence and nature of the pain, since the sensation of pain can be felt only by the person who has it
2. Our personal values and intuition about the trustworthiness of others is a valuable tool in identifying whether a person is lying about a pain	Personal values and intuition do not constitute a professional approach to the patient with pain. The patient's credibility is not on trial
3. Pain is largely an emotional or psychological problem, especially in the patient who is highly anxious or depressed	Having an emotional reaction to pain does not mean that pain is caused by an emotional problem. If anxiety or depression is alleviated, the intensity of pain will not necessarily be any less
4. Lying about the existence of pain, malingering, is common	Very few people who say they have pain are lying about it. Outright fabrication of pain is considered rare
5. The patient who obtains benefits or preferential treatment because of pain is receiving secondary gain and does not hurt as much as he or she says or may not hurt at all	The patient who uses pain to advantage is not the same as a malingerer and may still hurt as much as stated gain
6. All real pain has an identifiable physical cause	All pain is real, regardless of its cause. Almost all pain has both physical and mental components. Pure psychogenic pain is rare
7. Visible signs, either physiological or behavioural, accompany pain and can be used to verify its existence and severity	Even with severe pain, periods of physiological and behavioural adaptation occur, leading to periods of minimal or no signs of pain. Lack of pain expression does not necessarily mean lack of pain. How must the patient act for us to believe he or she has pain?
8. Comparable physical stimuli produce comparable pain in different people. The severity and duration of pain can be predicted accurately for everyone on the basis of the stimuli for pain	Comparable stimuli in different people do *not* produce the same intensities of pain. Comparable stimuli in different people will produce different intensities of pain that last different periods. There is no direct and invariant relationship between any stimulus and the perception of pain
9. People with pain should be taught to have a high tolerance for pain. The more prolonged the pain or the more experience a person has with pain, the better is the tolerance for pain	Pain tolerance is the individual's unique response, varying between patients and varying in the same patient from one situation to another. People with prolonged pain tend to have an increasingly low pain tolerance. Respect for the patient's pain tolerance is crucial for adequate pain control
10. When the patient reports pain relief following a placebo, this means that the patient is a malingerer or that the pain is psychogenic	There is not a shred of evidence anywhere in the literature to justify using a placebo to diagnose malingering or psychogenic pain

From McCaffrey and Beebe (1989), with permission.

and Pasero 1999). A VAS with points (either words or numbers) between the ends is known as a graphic rating scale (GRS). The patient makes a mark on the line appropriate to the level of pain she or he is experiencing. The scales may also be drawn vertically. The distance from the 'no pain' end is measured, and provides the patient's intensity score.

No pain _____ Pain as bad as it could be

Scores obtained on the VAS and GRS have been shown to correlate well with other measurements.

Visual analogue pain relief scale (VAPRS)

These are comparative scales that present the extremes in amount of relief achieved. According to Skevington (1995) this approach has the advantage that all patients start from the same baseline and consequently the size of the response does not depend on the initial severity of pain. However, a big disadvantage – which outweighs its usefulness – is the absence of options to demonstrate an increase in pain. Another limitation is the fact that individual variations are masked because the scale gives the impression that all patients start with the same level of pain (Skevington 1995).

No relief _____ Complete relief

Numerical rating scales

Numerical rating scales are a variation of VASs where subjects are asked to score their pain intensity from 0 to 10 or from 0 to 100. These scales are regarded as easier to score and analyse in many different pain settings. For example, in a study of 60 post-operative patients, Deloach et al (1998) found that a 0–10 NRS was easier to use than a VAS.

Simple descriptor scales

This is a list of adjectives such as no pain, mild, moderate, and severe pain that describe different levels of pain intensity. This is a very well-established way of assessing pain that is easily understood.

Picture scales

Picture scales were first developed by Frank et al (1982). The scale consists of eight line drawings of human faces experiencing different levels of pain. The drawings are presented randomly. A useful scale for children is the one developed by Beyer (1994) called the *Oucher*, this is a pictorial scale that makes use of happy and sad photographically represented faces for assessing pain intensity in children aged between 3 and 12 years. In addition to being ideally suited for use among children, pictorial scales are advantageous for the patient who cannot speak or understand English.

The unidimensional rating scales do not reflect the complexity of the pain experience. Reading (1984) suggests that over repeated trials patients may use single scales to reflect different components of their pain. This occurs because it is difficult for the VAS to distinguish between the intensity of sensory pain and the unpleasantness of affective pain. Attempts have been made to overcome this problem by making use of questionnaire methods in an attempt to reflect the multidimensional experience.

QUESTIONNAIRE METHODS

The McGill Pain Questionnaire (MPQ) (Melzack and Torgerson 1971) was developed from work demonstrating high agreement among patients, students and physicians on the meaning attached to pain adjectives. It consists of 78 adjectives arranged into groups. The questionnaire is intended to reflect three dimensions – sensory, affective and evaluative – with three remaining groups reflecting a sensory miscellaneous category.

The MPQ yields a number of indices: a *pain rating index* based on two types of numerical values that can be assigned to each word descriptor; the *number of words chosen*; and the *present pain intensity* based on a 1–5 intensity scale. Since its introduction the MPQ has been used extensively, and experience suggests that it provides precise information on the sensory, affective and evaluative aspects of pain experience as well as discriminating among different pain problems (Melzack 1975).

Researchers from various countries have translated the MPQ and tested its reliability and validity; it is currently available in a wide variety of languages. A shortened form of the MPQ (SF-MPQ) has been developed (Melzack 1987) for use in the clinical post-operative situation and research situations that require a more rapid acquisition of data than is possible with the standard MPQ. The data obtained with the SF-MPQ provide information on the sensory, affective and overall intensity of pain.

The brief pain inventory (BPI) has been well validated within research settings and has been found to be reasonably reliable in clinical settings (Cleeland et al 1994). It is available in a number of languages and focuses on pain in the past 24 hours. It consists of 9 questions that range from asking about common aches and pains to questions that attempt to identify the impact of pain on activities of daily living.

All the scales discussed above are valid measures but some scales are more appropriate for clinical practice than others. In terms of deciding what scales to use, research has shown that in addition to reliability and validity, pain scales should be simple, easy to use and comprehend and should also be liked by patients and staff.

METHODS OF MANAGING PAIN

PHYSICAL APPROACHES

Transcutaneous electrical nerve stimulation

Transcutaneous electrical nerve stimulation (TENS) is a small battery-operated pack that generates impulses via electrodes producing a continuous low-intensity electrical current to the skin. One of the most obvious predictions of the **gate control theory** was that stimulation of large-diameter fibres would inhibit pain. The practical implication of this is that increasing large-diameter fibre input to the spinal cord with vibration, acupuncture and electrical stimulation can inhibit upward transmission of pain impulses. TENS controls pain by stimulating the large fibres, closing the gate on the smaller-diameter pain fibres. Simultaneously, TENS is thought to stimulate the production of **endorphins**.

Acupuncture

Acupuncture is part of traditional Chinese medicine that involves the insertion of needles at specific points on the body. Acupuncture points were discovered and mapped thousands of years ago and the effects can be powerful enough to control severe pain (Schoen 1994). Acupuncture points do not necessarily have to be close to the source of the pain to be effective. The effects are produced by the release of endogenous opioids such as **enkephalins** (Heath 1997).

PHARMACOLOGICAL CONSIDERATIONS IN THE MANAGEMENT OF PAIN

It is only in recent years, as we have begun to understand the physiological processes that underlie pain, that drugs have begun to be designed with predictable analgesic activity.

Analgesics can be divided broadly into two groups, antiinflammatory and opioids, and these vary in effectiveness, site of action and incidence of side-effects.

Antiinflammatory analgesics

Paracetamol and aspirin are the most commonly used antiinflammatory analgesics. They have the common property of inhibiting prostaglandin synthesis and may have a more peripheral site of action. Paracetamol is used most commonly and, although it can cause liver damage in overdose, it is safe in normal dosage. Aspirin is also an effective analgesic but has many contraindications which relate primarily to its effects on thrombotic regulation.

Non-steroidal antiinflammatory drugs

Non-steroidal antiinflammatory drugs (NSAIDs) are a useful group of medicines for managing pain due to inflammation such as rheumatoid arthritis and osteoarthritis. NSAIDs are cyclo-oxygenase inhibitors and therefore reduce prostaglandin synthesis. According to Heath (1997) they act peripherally at the site of trauma and consequently are an effective adjuvant to opioid drugs without increasing unwanted side-effects. However, in the UK every year over 2000 people die as a result of upper gastrointestinal damage induced by NSAIDs (NICE 2001). NSAIDs are contraindicated in patients with renal impairment and also cause hypersensitivity reactions in situations of prolonged use. Of particular importance is the risk to patients who have asthma as aspirin can cause an exacerbation. People with asthma should not routinely use NSAIDs.

Opioid analgesics

Opioid analgesics are the most commonly prescribed drugs for surgical and other forms of intense acute and chronic pain. The term opioid is used to describe all drugs, natural and synthetic, which bind specifically to opioid receptors and exert an agonist action. The ability to bind to these receptors is antagonized by the opioid antagonist naloxone. It is now known that the opioid system comprises four distinct receptor subtypes: mu, kappa, delta and sigma. Mu receptors are of two kinds, m1 and m2; m1 is believed to mediate analgesia, whereas m2 receptors mediate the unwanted side-effects of respiratory depression, addiction and constipation (Melzack and Wall 1988).

Weak opioids

A number of agents related to morphine, for example codeine, dihydrocodeine and dextropropoxyphene, are used in an attempt to increase analgesia via the oral route whilst minimizing the unwanted side-effects. The main use of these drugs is for 'step up' or 'step down' treatment according to the analgesic ladder in the management of changing situations, either when simple analgesia ceases to be effective in a progressive condition or where the degree of pain no longer warrants strong opioids (Heath 1997).

Morphine

Despite the current availability of several new agonist/antagonist or partial agonist drugs, morphine – the pure agonist – remains the mainstay of the treatment of postoperative pain, sickle-cell crisis pain, cancer and other acute pain. It will be used as a practical example of the pharmacological properties of drugs of this type. Morphine is the most pharmacologically active constituent of opium; its use is dictated by intensity of pain and not brevity of prognosis (Twycross 1984). This means that morphine should be prescribed when a weaker narcotic fails to relieve pain.

Morphine and diamorphine (heroin) are agonists at mu receptors and also have some affinity for kappa receptors, although the affinity for mu receptors is nearly 100 times greater (Alexander and Hill 1988). Under some circumstances opioids may produce analgesia by a peripheral mechanism, and also act within the central nervous system.

Diamorphine is a derivative of morphine and its pharmacological properties are almost identical to those of morphine. It is readily absorbed by all routes of administration and its greater solubility allows larger doses to be administered in a single injection.

All morphine and other mu-selective opioid agonists are potent analgesics; they tend to induce euphoria and have a strong dependence liability, which makes these drugs subject to legal controls. Mu opioids are respiratory depressants and, in large doses, can cause heavy sedation. They can also produce nausea and vomiting, and cause constipation (Alexander and Hill 1988).

Morphine depresses the respiratory centre, making it less sensitive to carbon dioxide (the stimulus for normal respiration). The euphoria-inducing element of morphine is the reason for its strong addictive potential; however, there is little convincing evidence to suggest that the appropriate use of morphine to control severe pain leads to addiction. The incidence of addiction associated with therapeutic use of opiates in the adult population is generally overestimated by nursing staff (McCaffrey and Ferrell 1990).

Morphine and other mu opioids show reduced effectiveness if administered repeatedly at high doses; this is usually referred to as tolerance. When prolonged high-dose administration of mu opioids is stopped, a withdrawal syndrome develops. This can also be precipitated without stopping the opioid if a potent antagonist drug such as naloxone is given. Typically, withdrawal leads to sweating, cramps, diarrhoea, shivering and general malaise.

Alternatives to morphine

Pethidine

Pethidine is a synthetic compound that has a similar receptor-binding profile to morphine, being largely mu selective. In addition to the opioid properties shared with morphine, pethidine has atropine-like actions and is about one-eighth as potent as morphine. It has an established role in obstetrics because it is a mild stimulant of uterine contractions and appears to cause less respiratory depression in the newborn than morphine. It was also used historically to manage acute sickle-cell crisis pain but because of its short half-life and the toxic build-up of the metabolite, norpethidine, use of pethidine in this area is no longer tenable. Consequently pethidine is now contraindicated in the management of sickle-cell pain throughout the UK.

Fentanyl and alfentanil

These compounds are potent mu-selective agents and are chemically closely related to each other and to pethidine. Fentanyl is some 50–100 times more potent than morphine as an analgesic because of its lipid solubility. It has, however, a shorter duration of action. Alfentanil is similar to fentanyl but has a more rapid onset of action and an even shorter duration of action, it is therefore useful in the intra-operative period. Fentanyl has not been used generally for post-operative pain because doses that do not cause respiratory depression have a very short action. However, with the increased use of patient-controlled analgesia (PCA) its use in the management of post-operative pain is becoming more common (Mather and Owen 1988). Fentanyl is also useful in the management of breakthrough pain for patients who are already using opiod analgesics and in the management of patients who have chronic intractable pain. It can be administered either as a lozenge or a patch and individual dose adjustment is important in order to achieve the best possible pain relief with the least amount of side-effects.

Patient-controlled analgesia

From the above discussion it is clear that there is a wide range of potent medications for controlling pain, and the past four decades have seen a change in the focus of attention from seeking the perfect drug towards providing optimal drug delivery methods that integrate with the personal experience of the patient. Patient-controlled analgesia (PCA) offers an individualized method of drug delivery system, and also offers more precise control of pain.

The PCA system consists of a syringe pump and a timing device. The patient activates the system by pressing a button, causing a small dose of analgesic to be delivered into the venous system. Simultaneously a lockout device is activated, ensuring that another dose cannot be delivered until the first dose has had time to exert its full effect. Thus, PCA is currently the ultimate patient-centred pain management technique because it allows patients to determine when and how much analgesic they receive, and secondly it allows determination of a minimum blood drug concentration associated with effective analgesic concentration and minimum side-effects, despite great inter-patient variability.

Recent development of PCA technology appears to have followed two main streams. One is the development of increasingly sophisticated bedside drug delivery systems and the other is the production of smaller devices suitable for ambulatory use.

Patient-controlled analgesia as an efficient means of controlling post-operative pain

When compared to the conventional PRN (when required, nurse administered method) the active involvement of the patient offered by PCA has been found to provide more effective relief (O'Connor et al 1993, Thomas et al 1995). For example, O'Connor et al (1993) found that within the first 4 hours after an operation patients receiving intramuscular injections experienced 80% of the worst pain they could imagine, compared with 30% among the PCA groups. This efficacy is verified by Ballantyne et al (1993) who undertook a systematic review of studies evaluating the efficacy of PCA and found it to be associated with significantly better pain relief when compared to the more conventional method.

PCA is also associated with a reduction in the length of stay in hospital (Thomas et al 1993), with findings demonstrating that patients receiving PCA are discharged on average 2 days earlier than those having intramuscular injections. This suggests that PCA promotes recovery. An explanation for this is that PCA provides an increased sense of control, which promotes a sense of well-being (Thomas and Rose 1993). Research undertaken by Taylor et al (1996) was aimed at determining whether patients did experience enhanced personal control when using PCA. The research which used semi-structured interviews amongst post-operative patients found that PCA was not associated with the perception of enhanced control, rather patients valued PCA because it offered a means of avoiding the difficulty of disclosing pain or asking for analgesia within the nurse–patient relationship.

In addition to the focus on pain control, it is important to ensure that the patient receives adequate anti-emetic medication to prevent the continual nausea and vomiting that may be associated with PCA administration of opioids.

PSYCHOLOGICAL ASPECTS OF PCA

Although patients are generally satisfied with the effectiveness of relief obtained from PCA, effective analgesia may not necessarily be related to patient satisfaction. Some patients may prefer more nursing attention (Koh and Thomas 1994), whilst fear of overdose may result in under-use of PCA and the patient experiencing more pain than with intramuscular injections. The extent to which patients accept and use PCA is dependent on their attitudes and beliefs about pain and its relief – in other words, their psychology.

Whilst in general terms PCA does appear to be superior to intramuscular injections, this cannot be taken to mean that PCA functions optimally for all patients. For instance, Murphy et al (1993) found that a small proportion of surgical patients were unwilling to use PCA despite encouragement. Although psychological variables were not measured it is likely that this reluctance may have been influenced by psychological factors.

It is well recognized that psychological factors play a significant role in the perception and tolerance of pain as well as in the willingness to communicate the discomfort and distress caused by pain (Melzack and Wall 1988), and these factors are of utmost importance in relation to PCA (Thomas and Rose 1993). Research addressing the psychological issues concerning PCA is limited (Thomas et al 1995), but the implications from these studies suggest that, if a patient does not normally acknowledge a degree of personal control and responsibility for his or her own health, allocation to a PCA regimen may be a source of stress to the patient and prove less beneficial than more conventional methods.

PSYCHOLOGICAL APPROACHES TO PAIN MANAGEMENT

The psychological techniques that can be used in pain management are extensive and deserve the space of a whole chapter, if not a book, and I refer the reader to Gatchel and Turk (1996). The present discussion will be confined to the role of information and cognitive behavioural therapy (CBT). As outlined in the discussion of the gate control theory, there is a close relationship between physiological and psychological factors. Thus cognitive processes (i.e. the way we think) can affect the amount and quality of pain experienced by altering the influence of the spinal gate mechanism.

Information

Eccleston (1997) suggests that pain activity in the nervous system can be interpreted as a sudden increase in information that travels quickly to the brain where it is decoded and acted upon. The decoding is known as cognition (the meaning of the pain) and the action is the resultant behaviour. Information is extremely important in helping to appraise (give meaning to sensation) and manage pain. In the acute pain situation information is used to prepare people for what to expect, whilst in the chronic pain context information is best used to counteract unhelpful and inaccurate beliefs (Williams 1997). The provision of adequate information to a person who is about to undergo surgery reduces the uncertainty and the distress and degree of pain experienced in the post-operative period.

Some typical informational control techniques have informed patients about the sensations they are likely to experience and procedures involved in the situation (Boore 1978, Hayward 1975). The extent to which information is of value depends largely on the coping styles of the patients (i.e. their normal preference for information). Thus, if a person usually copes with stress by distraction, providing detailed information about what the operation entails, what it will feel like and what the sounds represent is likely to increase anxiety and subsequent pain.

Cognitive behavioural therapy

By far the most effective psychological approach used in pain management utilizes cognitive behavioural psychology. It seeks to influence patients' perception or appraisal of events and their behaviour by addressing their concerns at cognitive and behavioural levels. The cognitive aspect recognizes the importance of the individual's personal view of the experience. The behavioural portion emphasizes active performance-based strategies to reduce pain. Behaviourally oriented training recognizes that remedial efforts towards successful coping require the practice of relevant practical skills and thinking strategies.

The central features of the CBT perspective include:

- interest in the nature and modification of patients' thoughts, feelings, beliefs and behaviours
- some commitment to behaviour therapy procedures in promoting change (e.g. graded practice, homework assignments, relaxation and relapse prevention training).

Although CBT may result in a reduction in the frequency and intensity of pain, pain relief is not the primary goal. Rather, the aim is to help patients learn to live more effective and satisfying lives despite the presence of pain (Turk and Meichenbaum 1994) (see Box 8.2).

Studies evaluating the efficacy of CBT in chronic pain have consistently revealed that it is significantly more effective than an attention placebo or no-treatment control (Compass et al 1998, Keefe and Caldwell 1997, Thomas et al 1999, Turner and Jensen 1993). CBT reduces pain, distress and negative coping strategies, and it improves positive coping strategies, perceptions of internal control and pain self-efficacy. In a recent systematic review of 25 randomized controlled trials of CBT, Morley et al (2005) found that CBT was more effective in reducing pain and improving positive coping in patients who suffer with chronic pain than those in control conditions.

The main focus of the work in CBT is to get patients to understand the relationships between their beliefs about pain, their feelings and their behaviour. The aim is to teach patients to identify unhelpful thoughts that lead to negative feelings such as anger, anxiety and depression, and to modify them. This is achieved by a technique known as cognitive restructuring, whereby patients are taught to examine objectively whether such thoughts are accurate and justified by the evidence (Turner and Keefe 1999). Another important task of the therapist is to teach patients to keep a log of their thoughts. This is achieved by providing a record sheet with four columns, for identifying a particular event that triggers such thoughts, feelings and behavioural outcome. With respect to feelings, patients are asked to rate the intensity of accompanying emotion on a scale of 0–100%; in the example given in Box 8.3, feelings of sadness and depression are estimated to be 80%, indicating a very powerful sense of depression.

Thought monitoring is done as homework activity, and is useful in educating patients to distinguish between thoughts and feelings. As therapy progresses, the therapist works with the patient to determine whether negative thoughts are accurate and whether alternative interpretations are possible. For example, in response to the negative thought

'There is nothing I can do to relieve the pain', the therapist helps the patient to recognize that such a thought is incorrect because relaxation is something the patient can do to relieve the pain. The objective is to assist patients to recognize that negative thoughts are only one way of thinking about their situation and that with systematic examination of the evidence, more optimistic alternatives are possible.

Relaxation

Relaxation training appears to be an effective adjunctive treatment, used in comprehensive pain management programmes. Chief benefits include: the reduction of muscle tension and pain, a decrease in the fear associated with the anticipation of pain, and an increase in confidence in coping with pain. As relaxation training emphasizes self-control, many medical centres offer this training in an attempt to reduce the need for analgesic and anti-anxiety medication. In evaluating the efficacy of relaxation in adults with chronic pain, McCaffrey and Beebe (1989) reported that patients rated relaxation training to be more helpful than pharmacological treatments and counselling, but less helpful than physical therapy. According to Linton (1982), relaxation is helpful because it reduces tension in patients with chronic pain. Progressive muscle relaxation is the commonest relaxation strategy used in chronic pain situations and has been found to be effective in reducing pain, anxiety and disability at 1 and 4 months' follow-up (Seers 1997).

Imagery

Focusing on a pleasant image is a useful addition to relaxation. Images can involve ourselves, the outside world and images of ourselves in the world. However, in the context of CBT strategies, images using multiple senses (seeing, hearing and touching) are likely to be most effective (Turner and Keefe 1999). For example, the patient might imagine herself lying on a Caribbean beach, and in this imagery she can imagine seeing the deep blue-green of the sea, hear children's laughter as they play in the water, feel the sun on her face, and trail her fingers in the warm sand.

As people with chronic pain frequently have imagery of the part of their body that hurts, the therapist can guide the patient (guided imagery) to soothe the pain; for example: 'Imagine that the sun is acting as a heat pad to the painful part and soothing the pain away'.

Coping self statements

Positive statements such as 'I know that I can cope with this if I remain calm and relaxed' are very helpful in countering

---

Box 8.2 Primary objectives of cognitive behavioural treatment programmes as outlined by Turk and Meichenbaum (1994)

- To combat demoralization by assisting patients to change their view of their pain and suffering from overwhelming to manageable

- To teach patients that there are coping techniques and skills that can be used to help them adapt and respond to pain and the resultant problems

- To assist patients to reconceptualize their views of themselves from being passive, reactive and helpless to being active, resourceful and competent

- To help patients learn the associations between thoughts, feelings and their behaviour, and subsequently to identify and alter automatic, maladaptive patterns

- To teach patients specific coping skills and, moreover, when and how to utilize these more adaptive responses

- To bolster self-confidence and encourage patients to attribute successful outcomes to their own efforts

- To help patients anticipate problems proactively and generate solutions, thereby facilitating maintenance and generalization

---

Box 8.3 Example of thought monitoring

Event	Thought	Feeling	Behaviour outcome
Woke up with pain in right hip	There is nothing I can do to relieve the pain	Sadness, depression (80%)	Stayed in bed all day

negative thoughts such as those discussed above. As with all the strategies taught in CBT, coping self-statements need to be practised over several weeks in order that they become part of a repertoire of coping skills.

Group therapy

Although CBT has been established as individual therapy, group CBT is very popular in many chronic pain management programmes. The advantages of group over individualized approaches include more efficient allocation of professional resources and the value of support from others who have similar problems (Turner and Keefe 1999). However, all group programmes take account of the individual in the group, and goals for behavioural change are developed individually with each patient.

Maintenance of gains

An important component of CBT programmes is the prevention of relapse. To maintain positive benefits, the therapist works with patients to identify early signs of obstacles or high-risk situations and develop an action plan. Through the use of role play the patient rehearses how to cope in such situations.

SUMMARY

This chapter has considered the physiology, pharmacology and psychology of pain, which must all be taken into account when discussing pain and its control. The routine assessment of pain and its relief is an important component of any pain management strategy and, as the above discussion showed, there are many different methods of assessing pain. However, the use of a simple VAS in the absence of more comprehensive methods is recommended.

An important way of achieving effective pain control is through effective communication with the patient and the multidisciplinary team: Carr (1997) has argued that no one member of the team should assume responsibility for pain control. Therefore, the nurse needs to liaise closely with physicians, physiotherapists, psychologists and pharmacists. The development of newer methods of analgesic administration such as PCA has provided opportunities for greater relief compared with the traditional nurse-administered intramuscular injection method. Effective pain management should be seen as essential to the provision of good-quality care, but can occur only with accurate and regular assessment of the patient's pain.

REFERENCES

Alexander JJ, Hill RG (1988) Postoperative pain control. Oxford: Blackwell Scientific.

Anand KJS, Hickey PR (1987) Pain and its effects in the human neonate and fetus. New England Journal of Medicine 317(21): 1321–1329.

Ballantyne JC, Carr DB, Chalmers TC et al (1993) Postoperative patient-controlled analgesia: meta-analyses of initial randomized control trials. Journal of Clinical Anesthesia 5: 182–193.

Beck AT (1976) Cognitive therapy and the emotional disorders. New York: New American Library.

Beecher HK (1956) Relationship of significance of wound to pain experienced. Journal of American Medical Association 161: 1609–1613.

Belville JW, Forrest WH Jr, Miller E et al (1971) Influence of age on pain relief from analgesics. Journal of American Medical Association 217: 1835–1841.

Berkowitz BA, Ngai SH, Yang JC et al (1975) The disposition of morphine in surgical patients. Clinical Pharmacology and Therapeutics 17: 629–635.

Beyer J (1994) The Oucher: a pain intensity scale for children. In: Funk SG, Tornquist EM, Champagne MT et al, eds. Management of pain, fatigue and nausea. Basingstoke: Macmillan, p 35–45.

Bond MR (1979) Pain, its nature, analysis and treatment. Edinburgh: Churchill Livingstone.

Boore JRP (1978) Information a prescription for recovery. London: Royal College of Nursing.

Burns JW, Hodsman NBA, McLintock TT et al (1989) The influence of patient characteristics on the requirements for postoperative analgesia. Anaesthesia 44: 2–6.

Carr E (1997) Management of post-operative pain: problems and solutions. In: Thomas V, ed. Pain, its nature and management. London: Baillière Tindall, p 156–175.

Carr ECJ, Thomas VJ, Wilson-Barnet J (2005) Patient experiences of anxiety, depression and acute pain after surgery. International Journal of Nursing Studies 42: 521–530.

Cassell EJ (1982) The nature of suffering and the goals of medicine. Oxford: Oxford University Press.

Chapman CR (1984) New directions in the understanding and management of pain. Journal of Social Science and Medicine 19(12): 1261–1277.

Chapman CR (1989) Assessment of pain. In: Nimmo WS, Smith G, eds. Anaesthesia. London: Blackwells, p 1149–1165.

Cleeland CS, Gonin R, Hatfield A.K et al (1994) Pain and its treatment in outpatients with metastatic cancer, New England Journal of Medicine 330: 592–596.

Compass BE, Haaga DAF, Keefe FJ et al (1998) Sampling of empirically supported psychological treatments from health psychology: smoking, chronic pain, cancer and bulima nervosa. Journal of Consulting and Clinical Psychology 66: 89–112.

Copp LA (1974) The spectrum of suffering. American Journal of Nursing 74(3): 491–495.

Crombez G, Eccleston C, Baeyens F et al (1998) When somatic information threatens catastrophic thinking enhances attention interference. Pain 75: 187–198.

Daut RL, Cleeland CS (1982) The prevalence and severity of pain in cancer. Cancer 50: 99-108.

Davis P (1993) Opening up the gate control theory. Nursing Standard 7(45): 25–27.

Deloach U, Higgings MS, Caplan AB et al (1998) The visual analogue scale in the immediate post operative period: intrasubject variability and correlation with a numeric scale. Anesthesia and Analgesia 56: 102–106.

Donovan BD (1983) Patients' attitude to postoperative pain relief. Anaesthesia and Intensive Care 11(2): 125–129.

Eccleston C (1997) Pain and thinking: an introduction to cognitive psychology. In: Thomas V, ed. Pain, its nature and management. London: Baillière Tindall, p 35–53.

Eccleston C (2001) Role of psychology in pain management. British Journal of Anaesthesia 87(1): 144–152.

Eccleston C, Crombez G (1999) Pain demands attention: a cognitive-affective model of interruptive function of pain. Psychological Bulletin 125(3): 356–366.

Eccleston C, Mallesson PN, Clinch J et al (2003) Chronic pain in adolescents: evaluation of a programme of interdisciplinary cognitive behaviour therapy. Archives of Diseases in Childhood 88: 881–885.

Eland JM (1981) Minimising pain associated with pre-kindegarten intramuscular injections. Issues in Comprehensive Paediatric Nursing 5: 361–372.

Eland JM (1985) The role of the nurse in children's pain. In: Copp LA, ed. Recent advances in nursing: perspectives on pain. Edinburgh: Churchill Livingstone, p 24–45.

Flannery RB, Sos J, McGovern P (1987) Ethnicity as a factor in the expression of pain. Psychosomatics 22: 39–50.

Fordham M, Dunn V (1994) Alongside the person in pain: holistic care and nursing practice. London: Baillière Tindall.

Frank AJM, Moll JMH, Hort JF (1982) A comparison of three ways of measuring pain. Rheumatology and Rehabilitation 21: 211–217.

Frayling IM, Addison GM, Chatergee K et al (1990) Methaemoglobinaemia in children treated with prilocaine-lignocaine cream. British Medical Journal 310: 153–154.

Gatchel RJ, Turk DC (eds) (1996) Psychological approaches to pain management: a practitioners' handbook. New York: Guilford Press.

Gillies ML, Smith LN, Parry-Jones WJ (1999) Postoperative pain assessment and management in adolescents. Pain 79: 207–215.

Goodman JE, McGrath PJ (1991) The epidemiology of pain in children and adolescents: a review. Pain 46: 247–264.

Harrison A, Busabir AA, Al-Kaabi AO et al (1996) Does sharing a mother tongue affect how closely patients and nurses agree when rating pain, worry and knowledge? Journal of Advanced Nursing 24: 229–235.

Hayward J (1975) Information: a prescription against pain. The Study of Nursing Care Reports, series 2, no. 5. London: Royal College of Nursing.

Heath M (1997) The use of pharmacology in pain management. In: Thomas V, ed. Pain, its nature and management. London: Baillière Tindall, p 93–107.

Jackson T, Pope L, Nagasaka T et al (2005) The impact of threatening information about pain on coping and pain tolerance. British Journal of Health Psychology 10: 441–151.

Jensen MP, Karoly P (1991) Control beliefs, coping effort, and adjustment to chronic pain. Journal of Consulting and Clinical Psychology 59: 431–438.

Keefe FJ, Caldwell DS (1997) Cognitive behavioural control of arthritis pain. Medical Clinics of North America Advances in Rheumatology 81: 277–290.

Khun S, Cooke K, Collins M et al (1990) Perceptions of pain relief after surgery. British Medical Journal 300: 1687–1690.

Koh P, Thomas VJ (1994) Patient controlled analgesia: does time saved by PCA improve patient satisfaction with nursing care? Journal of Advanced Nursing 20: 61–70.

Larue F, Fontaine A, Colleau SM (1997) Underestimation and under-treatment of pain in HIV disease: multicentre study. British Medical Journal 31(44): 23–28.

Leinonen T, Leino-Kilpi H (1999) Research in perioperative nursing care. Journal of Clinical Nursing 8: 123–138.

Lim AT, Edis G, Kranz H et al (1983) Postoperative pain control: contribution of psychological factors and transcutaneous electrical stimulation. Pain 17: 179–188.

Linton SJ (1982) Applied relaxation as a method of coping with chronic pain: a therapist's guide. Scandinavian Journal of Behaviour Therapy 11: 161–174.

Lipton J, Marbach J (1984) Ethnicity in pain experience. Social Science and Medicine 19(12): 1279–1298.

Llewellyn N (1997) The management of children's pain. In: Thomas V, ed. Pain, its nature and management. London: Baillière Tindall, p 135–155.

Lorenz J, Beck H, Bromm B (1997) Cognitive performance, mood and experimental pain before and during morphine-induced analgesia in patients with chronic non-malignant pain. Pain 73: 369–375.

Mandler G (1972) Helplessness: theory and research in anxiety. In: Spielberger CD, ed. Anxiety: current trends in theory and research. New York: Academic Press, p 93–105.

Mather LE, Owen H (1988) The scientific basis of patient controlled analgesia. Anesthesia and Intensive Care 16(4): 427–446.

McCaffrey M, Beebe A (1989) Pain: clinical manual for nursing practice. St Louis, MO: CV Mosby.

McCaffrey M, Ferrell B (1990) Do you know a narcotic when you see one? Nursing 20: 62–63.

McCaffrey M, Pasero C (1999) Pain: clinical manual, 2nd edn. St Louis, MO: Mosby.

Meinhart NT, McCaffrey M (1983) Pain: a nursing approach to assessment and analysis. New York: Appleton Century-Crofts.

Melzack R (1975) The McGill Pain Questionnaire: major properties and scoring methods. Pain 1: 275–299.

Melzack R (1987) The short form McGill Pain Questionnaire. Pain 30: 191–197.

Melzack R, Dennis SG (1978) Neurophysiological foundations of pain. In: Sternbach RA, ed. The psychology of pain. New York: Raven Press, p 1–25.

Melzack R, Torgerson WS (1971) On the language of pain. Anesthesiology 34: 50–59.

Melzack R, Wall P (1965) Pain mechanism: a new theory. Science 150: 971–979.

Melzack R, Wall PD (1988) The challenge of pain. Harmondsworth: Penguin Books.

Miller JF, Shuter R (1984) Age, sex and race affect pain expression. American Journal of Nursing 9: 981.

Miller SM, Coombs C, Stoddard E (1989) Information, coping and control in patients undergoing surgery and stressful procedures. In: Steptoe A, Appels A, eds. Stress, personal control and health. Chichester: Wiley, p 107–129.

Mitchell RWD, Smith G (1989) The control of postoperative pain. British Journal of Anaesthesia 63: 147–158.

Morley S, Eccleston C, Williams A (2005) Review: cognitive and behaviour therapies are effective for chronic pain. Online. Available: ebmj.bmjjournals.com

Murphy DF, Grazioti P, Chalkiadias G et al (1993) Patient controlled analgesia for postoperative pain relief: a comparison with nurse controlled intravenous opioids. Abstracts of the

Seventh World Congress on Pain, 22–27 August. Seattle, WA: IASP Publications, p 393.

National Institute of Clinical Excellence (2001) Guidance on the use of cyclo-oxygenase Cox II selective inhibitors NICE: London

O'Connor M, Warwick P, Culpeper VE (1993) Evaluation of the effectiveness of an acute pain team. Abstracts of the Seventh World Congress on Pain, 22–27 August. Seattle, WA: IASP Publications, p 394.

Paice JA, Mahon SM, Faut-Callaghan M (1991) Factors associated with adequate pain control in hospitalised postsurgical patients diagnosed with cancer. Cancer Nursing 14: 298–305.

Peck CL (1986) Psychological factors in acute pain management. In: Cousins MJ, Phillips GD, eds. Acute pain management. Edinburgh: Churchill Livingstone, p 251–274.

Perguin CW, Hazebroek-Kampscheur AAJM, Hunfield JAM et al (2000) Pain in children and adolescents: a common experience. Pain 87: 51–58.

Perguin CW, Hazebroek-Kampscheur AAJM, Hunfield JAM et al (2001) Chronic pain among children and adolescents: Physicians consultation and medication use. Clinical Journal of Pain 16: 229–235.

Reading AE (1984) Testing pain mechanisms in persons in pain. In: Wall PD, Melzack R, eds. Textbook of Pain. Edinburgh: Churchill Livingstone, p 195–206.

Romano JM, Turner JA (1985) Chronic pain and depression: does the evidence support a relationship? Psychology Bulletin 97: 18–34.

Schoen AM (1994) Veterinary acupuncture, ancient art to modern medicine. Goleta, CA: American Veterinary Publications.

Seers K (1997) Chronic non-malignant pain: a community-based approach to management. In: Thomas V, ed. Pain, its nature and management. London: Baillière Tindall, p 221–237.

Skevington SM (1995) Psychology of pain. Chichester, UK: John Wiley.

Sloan PA, Donnelly MB, Schwartz RW et al (1996) Cancer pain assessment and management by housestaff. Pain 67: 475–481.

Spielberger CD (1966) Theory and research on anxiety. In: Spielberger CD, ed. Anxiety and behaviour. New York: Academic Press, p 3–21.

Spielberger CD (1973) Emotional reactions to surgery. Journal of Consulting and Clinical Psychology 40: 33–38.

Streltzer J, Wade TC (1981) The influence of cultural group on the undertreatment of postoperative pain. Psychosomatic Medicine 43: 397.

Taenzer PA, Melzack R, Jeans ME (1986) Influence of psychological factors on postoperative pain, mood and analgesic requirements. Pain 24: 331–342.

Taylor N, Hall GM, Salmon P (1996) Is patient controlled analgesia controlled by the patient? Social Science and Medicine 43(7): 1137–1143.

Thomas V, Heath M, Rose D et al (1995) Psychological characteristics and the effectiveness of patient controlled analgesia. British Journal of Anaesthesia 74: 271–276.

Thomas VJ (1991) Personality characteristics and the effectiveness of patient controlled analgesia. PhD thesis, Goldsmiths' College, London University.

Thomas VJ, Rose D (1991) Ethnic differences in the experience of pain. Social Science and Medicine 32: 1063–1066.

Thomas VJ, Rose D (1993) Patient controlled analgesia: a new method for old. Journal of Advanced Nursing 18: 719–726.

Thomas VJ, Dixon A, Milligan P (1999) Cognitive behaviour therapy for the management of sickle cell disease pain – an evaluation of a community based intervention. British Journal of Health Psychology 4(Part 3): 209–229.

Thomas VJ, Heath ML, Rose FD (1990) Effect of psychological variables and pain relief system on postoperative pain. British Journal of Anaesthesia 64: 388–389.

Thomas VJ, Rose FD, Heath ML et al (1993) A multidimensional comparison of nurse and patient controlled analgesia in the management of acute post surgical pain. Medical Science Research 21: 379–381.

Trijsburg RW, Jelicic M, van den Broek WW et al (1992) Behavioural treatment of needle phobia. Trijsburg voor Psychotherapie 18(6): 335–347.

Turk DC, Meichenbaum D (1994) A cognitive-behavioural approach to pain management. In: Wall PD, Melzack R, eds. Textbook of pain, 3rd edn. Edinburgh: Churchill Livingstone, p 1337–1348.

Turner J, Keefe FJ (1999) Cognitive behavioural therapy for chronic pain. In: Max M, ed. Pain: an updated review. Refresher course syllabus. Seattle, WA: IASP Press, p 523–535.

Turner JA, Jensen MP (1993) Efficacy of cognitive therapy for chronic low back pain. Pain 52: 169–177.

Twycross RG (1984) Narcotics. In: Wall PD, Melzack R, eds. Textbook of pain. Edinburgh: Churchill Livingstone, p 515–525.

Tyrer SP (1992) Psychiatric and psychological issues in different illnesses. In: Tyrer SP, ed. Psychology, psychiatry and chronic pain. Oxford: Butterworth Heinemann, p 57–69.

Tyrer SP, Capon M, Peterson DM et al (1989) The detection of psychiatric illness and psychological handicaps in a British pain clinic population. Pain 36: 63–74.

Unruh A, Ritchie J, Merskey H. (1999) Does gender affect appraisal of pain and pain coping strategies? Clinical Journal of Pain 15(1): 185–190.

Vlaeyen JWS, Kole-Snijders AMK, Boeren RGB et al (1995) Fear of movement (re) injury in chronic low back pain and its relation to behavioural performance. Pain 62: 262–272.

Walsh M (2005) Nurse practitioners: clinical skills and professional issues, 2nd edn. Oxford: Butterworth Heinemann.

Wells N (1994) Perceived control over pain: relation to distress and disability. Research in Nursing and Health 17: 295–302.

Williams AC de C (1997) Psychological techniques in pain management. In: Thomas V, ed. Pain, its nature and management. London: Baillière Tindall, p 108-124.

Woodrow KM, Friedman CD, Siegelbaub AB et al (1972) Pain tolerance: differences according to age, sex and race. Psychosomatic Medicine 34: 548–556.

FURTHER READING

Thomas VJ, ed. (1997) Pain, its nature and management. London: Baillière Tindall.

This textbook provides current, scientifically based, practical information for nurses, doctors and those working in professions allied to medicine. It focuses on certain pain conditions that are known to be problematic and to represent a challenge to management approaches. The contributors to the book come from different disciplines in clinical nursing, nurse education, psychology and medicine. This variety reflects the fact that successful pain management requires the combined efforts of the multidisciplinary pain team.

McCaffrey M, Pasero C (1999) Pain: clinical manual. St Louis, MO: Mosby.
This manual also provides up-to-date, scientifically based, practical information, presented in a clear manner that can be readily applied to a variety of pain populations. There are many patient examples and practical guidelines. It is written by two well-known nurses who are expert pain specialists.

Infection and disease

Mike Walsh

INTRODUCTION

Humans and animals are host to populations of micro-organisms that live on the skin and mucous membranes. Normally the human fetus lives in a sterile environment until birth, when the infant soon gains a complex flora of bacteria derived from maternal flora and surroundings. Certain species of bacteria regularly inhabit different parts of the body where they constitute the normal flora of the area.

Micro-organisms that are capable of causing disease make up only a tiny proportion of all the micro-organisms on earth. However, these are the ones of concern to us and they are termed *pathogens*. *Infection* occurs when an infectious agent multiplies within the body tissues causing adverse effects. The outcome of **infection** is determined by the ability of the micro-organism to invade and overcome the host's defence mechanisms. Infection affecting specific body systems is discussed in later chapters. This chapter concerns infection in general.

INFECTIOUS AGENTS

Micro-organisms that cause infection in humans include bacteria, viruses, fungi, protozoa and parasitic worms.

Bacteria are extremely diverse single-celled microscopic organisms. Bacterial cells have a simple structure and are termed *prokaryotic*. They are characterized by a rigid cell wall made up of a network of carbohydrates and amino acids, called *peptidoglycan*. As it is unique to bacterial cells, pepti-doglycan is a common target for antimicrobial drugs. When bacteria are viewed under a microscope they are found to occur in several distinct shapes such as round (cocci), oblong (bacillus), curved rod (vibrio) or spiral (spirochaete). Staining the cells with dye distinguishes two main groups: those that stain purple are called Gram-positive and those that do not are called Gram-negative.

Some bacteria, when exposed to adverse conditions, form spores by surrounding themselves with a resistant casing (e.g. *Clostridium tetani*). These spores are very difficult to destroy by heating and will survive being immersed in boiling water or the use of many chemical agents. This is an important factor to consider when decontaminating used equipment.

Bacteria multiply by simply dividing into two. This process can be so rapid that, under favourable conditions, a single bacterial cell can give rise to 1 million cells after only 6 hours. Specimens taken for bacteriological analysis are usually stored in special containers and at low temperatures to prevent such rapid multiplication.

Bacteria are present in most environments. The surface of the body is populated by a wide variety of micro-organisms – the **normal skin flora**. These organisms are *commensals*: they form a balance with their hosts, using them for growth and survival but not harming them. For example, the skin is a normal habitat of staphylococci, coliform bacilli are always present in the intestine, and lactobacilli inhabit the vagina. These commensal organisms may play an essential role in the body; for instance, **vitamin K**, which is necessary for **blood clotting**, is produced by the action of bacteria in the intestine. This commensal flora may cause disease if it gains access to another area of the body. For example, staphylococci may cause infection in surgical wounds and coliforms may cause urinary tract infection if they enter the bladder.

Other important organisms are rickettsiae, which are smaller than normal bacteria and are parasitic in that they can exist only within other cells. They are transmitted via tick or lice bites, producing diseases such as typhus. Chlamydia are small bacteria-like micro-organisms that also only grow inside cells, and *Chlamydia trachomatis* is the major cause of sexually transmitted infections in the developed world (see p. 154) and the main preventable cause of blindness in the developing world. Mycoplasmas are the smallest of all cells. They lack rigid cell walls and inhabit body fluids. *Mycoplasma pneumoniae* is a common cause of community-acquired pneumonia.

Viruses are small infectious agents ranging in size from 0.02 to 0.3 μm. They differ from other living organisms in that they are not cells but simply a piece of either **DNA** or **RNA** surrounded by a protein coat, and sometimes a lipid envelope. They are unable to reproduce themselves but are obligate parasites of living cells in plants, animals and even bacteria. Once inside the cell, they direct the host's metabolic machinery to reproduce themselves. New viruses are released from the cell by budding out of the membrane or by the virus causing the cell to rupture. The damage to the cells causes the symptoms of the disease in the host. Mutation of the cell's DNA can occur as a result of the activity of the virus within the cell which can lead to the development of malignancy. Cervical cancer is frequently associated with infection by the human papillomavirus (HPV). Some viruses may become integrated within the host cell genome and become established indefinitely. The initial symptoms of the invasion may disappear and the virus remains dormant, only to reactivate later and produce symptoms, as in herpes simplex infection.

The many varieties or strains of virus and their intracellular location have made effective therapy more difficult. Examples of viral diseases are the common cold, influenza, measles, mumps and acquired immune deficiency syndrome (**AIDS**).

Fungi are plants. They have complex, eukaryotic cells. Most are multicellular organisms that grow as interlacing filaments or chains. A disease caused by a fungus is in general called a *mycosis*, or the specific disease may be indicated by the suffix -osis, preceded by the name of the causative fungus. Thrush, ringworm and histoplasmosis are examples of mycotic disease.

Protozoa are single-celled organisms that belong to the animal kingdom and are more complex in structure and activity than bacteria. Diseases that are caused by protozoa include malaria, giardiasis, amoebic dysentery and trichomoniasis.

Parasites may also cause infection. The most common parasitic infections in the developed world are those caused by the roundworm, pinworm and tapeworm (examples of parasitic worms or helminths). However, parasitic infections are endemic in the developing world and a serious public health hazard. Increased travel to these regions requires nurses to be more aware of the potential infections that can occur, whilst nurses working in the developing world know only too well the contribution they make to the disease burden.

INTERACTION BETWEEN HOST AND INFECTIOUS AGENTS

The outcome of the interaction between micro-organisms and the host depends on the balance between the ability of the organism to establish infection and the host defence mechanisms. The ability of a micro-organism to invade and injure host tissue is termed *virulence*.

VIRULENCE

There are a number of ways in which micro-organisms can increase their virulence. To establish infection, the organism must first be able to enter and adhere to tissue in the host. Different species are able to invade specific tissues in the host. For example, *Neisseria meningitidis* attacks the meninges of the central nervous system, while *Neisseria gonorrhoeae* and *Chlamydia trachomatis* invade epithelial cells of the cervix.

Many bacteria protect themselves against phagocytic white blood cells (see p. 141) by covering the outside of their cell with a layer of gelatinous material. This *capsule* can also help the cell to adhere to surfaces (e.g. *Streptococcus pneumoniae*). Some bacteria protect themselves from attack by the immune system by multiplying within phagocytic cells themselves (e.g. *Mycobacterium tuberculosis* multiplies within macrophages), while some viruses may lie dormant within host cells for long periods of time. Herpes simplex may persist for long periods before producing signs of infection such as cold sores (HSV 1) and genital herpes (HSV 2).

Bacteria may also invade their host as a result of producing destructive substances known as *toxins* (e.g. haemolysins which destroy red blood cells). Some bacteria excrete exotoxins that give rise to serious illnesses. *Clostridium tetani*, for example, produces a toxin that, by acting on the nervous system, produces the muscular spasm associated with tetanus. Toxic shock syndrome is associated with the toxin released by *Staphylococcus aureus* when present in the vagina. Some bacteria secrete endotoxins into their cell walls. These are responsible for raised temperature and a feeling of general malaise. When bacteria are killed they may release these endotoxins. These are responsible for the syndrome of septic shock characterized by high temperatures and dangerously low blood pressure (hypotension).

HOST DEFENCES

The body has several different defences to protect it from invasion by microbes or other foreign material known as *antigens*. Non-specific defences act against all types of **antigen**. The specific immune response recognizes antigens previously encountered and mounts a rapid and very specific action against them.

Non-specific defences

Barriers

The **skin** is a protective barrier against most micro-organisms as long as it is intact; however, any breach such as an intravenous cannula site or a wound offers easy access for invading microbes. Mucous membranes are less resistant and may be penetrated by bacteria such as *Neisseria gonorrhoeae*, while organisms such as the influenza virus can invade mucosal cells.

Bactericidal substances in body fluids

Skin secretions contain fatty acids that inhibit the growth and survival of many pathogens. Mucous membranes secrete an external layer of mucus which traps infectious agents, preventing their adhesion to the epithelial cells. The mucus and trapped micro-organisms are propelled upwards and out of the body by ciliary movement (mucociliary flushing) in the respiratory tract and by coughing and sneezing.

Most body fluids have bactericidal activity. Lysozyme is present in all tissues and all body secretions except urine. It is present in high concentration in tears. It is an enzyme capable of damaging the peptidoglycan cell wall of bacteria, causing the cell to rupture and die.

Gastric juice, highly acidic at pH 2.0, is lethal for nearly all bacteria, although if large numbers of microbes are ingested they may be protected by the bulk of food eaten. The major exception to this rule is *Helicobacter pylori* which has successfully adapted to living in the stomach and is the major cause of peptic ulceration. *H. pylori* is able to burrow into the gastric mucosa to escape gastric acid; it deliberately causes inflammation of the stomach wall to lower acidity in the region by affecting hormonal regulation (via the hormones somatostatin and gastrin) of acid secretion (Blaser 2005). It also synthesises an enzyme (urease) which converts urea into alkaline ammonia to help neutralize the gastric acid (see p. 444). Breast milk and saliva contain lactoperoxidase, which inhibits multiplication of some bacteria. It also contains an antiviral agent (distinct from antibodies) that protects the mucosa against rotavirus infections.

Normal body flora

The commensals that form the **normal body flora** help to prevent colonization and infection by pathogens. Antimicrobial treatment for an infection often destroys commensals, leaving the way open for resistant strains of bacteria to flourish in their place.

Phagocytosis

Phagocytosis is the engulfment, killing and digestion of micro-organisms by white blood cells known as neutrophils, monocytes and macrophages, which originate from stem cells in the bone marrow (see p. 368).

Neutrophils are highly mobile cells present in the blood (sometimes known as polymorphonuclear leukocytes). They contain granules filled with potent chemicals that enable them to kill and digest micro-organisms.

Monocytes circulate in the blood and then migrate into tissues, where they develop into macrophages. They are found in connective tissues in the lungs, liver, spleen, brain and lymph nodes.

Macrophages play an important role in both the non-specific and specific defence mechanisms of the body. They rid the body of cell debris (micro-organisms and worn-out cells). The vital role played by macrophages in the immune responses and the development of inflammation is discussed below.

Complement

The **complement** system is a series of about 30 proteins that work to complement the activity of antibodies in destroying bacteria, either by facilitating phagocytosis or by puncturing bacterial cell membranes. It also aids in the elimination of antigen–antibody complexes from the body.

Complement proteins circulate in the blood in an inactive form. When the first of the series is activated by encountering a microbe, it sets in motion a cascade effect. As each protein is activated, it in turn acts on the next in a precise sequence that ends in the formation of the desired final protein.

In addition, this cascade has other consequences: the production of vasoactive substances by degranulation of mast cells and basophils, causes redness and swelling; the attraction of polymorphs to the area (chemotaxis); and the rendering of target cells attractive to phagocytes by making their outer surface more sticky which helps phagocytosis (opsonization).

Natural killer (NK) cells

These non-specific lymphocytes rid the body of what they perceive as foreign or non-self cells without having to recognize a specific antigen. They migrate from the lymphoid tissue to the site of inflammation or tumour growth where they destroy the pathogens, tumour cells or virus-infected cells.

The inflammatory response

Damage from any source (infection, trauma) sets in motion the **inflammatory response** which aims to limit the damage and promote healing. It involves both a vascular and cellular response.

The *vascular response* increases the blood supply to the affected area and hence the capillary blood pressure. This drives fluid out into the surrounding tissue (transudate). Meanwhile chemicals released by injured cells cause neighbouring cells in the epithelium of the capillary wall to relax, opening gaps between them which allows the escape of protein-rich fluid called exudate. This happens within a few minutes and has the beneficial effect of diluting localized toxins, facilitating the arrival of antibodies at the site of injury and causing pain which restricts movement of the injured part. A range of chemicals initiates this vascular response including histamine (from mast cells), serotonin (from platelets), the eicosanoids (synthesized via enzyme pathways) and nitric oxide (from mast cells).

The *cellular response* is characterized by the rapid arrival of neutrophils to phagocytose the infectious agent. They only survive a few hours but give the body a rapid response to invasion and injury. Macrophages appear later to mop up the debris, which consists of dead leucocytes, bacteria and necrotic tissue. If the infection is severe enough, pus may form (purulent inflammation).

The whole inflammatory process can be recognized by local swelling, redness, heat and pain. A plasma protein cascade that is particularly important in amplifying pain is known as the kinin cascade and leads to the formation of bradykinin. Pain is also amplified by the cyclooxygenase enzyme pathway (part of the eicosanoid system referred to above) which leads to the formation of prostaglandins. This pathway is the target of the non-steroidal antiinflammatory drugs (NSAIDS) such as ibuprofen which therefore give effective pain relief and reduce inflammation.

Host resistance to viruses

Interferon is an important component in the defence mechanism against viruses. When certain body cells – leucocytes, fibroblasts and T lymphocytes – are infected by some viruses, they respond by producing interferon, a group of small proteins that inhibit virus multiplication within the cells. These proteins work only on the species that produced them. Interleukins are types of interferons that have many functions and aid in stimulating the antibody response (play a role in the specific immune response).

Fever

Fever is a common manifestation of the inflammatory response and often indicates that infection is present. Various products of inflammation cause the hypothalamus to reset the body temperature to a higher level. These are known as endogenous pyrogens (such as tumour necrosis factor produced by activated macrophages and products of the cyclooxygenase pathway) and it is thought this is a defence against micro-organisms which ideally like a body temperature of only 37°C.

Specific defences
Anatomy of the immune system

The immune system consists of specialized cells and organs that are distributed throughout the body. The primary organs of the system are the bone marrow and the thymus, whereas the secondary organs include the lymph nodes, spleen and lymphatic tissue such as the tonsils.

The lymph nodes are connected by a network of small channels called **lymphatics**. Immune cells originate from the lymphoid stem cells of the bone marrow (Fig. 9.1) and differentiate into two distinct types known as T lymphocytes and B lymphocytes. The thymus gland houses the T lymphocytes which are involved in the *cell-mediated immune*

responses, whilst the B lymphocytes (which originate in the red bone marrow) migrate to the lymphoid tissues where they are responsible for the production of antibodies or immunoglobulins. This is known as the *humoral response*.

The T and B lymphocytes are transported by the blood and lymph vessels. The lymph nodes filter the lymph drained from the tissues, separating out antigens and exposing them to the cells of the immune system. The spleen, like the lymph nodes, contains both T- and B-cell areas and is particularly effective in filtering out particulate antigens such as micro-organisms. Removal of the spleen results in the loss of a significant part of the defences of the body.

The cells of the immune system must be able to recognize host cells to avoid attacking and destroying self tissue. A marker glycoprotein molecule on the surface of all host cells enables them to be distinguished from foreign non-self material. This is called *the major histocompatability complex* or MHC. It occurs in two forms, MHC I which occurs normally on every cell in the body and MHC II which only occurs on cells presenting an antigen (i.e. infected). The appearance of MHC II is a signal to the immune system and triggers either a cell or antibody mediated defence (see below). Autoimmune diseases, however, are caused by the failure of the immune cells to recognize normal healthy host tissue.

Cell-mediated response

When bacteria enter the body they are first ingested by macrophages. The bacterial antigen then appears on the surface of the macrophage where it is recognized by a corresponding T cell which binds with the antigen–macrophage complex. The T cell then starts to divide and produce a range of chemical mediators called *lymphokines*. The major lymphokines are interleukins and interferons, and these promote and coordinate the immune response.

Humoral or antibody mediated response

Antibodies are secreted by the B cells, with cooperation from helper and cytotoxic killer T cells (known as T4 and T8 respectively). B cells bind with the antigen that fits their receptors. They then multiply, producing identical clone cells, which differentiate into plasma cells. The plasma cells produce large quantities of antibodies specific to the antigen for several days until they die. The antibodies are released into the circulation where they interlock with matching antigens to form antigen–antibody complexes. These complexes stimulate phagocytic activity and activate complement to destroy the bacterial cell or toxin.

The antibody production declines as the infection is overcome, plasma cells die and the cytotoxic killer T8 cells exert their control. Some activated B cells not converted to plasma cells become *memory cells*, which are stored and respond later when stimulated by exposure to the same antigen.

Antibodies are immunoglobulin molecules. They are composed of four interlinked polypeptide chains (two long or heavy chains and two shorter, light chains), shaped to form a Y (Fig. 9.2). The sections at the tips of the Y arms, called the *variable* regions, are the specific antigen-combining sites.

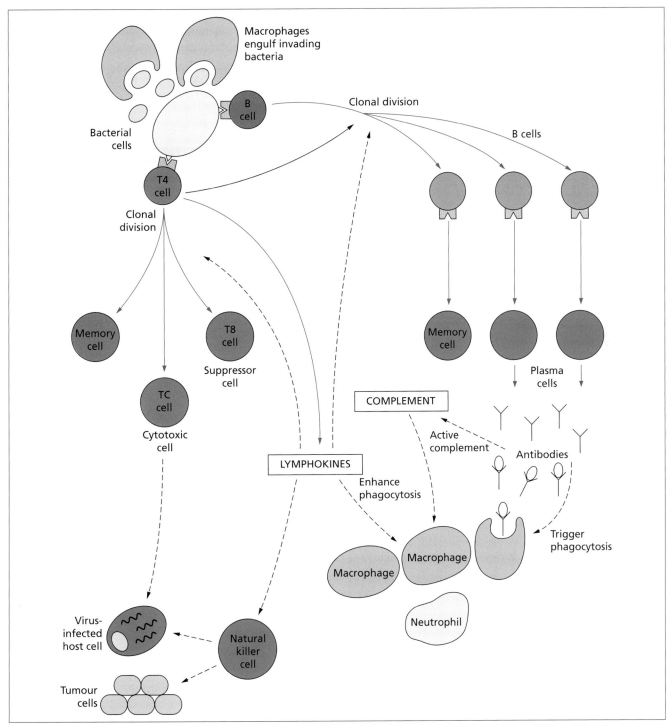

Figure 9.1 The specific immune response. The B cells, T cells and macrophages all interact to fend off the attack from invading microorganisms. Reproduced with permission from Wilson (1995).

The stem of the Y, called the *constant* region, links the antibody to complement and phagocytes. The major classes of immunoglobulins (Ig) or antibodies are labelled A, D, E, G and M, preceded by the symbol Ig (i.e. IgA, IgD, IgE, IgG and IgM) (Box 9.1).

On first exposure to an antigen there is a lag in response of a few days or weeks. IgM antibody is produced first, followed by IgG and IgA, or both. IgM levels soon decline. This is termed the *primary response*. On second exposure to the same antigen, months or even years later, antibodies are produced rapidly (the same amount of IgM but much more IgG). The prompt response is attributed to the persistence of memory cells for that specific antigen and is called the *secondary response*.

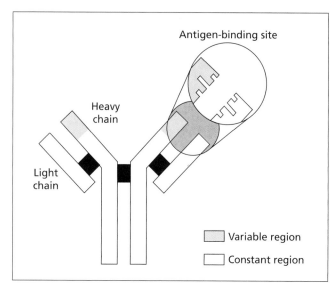

Figure 9.2 Structure of an antibody.

Box 9.1   The five major immunoglobulins

- *Immunoglobulin G (IgG)* is the most common antibody in the blood and is able to enter the tissues. It crosses the placenta and provides protection against infection to the fetus and newborn

- *Immunoglobulin M (IgM)* is large and tends to remain in the bloodstream where it produces an early line of attack against bacteria. It does not cross the placenta

- *Immunoglobulin A (IgA)* is found in saliva, tears, respiratory and gastrointestinal secretions, and colostrum, as well as the bloodstream. It protects the external body openings against invasion

- *Immunoglobulin E (IgE)* is associated with the symptoms of allergic responses

- *Immunoglobulin D (IgD)* function is unclear but maximum levels appear in childhood

---

THE COURSE OF AN INFECTIOUS DISEASE

The course of most infectious diseases extends over three phases: incubation, acute illness and convalescence.

The *incubation period* is the interval between the time the organism enters the body and the initial clinical manifestations of an infection. During this stage the organisms multiply and host defences are mounted to counter the infection. The patient is asymptomatic but may excrete the infectious agent. If the host defences overcome the causative organisms, there may be no signs or symptoms. Sometimes a person may continue to excrete the pathogen without symptoms of the disease for a period of time. In this situation the person is said to be a *carrier*.

The *acute illness* is the stage in which the disease reaches its full intensity. The duration of acute illness varies from a few hours to weeks. It is generally predictable for the specific disease.

Convalescence is the stage during which the clinical manifestations subside. Many infectious diseases are self-limiting and recovery takes place over a short, defined period of time.

TYPES OF INFECTION

Certain terms may be used to describe infection. *Local* means the infection remains confined to one area. A *systemic* infection is one in which the organisms are disseminated throughout the body. If a person becomes infected by another type of organism during the course of an infection, this is termed a *secondary* infection, and the initial one is referred to as the *primary*. An infection may be *acute*, that is an intense illness of short duration, or *chronic*.

The presence of bacteria in the blood is called *bacteraemia*, but where this is accompanied by symptoms, such as fever, rigors, or chills and hypertension, this is called *septicaemia*. *Toxaemia* implies a concentration of bacterial toxins in the blood.

CLINICAL CHARACTERISTICS OF INFECTION

During the incubation period, symptoms of infection are usually general and include headache and malaise. During the acute stage the following systemic and local symptoms may occur:

- fever, which may be preceded by chills
- an increase in the pulse and respiratory rates
- anorexia
- nausea and vomiting
- headache
- apathy and fatigue
- joint and muscle pain
- general malaise.

The patient may appear hot and flushed, and the tongue is frequently furred and dry. There may be enlargement and tenderness of the lymph nodes closest to the site of infection.

If the infection is local, the classical symptoms are redness and heat due to vasodilatation, swelling (oedema) due to increased vascular permeability, and pain caused by the release of chemical mediators and pressure from increased tissue fluid. These symptoms are due to the inflammatory response. Inflammation is always present with infection unless the patient's immune system is severely impaired. Infection, on the other hand, is not always present with inflammation as inflammation may be caused by chemical irritants, radiation or trauma, as well as by micro-organisms.

In addition to the common signs and symptoms described above, certain features characteristic of a specific infection may be present and may play an important role in the diagnosis. For example, certain infections cause a rash, while others may give rise to a marked increase in the level of a particular type of leucocyte.

DIAGNOSTIC PROCEDURES USED IN INFECTION

LEUCOCYTE COUNT AND DIFFERENTIAL

Some infections cause an increase in the number of white blood cells well above the normal (leukocytosis). An increase in a particular type of leucocyte is recognized as being characteristic of certain infections. Eosinophils for example phagocytose many types of parasitic worm and so a high eosinophil count could indicate parasitic infection. Eosinophil levels also become elevated during an allergic reaction.

ERYTHROCYTE SEDIMENTATION RATE

This is a non-specific test sometimes requested as part of the diagnostic investigation. The rate at which the red blood cells settle in a specimen of blood is increased in infection and inflammation.

IDENTIFICATION OF THE CAUSATIVE ORGANISM

To identify the organism responsible for an infection it must be isolated from the body tissue or secretion where it is causing the infection. This is done by the following methods:

1 *Direct examination* of a specimen of sputum, blood, spinal fluid, urine, faeces, discharge or of the scrapings from a lesion. These are stained and examined under the microscope for organisms. Appearance, shape and certain staining characteristics assist in identifying different organisms.
2 *Culturing* the causative organism by inoculation of the specimen into nutrient media and allowing time for the organisms to multiply.

A pure growth of the causative organism that is isolated is tested for susceptibility to appropriate antimicrobial drugs. The results of these tests form the basis for the selection of the most appropriate, effective drug to destroy the organisms.

ANTIBODY TESTS

A specimen of blood may be examined to determine the concentration of antibodies present; this is referred to as an *antibody titre*. Micro-organisms act as antigens, stimulating the production of specific antibodies, and these antibody titres rise as the disease progresses (e.g. *Legionella*). Tests to detect the presence of certain antigens or antibodies may also be carried out; a known antibody is used to determine the presence of a corresponding antigen, or a known anti-gen is used to detect antibodies. HIV testing for example, is based on antibody detection but the timing has to be correct for seroconversion to occur (the time it takes for a person, after infection, to develop antibodies which can be detected). This is generally taken as between 4 and 12 weeks, so if the person is tested too soon a false-negative result can occur (Black and Hawks 2005).

SKIN TESTS

The *Mantoux tuberculin skin test* is used to determine whether an individual is immune to *Mycobacterium tuberculosis*, the cause of tuberculosis. A small amount of protein derived from mycobacterium is injected into the skin on the surface of the forearm. Swelling and redness at the site of injection within 2–3 days indicates a positive reaction. This means the individual has or has had an infection by tubercle bacilli, acquired either naturally or following bacille Calmette–Guérin (BCG) vaccination. The test is considered negative if there is no reaction. If the first test is negative, it may be repeated 6 weeks later.

An alternative skin test, which is more commonly used in the UK is the multiple puncture test, or Heaf test. This is administered by use of a Heaf gun with a needle block of six needles that puncture the skin on firing. Puncture depth of the needles must be set to 2 mm for adults and children aged 2 years or more, and 1 mm for children under 2 years old.

The recommended site for testing is on the flexor surface of the left forearm at the junction of the upper one-third with the lower two-thirds, avoiding any eczematous areas. The skin is cleansed with an alcohol wipe only if it is visibly dirty, and is allowed to dry before undertaking the test. A small amount of tuberculin solution is dropped on to the skin at the standard test site. The Heaf gun is placed firmly on the solution and the handle is pressed until a click is heard, which indicates that the needles have been fired. Any excess fluid is wiped off the skin and the forearm checked for signs of the six puncture marks. The test is usually read at 7 days but can be read between 3 and 10 days. The Heaf test is graded 0–4 and depends upon the degree of induration: 0–1 is regarded as negative; those with a grade 2 reaction are considered positive if there is no history of BCG immunization, and should be referred to the chest clinic; those with a grade 3–4 reaction should be referred directly to chest clinic.

COLLECTION OF SPECIMENS

The examination of specimens in the laboratory plays an important part in the diagnosis and therapeutic management of an individual with infection. For accurate diagnosis it is particularly important that the sample represents the conditions that prevailed at the time of collection. The specimen must therefore not be allowed to deteriorate between collection and examination. When collecting specimens, these general procedures should be followed:

1 All specimens must be collected in a sterile, leak-proof container, which must be properly labelled with the patient's name and the source of the specimen, and submitted with a requisition form providing relevant clinical information, the date, time of collection, clinician's name and laboratory tests required. The container is usually sealed in a plastic bag to protect people handling it from contamination, should it leak.

2 The sample should be obtained from the site of infection and care must be taken to avoid contamination by normal body flora. The amount should be adequate for the number of tests required. (Check with the laboratory if unsure.)

3 Specimens should be collected before the administration of antimicrobials. If this is not possible, indicate on the request form which antibiotics have been given.

4 Specimen collection should be performed with care and tact to avoid harming the patient, causing discomfort or undue embarrassment. Where patients are expected to provide a specimen themselves, they should be given clear instructions.

5 Specimens should be stored in a cool place and delivered promptly to the laboratory. If delivery is delayed, some delicate pathogens will die. Anaerobes (organisms that grow in the absence of molecular oxygen) will die when exposed to air. In addition, the normal flora of the patient may overgrow the pathogens and inhibit or kill them.

Where the suspected cause of the infection is a virus, fungus or protozoon, different techniques for specimen collection may be required and the laboratory should be contacted for advice.

HEALTHCARE ACQUIRED INFECTION AND ANTIMICROBIAL RESISTANCE

There are three key aspects to the management of infection, all of which relate to the problems of healthcare acquired infection (HCAI) and antimicrobial resistance:

● Prevention of HCAI
● Administration of appropriate therapy if an infection is present
● Supporting the patient through the illness by alleviating symptoms and monitoring for complications.

PREVENTION OF HEALTHCARE ACQUIRED INFECTION

Winter (2005a) cites evidence that places the cost of HCAI in the UK alone at £1 billion per year and also suggests about 5000 deaths per year are attributable to HCAI. It is estimated that 10% of all UK NHS patients will develop an HCAI every year. Prevention is therefore crucial and the main principles involved are discussed in detail on page 149. These principles should be considered in light of the work of Cookson (2005) who considers key factors in the spread of HCAI (such as

methicillin-resistant *Staphylococcus aureus* (MRSA)), which include:

● Increased staff workloads reducing time available for infection control
● Fewer hospital beds mean patients have to be transferred between wards more frequently
● High rates of bed occupancy (100%) reduce time for cleaning and disinfection after discharge
● Reduced length of stay could be leading to patients being discharged with undiagnosed infections which they then re-introduce upon subsequent re-admission.

It is therefore salutary to note that the Health Protection Agency (HPA) were moved in December 2005 to put out an urgent press release concerning a recent survey into a serious HCAI called *Clostridium difficile* which causes inflammation of the bowel and diarrhoea and sometimes results in death (HPA 2005a). Haslett et al (2002) estimate that 20% of elderly patients in long-term care are infected with this bacterium; some are unaffected (carriers) while others become seriously ill. The reason for this paradox is unknown. What is known is that infection occurs after the normal bowel flora has been disturbed by antimicrobial use. It is therefore an opportunistic HCAI. The HPA survey showed that 38% of English NHS trusts do not have restrictions in place to prevent the inappropriate use of antibiotics which would minimize the risk of *C. difficile* infections, and over 33% indicated they had no ward that could be used to isolate a patient who had contracted this infection. Forty per cent stated they would *not* follow guidance in the event of an outbreak despite 25% reporting they had been forced to close wards in the previous 12 months as a result of an outbreak. This is serious enough in itself but if this is indicative of the attitude towards HCAI in general in some parts of the NHS, it is a disturbing finding. Nurses have a crucial role in preventing HCAI but NHS trusts also have to take the threat seriously as well.

ADMINISTRATION OF APPROPRIATE THERAPY

Antimicrobial therapy can be very effective, however, we are now seeing increasing numbers of micro-organisms developing resistance to medication, raising the spectre of a return to days before the first antibiotics were discovered.

Public attention has, in recent years, been grabbed by the problems associated with methicillin-resistant *Staphylococcus aureus* or MRSA. The first effective and non-toxic antimicrobial agent, penicillin, was discovered in the 1930s but by 1942, *Staph. aureus* was showing resistance to this drug (penicillin was called an *antibiotic* because it was produced from living material whereas the modern term antimicrobial refers to any drug regardless of its means of production). Methicillin became widely available in 1960 to treat resistant *Staph. aureus* but resistance to the new drug was rapidly reported and the term MRSA was coined. To make matters worse, MRSA organisms also showed resistance against most other cheap and commonly available antimicrobials. It was only in the late 1980s, however, that the frequency of MRSA reports began to increase to the level where it became a problem.

We need to consider how resistance arises. This can happen by chance mutations that accidentally confer resistance upon a particular organism, and subsequently the resistant organism thrives as the susceptible form is killed by antimicrobials. A more serious threat is posed by transferred resistance whereby plasmids within the bacteria carrying DNA may be shared between bacteria, thus spreading resistance. During the 1980s it was discovered that drug-resistant plasmids from bacteria infecting less advanced animals could be transferred to human bacteria (Winter 2005b). Strains of bacteria therefore emerge which are resistant either to specific antimicrobials or to many drugs (multiple drug resistant or MDR). In many cases the origin of the drug-resistant DNA was inappropriate use (insufficient dose, courses not completed or antimicrobials used when there was no need). As a consequence there is a constant race to develop new antimicrobials that will replace their older and increasingly ineffective predecessors.

The growing problem of drug resistance and HCAI forced the Department of Health (England) to introduce a compulsory MRSA surveillance scheme in 2001. Data from the Health Protection Agency shows cases of MRSA bacteraemia in English hospitals have averaged just over 7000 per year each year since (HPA 2006). If this is not bad enough we should look at the rest of Europe and see how badly the UK is doing compared to other countries. Leifer (2005) reports data showing that in the UK, the proportion of blood isolates of *Staph. aureus* that are methicillin resistant is 44% compared to countries such as Norway, Sweden and the Netherlands where the figure is only 1%, while Germany and the eastern European countries such as Poland achieve rates of 10 and 25%. Only Romania is significantly worse (50%). There are factors that have to be taken into account in looking at such statistics such as how rigorously MRSA is diagnosed and reported together with differences in hospital populations between countries; however, these are still worrying statistics.

MRSA is only part of the story as many other organisms are developing drug resistance. Resistance to ciprofloxacin in *Escherichia coli* has for example climbed from 6.7% in 2001 to 12.4% in 2003 while in *Neisseria gonorrhoeae* the figures are 3.1% and 9.8% respectively. Resistance to at least one first line drug in the treatment of tuberculosis was reported as 8.4% (HPA 2006) and the fear is of a multiple drug-resistant strain spreading west from Russia.

The key to the management of infection is the early recognition of symptoms and identification of the causative organism. The correct drug can then be administered before the organism is able to overwhelm the host's immune defences. Viruses exist within their host cells and there are very few antimicrobial agents that are effective against them. Treatment of viral infections mostly involves symptom con-

trol and supporting the patient through the acute phase of the illness, which in most cases is self-limiting. The cause of many common illnesses is usually viral and patients frequently attend primary care asking for 'antibiotics' to treat their coughs and colds. Nurses have a key role in preventing the development of drug resistance by explaining to patients that there is no effective antibiotic for their ailment as it is probably viral and therefore a prescription for an antibiotic is not going to be forthcoming.

SYMPTOM RELIEF AND MONITORING FOR COMPLICATIONS

Whether a patient is on antimicrobial therapy or not (due to the viral nature of their illness) the nurse can greatly help the patient in primary care with advice about symptom relief such as simple analgesia, rest, warmth, drinking plenty of fluids and staying at home to avoid spreading their infection. It is also important to tell the patient to return if their symptoms are not improving or getting worse as this could indicate complications such as a secondary infection.

ASSESSMENT OF INFECTION

The clinical signs of infection may be non-specific in the early stages, and include a general malaise, headache, anorexia and arthralgia. As the infection progresses, symptoms associated with the inflammatory response may develop. The patient should be examined for these signs and for other symptoms such as purulent discharge, productive cough or abnormal respiration. Often infection will be accompanied by fever and chills. Night sweats are associated with intermittent fevers. A careful medical history can help to identify the site of the infection, and questioning about contact with an ill person, animals or travel abroad may provide vital clues regarding its cause. In the elderly the signs and symptoms of infection may be abnormal. They may not develop a fever but can often present with a history of incontinence, confusion or falling related to an underlying infection.

Once an infection has been diagnosed, there are a number of effects it may have on the body which require close monitoring.

Pyrexia. A raised body temperature is commonly associated with infection. The effects of fever can be exhausting to the patient and deplete energy supplies, particularly if associated with violent shivering or rigors. The increase in metabolic rate associated with high fever may cause particular problems in the elderly as each increase of 1°C causes a 13% increase in oxygen demand. A patient who already has heart failure or pulmonary disease is therefore at increased risk. High fever in very young children (under 5 years) can cause seizures called febrile convulsions.

Dehydration. High fever, sweating and diarrhoea may result in excessive fluid loss from the body. This may be exacerbated by the inability to ingest fluids or food. Severe dehydration is particularly associated with gastrointestinal infection, especially in infants and the elderly, who are vulnerable to the effects of dehydration.

Respiratory problems. Viral infections may affect the immune defences of the lungs and render them more susceptible to invasion by other micro-organisms. Patients with impaired ability to clear their lungs of secretions, such as those with obstructive airway disease, are more susceptible to pulmonary infection.

Alteration in mucous membranes. The mucous membranes of the mouth are maintained by a constant flow of saliva, which removes bacteria and food debris. Saliva production is induced by chewing and is therefore reduced in the anorexic patient. The inability to ingest food and fluids, combined with fever and possibly nausea, can cause the mucous membranes to become dry and susceptible to secondary bacterial or fungal infection.

Nutritional imbalance. A severe infection may cause energy and protein depletion, particularly where a high fever increases the metabolic rate or the patient has experienced prolonged vomiting or diarrhoea.

Diarrhoea. This may be caused by the pathogen infecting the gastrointestinal tract or by an alteration in the normal flora of the bowel caused by antibiotic therapy. Children frequently manifest gastrointestinal symptoms when feverish. Severe diarrhoea may result in dehydration and cause considerable anguish and discomfort to the patient.

NURSING INTERVENTIONS

Planning the nursing care of a patient with infection depends on the nature of the infection. However, there are some general principles related to monitoring for complications of infection and symptom control that should be included in the plan of care.

Maintaining a normal body temperature

The **body temperature** of an infected patient requires regular assessment to monitor the progress of the infection and effect of treatment. Antiinflammatory medication such as aspirin or paracetamol may be prescribed, which will reduce body temperature. Efforts should be made to provide a cool environment by reducing the amount of bedclothes or providing a fan. Sweating may aggravate an itchy rash and this can be alleviated by bathing with warm water.

Maintaining fluid balance

The patient should be assessed for signs of dehydration. These may include dryness of the mucous membranes, concentrated urine, reduced urinary output and loss of skin turgor. Skin turgor can be evaluated by gently pinching the skin; in a dehydrated patient the skin will return only slowly to its normal position when released. Dehydration may also cause an imbalance in serum electrolytes which can be prevented by the use of oral rehydration solution, especially in hot climates. Intravenous fluids may be prescribed if the patient is vomiting or the dehydration is severe.

Maintaining normal respirations

Patients at high risk of developing pulmonary complications should be carefully monitored for altered chest movements, respiratory rate, cough and shortness of breath. Regular changing of position and early mobilization help to expand and remove secretions from the lungs. Fluid intake should be encouraged to thin the mucus and facilitate expectoration. If pulmonary function is poor, oxygenation may be indicated. The supply should be well humidified to prevent drying of secretions.

Maintaining healthy oral mucous membranes

The **mouth** should be examined regularly for signs of infection, dryness or cracking. Debris should be removed by regular cleaning using a toothbrush, toothpaste and water. Petroleum jelly can be applied to the lips to prevent cracking. The patient should be encouraged to eat, even small amounts, as soon as possible, to stimulate saliva production.

Maintaining nutrition

The nutritional status of the patient should be assessed and, where necessary, a high-protein diet provided to replace nutrients lost during the acute phase of the illness. The infection may cause loss of appetite so that meeting the preferences of the patient and providing frequent, small amounts of food may help to encourage intake. To minimize the energy demands on the body, as much rest as possible should be planned for the patient.

Maintaining bowel function

The colour, consistency and frequency of stool should be monitored. The presence of blood or mucus in the stool and history of vomiting, nausea and abdominal pain may also be of importance in the diagnosis of a gastrointestinal infection. Collection of faecal specimens for examination in the laboratory may be required.

Infection control precautions should be adhered to after contact with faeces to prevent cross-infection of other patients or staff.

Prescription and administration of antimicrobial agents

Nurses are becoming increasingly autonomous practitioners in this field and prescription policy in the UK is changing almost too quickly for a book such as this to keep pace with the changes. Suffice it to say we have a responsibility to follow guidelines and policies at all times in order to ensure patient safety, effective treatment and the prevention of drug resistance.

When administering antimicrobial drugs it is important to provide adequate constant serum and tissue levels of the antimicrobial agent. To achieve this, the nurse must administer the medications at the correct time and, if given intravenously, over the prescribed time interval (e.g. 20 min). Aminoglycoside drugs (e.g. gentamicin) in particular require careful monitoring of blood levels. They can be nephrotoxic and hepatotoxic if the concentration circulating in the blood is too high. It is important to space the administration of different antimicrobial agents so that a constant serum level of the specific drug is maintained and incompatible drugs are not mixed together.

When the patient is taking antimicrobial drugs at home or is being discharged from hospital with a prescription for these agents, it is important that the patient is instructed to complete the full course of the prescribed medication and given specific instructions as to when drugs are to be taken. Times are determined by assessing the patient's daily lifestyle. The nurse should explain that antimicrobial therapy should not be stopped when the patient feels better, as this may result in relapse or enable resistant strains to develop, and that medications prescribed for a previous illness should not be substituted.

PREVENTING THE SPREAD OF INFECTION

Excretions and secretions may contain pathogens that are easily transmitted, especially on the hands of staff. Gloves should always be worn for handling potentially infected body fluids from a patient with infection, and hands washed before providing care to another patient. Alcohol-based hand rubs provide an alternative and effective means of keeping hands clean. Gloves are not a substitute for handwashing, and if not removed, they are just as capable of transmitting infection to another patient, as are unwashed hands. Handwashing must, however, be effective which means being thorough, using an effective cleansing agent and also including careful drying afterwards to decrease skin surface microbe counts. *Staph. aureus* can be found in the noses of 20–30% of healthy people and thrives on human skin. It is readily spread by casual hand to nose contact and then hand to hand contact with another person. It is rarely spread by the droplet route (Collins and Hampton 2005). Equipment in contact with body fluids (e.g. commodes) may also transmit infection and should be carefully decontaminated before use by another patient.

It has been known for over 20 years that the following five procedures are commonly associated with HCAI (Storr et al 2005):

- care of urinary catheters
- care of vascular access devices
- support of pulmonary function
- surgical procedures
- hand hygiene and other standard precautions.

In the USA similar risk factors have been identified for action and a major campaign is targeting the prevention of central venous catheter infections, prevention of surgical site infections and ventilator-associated pneumonias (IHI 2005). Each target area is broken down into components, for example, preventing infection of surgical sites involves guideline-based use of prophylactic antimicrobials, appropriate hair removal and peri-operative blood glucose control.

Storr et al (2005) emphasize the importance of hand cleansing and the 'cleanyourhands' campaign involving placing hand rub dispensers at convenient multiple locations around healthcare facilities. However, this is not enough, as the author observed on a recent study trip to North America. In a large downtown general hospital I was struck by newly installed dispensers located in the main hallway, along all the public corridors, elevators and into the ward areas. At the end of my day there, I had not seen a single member of the public use any of them. Hand rub dispensers have to be used to be effective!

Ward nurses can play a key role in preventing HCAI by carrying out a thorough risk assessment on every patient admitted to their ward which should include (Storr et al 2005):

- Age (the older the patient the greater the risk)
- Medical history (immunocompromised, immunosuppressed?)
- Presence of invasive devices (catheters, IVI lines, etc.)
- Skin health (breaks in skin?)
- Antimicrobial use
- Previous surgery or hospital admissions (opportunity for infection)
- Mobility
- Length of stay
- Movement to other departments/wards within the hospital.

However, risk of an HCAI is not confined to hospitals. In primary care, nurses are caring for patients with higher levels of dependency and vulnerability after ever earlier discharge. Patients may be discharged unaware they are developing an HCAI or they may become infected in the community due to their increased vulnerability and poor health care practice by health professionals (Wilcox 2005). A particular concern for primary care nurses is uniform hygiene and the following guidelines from the RCN (2005) are equally valid in community and hospital settings:

- Change out of uniform at the end of a shift
- Assume contamination of work clothes at the end of a shift, however clean they may look
- Wash hands thoroughly after handling a used uniform
- Keep clean and dirty uniforms separate
- Do not handwash uniforms; this is an ineffective method of decontamination
- Do not enter commercial premises (e.g. shops) in uniform
- Minimize travel in uniform
- Know your employer's dress code and laundry guidance.

Isolation precautions

Some infections spread easily from person to person. In hospital, where patients may be particularly vulnerable, isolation precautions may be necessary to prevent transmission. These precautions include the use of protective clothing for contact with infectious material and the isolation of the patient from contact with others. The precautions are intended to prevent cross-infection of other patients and to protect healthcare providers from infection. The decision to use isolation precautions depends on the infecting organism, the site and symptoms of infection, and the presence of immunocompromised patients.

Various approaches to isolation have been recommended over the years. *Standard isolation precautions* (Box 9.2) have been recommended since 1996 (Garner 1996). These are precautions to be taken with all patients regardless of their presumed infection status or diagnosis. This system combines the major features of universal precautions (transmission of blood-borne infections) and body substance isolation (transmission of infections via moist body fluids). They apply to blood, all body fluids, secretions and excretions (except sweat) whether blood can be seen or not, non-intact skin and mucous membranes. Standard precautions are used in conjunction with transmission-based precautions (Box 9.3) when patients are known or suspected to have an infection or to be colonized with pathogens that are spread by the air-borne, droplet or contact route.

Patient isolation is sometimes necessary to reduce the risk of cross infection and it can affect individuals adversely. Isolation combined with the fear and stigma of infection can be extremely stressful. Some patients may become demanding, fussy or irritable, and the nurse must recognize these responses to isolation rather than label the patient as difficult. There can be a tendency to avoid visiting the patient because of the additional time required to put on protective clothing; this can increase the patient's fear and sense of isolation. The plan of care should, where possible, incorporate regular amounts of time spent with the isolated patient, and the precautions should be discontinued at the earliest opportunity.

As this book goes to press, the possible threat of a terrorist attack, using a biological agent such as smallpox, hangs in the air. More likely is the risk of a major global pandemic of flu (see p. 156). Isolation of households and whole communities, (quarantine) as a means of restricting the spread of the infective agent is being seriously studied as a means of reducing the harm that could be caused by such major public health hazards.

Box 9.2   Standard precautions

These precautions apply to blood, all body secretions and excretions, areas of broken skin, and mucous membranes:

- Always wash your hands thoroughly before and after patient contact. Use plain soap

- Wear gloves if your hands will or could come in contact with any of the above substances or objects, or objects that have been contaminated with them

- Wear a gown, eye protection and a mask during procedures that might generate droplets of these substances (e.g. surgery)

- Handle with great care equipment that has come into contact with these substances and follow cleaning and disinfecting procedures closely

- Follow procedures for handling contaminated equipment such as correct labelling and packaging

- Dispose of sharps carefully and intact immediately after use into an approved disposal box

- Place potentially infective patients in a single room and notify infection control

- Mouth-to-mouth resuscitation should be used only as a last resort

- These are basic principles that need to be interpreted for individual patients

From Springhouse Corporation (2000).

Box 9.3   Transmission-based precautions

These should be followed in addition to standard precautions when the patient is known or suspected of being infected with epidemiologically important pathogens that can be transmitted via air, droplet or contact with dry/other contaminated surfaces.

Airborne transmission-based precautions
- Nurse the patient in a single room that has monitored negative air pressure relative to surrounding area

- Limit movement in and out of the room

- Wear a face mask; this is controversial as some authors (e.g. Ward 2000) consider these to be of little value

Droplet transmission-based precautions
- Nurse the patient in a single room (negative air pressure and ventilation precautions are not necessary)

- Wear a mask when working with the patient

- Visitors are to remain at least 1 m away from the patient

- Avoid movement of the patient out of the room

- Consider extra precautions if a ventilator is needed

Contact transmission-based precautions
- Nurse the patient in a single room

- Wear gloves and a gown whenever in the room

- Avoid movement of the patient out of the room

From Springhouse Corporation (2000).

OCCURRENCE OF INFECTIOUS DISEASE IN POPULATIONS

Epidemiology is the study of the occurrence and distribution of a disease within populations. An *endemic* disease is constantly present at a static level within a given population. An *epidemic* occurs when there is a definite increase in the number of cases of the disease above the normal level. A *pandemic* occurs when the epidemic extends worldwide.

THE CHAIN OF INFECTION

Micro-organisms live and multiply in a *reservoir* from which they can transfer to a host. The reservoir may be in humans, animals or the environment. Viruses, in particular, are unable to replicate outside living cells and survive by passing from one human reservoir to another. Humans are a common reservoir of pathogenic micro-organisms. They may be a source of infection during the incubation period, acute stage or convalescence of the disease, or may carry pathogenic micro-organisms asymptomatically. Figure 9.3 illustrates stages in the transfer of pathogens between reservoir and host.

The normal flora of the body may cause disease when the host's resistance is lowered, or when the organisms are transferred to another area of the body where they are not normally found; for example, *Escherichia coli*, a commensal in the bowel, may cause urinary tract infection if it enters the bladder.

Organisms associated with animal reservoirs include salmonella, which commonly colonizes the intestines of poultry. A major cause of serious food poisoning are the toxins produced by *E. coli* type 0157. These lead to severe bleeding and inflammation of the intestine, and possible renal failure (Haslett et al 2002). Animals infested with parasites may be a source of disease if their flesh is eaten raw or cooked insufficiently (e.g. toxoplasmosis can be transmitted by eating cysts in undercooked meat). The most common environmental reservoirs are water, decaying organic matter and soil.

Mode of escape

The micro-organism leaves the host via a portal of exit. This may be the respiratory, alimentary or genitourinary tract, or via open lesions on the skin.

Mode of transmission

Direct spread involves transmitting the micro-organisms directly from the reservoir to the person (e.g. by sexual intercourse). *Indirect spread* requires an intermediary such as food, airborne particles, contaminated instruments or hands to pass the infection on.

Portal of entry to host

This may be through the respiratory, alimentary or genitourinary tracts, or via a break in the skin. In pregnancy the placenta normally acts as a barrier, preventing micro-organisms from reaching the fetus. However, some organisms

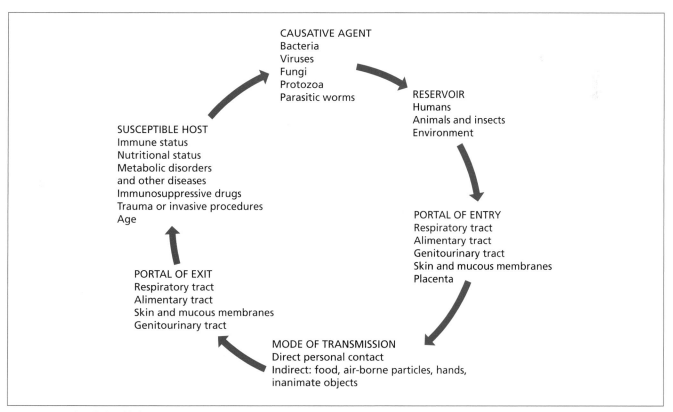

Figure 9.3 The chain of infection.

and viruses may cross to the placenta to cause infection in the fetus (e.g. syphilis).

FACTORS PREDISPOSING TO INFECTION

Factors that influence the host's resistance and susceptibility to infection include the following:

Age

Immunological maturity develops steadily during the first few years of life, and both humoral and cellular immunity are weak in infants.

Immune changes occur in pregnancy, probably related to depression of cell-mediated immunity. These changes may exacerbate underlying autoimmune diseases, such as lupus erythematosus, but have little effect on the incidence of infectious disease.

The incidence of autoimmune disease and cancer increase with ageing. The elderly are more susceptible to, and have a diminished capacity to combat, infection. The thymus gland begins to atrophy at about 45 years of age, resulting in a decreased production of its hormones which play a role in the differentiation of lymphocytes. There is an increase in the number of autoantibodies in the elderly, which is believed to contribute to the pathological changes that occur with ageing. The response to foreign antigens decreases and the elderly are not able to sustain resistance against infection.

Nutritional imbalances

Lymphoid tissue is vulnerable to excesses and deficiencies of many nutrients because of its rapid rate of proliferation. Protein and calorie deficiency can cause impaired cell-mediated immunity. Humoral immunity and phagocytosis are less affected. Inadequate dietary intake of vitamins A, B and folic acid, and of minerals such as zinc and iron, affect the components of the immune system. Without the required nutrients and energy, the production of antibodies, lymphocytes and the chemical mediators of the immune response is impaired.

Stress

Psychoneuroendocrine immunology is a developing field of study that looks at the interactions between immune function, neuroendocrine responses and life **stresses**.

Drugs

Immunosuppressive drugs are used to treat autoimmune disorders such as rheumatoid arthritis, glomerulonephritis and inflammatory bowel disease, to prevent rejection of transplanted tissue and to treat cancer. These include corticosteroids, cyclophosphamide and azathioprine. Some commonly used antibiotics may also impair immune function and increase susceptibility to infection by disrupting the normal flora. All drugs are capable of initiating a hypersensitivity reaction.

Other infections and underlying conditions

Some infections decrease the person's resistance to a secondary infection. The human immunodeficiency virus (HIV) depresses cell-mediated immunity and leaves the individual vulnerable to many opportunistic pathogens, which take advantage of the deficient immune response. Some underlying conditions affect the immune system and increase the patient's vulnerability to infection, for example carcinoma, leukaemia, liver and renal disease.

Invasive procedures and devices

These increase susceptibility to infection by bypassing defence mechanisms such as skin.

Local factors

Tissue that is poorly perfused by blood (e.g. lower legs in peripheral vascular disease) becomes hypoxic and more susceptible to invasion by micro-organisms. Skin lesions such as **pressure sores** and burns provide an exposed, moist area of tissue in which microbes can multiply.

PREVENTING HEALTHCARE ACQUIRED INFECTIONS

The importance of preventing HCAI has already been stressed. The nurse has a responsibility to practise and promote measures that will confine micro-organisms and prevent their spread to other persons.

WASTE DISPOSAL

Waste material contaminated with body fluids could expose those who handle it to infection, and safe disposal of this clinical waste ensures that this risk is minimized. The three major groups of *clinical waste* are: contaminated materials (e.g. dressings, swabs, incontinence pads), which must be discarded into yellow plastic bags; sharps instruments, needles and scalpels, which must be discarded into puncture-resistant sharps containers; and human tissue (e.g. placenta, amputated limbs) which must be segregated from other clinical waste and collected separately. Clinical waste must be disposed of by incineration. All other waste not considered contaminated or infectious is designated as household waste and can be discarded into black bags, for compaction and disposal at landfill sites (Health Services Advisory Committee 1999).

Staff who collect waste can be put at risk by the careless actions of others, for example by the disposal of sharps into plastic bags or overfilling waste bags which subsequently spill open. Waste bags or sharps containers should be sealed securely before being taken out of the clinical area. Bags should be marked with the point of origin to help identify any breakdown in the waste disposal procedure.

SHARPS: HANDLING AND DISPOSAL

Great care should be taken in the handling of sharps. There are five documented definite cases of occupationally acquired HIV infection amongst healthcare workers in the UK and a further 14 probable cases (HPA 2005b). In the UK, nurses have the highest risk of needlestick injuries with Watterson (2005) reporting 43% of all such injuries across 20 sites happening to registered nurses. Junior doctors were next with 17%. During 2004, the 20 sites involved reported a worrying 1990 needlestick injuries, 10% of which happened when putting disposable needles in 'safe' boxes. Watterson (2005) is particularly concerned at accidents happening because staff continue to re-sheath disposable needles after use despite explicit guidance not to do this.

During procedures where sharp instruments are passed between staff they should be placed in a receiver rather than passed directly from hand to hand.

Management of sharps injuries and other exposures to body fluid

Blood-borne viruses can be acquired through an injury with a contaminated sharp instrument or splashing of infected body fluid on to mucous membranes (eyes and mouth), or cut or broken skin. As it is difficult to identify carriers of blood-borne viruses and the source of the contaminated needle may be unknown, all such exposures must be followed up appropriately to minimize the risk of infection. This follow-up is normally carried out by the occupational health department, but by the A&E department outside office hours.

Hepatitis B vaccination

There is now an effective and safe vaccine against hepatitis B. It is recommended that all healthcare workers who have direct contact with body fluids or tissues should be immunized. Most people require a series of three injections to confer immunity and a booster dose every 3–5 years.

LINEN

Micro-organisms are physically removed from linen by detergent and water, and most are destroyed by the temperature of 71°C or more during the wash process. Some fabrics (e.g. patients' clothing) are damaged by high wash temperatures and are washed at a lower temperature with a chemical disinfectant added to the rinse cycle. Linen is usually sorted by laundry staff before washing. Their risk of acquiring infection can be reduced by the use of protective clothing, but guidance from the Department of Health recommends that potentially infectious linen should not be sorted before washing (NHS Executive 1995). This includes soiled linen from patients with enteric infections, blood-borne viruses and tuberculosis. Infected linen should be placed into a water-soluble plastic bag and distinguished from other linen by placing in a red outer bag. The water-soluble bag is placed directly into the washing machine, and splits open to release its contents once in contact with water.

Duvets used in clinical areas should be able to withstand a wash temperature of 71°C and should comply with Department of Health regulations on fire retardancy.

DECONTAMINATION OF EQUIPMENT

Equipment used between patients can present a risk of cross-infection if it is not adequately decontaminated between uses. The method of decontamination selected depends on how the equipment is used and the risk of transmission associated with it. *Sterilization* means a process that completely destroys micro-organisms, including their spores. *Disinfection* is intended to kill or remove pathogenic micro-organisms but will not destroy bacterial spores. *Cleaning with water and detergent* removes contamination physically and along with it many micro-organisms. Cleaning is an essential preparation for equipment prior to sterilization or disinfection, as the presence of organic matter reduces the effectiveness of sterilizing or disinfecting agents. Staff must wear protective clothing while carrying out cleaning and use a dedicated sink, not an ordinary handwash basin. Water must be *below* 45°C to prevent protein coagulation on the instruments being cleaned (NHS Estates 2004).

METHODS OF STERILIZATION

The most efficient method of sterilization is *autoclaving*. If atmospheric pressure is increased, water boils at a higher temperature, sufficient to destroy even bacterial spores. In most autoclaves a pressure of 104 kPa is used to produce steam at a temperature of 121°C. This will sterilize items in 15 minutes, although the autoclave cycle includes time taken to reach temperature and cool down. In central sterile supply departments, porous-load autoclaves are used to sterilize packed instruments. These create a vacuum in the chamber before the injection of steam and ensure that steam penetrates porous materials such as paper or linen wrappings. The simpler, bench-top autoclaves used in some wards, surgeries and clinics do not include a pre-vacuum stage and are therefore not suitable for the sterilization of wrapped instruments. In this type of autoclave the instruments must be separated so that steam can reach all the surfaces.

A few *chemicals* such as ethylene oxide gas or glutaraldehyde can be used to sterilize heat-sensitive equipment but this requires specialist facilities and precautions due to the hazardous nature of these substances. For example, glutaraldehyde must be handled wearing heavy-duty gloves and eye protection because it is highly irritant and can cause skin reactions and respiratory symptoms in those regularly exposed.

Packed instruments will remain sterile provided the wrapping remains dry and intact. Unwrapped instruments should be stored in a sterile or clean, covered container until required, but sterility cannot be guaranteed for more than a few hours.

METHODS OF DISINFECTION

As with sterilization, heat is the best method of disinfection because its effects are more predictable and more easily controlled than chemicals. Items can be *pasteurized* by heating to a temperature of between 65°C and 80°C, for between 5 and 10 minutes. This will destroy most micro-organisms but not spores. In the clinical setting, pasteurization is used to disinfect bedpans, linen and crockery. *Boiling* can be used to disinfect medium-risk equipment. Items should be immersed in water at 100°C and, once the water returns to boiling, timed for 5 minutes.

Chemicals are widely used for decontamination, although to be effective they must be used appropriately. This includes ensuring the dilution is correct (if too high the chemical may be corrosive, if too low it may be ineffective); selecting the correct chemical for the type of equipment and level of decontamination; and using freshly made solutions (diluted disinfectants are frequently unstable and cannot be stored for long periods). The time taken to destroy micro-organisms varies with different chemicals and microbes. Some (e.g. alcohol and hypochlorite) kill most microbes within a few minutes on clean surfaces. Others may take longer: immersion in glutaraldehyde for 1 hour is required to destroy some species of *Mycobacterium*.

Chemical disinfectants can be corrosive and equipment should be rinsed thoroughly after disinfection. Hypochlorites may damage some materials and should not be used to disinfect metal items or fabric. Many disinfectants are toxic and should always be handled wearing gloves and a plastic apron. Eye protection may also be necessary if there is a risk of splashing. Disinfectants are frequently used unnecessarily or inappropriately. Guidance on their use should be obtained by reference to the disinfection policy or by contacting the infection control nurse.

Cleaning

A surface that is clean and dry will not easily support the growth of micro-organisms, and floors, walls and furniture are not common sources of infection in hospital. Most of the micro-organisms on floors can be found in dust particles that settle on horizontal surfaces. A major aim of environmental cleaning is to remove this dust, either by the use of a vacuum cleaner or dust-control mop. These devices are designed to remove the dust with the minimum of disturbance to ensure it does not become air-borne. Mopping with detergent and water is of value when surfaces are soiled or exposed to spillages, for example toilets, bathrooms and kitchens. Mops need careful maintenance as they readily become heavily contaminated if allowed to stand in dirty water. They should be laundered regularly, and fresh detergent and water should be used for each cleaning task. Disinfectants will remove more bacteria from the floor than detergent but the effect is short lived and there are very few indications for their use. The frequency with which cleaning should be performed depends on the type of area and extent of use.

Nurses are commonly required to clean equipment such as washbowls, jugs and receivers. In all cleaning procedures it is advisable to wear gloves to protect the hands from contamination by micro-organisms and the effects of detergent. Efficient cleaning is possible only if detergent is used to break up and remove the grease and dirt. A clean disposable cloth and fresh water and detergent should be used for each task.

UNIVERSAL BLOOD AND BODY FLUID PRECAUTIONS

Concern about the risk to healthcare workers of acquiring **HIV** and the difficulties in identifying infected patients gave rise to the proposal that precautions to prevent the transmission of blood-borne viruses should be applied to all patients. There are three routes by which healthcare workers may acquire blood-borne viruses occupationally:

- inoculation of infected blood through the skin on a contaminated needle or other sharp instrument
- contamination of mucous membranes with infected body fluid
- contamination of cut or abraded skin with infected body fluid.

Universal precautions are aimed at avoiding direct contact with body fluids from all patients at all times. They incorporate the routine infection control measures already discussed together with the use of protective clothing when direct contact with body fluid is anticipated (Box 9.4).

Box 9.4 Universal blood and body fluid precautions

1 Wash hands with soap and water before and after procedures

2 Cover cuts and abrasions with a waterproof dressing

3. Wear gloves for direct contact with body fluid and mucous membranes

4 Wear eye protection and a mask where there is a risk of body fluid splashing into the face

5 Wear a plastic apron to protect from contamination with body fluid

6 Place sharps directly into puncture- and liquid-proof container, never re-sheathe, do not overfill container and close securely before disposal

7 Discard contaminated waste safely, either directly into the drainage system or into a clinical waste bag; use gloves to dispose of soiled linen into leak-proof bags

8 Decontaminate and disinfect equipment between patients

Source: WHO (2006).

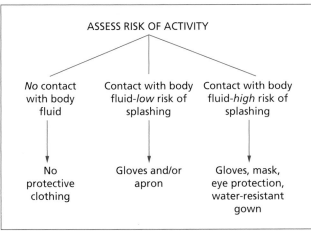

Figure 9.4 The selection of protective clothing: risk asessment. Reproduced with permission from Wilson (1995).

Box 9.5 Summary of key infection control measures

- Apply universal precautions
- Carry out frequent effective handwashing
- Ensure strict levels of environmental cleanliness
- Implement isolation measures as needed
- Liaise with the infection control team
- Act as a role model for patients and other staff to promote hygiene and infection control

From Clark (2000) British Journal of Nursing with permission from Mark Allen Publishing Ltd.

The selection of appropriate protective clothing depends on an assessment of the anticipated risk of exposure to body fluid during a particular procedure (Fig. 9.4). For example, assisting a patient to wash or recording their vital signs is unlikely to involve any direct contact with body fluid and therefore protective clothing is unnecessary. On the other hand, scrubbing contaminated instruments or performing a surgical procedure is likely to cause splashing of body fluid, and therefore eye protection, a mask, apron or gown and gloves need to be worn.

If universal precautions are applied consistently they also protect the patient from other pathogens since these are most likely to be found in body fluid and transmitted between patients on the hands of staff. The use of the same level of precaution with every patient helps to maintain patient confidentiality, which could otherwise be compromised with the use of precautions directed only at those suspected to be infected.

Key infection control measures are listed in Box 9.5.

PREVENTION AND CONTROL OF INFECTION IN THE GENERAL POPULATION

COMMUNITY MEASURES

In developed countries the incidence of major communicable diseases has been greatly reduced as a result of improved socioeconomic and environmental conditions, immunization programmes, and advances in epidemiology and medical treatments. In the community, measures to control infectious disease are directed at adequate sewage disposal and the provision of safe water and food supplies. Control of enteric diseases, such as typhoid fever and many other gastrointestinal infections, is largely dependent on these factors. Immunization programmes are also widely used to prevent and control the spread of many infectious diseases.

IMMUNIZATION

Vaccines can be used to protect against infection by stimulating the production of antibodies. When the individual is exposed to the micro-organism, the immune system can then respond quickly to prevent infection establishing.

Immunization schedules vary in different countries and in different areas depending on which diseases are more prevalent. Table 9.1 shows the recommended immunization schedule for children in the UK (DoH 1996). This service is provided by general practitioners and local health authorities, and is accessible to most individuals without cost.

Immunity induced artificially in this way becomes weaker over a period of months to years depending on the type of vaccine. As a result, reinforcing or booster doses of some vaccines are necessary. Records of immunization received and the date given should be kept by each individual for future reference. This is particularly important for healthcare workers, who may be exposed to a variety of infectious diseases at work and depend on vaccination for protection against infection.

In some instances it is possible to protect individuals who have been exposed to a pathogen by administering a booster dose of vaccine to enhance existing immunity. Rapid, short-term protection (passive immunity) can also be provided by the administration of specific antibodies (immunoglobulins). These will augment the body's immune system but will not provide lasting protection. For example, a patient who is not fully immunized against tetanus and who sustains a contaminated high-risk wound would be given a 250 IU injection of human tetanus immunoglobulin (HTIG) whilst a patient who was not even partially immunized would receive the same injection for any tetanus-prone wound (Newcombe 2004). Natural passive immunity occurs when IgG antibodies from a mother cross the placenta to the fetus and protect the newborn baby for the first few months of life. The term 'herd immunity' refers to a situation where such a critical mass of a population has been immunized that it is very

Table 9.1 Schedule for routine immunizations (NB Changes to this schedule are expected to be announced as this book goes to press.)

Age	Immunization	Dose
2, 3 and 4 months	Diphtheria, tetanus, pertussis, polio, Haemophilius influenzae (HIB)	1 injection
	Meningitis C	1 injection
Around 13 months	Measles, mumps rubella (MMR)	
3 years 4 months to 5 years	Diphtheria, tetanus, pertussis, polio	1 injection
	MMR	1 injection
13–18 years	Diphtheria, tetanus, polio	1 injection

Source: DoH (2004).

difficult for infection to spread to the very small proportion that is not immunized.

Many measures to control infectious disease in the community are controlled by legislation and are monitored by international, European Union (EU), national and environmental health departments or local government authorities. The World Health Organization (WHO), an agency of the United Nations, monitors outbreaks of infectious disease throughout the world and institutes appropriate prevention and control measures. They are currently watching very closely the development of a possible flu pandemic.

FLU PANDEMICS

As this book goes to press there is major concern about the growing threat of a pandemic, involving flu. Flu is of course a common viral illness and there is ample evidence that flu vaccination is very effective in preventing it. Demichelli et al (2004) have undertaken a major systematic review of 25 randomized-controlled trials involving almost 60 000 patients and demonstrated that whether flu is diagnosed clinically or serologically, vaccination is beneficial. The number needed to treat in these trials is typically in the range of 10 to 20 meaning that by vaccinating 10 to 20 people, one case of flu is prevented.

Flu is caused by a group of viruses called myxoviruses and there are three main groups: A, B and C. Groups B and C regularly infect humans and have never caused major problems. However, group A viruses infect a range of other animals rather than humans, especially poultry, pigs and water birds such as ducks. The problem for humans is the ability of the 'wild' A group to mutate and exchange genetic material with the human B and C strains to produce a new strain of a virus which infects humans, is readily passed from human to human and which our immune system is completely unfamiliar with. This happened in 1918, 1957 and 1968 producing pandemics in each of those years.

The 1918 pandemic was the worst. The first reported case was a recruit to the US Army in a training camp near Boston

and he reported sick on 7 September 1918. Within a year, this pandemic had killed 40 million people. More had died than in all the carnage of World War I. Remarkably, scientists have been able to track down remains of the killer virus from samples in medical museums such as the Royal London Hospital and the US Army Museum and by exhuming the graves of victims from an Innuit village in Alaska where 85% of the population died in a few days. As a result they have been able to reconstruct the viral RNA and entire viral genome of the 1918 killer. Findings include the knowledge that the virus bound itself to human cells in exactly the same way that the avian flu group attack bird cells. Work is taking place to create hybrid strains involving the 1918 genome and modern strains in order to study how it was so lethal. A striking finding in the 1918 outbreak was that young adults, at the peak of their fitness, were the most susceptible and likely to die (Taubenbarger et al 2005).

The relevance of this work today is that a new strain of avian flu has emerged in Asia which is starting to kill humans. It is called strain A (H5N1). The name is derived from two 'signature proteins' found on the viral surface, haemagglutinin (H) and neuraminidase (N). The former is known to have 15 subtypes and the latter has 9, consequently H5N1 just means types 5 and 1 of these subtypes respectively (Taubenberger et al 2005). So far it has not acquired the ability to spread from human to human; however, if it does (by mutation) the effects could be as disastrous as 1918 as our immune system probably could not cope with this unfamiliar virus. Predictions range all the way up to 1 person in 3 being infected and a global death toll in the tens or even hundreds of millions if this mutated H5N1 virus achieved its full potential for virulence.

Existing flu vaccines would be useless against this new strain. As nobody has ever been exposed to the new H5N1 strain each person would need two vaccinations with any new vaccine that could be developed, a primer and then a booster 4 weeks later. Current technology requires 6 months from isolating the necessary viral antigens to producing an effective vaccine so from the first appearance of a 'human to human' strain of H5N1 it would be at least 7 months before the first vaccines would be available, and then it would take a lot longer to produce sufficient to vaccinate whole populations (Gibbs and Soares 2005).

Tests on the H5N1 strain at present indicate it is sensitive to antiviral drugs known as neuraminidases and consequently governments are stockpiling these agents (e.g. Tamiflu) in the hope of successfully protecting key workers in the population. Making decisions about rationing these drugs when there is unlikely to be sufficient to treat everybody could be a dreadfully difficult task, especially if faced with public hysteria and panic.

Expert opinion and computer modelling indicates that rapid diagnosis and exchange of information concerning new cases coupled with isolation and quarantine measures for whole communities offers the best chance of holding the disease at bay long enough for limited supplies of antiviral agents to further restrict its spread. The aim is to hold the disease in check long enough for a vaccine to be developed and deployed to whole populations. Nurses will be crucial for both public education and vaccination programmes as this will require a massive primary healthcare effort. Secondary care in acute hospitals may well collapse under the burden of illness and death.

It may be that the H5N1 virus fails to mutate into a human transmissible virus or that if it does, its virulence will be so low that fatalities will be light. Then we will all have had a near miss as happened with the previously unknown SARS virus in 2002–2003, which, despite affecting 27 countries, only killed 800 people (Winter 2005c). However, if H5N1 does cross over into humans and achieves the levels of virulence that are predicted, the whole global community faces its biggest collective threat to health and well-being for at least a century, worse even than HIV. Sitting writing these words on a chilly January afternoon in 2006, I am very aware that avian flu has arrived on the doorstep of Europe with the first deaths just reported from Turkey. By the time you are reading this book it could all have blown over or you, as a nurse, could be in the front line of a battle that will kill more people that World War I or World War II.

SEXUALLY TRANSMITTED INFECTIONS

These are on the increase worldwide and young men aged 18–34 years are the most at risk. The health problem of greatest concern is HIV/AIDS but other sexually transmitted infections (STIs) still pose a significant health hazard.

HUMAN IMMUNODEFICIENCY VIRUS INFECTION

The **human immunodeficiency virus** (HIV) causes damage to the immune system. It is associated with a spectrum of disease, ultimately presenting as acquired immune deficiency syndrome (AIDS).

A disease or illness is shaped not only by its biological qualities but also by the cultural milieu in which it exists.

HIV is primarily a sexually transmitted infection and carries with it connotations of 'sin' and 'evil'. The myths and misconceptions about HIV and AIDS are widespread amongst the general public and healthcare professionals.

Pathophysiology

The genetic information of most organisms is composed of **DNA**, and complementary molecules of **RNA** are made as templates for protein production. HIV is a retrovirus: its genetic information is RNA but it has an enzyme called reverse transcriptase, which can synthesize DNA by using RNA as the pattern (Haslett et al 2002).

The primary target of the virus is the T4 or T helper cells of the immune system which carry a protein called **CD4** on their surface (CD4 lymphocytes) but it also infects macrophages, cells in the mucous membranes and the brain. Once HIV has invaded a cell, the reverse transcriptase converts its RNA to DNA, which is then integrated into the DNA of the host cell (Fig. 9.5).

HIV particles are then assembled in the cytoplasm of the cell and escape by budding through the cell membrane, killing the cell in the process. As increasing numbers of T4 cells are invaded and destroyed, the body's immune system is weakened, making the individual prone to a variety of opportunistic infections, malignant diseases and neuropsychiatric complications. There is a strong association between the number of CD4 T lymphocytes and the development of life-threatening illnesses (Table 9.2).

Transmission

HIV is transmitted by sexual intercourse, inoculation of infected body fluids through skin or on to mucous membranes, transplantation of tissues and transfusion of contaminated blood. It may also be transmitted from mother to baby, either through the placenta or during delivery. Transmission of HIV has occurred through blood, semen, vaginal fluids and occasionally breast milk.

Although HIV has been isolated in tears, urine and saliva, the concentration is extremely low and there is no documented evidence that the virus can be transmitted by these secretions. HIV cannot be transmitted through casual contact such as hugging, holding hands, crying, shared toilet seats, etc.

High-risk behaviours

The patterns of HIV infection and transmission vary in different parts of the world. In Africa and South America, transmission occurs mainly through heterosexual activity and by vertical transmission from mother to baby. The disease is now the leading cause of death in Africa, accounting for 20% of all deaths. Sub-Saharan Africa has witnessed 95% of deaths and over 13 million children have been orphaned. Adult infection rates are between 20 and 40% in most countries in this area. The disease spreads alarmingly throughout the world and over 4 million persons are estimated to be infected in India, for example. In North America and Europe

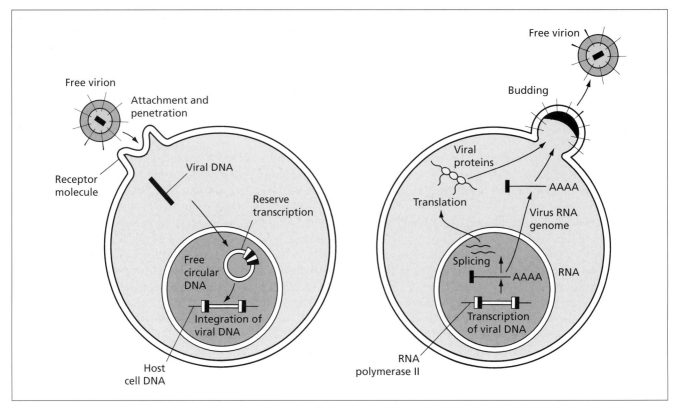

Figure 9.5   The life cycle of a retrovirus.

infection has occurred mostly amongst men who have sex with men (MSM) and injecting drug users while in other parts of the world such as China and Malaysia, injecting drug users (IDUs) make up the major group of infected persons.

The year 2004 saw record levels of new cases of HIV diagnosed in Scotland and Northern Ireland and in the UK overall there were estimated to be 58 300 people living with HIV, of whom 19 700 were unaware of their infection (HPA 2005c). For comparison, amongst men having syphilis tests in London, the prevalence of previously undiagnosed HIV in MSM was 4.7% whilst in heterosexual UK born men the same figure was 0.5%. This indicates it is still predominantly concentrated amongst MSM but is spreading slowly into the heterosexual population. Approximately 140 new HIV diagnoses were reported amongst IDUs in England and Wales during 2004 and the final death figure is expected to be just over 50. London remains the focus of IDU-related HIV with some 50% of UK newly diagnosed cases in 2004. Scotland accounted for approximately 36% of IDU-related HIV diagnoses in 1994; this figure has been reduced to 8% by 2004 indicating significant progress in harm limitation schemes.

It is important to recognize that it is *risk behaviours* that place an individual at risk of infection rather than association with a particular group. The major route of transmission remains by sexual intercourse, with specific sexual practices carrying varying degrees of risk.

HIV can also be transmitted by infected blood or blood products. The use of drugs or alcohol does not specifically put a person at risk, but sharing needles to inject drugs with someone who is infected is risky because small amounts of infected blood are transmitted in the injecting equipment. Individuals who suffer from clotting disorders, who require multiple infusions of clotting factor concentrates manufactured from the pooled plasma of thousands of donors, are also at risk of HIV infection. Routine screening for HIV antibodies and heat treatment that inactivates HIV have greatly reduced the risk of transmission by this route.

An infected health worker may transmit a blood-borne virus to a patient as a result of accidental injury during a procedure such as surgery or dental practice that resulted in blood entering the patient's open tissue. Health workers who are infected with HIV may therefore be advised to avoid performing invasive procedures.

Progression of HIV infection

The rate at which symptoms develop in people with **HIV** infection is unpredictable and varies a great deal between individuals. Some people may develop an acute illness 2–6 weeks after infection. Symptoms include fever, myalgia, arthralgia, headache, diarrhoea, sore throat, lymphadenopathy and a maculopapular rash. After about 3 months it is possible to detect antibodies to the virus in the blood; this is known as *seroconversion*.

In a small number of cases seroconversion may take 6 months or longer. The presence of infection is detected using a test called the enzyme-linked immunosorbent assay

Table 9.2 HIV classification: Center for Disease Control and Prevention (CDC) and World Health Organization (WHO) staging systems

CD4 Cell Categories	A Asymptomatic, acute HIV	B Symptomatic conditions	C AIDS-indicator conditions
The CDC system is based on the lowest documented CD4 count			
≥ 500 cells/μL	A1	B1	C1
200–499 cells/μL	A2	B2	C2
< 200 cells/μL	A3	B3	C3

Category B symptomatic conditions are symptomatic conditions occurring in an HIV-infected adult or adolescent that meet at least one of the following criteria:
a. The are attributed to HIV infection and/or indicate a defect in cell-mediated immunity
b. They are considered to have a clinical course complicated by HIV infection
Examples include oral or vaginal thrush, pelvic inflammatory disease, peripheral neuropathy, herpes zoster, idiopathic thrombocytopenic purpura
Category C AIDS indicator conditions include candidiasis of the respiratory tract, Kaposi sarcoma, extrapulmonary cryptococcosis, HIV-related encelopathy, pneumocystis carinii pneumonia, mycobacterium tuberculosis

The WHO system is based on clinical findings and is therefore of use where laboratory facilities are not available in the Developing World
Primary HIV infection
Asymptomatic, acute retroviral syndrome

Clinical stage 1
Asymptomatic, persistent generalized lymphadenopathy (PGL)

Clinical stage 2
Moderate weight loss, recurrent respiratory infections, herpes zoster, minor mucocutaneous problems such as oral ulcers

Clinical stage 3
Conditions which permit a presumptive diagnosis based on clinical signs and simple investigations. These include severe weight loss (> 10%), unexplained persistent diarrhoea and fever, oral thrush, pulmonary tuberculosis within last 2 years. Other suggestive conditions requiring confirmatory testing include unexplained anaemia, neutropenia or thrombocytopenia

Clinical stage 4
Conditions which permit a presumptive diagnosis based on clinical signs and simple investigations. Examples include Kaposi sarcoma, HIV-related encelopathy, *Pneumocystis carinii* pneumonia, mycobacterium tuberculosis (extrapulmonary), HIV wasting syndrome. Other suggestive conditions requiring confirmatory testing include extrapulmonary cryptococcosis and candidiasis of the respiratory tract

Source: AIDS Education and Training Centers National Resource Center (2006).

(ELISA antibody test) which detects antibodies to HIV in the serum.

Being tested for HIV can have far-reaching implications and place the individual under considerable stress. Issues include how the result may affect their sexual behaviour, potential problems with housing, insurance or employment, and people in whom they might confide if the test is positive. Inadequately prepared individuals may become extremely distressed, acutely anxious, severely depressed or suicidal. It is therefore crucial that the person receives professional counseling both before and after the test.

The counselor should act as a confidential listener, questioner and source of information and support. The pre-test counseling session is an opportunity to:

- provide information about HIV infection
- explore the risks and benefits of being tested (Box 9.6)
- discuss the meanings of the test (Box 9.7)
- help the individual to develop a plan to maximize the benefits and minimize risks.

It also gives the counsellor an opportunity to assess the individual's support system and provide some preventive education related to safer sexual practices and drug use.

The counselor can also put the individual in touch with support groups set up by people with HIV. These groups may run advice centres or alternative therapy clinics as well as providing opportunities to discuss issues with others in the same situation.

Box 9.6   Issues around testing for HIV

There are many things that need to be considered when planning to have an HIV test:

- It may be stressful not to know your HIV status

- Knowing whether you are HIV positive will help you make decisions about your future

- Early treatment of HIV can delay onset of AIDS and allow you to be well for many years, but it is not a cure

- You can protect yourself and your partner by following guidelines for safer sex and/or drug use

- The result may enable you to have sex with your partner without using condoms

- It may be stressful to know that you could become ill at any time if you test positive

- It can be difficult to tell friends, family and partners if you are HIV positive

- You may have difficulties obtaining a mortgage or insurance

- There may be strains on your relationship with your partner if you are HIV positive

- You will need advice from health professionals if you are considering pregnancy

HIV disease

Current data suggest that the majority of individuals infected with **HIV** will eventually become severely immunosuppressed and develop AIDS. There will be a preceding period of several years when they are only mildly symptomatic (stage B in Table 9.2). The main diseases associated with AIDS are unusual infections caused by micro-organisms that are not pathogenic in people with a competent immune system (*opportunistic infections*) and various cancers. A case definition of AIDS has been developed by the Centers for Disease Control in the USA and is recognized internationally (see Table 9.2). It is estimated that 40% of HIV-infected individuals will have reached stage C and developed AIDS 8 years after seroconversion, 95% after 15 years. They will remain infectious throughout the course of the disease, although they are probably more infectious during the latter stages. The progressive impairment of the immune response is caused by the gradual depletion of the CD4 T lymphocytes, which coordinate a number of important immune functions. There is a strong association between the number of CD4 T lymphocytes and the development of serious opportunistic illness. CD4 counts are used to monitor the progress of the disease and guide therapeutic management.

Usually the first clinical signs of infection are fevers, night sweats, skin rashes, diarrhoea, unexplained weight loss or respiratory symptoms (Haslett et al 2002). The type and extent of symptoms with which the individual presents will depend on the degree of immunodeficiency.

A debilitating syndrome of weight loss, diarrhoea, fever and night sweats may be caused directly by HIV or by secondary infection. The most common opportunistic infection in individuals with AIDS is *Pneumocystis carinii* pneumonia. The most common neoplasm is Kaposi's sarcoma, which is most likely to develop in homosexual or bisexual men. Tables 9.3 and 9.4 outline the common opportunistic infections and neoplasms associated with AIDS.

HIV disease in women and children

HIV infection may present differently in women, with many of the symptoms being focused on gynaecological problems such as persistent and virulent yeast infections, irregular menstrual periods, pelvic inflammatory disease and cervical cancer. Women often do not have the information they require to make informed decisions about safer sex, intimacy, childcare and reproductive rights. Because women have traditionally been care providers in society, they may neglect their own health because the needs of family and significant others appear more important.

The epidemic among women follows different patterns according to the geographical area. In parts of the world where the virus was first introduced in the heterosexual population (e.g. Africa), the ratio of male to female cases is close to 1:1. In Europe and North America, where the epidemic began in homosexual men and intravenous drug users, the ratio of male to female cases is steadily falling. In England and Scotland, during 2004, 0.1% of women born in the UK undergoing antenatal screening were estimated to have an undiagnosed HIV infection compared to 2.2% of women born in Africa. Women from Africa who attend genitourinary medicine (GUM) clinics in England (outside London) had an HIV infection rate of 8.2% during 2004, which bears out this global picture of HIV distribution between heterosexual and MSM populations (HPA 2005c). Worldwide, 5–10% of new infections occur in children, mostly during pregnancy, birth or breastfeeding (Haslett et al 2002).

The current evidence does not suggest that pregnancy accelerates progression of asymptomatic HIV infection to AIDS. However, it is possible that pregnancy may have adverse effects in women with advanced disease and low CD4 counts. Women who are HIV seropositive transmit the virus to their unborn child mainly at the time of birth, although about 20% of infections occur in utero. The risk of perinatal transmission can be significantly reduced by short course prophylaxis involving either single drug regimens of ZDV or nevirapine (see p. 163). Mother to child transmission rates average around 25–44% in developing countries and 13–25% in developed countries. Haslett et al (2002) suggest post-natal infection via breast feeding may account for the higher rates in developing countries. There is no difference in rates of prematurity or low birthweight in babies born to HIV-infected women. Women who are addicted to

Box 9.7   Facts about the HIV antibody test

The following factual information should be explained to patients before they undergo HIV testing.

- Human immunodeficiency virus (HIV) destroys the body's immune system and can leave you vulnerable to serious infections. HIV causes the disease known as AIDS. The antibody test detects the proteins called antibodies, which the body produces in response to an infection by HIV

- The standard test requires venous blood to be withdrawn via a needle placed in a vein in your arm. An alternative is the OraQuick Rapid HIV-1 Antibody Test, a test which has been developed in the USA and can be carried out on a fingerstick specimen of capillary blood. This test only detects Type 1 HIV, is not yet widely available but where it is used, a second confirmatory test is required for any positive finding (see below)

- When venous blood is tested, two tests are carried out (first the ELISA and then the Western Blot) and you must test positive to both to be designated HIV positive as sometimes a false positive can occur with just the one test. Whichever test is used, a positive result indicates that the antibody to HIV has been found in your blood.

A positive antibody test result means that:

- your blood sample has been tested more than once and the tests indicate that antibodies to the AIDS virus are present

- you have been infected with HIV, and therefore you should assume that you are capable of infecting others with HIV.

A positive test does *not* mean that:

- you have AIDS or an AIDS-related condition at present

- you will inevitably get AIDS or AIDS-related complex (ARC)

- you are immune to AIDS.

A negative antibody test result means that no antibodies to the AIDS virus have been found at this time. There are three possible explanations for this:

1 You have not been in contact with the virus.

2 You have come in contact with the virus, but have not become infected. Repeated exposure to the virus through high-risk behaviour greatly increases the likelihood of your becoming infected.

3 You have been infected with the virus but have not produced antibodies yet. It is estimated that the body normally takes 2–4 weeks to produce antibodies so a repeat test may be necessary. A small number of persons who become infected never produce antibodies.

A negative antibody test does *not* mean that:

- you are immune to the virus

- you have not been infected with the virus (you may have been infected and have not yet produced antibodies)

- you can carry on with high-risk behaviours without worrying about infection

All three of the above are wrong.

Sources: Lab Tests Online (2006), CDC (2006).

intravenous drugs, however, commonly have premature and low birthweight babies.

A child with HIV infection will live approximately 2 years from the time of diagnosis. Problems associated with infection are characterized by failure to thrive and delays in development. The child is particularly prone to recurrent bacterial infections, recurrent oral thrush and chronic diarrhoea (Box 9.8). Chronic parotid swelling and pulmonary lymphoid interstitial pneumonitis, thought to be linked to the Epstein–Barr virus, are found frequently in children with AIDS. The major cause of morbidity in these children is lung disease. Children do not acquire as many opportunistic infections as do adults, with the exception of *Pneumocystis carinii* pneumonia. Opportunistic infections presenting in the first year of life are associated with a higher mortality rate. Kaposi's sarcoma is seldom found in children. Children

Table 9.3 Common opportunistic infections in persons with AIDS

Cause	Usual site	Symptoms	Common diagnostic tests	Therapy
Protozoa				
1. Pneumocystis carinii	Lungs	Dry, non-productive cough, shortness of breath, fever, night sweats	Chest radiography, bronchoscopy	Trimethoprim Pentamidine Co-trimoxazole
2. Toxoplasma gondii	Brain	Headache, seizures, neurological deficits, behaviour changes, may lead to dementia	CT scan (head) MRI scanning	Sulfadiazine Pyrimethamine
3. Cryptosporidium	GI tract	Profuse, watery diarrhoea, dehydration, debility	Stool cultures	Spiramycin Antidiarrhoeals Antiperistaltics
Fungi				
4. Candida albicans	Mouth (thrush)	Dysphagia	Visible lesions scraped and cultured	Nystatin Clotrimazole
	Oesophagus	Dysphagia (oral candida may not be present)	Endoscopy with biopsy and culture of tissue	Ketoconazole Fluconazole
5. Cryptococcus	Brain	Headache, fever, confusion, behaviour changes	Lumbar puncture, bone marrow aspiration	Amphotericin B Neoformans
	Lungs	Non-specific cough or fever, dyspnoea	Chest radiography, sputum for culture, bronchoscopy with culture	Flucytosine
Viruses				
6. Cytomegalovirus	Eyes Lungs GI tract	Retinitis, loss of vision Cough, dyspnoea, fever Abdominal pain, ulcer, Gastrointestinal bleeding	Serology testing Bronchoscopy with biopsy and culture Endoscopy, colonoscopy	DHPG Foscamet Ganciclovir
	Spinal cord	Paraparesis, quadraparesis	Analysis of spinal fluid	
7. Herpes simplex virus	Skin	Painful cold sore clusters at mouth and perianal area	Histology and culture	Aciclovir
	Spinal cord	Paraparesis, quadraparesis	Analysis of spinal fluid	
Bacteria				
8. *Mycobacterium avium intracellulare*	Disseminated, many organs affected: liver, spleen, lungs, lymph nodes, bone marrow, GI tract	Fever, profuse sweating, productive cough, lymphadenopathy, diarrhoea, weight loss	Blood cultures, bone marrow aspiration, stool for acid-fast bacilli, endoscopy, colonoscopy with culture of biopsy tissue	Isoniazid Rifampicin Ethambutol Streptomycin Amikacin Biofazimine

Table 9.4 Secondary cancers common in patients with AIDS

Type	Site	Signs/symptoms	Diagnostic tests	Therapy
Kaposi's sarcoma	Skin Gastrointestinal (GI) tract Lungs	Multiple pink/purple/brown vascular lesions Usually asymptomatic Symptoms often same as pneumocystic pneumonia, unless pleural thickening or effusion present	Skin biopsy Endoscopy Chest radiography, bronchoscopy	Chemotherapy Radiation
Lymphomas	Brain Bone marrow GI tract	Neurological deficits according to site	CT scan Selective biopsy according to site	Radiation Chemotherapy

also present with neurological abnormalities such as acquired microcephaly, brisk tendon reflexes and abnormal electrophysiological findings. Developmental delays in motor, language and cognitive skills are also common. Some studies suggest the presence of HIV-induced embryopathy, while other studies conclude that there is not a consistently documented syndrome associated with HIV. Children with HIV infection are particularly susceptible to infectious diseases and should receive the routine immunizations outlined in Table 9.1. These vaccines are safe to give to children infected with HIV, provided the general contraindications to vaccination are not present (e.g. febrile illness, allergy to eggs (MMR), severe reaction to previous dose) (DoH 1996). HIV-positive individuals should not be given BCG vaccination against tuberculosis, or live vaccines such as yellow fever.

Intravenous drug users

Infection amongst intravenous drug users (IDUs) may be complicated by poverty and social factors. Traditionally, these individuals are distrustful of medical and government establishments, making the building of a therapeutic relationship, and interventions, extremely difficult. IDUs are also not as likely to belong to formal organizations, diminishing the power of influence available through collective action. Behavioural change may be made difficult by barriers such as low educational level, alienation from sources of accurate information, and the presence of a folklore belief system that supports the activities and values of intravenous drug use.

Intervention to stop transmission of HIV through sharing of needles ideally involves reaching individuals via drug treatment centres. In reality this is often difficult to accomplish. Ideally IDUs should be encouraged not to share dirty needles and syringes. In some centres this is being achieved by needle exchange programmes, where clean needles are issued when IDUs return their dirty ones. If needle exchange is not possible, the risk of infection can be reduced by disinfection of the needle and syringe by boiling or flushing through with bleach solution. A suitable solution can be made by diluting household bleach 1:10 with water, and the

Box 9.8 Major symptoms of AIDS in children

Infants

Failure to thrive, swollen lymph nodes, swollen abdomen due to enlargement of the liver and spleen, oral thrush, diarrhoea

Children over 1 year old

- *Mild*: abdominal swelling, dermatitis, recurring sinus and ear infections and parotid swelling developmental delays and regressions

- *Moderate*: pneumonitis, persistent oral thrush, frequent diarrhoea, fevers, hepatitis, kidney disease and chickenpox

- *Severe*: two serious bacterial infections in under 2 years (e.g. meningitis), fungal infection of the lungs or digestive tract, tumours, encephalopathy, pneumocystis carinii pneumonia (PCP)

Adolescents

Symptoms of HIV infection in teenagers may be similar to that of adults including a flu-like illness a month or so after infection. Symptoms found in children may also be present

Source: Children's Hospital Boston (2006).

needle and syringe should be flushed first in cold water until clear of blood.

Antiviral therapy

The main approach to therapy has been the use of drugs that are designed to block viral gene replication (nucleoside reverse transcriptase inhibitors or NRTIs and non-nucleoside reverse transcriptase inhibitors or NNRTIs) or target the enzyme responsible for assembling the newly copied genetic information (protease inhibitors or PIs). UK licensed examples of these drugs are:

- NRTIs: zidovudine, stavudine, abacavir
- NNRTIs: efavirenz, nevaripine
- PIs: nelfinavar,ritonavir.

The HIV virus can quickly develop resistance to the current medications, which has given rise to what is known as highly active antiretroviral therapy or HAART which involves using a combination of NRTIs. Combination therapy can be effective in maintaining health for long periods. Side-effects may be severe and adherence rates to HAART may be as low as 40–60% which only increases the development of resistant strains of HIV (Black and Hawks 2005). The cost of these drugs is prohibitive for developing countries, hence the drive to allow cheaper generic copies to be made available in the developing world where the need is greatest.

New drugs are continually being developed and tested, although access to drug trials is a controversial issue for patients.

The development of a vaccine to prevent HIV infection remains to be achieved. This is proving very difficult for many reasons, not the least of which is the ability of the virus to change and mutate very rapidly (termed 'genetic promiscuity'), which negates the benefits of any specific vaccine that may be developed as well as facilitating rapid resistance to effective anti-viral drugs. Clearly, the strongest weapon available against the virus is education and prevention.

GONORRHOEA

The specific organism causing gonorrhoea is *Neisseria gonorrhoeae*, which is transmitted almost exclusively by sexual intercourse and is found in the heterosexual and MSM populations. Anal or vaginal penetration, oral sex (both fellatio and cunninglingus) and ano-oral sex ('rimming') will all transmit the infection as can the use of various sex toys (Tyson 2005). The organism dies quickly when not harboured in the human body. The incidence of gonorrhoea is a key indicator for other STIs, including HIV, and is therefore closely monitored. Between 1995 and 2003 the number of newly diagnosed cases doubled in the UK although in 2004 there was an 11% decrease (to 22 335 new cases) compared to 2003. The highest incidence is in young adults, for example, 42% of women with gonorrhoea were under 20. Nurses involved in travel clinics should note that 10% of new infections are contracted overseas with Western Europe and the Caribbean being the two areas associated with the most infections (Tyson 2005).

Effects on the patient

Symptoms appear 2–10 days after the initial contact. In the male, urethritis occurs heralded by a purulent urethral discharge. Some itching and burning about the meatus are also present. The urethral meatus is red and oedematous. An ascending infection involving the prostate, seminal vesicles, bladder and epididymis may also occur. If adhesions develop, they may damage the urethra and duct system with consequent urethral stricture and infertility. Rectal infection is possible in gay men and is frequently asymptomatic, while infection of the pharynx may also occur due to unprotected oral-genital sex. Women may develop pelvic inflammatory disease and infertility as a result of an untreated infection.

Diagnosis is confirmed when the gonococcus is seen microscopically in smears or cultures taken from the site of infection. If urethral discharge is slight, the first urethral washings may be used. These are obtained by collecting the first portion of a voided urine specimen. The penis is not swabbed off before collecting the specimen.

Treatment

As in all cases of sexually transmitted disease, treatment should be carried out by specialist GUM departments because of the need for strict confidentiality, contact tracing, counseling and adherence to antimicrobial drug protocols to combat the growth of resistant strains, the first of which was identified in 1976. There are wide variations in resistance according to region of the UK with the north east of England having the highest rate of 36% in 2004 (compared to 3% in 2000) compared to neighbouring Yorkshire and Humberside with only 6% in 2004. As a result of the emergence of resistant strains, a single dose of cefixime (400 mg orally) or ceftriaxone (250 mg IM) is recommended for uncomplicated cases (Tyson 2005).

CHLAMYDIA

Chlamydia infection accounts for the single largest group of GUM attendances each year in the UK and male infection rates have dramatically increased from around 220 new cases per 100 000 population in 1995 to almost 1000 per 100 000 in 2004. Female rates have seen a similar rise and are now reaching close to 1100 new cases per 100 000. The age group with the highest infection rate in both sexes are the 16–19 year olds (HPA 2005). The spread of this infection indicates increasing risk taking in the sexual behaviour of young adults and with the threat of HIV lurking in the background, this is a major cause for concern. It is a similar story in other developed countries with 3.5 million new infections each year in the USA, of whom approximately 85% show no immediate symptoms. Concern at the spread of this infection in the UK has led to the establishment of an opportunistic screening programme that is currently being developed into a full national programme which is expected to be fully implemented by 2007 (Peate 2005).

The name chlamydia actually refers to a whole genus of bacteria whose pathological effects extend far beyond STI. *Chlamydia trachomatis* is a major cause of blindness in the developing world as well as STI in the developed world. The bacteria cause conjunctivitis that is exacerbated by the often hot and dusty conditions in developing countries. Lack of health care means that the simple treatment that could cure this disorder is lacking and consequently approximately 150 million people are infected in the developing world. As a result there is chronic infection, inflammation and irritation leading to corneal scarring and blindness, all of which could have been prevented. The result is approximately 6 million people who have gone blind in developing countries. Another strain of the genus, *Chlamydia pneumoniae,* is now thought to account for 10% of community-acquired pneumonia infections in the developed world and early research is suggesting this strain may even be involved in causing atherosclerosis (Ojcius et al 2005).

The genus chlamydia has the ability to induce epithelial cells (such as those of the genital tract or conjunctiva) to engulf them in little sacs called vacuoles. Normally cells destroy such a foreign interloper with lysozomes and display remnants of their molecular structure on the cell surface via the MHCII mechanism (see p. 142) alerting the immune system to the invader. Chlamydia have found a way of avoiding lysozome attack and can therefore live and multiply inside our cells without alerting the immune system, hence their insidious longevity in humans. They do little damage to cells apart from induce a slight inflammatory response with the result that many patients have little or no symptoms, especially if areas such as the uterus or anus are involved (Ojcius et al 2005). If the male urethra is infected there may be a slight soreness on micturition and a discharge although up to 50% of men are asymptomatic (Peate 2005) and women are often completely asymptomatic. However, pelvic inflammatory disease often develops over time as the infection spreads over the uterine endometrium and ascends into the fallopian tubes with serious consequences for the woman such as acute salpingitis or in the long term, fertility problems or a ruptured ectopic pregnancy (p. 795). Men may develop epididymitis or prostatitis if the infection is untreated.

As an STI, the infection frequently coexists with gonorrhoea but may persist as post-gonococcal urethritis following successful treatment of the gonorrhoea. This can make the patient anxious. Reassurance and teaching about the complaints are helpful in relieving anxiety.

Cultures for *Chlamydia trachomatis* are made from swabs of the anterior urethra and from first urethral washings. Doxycycline (7-day course) or azithromycin (single dose) is the antimicrobial of choice (BNF 2006). Recent sexual contacts are encouraged to come forward for investigation and treatment. After treatment (of both partners) abstinence from sexual intercourse is encouraged for at least 7 days and some consultants suggest that a condom should be used for a further 7 days. This is to prevent re-infection. If these guidelines are followed there is no need for repeat tests or follow up; the patient can consider him or herself to be cured of the infection.

VIRAL INFECTION (EXCLUDING HIV)

Anogenital herpes simplex

This is a very distressing condition and one of the most common STIs in the UK. Either HSV 1 or 2 may cause such an infection. Primary infection may be asymptomatic but the first symptoms are painful ulcers appearing within 7 days of infection, which rupture and then form a crust. Rectal ulcers may just produce pain whilst vaginal ulcers produce a vaginal discharge. The first stage lasts for up to 12 days and may be associated with systemic symptoms such as headache and malaise. Recurrent, less severe, attacks occur subsequently every few months. Unfortunately many patients may not realize they have been infected.

Human papillomavirus

Human papillomavirus (HPV) is the causative agent in condylomata acuminata, or genital warts. These warts may be confused with those of syphilis, but they are different: they are less flat and more cauliflower like. Perianal warts are usually confined to gay men. This viral infection was previously thought to be benign but recently some genotypes of the HPV (there are over 90 different types) have been associated with genital cancers in both men and women (e.g. cancer of the cervix, anus or penis).

The risk factors for acquiring the virus are early age at first intercourse (less than 17 years), multiple sexual partners, a history of STI, poor personal and sexual hygiene, a sexual partner with a similar history, a history of unprotected anal intercourse, and immunosuppression or immunodeficiency for any reason. Sexual intercourse is the major method of transmission.

Those presenting with external warts are screened for other sexually transmitted diseases which, if present, are treated. The partners of infected patients should also be examined and treated if necessary. External warts can be treated with podophyllin 10–25% in industrial spirit or tincture of benzoin. This caustic agent is applied with a cotton applicator and washed off 4 hours later. The surrounding skin is coated with petroleum jelly before application of the podophyllin, as this is a very irritant substance. The warts can also be treated with liquid nitrogen; the method of eradication will depend upon the practices of the local GUM clinic. Non-visible warts (areas of dysplasia associated with the HPV on the penis) are frequently vaporized with a carbon dioxide laser.

Hepatitis

Hepatitis B virus (HBV) is readily transmitted between MSM but rarely between heterosexual couples. It is found in semen, saliva and blood. As hepatitis B is a blood-borne infection it is a serious source of potential illness for anyone working in an occupation that brings them into contact with blood and body fluids. Hepatitis A is transmitted through contaminated water and food products. Hepatitis C is transmitted through blood and body fluids and tends to be transmitted through the sharing of needles, and needlestick injuries. Hepatitis D is only present in people who are also infected with Hepatitis B; it is uncommon in the UK and is mostly found in injecting drug users. It can be transmitted via sexual contact at the same time as Hepatitis B or it can be transmitted on its own if the patient is already infected with hepatitis B (Association of Medical Microbiologists 1993).

SYPHILIS

Syphilis is a serious disease and, fortunately, is much less common than gonorrhoea. The causative organism is the spirochaete *Treponema pallidum*. During 2004 there were 2254 new diagnoses in the UK, representing a 37% increase on 2003 and continuing a sharp upward trend in numbers seen since 2000 when the total was just over 200. Of particular note is that 88% of cases were male and over half of them MSM. There have been several reported localized severe outbreaks of syphilis during recent years in big cities such as Manchester and Newcastle, focused mostly on MSM (HPA 2005c).

Effects on the patient

Incubation is usually 14–28 days. In most cases the disease is spread by sexual intercourse. As with the gonococcus, the spirochaete does not survive outside the host. In the untreated condition, three stages are distinguished. The stages may overlap or be widely separated.

The *primary lesion* is a small, painless chancre or ulcer. It is deep and has indurated edges. Usually, this chancre heals spontaneously, giving the false impression that the disease is cured. This primary lesion appears most commonly on the penis of the male.

The *secondary stage* is usually characterized by a rash appearing over the body. The rash is usually accompanied by malaise and fever. In a short period the rash regresses and the patient enters the latent stages. *Latency* refers to the absence of symptoms in the infected individual. Progress of the disease in the individual seems to be arrested and only rarely can others be infected in this stage.

Three outcomes are now possible:

1 The patient proceeds immediately or after a delay of 10–30 years to the third stage.
2 The disease remains latent for the rest of the person's life.
3 A spontaneous cure occurs.

In the *tertiary stage* the bones, heart and central nervous system, including the brain, can be affected. Personality disorders arise and the typical ataxic gait of tertiary syphilis appears. A large, ulcerating necrotic lesion known as a *gumma* now occurs. Rarely is it seen in the genital tract, but it may occur on the vulva or in the testes. At this stage the disease may be arrested but not reversed.

Diagnosis is made by a careful history, clinical findings, and cultures or biopsies from the lesions. Treatment of early syphilis is with a 14-day course of procaine benzylpenicillin, doxycycline or erythromycin.

NURSING INTERVENTION

Most patients with an STI are treated on an outpatient basis; the person should be taught how to protect themselves and others. First, the nature and transmission of the infection need to be understood. No immunity develops and re-infection can occur easily. Strict personal and perineal hygiene should be observed. Handwashing following any handling of the genitalia is imperative as, for example, the gonococcus can be readily carried to the eye, which quickly becomes infected. Blindness may ensue if treatment is not received. Nurses in primary care should realize that STI can occur in those under 16 and can even be the consequence of sex abuse. It is therefore a child protection issue that *all* nurses who come into contact with children should be aware of.

Sexual intercourse is to be avoided until the infection has been treated successfully. All equipment must be sterilized following use, and dressings or swabs disposed of in a safe way. Syphilis may be transmitted by direct contamination of a laceration with living spirochaetes. For this reason, the routine use of universal body substance precautions will also control inadvertent transmission of this disease to health professionals. Once therapy has been initiated, the patient is usually non-infectious within 48 hours.

An STI is often very distressing to the patient. The patient may experience guilt feelings, and marital difficulties may arise when one partner infects the other. Infection carries a social stigma. For these reasons, confidentiality must be maintained by the nurse at all times; the issue is protected by law and the disease is reportable. Contacts must be identified and followed discreetly by the contact tracer. The contact tracer, by explaining the nature of the disease, usually obtains the patient's cooperation in identifying contacts. A great deal of tact and sensitivity is required as detailed information about sexual practices and partners needs to be obtained for the correct tests and treatment to be made available to those who need them. The interview requires privacy, reassurance of confidentiality, and is done while the patient is dressed, before the physical examination. The contact tracer should explain clearly to the patient the purpose of the questions and why they are necessary. In addition, the nurse should include STI in any lectures prepared on general health education in schools so that the population may become more aware of the signs and symptoms, the modes of transmission, and the safer sex practices needed to prevent spread of these diseases.

SAFER SEX GUIDELINES

Responsible sexual conduct, based on a healthy understanding of human sexuality, should be taught at every opportunity. The definition of responsible sexual conduct varies considerably. For some, it means complete abstinence from sexual intercourse or activity until permitted by religious or cultural laws; for others, a wide range of sexual practices is accepted and practised. However, low-risk sex practices should be known to all, and some safer sex guidelines follow:

1 *Reduce the number of sexual partners*. Abstinence is safe. Adolescents and adults should be encouraged to avoid

casual sexual encounters. Longer-term monogamous relationships with known sexual partners reduce the risks and opportunity for exposure. Within such a long-term relationship, the latitude available for sexual practices can be broader and still be considered safe from the threat of disease.

2 *Avoid the exchange of body fluids* by:
- using a condom during vaginal, anal and oral intercourse. Condoms have been shown to be effective barriers to bacterial and viral agents. Use each condom only once
- never using saliva as a lubricant. Use spermicides or water-soluble jelly
- not following or preceding anal intercourse with vaginal penetration without a change of condom
- using gentle sexual practices that avoid trauma to mucous membrane or skin
- avoiding other sexual practices such as oral-anal, oral-genital sex (without condom) as it is difficult to avoid the ingestion or exchange of body fluids or organisms. Gonorrhoea, hepatitis, HIV and other viruses can be transmitted in these ways
- avoiding prolonged wet (French) kissing unless with a partner whom you consider to be safe.

3 *Consider who your partner is.* If your partner is a total stranger what do you know about them? Sex is far riskier if they are an IDU or a person who has multiple casual sexual partners. They may even know they are infected and deliberately withhold such information from a casual partner who they do not expect to see again.

4 *Sex under the influence of alcohol is especially risky.* Precautions such as those listed above may be disregarded due to the disinhibiting effects of alcohol whilst pregnancy is also more likely.

SUMMARY

This chapter discussed the main causes of infection and key preventive measures. The interaction between host and microbe determines the likely development of infection. The care of a patient with an infection centres around supporting the person through the illness, alleviating symptoms, observing for complications and administering antimicrobial therapy.

In recent decades there has been a substantial reduction in many infectious diseases (e.g. measles, poliomyelitis and diphtheria). This has stemmed from increased knowledge about the interaction between host and microbial agent, the widespread use of immunization programmes and vigorous public health measures. Sadly this has not been the case in large parts of the developing world where HIV, malaria and TB exact a dreadful toll on human life.

The decline in the many familiar infections in the developed world has occurred at the same time as the growth of others such as HIV, HCAI and the threat of a global pandemic of flu. HIV is complicated not only by the seriousness of the illness, but also by the social and ethical challenges it provides. Care of the individual must focus not only upon the physical manifestations of the illness, but also upon the psychological and social effects. As a reliable vaccine for HIV lies a long way in the future, the only reliable mode of intervention is effective education, and hence prevention. The sophisticated health services of developed countries now face the consequences of increasing numbers of HCAIs and nurses must be aware of the risks to take steps to protect both the patient and themselves. Finally we all must be aware of the implications of a flu pandemic and face this threat together with our local communities, wherever we live in the world.

CASE This study is based upon a study presented by Gandhi et al (2002) and illustrates some of the main points covered in this chapter. The chapters on the respiratory system and substance misuse will provide useful further information.

David is a 36-year-old man who presents to the A&E department. He is thin, unshaven, sweaty (diaphoretic) and rather scruffily dressed. He complains of having become increasingly short of breath over the previous 2 weeks and has a cough which is producing green sputum. He wakes up at night sweaty and has begun to have episodes of severe shivering (rigors). The triage nurse assigns you to check his vital signs and you ask him to take off his jacket so you can check his BP. He is wearing a short-sleeved T-shirt underneath and you notice obvious injection sites around veins on both arms. What is the next question that you should ask him?

Your question:

When you ask about drug use his reply is 'Yes, I do IV smack, what's that got to do with my chest?' What is the correct reply to his question?

Your answer:

His vital signs are T 39.8, P116, BP 105/70, RR 22. What else should you measure right now?

Your answer:

Well done, you should measure his oxygen sats which are only 91% (on air).

You ask how long he has had his bad chest. He says '2 weeks' and then tells you he did actually present at the department about 10 days before and had a chest X-ray but he could not hang around waiting any longer as he needed to see his dealer as he was low on 'stuff'. He tells you his chest has been getting worse ever since and is really painful, especially on the right side, which he is holding in a protective way. You notice nicotine stains on his fingers and when you ask about them he says he gets through about 30 cigarettes a day and regularly drinks alcohol as well, mostly strong lagers. However, he has no idea how many units a week. He jokingly says 'Thought you would be more worried about the hard stuff' then laughs at his own joke, immediately regretting it as he coughs and grimaces.

With oxygen sats of 91% and obvious respiratory problems, what should you provide for him next?

Your answer:

Clerical staff supply his old notes and find the radiographs. You read the X-ray report and it states that he had a right lower lobe infiltrate (abnormal fluid accumulation in the tissue of the lower lobe of his right lung). The notes show that when first examined the doctor had queried a viral pneumonia and was waiting for the X-rays when the patient walked out of the department saying he had waited too long already. There is a note from a nurse stating she had told him to come back if things did not improve and to take paracetamol for his chest pain. He is not registered with a GP.

He is sent for another chest X-ray which now reveals a large right-sided pleural effusion with infiltrates into the right middle and lower lobes. (See p. 346 concerning pleural effusion).

Bloods are taken for a full blood count and a culture. He is able to produce a sputum specimen for lab analysis and this time agrees to stay in hospital so the on-call medical team admit him as an emergency. They are concerned that the effusion seen on X-ray represents a purulent effusion, i.e. fluid consisting of the debris of infection otherwise known as pus. This is called empyema and when it forms secondary to pneumonia the purulent effusion accumulates in the pleural space, progressively compromising breathing. If the physicians are correct, this needs urgent evacuation to facilitate his breathing.

If the fluid was found to be an exudate, what would this consist of? (clue, see p. 346). If it was a transudate what would that consist of?

Your answer:

An exudate could be due to infection (e.g. pneumonia) or cancer of the bronchus, for example, while a transudate may form due to chronic heart failure. A pulmonary embolism could form either a transudate or an exudate. An effusion can also be bloody indicating tissue trauma.

The lab phone later in the day to say his white cell count is 18×10^9/L (normal range 4.0–11.0). What is that telling you?

Your answer:

Shortly after admission a thoracentesis was performed with ultrasound guidance to ensure optimum positioning, and a light brown coloured fluid was aspirated which had a very high leucocyte count, consisting predominantly of neutrophils. What does this indicate?

Your answer:

An underwater seal drainage system was established to drain all the fluid and re-expand his right lung. Antimicrobial therapy was commenced.

Microbiology showed chains of Gram-positive cocci in the fluid. A follow up X-ray showed no pneumothorax, which is always a risk with a procedure such as this.

Pause for reflection

- Think of the consequences of patients walking away when diagnosis and treatment are incomplete (this happens in places like A&E and walk-in clinics). How might the situation have been handled to avoid the patient's self-discharge and the progressive deterioration in his condition that occurred over the next 2 weeks?
- What do you think might be the implications of his IV heroin use for hospital care?
- Prior to discharge what kind of topics might you raise with him in a health promotion discussion?

See Chapter 26 on substance misuse to check out your answers.

REFERENCES

AIDS Education and Training Centers National Resource Center (2006) HIV classification: CDC and WHO Staging Systems. Online. Available http://www.aidsetc.org

Association of Medical Microbiologists (1993) Viral hepatitis. Online. Available: http://www.amm.co.uk/newamm/files/factsabout/fa_virhep.htm 24 Feb 2006.

Black J, Hawks J (2005) Medical-surgical nursing, 7th edn. St Louis: Elsevier Saunders.

Blaser M (2005) An endangered species in the stomach. Scientific American 292(2): 24–31.

BNF (2006) British National Formulary; 51. London: BMA, RPS.

CDC (2006) Frequently asked questions about Ora Rapid HIV-1 Antibody Test. Online. Available: http://www.dcd.gov/hiv/resources/qa/print/oraqck/htm

Children's Hospital Boston (2006) My child has AIDS/HIV. Online. Available: http://www.childrenshospital/org/az/site550/printerfriendlypages5550PO.html

Clark L (2000) Antibiotic resistance, a growing and multifaceted problem. British Journal of Nursing 9(4): 225–230.

Collins F, Hampton S (2005) Hand washing and methicillin-resistant *Staphylococcus aureus*. British Journal of Nursing 14(13): 703–707.

Cookson B (2005) Methicillin-resistant *Staphylococcus aureus*: a modern epidemic. Evidence-Based Healthcare and Public Health 9(1): 1–3.

Demicheli V, Rivetti D, Deeks J (2004) Vaccination reduces the incidence of serologically confirmed influenza in healthy adults. Evidence Based Nursing 8(2): 47.

Department of Health (1996) Immunisation against infectious diseases. London: HMSO.

Department of Health (2004) Full immunisation schedule. Online. Available: http://www.immunisation.org.uk/article.php?id=97

Gandhi M, Bacon O, Caughey A (2002) Clinical cases in medicine. Malden, Mass: Blackwell Publishing.

Garner J (1996) Guidelines for isolation precautions in hospital. American Journal of Infection Control 24: 24–52.

Gibbs W, Soares C (2005) Preparing for a pandemic. Scientific American 293(5): 44–54.

Haslett C, Chilvers E, Boon N et al (2002) Davidson's principles and practice of medicine, 19th edn. Edinburgh: Churchill Livingstone.

Health Services Advisory Committee (1999) Safe disposal of clinical waste. London: HMSO.

HPA (2005a) Press release: healthcare agencies urge NHS to step up measures to minimise risk of patients contracting *Clostridium difficile*. Online. Available: http://www.hpa.org.uk/news/articles

HPA (2005b) HIV and AIDS: information and guidance on the occupational setting. Online. Available: http://www.hpa.org.uk/infections/topics

HPA (2005c) Mapping the issues; HIV and other STIs in the United Kingdom 2005. Online. Available: http://www.hpa.org.uk/publications/hiv

HPA (2006) Annual report of the HPA 2005; Common bacterial pathogens causing systemic infections. Online. Available: http://www.hpa.org.uk

IHI (2005) Institute for Healthcare Improvement; 100k Lives campaign. Online. Available: http://www.ihi.org/Programs/Campaign/

Lab Tests Online (2006) HIV Antibody. Online. Available: http://www.labtestonline.org/understanding.analytes/hiv_antibody/multiprint.html

Leifer D (2005) MRSA hotspots. Nursing Standard 19(52): 20–22.

Newcombe (2004) Treating and preventing tetanus in A&E. Emergency Nurse 12(6): 23–29.

NHS Executive (1995) Hospital laundry arrangements for used and infected linen. HSG(95)18. London: HMSO.

NHS Estates (2004) A protocol for the local decontamination of surgical instruments. London: Department of Health.

Ojcius D, Darville T, Bavoil P (2005) Can chlamydia be stopped? Scientific American 292(5): 54–61.

Peate I (2005) Physiological and general health effects of chlamydia on men. British Journal of Nursing 14(9): 1010–1013.

Royal College of Nursing (2005) Guidance on uniforms and clothing worn in the delivery of patient care. London: RCN.

Springhouse Corporation (2000) Nurse practitioners clinical companion. Springhouse, PA: Springhouse Corporation.

Storr J, Topley K, Privett S (2005) The ward nurse's role in infection control. Nursing Standard 19(41): 56–64.

Taubenberger J, Reid A, Fanning T (2005) Capturing a killer flu virus. Scientific American 292(1): 48–57.

Tyson M (2005) Guidance for first-line treatment of ano-genital gonorrhoea infection. British Journal of Nursing 14(12): 646–670.

Ward S (2000) Evidence based practice and infection control. British Journal of Nursing 9(5): 267–271.

Watterson L (2005) Sharp thinking. Nursing Standard 20(5): 20–22.

Wilcox A (2005) Preventing healthcare associated infections in primary care. Primary Health Care 15(8): 43–49.

Wilson J (1995) Infection control in clinical practice. London: Baillière Tindall.

Winter G (2005a) A bug's life. Nursing Standard 19(33): 16–18.

Winter G (2005b) Origin of the species. Nursing Standard 19(34): 24–25.

Winter G (2005c) Global virus alert. Nursing Standard; 19(44): 24–26.

World Health Organization (2006) Universal precautions including injection safety. Online. Available: http://www.who.int./hiv/topics/precautions/universal/en/print.html

USEFUL WEBSITES

Health Protection Agency: http://www.hpa.org.uk
US. Center for Disease Control: http://www.cdc.gov
World Health Organization: http://www.who.int

10 Clinical investigations

Susan Skinner

INTRODUCTION

Clinical investigations provide the essential information needed to assess health, potential health problems or disease. Within a formal healthcare setting, clinical investigations are associated with complex methods of testing but informal clinical investigations to monitor health are frequently taking place. Stepping on weighing scales in the home or noting the physical effect of exercise provide a value which, though rarely recorded, provide people with important information about the state of their health.

For nurses, the clinical investigation of a patient, or client, begins from the first point of contact, using both formal and informal methods of assessment. Using clinical expertise that has come from education and experience the nurse will make an informed appraisal of the patient's well-being. The visual assessment will give a strong impression of the patient's health and well-being. In addition, the nurse will listen to what the patient has to say and note the way in which the patient tells his or her story. The nurse will ultimately use all of his or her senses to collect information about the patient's physical, psychological and spiritual health, building a picture that may go beyond the rational information gained from more scientific methods of clinical investigations.

This clinical appraisal forms the foundation from which further clinical assessment, using science and technology can be planned. Technological advances in recent years have extended the precision and accuracy of clinical assessment. The complex equipment used for health screening and diagnostic purposes is constantly evolving to provide detailed clinical pictures. It must be remembered, though, that the use of this sophisticated technology follows the first examination and initial observations made by the nursing and medical staff. The equipment assists and extends the accumulation of information but it is the knowledgeable practitioner who initiates and steers the process, and ultimately interprets the results for each individual patient.

RATIONALE FOR CLINICAL INVESTIGATIONS

There should always be reasonable justification for requesting clinical investigations. When a clinical investigation is performed, there is a cost in time and money for both the patient and the health service. Anxiety is a probable additional cost to the well-being of patients while the investigation is performed and as they wait for the results. An increasing amount of guidance regarding the appropriate use of clinical investigations is being made available through the National Institute of Clinical Excellence (NICE). As a national body, NICE review evidence-based practice and provide guidance for best practice. Local and individual variations and preferences may still remain, especially when the clinical investigation relates to a difficult clinical problem. An example of this is the testing of pregnant women for vaginal Group B Streptococcus: NICE guidelines have been prepared for this but local policy variations on clinical testing continue to exist for the present.

In overview, clinical investigations can:

- provide a snapshot with which to assess the health of a patient at a given moment in time
- be used to preclude, or confirm, a suspected diagnosis following a physical examination
- monitor the clinical status of patients as they undergo therapeutic regimens, revealing trends in health and well-being
- be used to provide national health screening programmes with specified tests utilized for specified population groups. These are designed to confirm health, provide early diagnosis or alert patients to potential problems
- provide reliable information for analysis from the results gained from national screening programmes, giving indications of regional variations in the epidemiology of specific diseases.

ASSESSMENT AND CLINICAL INVESTIGATIONS

Few clinical investigations give sufficient information when interpreted in isolation. The results will need to be put into the context of other health indicators and the life as lived by the patient before any clinical decisions can be made with any certainty. The results must be evaluated using other physiological, psychological and social parameters that have an impact on the patient's health.

Lists of 'normal' reference values are commonly found in nursing textbooks and they provide useful guidelines to assess deviation from the norm. However, 'normal' values may be a matter of debate and there may be differences in acceptable normal values. It will always be necessary to familiarize yourself with the list of accepted values for clinical investigations carried out in the unit that you work in.

It must also be remembered that some values given as 'normal' may not apply to all of your patients. An example of this would be a child with congenital heart disease who has a 'normal' oxygen saturation monitor value of 92%. This compares poorly with the normal healthy oxygen saturation value, which is usually given as 99%. However, for this child a value of 92% is normal – and one the child learns to cope with.

The results of specific clinical assessments often have additional significance within a specialized hospital unit. It then becomes an essential issue of policy making to provide staff with reference lists of agreed acceptable values that are applicable only for use within that hospital unit.

Whenever an abnormal value is revealed during a clinical assessment the nurse must be aware that the results may reflect factors that are associated with the life that the patient leads rather than being a cause for concern. There are many influences acting on the body to produce deviations from expected norms. Some examples to be aware of are given below.

FOOD

The nutritional status of a patient has a strong influence on many tests. Dieting will produce a urine that tests positive for **ketones**, yet the presence of ketones in other circumstances (e.g. diabetes) would be a serious consideration when evaluating a patient's health. A further example is variation in **blood glucose** values, which occur naturally in response to meal times.

AGE

Ageing has a detrimental effect on all systems and tissues of the body. The person's age must always be considered when results are being interpreted (e.g. sex hormone levels).

DRUGS

Drugs are designed to interfere with or change physiological processes (see Ch. 6). It is therefore inevitable that they will have an impact on the results of some clinical investigations. An example of this is the decreased measured **prothrombin** time associated with oral contraceptive use.

TIME OF DAY

The importance of the biorhythms on hormone and other tissue secretions are a matter of current research. **Growth hormone** is an example of this. It is secreted in regular bursts at pre-set times throughout the day, with the largest burst of the hormone being secreted during the early part of sleep at night. As expected, the amount of growth hormone secreted and considered as a normal value will additionally be affected by the age of the patient.

BODY MASS

The measurement of body mass and the estimation of normal standard values will always have to be set within the considerations of age and sex. Many other additional influences will affect the measurements taken. These can include drug therapies, disturbances in metabolic rate, poor health and the appetite for food. Examples include the effects of long-term steroid therapy for a patient with inflammatory disease or young men who abuse unprescribed anabolic steroids for body building.

GEOGRAPHICAL AREA

Adaptation of patients to their local environment may affect the normal values expected to be returned, when clinical investigations are carried out. For example, the lower oxygen values in air at altitude will cause the local population to have **polycythaemia** (an increased number of circulating red blood cells). This adaption makes sufficient **haemoglobin** available at the **respiratory membranes** to keep oxygen values at an adequate level.

SPECIMENS

The conditions under which the specimen was taken, or the use of poor collection techniques, may cause the results to be unreliable. For example a blood sample that has been shaken about during transport can produce a high level of potassium when it is analysed at the laboratory. This is due to the haemolysis associated with the breakdown of red blood cells when they become damaged during transportation. Results therefore must be considered within the context of previously measured personal values or against previously measured baseline values. The nurse should use a process of individualized patient assessment and evaluation.

CARE OF PATIENTS NEEDING CLINICAL ASSESSMENT

Most of us have experienced the fear and uncertainty that arises when checks are made on our own health, or on the health of our family. Some outcomes can mean a complete alteration in the opportunities that life can offer and the patterning of everyday life. Some results may cause a difficulty in the relationships with loved ones; other positive results may have financial implications that can undermine the quality of a person's life. As nurses, we must not forget that the routine blood test may take on great significance for the patient, as it may be anything but 'routine' for that person. Nurses must be ready to give explanations, guidance and support. They should be aware of the place that the investigation has in the planned assessment and care of the patient, and be prepared to provide a complete explanation and give some indication of the significance of the results. It is important to give patients an explanation of the procedure before each investigation is carried out. The explanation must be in terms that makes meaning clear to each patient and in a format that helps with understanding, both as the explanation is given and when the patient considers what has been said at a later time. This clarification is important for giving patients guidance and maintaining their confidence throughout the investigative process. It is also an essential part of the process that allows patients to exercise *informed choice*. It is through the ability to understand the rationale of the clinical investigations, and the exercising of informed choice, that patients can become full partners in the planning of their care. They will be able to give *consent* for the procedures needed for the clinical investigations with increased confidence. The information given must contain the reasons why the investigations are necessary and the process of the procedure. Patients must be informed of the time at which the results will be available and how they will obtain them. If you are the nurse who is to carry out the investigation, it is essential that you give yourself time to prepare before meeting the patient. The patient will appreciate a nurse who appears unhurried and is able to give appropriate support when it is needed. This initial preparation will also help

should unexpected events occur while the investigation is taking place. If you are fully prepared, you can work with confidence. This helps both you and the patient.

Talk to the patient throughout the procedure, reporting the progress of the techniques you are using and assuring the patient that the clinical investigation is progressing as planned. Such reassurance is especially important if the patient is experiencing discomfort and is anxious that difficulties are occurring. If it is difficult for the nurse who is carrying out the procedure to talk to the patient, a colleague must be asked to stay with the patient to give the support that is needed. The reduction of patient anxiety must be a priority for all staff.

The nurse must try to keep the patient as calm and comfortable as possible throughout the procedure, as the results of some clinical investigations may be altered by the patient feeling anxious. An environment that helps the patient to relax is also important. The procedures necessary for the test may test the tolerance of the patient and it can become a difficult task for nurses to help the patient at such a personal level. The reduction of stress will improve the accuracy of many clinical investigations, especially those connected with the cardiovascular system. If the nurse observes that the patient is overly anxious, the patient should be allowed to recover his or her basal state before proceeding with the clinical assessment.

INFORMED CONSENT

All clinical investigations require the patient to have a clear understanding of the rationale for the test and the method of testing. This relies on adequate methods of communication to be used by clinical practitioners. Guidelines on informed consent to treatment drawn up by the UK Department of Health (2001a) state that a professional who carries out investigations on a patient before obtaining a valid consent makes that employee liable to legal action by the patient and also their professional body. These guidelines are very clear as to the meaning of 'valid' consent. Acquiescence to the procedure by a patient who does not understand why, or how, the clinical investigation is being performed is not valid consent. Valid consent requires that:

● permission to perform the clinical investigation is given voluntarily, without coercion from any source
● the person has the capacity to understand and retain the information given to them about the clinical investigation. When this is not possible, carers and parents are able to give permission for the clinical investigation to proceed as long as the proper legal and ethical guidelines indicated in the Department of Health document (Department of Health 2001a) are fully complied with
● sufficient, clear information has been given to the patient about the nature and purpose of the clinical investiga-

tion. Any misrepresentation within the explanation will invalidate any consent given by the patient.

The Code of Professional Practice (Nurse Midwifery Council 2004) for nurses confirms that nurses must comply with these Department of Health guidelines.

As the advocate for the patient in all care settings, a nurse will need to ensure that the patient has a full understanding of the clinical investigation before it is carried out, even if it is another practitioner carrying out the clinical investigation. The information that you give must be truthful and unbiased, especially when the patient has to use information to make a difficult choice. The clarity and impartiality of information is especially important when a patient is giving consent to a clinical investigation that may change the course of his or her life. An example of this would be a woman who feels in good health but is advised to have screening for hepatitis C virus. A positive result from the test would confer on her a state of poor health, which will inevitably alter her perception of her own well-being and sense of happiness in her life.

In all circumstances the patient must give written or verbal consent before any clinical investigation is undertaken. When it is not possible for the patient to understand the information the nurse must provide the information for the relative or carer, using the Department of Health (2001a) guidelines. When consenting to any investigative process the patient tacitly assumes that the person carrying out the test is competent and educated fully in the investigating procedure. This factor becomes important when the procedure is one that was originally performed by a doctor but has become part of a nurse's expanded role. Furlong and Glover (1998) argue that nurses should identify themselves as the lead practitioner in this situation as there may be legal questions to answer at a future date if the assumption was made by the patient that a doctor was performing the investigation.

GIVING INFORMATION

Consent to clinical investigations can be given by the patient only if adequate information is available for him or her to make informed choices. The relevant information must be delivered in an acceptable and understandable format. It is this information that will enable the patient to cope with the process of clinical investigation and its outcome (Lowry 1995). Commonly, the patient will learn from the medical team about the clinical investigations that they are advising the patient to give consent to. The anxiety induced from such a meeting with a clinician will interfere with the amount of information the patient can recall (Lloyd et al 1999). Anxiety regarding the circumstances of the meeting, the fear of bad news and the amount of information that needs to be assimilated by the patient interferes with both the recall and comprehension of the information. It is the nurse who provides the continuing care who is in the best

position to clarify the explanations for the patient. It is through the nurse providing a repetition of the facts and answering further questions that the patient is provided with a full rationale for the clinical explorations ordered.

Remembering full explanations in detail when they are given verbally is difficult for most people, and the difficulty is compounded for the patient when anxiety also becomes a barrier to listening and understanding. To help the patient with this, information leaflets to supplement the verbal explanation have become an essential tool for nurses. An information leaflet that is clearly and attractively written will provide a constant reference point and source of information for the patient. It has the additional benefit that it can be read at the patient's own speed and provide the starting point for further questions. These information leaflets should give a truthful account of the clinical investigation that they explain. A leaflet must not give a misleading account of the clinical investigation. It must be truthful when describing discomforts that are known to be expected during or after the investigation. If the information leaflet is found to be inaccurate or incomplete there may be detrimental consequences during the subsequent investigation and the patient's confidence in other written or verbal information issued from the same source will be reduced. Throughout this information-giving process the nurse must remain sensitive to the patient's ability to understand. The information may be given using unfamiliar words, either from the use of clinical terminology or not in the patient's first language. The written information may have been prepared without being tested for its reading age and may contain words and phrases that are beyond the ability of some people to read. The nurse must also make sure that conflicting information is not given at any point.

PATIENT ANXIETY AND CLINICAL INVESTIGATIONS

A 'routine' test may shatter the future hopes and ambitions of a patient. The results of the test may confirm a prognosis that is predictive of disability, sensory impairment or premature death. It may bring about circumstances that involve the patient adjusting his or her views on quality of life. This adaptation may become necessary in order that the patient can remain in control of events in his or her own future. The tests may cause difficulties in the relationships with those that the patient is closest to. The results of a simple, routine test performed by a nurse may lead the patient to face serious and complex difficulties. For example, a swab taken from a newborn baby with sticky eyes could produce a culture that grows the gonococcus bacterium. This is seen to have been contracted from the birth canal of the mother and can lead to a situation that is difficult to resolve at this most sensitive time. This swab result may have an impact not only on the lives of the parents but also on the early years and future life of the newborn baby.

PROFESSIONAL PREPARATIONS

It is essential that nurses understand the principles, process and purpose of all clinical investigations that they perform, or when they give assistance during testing by another clinician. The nurse must have an understanding of the principles of the normal physiology associated with the test or have knowledge of the anatomy of the system that is being assessed. A knowledge of normal physiology will give the foundations on which variations found during the assessment can be identified and understood.

The accuracy of the clinical investigations will be completely dependent on the care taken by the nurse to ensure all possibilities for error are eliminated. Technology, especially when it is utilized in the clinical setting, has the potential to produce erroneous readings through the poor technique of the operator. For this reason, when the initiation of medical or nursing interventions is dependent on the information taken from the clinical investigations, it is essential that nurses are given proper clinical supervision to ensure the accuracy of testing. It is essential that the nurses have all relevant knowledge and are supervised until the technique is seen to be performed safely and competently.

Evidence that this education and supervision has taken place is especially important when professional boundaries are crossed and the nurse takes on an expanded role in order to perform a clinical investigation. A formal training period must then be instituted. Essential theoretical knowledge and practice must be tested to ensure that the nurse is performing the investigation to defined criteria. Nurses should refuse to perform a clinical investigation when they have doubts regarding their own competency or when the procedure will breach their own level of expertise. It is part of a nurse's own professional practice development to assess him- or herself, against standards of competency and safe practice (Nurse Midwifery Council 2004).

Learning the practical skills attached to clinical investigations may be the most straightforward part of acquiring the new skill. Competence to perform the skill will also include the interface with the patient: the ability to answer questions with assurance and empathy, and to give the patient confidence. The nurse must also be able to provide information regarding the further actions that may be necessary based on the outcome of the assessment.

To be competent to perform clinical investigations is also to be fully aware of personal safety issues when the clinical investigation is carried out. Knowledge of the risk factors for both the patient and the nurse is essential. The nurse must make provision for appropriate safety precautions for both staff and the patient.

ESSENTIAL NURSING KNOWLEDGE RELATED TO CLINICAL INVESTIGATIONS

To help patients through any assessment process, nurses should ensure that they are secure in the following fundamental knowledge:

- They know exactly what is being measured and for what purpose; nurses must know the principles that lie behind the investigation
- They have knowledge of the assessment within the context of normal physiological function
- They have given thought to how the patient can be best prepared – physically, psychologically and emotionally – to be a positive participant in the process. This point is especially pertinent when caring for children and their parents
- They are aware of side-effects that can arise from the procedure associated with the clinical investigation and be prepared to prevent or counter effects if they occur
- Most clinical investigation procedures have the potential to harm the assessor or patient through the incorrect use of equipment or procedure. The nurse must know of any specific precautionary measures that must be taken when using the equipment. Be aware of the hazards and work only within prescribed guidelines and procedures
- Nurses must help the patient understand that the interpretation of the results of clinical investigations is not always an easy process and that conclusions cannot always be drawn from a single result. The results need to be considered using knowledge of a multiple of variables. These may include the:
  a) values being compared to the normal ranges supplied by your local guidelines, which may not equate to values shown in textbooks
  b) values recorded for the patient obtained when previously investigated
  c) values considered within the context of other clinical investigations that have an impact on the assessment taken
- To initiate a rapid response, nurses should ensure that a system of reporting is in place that allows the laboratory to alert staff immediately when the result obtained is life threatening for the patient.

PRE-PROCEDURE PREPARATION

Time spent preparing for the procedure will enhance its smooth operation. Plan ahead and think through the procedure carefully. Ensure that all necessary equipment has been collected. Examine the area where the investigation is to take place and ensure that the patient, and you, will remain comfortable throughout. It is particularly important that the investigator is not placed in a position that puts any strain on the back, even for a short period of time.

There must be optimal communication with the patient throughout the procedure so, as part of the preparation, ensure that any necessary aids to understanding are available. If the patient normally needs a hearing aid, make sure that they are wearing it. A translator may be necessary to allow you to communicate with the patient in a language that he or she can understand. Be additionally sensitive when the investigation requires the patient to comply with instructions that are not culturally comfortable. Be aware of the patient who has special problems associated with the investigation, for example an aversion to hypodermic needles. Alternative methods may need to be found for investigative purposes. Check that all specific preparatory test instructions have been complied with, e.g. the patient has complied with the food intake instructions prior to taking a sample of blood to assess cholesterol values or the instructions for bowel preparation prior to endoscopy.

Instructions and assurance must be given clearly throughout the procedure, using words that the patient is clearly able to understand. Listen to what the patient says to you while the clinical investigation is proceeding. Warn of discomforts or pain, and accept the patient's word when he or she describes the pain. Patients who feel that they are experiencing an unusual degree of pain, often are suffering from increased anxiety.

Accurate records must be made once the investigation has been completed.

CARE OF SPECIMENS

When you are the lead nurse associated with any clinical investigation, even when it is performed by other healthcare professionals, you must ensure that:

- the labels on all specimens are marked correctly and clearly
- the necessary precautions have been taken to ensure that it is a specimen that will produce valid results for the investigation
- if the specimen is to be transported, it is stored in the correct medium
- the specimen cannot be contaminated, or become a contaminant, in transit
- the forms that accompany the specimen are the correct type for the test ordered. These forms must be completed in full and contain all information requested. Omitting to complete the form may lead to a delay in the processing of the specimen. The writing must be in black ink for clear duplication of the result sheet
- the specimen is stored appropriately to avoid changes that will affect the result when it is known that a delay will occur before the specimen is assessed, for example newborn blood spot tests taken prior to the weekend when pathology laboratories are closed to routine tests.

PRINCIPLES BEHIND THE SPECIFIC TYPES OF CLINICAL INVESTIGATION

BLOOD TESTS

Specimens of blood are usually taken by venepuncture. When a small sample of blood is sufficient for testing (e.g. for capillary blood glucose measurement), a finger or heel prick will suffice.

Invasive procedures that break the integrity of blood vessels always carry risks for the patient. For this reason, the procedures must be carried out under the terms of locally agreed protocols. These will designate the:

- staff who are authorized to take blood from patients
- programme of education that sets standards of practice. Staff will need to prove that they practise safely and competently when taking blood for testing
- standards set for the procedure ensure the safety of the client and staff.

Technique

Introducing a foreign object into a blood vessel inevitably brings a risk of infection. Aseptic technique is essential when taking all specimens of blood.

The patient's arm must be relaxed throughout the process. Some patients find venepuncture a very uncomfortable process, so supports and pillows should be used to keep the arm placed correctly. The patient's arm should also be positioned to avoid placing any strain on the nurse's back as he or she leans over to take the blood sample.

Poor technique will produce an inaccurate blood result. The most reliable blood results come from a sample of blood that has been free flowing through a wide-diameter vein.

Occlusion of the vein through prolonged use of the tourniquet or a disease process will cause stasis of the blood in the vessel. The fluid content, electrolytes and the blood gases in a blood sample taken from this vessel will not be representative of the blood that is circulating in the rest of the body.

When blood does not flow freely from a finger or heel prick, it is a temptation to squeeze the finger or heel to encourage a drop of blood to form. This not only causes intravascular fluid to move from the surrounding tissues into the blood to give inaccurate values, but is also extremely painful for the patient. Devices are now developed to reduce the pain of skin puncture when heel and finger pricks are performed. These should be available for all patients who need to have regular samples of blood taken by this method, the most obvious example being patients with diabetes mellitus.

Blood in specimen bottles must be *inverted* for it to mix with the container fluid, rather than shaken. Shaking the blood will damage the red blood cells and cause haemolysis. The blood will not then provide a reliable sample for testing.

Firm and prolonged pressure must be applied to the puncture site to avoid haematoma formation. This is especially relevant when the patient is having blood clotting studies carried out or is on anticoagulant therapy.

Throughout the procedure, staff must be careful to avoid coming into direct contact with the patient's blood or acquiring a needlestick injury from a contaminated needle. A health and safety policy must be in place at locations where venepuncture is carried out to allow a rapid response if an accident happens.

Other factors that affect blood values

When an intravenous infusion is in progress, blood samples should be taken from the opposite arm. The presence of the infusion fluid in the vessels may affect the measured values.

Strenuous exercise causes excessive mobilization of white blood cells from the sides of blood vessels. The picture of blood taken immediately after exercise will show an artificially raised white cell value.

When considering blood results, remember that many things besides pathology can alter them, e.g. drugs, diurnal patterns, exercise, food intake, gender and genetic make-up.

URINE TESTING

Reliable results from any urine test can be obtained only when the urine has been collected in a clean, dry container. It is important to ensure that the specimen is uncontaminated by faeces, penile or vaginal discharge, or menstrual fluid.

Technique

Urine testing requires staff to have close contact with a potentially hazardous substance: urine. For personal protection you must wear gloves when dealing with all urine specimens – at all stages of the collection and testing. Always follow local policy and procedure. Urine must be tested soon after it is voided.

For routine testing, the early morning specimen is the best specimen to collect, for the following reasons:

1 Having fasted overnight, the urine collected in the bladder will not have the recent absorption of food components to affect the overall results.
2 If the urine test is to investigate the presence of a specific substance, the quantity of that substance will accumulate in the bladder overnight.
3 The lack of fluid intake by the patient overnight will reduce the water content of the urine. This less dilute urine will hold a greater concentration of the substances investigated by testing.

The exception to the above will be the testing of the first morning urine voided for glucose and ketones in diabetes. The early morning specimen of a diabetic patient will *not* give accurate values. This is because urine that has accumulated in the bladder overnight will not reflect the blood glucose and ketone values at the time of the urine test. The bladder will need to be emptied of the overnight urine and a specimen of fresh urine collected 1 hour later for testing.

When a nurse is collecting a specimen of urine for testing, part of the investigative procedure should include additional, pertinent, observations to give a clearer clinical picture of the patient. These observations will include:

- whether the patient reports pain or dysuria when passing urine
- whether the patient has difficulty starting the flow of urine

- how frequently the patient has to pass urine during a 24-hour period. Special note must be taken of the number of times the patient wakes during the night to use the toilet
- whether the patient has any signs of urinary incontinence.

The following observations should be made on the urine in addition to the values measured using a reagent stick:

- *The colour of the urine in the container*
  – The urine should be pale to golden yellow. A darker coloured urine may be the result of dehydration or a raised bilirubin level in the urine
  – A red-coloured urine is always alarming because of its association with blood, but a red colour may be caused by food dyes (e.g. beetroot) or harmless urates
  – Red urine may be a sign of the inherited disease porphyria
  – Injected dyes used for investigation purposes that are excreted through the kidney will also colour the urine. These dyes may be radioactive.
- *The presence of abnormal substances*
  – Urine should be clear when held up to the light
  – The nurse should look for signs of blood. It is important to observe whether the blood looks fresh, having entered the urine lower down in the excretory system, or is dark blood that may have been in the urine for some time. This observation will link with the reagent stick test for haemolysed or non-haemolysed blood. Fresh blood found in the urine will tend not to be haemolysed
  – Threads or casts will be visible in the urine when the urinary tract is inflamed or infected.
- *The smell of the urine*
  – The odour of the urine should not be offensive
  – **Infection** is the major cause of malodorous urine
  – Stale urine smells of ammonia.
- *Frothy urine* may indicate a high protein content.

Always label each urine specimen as the container is given to you. When more than one specimen is to be tested it is very easy to confuse the specimen and allocate the wrong results to patients.

For accurate testing, the reagent stick must be used exactly according to the instructions that are given. Delay in testing the urine, incorrect timing of test results or contamination of the reagent sticks will alter the results obtained.

Additional methods of obtaining a sample of urine

A specimen of urine taken from a *urinary catheter* will give fresh urine for testing almost as soon as it has left the bladder. In health, it will not contain any contaminants. A catheter specimen of urine must be drawn from the catheter tubing; a stale sample of urine drawn from the catheter bag will not provide accurate analysis or results. As the nurse will be entering a sterile area to remove the urine from the catheter tubing, it is essential to use aseptic technique for this procedure.

When an uncontaminated urine specimen is required from a patient who is not continent or is unable to comply with instructions, a *suprapubic aspiration* of urine from the bladder may be the only optional procedure. Following the palpation of a full bladder, a sterile needle is inserted into the bladder. It is inserted from a position just above the symphysis pubis and a specimen of urine is syringed back. The procedure will produce a sterile, uncontaminated specimen of urine.

A *mid-stream specimen* of urine is taken when urine is required for *culture and sensitivity* testing. The nurse and patient must work in cooperation to obtain a specimen of urine that is free from any contamination during collection. Before this urine collection, all areas of the external genitalia likely to come into contact with the urine must be washed free of contaminating organisms. The patient is instructed to produce an initial flow of urine, which is discarded. This initial urine will contain tissue debris from the **urethra** and the urinary meatus. The next, mid-part of the urine flow is collected in a sterile container. The patient then finishes emptying the bladder and this final specimen of urine is discarded.

The collected mid-stream specimen is put into a sterile container for immediate transport to the testing laboratory. Care must be taken by the nurse and the patient that only the outside of any sterile container is handled during the process so that contamination does not occur.

A *24-hour urine* collection may be needed. It is essential to follow local laboratory instructions when preparing for this test and while the test is underway. It is also important that, if a volume of urine is accidentally thrown away while the collection is in operation, staff admit this mistake or else the results of the test will be invalid.

SPECIMENS FOR CULTURE AND SENSITIVITY

The purpose of taking specimens for culture and sensitivity testing is to identify organisms that are colonizing a specified tissue and to identify the antibiotic that will destroy identified infecting bacteria.

When a swab or any other specimen is collected for investigation of culture and sensitivity, the sample sent for analysis must be completely uncontaminated during the collection process. Complex instructions may be required if the patient is to understand the collection protocol and to ensure that the specimen is not contaminated as it is taken or put into a container for transport, for example a mid-stream urine specimen. Infirmity or difficulty following instructions can make adhering to the protocol very difficult for the patient to carry out alone.

An aseptic technique must be used to obtain the specimen and the nurse should wear gloves when handling the specimen container, to avoid it being accidentally contami-

nated with infected material. Containers and lids must be handled only using the outside surfaces.

The specimen taken should not contain any other substance that could be contaminated by bacteria, other than found in the tested tissue, i.e. food particles. Swabs are taken from tissues to collect debris and discharge directly attributed to the infecting organism. Once collected, a transport medium should be used to transport the swab to a laboratory. The laboratory slip should contain a record of recent and current antibiotic therapy.

GRAM STAINING

Bacteria are classified into descriptive groups for identification. To identify the bacteria present on the specimen, laboratory slides are smeared with material from the collected sample. Having fixed the specimen onto the glass, colour dyes are dripped on to the slide and the bacteria that are present will take up the dye. The slides are then viewed under a microscope. Differentiation of the bacteria can then take place (Box 10.1).

CULTURES

In addition to identification by microscope, a sample of the collected material is put onto a culture medium. This allows the organisms to feed and multiply under ideal conditions. From this growth, definite identification of the invasive organisms can be made.

SENSITIVITY

Once the identification of the infecting organism has been isolated, it is exposed to various antibiotics. From this exposure the bacteria may show:

● resistance to an antibiotic – growth is not checked
● moderate susceptibility to the antibiotic – growth is slowed
● sensitivity to the antibiotic – the bacteria are destroyed.

Box 10.1 Microscopic differentiation of bacteria

Bacteria are typed according to the stain they have taken:

● Gram-positive organisms take the purple stain of gentian violet

● Gram-negative organisms take the red stain of eosin.

Bacteria are also typed according to their shape when seen under a microscope, for example:

● elongated-shaped bacteria are rods or bacilli

● round-shaped bacteria are cocci.

A bacterium is described as acid-fast when it stains with carbofusion after being washed with acid-alcohol solution.

The most effective antibiotic against the bacterial infection can then be recommended as treatment for the patient.

INVESTIGATION BY MEANS OF DIAGNOSTIC IMAGING

With the exception of endoscopy, the following investigations are usually conducted in a radiology department. Although radiographers are responsible for the technical aspect of these clinical investigations, the nurse will provide important preparatory and aftercare of patients. Patients' needs at this time are diverse, although there are commonalities between investigations. Patients will need to remain as comfortable as the investigation allows for the duration of the test. They will need to have appropriate methods of communication and information. The look of the technology used for these investigations can cause apprehension so the patient needs to feel fully informed, supported and safe.

ULTRASONOGRAPHY

The patient is prepared and positioned so that the technician is able to move an electrical transducer across the skin, over the designated organ. The impulses from the transducer are changed into ultrasound waves as they travel through the internal organs. When the wave hits an internal structure, it rebounds back to the skin. The wave is converted back to electrical impulses by the transducer. A computer analyses the incoming impulses and forms a visual image of the internal structures. The returned image can be processed rapidly, allowing the motion from a beating heart or from a fetus to be viewed on a monitor. Still pictures can be taken of the image as a record (see Fig. 10.1).

The clarity of the images returned will depend on the degree of pre-test preparation of the patient. Some organs require particular preparation to enhance the final pictures, and the instructions specified by the ultrasound scanning department must be followed. This preparation may give the patient some discomfort; for example, the patient may need a full bladder to give greater clarity to the image obtained. The area of skin over the site of the target organ is prepared for better penetration of the ultrasound waves. A gel is used to seal the contact between skin and the transducer to obtain a better view of the target organs.

The patient must be assured that this is not an invasive test and pre-test preparations must include a description of the test procedure.

RADIOGRAPHY

X-rays are used for screening and diagnostic purposes. They identify the presence of abnormal structures and lesions, and incorrect positioning of organs.

To form the required image, X-rays are aimed at the part of the body that needs investigation. As they pass through the body, the X-rays are interrupted in their track by the internal structures of the body. The X-rays that are blocked during their pathway through the body and do not reach the film make a white image on the film. X-rays that penetrate the whole width of the body form a black image. The picture that forms is a negative image of the internal tissues.

The penetration of the tissues by X-rays depends on the density of the structures that are impeding their progress. A diagnostic picture of the internal organs can be built up (see Fig. 10.2), knowing that:

- air and spaces within the body allow the uninterrupted passage of X-rays
- air-filled cavities (i.e. the lungs or flatus-filled intestines) look black on the radiograph
- organs and fatty tissues become a darker grey; the shade of grey is dependent on the ability of the X-rays to penetrate the tissue mass of the organ and reach the film
- water is a poor conductor of X-rays; structures with a high water content look light on the radiograph

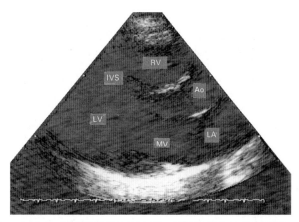

Figure 10.1 Ultrasonography: echocardiogram from a normal subject in two-dimensional long-axis view. The convention that shows the position of the transducer at the top of the paper causes the heart to appear 'upside down'. Ao, aorta; IVS, interventricular septum; LA, left atrium; LV, left ventricle; MV, mitral valve; RV, right ventricle. From Kumar and Clark (1994), with permission.

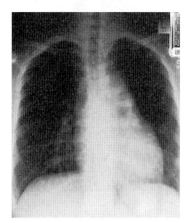

Figure 10.2 Chest radiograph. From Kumar and Clark (1994), with permission.

- bones are impenetrable to X-rays; they appear white on the radiograph.

Dyes or contrast media can be used to highlight tissues and organs that would normally be poorly defined on the radiograph. Dyes are given to form an impenetrable barrier to X-rays, usually forming a thin film on the inside of the organ. The white picture that appears in contrast against the black film allows features to be seen that would not normally be visible (Fig. 10.3). Patients normally need specific instructions for preparation when dyes or contrast media are to be used. Advice regarding aftercare may also be needed until the dye has been eliminated from the body. Any instructions from the radiography department must be complied with to avoid a poor image being produced and the patient having to return for a repeated procedure and additional exposure to X-rays.

Radiological investigation is not without risk as X-rays are a form of ionizing radiation capable of damaging cellular DNA. Repeated exposure to X-rays is known to cause cell damage and disease; the procedure can therefore be hazardous for patients and staff. Protective screens and clothing must be worn by staff who need to be in close proximity to X-rays. A badge that monitors exposure to radiation must be worn by staff who are in frequent contact with X-rays.

The damage that X-rays can do to rapidly dividing cells explains why a pregnant woman should not be exposed to X-rays. If the slightest risk of pregnancy exists, it is essential to avoid exposure to X-rays.

If you need to accompany a patient while radiography is being performed, you need to be supportive and informative. By encouraging the patient to relax and be still, you will ease them through the procedure and ultimately obtain a good image. When mobilization or communication with the patient is difficult, the radiographer will appreciate the knowledge of the patient brought by the nurse.

COMPUTED TOMOGRAPHY

Computed tomography (CT) uses X-rays to make three-dimensional pictures of cross-sections of the body (Fig. 10.4). An X-ray machine revolves in an arc around the body of the patient. The pictures received reflect the varying density of the tissues met by the X-rays as they travel between the skin and the X-ray detector. A computer interprets the images received. It translates the information into pictures to show cross-sectional views of the body. From these images, tumours and other lesions, tissue damage, haemorrhage and tissue atrophy can be visualized.

Contrast media can be used to improve the quality of the pictures. Contrast media may produce an allergic reaction in the patient, so the patient must be asked about any previous sensitive reactions. Full resuscitation equipment must be immediately available in case of an anaphylactic reaction. CT should not be used on a pregnant woman.

CT is a lengthy procedure and the patient is required to lie completely still while the images are produced. The patient must be safe and secure throughout, even in the midst of the technology that is surrounding them. Sedation may be needed to relax the patient and assist in keeping him or her motionless. Discussions with the patient are needed to explain the purpose of the investigation. Description of the equipment and the process may relieve some of the anxiety.

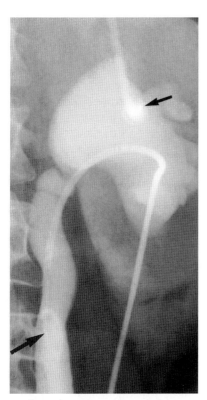

Figure 10.3   Radiography with contrast medium: antegrade pyelography via a percutaneous catheter (small arrow) of obstructed system. A percutaneous drainage catheter (large arrow) has been inserted. From Kumar and Clark (1994), with permission.

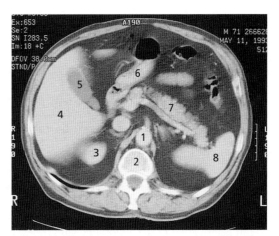

Figure 10.4   Computed tomogram of the normal abdomen at the level of the liver. 1, Aorta; 2, spine; 3, top of right kidney; 4, liver; 5, gallbladder; 6, stomach; 7, pancreas; 8, spleen. From Kumar and Clark (1994), with permission.

All metal objects and jewellery must be removed before the procedure. Further preparation of the patient before the investigation depends on instructions from the radiography department.

MAGNETIC RESONANCE IMAGING

With magnetic resonance imaging (MRI), the patient is placed in a strong magnetic field. Radio waves are used to initiate the release of electromagnetic energy from the body. It is this release of energy that provides the information from which a three-dimensional picture of the body can be represented.

IMAGING WITH RADIOACTIVE MATERIALS

These investigations are used to make an assessment of the activity of the organ under investigation. A radionuclide or a radioisotope is given to the patient, to be absorbed by the target organ. The radioactive material has an affinity with the organ to be tested and is taken into its tissues. The radioactive substance will act as a marker as it becomes part of the activity of the target organ.

A scanner is passed across the organ and a computer analyses the amount of radioactivity emanating from the scanned tissues. When high levels of radioactivity are recorded in one area, it is described as a 'hot spot'. A low level of radioactivity is a 'cold spot'. From this analysis, the size and outline of the structure can be assessed. The position of tumours, cysts and areas of non-functioning tissue can be outlined.

Discussion with the patient needs to take place before the test is performed. The patient needs to know the length of time that the test will take to perform, the preparations that need to be made and a description of the routine that will be followed during the test. The patient's own anxieties and queries must be addressed. The patient must also be advised that the radioactive substances will be excreted in the urine. To safeguard patients and staff from this radioactive waste, local guidelines and procedures must be followed. Subsequent to investigations, precautions must be in place when the patient uses the toilet or when there is a need to dispose of a used bedpan or commode.

ENDOSCOPY

Endoscopes have been developed to give direct access and visibility within the hollow structures of the body. Each type of endoscope is designed to enter a specified body cavity. Once in place, the operator has a direct view for examination purposes. From this biopsies can be taken via the endoscope, and cautery and other local treatments can be performed. A camera can be attached to the endoscope, and the examination findings can be recorded as photographs or on video.

Endoscopy is an uncomfortable procedure if it is performed when the patient is fully conscious. Analgesia, sedation and local anaesthetics will help the patient to cope with the procedure, but some endoscopies need to be performed under general anaesthesia, e.g. laparoscopy and arthroscopy.

The preparation of the patient will vary according to the area of body that is to be examined by endoscope. Guidelines for preparation will be set by the department that is to perform the endoscopy. The patient will need to feel supported by the nursing staff as the idea of these tests can be daunting and stressful.

After the procedure is completed the nurse must be certain that the endoscopy has not caused bleeding, either by perforating an organ or through taking biopsies. Analgesia should be given for pain or discomfort experienced as a result of the examination.

When a local anaesthetic has been given to abolish the gag reflex prior to endoscopic examination, food and fluids must be withheld until the reflex returns.

GENETIC TESTING

These clinical investigations provide information that has an impact not only on the patient who consents to the assessment, but on that person's family through generations to come. This brings challenges to nursing as the issues that may be raised from the tests will be complex. The nurse is the person who is best placed to provide a continuing dialogue with the patient, who will need time to appreciate fully the results of the genetic testing and to evaluate the impact of the results on present and future family members.

Genetic assessments, especially predictive or carrier testing, will present the patient with difficult ethical problems to answer. Patients may feel a duty to comply with testing to protect the well-being of future generations of the family (Hallowell 1999). This altruistic motive for testing will not protect the patient from the psychosocial difficulties that may arise as a result of the testing. Nurses will need to be at the forefront in helping patients to find a way through the complex questions that will inevitably become part of the follow-through of the process. Counseling will need to be offered to patients before the test is carried out to help them come to terms with the results.

The questions that are associated with this type of testing are also profound. The ability to look for genetic markers that predict the onset of future disease, especially if this information is gathered from a baby or child, could have an impact on the person's total life experiences. Nurses must reflect on these issues as the technology is introduced, and they must add their voices to the debate. The nurse will be a key person who can help prepare the way for the impact of genetic testing as each new development provides a new frontier of clinical assessment. The results of each test will affect patients, their families and society. It is this holistic view of patient care that gives the nurse a powerful position in the debate.

NATIONAL SCREENING PROGRAMMES

Even in health, clinical investigations are becoming integrated into every stage of life. The strategic view of health care has shifted with the changing of the century. National healthcare planning is now emphasising the maintenance of good health rather than the restoration of health following sickness (DoH 1999). Health education, disease prevention and the growing requirement for national health screening programmes are prevalent in the community, promoting good public health awareness. As well as being the diagnostic tools that provide answers when disease becomes apparent, clinical investigations are now used more widely to monitor health through screening programmes. The motives behind health screening could be described as impeccable, but screening does require that a 'healthy' person has to contemplate the possibility of 'ill-health' for a short time, and this brings with it uncertainty and anxiety. This may cause people to resist participating in health screening.

From directives given in the National Service Frameworks, devised by the Department of Health, the UK government has devised a programme of health checks from before birth until old age, according to individual needs.

The screening tests are constantly being evaluated, revised and updated. The clinical investigations selected for any screening programme must meet the stated criteria set by the National Screening Committee (DoH 2000). In essence the clinical investigation used for routine health screening must be a reliable test for an important health problem that can be treated effectively. The method of testing should be safe and uncomplicated and acceptable to the screened population.

Some health screening has been in place for many years but this was primarily to detect disease during a specific time of life, i.e. pregnancy. Monitoring an apparently healthy community using clinical investigations for screening purposes needs a different perspective. The screening programme has been devised to prevent poor health. It provides each individual with information about the state of their health and, where possible, provides appropriate health education to maintain health. The national screening programme consists of five screening programmes to suit population groups; antenatal, child, men, women and the older person, but in reality these five programmes are integrated into an overarching national public health programme, because the health of each population group does not stand in isolation. It is impossible to separate a woman's health from her antenatal checks or the health of her child, and the health of the child will have a strong influence on their health as an adult.

The screening process may introduce anxiety when it is not necessary. A patient who voluntarily decides to have the health assessment should be welcomed into a positive and welcoming environment. The service should also ensure that the client has to wait as short a time as possible for the test results to be returned (see Box 10.2).

Box 10.2   Screening pregnant women for HIV

The government would like all women to voluntarily be tested for HIV during the antenatal period of pregnancy. HIV testing has always been a sensitive issue because a positive result confers physiological, sociological and psychological problems on to the patient. The Department of Health (1996) produced guidelines for practice to help promote testing for HIV. The guidelines lay down standards of care that must be adhered to when HIV testing is offered.

The guidelines state that:

- the woman must give explicit consent to testing

- this consent must be obtained after appropriate pre-test discussion and information

- the woman must understand the purpose of the test, its benefits and problems for herself, partner and unborn child

- the woman must be told, at testing, when the results will be available

- the results must be confidential to the woman

- the results of the test will not affect the woman's right to determine the outcome of the pregnancy or the care of the child.

Needless anxiety occurs when false-positive results arise and re-testing is required to find that no disease is present. Equally disease can develop following a negative result and this is known as a false-negative. The report of the screening committee (DoH 2000) recognizes the anxiety that health screening can cause but argues that despite the distress that is caused, the screening programmes do help to preserve or regain health as well as reduce the mortality rate associated with breast cancer and cervical cancer.

The use of specified clinical investigations, accurately taken at the appropriate time, has provided the monitoring systems by which the nation's health can be improved. New screening methods are being introduced on a regular basis. Tests that have been in place for some years have been evaluated and expanded, i.e. the newborn Guthrie test for phenylketonuria has been renamed the blood spot test as the test now screens for other diseases that are detectable during the first weeks of life. Testing for the presence of the human immunodeficiency virus (HIV) is now a routine blood test during the antenatal period.

The results of the clinical investigations provided by health screening programmes will also give important information on the health of the whole population. Analysis of the data will show regional differences in the nation's health, and indicate where there are rising, or falling, trends in specific health conditions. Resources can then be directed to areas where they are most needed for health education or prevention.

GIVING UNWELCOME NEWS

Giving bad news to the patient, even when it follows the most minor investigation, is always difficult. The nurse who has most information and is able to answer all the patient's questions with confidence must give the results. The information will be better assimilated and accepted by the patient if the nurse knows the patient well enough to provide continuous assessment of the patient's reaction as the news is given, and is able to respond appropriately.

When the results of the clinical investigation indicate that the patient will need to be given the results in the most sensitive way possible, it is important to be fully prepared for the meeting.

The meeting must take place in a room that does not allow interruptions to conversation and where all participants can sit comfortably, with the chairs positioned to allow good eye contact to be maintained. If possible, a close relative should also listen to what is said. The giving of information must not be hurried. Time is needed for the patient to adjust his or her self-perceptions – from a well person in command of his or her own destiny to a person who has to adjust to being 'unwell', living within the limitations that this may bring.

The professionalism and behaviour of the nurse imparting difficult news must assist the feeling of trust that the patient needs to experience in the healthcare system. The patient must leave the room feeling that he or she will receive optimal care through this most difficult time. The patient must also know the options available (informed choice) and be comfortable with the selected pathway of treatment and care (informed consent).

Nurses need peer support to give their best to their patients at this time, to help them manage these situations effectively and with expertise. A nurse should be able to recognize pertinent non-verbal and verbal signs that indicate how the patient is receiving the information, and recognize the use of coping mechanisms to reduce the impact of the news.

A written record of the information given and the patient's responses must be kept to allow other staff to continue with the support of the patient. Conflicting advice or information at this time is not acceptable to the patient.

SUMMARY

Technology will continue to offer increasingly accurate measurements of biochemical values and more precise imaging of body tissues and structures. Entirely new clinical investigations that offer new dimensions in assessment will come from work developed from research into genetic and chromosome studies. Patients often report that it is the 'not knowing' that increases worry. Clinical investigations are part of that 'not knowing' process. The investigations are carried out to make clinical conditions known and visible. The process of clinical investigation will exacerbate anxieties until the results confirm the fear or give joyous relief. Nurses are with patients throughout the clinical investigation process. They cannot change the outcome of the tests, but they can provide patients with information and positive support. As patients gain confidence in the care that they receive during the process of clinical investigation, they will face future treatments with more confidence, which will ultimately help them deal with their illness more positively.

CASE A 25-year-old woman, Miss H. who has a past history of intravenous drug misuse is considering becoming pregnant in the near future. Before she conceives the baby she is anxious to know her HIV status. Her partner does not want her to have the HIV blood test and is very insistent that she does not have this investigation. She came for advice as she wants to dispel her growing anxiety about her HIV status before her pregnancy, or be prepared to make further very important decisions about her life. It was made very clear to her that her decision to take the test was hers alone. Her partner had no right even to know whether the test was performed. She was counseled about the implications and practicalities of taking the test. She was asked to consider the changes that would happen in her life if the test was positive. Her partner would need to be told as they had a sexual relationship. It was also suggested that his negative response to her taking the test could come from his own insecurity about having contracted HIV. Miss H decided to go ahead with the HIV test. Confidentiality forbids that I disclose the result.

CRITICAL INCIDENT

You are caring for a woman aged 86 years. She lives on her own and, other than being a little forgetful, she copes very well. She has a hearing problem but she is not comfortable wearing a hearing aid. She tells you that she has needed to pass urine every 2 hours for the past 4 days. You suspect that she has a urinary tract infection. A mid-stream urine test for culture and sensitivity is ordered for her. You attempt to explain to her the process of collecting the urine but she has considerable difficulty understanding the process. Using reflective questions, consider how you might overcome this patient's (and your) difficulty.

CASE Reflection

Mr Wilson has claustrophobia. He does not like travelling in lifts and needs to be able to look through a window while sitting in his bed or chair, in your hospital ward. An MRI scan has been arranged for him and this has made him extremely anxious as he knows that he will be in a confined space for the duration of the investigation. He is thinking of asking for the investigation to be cancelled. How would you help Mr Wilson?

REFERENCES

Department of Health (1996) Guidelines for pre-test discussion on HIV testing. London: DoH.

Department of Health (1999) Saving lives: our healthier nation. London: HMSO.

Department of Health (2000) Second report of the UK National Screening Committee. Department of Health, Social Services and Public Safety, Northern Ireland. The Welsh Assembly. The Scottish Executive. London: DoH.

Department of Health (2001a) Reference guide to consent for examination or treatment. London: HMSO. Online. Available: http://www.doh.gov.uk/consent

Department of Health (2001b) Second report of the UK National Screening Committee. London. Online. Available: http://www.nsc.nhs.uk/

Furlong S, Glover D (1998) Consent, equity and ethics in new nursing. Nursing Times 94(38): 52–53.

Hallowell N (1999) Doing the right thing: genetic risk and responsibility. Sociology of Health and Illness. A Journal of Medical Sociology 21(5): 597–621.

Kumar P, Clark M (1994) Clinical medicine. London: Ballière Tindall.

Lloyd AJ, Hayes PD, London NJM et al (1999) Patients' ability to recall risk association with treatment options. Lancet 353: 645.

Lowry M (1995) Knowledge that reduces anxiety: creating patient information leaflets. Professional Nurse 10(5): 318–320.

Nursing and Midwifery Council (NMC) (2004) The NMC code of professional conduct: standards for conduct, performance and ethics. London: NMC.

FURTHER READING

Department of Health (1998) National Service Frameworks London: HMSO. Online. Available: http://www.doh.gov.uk

Department of Health (1999) Choosing health. London: HMSO. *This document continues the work of the original Department of Health document* Our Healthier Nation. *It indicates where the government priorities are for ensuring the future health of the population and it indicates to the reader where there is a need for health screening programmes and clinical testing.*

Department of Health (2004) Choosing health. London: HMSO. Online. Available: http://www.doh.gov.uk

Department of Health internet site. Online. Available: http://www.doh.gov.uk
This website is full of information related to patient care and health professionals.

Fuller J, Shaller-Ayres J (2000) Health assessment: a nursing approach, 3rd edn. Philadelphia, PA: Lippincott.
This book is well laid out for the reader to view and access information. The colour pictures and diagrams give additional clarity to the text. It is a detailed text but an interesting book to access.

National Institute for Clinical Excellence (NICE). Online. Available: http:// www.nice.org.uk
This website provides the national guidelines for best clinical practice following a thorough review of the evidence.

Royal College of Nursing (1995) Never going to be easy: giving bad news. RCN Nursing Update. Nursing Standard 9(50).

Royal College of Nursing (2004) Sheet 2 day surgery information. Patient information and the role of the Carer. Online. Available: http://www.rcn.org.uk

Skinner S (1995) Understanding clinical investigations. London: Baillière Tindall.
This book provides a clear explanation of all common clinical investigations. Using tables, flowcharts and short notes, it clarifies the underlying principles of each investigation, shows where it links to normal physiology and indicates how disease can alter the results. It also provides links to other clinical investigations that may be useful when a particular investigation shows abnormal results.
This book contains detailed information on all the clinical investigations that a nurse is likely to meet in practice.

Skirton H (1995) Psychological implications of advances in genetics – 1. Carrier testing. Professional Nurse 10(8): 496–498.

Winchester A (1999) Sharing bad news. Nursing Standard 13(26): 48–52.

Yeo H (1998) Informed consent in the neonatal unit: the ethical and legal rights of parents. Journal of Neonatal Nursing 4(4): 17.

SECTION 3

Specific patient groups

INTRODUCTION

This is the final and largest section of the book and involves a systematic review of the human body and the various problems that can turn a person into a patient. In reading these chapters remember that most of the person's career as a patient takes place outside the hospital, at home with friends and family supported by the primary healthcare team. You should also remember that it is not uncommon for patients to have more than one problem at once, a tendency that increases with age. In using the book, therefore, you will find it helpful to think of patients that you have cared for at any given time. You will also find that you may well have to refer to more than one chapter in this section, and of course refer back to the previous sections on clinical principles. Complicated? Yes it is, but that reflects the complexity of clinical practice and a very important skill you will develop in your education is the ability to think of the whole rather than just the component parts. Being able to see the big picture is the hallmark of quality nursing care and is the key skill that helps mark out the unique contribution of the registered nurse to patient care.

11 Caring for the patient with cancer

Miriam Rowswell

INTRODUCTION

THE NATURE OF CANCER

Cancer is not only a disease but also a series of experiences that profoundly affect the daily life of both the individual who has the cancer and those who share the experience with them. Cancer is a collective term for many different diseases, each carrying a different prognosis and with a variety of consequences for the individuals concerned. While many are very serious and potentially life-threatening, advances in combining the main treatment modalities of surgery, radiotherapy, and chemotherapy have resulted in the effective management of clinical manifestations, over variable periods of time. In other cases, the initial treatment effects a permanent cure with no recurrence of the primary disease within an individual lifespan. New treatments using biological therapies and stem cell technology offer prospects for further advances in the management of many cancers. Increasingly, cancer may be considered to be a chronic disease and the course of the disease can be understood as a journey (National Cancer Alliance 1996) that people undertake from diagnosis, through varying amounts of treatment aimed to eradicate disease or to provide effective control and symptom management in advanced disease. At all stages of the journey, people need support and care from nurses and other healthcare professionals who are knowledgeable about the causation and prevention of cancer, therapeutic regimens and supportive care, and the physiological and psychological impact of cancer.

CARCINOGENESIS

In order to begin to understand cancer, it is necessary to have a thorough knowledge of the normal functioning of the cell and **cell division**. Although there has been an increase in knowledge and understanding of cancer based on recent advances in molecular biology and genetics, the exact cause of many human cancers remains unknown. A number of mechanisms occur over time causing abnormalities in cell growth and cell division, which eventually lead to the development of a cancer. Cancer is essentially a genetic disease which results from one or, more likely, a series of mutations in the DNA of genes which control differentiation, repair and cell death. This malignant transformation, known as *carcinogenesis* begins with genetic alteration of the cell. This occurs through errors in the replication of **DNA**, leading to mutations of various types:

- point mutations involve the deletion, substitution or addition of one or a few bases of DNA (e.g. a codon)
- genomic mutations involve the deletion, substitution or addition of a larger strand of DNA
- chromosomal mutations involve the same disorders of long segments of DNA.

The majority of cancers arise as a result of these *somatic* mutations but a small percentage of cancers, less than 5%, result from inherited mutations in the germ cells.

The second stage of the process, or *progression*, occurs as a result of deregulation of the normal functions of the cell. This is caused by *oncogenes*, mutated forms of protooncogenes, which commonly have an important cell regulatory function. Oncogenes can cause excessive cell multiplication by 'switching on' the cell's own growth cycle in the absence of, or by over stimulation of normal growth factors. This is often combined with a loss of *tumour suppressor gene* activity, the normal function of which is to inhibit cell proliferation and growth. Another mechanism that exists to prevent uncontrolled cell division is the process of *apoptosis* or cell death via the protein p53. Disruptions in the gene involved in the p53 protein may mean that abnormal cells can avoid cell death, and continue to divide and replicate. Cancer cells are also found to produce an enzyme called telomerase that is virtually absent in mature cells. Telomeres are DNA segments at the end of chromosomes that shorten each time the cell divides. When the telomeres are shortened to a critical length the normal cell stops dividing but the telomerase enzyme produced in cancerous cells repairs the telomere enabling proliferation to continue.

When these various control mechanisms either alter or fail, abnormal tissue growth occurs. This multi-step process (Fig. 11.1) explains why cancer is in the most part associated with older people and why inheritance of a mutation conferring cancer susceptibility results in cancer presenting at a younger age because the process has effectively skipped one or two steps. Controversy has centred on the question of what initiates the transformation in the DNA of a cell necessary to cause cancer. Genetic, chemical, physical and hormonal factors together with viral agents have all been implicated as components of carcinogenesis.

Single gene disorders are known to predispose to cancers of the haematopoietic and lymphoreticular system. Risks among first-degree relatives of patients with certain cancers have been shown to be statistically higher than in comparable control families or in the general population. The influences of environmental factors have been difficult to separate from a possible genetic aetiological component but, in general, these familial patterns appear to reflect the genetically transmitted susceptibility to neoplasia. For example, a female carrier of the *BRCA1* or the *BRCA2* gene mutation has a 40–85% lifetime expectancy of the development of breast cancer, depending on ethnic background (Ford et al 1998). Furthermore there is some evidence that inheritance of these specific gene mutations also increase risk of ovarian cancer, prostate cancer and pancreatic cancer. It is hoped that further research on oncogenes, which have the potential to cause cancer when activated, will provide answers to the aetiology of cancer and lead to more effective preventive, diagnostic and treatment techniques.

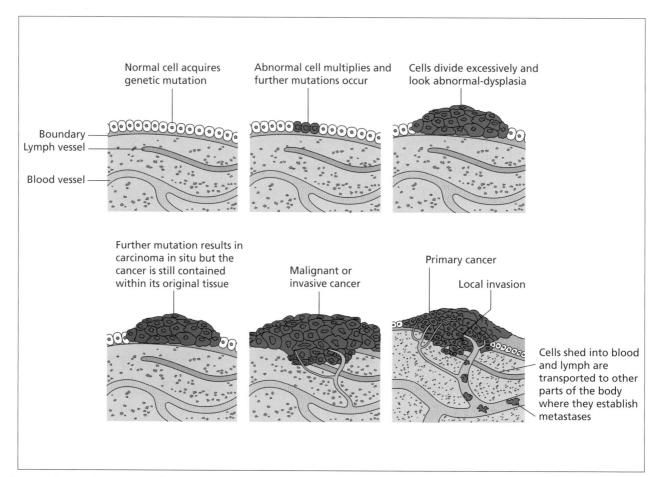

Figure 11.1 The development of cancer – a multistep process.

An excessive concentration of certain hormones appears to influence the change of some normal cells to malignant ones. Such cancers are said to be *hormone dependent* and manifest changes in growth activity when the concentration of particular hormones is altered. For instance, the ovarian oestrogenic hormones favour the growth of some breast cancers, while androgens (male hormones) tend to suppress their progress. Whether the hormone is the primary incitant in hormone-supported cancer in humans or whether it simply produces a tissue susceptibility to viral, chemical or physical carcinogens is not clear.

CAUSATIVE FACTORS

The development of most cancer diseases is due to or enhanced by some factors in the environment. Certain chemical and physical agents and some viruses are recognized to have a causative or contributory role. Carcinogenic chemical agents include asbestos, vinyl chlorides, aniline dyes and benzene. Many of these have been recognized as a result of the high incidence of cancer associated with occupational exposure to the specific chemical. For example, persons working with an aniline dye, which may be absorbed through the skin and excreted in the urine, show a high incidence of urinary bladder cancer. A causative relationship has also been established between inhalation of asbestos dust and mesothelioma lung cancer. Insecticides and herbicides are highly suspect, and animal growth-stimulating hormones and some food additives are being investigated as potential carcinogens. Cigarette smoking as a cause of cancer of the respiratory tract, and a contributor to cancer of the bladder, has also been well documented. Air pollutants and involuntary or passive smoking are also suspect, especially in relation to lung cancer. Research has indicated that there is usually a relatively long latent period between exposure to chemical carcinogens and the development of cancer.

Diet has also been implicated as a possible factor in tumour induction. To date, epidemiological and animal studies have provided the bulk of available information. High levels of dietary fat, nitrosamines and coffee, and deficiencies of fibre and certain micronutrients (e.g. vitamins A and C, riboflavin and selenium) in the diet, have been associated with the development of cancers in humans (World Cancer Research Fund 1997).

Significant physical carcinogens include excessive exposure to the sun's rays, radiation and chronic irritation. A large proportion of skin cancers are attributed to excessive exposure to the sun's rays. Fair-skinned individuals with less natural pigmentation of the skin, and those whose occupation keeps them outdoors (e.g. farmers), appear to be more susceptible to neoplastic changes in the dermal cells as a result of excessive sun exposure. X-rays and radioactive substances have proved beneficial in the diagnosis and treatment of some diseases, but repeated radiation exposure may lead to malignant neoplasia. The adverse effects may not be seen for a long period after irradiation, as the effects can be cumulative. Repeated exposures to even very low doses may eventually be of pathological significance, hence the importance of radiological protection measures for all staff working in diagnostic radiography departments.

Chronic irritation of an area and repeated tissue destruction and repair are also thought to be contributory factors in the development of cancer explaining why people with chronic inflammatory bowel diseases are at greater risk of developing bowel cancer.

Scientists have established that various types of RNA and DNA tumour viruses produce some forms of malignant neoplasia in experimental animals. The successful isolation of human viruses in some patients with leukaemia strongly supports the aetiological role of viruses in malignant disease, but the exact viral action in producing cancer is not known. Viruses are suspected in the development of some forms of leukaemia, lymphoma and nasopharyngeal cancer, as well as primary liver cancers. Viruses are known to cause warts and mucosal papillomas in humans and the human papilloma virus (HPV) (Types 16 and 18) are thought to account for around 70% of cases of cervical cancer. A vaccine against four HPV strains (Gardasil) has recently been licensed and offers the prospect of a new way to combat cervical cancer.

Knowledge surrounding the complexity of the immune system and the immune response is of increasing importance in understanding the development and spread of cancer. Considerable attention and support is being given to the concept that the abnormal cells contain substances that are foreign to the host's normal body cells and are therefore antigenic. These antigens prompt an immune response in the host that controls the development, growth and spread of the disease. There is evidence that spontaneous regression and disappearance of cancers have occurred when the host's immune mechanisms have destroyed the cancer cells. If the host's immune response is deficient, the abnormal cells multiply rapidly, invade surrounding tissues and spread to distant areas. It has been observed that there is a higher incidence of cancer in persons with an inadequate immune response, which may be due partly to primary immunodeficiency disease, immunosuppressive drugs, radiation exposure or the ageing process.

The role of the immune system in the development of cancer is not fully understood, yet it is known that cancer 'runs in families' and that some families appear to have a greater prevalence and therefore each individual has an increased risk of contracting cancer. Tumour immunity is mediated by a variety of immune mechanisms, including humoral antibodies, T and B-lymphocytes, killer (K) lymphoid cells, natural killer (NK) cells (which can act on tumour cells without specific immunization) and macrophages. Investigation of immune factors in cancer continues, with the hope of determining why the patient's defence mechanisms fail and of providing information that aids in cancer prevention, detection and treatment (Gore and Riches 1995).

STRESS AND CANCER

Stress is difficult to define and there is no firm evidence that stress has a direct causal effect. Prolonged high levels of glucocorticoid secretion do produce changes in the immune and inflammatory responses of the body. Depressed cellular immunity appears to result in impaired surveillance for abnormal cells and thus malignant cells are able to multiply and spread. Whilst more research is needed to determine if there is any relationship between psychological stress and cancer occurrence or cancer progression, it makes sense to avoid developing unhealthy behaviours that may result from prolonged stress.

DIFFERENCES BETWEEN BENIGN AND MALIGNANT GROWTHS

Cancer often presents as a lump or *tumour*, which may be palpable or detectable only via a radiograph or scan. In the vast majority of cases, the lump will be *benign*; new growths (neoplasms) or tumours that are benign are a frequent occurrence. They do not generally pose a threat to life unless in an anatomically difficult position, such as the brain or spinal column, in which case there may be serious effects on neighbouring structures through obstruction of blood vessels and pressure. The growth of a benign neoplasm is slow and tends to be expansive rather than invasive; the mass remains localized and is frequently encapsulated, and the cells may show little abnormality compared with those of the normal tissue from which they originated. Some benign lesions tend to become malignant if left untreated; examples are polyps in the intestine, papillomas of the bladder and larynx, and pigmented moles. Furthermore, some tissues may display cytological changes of malignancy but without any invasion of other structures (e.g. carcinoma in situ of the cervix). Benign tumours do not spread to other sites and it is usually possible to eradicate all disease by surgical removal of the mass. In contrast, *malignant* tumours or cancers are a distinct threat to life because of their ability to proliferate destructively into surrounding tissue and to other parts of the body. Table 11.1 summarizes some of the differences between benign and malignant tumours.

Cancer may develop from any type of cell and in any body part or organ. It begins as a *localized* disease, but over a period of time will spread and *invade* surrounding tissues. In the more advanced stages of the disease, cells become detached from the neoplasm and are carried by lymph or blood vessels to other parts of the body, where more cancer develops (see Fig. 11.1). Malignant cells may also spread by *implantation* or seeding within a body cavity. The serous fluid in the pleural or peritoneal cavities carries the tumour cells through the cavity. Cells carried in the lymph may be trapped in lymph nodes near the original site, producing disease in the nodes and causing what is known as *regional involvement*. Eventually these areas of disease disseminate cancer cells to other parts; this process is described as *metastasis*. Some tumours, such as basal cell carcinomas and gliomas, rarely metastasize, whereas others, such as melanomas and lung carcinomas, metastasize widely and are less invasive. Specific and predictable patterns of lymphatic and/or haematogenous spread have been identified clinically for many tumours. For example, testicular tumours generally favour the lymphatics as an initial route of spread. Once entry into the lymphatic channels has occurred, vascular spread follows: the lungs are the most common distant target organ for this particular tumour.

Many tumours have been observed to have unique patterns of metastasis that may include not only those common target organs but some more unusual sites as well. It was once thought that metastasis was a chaotic random event (Dudjak 1992, Vile 1995). However, it appears that the preferential distribution of metastasis is not random but is probably related to tumour cell characteristics that promote growth in some organs and not in others. Certain properties on the surfaces of tumour cells are probably responsible for

Table 11.1 Differences between benign and malignant tumours

	Benign	Malignant
Cells	Relatively normal and mature	Little resemblance to normal; poorly differentiated, atypical in size and shape, non-uniform and immature
Growth	Slow and restricted. Non-invasive of surrounding tissue; expansive, pushing aside normal tissue	Usually rapid and unrestricted. Invasive of surrounding tissue
Spread	Remains localized. Usually encapsulated	Metastasizes via blood and lymph streams
Recurrence	Rarely recurs	Frequently recurs
Threat to host	Prognosis favourable. The effect depends on the size and location. May cause pressure on vital organs or obstruct a passageway, which is usually corrected by surgical excision of neoplasm	Threatens life by reason of its local destructive proliferation and formation of secondary neoplasms in other structures. Prognosis more favourable with early diagnosis and treatment, when cells show less departure from the normal and there is no metastasis

the organ specificity of metastatic cells. In addition, it is thought that, although tumour cells may lodge in the capillary beds of multiple organs, certain micro environmental characteristics determine whether tumour growth will be supported. Furthermore, as many as 70% of individuals will have *micrometastases* (disease that is not yet detectable at diagnosis) and this has major implications when planning treatment (Davidson and Sacks 1995).

INCIDENCE AND TRENDS

In the UK, it is estimated that 1 in 3 people will develop cancer during their lifetime. Cancer tends to be diagnosed in later life as 64% of all new cases are diagnosed in people aged 65 years or over (Cancer Research UK 2005a). Cancer accounts for an increasing number of deaths – second only to heart disease in the UK. The factors that contribute to this include:

- a greater number of people living to an older age
- the increased risk of developing certain cancers due to prolonged exposure to specific carcinogens (e.g. cigarette smoke, environmental pollutants)

- increased identification through new and improved diagnostic procedures
- a decrease in deaths from acute infectious diseases.

Cancer incidence refers to the number of new cancer cases arising in a specified period of time. Although there are over 200 different cancers, four types of cancer predominate. These are breast, lung, colorectal and prostate cancers which together amount to more than 50% of all cancers diagnosed. The mortality attributable to these and other common cancers for both men and women are shown in Figure 11.2.

Cancer *prevalence* refers to the number of people with a history of cancer who are alive at any given time and it is estimated that this applies to approximately 1% of the population. Many of these individuals will be elderly, often with other medical conditions as well as cancer, and thus requiring care and support in both hospital and community.

Worldwide, 10.9 million people are diagnosed with cancer every year. Although cancer causes on average about 12% of deaths this percentage ranges from 4% in Africa to 19% in Europe and 23% in the USA. Cancers of the lung, stomach and liver are the most common cause of cancer deaths worldwide (Cancer Research UK 2006).

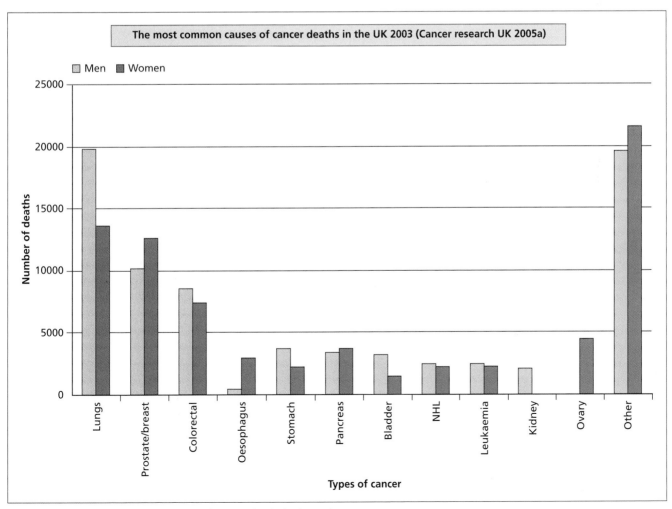

Figure 11.2 The most common causes of cancer deaths in the UK in 2003.

PREVENTION AND EARLY DETECTION OF CANCER

Some cancers can be prevented by the avoidance of recognized carcinogens and by altering health behaviours. *Primary prevention* of cancer is activity taken to prevent the occurrence or reduce the risk of cancer in healthy persons. Activities in this area of health promotion include identifying risk factors for individuals and groups; counseling regarding risk factor reduction; facilitating lifestyle changes; and implementing cancer prevention programmes. In recent years, government bodies and cancer organizations have instituted intensive campaigns to alert the public to high-risk factors and to behaviour changes that may modify their risk of developing cancer. In the UK, the National Cancer Plan (DoH 2000) identifies both strategies and resources for increasing prevention such as smoking cessation programmes and the 'five a day' fruit and vegetable scheme for schools. Campaigns aimed at promoting risk reduction behaviours (Cancer Research UK 2005b) suggest that adopting healthy behaviours, whilst emphasizing the positive benefits to health more generally, could prevent more than half of all cancers. Individuals are encouraged to:

- stop smoking
- stay in shape
- eat and drink healthily
- be sun smart
- look after number one.

Of particular concern is the growing evidence that being obese or overweight is linked to an increased risk of developing cancer (Bianchini et al 2002), especially since the number of people who fall into an obese category on the basis of their body mass index has trebled in the last 20 years.

In occupations where carcinogenic substances, such as asbestos, chromium, ether, vinyl chloride and benzene, are used, regulations are necessary to protect employees and communities from carcinogenic hazards. In addition to protective measures for those in a high-risk situation, workers need to develop an understanding of the risks and the precautions that should be observed. They should be aware of early symptoms that must be reported promptly, and receive regular examinations. Some industries may produce and release hazardous substances that could affect many citizens in the community. Governments are becoming more aware of such hazards and are requiring protective measures to be taken. Individuals who develop cancer as a result of industrial exposure may be eligible to receive compensation via government compensation schemes. For example people who develop mesothelioma, a malignancy of the pleura or peritoneum, caused by occupational exposure to asbestos may apply for a lump sum if they are in receipt of industrial injuries disablement benefit or make a civil claim for compensation from insurers of the company responsible for their exposure.

Secondary cancer prevention is focused on early diagnosis, of which early detection and screening are the major components. Screening and detection programmes are concentrated on some of the most common cancers, including cancers of the breast, cervix, colon and rectum, prostate, skin and oropharynx. Pre-cancerous lesions or cancers that are detected early and remain localized are more likely to be treated successfully. Delay in detection and treatment diminishes the chance of cure and survival, because it permits the growing tumour to invade surrounding tissues and metastasize to other areas of the body.

National screening programmes for breast cancer and cervical cancer target specific groups of apparently healthy women in order to detect those who either have or are at high risk of developing cancer. These individuals are then offered treatment. Screening raises some interesting ethical issues in relation to both false-negative (where the test is negative but a cancer is present) and false-positive results (the test is positive but a cancer is not present) and also because it is probable that some individuals may be over-treated as a result of positive findings. This is arguably the case for women with very small breast cancers and ductal carcinomas in situ detected by mammography, although it is hoped ongoing clinical trials will determine the best management strategy for these lesions. Taking a Papanicalaou smear to obtain a specimen of cervical cells that are then examined microscopically has long been the basis of screening to detect cervical abnormalities. A change to liquid-based cytology is currently being implemented. This is expected to reduce the percentage of inadequate smears taken from 9% to less than 2% (NHS Cancer Screening Programmes 2006). In addition, testing for the presence of HPV which is known to be associated with invasive cervical cancers will, in the future, enable those women with mild cervical abnormalities, but who are at high risk of developing invasive cancer, to be identified for intensive surveillance. A new national screening programme for bowel cancer is due to commence in 2006. People between the ages of 60 and 69 years will be screened every 2 years by means of a stool-testing kit designed to detect faecal occult blood. This will be sent to members of the public through the post and returned to a screening laboratory for analysis. Those individuals found to have evidence of occult bleeding will be offered colonoscopy at a local screening centre. It is anticipated that only 1 in 10 individuals requiring a colonoscopy is likely to have bowel cancer diagnosed.

Screening for prostate cancer is not currently part of a national screening programme. This is because controversy exists concerning the value of the prostate specific antigen (PSA) test and because of uncertainty about the best treatment for early prostate cancer (Law 2004). Despite this level of doubt, increasing numbers of men are being diagnosed with prostate cancer as a result of PSA testing. Many prostate cancers grow slowly and if left untreated may not cause problems; for some men a safe option is for active monitoring through regular PSA testing rather than radical treatment.

Seven important early symptoms of cancer that are stressed in public education programmes are:

1 Unusual bleeding or discharge from any body orifice
2 A lump or thickening in the breast or elsewhere

3 A sore that does not heal
4 A persistent change in bowel or bladder habits
5 A persistent cough or hoarseness
6 Indigestion or difficulty in swallowing
7 An obvious change in a wart or mole.

Whilst any of these may have a perfectly benign cause, awareness of these seven signs, knowledge of the environmental and lifestyle factors that predispose to cancer, and access to community resources for information and advice, provide opportunities for individuals to be well informed. However, the uptake and utilization of screening and other services aimed at early detection is also influenced by the beliefs and attitudes of individuals and groups. For example, the uptake of breast and cervical cancer screening in many Asian communities has been found to be much lower than that in the general population (Thomas et al 2005). Targeted education among Asian women and their community leaders to address cultural taboos about cancer may help to increase the number of women attending for screening.

DIAGNOSIS AND STAGING OF CANCER

Unless discovered through routine screening procedures, most cancers remain undetected until the patient begins to experience signs and symptoms secondary to the cancer, such as unexplained weight loss, pain, fatigue or any of the signs listed above. To assist GPs in identifying those patients in whom cancer is a possibility, clinical guidelines have been produced by the National Institute for Clinical Excellence (NICE 2005).

Accurate and speedy diagnosis is essential to ensure an appropriate and effective treatment approach. As part of the National Cancer Plan (DoH 2000), measures have been introduced to reassure the public that signs and symptoms indicative of cancer will be seen and treated urgently. A specialist now sees all cases of suspected cancer urgently referred by GPs within 2 weeks of referral. Cancers diagnosed as a result are treated within 62 days and cancers diagnosed by any other route should be treated within 31 days of a decision to treat being agreed with the patient. To achieve these targets many trusts have adopted greater multi-professional working with specialist nurses or nurse practitioners taking on roles that were previously exclusively medical. For example, when attending a hospital for investigation of rectal bleeding or haematuria, it may be the nurse who performs the flexible sigmoidoscopy or cystoscopy, who gives the patient either reassurance or a provisional diagnosis, and who initially discusses the treatment options. The speed with which patients are now diagnosed and offered their first treatment is reassuring for many; however, it can be alarming for others, as it may allow little opportunity to digest the diagnosis after the initial shock or to fully consider all the implications of the various treatment options. There is some evidence reported by Brennan (2004) that if patients have insufficient time to prepare themselves for a cancer diagnosis, this can result in higher levels of depression after treatment.

The impact of a diagnosis of cancer is profound, as is the way it is conveyed to the patient and reactions to the initial shock may include disbelief, acute distress or downright denial. Northouse (1984), in a study of patients with breast cancer, discovered that many viewed the period between investigations and starting treatment as being more stressful than actually being on treatment.

A wide variety of diagnostic procedures may be used in determining the presence, type and extent of a cancer. The detection and staging of cancers through imaging techniques has become progressively more sophisticated and of greater diagnostic value with the introduction of new techniques. Common tumour imaging techniques are listed below and are described more fully in Chapter 10:

- plain radiography
- angiography
- mammography
- barium studies
- computed tomography (CT)
- ultrasonography
- nuclear medicine imaging
- magnetic resonance imaging (MRI)
- positron emission tomograpy (PET).

BIOPSY AND HISTOLOGICAL EXAMINATIONS

Progressive refinement of equipment and techniques enables a great deal of information to be gained with minimal invasion, but eventually a sample of tissue is required.

A biopsy obtains tissue for histological examination and thereby allows a pathological diagnosis. The confirmation or exclusion of malignancy is the most common indication for biopsy; however, inflammatory and infective tissue may also have characteristic microscopic appearances. When malignant tissue is found, the type of cancer and the degree of differentiation of the cells can be determined. Samples of tissue may be obtained by aspiration or core biopsy (a technique that involves removing a small plug of tissue using a needle and syringe) or by open excision of a section of tissue under local or general anaesthesia. For lesions that are impalpable, biopsies can be performed under CT or ultrasound guidance.

Clonogenic assay involves the growth of human tumour cells on a special culture medium to predict specific chemotherapy suitable for the individual patient. Such translational research involving culture and sensitivity assays of human tumour cell responsiveness to chemotherapeutic agents provides a potential for increasingly individualized therapy for patients.

Exfoliative cytological tests involve the microscopic examination of smears of secretion or fluid taken from a body cavity. Cells are shed continuously from the epithelial surface tissue of the body cavities; this process is referred to as exfoliation or desquamation. Neoplastic cells may be detected before there are any other recognizable signs or symptoms, resulting in successful early treatment. Specimens may be taken from the cervix, vagina, respiratory tract, mouth, oesophagus, stomach, urinary tract, prostate, and the pleural and peritoneal cavities.

ENDOSCOPY

By inserting an endoscope into a body passage, the area can be inspected directly and a biopsy obtained. This method of examination may be used in the larynx, bronchus, oesophagus, stomach, colon, sigmoid, uterus, rectum and bladder.

LABORATORY STUDIES

Some haematological and serological tests are used to refine the diagnosis or to follow the progress of the malignancy. For example, the serum acid phosphatase level is used in investigation for carcinoma of the prostate; it is raised when the disease is present. Blood and plasma cell evaluations are important in diagnosis and assessment of malignant disease of the bone marrow and reticuloendothelial system and are discussed in Chapter 14.

TUMOUR MARKERS

Tumour markers are substances produced by tumours or by the host in response to the presence of tumour. Tumour markers are useful in staging disease, following response to treatment and identifying recurrent disease. A broad range of tumour markers exists, including antigens, antibodies, genes, enzymes and hormones. Limitations in the clinical usefulness of most tumour markers are the lack of sensitivity and lack of proportionality, i.e. presentations of the marker are irregular or fail to reflect the true tumour burden.

Some of the more useful markers used today are:

- human chorionic gonadotrophin (HCG), the level of which is raised in women with choriocarcinoma and in men with testicular carcinoma; HCG is useful in following tumour size and in detecting recurrent disease
- cancer antigen 125 (CA-125) is present in many women with ovarian cancer; it is proportional to tumour burden and is used to follow patients with disease and in detecting recurrence
- alpha fetoprotein (AFP) is present in cases of testicular teratomas
- carcinoembryonic antigen (CEA) can be evidence of bowel, ovarian and pancreatic cancers
- cancer antigen 19-9 (CA 19-9) is found in cases of pancreatic cancer.

Once all available information has been obtained, it is possible to classify the cancer and confirm its grade and stage.

CANCER CLASSIFICATION: GRADING AND STAGING

All cancers have certain common characteristics, but there are also marked differences between one type and another because of the type of tissue involved, the location, and the degree to which the cancer cells depart from normal. They also differ as to signs and symptoms, effects on the host, rate of growth and patterns of metastasis, form of treatment used, and the response to treatment. Cancers are classified according to the type of **tissue** or cells from which they arise. There are four main tissue types, epithelial, connective, haemopoietic/lymphoid and neural which give rise to the majority of cancers. These, and some examples of tumours arising from them, are outlined in Figure 11.3. In addition, there are some cancers whose origin is uncertain, and some whose cells are undifferentiated and bear no resemblance to any normal tissue. These are called anaplastic tumours.

Cancers are histologically *graded*, based on their microscopic appearance, using a numerical system of three or four grades, with the higher numbers indicating a greater degree of undifferentiation and a tumour that tends to behave more aggressively.

Staging refers to the clinical evaluation of the extent of the cancer. A small localized cancer is at an early stage whereas an extensive cancer that has spread to distant parts of the body is likely to be at an advanced stage and be more difficult to cure. As well as providing an indication of the likely outcome or prognosis of the disease, staging is very important in individualizing treatment options. Internationally recognized classification systems are used to facilitate commonality of approach in diagnosis and treatment. An example of this is the TNM system (Hermanek et al 1997) which has been developed cooperatively by the International Union Against Cancer (UICC) and the American Joint Committee for Cancer Staging (AJCCS). The TNM staging system uses the initials T, N and M each followed by a number to take account of primary tumour size (T1–4), local and regional lymph node involvement (N0–3), and evidence and extent of metastatic deposits (M0 or 1). Other systems use Roman numerals I–IV or capital letters often to indicate the stage. An example of the staging for prostate cancer is given in Table 11.2. The staging of a cancer may change as more information becomes available either radiologically or from microscopic evaluation of tissues following surgical removal.

Despite an increasingly sophisticated range of techniques to assist the process of diagnosis, there are occasions when it is impossible to detect the primary site or differentiate between a primary or secondary deposit.

In recent years there has been a move to ensure that cancer patients receive optimal treatment for their disease delivered by specialists in their type of cancer. The services and treatments that should be available for patients with specific types of cancer are outlined in a series of guidance documents produced by NICE on the basis of best available evidence. Central to these recommendations is the concept of the specialist multidisciplinary team (MDT) for a particular

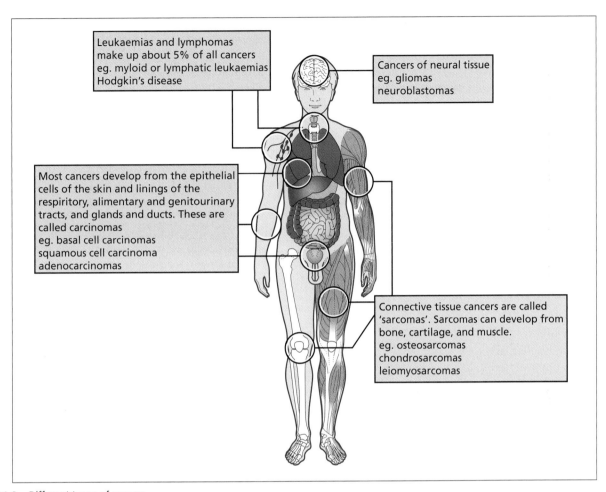

Figure 11.3 Different types of cancer.

Overall stage	Description	TNM classification
Stage I	Cancer is very small and completely inside the prostate gland. It is an incidental finding at TURP	T1 N0 M0
Stage II	Cancer is confined to the prostate gland but may show up on scans and may be felt on rectal examination or be found as a result of raised PSA. More than 5% of tissue is cancerous	T1 N0 M0 T2 N0 M0
Stage III	Cancer has spread outside the prostate capsule and may have grown into the seminal vesicles but not the lymph nodes	T3 N0 M0
Stage IV	Cancer has spread to other organs such as the rectum or bladder or pelvic wall or Has spread to lymph nodes or Cancer has spread to other parts of the body such as bones or lungs	T4 N0 M 0 T1–4 N1 M0 T1–4 N1–3 M!

Table 11.2 Stage and corresponding TNM classification for prostate cancer

cancer site (e.g. head and neck or urological cancer) consisting of surgeons, oncologists, radiologists, pathologists and increasingly specialist nurses. The role of the nurse in influencing decision-making at this stage is vital as she or he may be the only team member with extensive knowledge of an individual patient's situation and preferences.

The period of diagnosis and staging can be extremely stressful and is the beginning of the journey through treatment and, hopefully, to recovery. There is increasing evid-ence to suggest that people who are newly diagnosed with cancer have a strong need for information and to be in-volved in the decision-making process. In a study by Beaver et al (1996), it was identified that the extent of desire for active participation varied considerably, although there was a uniform desire for information. The role of nursing is central at all stages of the journey and involves participation in the delivery of care and monitoring individual responses to treatment.

TREATMENT OF CANCER

Once a diagnosis has been made, a combination of treatment approaches is used to maximize the likelihood of a cure. The concept of cure in cancer is expressed in terms of 5-year survival from initial diagnosis and treatment. Surgery has been the mainstay of treatment for solid tumours, but increasingly surgery is used in combination with chemotherapy and radiotherapy. It is now known that some tumours are far more sensitive to particular therapies. The developing knowledge around chemotherapy and radiotherapy sensitivities enables the development of treatment protocols that are designed for specific tumours and disease stage in order to achieve maximum effect. All treatments need to balance the likelihood of survival against attendant levels of toxicity, and patients need to be fully informed about treatment choices and likely outcomes. Treatment decisions in physiological terms are made on the basis of:

- tumour location
- growth rate
- metastatic potential
- general physical status.

Increasingly, quality-of-life issues and personal preference form part of the dialogue between the individual and the cancer team (Degner et al 1997, Langenhoff et al 2001). However, there is evidence to suggest that individuals may be strongly in favour of undergoing radical treatment, regardless of side-effects, despite the reservations of healthcare professionals (Slevin et al 1990).

SURGERY

The role of surgery in the treatment of cancer includes tissue diagnosis through biopsy; staging of disease; curative treatment through excision; amputation or surgical diversion; palliation; and reconstruction. Around 60% of cancer patients continue to undergo some sort of surgical procedure but new surgical, anaesthetic and critical care techniques, and use of equipment such as lasers and scopes and new technology, have resulted in the field of surgical oncology offering simultaneously more complex and less invasive procedures.

Types of procedure
Diagnostic procedures
Establishing a tissue diagnosis through biopsy can be done by *incisional* biopsy, where a small portion of tissue is removed and examined, or by *excisional* biopsy, whereby the whole tumour is removed (e.g. full or partial removal of a breast lump, usually under general anaesthesia). Needle biopsies use a needle to aspirate fluid or tissue and are easily done under local anaesthesia. Biopsy is increasingly performed in conjunction with radiological procedures such as a CT scan, which allows precise placement of the biopsy needle.

Endoscopy allows visualization of potentially cancerous lesions and biopsy without the need for invasive surgery and often using sedation rather than a general anaesthetic. Although advances in imaging and endoscopic procedures have largely precluded the need for it, surgery can be utilized to obtain a histological diagnosis and to determine the stage of disease where other diagnostic methods are unsatisfactory. A diagnostic laparotomy is an example of this, as is examination under anaesthetic (EUA) used to evaluate gynaecological and head and neck cancers. Surgery may also be used to excise 'bulky' disease, for example residual lymphatic tissues that have been treated by chemotherapy or radiotherapy or to establish that there is no focus of active disease left.

Curative surgery
Surgery is still a definitive treatment for many cancers, particularly solid tumours, and curative surgery needs to encompass both removal of the tumour mass and a safe margin of healthy tissue around it. Cancer in situ can be treated with cryosurgery, endoscopy or carbon dioxide laser. Many cancers can be removed and cured by local excision (e.g. skin cancers). Others require more radical block dissections involving not just removal of tumour, but also regional lymph nodes and any other involved contiguous structures. Examples are radical neck dissection, radical mastectomy and radical hysterectomy (Wertheim's hysterectomy). Within the abdomen and pelvis, radical excisions may involve diversions of bladder or bowel and creation of stomas. Such radical surgery inevitably results in some level of functional disruption that may cause both physical and/or psychological morbidity for the individual as they strive to adjust. A desire to preserve both form and function has led to a reduction in the scale of surgery performed. A radical trachelectomy, offered as an alternative option to radical hysterectomy for some women with early cervical cancer who wish to preserve their uterus in order to carry a baby is an example of this, although it is still complex surgery.

Sentinel node biopsy (SNB) is a relatively new technique used to reduce the need for axillary lymph node clearance during surgery for breast cancer. The sentinel node is the first lymph node to which a tumour drains and acts as a gatekeeper. If cancer is present in this node then it is likely that other nodes will be involved. Prior to surgery a small dose of radioactive labelled technetium is injected near the tumour site and at surgery a blue dye is injected into the tumour site. This allows the sentinel node or nodes to be identified both visually and by use of a Geiger counter. These nodes are then removed and examined by the pathologist for evidence of cancer cells during the surgery. If clear of cancer no further removal of nodes is required and this reduces the risk of post-operative complications, improves arm and shoulder mobility and reduces the risk of subsequent lymphoedema (Mansel et al 2004). SNB also has a role in surgery for malignant melanomas and is being evaluated in others such as vulval cancer. Increasingly, surgery is used in combination with other treatment modalities, and this may affect the timing and extent of the operation (Davidson and Sacks 1995).

Adjuvant surgery is used to remove residual masses in radio or chemosensitive tumours such as osteosarcomas and testicular teratomas. Wound healing may be a problem in these situations if there has been previous radiotherapy, and an individual's suitability for anaesthetic may be affected if their respiratory function has been reduced by certain chemotherapy drugs (e.g. bleomycin).

Prophylactic surgery

Surgery has a limited but important role in preventing the development of cancer, for example removal of the colon in the case of familial polyposis coli and hereditary non-polyposis colorectal cancer (Church 1996). Rather more controversial is the issue of prophylactic mastectomy for women with a high risk of developing breast cancer due to the inherited BRCA1 or BRCA2 gene and oophorectomy for women with a familial history of ovarian cancer. Here, the potential efficacy of the operation needs to be balanced against the impact on self-image, sexuality and a variety of psychosocial factors (Hartmann et al 1999).

Ablative surgery

Ablative surgery may be undertaken to remove hormonal influences on tumour growth through procedures such as oophorectomy, adrenalectomy and orchidectomy.

Palliative surgery

Palliative surgery is performed to improve the quality of life for the patient, rather than as a curative procedure. Examples of palliative surgery include neurosurgical management of pain (e.g. cordotomy, nerve blocks) and pinning of pathological fractures. It may also be used to bypass or relieve an obstruction such as in the bowel, which is a common complication of advanced ovarian cancer, or in the oesophagus in which case a stent may be inserted. Surgical management may facilitate control of local disease such as fungating wounds and often plays a role in the management of oncological emergencies such as haemorrhage and spinal cord compression. Single metastases in the liver, lungs or brain may also be removed surgically in certain cases.

Reconstructive surgery

In recent years, major advances and improvements have been made in reconstructive surgery. Reconstruction utilizing skin, muscle and bone grafting and insertion of prosthetic devices is now often done simultaneously with the excisional procedure. These advances have dramatically improved the appearance and functioning of patients undergoing head and neck, orthopaedic, and radical abdominal and pelvic operations. Reconstructive breast surgery is an option for women who have had a mastectomy (Neill et al 1998) and may be offered at the same time as the initial surgery.

Supportive surgery

Supportive surgery is carried out to provide venous access for chemotherapy, or to provide a means for providing nutrition such as formation of a percutaneous endoscopic gastrostomy (PEG).

Caring for people undergoing surgery

Caring for people undergoing surgical treatment for cancer offers unique challenges and requires understanding of the emotional and psychosocial impact of a cancer diagnosis and the ability to provide high-quality technical supportive care. In the diagnostic phase, people are frequently and understandably anxious, and need opportunities to express their fears. They also require information regarding diagnostic procedures and the possible treatment options should a diagnosis of cancer be confirmed

Patients undergoing surgery for cancer; particularly as a result of head and neck, gastrointestinal or ovarian cancer, are frequently nutritionally compromised which increases the risk of a variety of post-surgical complications. Liaison with dieticians and the wider inter-professional team may be required in order to maintain the patient's nutritional state. Patients with cancer are more susceptible to developing DVTs than patients undergoing surgery for benign disease and therefore DVT prophylaxis is essential. As previously indicated the majority of patients diagnosed with cancer are aged 65 years or more and many will have other medical conditions such as diabetes, hypertension and pulmonary disease to be taken into account when considering their surgical management.

The person who is receiving definitive treatment may experience radical changes in functioning and/or appearance as a result of surgery. Such treatment may occur very soon after diagnosis, when patients are only just beginning to cope with the impact of diagnosis on physical and emotional health. Nursing involvement needs to take account of this and include exploration of reactions and concerns, the provision of information on disease and treatment, and teaching for self-care in relation to post-operative recovery and alterations in functioning. The timing and manner of information giving are important factors in developing a therapeutic relationship between nurse and patient. Equally important is comprehensive discharge planning and referral to other healthcare professionals such as dieticians, occupational therapists, physiotherapists and speech and language therapists. Increasingly, people with cancer have access to a range of clinical nurse specialists with specific expertise, such as breast care nurses, colorectal nurses, and head and neck specialist nurses who embrace the role of key worker and are a point of contact with the wider multidisciplinary team. They frequently coordinate services, provide information, education and support and communicate not only with the patient and carers but also with health and social care professionals by working across primary, secondary and tertiary care boundaries. Local support groups, charities and voluntary organizations may also be helpful in enabling individuals to cope with cancer and lifestyle adaptation. Some people may have specific and ongoing needs for specialist equipment and rehabilitation, for example those who have undergone amputation or stoma formation. With progressively shorter stays in hospital, nursing is playing an increasingly important role in planning and coordinating continuing care in the community, as many cancer treatments move from an inpatient to an outpatient basis. While many people may value this, Fallowfield (1998) notes that, for some women with breast cancer, early discharge may not be so helpful because the woman has to make many physiological and psychological adaptations in relative isolation.

CHEMOTHERAPY

Chemotherapy is the use of chemicals (cytotoxic agents) in the treatment of cancer. Essentially, these are drugs that work by disrupting cellular replication, either by inhibiting the synthesis of DNA or by otherwise damaging the DNA. Although a more recent development in cancer care, this modality is now well established and is becoming an increasingly prominent treatment.

History and development

The development of chemotherapy as a treatment modality began with the observation that soldiers exposed to nitrogen mustard gas in World War I experienced bone marrow hyperplasia and atrophy of the lymph glands. In following years nitrogen mustard was developed as a chemical and, when given to patients with lymphoma, resulted in short-term therapeutic responses. In the late 1940s nitrogen mustard and methotrexate were the first two drugs recognized as chemotherapeutic agents. Since then, many thousands of chemicals have been tested for antitumour effects; currently there are several dozen chemotherapeutic agents commonly used in the treatment of cancer.

Role of chemotherapy in the treatment of cancer

Chemotherapy is increasingly being used in combination with other modalities in the treatments of all forms of cancer. As a systemic therapy, it is used primarily for primary or secondary disease that is disseminated throughout the body. However, it may also be used locally, as for example in the instillation of cytotoxic agents directly into the bladder for the treatment of superficial tumours. For chemosensitive cancers such as Hodgkin's disease, testicular cancer, acute lymphocytic leukaemia in children, Ewing's sarcoma and choriocarcinoma, chemotherapy is a primary and potentially curative mode of treatment and is the *definitive* treatment. When patients have relapsed after being treated with another modality, the term *salvage* chemotherapy is sometimes used to describe the subsequent treatment that will hopefully result in regaining control of disease. *Adjuvant* chemotherapy is the term used when cytotoxic drugs are used after removal of the primary tumour to destroy any micrometastatic disease, and this is an approach commonly used in the management of breast cancer. *Neoadjuvant* chemotherapy refers to the use of cytotoxic therapy to reduce or 'debulk' the size of a primary tumour, effectively downstaging the cancer to make it more easily resectable. Patients whose cancers cannot be controlled or cured may

benefit from *palliative* chemotherapy, which may be effective in shrinking the tumour mass, thus relieving obstruction or pressure on nerves or the lymphatic system. In this way, pain or other distressing symptoms may be managed and controlled more effectively.

Principles of action and treatment regimens

An understanding of the sequence of phases through which cells must pass as they replicate is fundamental to an understanding of how cytotoxic drugs act and the principles of cytotoxic chemotherapy treatment regimens.

Some drugs are *cell cycle specific*, i.e. they sustain their major cytotoxic effect during a particular phase of the **cell cycle**, such as mitosis, whereas others work throughout the cell cycle and are therefore *cell cycle-non-specific*. Cell cycle-non-specific agents act on resting and dividing cells, making the cells unable to divide or repair damage. Cancer cells that are in the process of reproducing are most likely to be affected, but normal cells are affected too. The effects are most obvious on rapidly dividing cells such as those of hair, mucous membranes and the haemopoietic system. However, normal cells are better able to recover. The timing of courses of chemotherapy is designed to exploit this ability of normal cells to recover whilst maximizing malignant cell death.

The method and duration of action of individual agents has important implications for the combination of drugs used in chemotherapeutic treatment regimens. Drugs may be given as single agents, but they are more frequently given in combination to maximize the effect on malignant cells. Unfortunately the value of any cytotoxic agent may be limited by development of tumour resistance, resulting in little or no response to drug therapy.

Classification of chemotherapeutic agents

Cytotoxic drugs may be classified as alkylating agents, antimetabolites, plant alkaloids, topoisomerase inhibitors; antitumour antibiotics, hormones, steroids, or miscellaneous agents. Commonly used cytotoxic drugs are listed in Table 11.3.

Alkylating agents, also known as antimitotic drugs, act within the nucleus of the cell and alter the DNA molecules causing cross links which prevent the DNA strands from separating resulting in inhibition of cell growth and reproduction. Their activity is not specific to any one stage of the cell cycle, although reproducing cells are more vulnerable. Many of the well-established anti-cancer drugs including the platinum-based compounds, the nitrogen mustard derivatives and nitrosureas, are included in this category.

Antimetabolites resemble substances that are essential to cellular activities, and which are therefore taken up by cells. These preparations are sufficiently different from normal metabolites to alter metabolism and inhibit growth and prevent production of new DNA. They function at a specific phase of the life cycle of the cell.

The *plant alkaloids* currently in use are vinca alkaloids derived from periwinkle plants and taxanes first isolated from the Pacific yew tree. These agents block cell division

Table 11.3 Commonly used cytotoxic drugs

Alkylating agents	Cytotoxic antibiotics	Antimetabolites	Plant alkaloids	Miscellaneous
cyclophosphamide	doxorubicin	methotrexate	vinblastine	crisantaspase
ifosphamide	epirubicin	cytarabine	vincristine	
chlorambucil	daunorubicin	fludarabine	vindesine	
dacarbazine	mitoxantrone	gemcitabine	vinorelbine	
melphalan	bleomycin	fluorouracil	paclitaxel	
busulphan	mitomycin	capecitabine	docetaxel	
lomustine	dactinomycin	mercaptopurine	etoposide	
carmustine	idarubicin	tioguanine	irinitecan	
temozolomide	tegafur		topotecan	
treosulphan	premetreted			
thiptepa	raltitrexed			
procabazine				
cisplatin				
carboplatin				
oxaliplatin				

during mitosis by preventing microtubule formation and function. Other plant derivatives are the topoisomerase inhibitors. They include camptothecins derived from the Chinese tree Camptotheca accuminata and podophyllotoxins primarily obtained from the Mayapple plant. Topoimerase enzymes control the manipulation of the structure of the DNA and inhibitors of these enzymes interfere with both transcription and replication of DNA.

Certain *antibiotics* have been found to be of value in inhibiting some types of neoplastic cells. They act by interfering with DNA and/or RNA synthesis of the cells. Included in this group of cytotoxic drugs are the anthracyclines and agents like bleomycin and mitomycin.

Hormones are used in the treatment of cancer on the basis that receptors for specific hormones needed for cell growth are found on the surface of some tumours. Hormone therapy can work by stopping production of a particular hormone, blocking the receptor or by substituting a chemically similar but inactive agent for the active hormone.

Clinical trials

New drugs are introduced frequently, and the search continues for a drug that will be selective and prove toxic to malignant cells without damaging normal tissues. The clinical evaluation of drugs has three clearly defined phases:

- *Phase I*: assessment of maximum tolerated dose, best route of administration and side-effects
- *Phase II*: assessment of the efficacy of treatment in a group of patients with a single tumour type

- *Phase III*: the drug is tested in clinical trials against existing drugs or other forms of treatment.

In all forms of chemotherapy treatment, and especially when drugs are being administered within a clinical trial, informed consent is essential. Patients require sufficient information to make an informed choice and nurses have an obligation to ensure that this is available in a form that is accessible to patients with different information needs.

Administration of chemotherapy

Chemotherapeutic agents may be administered by a variety of routes: oral, intravenous, intrathecal and intracavitary are the routes most commonly used but occasionally topical, intramuscular, and subcutaneous administration may be appropriate. Whatever route is used the nurse administering chemotherapy must be competent to undertake the tasks involved. These include the assessment of the patient's fitness for treatment, the checking of the drugs against the prescription, provision of patient information, delivery of the drug and education of the patient with regard to side-effects and lifestyle, all of which require the nurse to have thorough knowledge and understanding of the agents being used and their potential toxicities.

Preparation, handling and disposal

Cytotoxic drugs work directly or indirectly to cause cell death and may be mutagenic, teratogenic and carcinogenic. Their inherent toxicity has led to concerns over the potential hazard to health workers and other personnel exposed to them. It is therefore essential that safe practices and high standards of care be maintained when handling these drugs. The Health and Safety at Work Act 1974; Control of Substances Hazardous to Health regulations (COSHH 2002) and The Health and Safety Executive guidelines (HSE 2003) provide a framework for the management and containment of risk associated with cytotoxic agents. Guidelines produced by the Royal College of Nursing (Goodman1998) give specific guidance for nurses involved in chemotherapy administration. Specific local guidelines and policies as to the prescription, preparation, handling, administration and disposal of cytotoxic agents should be developed by the nursing and pharmacy staff of individual trusts. Such policies are needed for protection of community staff as well as hospitals as more chemotherapy is being administered in the patient's home.

Current safety guidelines for the preparation of chemotherapeutic agents recommend the use of a laminar airflow hood and protective clothing in order to prevent exposure of the person preparing the drugs. Personnel who are administering chemotherapy must also take precautions to prevent self-exposure or environmental contamination (see management and awareness of the risks of cytotoxics (marc) in Sewell et al 2003). As a minimum, personnel administering chemotherapy should wear a plastic apron and nitrile synthetic rubber gloves, although no glove is completely impervious to cytotoxic drugs. All materials used in the preparation and administration of chemotherapeutic agents must be disposed of as biohazardous waste and spillage kits should be available in all areas where cytotoxic drugs are administered in the event of accidental contamination. Following the administration of the prescribed agents, the patient's body fluids will contain metabolic waste products for up to 7 days. These should be regarded as potentially hazardous and nurses should employ safe handling techniques when involved in direct patient care bearing in mind that body fluids will be most hazardous in the first 24 hours (Allwood et al 2002).

Cytotoxic drugs are most commonly administered by *intravenous* injection or infusion because it enables rapid and reliable delivery to the tumour site and rapid dilution of the drug, reducing the potential for local irritation and tissue damage. Cannulation requires careful selection of the vein because of the need for repeated administration. Many chemotherapeutic agents are extremely irritating to tissue and may cause thrombosis of the vein. Some agents (vesicants) may cause necrosis of tissue if infiltration occurs. Agents classified as irritants will cause irritation in the vein and pain if not diluted sufficiently before administration, and if infiltrated into the tissue will cause pain without necrosis. The injection site should be observed frequently for signs of redness or swelling and the patient questioned as to pain, tenderness or burning. Prompt identification and management of site infiltration or *extravasation* is important to prevent excessive and unnecessary tissue damage. Extravasation of a vesicant drug is an acute emergency, and treatment includes the administration of specific antidotes

for the drug and the application of ice packs to the site to decrease the spread of the drug. Nursing actions taken need to be fully documented and the incident fully recorded and reported (How and Brown 1998).

With the development and widespread use of more orally administered cytotoxic drugs, like capecitabine, there is a potential that these drugs are perceived to be safer than those given parenterally. The need for precautions with capsules, tablets and liquids in terms of handing and storage is as important as with parenteral administration and the requirement for effective patient education and monitoring is possibly greater (Gerbrecht and Kangas 2004).

Intrathecal chemotherapy may be given where there are tumour cells in the central nervous system (CNS) or to prevent this. Chemotherapy given by other routes is not usually able to cross the blood–brain barrier, and therefore tumour cells present in the CNS are unaffected by the drug. Presence of tumour cells in the CNS is determined by examination of spinal fluid. Intrathecal therapy may also be given prophylacticly to patients with leukaemia who are at high risk for development of CNS disease. This type of therapy is given either by lumbar puncture or through a ventricular reservoir called an Ommaya reservoir, which is surgically implanted in the right frontal region of the skull. Following incidents where drugs intended for intravenous use have been accidentally administered intrathecally with devastating consequences, national guidance on the use of intrathecal chemotherapy has been produced (DoH 2003) and it is essential that these guidelines are rigorously applied. Only nurses who have been assessed as competent may check the drugs with a doctor prior to the administration of chemotherapy intrathecally. All staff members have a duty to challenge any practice that deviates from local and nationally recommended practice to protect patient safety.

Intracavitary administration of chemotherapeutic agents is usually done following aspiration of fluid from a body compartment such as the intrapleural space or the peritoneal cavity. Patients who develop malignant pleural effusions may have chemotherapy instilled in the pleural cavity through a thoracotomy tube. The resulting sclerotic changes in the lining of the pleural cavity may prevent the reaccumulation of fluid in the pleural space. Intraperitoneal chemotherapy allows direct contact of the drugs with the tumour in the peritoneal cavity. Direct delivery of the chemotherapy to tumour cells maximizes the effect of the chemotherapy while minimizing the systemic side-effects of the drugs. Intraperitoneal chemotherapy is most commonly used in the treatment of ovarian cancer. Intracavitary chemotherapy is very commonly used to control superficial bladder tumours through instillation of drugs following surgical excision.

Devices for the administration of chemotherapy

For patients receiving long-term or repeated courses of chemotherapy, a right arterial catheter may be inserted through the chest wall and into a large vein. A portion of the catheter remains outside the body and the exit site is covered with an occlusive dressing. The greater blood volume in the large vein and the right atrium dilutes the medication, and thus decreases irritation to the vessel walls. The risk of extravasation into tissue is decreased and the peripheral veins are preserved. A right atrial catheter such as a Hickman catheter allows for greater patient mobility as it can be left in indefinitely and sealed with a cap between treatments. These may be single, double or triple lumen, and are either open or closed (e.g. Groshong type with a slit valve), and thus venous access is assured for chemotherapy, intravenous fluids and medications, as well as blood products. Patency of the line is maintained by flushing the line regularly with a solution of heparin or saline according to local policy.

Peripherally inserted central catheters (PICCs) are inserted via the antecubital fossa and threaded through the veins of the upper arm until the tip rests in the superior vena cava. PICCs do not require a surgical procedure for insertion, and therefore insertion is frequently carried out by experienced nurses (Gabriel 1996). PICCs are ideal for short-term venous access but, as with other central venous devices, they do require the patient and/or carers to take on much of the maintenance of the device themselves with appropriate guidance and support. An alternative to central venous catheters is the use of totally implanted central venous ports. These ports are implanted under the subcutaneous tissue and the catheter attached to the port is inserted into a central vein. Access to the port is established by inserting a needle through the skin down into the port. As with the external catheters, patency is maintained by flushing with heparin before the needle is removed from the port. Ports require flushing only once a month. Implanted ports are advantageous to patients as much less self-care is required. There is no need for a dressing and there is no interference in activities of daily living as a result of having a port. Although not widely used, implanted ports are also available for implantation in the small veins of the forearm.

Ambulatory chemotherapy

The development of a range of venous access devices and more effective agents and regimens for managing side-effects has enabled many more people to receive chemotherapy at home (Dougherty et al 1998). For many patients, this may foster independence and a greater sense of control, but for others the absence of immediate access to clinical staff may be anxiety provoking. Careful consideration needs to be given to the patient's individual circumstances and needs, and a good learning programme established. Caring for people who are receiving chemotherapy, regardless of the setting, requires nurses to have a high level of technical skill and knowledge, and understanding of psychosocial and physiological responses to disease and treatments. Box 11.1 summaries the nursing care measures associated with administration of chemotherapy.

Side-effects and toxicities

Because chemotherapy has a systemic action, it affects the growth and division of both cancer cells and normal cells.

Consequently, a wide variety of generalized side-effects and toxicities are associated with chemotherapeutic agents. As the side-effects vary with different drugs, it is essential that the nurse knows the chemotherapeutic agent given, the possible side-effects of that particular drug, their significance, and how they are manifested. Details of all these drugs and common combinations are beyond the scope of this chapter and the reader should consult relevant data sheets for specific information. Treatment regimens are carefully selected based on the nature, size and extent of the tumour and the age, general health and performance status of the individual. Doses are calculated according to body surface area and therefore accurate height and weight measurements are essential, and weight change during treatment should be recorded and reported. Dose reductions during a course of treatment may be required if toxicity is significant or if, for example, renal function is poor. As well as assessing the patient holistically, and in relation to general and specific drug toxicities, specific blood parameters are monitored prior to each treatment.

The side-effects that are most commonly experienced by patients receiving chemotherapy include:

- bone marrow depression, leading to leucopenia, thrombocytopenia and **anaemia**
- mucositis
- **nausea and vomiting**
- **diarrhoea and constipation**
- hair loss (alopecia)
- fatigue.

A more detailed discussion of these, along with appropriate nursing interventions, can be found on page 215. For patients who undergo chemotherapy whilst of reproductive age, fertility issues may be of great significance and should be acknowledged and discussed. Alkylating agents are the drugs most likely to cause infertility and this risk is highest for women over 35 years of age. Sperm banking is an option for men but for women the value of cryopreserving ovarian tissue remains a subject for further evaluation. Sperm production can recommence within months of completing treatment but may not resume for a number of years depending on the level of damage to stem cells in the testes. This will vary according to the drugs given, dosage and the treatment schedule. Contraceptive precautions should be taken by men and women during active treatment to prevent pregnancy because of the potential teratogenic risk to any fetus conceived. Use of a barrier method of contraception during intercourse is advisable because of the risk of secreting small amounts of an active drug in ejaculate and vaginal secretions. The more general effects of chemotherapy on sexuality are discussed later in this chapter.

Second primary malignancy

A rare long-term complication of cancer treatment is the development of a second primary malignancy. This has been documented in relation to patients treated as children and young adults with chemotherapy for a variety of tumours.

> **Box 11.1** Nursing care of the person having chemotherapy or biological therapy
>
> **Goals**
> - The patient will express satisfaction with the level of information and support provided
> - The drugs will be administered safely and side-effects will be prevented or minimized.
>
> **Preparation prior to a course of treatment and each cycle**
> - Observe for the presence and severity of symptoms and report these accordingly
> - Provide verbal and written information and reassurance reinforcing explanation of the specific agent, including mode of action, method of administration, side-effects and self-care strategies
> - Encourage and answer questions
> - Provide support and clarification of information to assist in decision-making process
> - Include family or significant others in teaching session
> - Help the patient to anticipate potential side-effects and suggest strategies to manage these
> - Educate the patient and family to report subtle symptom changes
> - Participate with other team members in evaluating the patient's understanding of and ability to participate in a clinical trial
> - Provide 24 hour contact details
> - Assess the need for support (physical and/or emotional) and make appropriate referrals
> - Monitor the patient for weight gain/loss and inform doctors so that dose modification can be made
> - Assess the most suitable method of venous access for the patient having i.v. therapies.
>
> **Administration of agents**
> - Ensure all relevant pre-treatment checks (haematological, renal, etc.) have been completed and are within normal parameters
> - Select and assemble appropriate equipment and infusion fluids for the drugs being administered
> - Ensure that emergency equipment and drugs to manage possible toxicities are readily accessible
> - Establish patency of existing venous access or cannulate and establish any prehydration
> - Follow verification procedures
> - Administer pre-medications of antiemetics/steroids/antihistamines
> - Administer chemotherapy or biological therapy agents as a bolus injection or infusion, taking into account guidelines relating to vesicant drugs
> - Observe and monitor the patient for immediate effects, allergic reactions, indications of extravasation, etc.
> - Manage immediate side-effects – hypersensitivity reactions, chills, pain, nausea
> - Provide distraction or diversional activities such as hand or foot massage
> - On completion, dispose of equipment and waste safely
> - Assess the patient's need for ongoing support and provide medication to take home
> - Complete all relevant documentation.

Use of alkylating agents appears to produce the most risk of this. Combination treatment with chemotherapy and radiotherapy may also influence this process, although the exact mechanism is not fully understood. Patients treated for Hodgkin's disease by radiotherapy to the chest wall have been found to be at increased risk of developing breast cancer. Treatment regimens are under continuous review to maximize the anti-tumour effect and minimize exposure to treatments that may induce a second cancer.

Stem cell transplantation
Conventional treatment of cancer consists of the use of surgery, chemotherapy and/or radiation therapy to eradicate all tumour cells. Doses of chemotherapy and/or radiation

therapy are often limited because of toxicity to the patient's bone marrow. Many believe that if bone marrow toxicity could somehow be minimized, chemotherapeutic doses could be increased to levels that would cure the patient of the malignancy. If the patient's own haematopoetic stem cells from bone marrow or peripheral blood or those of a compatible donor could be introduced into the body and successfully engrafted, then doses far higher than those used conventionally might become possible. This is the rationale for haematopoeitic stem cell transplantation (HSCT), which has evolved over the past 30 years from an experimental procedure to an established and effective treatment for selected patients. HSCT is now being used as a treatment for an expanding list of malignant and non-malignant haematological diseases. It is also used in the treatment of metabolic disorders such as Batten's disease.

There are three sources of stem cell transplant:

1 Autologous – patient's own – harvested from peripheral blood or bone marrow
2 Syngeneic – from an identical twin
3 Allogeneic – usually from a sibling or other close relative but occasionally from an unrelated, but tissue-type-identical, donor. In this case and, as with any other organ transplant, histocompatibility testing must be carried out using human leucocyte antigen (HLA) typing and the mixed lymphocyte culture (MLC).

For a fuller discussion of HSCT and the care of patients with haematological disorders, see Chapter 14.

Biological response modifier therapy

Biological response modifiers (BRM) are a form of treatment designed to strengthen the patient's biological response to tumour cells. This type of therapy began with the use of the bacterial agents bacillus Calmette-Guérin (BCG) and *Corynebacterium parvum* (*C. parvum*) which were inoculated to stimulate the immune system. Current therapies are based on a greater understanding of manipulating the immune system using a variety of naturally occurring molecules that are capable of influencing the immune response and incorporating these into cancer treatment. These agents include interferons, interleukins, colony-stimulating factors, tumour necrosis factor and monoclonal antibodies. Depending on the BRM, this may occur by:

● stopping or suppressing cancer growth
● making cancer cells more recognisable to the immune system
● boosting the immune system's killing power
● enhancing repair or replacement of cells destroyed by chemotherapy or radiotherapy.

As a result of advances in recombinant DNA technology, highly purified BRMs are now produced in large quantities and are available for use in cancer therapy. BRMs are unique in their ability to regulate or enhance the immune response. In contrast to chemotherapeutic agents and radiation

therapy, which exert a direct effect on cancer cells, BRMs activate the body's natural defences with a potentially greater antineoplastic activity and reduced toxicity. However, despite a great deal of initial interest and much experimental evidence, therapeutic use has been slow to develop.

Monoclonal antibodies are a particular type of targeted biological therapy produced by cloning the antibodies produced in response to specific antigens expressed on the surface of cancer cells. This is achieved by injecting human cancer cell antigens into mice to produce antibodies. The mouse plasma cells are then fused with a laboratory grown myeloma cell line to produce a hybridoma which can indefinitely produce quantities of antibody. Several such agents have been developed and are in use therapeutically mainly for haematological malignancies (e.g. rituximab). Trastuzumab (Herceptin) is the first monoclonal antibody to be licensed for treating a solid tumour. It binds to HER2 a receptor for epidermal growth factor that is found on some breast cancers.

Cancers need a blood supply to grow and many appear to produce growth factors which stimulate the development of new blood vessels. Angiogenesis inhibitors are another type of targeted therapy aimed at preventing the formation of these new blood vessels by solid tumours in response to vascular endothelial growth factor. Bevacizumab is an example of monoclonal antibody which targets this growth factor and which appears to have some activity in colorectal cancer. Thalidomide is also under evaluation as a drug that acts as an angiogenesis inhibitor. Other new biological therapies include drugs, such as imatinib and bortezomib, which target tumour growth at a molecular level by blocking the activity of specific growth factor receptors.

Experimental work continues on developing therapeutic vaccines by using irradiated autologous and allogeneic tumour combined with various biological stimulants (e.g. BCG) but so far with little success. Melanoma is one form of cancer that is potentially amenable to treatment with vaccines because it has an intrinsic immunogenicity (i.e. an ability to generate an immune response in the individual). The full potential of these agents is yet to be realized, but with increasing knowledge and understanding of molecular and vaccine biology, future developments are anticipated.

A complete account of the immune system and how it relates to BRM therapy is beyond the scope of this chapter, but Table 11.4 summarizes the principal actions, potential indications, and commonly reported toxicities and side-effects for several of the BRMs. Because the majority of BRMs are still under investigation, this information continues to evolve.

The side-effects associated with BRMs are variable in their onset and intensity. Side-effects and toxicities vary with the agent, the dosage schedule, the dose and the patient. It is important to note that not all BRMs, or even the same BRM at the same dose, produce the same side-effects. The side-effect most unique to BRM therapy is a set of symptoms collectively known as flu-like syndrome. These symptoms include fever, chills and rigors, fatigue, anorexia, hypotension,

Table 11.4 Biological response modifier therapy: actions, potential indications and side-effects

Postulated mechanism of action	Potential indications	Toxicity and side-effects
Colony stimulating factors (CSFs) GM-CSF: stimulates production of neutrophils, macrophages, eosinophils and, in the presence of erythropoietin, red blood cells G-CSF: stimulates neutrophil production M-CSF: stimulates macrophage production EPO (erythropoietin): stimulates maturation of erythrocytes	Not directly tumoricidal. Research indicates they may be useful for cancer treatment because they: • decrease duration of neutropenia that often results from chemotherapy • enable higher doses of chemotherapy to be given since CSFs can alter the dose-related toxicity of myelosuppression • decrease bone marrow recovery time following bone marrow transplants or radiation therapy-related suppression of marrow. In clinical studies, CSFs have shown activity in the treatment of leukaemias, including chronic lymphocytic leukaemia, hairy cell leukaemia, myelodysplastic syndrome, and neutropenia secondary to chemotherapy	Flu-like syndrome: fever, chills, fatigue/weakness, myalgia/arthralgia, headache Gastrointestinal: nausea, diarrhoea, vomiting, anorexia Other: facial flushing
Tumour necrosis factor (TNF) *In vitro*: binds to receptors on tumour cells and is directly tumoricidal or tumoristatic *In vivo*: precise mechanism of action is unclear. TNF may be directly cytotoxic or it may cause vascular endothelial damage in tumour capillaries resulting in haemorrhage and necrosis of tumour cells. TNF may also work through immune cell activation as it has been found to augment natural killer T-cell activity and to enhance B-cell proliferation	Many clinical trials are underway to determine the efficacy of TNF. TNF may be helpful in treating metastatic adenocarcinomas including colorectal, hepatic and bladder carcinomas	Flu-like syndrome: fever, chills, fatigue/weakness, myalgia/arthralgia, back pain Gastrointestinal: nausea, vomiting, diarrhoea, anorexia Non-specific: severe pain at tumour site
Monoclonal antibodies (MAbs) Application of MAbs is based on the knowledge that all cells (including tumour cells) have antigens present on their surface that are specific to that cell type. MAbs may be used alone or bound to radioisotopes, toxins or chemotherapeutic drugs to stain, destroy or identity cells with specific antigens on their cell surface	May be used in the treatment of cancer as well as for diagnostic purposes In clinical trials MAbs have shown activity in the treatment of leukaemia, lymphoma, metastatic breast and colorectal cancer, ovarian, renal, bladder and prostate cancer Examples of MAbs in clinical use include: Rituximab; Trastuzumab; Alemtuzumab; Cetuximab; Bevacizumab	Flu-like syndrome: fever, chills, headache, fatigue, malaise, myalgia Gastrointestinal: nausea, diarrhoea, vomiting Skin: generalized erythema, urticaria, pruritus Tumour pain Anaphylaxis (rare, but severe and life-threatening) Cardiotoxicity and other specific toxicities are associated with individual agents

(continued)

Table 11.4 *Cont'd*

Postulated mechanism of action	Potential indications	Toxicity and side-effects
Interferons (IFNs)		
Antiviral: IFNs stimulate cells infected with viruses to produce proteins that interfere with viral replication *Antiproliferative*: IFNs slow the reproduction of cells. Although the mechanisms are not well understood, possible contributing factors include inhibition of DNA and protein synthesis of cancer cells and prolongation of the cell cycle *Immunomodulatory*: depending on the type of IFN, different aspects of the immune system are stimulated or augmented. Examples include: T-cell activation, increased phagocytic and cytotoxic activity of macrophages and mature natural killer cells	Have shown some activity in the treatment of hairy cell leukaemia, AIDS-related Kaposi's sarcoma, multiple myeloma, nodular cutaneous T-cell lymphoma, chronic granulocytic leukaemia, malignant malanoma and kidney cancer	Flu-like syndrome: fever, chills, headache, fatigue, malaise, myalgia Gastrointestinal: nausea, diarrhoea, vomiting, anorexia, taste alterations, xerostomia Neurological/psychological: paraesthesia, mild confusion, somnolence, irritability, poor concentration Haematological: neutropenia and thrombocytopenia Cardiovascular: arrhythmias and blood pressure Reproductive: fertility
Interleukins (ILs)		
Interleukins are among the most important regulatory substances produced by lymphocytes and monocytes. Seven types of IL have been isolated and identified; however, other than IL-1, IL-2, IL-3 and more recently IL-4, little is known about their biological effects. Much work is still taking place in clinical trials. The ILs appear to act by causing proliferation and stimulation of T and B lymphocytes, assisting in the synthesis and secretion of lymphokines (e.g. interferon, CSFs) and/or enhancing natural killer T-cell activity	Have shown limited activity in the treatment of metastatic renal cell carcinoma, malignant melanoma and non-Hodgkin lymphomas	Administration of interleukin results in multisystem toxicities that may be life threatening Toxicities are related to dose and schedule Flu-like syndrome: fever, chills, headache, fatigue, malaise, myalgia Gastrointestinal: nausea, diarrhoea, vomiting, anorexia, taste alterations, xerostomia Skin: dryness, erythematous rash, pruritus, desquamation Neurological/psychological: confusion, irritability, impaired memory, sleep disturbances, depression Cardiovascular: capillary leak syndrome, peripheral oedema, ascites, arrhythmias, hypotension Pulmonary: dyspnoea, pulmonary oedema, ascites, arrhythmias, hypotension Renal: oliguria, anuria, azotaemia, increased serum creatinine and blood urea nitrogen levels

GM-CSF, granulocyte–macrophage colony stimulating factor.
G-CSF, granulocyte colony stimulating factor.

myalgia, arthralgia and headache, and managing these side-effects represents a major challenge for both nurses and patients. Collectively, BRMs have the potential to manifest toxicities in virtually every body system. Box 11.1 outlines nursing care for patients receiving biological therapies.

RADIOTHERAPY

Radiotherapy is the controlled use of ionizing radiation, which damages cellular DNA and thus causes cell death. Radiotherapy for cancer has been used for over 100 years but in the early era of radiotherapy, it was a rather crude treatment as little was known or understood about the effects of radiation on tissues or about therapeutic doses. Since that time, research has greatly expanded the knowledge and development of radiation as a highly effective treatment modality for cancer. Today, radiotherapy is precisely calculated to deliver the correct dose to the area treated, while sparing the surrounding normal tissues. However, fears, misunderstandings and myths about radiotherapy still persist and therefore an important aspect of care is to provide accurate information about treatment while encouraging the expression of any anxieties or concerns. Radiotherapy is one of the three most commonly used cancer treatment modalities, with over 50% of cancer patients having radiotherapy as some part of their treatment.

The aim of radiotherapy may be *curative*, as in treatments for skin cancer, carcinoma of the cervix or Hodgkin's disease. Radiotherapy may also be given as adjuvant treatment following surgery or neoadjuvant treatment prior to surgery. Where cure or eradication is not possible, control of the cancer for periods ranging from months to years may be the aim. Recurrent breast cancer, some soft tissue sarcomas and lung cancer are examples of cancer controlled by radiotherapy in combination with surgery or chemotherapy. *Palliation* may be another goal of radiotherapy. Relief of pain, ulceration or bleeding, prevention of pathological fractures, and return of mobility can be achieved with radiation to metastatic lesions from a variety of tumours including breast, lung and prostate tumours. Palliative radiotherapy is also given for the relief of CNS symptoms caused by brain metastases or spinal cord compression. Haemorrhage, ulceration and fungating lesions can be reduced effectively, and in some cases eliminated, by palliative radiotherapy. It may also be used to prevent the emergence of potentially symptomatic lesions before they become a problem. Examples include the treatment of a mediastinal mass that threatens to produce superior vena cava obstruction and treatment of a vertebral lesion when spinal cord compression is impending.

The type, duration and method of delivery of radiotherapy will depend upon many factors and is tailored to individual requirements. Curative regimens may continue over many weeks and be very exhausting for the patient, whereas doses given for palliation may be very low and are sometimes delivered in a single treatment.

Principles of action

Radiation is given in the form of X-ray photons, electrons or gamma rays. When a radiation beam strikes an atom, it frees electrons from that atom – a process known as *ionization*. This process requires energy, and this comes from the radiation beam or *source*. Energy is thus transferred to the newly-released electrons which then interact with neighbouring atoms and cause further ionizations, until all energy is dissipated. It is this ionization that accounts for the biological and chemical changes resulting from radiotherapy treatments. Cellular function is disrupted first by damage to the DNA so that the cell is unable to repair itself, and secondly through the formation of free radicals which disrupt the chromosome structure. The radiation affects both cancer and normal cells, but the normal cells are more able to recover. The principles of the cellular response to radiation may be summarized as the four Rs:

- *Repair* – of sublethal damage by some cells between fractions. Some cells are able to repair themselves, but not all
- *Redistribution* – cells enter different phases of the cell cycle including resting cells which re-enter the cell cycle
- *Repopulation* – cells move into spaces and become less hypoxic
- *Reoxygenation* – as the total cell population becomes depleted, those that are left have more space, become better oxygenated and are therefore more susceptible to radiation.

This response forms the basis of radiotherapy treatments that are planned to give the maximum dose to the tumour with minimal effects on normal tissues. The radiation dose is defined as the amount of energy absorbed per unit mass of tissue and is measured in Gray (Gy). The total treatment dose is delivered in fractions: the small, sub-lethal damage that occurs after each fraction allows normal cells to be repaired before the next fraction of treatment.

There is considerable variability in the degree of radiosensitivity of different tissues, with eyes, lungs, ovaries and testes being very sensitive and others, such as bone, connective tissue, liver, and thyroid, less so. The least radiosensitive tissues are those that are composed of cells that divide infrequently, such as brain, spinal cord and muscle. A number of chemical and thermal modifiers of radiation are currently being studied in clinical trials. Developments in such approaches could make many tumours that are now considered radioresistant more amenable to control with radiotherapy. An increasing number of protocols now combine radiotherapy and chemotherapy, for example in patients with advanced head and neck cancer or for cervical cancer.

Methods of administration

The ionizing beams used in radiotherapy are either electrically produced or come from naturally occurring or manufactured radioisotopes. The use of external-beam irradiation is often referred to as *teletherapy* and most commonly it is delivered by a linear accelerator machine (linac) which is used to direct a beam of high-energy photons or electrons to the site to be treated. The dose of radiotherapy that can be given to the cancer or tissue being treated is maximized by using two or more radiation fields which enables the maximum radiation dose to be delivered where the beams intersect at the target site.

Accuracy is essential to avoid irradiating normal tissue and vital structures as much as is possible. Treatment planning is a meticulous and often lengthy affair, using a *simulator* machine and frequently CT to enhance the accuracy of the planned tumour dose. When the final plans have been made, it is important that the same dose is delivered at each treatment. This is achieved by the positioning of the treatment source with reference to body contours and ensuring

that this is consistent at each treatment. The treatment area is usually marked by a small tattoo on the skin and the person needs to remain completely still during the actual treatment. When sensitive structures are adjacent to the treatment area as is the case when irradiating the head and neck area, it is necessary to immobilize the individual and thus the treatment area further by use of a plastic shell. The moulding of this shell may be a particularly traumatic aspect of the planning and subsequent treatment period, and is probably beyond most people's previous knowledge and experience. Careful preparation and exploration of individual fears or concerns is vital at all stages, with continual review and reassessment once treatment has started.

External-beam radiotherapy is delivered via a series of fractionated doses and the conventional fractionation is in 2-Gy treatment doses. This is usually delivered 5 days per week over a 4 to 6-week period, depending on the total dose required. However, there is some research evidence to suggest that some tumours have the opportunity to grow whilst treatment is being delivered. For this reason there is interest in *continuous hyperfractionated accelerated radiotherapy* (CHART), which uses two or three treatment fractions in a day over a shorter period of time overall (e.g. 2–3 weeks). Hall (1995) emphasizes the importance of patient education and understanding of potential side-effects in enabling patients to tolerate such treatment regimens.

Another form of treatment involves the use of *sealed* radioactive sources, which are placed close to a tumour; this is called *brachytherapy*. In this case, a high dose of radiation is received by the tumour and less by the surrounding tissues. Sources can be temporarily implanted directly into small tumours (such as those in the tongue, lip or breast) in the form of interstitial treatment; placed in body cavities via the use of applicators (as in intracavitary treatments for cervical and uterine cancers) or placed intraluminally for cancers of the bronchus or oesophagus. Some radioisotopes or *unsealed* sources may be administered orally or parenterally, for example iodine-131 for the treatment of thyroid tumours and strontium-89 for multiple bony metastases.

Low dose interstitial brachytherapy for localized prostate cancers may also be delivered by the permanent implantation of 50–100 small radioactive pellets or seeds containing radioactive iodine or palladium into the prostate gland. These seeds emit radiation at a low dose over a period of months and are virtually inactive after a year. Because the prostate gland absorbs the majority of radiation dose, patients can be discharged the same day with minimal restrictions.

Radiation safety principles

All hospitals and other institutions that use X-ray equipment and other radioactive sources operate within national guidelines and local policies for radiation protection. Hospitals that have extensive equipment and facilities for radiotherapy treatment will have a medical physics department and radiation protection team who are responsible for the maintenance and storage of equipment and radioactive sources. There will also be a radiation protection service, which, amongst other activities, monitors the amount of radiation to which therapy radiographers, nurses and other workers are exposed. Personnel are provided with monitoring badges that measure the amount of radiation exposure. The dose received is calculated at regular intervals, with records kept of the cumulative dose. The badge itself provides no protection at all; it simply measures exposure. In order to ensure accurate reading, the badge should be worn only by the designated individual, kept within the working environment and changed at the designated time.

When caring for people using an internal source of radiation, all precautions need to be taken to reduce exposure to radiation. Three principles are important in taking adequate radiation precautions:

● *Time* – spend as little time as possible near the source
● *Distance* – keep as far away as possible from the source
● *Shielding* – protect self and the environment.

The principle of *shielding* is more readily employed in the handling of displaced radioactive sources, excreta collection and disposal, and disposal of linen, dressings and equipment contaminated with radioactive solutions. Because shielding from gamma radiation requires 6-mm thick lead or 10-cm thick concrete, it is usually impractical to expect that much physical care can be given from behind such a shield. The lead aprons used in diagnostic radiology are not of sufficient thickness to stop gamma rays and cannot protect the caregiver from exposure when caring for individuals with radium or caesium sources. For example, in the rooms of patients with encapsulated sources there should be a special container into which the sources can be placed if they become dislodged. If a source does dislodge, nurses must use 12-inch forceps and not the hands to place it in the container provided. Contaminated linen, equipment, dressings and excreta are usually a safety hazard only when metabolized radiation therapy is employed (e.g. iodine-131). The decontamination of these items is necessary before disposal or reuse.

Hospitals that offer brachytherapy treatments should have specially designed facilities that offer a high degree of protection to staff and other patients and where patients can stay for the duration of treatment. The extent of safety precautions that are necessary during use of internal sources is dictated by the energy of the isotope. The widespread use of remote afterloading equipment such as the high dose rate or low dose rate Selectron machine, allows sources to be transferred automatically to and from pre-placed applicators at the push of a button and has eliminated the need for nurses to restrict time spent in contact with the patient. However, necessary care should be well planned and expedited to minimize the time spent at the bedside, while still providing for the person's needs so that treatment times are not prolonged.

Effects of radiation on body tissues and organ systems

Several specific components determine the effect of radiation on tissues: the *dose*, the fractionation, time and volume,

and the area treated. Dose–time–volume interrelationships are as follows: (1) the greater the dose, the shorter the time of onset of any reaction; and (2) the larger the treatment area, the more potentially severe the reaction.

Except for those systemic effects that are described below, radiation side-effects are seen only in the tissues and organ systems that are within or immediately adjacent to the treatment field. Thus, an individual receiving treatment to the mediastinum will not develop radiation-induced diarrhoea, nor will an individual receiving treatment to an abdominal field lose scalp hair. Similarly, individuals undergoing brachytherapy will develop reactions to treatment that vary with the site, dose, volume and energy of the source. Side-effects from radiation will vary from individual to individual and therefore careful monitoring and an individualized plan of care needs to be developed and implemented.

Both the immediate or *acute* effects of treatment and the *late* effects must be considered in any discussion of the effect of radiation on tissues. In general, acute effects are seen within the first 6 months after treatment and are due to cell damage in which mitotic activity is altered in some way. If acute effects are not reversible, late or permanent tissue changes occur. These late effects can be attributed to the organism's attempt to heal or repair the damage caused by the radiation. These may be quite debilitating and cause a great deal of distress, such as brachial plexus damage following treatment for breast cancer (Ash 1999).

General side-effects of radiotherapy

The skin

The outer layer of skin (epidermis) is composed of several layers of cells, with mature non-dividing cells at the surface and proliferating cells at the base. Normal mature cells are constantly being shed from the skin surface and replaced by new cells from the basal layer. This continuous state of reproductive activity accounts for the high radiosensitivity of skin. Although the skin may be the primary site of radiation (as in skin cancer), it is also irradiated when any other site within the body is treated because radiation must pass through whatever tissues it encounters before reaching the target site. To assess pathophysiological changes and plan care accordingly, it is helpful to think in terms of cross-sectional anatomy. The entry point for external radiation is known as the *portal*. The radiation then passes through all tissues and organs encompassed in the treatment volume, and *exits* on the opposite side of the body.

Acute radiation reactions begin after a dose of 4–5 Gy, but evidence of skin damage is not normally visible until 10–14 days into treatment coinciding with the time it takes for the cells to migrate from the basal layer to the surface. For a similar reason skin reactions will not reach a peak until after the completion of treatment and will not start to improve until about 2 weeks after treatment has finished. Depending on the site irradiated and equipment used, skin at the exit site may also be affected.

Radiation skin reactions are caused by the inflammatory response that results from the breakdown of basal cells in the epidermis. The skin initially compensates by trying to replace damaged cells through increased mitotic activity. Radiotherapy skin reactions may be classified on a scale of 0–3 (see Table 11.5), healing may be slow, but is usually complete and leaves minimal evidence of the acute damage except for the changes in pigmentation due to destruction of melanocytes. In the longer term, and depending on the dose the skin has been exposed to, there may be some fibrosis of underlying collagen leading to indentation and occasionally telangiectasia is evident (visible spidery red lines on the skin surface which are dilated capillaries caused by fibrosis of the blood vessels).

Sebaceous glands and sweat glands within the treatment area are also damaged by radiotherapy and their function may be reduced or stop altogether. Irradiated skin will remain susceptible to delayed healing and this should be taken into account if there is subsequent surgery within the area exposed to radiation.

It is important to note in certain areas such as the head and neck, breast and chest wall, that skin is more commonly affected because treatment is targeted at tissue just below the surface. Areas containing skin folds such as the groin, gluteal fold, axilla and under the breasts, also exhibit a greater and often earlier reaction to radiation owing to the natural warmth, moistness and friction in these areas. An inappropriate term for this type of reaction is a radiation 'burn', as this term implies accidental or unexpected damage, neither of which should take place in a controlled therapeutic setting. Ulceration and necrosis are very rare complications with modern skin sparing radiotherapy machines and techniques.

Hair

Radiation affects all rapidly growing cells; the hair roots are no exception. Hair, after receiving threshold doses, becomes loose and may be pulled out painlessly or fall out spontaneously. This will apply to body hair within a treatment field as well as hair on the head. Generally hair loss occurs during treatment or shortly thereafter and re-growth generally occurs in 2–3 months. Hair loss may be permanent if high doses of radiation are given to the area. The loss of head hair (alopecia) is traumatic to most people regardless of whether they are prepared for this change in body image. The needless fear of this loss is equally traumatic, and if patients are receiving treatments to areas that do not include the scalp they should be reassured that hair loss will not occur as a result of treatment.

Haematopoietic system

Bone marrow and lymphoid tissues are highly radiosensitive. The greatest effect is on the stem cells, while mature non-dividing blood cells in the circulating bloodstream are relatively insensitive to radiation. When large areas of bone marrow in the adult are irradiated, including the ilia, vertebrae, ribs, skull, long bones and sternum, the number of circulating mature red blood cells, white blood cells and platelets decreases because production is suppressed. This reaction is more severe if previous or concomitant chemo-

Table 11.5 Assessment and management of radiotherapy skin reactions

Score	Description	Characteristics	Management
RTOG 0	No visible change		Advise to follow basic skin care guidelines Aqueous cream may be applied to promote comfort
RTOG 1	Faint or dull erythema	Pink, itching, warm, twinges similar to moderate sunburn	As above Use of aqueous cream is encouraged to soothe and moisturize
RTOG 2a	Tender or bright erythema with/without dry desquamation	Redness, tender, hot Very itchy, scaly and peeling similar to severe sunburn	As above Sparing use of a mild topical steroid cream such as hydrocortisone 1% may reduce itching but should be discontinued if the skin breaks or if there are signs of infection
RTOG 2b	Patchy moist desquamation, moderate oedema	Bright red patches, peeling oozing and painful	Continue as above for intact areas of the field Dress areas of moist desquamation using hydrogel, hydrocolloid or alginate dressings Dressings will need to be removed during treatment delivery Avoid adhesive and adherent dressings and use of tape to secure dressings as these may cause pain and epidermal stripping; tubular bandages or Netelast is preferable
RTOG 3	Confluent moist desquamation, pitting oedema	Extensive inflammation, blistered and sloughy There may be large amounts of exudate	As above Observe daily for signs of infection (sticky yellow/green increasing exudates and malodour, oedema and redness) Immuno-compromised patients may not demonstrate classic signs Topical antimicrobial dressings may be used but must not leave any residue on the treatment field that could interfere with the radiation dose (refer to manufacturer's information) Cellulitis spreading beyond the treatment field may require systemic antibiotics

therapy has been given. It is sometimes necessary to interrupt treatment for a few days to allow the bone marrow to recover.

Gastrointestinal system

The gastrointestinal tract, from mouth to rectum, is lined with mucous membrane that contains layers of cells. A large proportion of these cells are undifferentiated and mitotic, and are thus extremely sensitive to radiation. Oral mucous membranes may develop mucositis, usually after 2–3 weeks of fractionated radiation therapy. The mucous membrane will initially have increased redness, which will progress to yellowish-white patches. These patches will eventually become a pseudomembrane covering large areas of the mucosa. Salivary function is altered, and the patient may experience soreness, pain on swallowing, hoarseness, dryness, or changes in the sense of taste. If the oesophagus, stomach or bowel are within the irradiated field, the patient

may experience nausea, vomiting or diarrhoea. When the oesophagus is within the field, painful swallowing, dryness and spasms may occur. Abdominal irradiation is frequently associated with nausea, with greater exposures causing vomiting, abdominal cramping and diarrhoea. These can lead to electrolyte imbalances, dehydration and weight loss. If the anal sphincter is in the field of radiation, the distressing symptom of tenesmus (painful ineffectual straining) also sometimes occurs.

Respiratory system

Acute radiation pneumonitis may be asymptomatic or cause a hacking cough or mild chest discomfort. With moderate levels of radiation, acute changes such as shortness of breath may subside after 3–4 weeks. Large doses (75% of lung tissue exposed to 20 Gy or more) will often cause permanent damage, with the degree of disability related to the amount and condition of remaining untreated lung tissue.

Reproductive system

The germinal cells of the testes are very sensitive to even small doses of radiation. Small doses will cause temporary halting of sperm production; 5–10 Gy will probably cause permanent sterility. The secretion of testosterone is not affected, thus sexual characteristics are unchanged. It is possible to shield the testes from radiation damage in many cases.

Radiation to the ovaries produces either temporary or permanent sterility, depending on the age of the person being treated and the dose of radiation. Permanent sterilization will occur at doses of 6–12 Gy, and older women are sterilized at lower doses than younger women. In addition to sterility, hormonal changes (especially loss of oestrogen production) and early menopause may occur. The ovaries can be surgically repositioned in some patients to reduce ovarian exposure during pelvic radiation, a procedure known as oophoropexy.

Systemic effects

Generalized symptoms that commonly appear during radiation treatment are fatigue, weakness, headache, nausea and anorexia. These symptoms are more frequently discussed in the nursing literature than the medical literature, and their aetiology is not well understood. One suggested cause of generalized symptoms is the rapid breakdown of cells destroyed by radiation. Cell breakdown would release toxic metabolites and end-products, which accumulate faster than they can be excreted. These chemicals may act as toxic foreign proteins, causing some degree of shock. Others suggest that these symptoms result from an increased metabolic rate, from the body's attempt to restore homeostasis, or from the emotional stresses of daily treatment for a life-threatening illness.

Late effects

These complications may appear several months to a few years after the completion of treatment. Most late complications reflect diminished vascular supply and increased fibrosis in heavily irradiated areas. Unlike acute reactions, these complications are often chronic, and nursing management is symptomatic and based on the degree of functional impairment. The late complications of radiation therapy are summarized in Table 11.6.

Caring for people receiving external radiation therapy

During a course of radiation therapy, certain treatment-related side-effects can be expected to develop, most of which are site-specific as well as dependent on volume, dose fractionation, total dose and individual differences. Many symptoms do not develop until approximately 10–14 days after the start of treatment, and some do not subside until 2 weeks or more after treatment has ended. Patients need to be assessed regularly while on treatment. In particular, the skin over the area receiving radiation as well as the exit portal needs to be examined regularly, and discussions held about fatigue, weakness and nutritional problems.

The care management described in the following sections reflects the general consensus from the literature and the current evidence base for practice. A particularly useful text for further reading is *The Royal Marsden Manual of Clinical Nursing Procedures* (Dougherty and Lister 2004). Specific approaches and treatments may vary from institution to institution, and between different medical practitioners.

Skin reactions

Guidance on radiotherapy skin care is often based on local protocols and practice and published research evidence is limited. The Royal College of Radiographers (Glean et al 2001) and NHS Quality Improvement Scotland (2004) have produced skin care guidelines based on a consensus view of best practice that is aimed at minimizing symptoms and promoting comfort. Assessment of the patient's risk of developing skin reactions, patient education; regular review and implementation of appropriate management strategies, are the key to success. Risk factors to be considered prior to commencing treatment are outlined in Table 11.7. Information for patients should be provided both verbally and in written form explaining the nature and potential for skin reactions, their management and self-care strategies. Basic skin care advice that may be incorporated into patient information is summarized in Box 11.2. Recommendations for the management of radiotherapy skin reactions are based on using an assessment tool developed by the Radiation Therapy Oncology Group (Glean et al 2001) and follows the principles of moist wound healing (see Table 11.5).

Bone marrow depression

When large volumes of active bone marrow are irradiated (especially the pelvis or spine in the adult), the effect on the marrow can be quite significant. Other areas of concern when large fields are treated include the sternum, ribs, long bones and skull. During simulation and treatment planning, provision is made for shielding as much of this active marrow as possible without compromising the treatment; thus the majority of people receiving therapy are able to tolerate a course of treatment without experiencing bone marrow

Table 11. 6　Late or delayed effects of radiation therapy

Tissue	Result
Skin	Fibrosis, atrophy and pigmentation changes over irradiated areas; telangiectasia Acute recall reaction may occur after the administration of certain antineoplastic drugs such as dactinomycin
Gastrointestinal system	Oral fibrosis, decreased taste acuity or the loss of taste sensation, xerostomia, dental caries Chronic enteritis, intestinal fistula formation
Lung	Radiation pneumonitis
Blood and bone marrow	Anaemia Leukaemia
Eyes	Cataracts
Thyroid	Hypothyroidism Thyroid cancer
Reproductive system	Temporary or permanent sterility Premature menopause in women Fertility may return to normal depending on the dose of irradiation administered to the gametes and age
Urinary system (bladder)	Reduced capacity Chronic bleeding
Central nervous system	Transient or widespread demyelination

Table 11.7　Risk factors for developing radiotherapy skin reactions

Intrinsic/patient factors	Extrinsic factors
Age (rate of cell division in the epidermis decreases with age causing thinning of the epidermis) Skin diversity due to ethnic origin, previous extensive exposure to UV light; radiation or hormonal status Co-existing disease, e.g. diabetes, psoriasis Nutritional status Obesity Smoking	Energy of the beam used (orthovoltage beams cause the most skin reactions) Volume of tissue irradiated Fractionation Total dose Site of entry and exit beams Radiotherapy given in combination with chemotherapy Application of chemical irritants, e.g. deodorant or perfume and aftershave Mechanical irritation – anything causing friction Thermal irritation – from use of ice packs or heat

depression. Nonetheless, a full blood cell count needs to be done at regular intervals for all individuals receiving radiation therapy. Particular attention should be paid to this when individuals are receiving concomitant chemotherapy or have had extensive chemotherapy before irradiation. The nursing management of bone marrow depression is discussed later in this chapter and is outlined in Box 11.3.

Xerostomia

Xerostomia (dry mouth) may result from radiation to the salivary glands or portions of them. Xerostomia results in difficulty talking, eating and swallowing, and can be very distressing (Feber 1995). It also predisposes the individual to a variety of other oral problems. Although artificial salivas are available and pilocarpine tablets may be of value in stimulating residual salivary function, simple measures such as frequent sips of drinks or chewing sugar-free chewing gum may be equally effective.

Radiation caries

Although it is a potential late effect of irradiation to the mouth and oropharynx, radiation caries can be greatly reduced or avoided by proper care before, during and after a course of treatment. Absence of, or a decrease in saliva and the altered pH produced by treatment promote tooth decay. Before the start of therapy, a thorough dental examination

Box 11.2 Skin care advice for the person receiving radiotherapy

Goal

The person will experience minimal skin irritation in the affected areas (entry and exit sites)

Type of irritant to be avoided	Recommendations
Mechanical	Minimize friction during bathing/showering; shower gently; avoid rubbing the area with a washcloth or towel; pat dry with a soft clean towel
	Use an electric shaver rather than wet shaving
	Wear loose fitting, natural fibre, soft clothing
	Following mastectomy a soft prosthesis should be worn during treatment
	When the scalp is irradiated hair should be very gently combed/brushed
	Avoid scratching, rubbing or massaging skin
	Avoid use of adhesive tape on the area
Chemical	Use unperfumed soap/shampoo and rinse off thoroughly
	Avoid applying any deodorant and all perfumed products to the treatment area
	Use a mild detergent to wash clothing
	Apply only products recommended by radiotherapy team.
	Avoid use of wax or hair-removing creams; perming or colouring agents that may come into contact with the area of irradiated skin
Thermal	Use tepid/warm water on the area
	Avoid exposure to extremes of temperature
	Avoid direct application of heat or cold to the area (e.g. use of a hair dryer when the head is treated)
	Any cream or gel applied to the area should be used at room temperature
Sun exposure	Protect the area from direct sun exposure during treatment and until any reaction has settled
	Use a high factor sun block – at least SPF factor 15 or above
Swimming	Caution should be taken and some centres may advise against this as chlorine in the water has a drying effect on the skin
	Shower after swimming

and prophylaxis should be carried out. If extensive decay and general poor dentition exist, full mouth extraction is usually the treatment of choice. However, if teeth are in good repair, a vigorous preventive programme should be initiated to protect them from the late effects of radiation. This would include brushing the teeth with a soft-bristled brush several times a day, and a daily application of fluoride gel.

Oesophagitis and dysphagia

When the oesophagus is located in the treatment field, inflammation and ulceration of the mucous membranes may occur. This condition produces difficulty in swallowing as well as a great deal of discomfort, which patients experience as a severe and constant pain located in the substernal area. Management focuses on the need to provide relief from pain and the maintenance of nutritional status which in severe cases may necessitate tube or PEG feeding.

Tenesmus, cystitis, urethritis

Although infrequent, tenesmus, cystitis and urethritis do occur in some individuals receiving pelvic irradiation. Tenesmus of the anal or urinary sphincter produces a persistent sensation of the need to evacuate the bowel or bladder. Relief can sometimes be obtained from gastrointestinal and urinary

antispasmodic and anticholinergic agents. The problem may persist, however, until after the course of treatment has ended. Cystitis and urethritis resulting from radiation to the bladder areas are distressing to the person being treated. A clean voided urine specimen for culture and sensitivity should be obtained and appropriate antibiotic therapy instituted if indicated. Usually, infection is not found and treatment consists of urinary antispasmodics for symptomatic relief. A high fluid intake is encouraged.

Other more general side-effects of mucositis, nausea and vomiting, diarrhoea, anorexia and fatigue are considered later in the chapter.

Caring for people receiving brachytherapy

Patients who are receiving brachytherapy need a careful and detailed explanation of the treatment and subsequent care required. The goals of treatment are concerned with:

● assessment of the patient's suitability for the treatment
● radiation protection measures
● the need to promote patient comfort
● management of immediate and late side-effects
● psychological support.

Patients need to know what they will experience when the radiation source is applied or administered and removed, and any restrictions on physical activities need to be explained and planned for. Patients having intracavitary or interstitial treatment will be confined to bed during treatment. High-dose-rate treatment takes just a few minutes and the patient may just be sedated during treatment but low-dose-rate treatment may require 1–2 days of treatment in bed. These patients will be catheterized and may need both analgesia and sedation as the implants and applicators are quite uncomfortable. Analgesia should always be available prior to removal of applicators and gynaecological packing. Other medication may be required to control symptoms of nausea and vomiting and to prevent bowel motions (for gynaecological patients). Patients also need to be prepared for inactivity and have access to TV, radio or other suitable diversional activities. The need for physiological monitoring is governed by the patient's condition but is normally kept to a minimum. The position of applicators and implants should be checked at regular intervals to ensure they have not become dislodged. If this should occur the appropriate staff should be notified immediately and radiation safety procedures followed. Case 11.1 describes the care of a patient having Selectron treatment.

CASE Aretha Oluwale is a 54-year-old married nursery assistant who was diagnosed with stage III cervical cancer. Aretha had a 5-week course of external beam radiotherapy combined with cisplatin chemotherapy and was booked for one intracavitary treatment on the low dose rate Selectron machine. Aretha was extremely apprehensive about this. She had spoken to other women in the clinic who described the experience as being very unpleasant. The clinical nurse specialist explained the procedure involved in detail and showed Aretha the room where she would have the treatment and the machine to which she would be connected. As well as encouraging questions at the time she offered Aretha a leaflet about the treatment and stressed that she was available by phone if she had any further queries or worries.

When Aretha was admitted the nurses checked that she understood that whilst treatment was in progress they would be unable to enter the room, but that they would be able to see her via the CCTV and speak on an intercom link. They explained again how the radioactive sources would be transferred from the machine into the applicators that would be inserted in theatre and also that the treatment would be interrupted as little as possible in order not to prolong the treatment time. Aretha was very tearful as her husband left as she would not see him until the treatment was over.

As she had been experiencing quite a lot of diarrhoea since finishing external radiotherapy the doctor wrote her up for codeine to prevent her having a bowel motion during treatment. Later that day Aretha went to theatre and had three applicators inserted, one into her uterus and two positioned in the vagina. These were clamped together and

held in place by packing. After an X-ray to check they were correctly positioned Aretha was brought back to her room feeling very groggy and disorientated. She was conscious of discomfort and deep pressure within her pelvis and was reassured that she had a catheter in place to drain urine. After she had been given analgesia, Aretha was connected to the machine and before the nurses left the room they checked that Aretha had everything she needed within easy reach including plenty of drinks, her glasses, the call bell, books, CD player, watch and a sick bowl. After they left the room Aretha heard some noises from the machine outside and knew her treatment had started.

The time passed very slowly and Aretha found her inability to move around in bed very distressing. It made her feel panicky at times and she tried to listen to relaxation tapes to keep her anxiety under control. Every 4 hours the nurses stopped the treatment to check the applicators and to help her change her position and relieve the pressure on her back. They gave Aretha regular analgesia for backache and a sleeping pill, although she was very worried about accidentally dislodging the applicators and slept very little. Unfortunately there was no video or DVD player available but Aretha had access to Patientline so was able to watch TV and speak to her husband and daughter at regular intervals. Aretha didn't feel much like eating but kept up her fluid intake as she had been advised.

When the treatment ended the nurses offered Aretha the use of Entonox or a pain-relieving injection prior to removing the applicators. Aretha opted for the Entonox and the packing and applicators were removed without difficulty, although Aretha was most surprised at the length of packing used. She was relieved to be able to get up and have a shower. Aretha was allowed home once she was passing urine normally, although she was warned that she might experience transient discomfort when urinating for a couple of days. Before she went home the nurse specialist gave Aretha a set of vaginal dilators and explained how to use these to prevent the formation of vaginal adhesions. A few days later the nurse specialist rang Aretha to check all was well. During her follow-up appointment Aretha was reassured that she could start having intercourse again as soon as she felt ready and was encouraged to voice any concerns that she had.

Twelve months on Aretha is well, although she still experiences bouts of diarrhoea and colicky pain as a result of the radiotherapy. She had a brief scare when she noticed some spotting after intercourse (her original presenting symptom) but was reassured at the time and following a vaginal examination, that this was likely to have been due to vaginal adhesions, not disease and she was encouraged to recommence using her dilators regularly.

Patients who are being treated with unsealed sources such as iodine-131 will be confined to their treatment room but are able to mobilize and should have access to their own toilet and washing facilities. Education will involve advice over personal hygiene and explaining the need for a minimum of personal items, jewellery, etc., to be brought into the treatment area, as these may become contaminated. Urine is especially radioactive and the toilet should be flushed twice after use and hands washed thoroughly. Showering at least once a day removes radioactive perspiration. Disposable crockery and cutlery are provided and used bed linen must be monitored for radioactive contamination before going to the laundry. Nurses attending to these patients must wear disposable gloves, overshoes and protective clothing and use a digital dosimeter to record the amount of radiation received. Care should be kept to a minimum to reduce exposure and the principles of time, distance and shielding applied with responsibilities being shared amongst staff on duty. Medication may be required to control diarrhoea or vomiting as this could result in a contamination problem as well as being distressing. Patients will be assessed individually prior to discharge by medical physics staff and given specific advice regarding precautions to be observed. Medical physics will also be responsible for checking the room for contamination before cleaning takes place.

Patients who have internal sources of radiation are usually very sensitive to the fact that they can cause harm to others. This causes an increase in anxiety, especially as they have no way of detecting that this harm is occurring. They are also anxious about the harm the radiation is doing to their own normal tissues. Explaining the controls designed to protect others and also clarifying and reinforcing information about treatments and side-effects may allay this anxiety. It is also important for patients to know that they are no longer radioactive once a radioactive source has been removed.

Family members also often have a difficult time during internal radiation because of the enforced separation. Again, increased information and support may be helpful in allaying concerns and fears. Some family members may find it difficult to contemplate exposure to radiation despite explanations of radiation protection measures, in which case telephone communication can be encouraged.

COMPLEMENTARY THERAPIES

The term 'complementary' has been used widely in recent years to encompass any and all therapies that may be described as being outside orthodox or conventional medical practice. Other words used include; alternative, traditional, natural, fringe and unorthodox, and even in some instances quack. The term 'unproven methods' is used in many medical papers, reflecting the concern of many orthodox medical practitioners that most of the therapies are 'unproven' by scientific research methods. Generally, 'complementary therapies' may be viewed as those that are used *alongside* orthodox medical treatments and 'alternative therapies' as those that are used *instead* of conventional treatment approaches.

Whatever terminology is used, it is clear that there is an increasing interest in the use of the wide range of alternative and complementary therapies that are available. Some may be formulated specifically for the person with cancer, whereas others have wide application in both health and illness. To differing degrees, all therapies aim to enhance health and well-being by stimulating the self-healing capacities of the body. Such therapies include dietary manipulation, herbal medicines, immunizations, vitamin therapies and psychological techniques. People who seek these treatments are often terminally ill and may be particularly attracted to therapies that appear to offer the possibility of respite, or even cure. Often the drive to try alternative treatment regimens, which may be quite rigorous and demanding, comes from the family or significant others. While a patient may not experience any physical harm from this type of therapy, they may be at risk of being given unrealistic hope, leading to emotional distress, and of being financially burdened by the high cost of some therapies.

Some people may turn to unproven methods because of dissatisfaction with conventional medical treatment. There is often a degree of tension between conventional and unconventional practitioners, with the former believing that the latter are of no proven value and that they may lead patients to abandon potentially effective treatment regimens. Conversely, promoters of unproven methods may attack the medical and scientific community and be reluctant to share information about the methods employed. In either case, practitioners may be equally dogmatic, and perhaps a more constructive approach is to seek to combine elements from both as illustrated in Case 11.2.

CASE Jane Miller is 48 and a freelance translator who was diagnosed 3 years previously with bowel cancer. She initially presented to her GP with right-sided abdominal pain and sickness and whilst awaiting an urgent appointment to see a hospital consultant, ended up in A&E because of the severity of pain she was experiencing. Jane made a very good recovery from a right-sided hemicolectomy and was discharged 5 days post surgery. Histology showed a Duke's Stage C cancer of the caecum and Jane commenced adjuvant chemotherapy of irinotecan with 5 flurouracil (modified de Gramont regimen) which Jane found very difficult to tolerate. This regimen involved having 12 treatments over 6 months with the drugs being given via a PICC line and a Baxter infusor which allowed Jane to be at home during the 5FU infusion. Her main problems were: nausea which she describes as being horrid and different to anything she had experienced before and overwhelming fatigue which lasted virtually throughout the cycle. She experienced slight mouth soreness which was mainly a result of cracks in the corners of her mouth (angular chelitis) but her blood count remained satisfactory throughout the course. Jane lost all her hair on this treatment and was surprised to find it grew back wavy.

Unfortunately a CT scan 6 months later showed evidence of both peritoneal spread and liver metastases. At this stage, Jane with the support of her husband, opted to try a nutritional therapy, the Plaskett diet (a vegan diet with lots of fresh juices), which she tried for 3 months. The disease continued to progress unabated and Jane then agreed to have two courses of oxaliplatin chemotherapy which she found more tolerable than the irinotecan. The oxaliplatin gave her pins and needles in her feet. It also failed to demonstrate a response in terms of a reduction in the size of the mass in her pelvis or in the liver deposits and Jane is now on a combination of capecitabine which she will take for 14 days and oxaliplatin given on day one of a 3-week cycle. She expects to have an ultrasound after the second cycle to assess response.

Jane is fully aware that her disease is beyond cure and thinks she might be tempted to take her chances with another alternative therapy if there is no response. She has very little pain at present and takes oromorph 10–20 mgs p.r.n. Until Jane developed cancer she and her partner Jonathon had little interest in alternative therapies. Jonathon has done a lot of research on the internet and has encouraged and supported Jane in her use of nutritional therapy. She currently takes a variety of dietary supplements and uses phenergan and fish oils to combat nausea. She avoids steroid drugs and for this reason only takes granisetron as a pre-medication prior to chemotherapy. Both Jane and Jonathon find the nutritional advice given by hospital dieticians, with its focus on the need to maintain weight with a high protein and calorie intake, disappointing. They would like to have been given more dietary advice about foods that may themselves directly inhibit cancer cell growth. Fortunately Jane's oncologist has been very supportive of their request. Jane has continued to work when she can and is grateful that Jonathon runs his business from home and they have no financial difficulties. They have no children but Jane's mother and brother and family live locally and are very supportive.

If Jane decides to have no more chemotherapy, she and Jonathon may consider referral to her local hospice which offers patients and carers an individualized 6-week programme designed to support people coming to terms with metastatic and untreatable disease through a combination of psychological, physical or complementary therapies.

The Foundation for Integrated Health (Tavares 2003) outlines guidance for taking forward the integration of complementary and alternative therapies into mainstream health care. It is becoming increasingly common practice for patients to be offered complementary therapies such as aromatherapy, reflexology and massage whilst undergoing chemotherapy and radiotherapy. Patients having therapies on NHS premises should be reassured that their therapists are operating within a clinical governance framework whereas provision outside of the NHS or hospice setting is largely unregulated.

There are many problems inherent in research into the effectiveness of complementary therapies. Conventional medicine tends to utilize the experimental design approach and incorporates such techniques as randomized controlled trials. However, this approach is not always helpful or possible in assessing the varied and individual response to

therapies. Research methods that utilize or incorporate a qualitative approach may be more useful here (Corner and Harewood 2004). The difficulty of uncontrolled variables is a major challenge to researchers in this area and there has been limited rigorous evaluation of complementary therapies for people with cancer. Fellowes et al (2005) found some evidence of benefit for cancer patients in terms of well-being, reduction in anxiety, pain and nausea with aromatherapy and massage.

To become a competent practitioner in most of these therapies, several years of training and practice is required. However, some essential elements of certain of these practices may be successfully incorporated into nursing practice and there is growing enthusiasm for this among many nurses. Some health authorities have developed operational policies to clarify roles and responsibilities, and to ensure good standards of practice.

It is understandable that, when faced with a potentially life-threatening disease, a person may seek out any avenue that appears to offer hope, comfort and even survival. For many individuals, complementary therapies and alternative treatments offer an opportunity to regain some choice and control over a life disrupted by disease and the unpleasant side-effects of conventional treatment. Through knowledge and understanding about alternative and complementary therapies, and empathic discussion, nurses may play a key role in guiding the patient away from desperate measures and towards helpful coping strategies and supportive therapies.

NURSING ASSESSMENT AND MANAGEMENT OF DISEASE AND TREATMENT-RELATED PROBLEMS

There is a wide range of treatment and disease-related problems in cancer, and these are discussed in this section along with suggestions for appropriate nursing management strategies. Although some needs and problems appear to be primarily physical, all aspects of cancer care and treatment also have psychosocial and emotional dimensions. Through an understanding of the meaning and significance of cancer-related problems, nurses can work in partnership with individuals to explore and identify effective coping strategies.

BONE MARROW DEPRESSION

Leucopenia is the depletion of white blood cells that often develops as a result of chemotherapy and sometimes radiotherapy, and that makes the patient very susceptible to infection. The risk of infection increases as the white cell count falls and following chemotherapy the count tends to fall to a nadir around 7–14 days post-treatment. Patients having chemotherapy should be given details by their chemotherapy nurse of who to contact at any time if they feel unwell and should also be informed about the signs and symptoms that are indicative of infection. Delay in starting antibiotic treatment can have serious implications. The greatest risk is associated with a neutrophil count of less than 0.5×10^9/L. A decrease in neutrophils to this level or below indicates the need for urgent measures to be instituted to minimize the risk of infection. These include the use of protective isolation facilities and processes to protect the patient from sources of infection. Regimens vary from centre to centre, but broadly include dietary restrictions, effective personal and oral hygiene, and the administration of various prophylactic pharmaceutical agents. The use of invasive procedures, and breaks in the normal protective mechanism such as the skin and mucous membranes, may precipitate infection.

Patients with severe and prolonged neutropenia, with a neutrophil count of 0.1×10^9/L or below, are in a potentially life-threatening situation through the potential to develop septicaemia or septic shock, which carries a significant mortality. The most common sites of infection are the respiratory tract, alimentary tract, skin and genitourinary tract. An increase in temperature above 38°C is the most common sign of infection in a neutropenic patient, although in some cases fever may be absent. Other features that may be indicative of neutropenic sepsis include shaking, irritability, confusion, drowsiness, hypotension and tachycardia which if untreated may lead to circulatory collapse.

In most situations, intravenous antimicrobial treatment is initiated immediately and continued until the patient is apyrexial and the bone marrow has recovered. Blood cultures will be taken and immediate action instigated to maintain adequate tissue perfusion with fluids oxygen and plasma expanders. Intensive support may be required and this is likely to be a very distressing experience for both patients and their families. Administration of colony-stimulating factors may assist the process of recovery where leucopenia is profound and prolonged.

Anaemia may be manifested by weakness, tiredness, pallor and shortness of breath. Chemotherapy-induced anaemia is usually a gradual process and may not be evident for several weeks after initiating chemotherapy. If patients are symptomatic due to anaemia, a transfusion of packed red cells will be given to alleviate symptoms whilst the marrow recovers. Recombinant human erythropoietin may be prescribed to shorten periods of extended anaemia.

Thrombocytopenia increases the risk of the patient bleeding because of the impairment of the blood clotting process. Signs of thrombocytopenia include ecchymoses, petechiae, blood in the urine or stool, vaginal bleeding or evidence of bleeding in other organs or systems. The sclera is a common site of haemorrhage. When the platelet count drops below 50×10^9/L spontaneous haemorrhage may occur, and this risk increases when the counts drop below 20×10^9/L. Platelet transfusions are given to support the patient until his or her own bone marrow starts to produce adequate numbers of platelets.

Nursing management of patients with bone marrow depression includes prevention and management of infection and bleeding, patient education, close monitoring, and implementation of preventive nursing care measures. These are outlined in Box 11.3.

Box 11.3 Nursing care of the person with bone marrow depression

Leucopenia and infection

Assessment

Assess the patient for signs and symptoms of infection:

- Monitor for signs and symptoms of sepsis.

- Fever > 38°C, hypotension, tachycardia, increased respiratory rate; chills, cold clammy extremities; irritability and restlessness

- Monitor the respiratory and genitourinary systems, skin and mucous membranes, and sites of peripheral and central venous catheters for infection

- Monitor white blood cell counts and the differential regularly. A neutrophil count of less than 0.5×10^9/L greatly increases the risk of infection

Patient problems and goals

- The major problem is the potential for infection, and consequently the goal is that the person will not develop infection

- The patient/carer knows the signs and symptoms of infection and is able to monitor and report on them

- The patient/carer will notify the appropriate member of the health team when symptoms occur

- The patient will be protected from nosocomial infection during the period of hospitalization

Nursing intervention

1 Provide effective patient education and information on signs and symptoms of infection, self-care measures, how to take an oral temperature, and 24-hour contact details to notify healthcare providers if infection is suspected

(continued)

Box 11.3 *Cont'd*

2 Minimize exposure to potential sources of infection:
   a) avoid crowds and persons with infectious diseases
   b) stagnant water (flower vases, respiratory equipment, humidifiers)
   c) faeces of animals

3 Instruct the patient in maintaining good hygiene:
   a) handwashing after toileting and before meals
   b) daily shower or bath

4 Maintain integrity of skin and mucous membranes:
   a) prevent injury of rectal mucosa by avoiding enemas, suppositories and rectal thermometers
   b) promote oral hygiene and prevent injury to oral mucosa by using a soft toothbrush
   c) use an electric razor
   d) avoid injections if at all possible

5 Avoid use of invasive equipment such as indwelling urinary catheters

6 When severely neutropenic (neutrophils less than 0.5×10^9/L) protective measures are required:
   a) institute protective isolation, e.g. single room
   b) strict handwashing before and after caring for neutropenic patients
   c) keep equipment for sole use of patient and maintain cleanliness of the room
   d) consider need for diet that avoids high-risk foods (soft ripened cheeses, uncooked eggs, raw fish and meat products, unpasteurized milk and dairy products, salads, etc.)

7 Administer antibiotics, antifungal and antiviral agents on time

8 Monitor temperature 4-hourly or more frequently as indicated

9 Take swabs from any suspect lesions, urine sputum and stool specimens and blood as required for culture and sensitivity

Thrombocytopenia and bleeding
Assessment
● Monitor the platelet count daily

● Monitor for signs and symptoms of bleeding, especially petechiae, bleeding gums, bruising, epistaxis, blood in urine, stool, emesis, heavy menstruation, intracranial bleeding, oozing from i.v. sites or other wounds

Patient problems and goals
● The principal potential problem is that of bleeding and the patient goal is therefore that bleeding will not occur

● The patient/carer can identify measures to prevent bleeding

● Signs and symptoms of minor and serious bleeding will be detected and reported

Nursing intervention
1 Avoid use of medications that alter platelet production and function, i.e. aspirin and aspirin-containing products, anticoagulants, non-steroidal antiinflammatory agents

2 When the platelet count is $< 50 \times 10^9$/L institute measures to prevent trauma and possible bleeding:
   a) avoid activities that could cause physical injury, e.g. contact sports
   b) use electric razors to shave, and soft tooth brush
   c) avoid rectal trauma, including enemas, suppositories, rectal temperature
   d) blowing of the nose should be gentle to avoid epistaxis

3 Avoid injections. If necessary, use a small needle and apply pressure after the injection for 3–5 minutes or until bleeding stops

4 Minimize venepunctures as much as possible

5 Observe for evidence of bleeding from open lesions, gums, urine, stools and sputum. Check for any areas of bruising or petichiae

6 Administer platelet transfusions as prescribed

GASTROINTESTINAL PROBLEMS

Nausea and vomiting

Nausea and vomiting are two of the most common and distressing sequelae of cancer and cancer therapy and inadequate control of nausea and vomiting results in complications such as dehydration, anorexia, malnutrition and metabolic disturbances. Nausea and vomiting results from stimulation of the vomiting centre in the brainstem and by a variety of mechanisms and these are shown in Figure 11.4. An understanding of these mechanisms assists in the choice of an appropriate medication.

The distress associated with nausea and vomiting is one of the most feared and disruptive side-effects of chemotherapy, to the extent that it may cause patients to be unable or unwilling to continue treatment (Rhodes et al 1995, Richardson 1991). Different cytotoxic agents have different emetogenic potential, so knowledge of these and details of patients' specific chemotherapy regimens are an essential part of the assessment process. In recent years there has been increased effort to develop pharmacological and non-pharmacological methods to prevent and control nausea and vomiting. In particular, the 5HT3 antagonists, (e.g. ondansetron and granisetron) have had a significant effect in minimizing acute chemotherapy-induced nausea and vomiting. Locally agreed protocols for anti-emetic use, include combinations of domperidone, metoclopramide, dexamethasone, 5HT3 antagonists and lorazepam based on the emetogenic potential of the chemotherapy regimen. Of particular concern is the need to avoid the development of anticipatory nausea and vomiting, which is caused by a conditioned response to stimuli associated with chemotherapy administration, such as the smell of the unit. The key to this is to prevent nausea and vomiting effectively from the beginning of treatment.

The symptoms of nausea and vomiting may result from a wide variety of physiological causes other than cancer chemotherapy. Causes include mechanical obstruction of the gastrointestinal tract, increased intracerebral pressure as a result of the tumour, fluid and electrolyte imbalances (hypercalcaemia, hyponatraemia, hypokalaemia, volume depletion), pharmacological agents (antibiotics, narcotics) and radiation therapy (particularly to the abdomen, pelvis, back and brain).

The majority of patients having radiotherapy experience little or no difficulty with this side-effect. When nausea does occur, it can usually be controlled by anti-emetics administered on a regular schedule and by adjusting the eating pattern so that treatment is given when the stomach

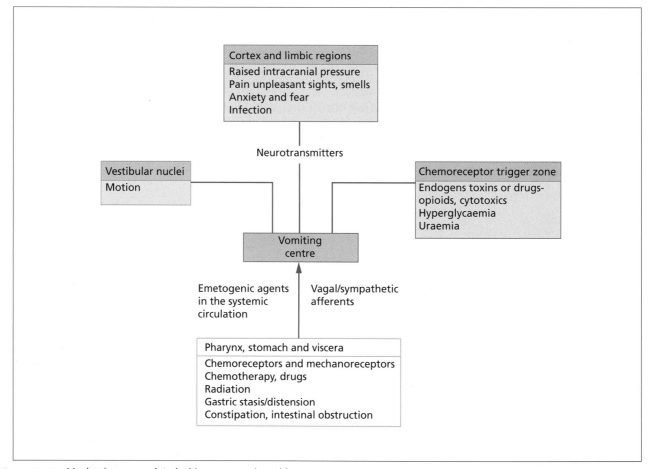

Figure 11.4 Mechanisms associated with nausea and vomiting.

is relatively empty. Delaying intake of a full meal until 3–4 hours after treatment is also helpful because nausea, if it occurs, will usually appear 1–3 hours after treatment.

Pharmacological management is based on the selection of an anti-emetic based on the likely cause, e.g. a prokinetic for gastric stasis, dexamethasone and cyclizine for raised intra-cranial pressure, haloperidol or a phenothiazine for morphine or hypercalcaemia-induced vomiting. Many of these drugs may be administered subcutaneously via a syringe driver when the patient is vomiting. Nursing care is directed at the prevention and active management of nausea and vomiting, and Richardson (1991) advocates the value of encouraging individuals to develop effective self-care strategies. Other interventions focus on the management of nutrition, hydration and comfort while the patient experiences nausea or vomiting.

Mucositis (stomatitis)

The terms *mucositis* and *stomatitis* are often used interchangeably to describe the inflammation, desquamation and ulceration of the oral mucous membrane that occurs as a result of either systemic chemotherapy or localized radiotherapy. The mucous membranes of the oral cavity sustain a great degree of trauma on a daily basis. The cells of these tissues must be highly proliferative to replace those that are continually damaged by thermal, mechanical, chemical and microbiological stressors. The fast-growing epithelial cells of the mouth and gastrointestinal tract are particularly susceptible to damage by chemotherapy and radiotherapy, firstly by direct action on cell metabolism and replication, and secondly indirectly as a result of generalized bone marrow suppression and increased susceptibility to infection and bleeding. Factors such as poor nutritional status, poor oral hygiene, or any other factor that causes dryness and/or trauma of the mucous membranes, increase the severity and the duration of mucositis. Loss of saliva, or *xerostomia*, exacerbates other problems and is a key problem, particularly for patients undergoing radiotherapy to the head and neck (see Case 11.3). *Oesophagitis* may also develop if the effects of treatment result in damaging or destroying epithelial cells in the oesophagus. As Gamble (1998) noted, the distress of mucositis is often underestimated and patients require considerable support to cope with symptoms. Nursing care is directed at managing comfort, nutrition and hydration, preventing infection and promoting oral hygiene.

CASE Ray Smith is a 41-year-old chef who lives on his own in rented accommodation. Until recently he worked as a chef in a small hotel but had been unable to work since he developed double vision in one eye. He was originally referred to the ophthalmic services but eventually his problem was identified as being a squamous cell carcinoma of the post-nasal space and Ray was referred to his local cancer centre for treatment. Although Ray has smoked since he was 12 he has never been a heavy drinker. Ray underwent examination under anaesthetic when biopsies were taken

and also had CT and MRI scans to determine the extent of his tumour. The tumour appears to be extensive and is already causing compression of two cranial nerves.

Following multidisciplinary team (MDT) discussion, chemo/radiation was recommended as the best treatment option. Whilst understandably devastated by this news Ray has been swept along in preparations for treatment. As part of this Ray had a consultation with the dental surgeon and this resulted in all but six of his teeth being extracted because they were in a poor state and potentially an infection risk during treatment. In addition this work was undertaken to prevent the possibility of a late side-effect of bone necrosis post radiotherapy as a result of dental treatment. This has already compromised his dietary intake and he will not be able to have dentures fitted until all the treatment is completed. Following his extractions, Ray was admitted overnight and had a PEG feeding tube inserted in preparation for treatment. He will be admitted for a 4-day course of cisplatin, 5flourouracil and docetaxel chemotherapy given as an inpatient and expects to have two or three courses prior to commencing radiotherapy. During this time he will be planned for radiotherapy treatment which will involve the construction of a semi-rigid shell to immobilize his head and neck during treatment. Two courses of cisplatin chemotherapy will be given during the first and fourth weeks of the radiotherapy treatment. This acts to make the cancer more radiosensitive.

Because of his age and because Ray has no children, discussions about the side-effects of chemotherapy had to include the possible effect on his fertility. Ray decided not to explore sperm banking as he has no current partner and his sperm count may recover post treatment. During this time his clinical nurse specialist (CNS) has been a vital link with the MDT team coordinating the preparations but also supporting Ray through the enormity of the emotional turmoil he is experiencing. He has an elderly mother who is his next of kin and few close friends.

The radiotherapy will cause swelling and inflammation resulting in both external skin soreness and mucositis which will cause pain and difficulty swallowing. Reduction in the quantity of saliva produced and its texture is also likely to contribute to swallowing problems. The CNS, therapy radiographers, dietician and clinical nutrition team will monitor Ray's weight and nutrition very closely throughout his treatment aiming to prevent dramatic weight loss and maintain his protein and calorie intake to promote healing. Ray will be especially vulnerable because he will have to learn to cope with his PEG feeds alone. It will be important for Ray to keep using the muscles of his mouth and throat by swallowing, even if using the PEG for feeding, as this will help to prevent swallowing difficulties post treatment. His CNS will liaise closely with his primary care team and he will be referred to the district nursing service for support. Because Ray will be off sick and unable to work for a period of months he has financial concerns and his CNS will assist Ray in claiming benefits he is entitled to and will apply on his behalf to Macmillan Cancer Support to assist with travelling and additional costs.

Careful assessment of the oral cavity is essential when mucositis is an expected side-effect of treatment. Eilers (2004) oral assessment guide has formed the basis of many subsequent assessment tools, all of which include; inspection of the lips, mucous membranes, gingiva and tongue for evidence of inflammation, desquamation, ulcers and infection, as well as moistness and evidence of debris. The amount and viscosity of the saliva needs to be noted as it becomes thick, ropy and viscous with severe mucositis, contributing to the dryness of the oral cavity and difficulty in eating. The patient's ability to eat, speak, swallow or wear dentures may be severely impaired. While the patient may experience mild burning at the onset of stomatitis, managed by topical measures, a severe case is extremely painful and may require systemic opioid analgesic management – orally, or by continuous subcutaneous infusion. One strategy that has been suggested for the prevention of the mucositis associated with 5FU chemotherapy involves the sucking of ice prior to and during administration of the chemotherapy (Nikoletti et al 2005).

Infection is a potentially serious problem when mouth ulcerations exist. The fungus *Candida albicans* is frequently the cause of lesions and inflammation, or may be a secondary infection when the oral mucosa is damaged by chemotherapy or radiation. Candidiasis presents as white patches on the tongue and buccal mucosa. When the patches are scraped off, a reddened ulcerated surface is apparent. Herpes simplex infection on the lips develops into painful vesicles that rupture and become encrusted. Gram-negative infections may occur in the mouth, as can *Pseudomonas* infections. The risk of systemic infection is of great concern. Ulcerated areas act as a port of entry for pathological organisms into the body, which may cause sepsis. Therefore, maintenance of good oral hygiene during periods of mucositis is essential in order to minimize the risk of infection. Wood (2004) claims that mouth care is still often carried out in a ritualized manner by staff lacking the appropriate knowledge and skills. This article and that of Cooley (2002) provide a very useful review of best practice in oral health care for cancer patients. Specific nursing measures in the care of the patient with mucositis are outlined in Box 11. 4.

Taste alterations

Alterations in taste can occur as a result of cancer treatment. The types of taste alterations include *dysgeusia*, which is an unpleasant taste perception; *ageusia*, an absence of taste; and *hypogeusia*, a decrease in the acuity of taste sensation.

Surgical treatment for cancer in the oral cavity, particularly the tongue, salivary glands, nasal area and trachea, may cause hypogeusia and ageusia. Mucositis and infections in the oral cavity may also contribute to alterations in taste. Taste alterations caused by chemotherapy include metallic and bitter taste sensations, and an increased threshold for the sweet sensation. The chemotherapy agents most commonly associated with taste alterations include cyclophosphamide, nitrogen mustard, 5-fluorouracil, vin-

cristine, methotrexate and dacarbazine. Taste alterations vary widely amongst patients in terms of severity and duration. Changes due to chemotherapy and radiation usually return to normal within weeks to months.

Nursing care is directed towards maintaining nutrition and hydration, and assisting patients to adapt their diet during periods of taste alteration. Patients at high risk should be prepared for the eventuality of taste alteration and self-care strategies for management suggested. This may include temporarily eliminating certain foods, experimenting with seasonings and flavourings, marinades and sauces to enhance or disguise unpleasant tastes and using citrus juices to mask metallic tastes and stimulate saliva production. It is important to assess for the presence of taste changes and contributory factors such as xerostomia, poor oral hygiene and oral infections. In addition it is important to assess for the impact on nutritional intake and to inform patients of this possibility in order to help the patient cope with taste alterations. Good oral hygiene should be encouraged.

Anorexia, weight loss and cachexia

Anorexia and *weight loss* are common problems for many patients with cancer. During radiotherapy, anorexia is probably related to the presence of the waste products of tissue destruction. Many factors may contribute to anorexia including, surgery, side-effects of therapy, nausea, taste changes, pain, fatigue, stomatitis, anaemia, inactivity, medications, alterations in the person's ability to ingest and digest foods, and psychological factors. Weight loss is also related to an increased demand of the tumour on host tissue, resulting in loss largely from muscle rather than fatty tissue. The combination of changes in metabolism and inadequate intake results in nutritional deficiencies that impair the body's ability to repair and heal, as well as affecting the patient's quality of life. Whilst the cause often cannot be identified clearly, the symptom must be treated by using a variety of strategies to encourage adequate intake. A self-perpetuating cycle of anorexia, weight loss, weakness, inactivity and more anorexia may develop if the symptom is untreated. Fluid intake should be encouraged to promote elimination of the products of tissue breakdown.

Cachexia involves both weight loss and anorexia, and is the wasting syndrome that is often associated with advanced cancer. Although not inevitable, many people with cancer are affected by it, particularly those with gastrointestinal and lung cancers. Unfortunately it has been something of a poor relation in cancer care yet is a significant factor in the morbidity of many cancers. Holmes (2002) reports that the reasons for metabolic changes associated with cachexia are complex, multifaceted and as yet unclear, although current theories implicate the role of cytokines.

Comprehensive assessment as to the nature, cause and consequences of nutritional deficiencies is essential and should include a history of any weight changes and the time within which this has occurred together with calculation of

Box 11.4   Nursing care of the person at risk of mucositis

Assessment
- Identify patients at risk of mucositis as a result of oral cancers, systemic chemotherapy, local radiotherapy, immunosuppression, impaired nutrition and drug therapy

- Determine if the patient smokes and offer smoking cessation advice if appropriate

- Assess the lips and oral cavity regularly using a light source and tongue depressor:
    - inspect lips, tongue gums and mucous membranes for red inflamed areas, ulcerations, bleeding and oedema
    - note degree of moistness of tissues; amount and viscosity of saliva
    - note presence of pain, difficulty eating or swallowing, difficulty talking
    - assess for evidence of infection (fungal, viral, bacterial), particularly in areas of ulceration, and on the tongue and palate
    - document findings, for example using Eilers assessment tool

Patient problems and goals
- The patient will be able to express an understanding of the need for oral hygiene measures and perform them after meals and at bedtime

- When the problem of mucositis occurs the goal should be that the patient will have a normal oral mucosa and experience no discomfort

Nursing interventions
1 Teach the patient a basic oral hygiene regimen or assist if the patient is dependent to:
   a) undertake self-inspection of the mouth and oral cavity
   b) follow regimen of brushing teeth with a soft toothbrush and flouride toothpaste four times a day or every 4 hours while awake
   c) remove and brush dentures and rinse mouth with clorhexidine mouthwash four times a day
   d) apply aqueous cream or yellow soft paraffin to lips to moisten if required

2 For patients at high risk or with evidence of mucositis:
   a) assess daily and increase frequency of mouth care to 2 hourly
   b) use recommended mouthwash after meals and before bed
   c) avoid commercial mouthwashes as they contain alcohol and are drying and irritating to oral mucosa. Do not use lemon and glycerin as this is drying and irritating
   d) provide regular analgesia as required, e.g. benzydamine mouthwash or spray, protective gels, local or systemic analgesia
   e) sip water for dry mouth or consider artificial saliva replacement
   f) provide topical antifungal and/or antiviral treatments as required. Allow 30 minutes between mouthwashes and antifungal application
   g) for haemorrhagic mucositis
       - irrigate mouth with normal saline
       - check platelet count and clotting screen

3 For patients at high risk and/or with evidence of severe mucositis:
   a) increase frequency of mouth care advised in 2 above to 1–2 hourly
   b) treat specific problems as necessary as indicated in 2d to 2g above
   c) very severe pain may require administration of oral, i.v. or subcutaneous infusion of morphine or diamorphine

4 Promote adequate hydration and nutrition:
   a) alter diet to soft or liquid to reduce mechanical irritation
   b) avoid salty, spicy, acidic or hot foods as they are chemically irritating
   c) try high-protein nutritional supplements
   d) maintain hydration of 3000 mL per day. If the patient is unable to swallow, intravenous hydration may be necessary

5 Consider referral to:
   - a speech and language therapist for swallowing difficulties
   - a dietician for weight loss of > 10% of usual body weight
   - oral hygienist for patients unable to maintain good mouth care

body mass index and a food diary. This will enable realistic goals of care to be determined. Nutritional goals are aimed at:

- Preventing or reversing nutritional deficiencies
- Energy conservation and preservation of lean body mass
- Minimizing nutrition-related side-effects
- Maximizing quality of life.

If patients are able to eat, food intake and nutrition status may be enhanced by:

- offering frequent small meals with snacks or drinks in between
- encouraging choice of favourite foods, particularly those that have a high protein content
- fortifying foods to increase their nutritional value – adding extra milk, cream and cheese
- adjusting timing of meals to reflect changes in appetite during the day enabling the patient to eat when they are hungry
- using anti-emetics and analgesics effectively
- maintaining good oral hygiene
- using alcohol or other appetite stimulants, e.g. megestrol acetate
- ensuring the environment is pleasant
- reducing unnecessary physical activities.

Commercial food supplements are frequently employed and, where this is not possible, enteral feeding via a nasogastric or percutaneous gastrostomy route may be used. Patients with head and neck cancers undergoing chemo-radiation and patients with oesophageal cancers frequently need feeding through inserted PEG feeding tubes to ensure nutritional intake is adequate during treatment. Parenteral (intravenous) feeding may also be an option, particularly as an adjunct to major surgery, although its general use in cancer care is controversial.

As well as being a physiological necessity, eating and drinking have a wider social significance, and the inability to engage in these activities represents a significant loss for both the individual and their carers. Jones et al (1993) interviewed 207 bereaved carers and identified that there were 144 instances where concerns about anorexia or weight loss were voiced. Any interventions that enhance comfort and enjoyment may result in a significant enhancement of quality of life.

Constipation

Constipation may be induced by a variety of causes, including nutritional deficits, particularly a lack of fibre, immobility, the disease process, such as spinal cord compression, hypercalcaemia or intestinal obstruction or by administration of opioid analgesia or the chemotherapeutic agents, vincristine and vinblastine. The vinca alkaloids cause smooth muscle neurotoxicity and consequences in the bowel range from mild constipation to paralytic ileus. Chemotherapy is usually interrupted during periods of ileus. A number of drugs especially opioids, tricyclic antidepressants, and antispasmodics cause constipation due to their effect on the bowel as do the 5 HT3 antagonists used to reduce chemotherapy-induced nausea and vomiting. Regular administration of stool softeners and stimulants or osmotic laxatives together with judicious use of suppositories and enemas will help to prevent constipation, as will an increase in fluid and fibre intake. This, of course, may be difficult if the patient is also experiencing mucositis and other gastro-intestinal symptoms, and thorough assessment and planning of appropriate interventions will be required. In its turn untreated constipation can cause abdominal pain, nausea and/or vomiting, intestinal obstruction and urinary retention. When intestinal obstruction is suspected, faecal stimulants and osmotic laxatives should be avoided.

Diarrhoea

Diarrhoea may cause fluid and electrolyte imbalances and contribute to the weakness and fatigue that patients experience. Nutrition may be severely hampered. Diarrhoea is also irritating to the perianal skin surfaces and may cause skin breakdown. It is a common temporary sequela of a number of chemotherapy drugs and occurs with radiation therapy to the abdomen and pelvis after a dose of about 20 Gy has been given. However, following radiotherapy, the effect may be prolonged or indefinite and may even develop months or years later with severe and debilitating effects on quality of life. Some individuals experience only an increase in their usual number of bowel movements, whereas others develop loose, watery stools and intestinal cramping. Nursing actions are focused on maintaining adequate hydration and nutrition, promoting comfort and hygiene, and returning bowel function to normal. Specific nursing care measures for the patient with diarrhoea include: maintaining fluid intake at a minimum of 3000 mL per day, a low-residue diet (e.g. starchy foods, white bread, bananas or apples, and avoiding caffeine, whole grains, high fibre, most fruits and juices, and fried, spicy or pickled meats), care of the perianal region and use of an anti-diarrhoeal medication such as loperamide or codeine phosphate.

ALOPECIA

Alopecia, or hair loss, is a side-effect of radiotherapy to the head, when some of the loss may be permanent, and of cytotoxic chemotherapy, when the loss may be total but is temporary. The degree of toxicity of different drugs in this regard varies but, as many are used in combination, hair loss is a frequent consequence of many regimens. The psychological impact of this may vary between individuals but is frequently considerable because of the visibility of the change as Batchelor (2001) noted, in a review of alopecia. Hair is also of cultural significance to certain ethnic groups, for example, people from the Sikh community and its loss may be equally distressing to both men and women. It is a visible and long-lasting sign of treatment for a disease that individuals might otherwise wish to keep private, or share only with a chosen few. On a practical level, the protective functions of hair are also lost (i.e. conservation of heat, protection from the sun, and the filtering out of air-borne particles from the eyes and nose). Scalp cooling may be offered to patients having chemotherapy, although this works only for certain drugs and is not effective in all cases. Scalp cooling acts by constricting blood vessels supplying the hair follicles thereby reducing circulation and therefore uptake of the drug within the hair follicle. It can be quite a lengthy and uncomfortable process, so careful assessment and evaluation is required (Dougherty 1995). Use of scalp cooling techniques are limited to patients with solid tumours and who are receiving specific cytotoxic drugs or regimens. Results are variable but for some patients even a chance of reduction in hair loss is more acceptable than certain complete hair loss. As intimated, patients should be assessed on a case by case basis as some will undoubtedly find the additional time and discomfort involved in the procedure unacceptable for limited benefit whilst others will opt for any chance of retaining hair. Dougherty (2004) makes the point that in published studies of scalp cooling, comparisons have been difficult due to the multitude of variables, small samples and lack of RCTs.

Nursing care aims to help patients prepare for hair loss and to suggest effective coping and self-care strategies to manage the changes in body image and self-concept. Patients need to be warned when to expect hair loss and to understand that when regrowth occurs it may differ in colour and texture. Wigs should be arranged in advance of hair loss so they can be matched to natural hair in colour and style if so wished. For individuals with long hair, cutting it before hair loss occurs may help to reduce the physical impact. When hair has been lost, care for the scalp includes gentle cleansing and moisturizing unless contra-indicated during radiotherapy. The scalp will need protection from extremes of both heat and cold until hair has regrown and in addition, chemical colorants and perms should also be avoided for at least 6 months. If a wig is unacceptable or uncomfortable, hats, scarves and turbans may be used as alternative head wear. If eyebrows and eyelashes are also lost then cosmetic techniques can be suggested.

FATIGUE

Fatigue or a profound lack of energy is a symptom that occurs frequently and is experienced by virtually every person with cancer (Richardson 1995). It may precede or accompany the illness; it may serve as a marker of disease progression and recurrence. A multitude of factors contribute to fatigue, including anaemia, surgery, chemotherapy, radiotherapy, disturbances in sleep and rest patterns, inadequate nutrition, mood disturbances and symptom distress.

Fatigue in patients with cancer is a complex phenomenon and clearly involves physical, psychological and emotional elements. Nursing interventions focus on exploring individual experiences and on ameliorating and devising strategies to adapt lifestyle, conserve energy, maintain optimum activity, and promote adequate nutrition and rest (Ream and Stone 2004). Specific nursing care measures for patients experiencing fatigue are outlined in Box 11.5.

Box 11.5   Nursing care of the person with fatigue

Assessment
- Assess factors that may be contributing to fatigue: anaemia, nutrition, sleep/rest patterns, treatment, symptom distress

- Assess pattern of fatigue: onset, duration, severity, ameliorating and exacerbating factors, and impact on lifestyle

Patient problems and goals
- The problem of fatigue leads to the setting of a goal, in conjunction with the patient, that the patient will achieve adequate periods of rest in order to pursue key interests and activities

Nursing intervention
1. Provide reassurance that fatigue is a common side-effect of cancer treatment and not an indication of disease progression

2. Correct underlying anaemia through the use of blood transfusion, erythropoetin; provide dietary advise on maintaining adequate intake of iron and vitamins

3. Assist the patient to prioritize key activities and schedule these according to energy levels, interspersing periods of activity with periods of rest

4. Promote adequate rest and sleep pattern. Meditation, progressive muscle relaxation and guided imaging may promote relaxation and increase energy

5. Explore taking light exercise several times a week as there is some evidence that this can reduce levels of fatigue and enhance well-being

6. Encourage patients to accept offers of assistance from friends and family with chores and tasks at home and delegate within the workplace

BREATHLESSNESS

Breathlessness (dyspnoea) is an uncomfortable awareness of breathing and serves as a stimulus for actions that may relieve respiratory insufficiency, such as clearing the airway, removing constrictive clothing or breathing rapidly and deeply. Whilst the symptom should be viewed first as a warning of disease and a signal to investigate and treat the underlying medical condition, breathlessness is a discomfort that can be relieved regardless of its pathophysiological basis.

Breathlessness is experienced as a result of many underlying conditions that may coexist in people with cancer. Respiratory failure, particularly pneumonia, is a frequent cause of death among patients with cancer, and breathlessness may also occur in a variety of other terminal conditions (e.g. sepsis, cardiac failure or severe anaemia). Specific causes of breathlessness for people with cancer are largely related to primary or secondary tumours that result in obstruction to the upper airways, pleural effusion (fluid in the pleural cavity) or a generalized lymphangitis within the lungs.

Whenever possible, the root cause should be investigated and may be treated by surgery, radiotherapy or chemotherapy. Otherwise, drug treatment with bronchodilators may help to alleviate acute episodes. Opioids are often helpful in easing the subjective sensation of breathlessness and may be combined with an anxiolytic to reduce the panic of an acute episode. Physiotherapy, which assists with the removal of secretions, nebulized saline and techniques to encourage diaphragmatic breathing are helpful. Corner et al (1995b) proposed a model for the management of breathlessness which views the functional, emotional and sensory elements as inseparable and which employs a variety of non-pharmacological measures to enhance coping skills.

Breathlessness is a frightening experience and patients may fear they will choke or will just stop breathing and die. Patients may experience panic attacks and extreme anxiety,

---

Box 11.6 Suggested nursing interventions for the person experiencing breathlessness

Assessment
- Take a history to establish speed of onset and associated symptoms – pain, cough, wheeze
- A visual analogue scale may be helpful in assessing severity
- Identify factors that ameliorate or exacerbate breathlessness
- Establish ability to perform activities of daily living
- Explore the level of anxiety and fear particularly around fear of sudden death

Patient problems and goals
- The problem of breathlessness leads to the setting of a goal, in conjunction with the patient, that the patient will regain a sense of control over breathing patterns; maximize functional capacity and report reduction in fear and panic

Nursing interventions
1. Assist in administration of drug treatments that may be helpful in certain situations (nebulized saline to reduce tenacious secretions, opioids to ease subjective sensation of breathlessness, anxiolytics, steroids, antibiotics, bronchodilators and oxygen therapy) and drainage and pluerodesis for pleural effusions
2. Encourage the prioritization of activities, and pace and plan activities in advance to minimize expenditure of effort
3. Assist patients in finding positions that provide for maximal lung expansion, e.g. sitting or sleeping in an upright position
4. Liaise with physiotherapist regarding chest physiotherapy and breathing retraining techniques to encourage diaphragmatic breathing and pursed lip breathing
5. Include planned rest periods, particularly with more demanding activities, which should be scheduled at hours of the day when breathing is the easiest
6. Review exertion caused by eating and suggest smaller, more frequent, meals of soft, easy-to-chew foods
7. Improve air circulation with fans; open windows
8. Maintain adequate humidity to decrease dry airway and thick secretions
9. Spend time with patient to understand the impact and meaning of breathlessness for them and their carers
10. Provide information on causation and significance of symptoms
11. Teach progressive muscle relaxation and visualization techniques. Complementary therapies may benefit some patients

which exacerbate the physiological impairment and lead to even more dysfunctional breathing patterns. The experience of being with someone who is acutely breathless is also extremely frightening, particularly in the home or other areas without immediate access to medical or nursing services. Suggested nursing measures for the patient experiencing breathlessness are listed in Box 11.6.

PAIN

Pain is the symptom most frequently associated with cancer and is one of the most feared consequences of the disease and treatment. The assessment and management of pain and other symptoms in patients with cancer is one of the major activities in cancer care, with Hanks (2005) reporting pain to be a problem for 30–40% of patients undergoing curative treatments and in 70–90% of patients with advanced disease. Effective pain management involves sound knowledge of the pathophysiology of cancer pain, pain assessment strategies and pain management principles, including the use of pharmaceutical and non-pharmaceutical measures.

Definition and description

Even though a person may experience pain and knows how it feels to hurt, it is difficult for both the observer and the sufferer to define and describe pain adequately. Pain is commonly divided into two subtypes: acute and chronic. Acute pain is characterized by a well-defined time of onset and is associated with subjective and objective signs indicating activation of the sympathetic nervous system (e.g. sweating, paleness, tachycardia, hypertension, grimacing, crying and anxiety). Chronic pain, on the other hand, is defined as the persistence of pain for longer than 6 months. In general, the onset of chronic pain is less well defined. In addition, patients with chronic pain no longer exhibit the signs and symptoms usually associated with pain. In fact, the patient with chronic pain often shows very few signs of distress; often the suffering is hidden beneath a brave, stoical face. After long periods of unrelieved pain, the face no longer reveals anxiety – but exhaustion and depression. The lack of outwardly obvious signs and the depressed, sleepy face is often misinterpreted and the patient's complaints of severe pain discounted.

Patients with cancer may experience acute pain, chronic pain, or acute pain superimposed on chronic pain. The type of pain experienced is determined by the stage of the disease; the type of treatment the patient is receiving, and any other predisposing medical or surgical conditions.

Nature of cancer pain and pain pathways

In order to focus attention on the complexity of pain as a somatic and psychological experience, Saunders and Baines (1983) introduced the notion of 'total pain'. The suffering experienced by the patient with cancer pain is derived from a variety of sources. Anger, anxiety, depression, isolation, fearful memories, boredom and other psychosocial factors can lower a patient's pain threshold. On the other hand, a positive outlook, a supportive family, empathy from nurses and doctor, forgiveness, diversion and sleep may raise the pain threshold and decrease the pain experience. An understanding of pain pathways and pain control mechanisms is essential to the understanding of cancer pain management, and these are outlined in Chapter 8.

Aetiology of cancer pain

As shown in Box 11.7, the pain of cancer can have multiple causes, including the cancer itself, the treatment, and concomitant non-malignant disease or factors unrelated to the cancer or therapy. Most pain arises from stimulation of nociceptive nerve endings; however, neuropathic pain is a feature of nerve compression or nerve irritation caused by expansion or infiltration by the cancer. This gives rise to pain that is characteristically described as having burning, shooting or electric shock type qualities.

Assessment

The phase of assessment is possibly one of the most important steps in good pain management, and accurate assessment is based on trust; McCaffrey (1979) stresses the importance of trust and belief in the patient's report of the severity and nature of the pain. As Lanceley (1995) noted, pain is deeply personal and the extent of the disease shown on examination of a radiograph or scan does not necessarily

---

Box 11.7 Pain syndromes in people with cancer

Pain caused by cancer
- Metastatic bone disease
- Compression or infiltration of nervous structures
- Compression or infiltration of veins, arteries, lymphatics
- Rapid tumour growth causing stretching of pain-sensitive structures
- Obstruction of a hollow viscus, such as bowel
- Ulceration of pain-sensitive mucosal surfaces

Pain caused by anticancer therapy
- Surgery
- Chemotherapy, e.g. mucositis
- Radiation therapy

Coincidental pain
- General debility
- Joint stiffness
- Pressure sores
- Constipation

reveal the extent of the pain. Lack of belief can accentuate the patient's feelings of helplessness and hopelessness, and may also lead to stoical under-reporting or anxious over-reporting of the experience. Either reaction aggravates the spiral of mistrust, anxiety and pain. At the initial pain interview and as part of an ongoing nursing assessment, it is important to explore the key elements of a pain history, as outlined in Box 11.8 utilizing the PQRST symptom analysis tool. A feature of cancer pain is that pain may be due to more than one cause and may be present in more than one part of the body. For this reason it is useful to use a body outline to record the location of different pains.

Measurement of pain

Although the experience of pain is not open to direct external measurement, several instruments have been developed to assist the patient in describing the intensity of pain. Measurement tools are advantageous because they facilitate clarity and consistency in interpretation and communication of the pain and quantification of the effectiveness of an intervention. For example, if a patient's pain is the most severe at a rating of 9 and 2 hours after analgesia it is still at 7, it is evident that more effective interventions are needed. Verbal or written statements of a patient's exact numerical pain ratings are likely to be more consistently reported among health team members than a word description, such as 'a lot of pain'. Examples of some instruments are given in Chapter 8.

The type of scale used is less important than:

- the consistency with which it is used
- the patient's understanding of the scale

Box 11.8 Key components of the pain history

Provocation/palliation
- What brings on the pain?
- What relieves the pain?
- When did it start?

Quality
- Describe the pain in your own words (e.g. dull, sharp, aching, throbbing, burning)

Region/radiation
- Location of pain. Does it spread anywhere? Use a body outline to document this

Severity
- How severe is the pain? (Consider using an instrument such as a vertical or linear visual analogue rating scale to assist the patient in describing the intensity of pain and to track response to pain management strategies over time. (see Fig. 11.3 and Ch. 8)

Timing
- How long have you had it?
- Does it come and go, or is it always there?
- How long does each spasm last?

In addition to the PQRST analysis, the following should also be ascertained

Impact of pain on daily life
- Sleep – does pain disturb your sleep? (note: patients with pain may adapt to the pain so that they can sleep)
- Mood – does the pain cause you to be depressed or discouraged?
- Activity – how has pain affected your activities (mobility, self-care, job, social life, etc.)?

Explore knowledge and/or fears about use of analgesics to treat chronic pain as follows.

Meaning of pain
- What does the patient think is causing the pain?
- What does the patient think should be done about it?

Previous therapies
- Which drugs (or other therapies) have helped and which have failed to relieve the pain? Analgesic history should include: dose, frequency, regular or p.r.n., the patient's view of drug efficacy, duration of use, side-effects, reason for discontinuation

---

the clarity with which the scale assigns a score to the pain experience.

For example, a rating of 5 is meaningless unless it is followed by a statement of the scale used, for example: 5 on a scale of 0–10 (0 = no pain, 10 = worst pain), or 5 on a scale of 0 – 5 (0 = no pain, 5 = worst pain).

Some patients are unable to use a numerical scale to rate their pain; the numbers do not make sense to them or it is too hard for them to apply numbers to their experience. In this case, it may be more helpful for the patient to use a verbal rating, visual analogue or picture rating scale, but this needs to be consistently used by the healthcare team so that characteristics of the patient's pain can be recorded or tracked and the response to therapy monitored. Not keeping pain records when dealing with a patient in pain is like trying to treat hypertension without recording blood pressure.

A flow sheet allows ongoing evaluation of pain. The only safe and effective way to administer an analgesic is to monitor the patient's response to the medication and make changes based on these responses. The flow sheet is a tool that allows quick documentation of such responses along with easy retrieval of information for continuous evaluation. An example of a flow sheet that may be used by the patient or by the nurse is given in Figure 11.5.

PHARMACOTHERAPEUTICS

Administration of systemic analgesics, psychotropic drugs and antiinflammatory agents is probably the most practical and widely used method for relieving cancer pain. Twycross and Lack (1990) have suggested a realistic clinical plan for 'graded pain relief': initially, a pain-free, sleepful night; next, comfort at rest in bed or a chair during the day; and finally, freedom from pain on movement.

The choice of analgesic will depend partly on whether the individual is suffering chronic or acute pain, or a combination of both. Acute pain in a person with cancer (e.g. post-operative, recent fracture, painful diagnostic procedure) might call for an intramuscular injection of a standard dose of a relatively short-acting opioid. Further analgesia would be administered on an as needed (p.r.n.) basis because pain intensity is likely to change rapidly. However, if the individual is already taking large amounts of opioid analgesia for chronic pain, this would need to be taken into account in an acute situation.

Chronic cancer pain, on the other hand, demands a different approach. Analgesics should be given regularly (around the clock) with the dose and choice of medication matched to pain intensity. Pain severity is determined by listening to the patient's report of pain and observing the degree of relief obtained from previously administered drugs.

NAME _____

Date/time	Pain rating on a scale of _____	Respiratory rate	Accompanying symptoms/ level of consciousness/ other observations	Analgesic

Code key for accompanying symptoms:

1 Nausea	3 Vomiting	5 Constipation	7 Drowsiness
2 Confusion	4 Halucinations	6 Fatigue/weakness	

Figure 11.5 Pain flow chart.

As part of the Worldwide Cancer Pain Relief Programme, the World Health Organization (WHO 1986) has advocated a three-step analgesic ladder. This concept is illustrated in Figure 11.6. In patients with very severe pain, it may be necessary to administer high doses of strong opioids initially, with or without other adjuvant drugs. The National Council for Hospice and Specialist Palliative Care Services (2003) has produced some useful guidelines for the management of cancer pain. It sets out the aims of cancer pain management as being to:

- achieve a level of pain control that is acceptable to the individual
- assess the pain and evaluate the effectiveness of pain management promptly
- be aware of the component of total pain
- relieve pain at night and at rest and on movement
- provide up-to-date information on use of pain-relieving drugs to patients and their carers
- To provide support and encouragement to the caregivers of patients with cancer pain.

PRINCIPLES OF THERAPY

1 *Use the oral route whenever possible.* The oral administration of opioids gives more consistent and prolonged analgesia, and avoids the toxicity that may occur with parenteral administration. The oral route eliminates parenteral injections, enables the patient to maintain control of the drugs and allows mobility for home care and travel. When injections are required, subcutaneous administration of morphine, either continuously via a syringe driver or by regular intermittent injection, should be used in preference to the intramuscular route, as it is much less painful for the patient.

2 *'Round the clock' dosing.* The duration of analgesic action of most narcotic drugs is 4–6 hours; therefore, control of chronic pain requires 4–6 doses spaced equally throughout the 24-hour period.

3 *Never use 'as needed' dosing.* Continuous pain requires continuous analgesia and the aim of therapy is to prevent the resurgence of pain rather than repeatedly to treat it. This anticipation breaks the vicious cycle of pain–despair–more pain, which causes dose escalation. While p.r.n.

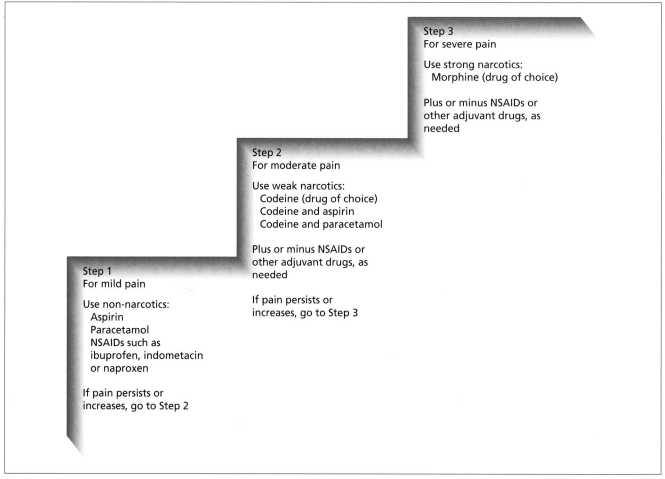

Figure 11.6   The analgesic ladder.

orders may be needed for 'breakthrough' pain, the basis of control must be regular scheduling. The individual and family members will need advice and information about the rationale for using a preventive approach.

4 *Wake the patient.* A patient with chronic pain often sleeps despite severe pain. Sleep does not indicate pain control. On initiating therapy, the patient should be woken until pain has been consistently controlled for 2–3 days and their confidence has been restored. Once pain is well controlled, some centres give a larger dose at bedtime (e.g. one and a half times or twice the daytime dose), often allowing the patient to sleep throughout the night free of pain.

5 *Titrate the dose individually.* There is no standard or set dose of opioids in cancer pain, and there is great variation between individuals in analgesic efficacy. The correct dose is that which gives pain relief for at least 3 hours, or preferably 4 hours or more. As pain changes through various stages of disease and treatment, the dosage must be adjusted to match pain intensity.

6 *Consult.* Consult with nursing and medical experts in pain management when usual interventions are unsatisfactory and before pain becomes intractable.

Many myths persist about the use of morphine for cancer pain which may lead to reluctance to prescribe it. These include both lay and professional beliefs that it may cause addiction, respiratory depression, and that its use indicates imminent death. Such fears should be addressed by effective education and information giving by palliative care experts.

CO-ANALGESICS

Several drugs, while not true analgesics in the pharmacological sense, act to relieve pain, either alone or in combination with analgesics. These co-analgesics may be used in the treatment of all types of cancer pain but are particularly important for pain that is relatively unresponsive to morphine. Even when a narcotic is being used, the addition of a co-analgesic may often result in better pain control with fewer side-effects. Examples of co-analgesics include the steroids (e.g. prednisolone, dexamethasone), non-steroidal anti-inflammatory drugs, bisphosphonates (e.g. pamidronate or zoledronic acid) for bone pain and tricyclic antidepressants (e.g. amitriptyline) or anti-convulsants (e.g. carbamazepine or gabapentin) for neuropathic pain.

It should be noted that, to gain effective relief, the required dosage for all drugs may differ from that which doctors and nurses are accustomed to prescribing and administering in other areas of clinical practice.

NON-PHARMACOLOGICAL MEASURES

Cancer pain usually requires systemic analgesic therapy. However, in many situations non-drug measures may be extremely important adjuncts. Box 11.9 lists some of the co-analgesic and non-pharmacological measures that may be helpful in relieving cancer pain.

It is very important periodically to reassess the adequacy of pain control and to consider reasons for loss of previously adequate control. Cancer pain is seldom static: new pains develop and old pains re-emerge. Changes in the site or intensity of pain require thorough reassessment and review, not just an increase in the dose of the current analgesia.

CONTROL OF OPIOID SIDE-EFFECTS

Constipation

If not carefully monitored and prevented, constipation may be just as difficult to control as the pain itself and it occurs in 40–90% of patients on opiate analgesia. The constipation associated with opioids occurs because the morphine binds to receptors in the gastrointestinal tract, causing decreased peristalsis and diminished secretions (Campbell et al 2001). In patients with cancer, decreased liquid intake, less exercise and a low-fibre diet all aggravate the problem. As in pain control, the aim of bowel care should be to prevent rather than treat the problem. It is recommended that all patients should be prescribed both softening and stimulant laxatives when commencing on opioid analgesia for moderate to severe pain.

Nausea and vomiting

When opioids are initiated, nausea and vomiting may occur as a side-effect. When commencing oral morphine, a prescription for an antiemetic (e.g. haloperidol, cyclizine or metaclopromide) should be obtained in case nausea or vomiting should develop. The risk of nausea and vomiting often decreases a week or two after morphine is started, so that for some people the antiemetic may be phased out.

Drowsiness and sedation

Transient sedation frequently occurs when morphine treatment is started. This is partly a direct drug effect on the CNS, but the exhaustion and sleep deprivation as a result of chronic pain are other major factors. When pain is finally relieved, the patient may sleep for long periods, but general drowsiness usually clears 2–5 days after a steady dose is achieved. Continuing drowsiness may indicate a need to decrease the dose, switch to another opioid and/or add less sedating co-analgesics. Sedation may also be a sign of disease progression and is not always a side-effect of therapy. It is important to explain to patients and their family that sedation may be a problem for the first few days but that this should be temporary.

LYMPHOEDEMA

Lymphoedema is a swelling resulting from the excess accumulation of fluid in the tissues and is caused by inadequate lymph drainage. It is often accompanied by inflammation and fibrosis. Cancer-related lymphoedema can be secondary to obstruction by tumour or caused by destruction or removal of lymphatics by surgery or radiotherapy. Upper limb lymphoedema is associated most frequently with breast cancer

Box 11.9 Co-analgesics and non-pharmacological measures in cancer pain

For bone pain

- Full doses of non-steroidal antiinflammatory drugs (e.g. indometacin, diclofenac, naproxen, aspirin), if tolerated. Gastric protection is required for patients on steroids or with other risk factors

- Radiotherapy – usually to specific sites of localized metastasis, but in widespread disease, upper or lower hemi-body irradiation may be given

- Bisphosphonates (e.g. pamidronate, clodronate, zoledronic acid)

- Orthopaedic surgery for pathological fractures

For neuropathic pain due to nerve compression or nerve destruction

- Corticosteroids

- Anaesthetic nerve blocks

- Transcutaneous electrical nerve stimulation (TENS)

- Anticonvulsants

- Tricyclic antidepressants (e.g. amitriptyline)

- NMDA receptor channel blockers (e.g. ketamine)

- TENS

Abdominal colic
- Antispasmodics

Muscle spasm
- Muscle relaxants

Other modalities
- Positioning

- Massage, warm or cold compresses

- Air fluidized therapy (e.g. Clinitron bed)

- Physiotherapy and occupational therapy; collars, corsets, splints, slings (for extra support), elastic stockings, compression cuffs transfer aids, walking aids, hydrotherapy, etc.

- Distraction, relaxation, imagery

(Note: The response to these modalities may be limited when used alone, but they can be useful when most pain has been controlled by other means, as above.)

especially in women who have undergone axillary dissection and/or radiotherapy. Lymphoedema also occurs in patients with gynaecological tumours, melanomas, cancers of the prostate and head and neck cancers, and may develop some years after treatment as a result of minor trauma or infection. Severe lymphoedema is a very debilitating condition restricting the mobility and function of the limb affected, causing pain and discomfort and distress from altered body image. Complications of lymphoedema are lymphorrhoea and acute inflammatory episodes which may necessitate hospitalization. Patients at risk should be given advice on simple precautions to prevent lymphoedema such as avoiding injuries, infections, and insect bites; using the unaffected limb for blood pressure monitoring and venepuncture. Treatment of the condition at an early stage can prevent progression and maintain the functional integrity of the limb. The cornerstones of management are good skin care, exercise, compression hosiery and multi-layered bandaging, or in severe cases, manual lymphatic drainage (Woods 2004).

MALIGNANT EFFUSIONS

A malignant effusion is an abnormal collection of fluid in the peritoneal or pleural space caused by overproduction of fluid or obstruction of lymphatic channels by tumour. Both have a tendency to re-occur. Malignant ascites is associated with intraperitoneal disease and is frequently seen in cancer of the ovary where it is often a presenting symptom with abdominal distension causing pain, breathlessness, leg oedema and an inability to eat due to pressure on the stomach. It is also a symptom of advanced disease when management focuses on keeping the patient comfortable through repeated abdominal paracentesis and use of the diuretic spironolactone. Large volumes of fluid may be drained off and this must be done with some care to avoid fluid and protein depletion. Malignant pleural effusions are a feature of advanced cancer and a common cause of breathlessness. Large symptomatic effusions are drained or aspirated and pleurodesis may be achieved by injecting a chemotherapy agent such as bleomycin or other sclerosing agents.

Patients who develop malignant effusions will need information and support to come to terms with the recurring nature of these problems. They will also need, support, observation and monitoring during procedures designed to alleviate their discomfort.

MANAGEMENT OF ONCOLOGICAL EMERGENCIES

Patients with cancer of all types may present with emergency conditions related to their disease or treatment. The appropriate management will depend upon the nature of the underlying disease, previous therapy and likely long-term prognosis (Falk and Fallon 1997).

Tumour lysis syndrome
Tumour lysis syndrome can occur in the treatment of tumours that have a large number of tumour cells, such as acute leukaemia or lymphoma, which are very sensitive to chemotherapy. As large numbers of malignant cells are killed by the chemotherapy, cell lysis releases large amounts of nucleic acids and intracellular ions into the bloodstream. This can cause *hyperuricaemia* (raised levels of uric acid in the blood) which, when excessive, leads to *hyperuricaemic nephropathy* and severely affects renal function. Other metabolic imbalances such as hyperkalaemia, hyperphosphataemia and hypocalcaemia may also occur as a result of massive cell lysis. Additional risk factors exist for those who are over the age of 65 years, those who have pre-existing renal disease, and those who are being treated with nephrotoxic drugs. Prophylactic treatment includes careful monitoring of renal function and biochemical parameters in conjunction with increased fluid administration, diuresis, alkalinization of the urine and administration of the drug allopurinol.

Hypersensitivity reactions
Hypersensitivity reactions may occur in response to some chemotherapeutic agents or biological response modifiers, which stimulate the body's immune response producing an anaphylactoid reaction or severe *anaphylaxis*. Risk factors include use of drugs commonly known to cause such reactions, e.g. paclitaxel, etoposide, cisplatin, bleomycin and l-asparaginase and monoclonal antibodies. Reactions may occur without prior exposure to the drug. It is always good practice to ask patients about their allergy history, as a history of other allergic conditions may be a predisposing factor. Prophylactic medication with antihistamines and corticosteroids should be given with high-risk drugs, and emergency equipment and drugs should always be in the immediate vicinity when such chemotherapy is being administered.

Hypercalcaemia
Hypercalcaemia is a potentially fatal metabolic condition that occurs in approximately 8–20% of patients with cancer. Hypercalcaemia is caused by increased bone resorption, which results from tumour invasion of bone, increased levels of parathyroid hormone, prostaglandin or osteoclast-activating factors. Patients at greatest risk are those with bone metastases (commonly from breast, prostate, lung or renal tumours) or multiple myeloma which cause extensive bone destruction and release of calcium into the extracellular fluid.

The effects of hypercalcaemia in the body are seen in the gastrointestinal, neuromuscular, cardiac and renal systems. Gastrointestinal changes include anorexia, nausea, vomiting, constipation, abdominal pain and dehydration. Neuromuscular changes are confusion, lethargy, convulsion and hyporeflexia. The heart may be affected, leading to rhythm disturbances such as bradycardia and tachycardia. Polyuria, polydipsia and renal failure are signs of renal dysfunction. Diagnostic studies will show a raised corrected serum calcium level (normal values 2.13–2.63 mmol/L). A calcium level over 3.0 mmol/L requires emergency interventions, which include:

- rapid hydration, in order to promote renal excretion of calcium, and diuretic therapy
- intravenous bisphosphonates (e.g. pamidronate, clodronate, zoledronic acid), which inhibit the release of bone calcium
- calcitonin, which inhibits bone resorption and promotes urinary excretion
- steroids, which decrease the release of cytokines that can stimulate osteoclastic activity
- Bisphosphonate therapy may be continued every 3–4 weeks in patients at risk of bone complications.

Specific nursing care measures are related to prescribed treatment regimens and include close monitoring of fluid intake and output, weight, oedema, respiratory distress, confusion and disorientation, maintenance of personal hygiene and elimination, and the overall enhancement of comfort.

The urgency of the treatment depends not only on the serum calcium level but also on an assessment of the individual's general health, symptoms and overall prognosis. In some circumstances, acute treatment may not be appropriate, and treatment and care will be related to effective symptom control and helping the patient and family to cope with issues related to death and dying. As current rehydration regimens are shorter than previously, patients will spend less time in an acute setting. This may be an advantage for many patients, particularly those with a poor prognosis, but it also makes significant care demands on family and community-based services. Monitoring of early signs and symptoms of recurrence of hypercalcaemia is an important aspect of care, and patients, families and carers will need advice and information regarding significant signs and symptoms. An oral fluid intake of 3 L per day is required to maintain hydration and promote the excretion of calcium. Assessment of practical and social support requirements, and liaison with other care agencies, is necessary to ensure that patients and their families feel secure and supported.

Spinal cord compression

Spinal cord compression is caused by either primary or, more frequently, secondary tumours which lead to vertebral destruction and compression of the spinal cord or cauda equina. The resultant impairment of venous return and arterial flow leads to ischaemia and subsequent destruction of neurological tissue.

Metastatic spinal tumours of the breast, lung and prostate are the most common cancers causing cord compression, accounting for over 50% of instances (Heys et al 1997). Signs and symptoms frequently begin with a history of back pain close to the site of compression, which is tender on palpation. The pain may radiate along the distribution of the nerve root, is not relieved by lying down, and is exacerbated by coughing or straight leg lifting. Motor weakness (weakness, foot drop, ataxia), sensory loss (paraesthesia, numbness, tingling), and abnormal bladder and bowel sphincter control then follow. Although the pain tends to increase gradually, neurological deficits rapidly evolve into paraplegia. The degree of sensory and motor loss is dependent on the level of the cord compression. The thoracic spine is the area most frequently affected (70%) followed by the lumbar and then the cervical spine. Diagnosis is made through both clinical signs and radiological investigation.

Early detection is vitally important, and treatment must be instituted rapidly to preserve as much neurological function as possible. Radiation therapy, surgical decompression or a combination of both may be recommended. Steroids are used immediately after diagnosis to decrease inflammation, relieve pain and increase neurological function. Chemotherapy may be used for extremely chemosensitive tumours (e.g. lymphomas), where a rapid effect may be seen.

Nursing care includes monitoring and evaluation of neurological status (sensory and motor function), vital signs and degree of pain. Assistance with self-care may be necessary if the patient is experiencing motor and sensory deficits. Assessment of skin integrity and the institution of measures to prevent skin breakdown are essential in patients experiencing sensory and motor deficits. Maintenance of regular bowel habits may require starting a bowel maintenance regimen (laxatives and suppositories). Loss of voluntary micturition control may result in distension, retention, urinary overflow and urinary tract infections. Patients may require intermittent catheterization if they are unable to void. Checking of residual urine after voiding is

necessary. Rehabilitation following the acute phase will be indicated if the patient suffers permanent deficits and may involve home modifications after occupational therapy and physiotherapy assessment.

Superior vena cava obstruction

Superior vena cava obstruction is a rare but distressing complication of primary or secondary disease in the thoracic cavity. Pressure from tumours or enlarged lymph nodes causes partial or complete obstruction of the vena cava, resulting in venous congestion in the head, arms and upper chest. The onset is usually insidious with the patient reporting increasing breathlessness, feelings of fullness in the head and neck, and upper body swelling. As the symptoms become more acute there may be stridor, cough, hoarseness, facial swelling and progressive cyanosis, a situation that is distressing and frightening for patient, family and carers. Radiotherapy is often the treatment of choice, and usually starts with one or more high doses followed by a course of lower doses, depending on tumour histology and clinical signs. Chemotherapy may be useful for chemosensitive tumours and is often used in combination with radiotherapy.

Nursing care is related to assistance with medical interventions, the alleviation of symptoms, and the provision of information and psychological support.

Other emergencies

Other emergencies may occur related to the cardiovascular system (e.g. cardiac tamponade, pericarditis). Erosion of major arteries may result in sudden catastrophic haemorrhage unless vascular surgery can be undertaken very swiftly.

A rare but life-threatening and distressing emergency is that of upper airway obstruction. Gradual onset may be followed by symptoms of acute breathlessness and stridor. A combination of radiotherapy and steroids is usually the most effective form of treatment, or possibly laser therapy to an obstructing lesion in the trachea.

In any such emergency, a combination of efficient clinical skills and a calm, empathic approach is required to help alleviate the distress and anxiety of the patient and the concerns of family and friends.

COMMON ISSUES IN COPING WITH CANCER

Coping with cancer is a complex, multidimensional and ongoing process for the person with cancer and their family. From discovery of disease, through complex treatment regimens, rehabilitation and dying, many challenges are faced by individuals and their caregivers. There is an increasing awareness that, in addition to quality medical care, patients need emotional care and support and an opportunity to express feelings and responses to the experience of cancer. An individual's perception of the threat posed by their disease is an important factor in determining their adjustment to it. The possibility that positive mental attitude may have a significant effect on disease outcome, particularly in patients with early non-metastatic cancers was suggested by Greer et al (1990). A more recent systematic review of studies examining the effects of various psychological coping styles on survival and recurrence of cancer has found the evidence to be inconsistent (Petticrew et al 2002) and patients should not feel under any pressure to adopt any particular coping mechanism in the absence of further research.

Grief and loss

Grieving by the person with cancer may be due to the loss of a body part or body function, loss of independence, loss of role in the family and/or society, and the threat to life. The loss may be partial or complete, temporary or permanent, but the meaning to the individual will, to a large extent, depend on personal beliefs, characteristics and circumstances. There is a great need to make sense of things and to find ways to adapt to the change and disruption to life, however devastating and fundamentally unacceptable. In advanced cancer, adjustment to imminent death is clearly a major focus of the grief, but other issues that cause distress may be related to the loss of independence or the effect that illness and death will have on the family. The work of Kubler-Ross (1973) was introduced in Chapter 4 and has had a major influence on shaping thinking and understanding about grieving. Five stages of grieving are described by Kubler-Ross:

1 denial
2 anger
3 bargaining
4 depression
5 acceptance.

It is recognized that these categories are neither mutually exclusive nor sequential. Behaviours characteristic of the various stages include: shock, disbelief, denial, crying, rage, frustration, anger, sorrow, detachment, acceptance, calmness, and return to realistic functioning and reattachment. Similarly, individuals do not necessarily move through these phases progressively or within a given period of time but fluctuate in their reactions, varying in the time spent in any given phase.

This and other theories of grief such as that of Parkes (1996) who describes phases or psychological transitions and Worden (1991) who defined tasks of grief work, have been criticized as being over simplistic and too focused on the ultimate goal of 'acceptance' and recovery. The implication being that if this is not achieved the person has somehow failed. The danger of labelling of behaviours in this way is that it may lead to stereotyping of patient responses and superficial understanding of complex phenomena. However, it can provide a framework for guiding understanding of what is happening to the individual and their significant others.

The extent to which there is *openness* about progress and care management issues at all stages of the cancer journey may vary considerably depending on the individual practitioners involved and the practice and culture of the care environment. In particular, the transition from active to palliative care and communication about death and dying still appear to be very challenging for many nurses and doctors. In their early and significant work, Glaser and Strauss (1968) proposed the concept of the 'dying trajectory' and the notions of certain and uncertain death at known or unknown times. The extent to which imminent death was acknowledged or discussed, they described as 'open' or 'closed' awareness and this was perceived to be orchestrated and maintained by staff. As a result, the support required by individual patients to develop effective coping styles was often not forthcoming. Although there is now more openness it is still an area of complexity and difficulty, and it is therefore not surprising that nurses may find such communication problematic (Wilkinson 1991). Acknowledging the reality of the situation, providing opportunities for listening, quiet discussion and the use of touch may help the individual to express feelings of grief, sorrow, anger or frustration.

Grieving is a normal process that requires understanding and support, but rarely direct intervention. Counseling and help from skilled, experienced workers may be necessary when grieving is delayed or one stage is prolonged, or the patient is not able to resolve grief. Problems may also arise when the patient and family members are at different stages of the grieving process at a given time. They may require help to understand the responses and feelings of one another and why conflicting emotions are occurring.

Need for information and knowledge

Advances in cancer treatment are encouraging: patients are living longer and the occurrence and duration of remissions of the disease are increasing. The period of hospitalization for most people with cancer is relatively short in relation to the overall illness experience. Responsibility for day-to-day care then rests to a large extent with the individual and the family, who require knowledge, skills and resources to manage the person's home care successfully. Understanding of the plan of care and reasons for it also facilitates patient and family participation in decision-making regarding treatment and care, and provides them with a sense of control and involvement in what is happening to them.

A teaching plan for the patient needs to take into account the patient's and family's perspectives. What are their major concerns about hospital and homecare management? What knowledge and skills do they possess? What resources exist within the family and neighbourhood? What healthcare and social services are available in the community? How does the patient learn best? What barriers exist to learning?

Teaching sessions may need to include supervised practise of care as well as information giving, so that the appropriate knowledge and skills are developed to enable procedures to be carried out safely and effectively.

Written information given to the patient and family enhances learning and facilitates recall. The use of a variety of formats including CD-ROMs, DVDs, videos, slides and pictures helps the patient and family to envisage a technique or problem being discussed. Patients and family members may need advice and help to navigate the variety of resources now available to them, especially via the internet. Balmer (2005) found that patients were often unable to access the kind of information they needed from the media because it tended to be too technical or was designed to be newsworthy. Some patients may still decline offers of written information or may prefer information to be customized to their particular situation rather than generic; others will be armed with knowledge they have gained from internet websites not all of which may be reliable sources. Group sessions may be useful to provide basic information and to promote sharing and discussion of experiences, but all patients and families require some individualized sessions to explore issues that are unique to their particular situation.

An holistic assessment and review of actual and potential problems needs to be undertaken at key points of the patient's cancer journey and referral made to the primary care team and other agencies where appropriate. The single assessment process offers an opportunity for these assessments to be brought together (Richardson et al 2005). In most areas, specialist nursing services and hospital or community-based symptom control teams are available to advise and support patients and the staff involved in home care. In some localities, cancer patients with complex needs due either to their cancer diagnosis or other underlying chronic disease may be referred to community matrons for proactive case management. A variety of programmes promoting self management for people with chronic conditions including cancer are available including expert patient schemes and Learning to Live with Cancer courses (Van Der Molen and Hutchison 1999).

Sexual and reproductive changes

The experience of cancer and its subsequent treatment inevitably affects an individual's sexuality to a greater or lesser extent. This may be as a result of altered body structure and function resulting from the disease process and/or therapy; change in self-concept, body image or sense of attractiveness; lack of knowledge or understanding of the effects of the treatment or the disease; and prolonged hospitalization and its associated lack of privacy.

Reproductive capabilities will be directly affected if there is surgical removal of the uterus, ovaries or testes, but surgery that involves the colon, rectum and genitourinary structures may also cause physiological changes such as impotence, retrograde or lack of ejaculation, dyspareunia, sterility and decreased libido. Chemotherapy and radiotherapy can cause changes in function in relation to sexual response, fertility and fetal development. Sperm banking can be offered to men whose treatment plan may result in sterility. Effective contraception is advisable during and for up to 2 years following treatment to avoid not only the teratogenic effects of treatment but also to ensure the disease is under control.

Fatigue, pain, decreased physical mobility, sterility, impotence and alterations in body structures resulting from the cancer or therapy may be barriers to sexual expression. Other factors including the pharmacological effects of medications and psychological factors such as fear and anxiety and clinical depression may affect sexual functioning (Hughes 2000). Confrontation with a potentially fatal disease may expose previous sexual and relationship difficulties, but it can also provide an opportunity for couples and individuals to reassess their values and relationship. They may find that sexual expression enhances the feelings of being alive and human, and that it may serve to allay fears and provide comfort to both partners.

Open communication regarding sexuality is enhanced when trust and respect are part of the nurse–patient relationship. Unfortunately there is evidence to suggest that many nurses and doctors continue to be embarrassed or uncomfortable in discussing aspects of sexuality (Katz 2005). Continuing professional development could provide opportunities for nurses to explore personal feelings and constraints, and develop effective approaches in this sensitive area.

General approaches that are helpful are:

- conveying a willingness to discuss the topic and providing privacy
- exploring physical and psychological issues related to disease and treatment
- providing accurate and manageable information and correcting any misinformation
- using open questions to explore and elicit fears and concerns.

Some patients and their partners may require specific information on measures available to compensate for the changes resulting from the disease or treatment (e.g. use of a lubricating gel when vaginal secretions are decreased; alternative positions and ways of expressing physical love). Complex problems may be referred to an appropriate specialist who can provide counseling and support for the patient and partner. The PLISSIT (permission, limited information, specific suggestions and intensive therapy) model provides a useful framework for nurses to use when assessing sexual concerns and its use in relation to cancer patients is described by Hughes (2000) and also by Holmes (2005).

Altered body image and self-concept

Physical changes may result from the cancer itself, surgical removal of a body part, or the effects of chemotherapy or radiation treatment. The loss of a limb, a mastectomy, mandibular resection, loss of hair, changes in skin pigmentation, skin rashes and weight loss are examples of visible changes in the body with which many cancer patients are faced.

Body image is concerned with both body perception and body attitudes. Actual changes in body structure and function can be assessed objectively, but how the individual perceives these changes and how they influence his or her responses is entirely subjective and thus difficult to measure. The patient with a disturbance in body image may exhibit:

- decreased socialization
- denial of the changes and avoidance of looking at the affected body part or of looking into a mirror
- refusal to touch the affected part
- avoidance of physical contact with close family members or friends
- expression of fears of rejection
- expression of feelings of hopelessness and helplessness
- preoccupation with the change.

Grieving for the lost part or previous physical appearance occurs before the patient can adjust to the changes, whether they are temporary, permanent, actual or perceived. Acceptance and understanding of this and exploration of the meaning of the loss to the individual concerned will be helpful in establishing rapport and empathy.

The cause of the physical changes and what may be expected should be explained and personal fears and concerns explored. Practical suggestions as to how physical changes and appearance may be managed are useful and these may involve the use of make-up, wearing a wig, or using clothing to cover defects or scars, so long as this is acceptable to them. However, over-concentration on practicalities may conceal the need to explore and develop more cognitive strategies to deal with the loss and facilitate adjustment. Greer and Moorey (1997) advocate the notion of 'adjuvant' psychological therapy to provide individuals with a different range of skills and support in order to address the impact of disease and treatment. Other practitioners advocate the value of therapeutic touch and in particular massage therapy in helping individuals to experience their body in a more positive way, particularly those who have undergone mutilating surgery (Corner et al 1995a).

PSYCHOSOCIAL AND EMOTIONAL RESPONSES

The experience of cancer may evoke a range of complex emotional and behavioural responses. Good communication and interpersonal skills will always be effective in developing empathy and enhancing patient care. Some patients' needs may be beyond the experience of the general nurse and the need for specialist help should be recognized and facilitated. The NICE guidelines *Improving Supportive and Palliative Care for Adults with Cancer* (NICE 2004) recommend four levels of psychological assessment and intervention as well a acknowledging the ability of patients themselves to meet their needs for psychosocial support from a range of sources. Level one involves all staff directly responsible for patient care, level two involves the ability to screen for psychological distress, level three requires trained and accredited professionals to differentiate between moderate and severe levels of psychological need and level four involves mental health specialists who can assess patients who have complex problems such as personality disorders or psychotic illness. The patient may experience a number of emotional responses to their illness and it is important to consider the ways in which the nurse may offer support and assistance.

Anger and hostility

Anger is a common and appropriate response to the insults imposed by cancer and its treatment on bodily and personal integrity. Anger can have enormous adaptive value, allowing patients to mobilize inner resources of strength, determination and hope. Adaptive anger is generally not directed at anyone in particular. Dysfunctional anger, on the other hand, is more diffuse and intense, and may feel out of control to the patient. Dysfunctional expressions of anger may include self-destructive behaviour, refusal of treatment, and displacement onto family members, healthcare providers and others. Such exaggerated anger can isolate the patient from important sources of personal support. Providing quality nursing care to an angry patient is not easy and nurses may become afraid and defensive, and withdraw. This increases the patient's anger and a vicious circle begins. The patient manifesting anger is not likely to feel grateful or express gratitude for the care given and it can be difficult to accept and tolerate the anger and work with the patient to clarify and validate its sources. However, because anger is usually a defence against deeper feelings of hurt and fear, an understanding of this will enable nurses to work gently and compassionately towards strategies for resolution.

The patient needs to be encouraged to move beyond the anger to problem-solving strategies in order to cope with the situation that caused the feelings; however, these actions will not magically eliminate the patient's feelings of anger. The patient will continue to need to express anger as it is experienced.

Some patients are so angry that trust is not possible. This usually occurs when the anger is not dealt with and a very unhealthy system of interaction develops. Some patients have had such negative experiences in other institutions or situations that trust develops very slowly, if at all. Giving as much choice and control as possible, rather than setting strict limits, and providing continuity of care via a named nurse or key worker may be helpful.

Anxiety and fear

Anxiety has been described, with depression, as the most common psychosocial reaction experienced by persons with cancer (Lynch 1995). Anxiety is an unpleasant feeling of dread, and may be caused by an unconscious conflict between an underlying drive and the reality of the environment. The anxious person is unaware of the specific cause of his or her feelings. Anxiety is a different emotion from fear. Fear is an unpleasant feeling caused by a threat in the environment that is specific and can be identified.

Patients with cancer are justifiably fearful and anxious about many things: pain, death, abandonment, dependency, and recurrence. Some fears are based on inaccurate information and can be relieved by providing that information. Other fears, such as the anticipation of unrelieved pain, require exploration and reassurance where possible, along with a description of measures that will be taken to provide for the relief of pain.

Death is a real possibility for many patients and, as identified above, both staff and patients may find it difficult to discuss death openly. Anxieties about the actuality of death are hard to allay, but the anxiety may be related more to the process of dying than to death itself. Patients may fear that they will be abandoned, and exploration of particular fears and concerns, along with information about services and facilities available, may be helpful.

Depression

Depression, sadness, despair and hopelessness in response to losses can be thought of as natural consequences of the actual or potential disruption of a close attachment or important goals. As cancer represents the potential loss of not only life, but also of body parts and functions, roles and relationships, depression has been identified as one of the most common responses to cancer.

The depressed patient often moves, thinks and speaks slowly; motivation and energy are often very low. Patients who are extremely depressed have little desire or energy to express feelings or make decisions. People tend to either avoid the depressed person or attempt to 'cheer them up' with happy, bubbly, enthusiastic talk: both actions may drive patients further within themselves. A better strategy is to try to encourage patients to talk about their thoughts and feelings. If very withdrawn, remaining silently with the patient for periods interspersed throughout the day can sometimes be helpful.

Sometimes patients can feel very depressed and conceal the feeling behind a facade of 'normal' or even excessively happy behaviour. This type of depression is a serious drain on the patient's available energy. Signs of this depression will be much more subtle but many of these patients admit to feeling depressed if asked. One of the difficulties in detecting depression in people with cancer is disentangling the symptoms of depression from those of the disease or its treatment.

Various psychological therapies, with or without antidepressant medication, may be used to manage depression. For some individuals, a sense of greater well-being may be induced through use of complementary therapies such as massage, art therapy, reflexology or relaxation.

Uncertainty and loss of control

The uncertainty and lack of predictability of the course of terminal illness can create enormous stresses. Most people are accustomed to a certain amount of predictability in their daily lives and in the way their bodies function. Cancer creates havoc. How will treatment turn out? When will new symptoms develop? How and when will death come? Uncertainty places enormous constraints and demands on the patient and those close to them.

The feeling that one's internal environment is out of control often generates a frightening sensation of helplessness and vulnerability. Deep shame may arise from concerns about loss of physiological control. Some patients fear that they will not be able to control their emotions under the stress of cancer.

Serious illness such as cancer often serves to diminish, at least temporarily, a patient's sphere of control. In addition, the patient is often required to give up certain usual roles and responsibilities and to accept the care of others. For patients whose self-esteem and sense of personal worth derives from attending to others, the need to be taken care of may cause great conflict. In addition, work, finances and family issues may be negotiated without the patient's involvement. It is hard for individuals to maintain any sense of 'health' when being treated for cancer, even when the treatment is aimed at cure. McWilliam et al (1996) explored the effectiveness of a health promotion intervention for people with chronic illnesses, including cancer, and found that individuals employed a number of strategies to promote a sense of health. These included drawing on friends and family, maintaining a sense of control, and reframing expectations of life and self.

Family issues

The patient's family suffers as a result of temporary or permanent changes in the patient's capacity to fulfil family and career roles. There is increased stress on family members with role transitions, and changes in responsibilities (Flanagan 2001). Family members may feel despair, isolation, vulnerability and helplessness, uncertainty, confusion and shock (Hilton 1993, Northouse and Peters-Golden 1993). They may feel excluded from care as professional caregivers focus on the care of the patient. Families may encounter difficulty in obtaining information from professionals and communication within the family may be affected. It is common that family members are unsure how to discuss a diagnosis of cancer and this can result in emotional tension exhibited as anxiety, agitation or guilt. A sense of helplessness and loss of control is common at this time.

The family may gradually adjust to changes in roles and lifestyles, and may begin to learn to live with uncertainty. Changing role responsibilities in the family may cause the patient to feel dependent on others and to worry about being a burden. Meanwhile other family members may have had little preparation to assume various roles within the family structure such as parenting or managing the finances. Financial resources may be affected by the loss of ability to work and the needs of well family members may be neglected because of the focus on the ill member. Coping with uncertainty about the future is a challenge for all family members. Some families may have open communication about fears and uncertainties, whereas others may be closed in order to try to prevent worry.

If the patient reaches a terminal phase the family are faced with the issues of providing care and support to the dying person, communicating about death among family members, and with feelings of loss and separation. Very little discussion about death may occur among family members, which may be an effective coping mechanism for some people. Caring for the dying family member may cause considerable strain on the family. Families have learning needs in terms of physical aspects of care, pain control and increased dependency. Feelings of grief and loss are paramount at this time and the family may feel helpless, abandoned and anxious.

Nurses can help families at this time by providing assistance, support and information. The family can be informed of available community resources for patient care and social services. Referral for counseling may be appropriate when the family is facing long-term disruption and when the ability of the family to cope is actually or potentially inadequate. Family members are encouraged to seek help from those they consider to be helpful and appropriate for them. Continuing help and support should be readily available from the nurse, doctor, social worker, pastoral counselor, hospital chaplain, friends and relatives. Continuity in those giving care does much to facilitate communication and long-term planning.

It is important that family members spend time together as well as resuming socialization outside the home. In the hospital setting, measures need to be taken to provide privacy and opportunities for the family to be together as a unit.

CARE OF THE PATIENT WITH ADVANCED CANCER

The care of the patient with advanced cancer in the terminal phase of their disease is directed towards the relief of symptoms and improving the quality of life, as opposed to quantity of life. Palliative care seeks to provide a holistic approach, focusing not only on the physical symptoms of disease but also the psychosocial and spiritual needs of the patient, and extending this care to the family and significant others. Care may be provided within an institution (i.e. hospital, nursing home, or hospice) or within the home. Increasingly, patients may experience care in all these settings at various times, depending on symptoms and therapy needs, and the availability of support systems and carers. It is important to establish the individual's preference for end-of-life care and to facilitate this whenever possible by advance planning. Many GP practices have registers of their patients who have advanced cancer and aim to proactively manage care through use of the Gold Standards framework (Thomas 2003). This focuses on the key areas of:

- communication
- coordination
- control of symptoms
- continuity including out of hours
- continued learning
- carer support
- care in the dying phase.

The aims of the Gold Standards are to:

- keep patients' symptoms controlled
- enable them to die where they choose
- prevent fewer crises and admissions to hospital by anticipating problems and planning for these in advance
- provide support for carers
- improve teamwork.

There are a number of symptoms that are common to patients with advanced disease, related largely to alterations in comfort and physical or psychosocial distress. Pain is an important issue in advanced cancer, and is a feature of the terminal phase of illness for many people. The increasing severity of pain may be perceived as signifying advance of the cancer to some patients and their families. The pain contributes to the physiological and psychological factors that, in turn, enhance its severity. Loss of sleep and rest due to pain increases the patient's fatigue. Anorexia, nausea and vomiting associated with the pain contribute to nutritional deficiencies and weight loss. Mobility is restricted by the pain, increasing the potential for skin breakdown, constipation, muscle weakness and chest complications. The patient may exhibit anxiety, irritability, anger and withdrawal. Adequate pain control requires the cooperative efforts of the patient and the care team, and is a central goal of palliative care.

Opioid drugs are usually the first choice for most forms of severe cancer pain, with or without other adjuvant drugs. Concurrent administration of oral laxatives and careful monitoring of bowel movements is necessary to avoid opioid-induced constipation. This largely avoidable condition is a cause of great distress to patients and is a common cause of admission to hospice or hospital.

Even in the terminal phase of disease, many pathological processes can be modified through the selective use of mainstream cancer therapies. Radiotherapy is particularly helpful for the treatment of bone pain and for reducing a tumour mass that is causing pain and pressure symptoms. Occasionally chemotherapy may be useful in reducing tumour bulk and associated pain, but the value of this would need to be weighed against side-effects such as hair loss, weakness and the general malaise associated with most forms of chemotherapy. Surgical interventions such as wound debridement, bypassing of abdominal obstruction, and the fixation of fractures are all commonly undertaken for patients with advanced disease. Again, careful consideration needs to be given to the possible consequences of such interventions, for instance anaesthetic risks, impaired healing due to malignancy and malnutrition, and full informed consent obtained.

People who are terminally ill respond and cope in a variety of ways. They are grieving for a range of actual and potential losses, while still trying to maintain hope. While the hope is not likely to be for a cure, hope remains to achieve short-term goals, to have a painless death, or to participate in a particular event or family occasion.

Frequent emotional responses are denial, anxiety, fear, depression, withdrawal, acceptance, resignation and anger. Denial may assist the individual to protect himself or herself from the painful reality of dying and to preserve hope. There are certainly degrees of denial and, while it is a useful protective response, it may also interfere with problem solving and communication between patient and family or patient and caregivers. Fear is a response to perceived danger, whereas anxiety is a feeling of distress and discomfort. Sources of anxiety for the patient may be spiritual in nature, fear of death, or fear of the dying process and what may be ahead. The person may respond to a terminal illness by withdrawal and depression as he or she disengages from relationships and surroundings. Acceptance and resignation to disease may fluctuate over time. They are dynamic in nature and may be observed in concert with other responses. Sadness and a sense of aloneness may be apparent at this time. Anger may be felt in response to actual and expected losses, and sometimes to the helplessness that patients experience.

The experiences of families caring for individuals in the terminal phase of illness were explored in a study by Addington-Hall and McArthur (1995). Families described a number of symptoms that caused distress to a greater or lesser extent, and pain was reported as being 'very distressing' for over 60%. Other items that caused distress were breathlessness, dry mouth or thirst, nausea and vomiting, loss of appetite, and constipation. Over half reported that they were unable to get all the information about their dying relative that they needed. Families want to be assured of patient comfort and may wish to be physically close to the dying person and to spend as much time as possible with them. The Liverpool Care Pathway for the Dying Patient (Ellershaw and Wilkinson 2003) is a valuable integrated care pathway designed to allow hospice principles of caring for dying patients to be utilized in other care settings including acute wards.

Following death, the withdrawal of contact with health professionals such as the community nursing services may be an additional loss for those who are left behind. Referral to specialist bereavement counseling services may be appropriate for some individuals to provide support and guidance during the period of mourning and reorganization.

Caring for people who are dying is extremely demanding and nurses need to be realistic about how far they can actually help and support family caregivers in their grief and loss. Strategies to prevent care fatigue and to foster positive personal coping behaviours need to be addressed at an individual and an organizational level (Mathers 1995).

Spiritual issues

Cawley (1997) suggests that spirituality may be beyond standard definition or expression in words but involves the individual's attempt to find meaning and purpose in life and encompasses the concepts of faith, hope and love. Kim et al (1984) view distress of the human spirit as a disruption in the life principle that pervades a person's entire being and that integrates and transcends their biological and psychological nature. Factors related to the spiritual distress of the patient with cancer may include: challenged belief and value system, loss of sense of purpose, a feeling of remoteness from God, loss of faith, questioning of the moral–ethical nature of therapy, a sense of guilt or shame, intense mental suffering, unresolved feelings about death, and anger toward God.

Expression of distress of the human spirit is very individualized. Behaviours that may indicate spiritual distress include: struggles with the meaning of life and death, seeking of spiritual assistance, expressions of anger and/or guilt, crying, withdrawal, sleep disturbances, questioning the meaning of suffering, fear of ability to endure suffering, views of illness as a punishment from God, questioning or refusing therapy, and seeking unorthodox therapy (Kim and Moritz 1982).

Some patients may find the confrontation with their values and religious beliefs to be a rewarding and reassuring experience, but for others it may be a source of considerable distress. Helping a person to address the spiritual aspects of their life offers a unique but, for many, a very challenging opportunity. Burnard (1993) emphasizes the need for nurses to explore their own beliefs and understanding about spirituality before seeking to embark on this with others. The assessment of spiritual care needs is an important area of care, but Ross (1997) suggests that nurses often neglect this, possibly as a result of varying degrees of spiritual distress on their own account.

Recognizing spiritual distress in others should be within the scope of all nurses' professional practice, but realistically there may be different levels of comfort and expertise in encouraging the patient to express feelings of support or conflict related to spiritual needs. Issues raised may challenge the nurse to respond in ways that that are flexible, non-judgemental and possibly at odds with their own belief systems. If the person has a particular religious observance, a religious adviser known and respected by the patient may be a more appropriate person to explore these issues. In general terms, the practice of religious observances can be facilitated by providing privacy for prayers or personal discussions, encouraging attendance at a place of worship, or arranging for visits and observances at the bedside.

REHABILITATION

Until recently, the term 'cancer rehabilitation' was seldom found in cancer nursing literature. Perhaps the view of cancer as a terminal disease has conflicted with the concept of rehabilitation. Often, little thought is given to rehabilitation of the patient with cancer compared with those with other conditions such as cardiac disease or stroke, with needs not therefore identified or resources allocated. However, improvements in early detection, treatment and supportive care have led to an increased number of people surviving and living with cancer.

Rehabilitation is a process that maintains or restores a person to an optimal level of functioning and effectiveness within the limitations of their disease or disability in terms of their physical, mental, emotional, social and economic potential. It affords an opportunity to redefine what a meaningful life is. A variety of disease and cancer treatment-related problems amenable to rehabilitation approaches have been identified, including decreased mobility, problems with activities of daily living (including weakness), pain, nutritional problems, financial and vocational problems, appearance, lymphoedema, respiratory difficulties, swallowing disorders, communication, transportation, and difficulties in individual and family psychological adjustment.

The rehabilitation team may include a doctor, rehabilitation nurse, specialist nurses (e.g. breast or stoma care nurse), physiotherapist, occupational therapist, speech and language therapist, orthoptist, prosthetist, vocational counselor, nutritionist, psychologist, social worker and minister of religion. Not every, or even most, patients will need all the resources available. However, it would seem likely that almost all people with cancer will need the services of at least one of the team members at some stage during the cancer experience.

Assessment of needs and goal setting are key aspects of rehabilitation, centred around an individual's functional ability. The aim is to foster independence through positive adaptation to the changing circumstances imposed by the disease or treatment.

The assessment and interventions relative to many of the rehabilitation needs of people with cancer have been addressed in other sections of this chapter. The principles and philosophy of rehabilitation should be an integral part of cancer care practice.

SURVIVORSHIP

Early detection and effective multimodal therapies have increased significantly the numbers of cancer survivors. Historically, cancer survivors have been defined as individuals 'cured' of their disease, with the 'cured' state commencing 5 years after diagnosis. The burgeoning population of survivors has given emphasis to the need to address quality of survival and the psychosocial consequences of cancer and its treatment. Long-term survivors may experience problems ranging from minor short-term difficulties to major psychosocial crises.

Fear of recurrence is probably the most common concern for all cancer survivors. Fear of relapse may present in a variety of forms, ranging from general uneasiness about the aetiology of mild to moderate or intermittent symptoms, to pronounced anxiety that interferes with daily life. As time passes, anxiety concerning recurrence may decrease, although a heightened sense of vulnerability to illness is often a feature of the survivor's experience. Not knowing when and whether cancer will reappear often negatively affects the survivor's sense of control over his or her life (Burnet and Robinson 2000).

The need for close, ongoing evaluation after the cessation of therapy mandates an ongoing relationship between the patient and the healthcare team. These relationships may engender both ambivalence and anxiety. As patients are nearing the end of treatment, they may feel elated over the prospect of discontinuing therapy, while at the same time being fearful of distancing themselves from the team that has helped them to get to this extended survival stage. Fear of detecting recurrence or other problems can lead to hypochondriasis, avoidance of doctors and pronounced anxiety about attending follow-up examinations.

Attempts to minimize memories of the treatment experience and to return to usual life tasks may not be easy. The transition from a sick role to a healthy role may be challenged by physical symptoms, negative expectations from those within the patient's work and social circle, and social stigma. The survivor's family may also worry about the possibility of relapse and the difficulties of social reintegration, and may respond with over-protectiveness and pervasive anxiety. On the other hand, family members may be hesitant to discuss mutual concerns about the recurrence of cancer because these concerns can trigger their own sense of insecurity about the future. Many survivors encounter ongoing socioeconomic impediments to full recovery, including difficulties regaining financial and work-related stability.

Because of the prevailing perception that cancer results in a painful, lingering death, most patients' immediate reaction to the diagnosis is the expectation of a shortened lifespan. Once successful completion of therapy is achieved, hope for continued survival often supersedes thoughts of death. Many survivors experience a greater appreciation of life and a greater sense of generalized well-being.

The availability of wellness-oriented follow-up clinics, education, counseling and supportive services, as well as advocacy, community action and policy development, are crucial to the achievement of quality survival. Further research is required to identify needs, and to develop and evaluate model programmes encompassing both professional and peer support.

SUMMARY

Although cancer remains a major healthcare problem and a very threatening, isolating illness for the patient and family to confront individually, significant progress continues to be made in the diagnosis, treatment and control of the numerous forms of cancer. New approaches to early diagnosis of cancer, new techniques to treat cancer, new measures to ameliorate distressing manifestations of cancer and its treatment, and new approaches to improve the quality of life for cancer survivors will continue to emerge.

Cancer nursing is integral to all these developments and, as such, will continue to be one of the most challenging fields in health care. This chapter has sought to provide an overview of the nature, treatment and experience of cancer, and of the many ways in which nurses may be involved in providing care and supporting individuals at all stages of the cancer journey. As the body of scientific knowledge and nursing knowledge continues to expand, there are new opportunities for nurses in this field such as nurse prescribing and the development of advanced nursing roles in clinical practice.

Peer review and clinical audit provides an opportunity for nurses and other staff to evaluate and monitor service provision. Reflection on practice is an increasing feature of professional nursing, and Johns (1996) believes that reflection offers nurses an opportunity to explore and develop greater understanding about the experience of practice and to reaffirm caring values. As this could be a difficult or painful process at times, an effective and accessible system of clinical supervision needs to be available.

Recent policy initiatives have also led to the rapid expansion of specialist nursing roles in many aspects of cancer care. In line with policy directives, these tend to be related to site-specific diseases (e.g. breast, lung, colorectal, gynaecology, head and neck), and the requirements of the roles may vary considerably depending on location and individual perceptions. However, a common feature of all is the recognition of the specialist nurse as a pivotal member of the multidisciplinary team. Such roles provide for increased levels of support to be offered to people with cancer and the opportunities for nurses to pursue research and provide an evidence base for practice. Standards for the education and training for these specialist roles and for chemotherapy nurses have been defined by the Manual for Cancer Services (DoH 2004), however, it must be acknowledged that the majority of cancer care is still provided by general nurses in hospitals and in community settings.

There is increasing interest in all aspects of practice development in cancer care particularly that which actively involves the perceptions and experiences of healthcare users in shaping services. Caring for people with cancer is complex and challenging but is also extremely rewarding, as it offers so many opportunities not only to enhance the experience of patients but also for the personal and professional growth and development of the nurses involved in this field of work.

REFERENCES

Addington-Hall J, McArthur M (1995) Dying from cancer – results of a national population-based investigation. Palliative Medicine 9: 295–305.

Allwood M, Stanley A, Wright P (eds) (2002) The cytotoxic handbook, 4th edn. Oxford: Radcliffe Medical Press.

Ash DV (1999) Breast irradiation injury litigation and RAGE. Clinical Oncology 11: 138–139.

Balmer C (2005) The information requirements of people with cancer. Cancer Nursing 28(1): 36–44.

Batchelor D (2001) Hair and cancer chemotherapy:consequences and nursing care – a literature survey. European Journal of Cancer Care 10: 147–163.

Beaver K, Luker K, Glynn Owens R et al (1996) Treatment decision making in women newly diagnosed with breast cancer. Cancer Nursing 19: 8–19.

Bianchini F, Kaaks R, Vainio H (2002) Overweight, obesity and cancer risk. The Lancet Oncology 3 (9): 565–574.

Brennan J (2004) Cancer in context: a practical guide to supportive care. Oxford: OUP.

Burnard P (1993) Giving spiritual care. Journal of Community Nursing 1: 16–18.

Burnet NG, Robinson L (2000) Psychosocial impact of recurrent cancer. European Journal of Oncology Nursing 4(1): 29–38.

Campbell T, Draper S, Reid J et al (2001) The management of constipation in people with advanced cancer. International Journal of Palliative Nursing 7(3): 100–119.

Cancer Research UK (2005a) UK cancer incidence statistics by age. Online. Available: http://info.cancerresearchuk.org/cancerstats/incidence/age/

Cancer Research UK (2005b) Reduce the risk. Online .Available: http://info.cancerresearchuk.org/healthyliving/reducetherisk/

Cancer Research UK (2006) Cancer worldwide – the global picture. Online. Available: http://info.cancerresearchuk.org/cancerstats/geographic/world/?a=5441

Cawley N (1997) An exploration of the concept of spirituality. International Journal of Palliative Care 3: 31–36.

Church JM (1996) Prophylactic colectomy in patients with hereditary nonpolyposis colectal cancer. Annals of Medicine 28: 479–482.

Control of substances hazardous to health (2002) The control of substances hazardous to health regulations 2002. Approved code of practice and guidance L5, 4th edn. Sudbury: HSE Books.

Cooley C (2002) Oral health: basic or essential care? Cancer Nursing Practice 1(3): 33–40.

Corner J, Cawley N, Hildebrand S (1995a) An evaluation of the use of massage and massage with essential oils on the well-being of cancer patients. International Journal of Palliative Care Nursing 1: 67–73.

Corner J, Harewood J(2004) Exploring the use of complementary and alternative medicine by people with cancer. Nursing Times research 9(2): 101–109.

Corner J, Plant H, Warner L (1995b) Developing a nursing approach to managing dyspnoea in lung cancer. International Journal of Palliative Care Nursing 1: 5–11.

Davidson T, Sacks NPM (1995) Principles of surgical oncology. In: Horwich A, ed. Oncology: a multidisciplinary textbook. London: Chapman & Hall, p 101–115.

Degner L, Khristjanson L, Bowman D et al (1997) Information needs and decisional preferences in women with breast cancer. Journal of the American Medical Association 112(18): 1485–1497.

Department of Health (2000) National cancer plan. London: The Stationery Office.

Department of Health (2003) HSC 2003/010 Updated national guidance on the safe administration of intrathecal chemotherapy Annex A. London: DH Publications.

Department of Health (2004) The Manual for cancer services. Online. Available: http://www.cquins.nhs.uk

Dietz J (1981) Rehabilitation oncology. New York: Wiley.

Dougherty L (1995) Scalp cooling to prevent hair loss in chemotherapy. Professional Nurse 11: 507–509.

Dougherty L (2004) Scalp cooling. In: Dougherty L, Lister S, eds. The Royal Marsden Hospital manual of clinical nursing procedures, 6th edn. Oxford: Blackwell.

Dougherty L, Lister S, eds (2004) The Royal Marsden Hospital manual of clinical nursing procedures, 6th edn. Oxford: Blackwell.

Dougherty L, Viner C, Young J (1998) Establishing ambulatory chemotherapy at home. Professional Nurse 13: 356–358.

Dudjak L (1992) Cancer metastasis. Seminars in Oncology Nursing 8(1): 40–50.

Eilers J (2004) Nursing interventions and supportive care for the prevention and treatment of oral mucositis associated with cancer treatment. Oncology Nursing Forum 31(4) Supp:13–23.

Ellershaw J, Wilkinson S (2003) Care of the dying. A pathway to excellence. Oxford: Oxford University Press.

Falk S, Fallon M (1997) ABC of palliative care: emergencies. British Medical Journal 315: 1525–1528.

Fallowfield L (1998) Early discharge after surgery for breast cancer: might not be applicable to most patients. British Medical Journal 317: 1264–1265 (editorial).

Feber T (1995) Mouth care for patients receiving oral irradiation. Professional Nurse 10(10): 666–669.

Fellowes D, Barnes K, Wilkinson S (2005) Aromatherapy and massage for symptom relief in patients with cancer. The Cochrane Library, No 4 (CD002287). Online. Available: http://www.mrw.interscience.wiley.com/Cochrane/clsysrev/articl e/CD002287/toc.html

Flanagan J (2001) Clinically effective cancer care: working with families. European Journal of Oncology nursing 5(3): 174–179.

Ford D, Easton DF, Stratton MR et al (1998) Genetic heterogeneity and penetrance analysis of the BRCA1 and BRCA2 genes in breast cancer families. American Journal of Human Genetics 62: 676–689.

Gabriel J (1996) Peripherally inserted central catheters: expanding UK nurses' practice. British Journal of Nursing 5: 71–74.

Gamble K (1998) Communication and information: the experience of radiotherapy patients. European Journal of Cancer Care 5: 153–158.

Gerbrecht B, Kangas T (2004) Implications of capecitabine (Xeloda) for cancer nursing practice. European Journal of Oncology Nursing 8: S63–71.

Glaser B, Strauss AL (1968) Time for dying. Chicago: Aldine.

Glean E, Edwards S, Faithfull S (2001) Intervention for acute radioterapy induced skin reactions in cancer patients: The development of a clinical guideline recommended for use by the College of Radiographers. Journal of Radiotherapy in Practice, 2(2): 75–84.

Goodman I (ed) (1998) Clinical practice guidelines: the administration of cytotoxic chemotherapy. Recommendations. Harrow: Nursing Standard Publications.

Gore M, Riches PM, eds. (1995) Immunotherapy of cancer. Oxford: Churchill Livingstone.

Greer S, Moorey S (1997) Adjuvant psychological therapy for cancer patients. Palliative Medicine 11(3): 240–244.

Greer S, Morris T, Pettingale KW et al (1990) Psychological response to breast cancer and 15 year outcome. Lancet 335: 49–50.

Hall D (1995) New ideas on fractionation and accelerated radiotherapy. Nursing Times 91(12): 42–43.

Hanks GW (2005) Pain relief in cancer: recent developments. Cancer Nursing Practice March Supp: 12–15.

Hartman LC, Shaid DJ, Woods JE et al (1999) Efficacy of bilateral prophylactic mastectomy in women with a family history of breast cancer. New England Journal of Medicine 340: 77–84.

Health and Safety Executive (2003) Safe handling of cytoxic drugs. HSE Information Shett MISC615. Online. Available: http://www.hse.gov.uk/pubns/misc615pdf

Hermanek O, Hutter RUP, Sobin LH, eds (1997) UICC TMN atlas, 4th edn. Berlin: Springer.

Herth K (1990) Fostering hope in terminally ill people. Journal of Advanced Nursing 18: 538–548.

Heys SP, Currie D, Eremin O (1997) The management of patients with advanced cancer III. European Journal of Surgical Oncology 23: 361–365.

Hilton BA (1993) Issues, problems and challenges for families coping with breast cancer. Seminars in Oncology Nursing 9(2): 88–100.

Holmes S (2002) Nutrition and cancer. Cancer Nursing practice 1 (5): 31–38.

Holmes L (2005) Sexuality in gynaecological cancer patients. Cancer Nursing Practice 4(6): 35–39.

How C, Brown J (1998) Extravasation of cytotoxic chemotherapy from peripheral veins. European Journal of Oncology Nursing 2: 51–58.

Hughes MK (2000) sexuality and the cancer survivor – a silent coexistence. Cancer Nursing 23(6): 477–482.

Johns C (1996) Visualising and realising caring in practice through guided reflection. Journal of Advanced Nursing 24: 1135–1143.

Jones R, Hansford J, Fiske J (1993) Death from cancer at home: the carer's perspective. British Medical Journal 306: 249–251.

Katz A (2005) The art of oncology:when the tumour is not the target. The sounds of silence: sexuality information for cancer patients. Journal of Clinical Oncology 23(1): 238–241.

Kim MJ, Moritz DA, eds (1982) Classification of nursing diagnosis. New York: McGraw-Hill.

Kim MJ, McFarland GK, McLaine AM (1984) Pocket guide to nursing diagnosis. St Louis, MO: Mosby.

Kubler-Ross E (1973) On death and dying. New York: Macmillan.

Lanceley A (1995) Wider issues in pain management. European Journal of Cancer Care 4: 153–157.

Langenhoff BS, Krabbe PFM, Wobbes T et al (2001) Quality of life as an outcome measure in surgical oncology. British Journal of Surgery 88(5): 643–652.

Law M (2004) Screening without evidence of efficacy. Bristish Medical Journal 328: 301–302. Online. Available: http://www.bmj.com 7 February 2004.

Lynch M (1995) The assessment and prevalence of affective disorders in advanced cancer. Journal of Palliative Care 11: 10–18.

McCaffrey M (1979) Nursing management of the patient with pain. Philadelphia: Lippincott.

McWilliam CL, Stewart M, Brown JB et al (1996) Creating health with chronic illness. Advances in Nursing Science 18: 1–15.

Mansel R E, Goyal A, Newcombe R G (2004) Objective assessment of lymphedema, shoulder function and sensory deficit after sentinel node biopsy for invasive breast cancer: ALMANAC trial. Breast Cancer Research and Treatment 88 Supp 1:S12.

Mathers P (1995) Learning to cope with the stress of palliative care. In: Penson J, Fisher R, eds. Palliative care for people with cancer, 2nd edn. London: Arnold, p 296–308.

National Cancer Alliance (1996) 'Patient-centred services?' What patients say. Oxford: NCA.

National Council for Hospice and Specialist Palliative Care Services (2003) Guidance for managing cancer pain in adults. London: National council for Hospice and Specialist Palliative Care Services.

National Institute for Clinical Excellence (2004) Improving supportive and palliative care for adults with cancer: the manual. London: National Institute for Clinical Excellence.

National Institute for Clinical Excellence (2005) Referral guidelines for suspected cancer. Clinical guideline 27. London: National Institute for Clinical Excellence.

NHS Cancer Screening Programmes 2006 NHS cervical screening programme. Online. Available: http://www.cancerscreeening.org.uk/cervical/lbc.html 1 Aug 2006.

Neill KM, Armstrong N, Burnet CB (1998) Choosing reconstruction after mastectomy – a qualitative analysis. Oncology Nursing Forum 25: 743–750.

NHS Quality Improvement Scotland (2004) Skincare for patients receiving radiotherapy. NHS Quality Improvement Scotland, Edinburgh. Online. Available: http://wwwnhshealthquality.org/nhsquis/files

Nikoletti S, Hyde S, Shaw T et al (2005) Comparison of plain ice or flavoured ice to prevent oral mucositis associated with 5 flourouracil. Journal of Clinical Nursing 14(6): 750–753.

Northouse L (1984a) Mastectomy patients and the fear of cancer recurrence. Cancer Nursing 4: 213–220.

Northouse LL, Peters-Golden H (1993) Cancer and the family: strategies to assist spouses. Seminars in Oncology Nursing 9(2): 74–82.

Parkes CM (1996) Bereavement;studies of grief in adult life, 3rd edn. London: Routledge.

Petticrew M, Bell R, Hunter D (2002) Influence of psychological coping on survival and recurrence in people with cancer: systematic review. British Medical Journal 325 (7372): 1066.

Ream E, Stone P (2004) Clinical interventions for fatigue. In: Armes J, Krishnasamy M, Higginson I, eds. Fatigue in cancer. Oxford: Oxford University Press.

Rhodes V, Johnson M, McDaniel R (1995) Nausea, vomiting and retching: the management of the symptom experience. Seminars in Oncology Nursing 11: 256–265.

Richardson A (1991) Theories of self-care; their relevance to chemotherapy-induced nausea and vomiting. Journal of Advanced Nursing 16: 671–676.

Richardson A (1995) Fatigue in cancer patients: a review of the literature. European Journal of Cancer Care 4: 20–32.

Richardson A, Sitzia J, Brown V et al (2005) Patients' needs assessment tools in cancer care: principles and practice. London: King's College London.

Ross L (1997) The nurse's role in assessing and responding to patients' spiritual needs. International Journal of Palliative Care 3: 37–41.

Saunders C, Baines M (1983) Living with dying. Oxford: Oxford University Press.

Sewell G, Cooper C, Robson G et al (2003) Marc guidelines. Selection and use of personal protective equipment (PPE) to minimise cytotoxic exposure. Online. Available: http://www.marcguidelines.com/templates/guidelineview.aspx?navigation=142 3 Jan 2006.

Slevin ML, Strubbs L, Plant HJ et al (1990) Attitudes to chemotherapy: comparing views of patients with cancer to those of doctors, nurses and the general public. British Medical Journal 300: 1458–1460.

Tavares M (2003) National guidelines for the use of complementary therapies in supportive and palliative care. The Prince of Wales Foundation for Integrated Health and the National Council for Hospice and Specialist Palliative Care Services. London: The Prince of Wales Foundation for Integrated Health.

Thomas K (2003) The gold standards framework in community palliative care. European Journal of Palliative Care 10(3): 113–115.

Thomas VN, Saleem T, Abraham R (2005) Barriers to effective uptake of screening among black and ethnic minority groups. International Journal of Palliative Nursing 11(11): 562–571.

Twycross RG (1997) Introducing palliative care, 2nd edn. Oxford: Radcliffe.

Twycross RG, Lack S (1990) Therapeutics in terminal care. Edinburgh: Churchill Livingstone.

Van Der Molen B, Hutchison G (1999) Learning to live with cancer: the UK experience of a European patient education and support programme. European Journal of Cancer Care 8: 170–173.

Vile R (1995) The metastatic cascade. In: Vile R. Cancer metastasis: from mechanisms to therapy. Chichester: John Wiley, p 1–20.

Wilkinson S (1991) Factors which influence how nurses communicate with cancer patients. Journal of Advanced Nursing 16: 677–688.

Wood A (2004) Mouth care and ritualistic practice. Cancer Nursing Practice 3(4): 34–39.

Woods M (2004) Causes and treatment of early lymphoedema . Cancer Nursing practice 3(5): 25–30.

Worden W (1991) Grief counselling and grief therapy, 2nd edn. London: Tavistock/Routledge.

World Cancer Research Fund (1997) Food, nutrition and the prevention of cancer: a global perspective. Washington: American Institute for Cancer Research.

World Health Organization (1986) Cancer pain relief. Geneva: WHO.

FURTHER READING

Brennan J (2004) Cancer in context: a practical guide to supportive care. Oxford: OUP.

Offers useful perspectives on the impact of a cancer diagnosis, not only for individual patients but also their families, partners and carers. Looks at the social and cultural context of cancer and examines the effects of caring for cancer patients on health professionals.

Brighton D, Wood M (2005) The Royal Marsden Hospital handbook of cancer chemotherapy. Edinburgh: Elsevier Churchill Livingstone

A resource both on general chemotherapy and chemotherapy specific to individual cancer sites.

Faithful S, Wells M (2003) Supportive care in radiotherapy. Edinburgh: Churchill Livingstone.

Reviews the challenges of caring for patients having radiotherapy and the management of problems associated with radiotherapy.

Kearney N, Richardson A (2006) Nursing patients with cancer: principles and practice. Edinburgh: Elsevier Churchill Livingstone.
A book that comprehensively covers all the main areas of caring for cancer patients and which integrates physiological, psychological and sociological aspects.
Souhami R, Tobias J (2005) Cancer and its management, 5th edn. Oxford: Blackwell Science.
A useful 'all round' text primarily on the medical management of cancer.

Twycross R, Wilcock A (2001) Symptom management in advanced cancer, 3rd edn. Oxford: Radcliffe.
Information and advice on the management of a wide range of symptoms.

USEFUL WEBSITE

http://www.cancerbacup.org.uk
Information for patients and professionals on all aspects of cancer.

12 Caring for the patient with a cardiovascular disorder

Alison Crumbie

INTRODUCTION

The care of people with a cardiovascular disorder utilizes a significant amount of nursing skill and resources. This is because cardiovascular disease remains one of the highest causes of morbidity and mortality in the world (WHO 2005). The World Health Organization estimates that currently, cardiovascular disease is a major cause of death worldwide, second only to infectious and parasitic diseases (WHO 2005). In the UK there are 2.6 million people who have coronary heart disease (CHD), approximately 660 000 people who live with heart failure and 65 000 people experienced a premature death in 2003 as a result of CHD (British Heart Foundation 2004). The UK's age standardized mortality rate for cardiovascular disease of 181 per 100 000 compares with the USA at 187 per 100 000, Spain at 137 per 100 000, China at 291 per 100 000 and India at 428 per 100 000 (WHO 2006a). Many conditions are chronic rather than curable, and in recent years nursing has adapted to more closely monitor and augment the health status of those with a cardiovascular condition. This has included the emergence of nurse-led clinics in the community and hospital settings, chest pain clinics and nurse-led thrombolysis. The latter allows specially trained nursing staff to administer thrombolytic (clot-busting) drugs to a set protocol when a patient is suffering a myocardial infarction (MI) owing to a blocked coronary artery. Such innovative approaches to traditional practice illustrate how nursing is developing and adapting to meet the needs of patients more fully. The government-initiated National Service Framework for Coronary Heart Disease, released in 2000, endorsed such practice, providing set standards to encourage the implementation of evidence-based practice and more equitable access to definitive treatments and care.

CIRCULATION

Normal cellular activity is dependent upon a constant supply of oxygen, nutrients and certain chemicals, as well as the removal of metabolic waste products. Specialized organs are necessary for the processes of oxygenation, nutrition and excretion, as well as a transportation system between these organs and cells throughout the body. This transportation of materials to and from tissue cells by the propulsion of blood through a closed system of tubes is the process referred to as circulation.

CIRCULATORY STRUCTURES

The circulatory system consists of the heart and the vascular system.

Heart
The **heart** is a hollow, cone-shaped, muscular organ lying obliquely in the thoracic cavity. Approximately two-thirds of it is situated to the left of the midline. The upper border (or base) lies just below the second rib. The lower border (or apex) is directed downward, forward and to the left, and lies on the diaphragm at the level of the fifth intercostal space in the left midclavicular line.

Pericardium

The **pericardium** is a strong, non-distensible sac which loosely encloses the heart and attaches to the large blood vessels at the base of the heart and to the diaphragm at the apex. Although the pericardial sac is firm and considered non-extensible, it does extend in response to the gradual, sustained stretching imposed by enlargement of the heart (*hypertrophy*).

Heart walls

The **walls of the heart** are composed of three layers of tissue:

1 The *epicardium* forms the outer layer of the heart and is the visceral layer of the pericardium.
2 The *myocardium* is the middle layer of tissue. This is composed of involuntary striated muscle fibres which interlace, branch and anastomose. This layer of muscle is responsible for the heart's contractile force.
3 The *endocardium* is a thin layer of endothelial cells lining the interior surface of the heart's chambers which covers the heart's valves. This layer creates a smooth surface, reducing friction between moving blood and the walls of the heart.

Heart chambers

The right and left sides of the heart each consist of two **chambers**, an *atrium*, which receives incoming blood, and a *ventricle*, which ejects blood into the arteries.

The atrial myocardium is much thinner than that of the ventricles, and the left ventricular wall is thicker than that of the right. This difference is related to the fact that the atria are required to deliver the blood only to the ventricles.

The right ventricle pumps blood through the lungs to the left atrium, forming the circuit referred to as the *pulmonary circulatory system*. The left ventricle must provide sufficient force to carry blood through all parts of the body and return it to the right atrium. This latter circuit is referred to as the *systemic circulatory system*.

Cardiac valves

Normal circulation requires the flow of the blood in one direction only. This is maintained in the heart by a set of four **valves**: two atrioventricular and two semilunar.

The right atrioventricular (AV) valve is located between the right atrium and ventricle. It has three cusps and is called the *tricuspid valve* (Fig. 12.1). The left AV valve, situated between the left atrium and ventricle, has two cusps and is called the *mitral valve*. These valves open into the ventricles but are prevented from opening into the atria by fine tendinous cords (*chordae tendineae*).

The *semilunar valves* guard the openings from the ventricles into the pulmonary artery and aorta, and are called the pulmonary and aortic valves, respectively. Each consists of three pocket-like pouches arranged around the origin of the artery, with the free borders being distal to the ventricle.

Electrical conduction system

The heart is a unique organ because it has an electrical **conduction** system to maintain its rate and rhythm of activity.

The *sinoatrial (SA) node* is a small mass of specialized tissue located in the upper portion of the right atrium near the superior vena cava inlet (Fig. 12.2). It is responsible for initiating impulses for a rhythmic heartbeat.

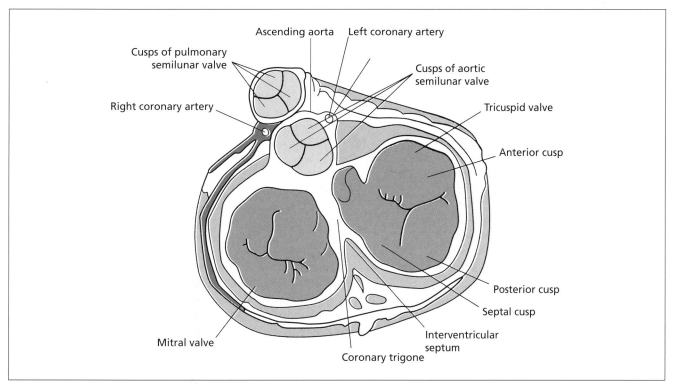

Figure 12.1 The valves of the heart.

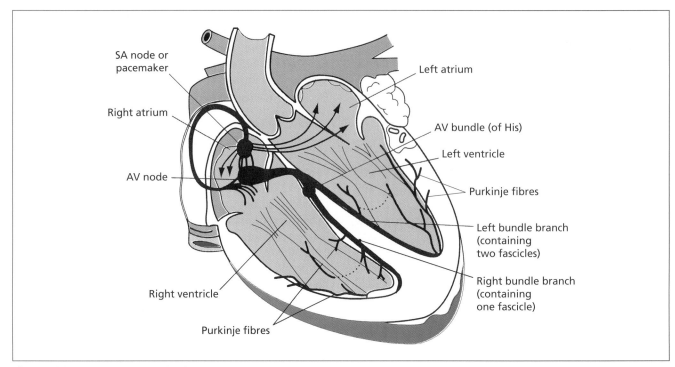

Figure 12.2 The electrical conduction system.

The *atrioventricular (AV) node* lies in the lower part of the right atrium in the interatrial septum. It conducts electrical impulses from the atria to the ventricles. A bundle of fibres called the *bundle of His* proceeds from junctional tissue at the AV node into the ventricular septum, where it divides into two, forming the left and right bundle branches. The left bundle branch further divides into the anterior (superior) and posterior (inferior) divisions (Fig. 12.2). As it descends, each bundle branch gives rise to a network of fine fibres which are known as the *Purkinje fibres*. They are distributed to the ventricular myocardial cells.

Coronary artery system

The **coronary artery system** (Fig. 12.3) provides the myocardium with its blood supply. There are two main coronary arteries, the left and right. The left main coronary artery divides into the anterior descending artery (LAD) and the circumflex artery. The large arteries divide and subdivide to form a network of smaller arteries and capillaries throughout the heart muscle. The blood is returned to the right atrium through a system of progressively enlarging veins which terminate in the coronary sinus.

The **myocardium** requires a large blood supply because it must work continuously and adapt its activity to the varying needs of tissues throughout the body. The coronary vessels dilate to increase the supply when demands are increased. They also dilate when there is an increase in the carbon dioxide concentration of the blood and a decrease in the pH.

Vascular system

The blood travels from the heart through arteries, arterioles, capillaries and veins back to the heart (Fig. 12.4). The structure of each type of vessel is modified according to its function and location.

Arteries and arterioles

The large **arteries** carry blood away from the heart, and branch and subdivide many times. Their structure varies with their size, the larger ones being more elastic and less muscular. Elasticity is an important property of these vessels; with the ejection of blood from the heart, the vessel distends and on recoil exerts a slight pressure on the contained fluid, helping to force it forward. If resistance is offered to the flow of the blood, normally the arteries can stretch to accommodate the increased volume of blood, and the pressure of the blood remains within the normal range.

The smallest arteries emerge as arterioles, which have walls composed mainly of a well-developed muscular coat over the endothelium. The muscle tissue may contract or relax to decrease or increase the amount of blood passing through the arterioles (vasoconstriction or vasodilatation). This feature of the arterioles gives them an important role in determining arterial blood pressure and in controlling the blood flow into the capillaries.

Capillaries

Each arteriole channels its content into microscopic endothelial tubes, the **capillaries**, which anastomose with one another to form a capillary bed. The exchange of fluids, gases and nutrients to maintain and regulate cell activity takes place as the blood passes through the thin capillary walls, usually by diffusion.

The number of capillaries through which blood is passing at any given time is adjusted locally to meet the needs of the

Figure 12.3   The coronary artery system.

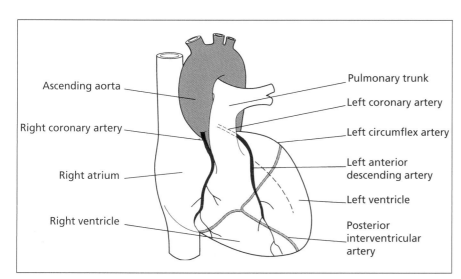

Ascending aorta

Right coronary artery

Right atrium

Right ventricle

Pulmonary trunk

Left coronary artery

Left circumflex artery

Left anterior descending artery

Left ventricle

Posterior interventricular artery

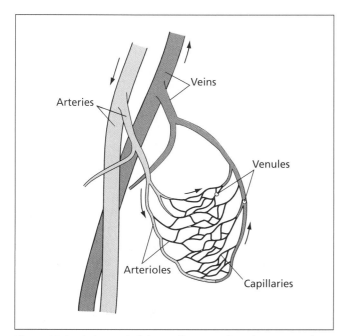

Veins

Arteries

Venules

Arterioles

Capillaries

Figure 12.4   Artery–arteriole–capillary–venule–vein sequence in the circulation.

tissues in the area. A small proportion of the blood is located in the capillaries in resting states; the volume increases as tissue activity increases. This adjustment is possible because some capillaries have at their origin a ring of plain muscular tissue which forms a pre-capillary sphincter allowing for closure of its capillaries when they are not needed.

Venules and veins
The collecting part of the vascular system originates in venules which drain the capillaries and progressively unite and enlarge to form **veins**. They differ from arteries in several ways: (1) they carry blood toward the heart; (2) their walls are much thinner and less elastic with the result that they collapse when empty; (3) the contained blood is under a much lower pressure; and (4) many of the veins have valves.

The structure of veins changes as they increase in size; more muscle and fibrous tissue appear in the walls but, in comparison with arteries, the muscle fibres are sparse. The thinner walls of the veins are readily compressed by skeletal muscle contraction; this assists the blood along its course toward the heart. Backflow toward the capillaries is prevented by one-way valves.

PHYSIOLOGY OF CIRCULATION

Normal circulation through the cardiovascular system is dependent upon an appropriate pressure gradient throughout the system, an adequate volume of blood, a closed system of unobstructed tubes and a set of valves to ensure flow in one direction only.

ROLE OF THE HEART IN CIRCULATION

The pressure that drives the blood through the circulatory system originates in the heart and is augmented slightly by the elastic recoil of the large arteries. A continuous succession of alternate myocardial contractions and relaxations, occurring rhythmically on an average of 60–70 times per minute, pumps the blood through the body.

Impulse origin and conduction in heart contraction

The cells of the myocardium are of two types: those that contract when stimulated and those that originate and conduct impulses. The ability to originate and conduct impulses is referred to as the *electrical activity* of the heart. The heart has three electrical properties:

1 *Automaticity*, or the ability to initiate an electrical impulse.
2 *Excitability*, or the ability to respond to an electrical impulse.
3 *Conductivity*, or the ability to transmit an impulse from one cell to another.

Contraction of the myocardium is dependent upon impulses that arise within the myocardium itself. The structures capable of generating and conducting impulses within the myocardium form the *conduction system*. They are the SA node, tracts of conducting fibres originating with the SA node, the AV node, the bundle of His, bundle branches and the Purkinje fibres.

The rate at which impulses are normally fired varies in the different areas: the SA node originates approximately 60–80 impulses per minute and is referred to as the dominant pacemaker. Impulses arising in the SA node are quickly conducted through the atria, initiating their contraction. At the same time, impulses are transmitted to the AV node where they are delayed; this delay allows for completion of atrial emptying and ventricular filling. From the AV node and junctional tissue they travel through the bundle of His and along the right and left bundle branches and the widely distributed Purkinje fibres to the ventricular contractile fibres, initiating their contraction.

Electrophysiology

Electrical currents in cardiac cells are produced by ion movement across the cell membrane. There is a marked difference in the intracellular and extracellular concentrations of ions, the most important of which are sodium and potassium. During the resting state the inside of the cardiac cell is negatively charged while the outside is positively charged, and the membrane is referred to as *polarized*.

During *depolarization*, the cell membrane becomes permeable to sodium ions, which rapidly shift inside the cell. This sudden influx of sodium reverses the transmembrane potential and potassium ions move out of the cell.

Repolarization, or return to the normal resting potential, occurs as the inside of the cell gradually resumes its negative electrical charge. During this time a stimulus of greater than normal intensity could reactivate the cell. There is then a period of stable resting potential which remains until the next wave of excitation.

During **depolarization**, ions move into and out of the cell because of differences in concentration gradients on either side of the cell membrane. During repolarization, however, an active transport system is required to pump out the sodium ions that have entered the cell and to pump in an equivalent amount of potassium ions. This mechanism is known as the 'sodium pump' and requires energy.

The cardiac cycle

The succession of events that occurs with each heart beat is called **the cardiac cycle**. This consists of the relaxation and contraction of the atria and ventricles, and the opening and closing of the cardiac valves, in a sequence that permits the filling and emptying of the heart chambers. Contraction of the atria or ventricles is called *systole*; their relaxation is known as *diastole*.

At the start of the cardiac cycle, the atria in diastole fill with blood received from their inlet vessels. In the early part of the relaxation period, the AV valves are closed, but as pressure builds up in the atria it becomes greater than that in the ventricles, forcing the AV valves open, and the blood starts to flow through into the ventricles. Atrial diastole is followed in a fraction of a second by contraction (atrial systole), to complete the emptying of the two upper chambers, and the atria again enter their diastole.

During the filling and contraction of the ventricles the blood floats the AV valve cusps up, closing off the AV openings and preventing a regurgitation of blood into the atria. In order to receive the blood from the atria, the ventricles must be in diastole and, at this time, the semilunar valves are closed. With ventricular filling, the intraventricular pressure builds up until it exceeds that in the aorta and pulmonary artery, with the result that the semilunar valves open, allowing blood to flow into the arteries. The ventricular muscle contracts, and the ventricles are emptied.

During ventricular systole, the papillary muscles also contract, exerting tension on the fine tendons (chordae tendineae) inserted on the AV valve cusps. This prevents the cusps from opening into the atria. If this control were not placed on the AV valves, there would be a backflow into the atria, especially with the ventricular contraction. The ventricles relax following their systole and emptying. This results in the pressure being greater in the arteries than in the ventricles, thus potentially allowing the backflow of blood into the ventricles. Closure of the semilunar valves prevents blood from re-entering the ventricles. The cardiac cycle is now completed.

The cycle in a heart beating approximately 70 times per minute is completed in 0.7–0.8 s. The length of each phase of the cycle varies: atrial diastole lasts approximately 0.7 s, whereas its systole is approximately 0.1 s. Ventricular diastole is about 0.4–0.5 s, and its systole takes about 0.3 s. Following the ventricular contraction there is a brief period, approximately 0.4 s, in which the entire myocardium is relaxed. The ventricular diastole overlaps the atrial diastole.

Cardiac output

The performance of the heart as a pump can be described in terms of **cardiac output** (CO). This is the volume of blood pumped by each ventricle in 1 minute. It is equal to the stroke volume (SV) or the volume of blood pumped by a ventricle in one beat, multiplied by the number of heart beats in a minute (the heart rate; HR). In an adult, the CO varies from 4 to 8 litres per minute, and the SV averages 60–80 mL. Thus, *cardiac output* is dependent on *heart rate* and *stroke volume* (CO = SV × HR).

Heart rate

The number of heart beats per minute varies in different people and under different conditions. The average normal rate for an adult is 70 beats per minute, but it may range from 60 to 90. Several factors influence the **heart rate**. In the infant a rate of 110–130 is normal. It becomes progressively slower as the child grows older; by the early teens it is usually about 80. Muscular exertion produces a marked increase, especially in an individual unaccustomed to physical exercise. The rate usually increases during emotional reactions, with fever, and in the lower atmospheric pressures found at high altitudes.

Stroke volume

Stroke volume is influenced by preload, contractility and afterload.

Preload This is the pressure of blood contained in the ventricle at the end of diastole. Another term to describe this pressure is *left ventricular end-diastolic pressure*, which is related to the volume of blood in the ventricle at the end of diastole.

Contractility The **contractile** or inotropic state of the myocardium is the ability of the heart to contract. If the heart is undamaged and is in a condition to respond, the strength of the heart beat is determined mainly by the length of the muscle fibres when contraction begins. Stretching of muscle fibres, within limits, increases the strength of their contraction. The length or stretching of the myocardial fibres is dependent upon the volume of blood entering the heart. This principle is known as *Starling's law of the heart*.

The inotropic state of the heart is also affected by local and circulating catecholamines, the rate and rhythm of ventricular contractions, physiological depressants such as acidosis or myocardial hypoxia, the amount of ventricular substance and certain drugs such as digoxin and/or caffeine.

Afterload Afterload describes the force against which the ventricle is working, or the resistance to the ejection of blood. This resistance is also called *impedance* and is reflected in the tension that ventricular muscle develops during systole.

Cardiac reserve

The ability of the heart to increase its output commensurate with increased tissue activity and needs is called **cardiac reserve**. The normal heart is capable of forwarding the volume of blood delivered to it and of responding to an increased demand without difficulty. It does this without causing prolonged breathlessness, tachycardia or palpitations.

For example, in strenuous exertion, the cardiac output may increase to a volume 13 times greater than the output during rest. This is achieved by an increase in the heart rate and stroke volume. An increase in the cardiac output also occurs in high environmental temperature, emotional responses such as fear, anger or other excitement, after a heavy meal and in the later months of pregnancy.

Regulation of cardiac activity

Certain **nervous**, chemical and mechanical factors play an important role in the action of the heart.

Nervous influence

The heart muscle is capable of generating its own impulses for contraction, but nerve impulses from the parasympathetic and sympathetic divisions of the autonomic nervous system may modify the rate and strength of the contractions. Vagal or parasympathetic innervation has an inhibitory effect on cardiac activity; it slows the heart rate and decreases the force of the atrial contraction by reducing the excitability of the pacemaker (SA node) and the conductivity of the AV node and conducting system. Sympathetic stimulation increases the heart rate and the strength of heart contractions.

Chemical influence

Normal, rhythmic heart contractions are greatly dependent upon an optimal concentration of potassium, sodium and calcium in the extracellular fluid. These minerals play an important role in the excitability of the cardiac muscle cells and their contraction.

Other chemicals of significance in heart action are oxygen and carbon dioxide. The chemoreceptors in the carotid and aortic bodies respond to lack of oxygen, increases in carbon dioxide and acidaemia. In emergency situations anoxia results in sympathetic effects causing an increase in the heart rate and blood pressure. In addition to the chemoreceptors the heart muscle is also responsive to oxygen levels. The myocardium is much more sensitive to oxygen lack than skeletal muscle. If the lack of oxygen progresses unabated the pulse becomes rapid, weak and irregular. With an excess of carbon dioxide in the blood, as may occur in respiratory insufficiency, heart action can gradually become impaired. Conduction is slowed, the relaxation period is prolonged and the contraction is briefer than normal.

Mechanical influence

The stretching of the myocardial fibres by the volume of blood entering the chambers has an influence on cardiac activity. Stretching of muscle fibres increases the strength of their contraction. However, the principal mechanical influence on cardiac activity is the stretching of the arterial walls particularly in the aortic arch and the carotid artery. The barroreceptors in the tunica adventitia of the aortic arch and the carotid artery respond to the degree of stretch in the arteries resulting in increased firing of nerve impulses to the cardiovascular centre in the brain. This produces a negative feedback and there is a reduced sympathetic discharge producing vasodilation and a decreased force and rate of contraction in the heart.

BLOOD PRESSURE AND PULSE

Blood pressure

Blood pressure may be defined as the pressure exerted laterally on the walls of the blood vessels. It varies in different parts of the circulatory system, being greatest in the large arteries, with a progressive decrease as the blood continues on through the smaller arteries, arterioles, capillaries and veins. The pressure is highest in the aorta and lowest in the large caval veins that enter the heart. Blood pressure at any point in the vascular system is dependent upon the force with which the heart pumps the blood out of the ventricles, the volume of blood in the system, the elasticity of the arteries, and the amount of resistance to the flow of the blood from one portion of the circulatory system to the next.

Arterial blood pressure

The blood pressure of greatest clinical interest is that in the arteries. The pulsatile nature of heart activity causes fluctuations in the pressure. With each contraction of the left ventricle a volume of blood is pumped into the aorta, which is already filled with blood. This causes an appreciable increase in the pressure of the blood and stretches the aortic walls. The higher pressure produced by the ventricular systole is referred to as the *systolic blood pressure*. The lower pressure that occurs during the ventricular diastole is dependent upon the recoil of the large arteries and is known as the *diastolic blood pressure*. The difference between these two pressures is called the *pulse pressure*. Pulse pressure varies inversely with the elasticity of the arteries. Rigid vessels with a loss of ability to distend and recoil produce a higher systolic pressure and a lower diastolic pressure, resulting in an increased pulse pressure.

Factors that determine arterial blood pressure Arterial blood pressure is influenced by the strength of the heart beat, volume of blood, elasticity of the vessels and the resistance offered to the flow of blood. Resistance offered to the flow of blood is dependent mainly on the calibre of the arteries and the viscosity of the blood.

Normal variations in arterial blood pressure occur under the influence of factors such as exercise and emotion.

During infancy and childhood, blood pressure is lower than later in life. In the newborn infant systolic pressure is approximately 55–90 mmHg; the diastolic is approximately 40–55 mmHg. This gradually increases throughout childhood, reaching adult level about puberty. Usually in the fifties, the systolic pressure begins to show a slight increase, which progresses with age – corresponding to the loss of elasticity and thickening of the walls of the arteries characteristic of the ageing process.

Physical exertion is accompanied by a rise in the arterial blood pressure due to the increased venous return and the increased production of metabolites such as carbon dioxide and lactic acid. The systolic pressure may increase by as much as 60–70 mmHg in strenuous exercise.

Emotions may also cause an increase in blood pressure: the more excited, anxious, angry or fearful a person becomes, the higher the blood pressure goes. Vasoconstriction is increased due to sympathetic innervation and the release of adrenaline (epinephrine) into the bloodstream.

Blood pressure increases with increased bodyweight, especially after middle age. This is of significance in our present-day society in which obesity and hypertension have a high incidence.

Venous blood pressure

The pressure of the blood is reduced slowly but progressively from the time it leaves the capillaries until it reaches the right atrium.

Venous blood pressure is influenced by cardiac strength, blood volume, respirations and posture. The blood enters the venous system under a pressure of approximately 10 mmHg. The walls of the veins continue to offer some resistance and the blood, particularly in the lower parts of the body, must travel a considerable distance before reaching the heart. The laws of physics tell us that pressure is inversely proportional to frictional resistance and the length of the tube. As a result, venous blood pressure is dissipated progressively, and by the time it reaches the right atrium is very low: 0–10 cmH$_2$O (0–1 mmHg). Obviously, if the left ventricular systole is weak and the blood starts out at a lower than normal arterial pressure, it will tend to move more slowly in the veins towards the heart.

Pulse

Each ventricular contraction ejects a volume of blood into the aorta, producing an increase in the blood pressure which causes an expansion of the artery. During ventricular diastole, the elastic recoil of the aorta moves the blood into the next portion of the artery, which stretches and then recoils. This alternating expansion and recoil spreads along the whole arterial system, producing a pulse wave. Each pulsation corresponds to a heart beat and is the result of the impact of the ejected volume of blood on the arterial wall. The pulsations occur in the arteries of the pulmonary circulatory system as well as in the systemic circulation.

PREVENTION OF CARDIOVASCULAR DISORDERS

In the UK, cardiovascular disease is a national health problem of considerable proportions. This is particularly true now that an increasing proportion of the population is over the age of 60 years, an age group with a high prevalence of cardiovascular disease in which the incidence amongst women approaches that in men. Cardiovascular disease is also the main cause of premature death and morbidity in the UK. Approximately half of the deaths from cardiovascular disease in the UK each year are from coronary heart disease. The term **coronary heart disease** (CHD) encompasses a group of clinical conditions ranging from asymptomatic disease to angina, acute myocardial infarction (MI) and sudden death. *Ischaemic heart disease* (IHD) is the official term used in the International Classification of Diseases; it is virtually synonymous with coronary heart disease.

The World Health Organization (2005) reports that mortality due to cardiovascular disease is steadily falling and is due to be overtaken by HIV/AIDs as the second major cause of mortality by the year 2030 (infectious and parasitic disease remaining as the number one major cause of death). In accordance with this estimate in the UK, death rates have been falling over the last 10 years (by 37% for people under the age of 75 and by 44% for people under the age of

65 years). Nonetheless, CHD remains an underlying cause of a substantial number of hospital admissions and one in five men and one in six women die from CHD, with CHD causing more than 114 000 deaths in the UK in 2003 (British Heart Foundation 2004). Myocardial infarction (heart attack) and sudden death are the most conspicuous manifestations of the problem, but far more people suffer less dramatic but still significant consequences including chest pain (angina), syncope, decreased exercise tolerance, anxiety and other psychological complications. Side-effects and the consequences of treatment can also cause problems for some. Reduced mobility, for example, may result in a loss of previous lifestyle affecting all aspects of daily life including work, social activities, roles within the family and financial security. The social and economic consequences of the disorder are thus far reaching and extend beyond the personal effects on those who suffer and their families. It has been estimated that the total economic burden of cardiovascular disease (CVD) is now £14 750 million each year and for coronary heart disease £3500 million with the total economic cost, including lost work days and the cost of informal care, exceeding £26 billion for CVD (British Heart Foundation 2004). Virtually every man, woman and child in the UK will be affected in some way by heart disease as a consequence of knowing or being related to a sufferer or being a sufferer themselves.

Not surprisingly, CHD is a significant feature in government health policy. The White Paper *Saving Lives: Our Healthier Nation* has set targets for a 40% reduction in deaths from CHD and cerebrovascular accident (CVA) in those under 75 years of age by the year 2010 (DoH 2000a). In addition the National Service Framework for Coronary Heart Disease (DoH 2000b) has created a 10-year programme for improving services for CHD. Standards have been set for the whole of CHD-related care, from cardiac health promotion, emergency care, specialist cardiology services and surgery through to rehabilitation.

THE NURSE'S ROLE IN PREVENTION OF CARDIOVASCULAR DISORDERS

The nurse has many opportunities to contribute to the prevention of cardiovascular disorders. Whether the work is in the hospital, clinic, home, industry or school, the role may be participation in health screening, education or provision of care. In addition, the emerging roles of nurse consultant and nurse-led clinics offer greater autonomy in the practice area of cardiovascular nursing. In order to recognize and fulfil responsibilities in the preventive programme, the nurse must be informed and must make a personal effort to keep abreast of new knowledge. In addition to an understanding of the role of the heart in supplying all the cells throughout the body with materials essential to their survival and activities, a knowledge of how this function may be impaired by various pathological processes is necessary. This information serves as the basis

for the recognition of excessive demands on the heart and circulation, significant signs and symptoms, and the need for medical attention. It also provides the basis for explanations and appropriate health education as well as for the planning and provision of safe and effective care.

Risk factors have been identified in large-scale epidemiological studies as clinical variables that are statistically associated with the manifestation of heart disease, particularly ischaemic heart disease (IHD). These factors are involved in the pathogenesis of atherosclerosis of the coronary arteries. The presence of multiple risk factors increases exponentially the likelihood of developing IHD, although individuals may live for many years with multiple risk factors and no manifestations of heart disease.

The nurse can play a very important role in facilitating health promotion, assessing potentially detrimental health patterns, and identifying and undertaking strategies to prevent or correct these behaviours.

Risk factors for ischaemic heart disease

Risk factors can be classified as either *non-modifiable*, such as age, sex, family history and culture, or *modifiable*, such as hypertension, hyperlipidaemia, cigarette smoking, diabetes mellitus, obesity, lack of physical activity, excessive alcohol and stress.

Nurses need to be aware of the far-reaching psychological and social consequences of cardiovascular disease, both for the individual and for their partners and families. Individuals may be aware that they are at risk, but having the ability to change their lifestyle is dependent on a variety of factors, including: their perception of the significance of the problem; their belief that action they take will reduce the risk; self-esteem; role within the family and society; time and financial constraints and support from others. Nurses need to consider their role in health education (see Ch. 1). Providing the patient with all the facts is not in itself a guarantee of them changing to and maintaining a healthy lifestyle. The individual needs to be able to make an informed choice about his or her own behaviour with the support of the healthcare team. The attitude of the nurse is likely to be important here. It may be necessary to prioritize risk factors in order to make compliance more likely. Someone who is overweight and smokes may be more likely to succeed in making appropriate changes if they are advised to concentrate on stopping smoking initially, even though this may lead to an initial weight gain.

Non-modifiable risk factors

Age Ischaemic heart disease is more prevalent in older people. Thus, the older the individual, the greater the likelihood of developing cardiovascular disease.

Sex Men have a higher incidence of IHD than women, although this difference diminishes as age increases. Women have a dramatically increased incidence of IHD after the menopause.

Family history   Family history is significant if first degree relatives have a history of IHD below the age of 55 years for men and 65 years for women. A history of IHD among blood relatives is associated with a poorer prognosis when it develops.

Culture   In the 1980s, it became clear that mortality from CHD differed significantly between ethnic groups in England and Wales. More recent figures still illustrate that southern Asians (people from India, Bangladesh, Pakistan and Sri Lanka) demonstrate a much higher premature death rate from CHD than average. The rate is 46% higher in men and 51% higher in women (British Heart Foundation 2004). Interestingly, in the African-Caribbean population the incidence of premature death from CHD is lower than average, (around half the rate found in the general population for men and two-thirds for women), although the presence of cerebrovascular accident (CVA), hypertension and diabetes is high (British Heart Foundation 2004). Other groups with an increased mortality rate include Irish, Scottish and Polish-born immigrants (Balarajan 1991).

Modifiable risk factors
The modifiable risk factors known to play a part in ischaemic heart disease include:

- cigarette smoking
- hyperlipidaemia
- hypertension
- diabetes mellitus
- obesity
- lack of physical activity
- high alcohol intake.

Hypertension   Raised systolic and diastolic blood pressure is a significant risk factor for cardiovascular disease including IHD, CVA and heart failure. It is estimated that 11% of all disease burden is due to raised blood pressure and that 50% of CHD and 75% of stroke is due to raised systolic blood pressure (British Heart Foundation 2004). Discussion of the nurse's role in the management of hypertension can be found later in this chapter.

Hyperlipidaemia   Blood lipids include cholesterol, triglycerides, phospholipids and free fatty acids. Cholesterol and triglycerides are of clinical significance and are transported in plasma as lipoproteins. There are four major classes of lipoproteins, containing varying proportions of protein and the three blood lipids:

1 *Chylomicrons* are mainly of dietary origin and are 85% triglycerides.
2 Very low-density lipoproteins (VLDLs) contain 50% triglycerides.
3 Low-density lipoproteins (LDLs) carry 75% of the total plasma cholesterol.
4 High-density lipoproteins (HDLs) remove excess cholesterol from body cells and transport it to the liver for elimination.

High levels of HDLs protect against the development of coronary atherosclerosis, although it is uncertain how this occurs (Tortora and Grabowski 2000).

Hyperlipidaemia (or hypercholesterolaemia) may be secondary to another disease such as obstructive liver disease, due to an excessive intake of saturated fats and cholesterol in the diet, or may result from a primary or familial disorder. Hyperlipidaemia can be detected by blood sampling. Control of hypercholesterolaemia is directed toward lowering the serum cholesterol levels by medications and diet.

By modifying the dietary intake of fats, carbohydrate and calories, the blood lipid levels of most patients with primary hyperlipidaemia can be lowered. The contribution of diet to the prevention of coronary atherosclerosis is controversial but evidence suggests that this approach might be worthwhile.

Long-term treatment with lipid-lowering drugs has been shown to improve the survival rate of patients with IHD (Scandinavian Simvastatin Survival Study Group 1994) and to prevent CHD and non-fatal stroke when used in patients who are hypertensive (Sever PS et al 2003). Lipid-lowering therapy is usually with a drug called a statin of which atorvastatin, rosuvastatin and simvastatin are examples. The aim should be to lower the cholesterol concentration to less than 5 mmol/L and the LDL to below 3 mmol/L or by 30%, whichever is the greater, as recommended in the National Service Framework for Coronary Heart Disease (DoH 2000b). The British Hypertension Society Guidelines have a different standard and recommend a reduction in total cholesterol to 4 mmol/L or below and LDL to 2 mmol/L or below or 25% reduction or 30% reduction in total cholesterol or low density lipoprotein respectively, whichever is the greater for both primary and secondary prevention of CVD (Williams et al 2004).

In addition to lipid-lowering medication the patient should be given advice about diet. The purpose of this might be to help with weight reduction, help prevent further increases in weight or to help reduce cholesterol. Current guidelines on an appropriate diet to maintain a healthy heart include the following (Daniels 2002):

- Reducing the level of fat eaten and replacing some saturated fats with polyunsaturated and monounsaturated fats. This can be achieved by eating more starchy foods such as pasta, bread, rice, cereals and potatoes. A high-fibre diet will also reduce the amount of cholesterol absorbed from the intestine into the blood. The stanols and sterols found in 'cholesterol lowering' spreads can be beneficial
- Eating at least five portions of fruit and vegetables a day. These should be of different types
- Eating fish at least three times a week including one portion of an oily fish such as mackerel, pilchards, salmon or herrings
- Reducing the amount of salt consumed. There is a clear link between a high salt intake and high blood pressure.

As a nation we eat about 10 g of salt per day; this should be at least halved. Salt is found in many foods, but notably processed foods, ready-made meals, and snacks such as crisps and peanuts. Food labelling for salt is complex because it may appear as 'sodium' and contain other chemicals such as sodium bicarbonate. A sodium content of less than 0.2 g per 100 g on the label is generally recommended (Hatchett 2001)

● Keeping a healthy weight. This will reduce the workload on the heart and help to reduce any hypertension
● Choosing soluble fibre-containing foods such as oats porridge, pulses, beans and lentils
● Eating regular meals rather than missing meals and then being tempted to snack on high-fat foods

Dietary education is a combined function of the patient, doctor, nurse and dietician. The dietician is the primary person involved if the diet is complex, but the nurse also needs to be informed so that teaching can be reinforced. Some patients may require much support and understanding to continue on their diets, especially if drastic changes in eating habits are needed. Adherence will probably be greater if the diet is adjusted as much as possible to individual tastes.

Involving the spouse or the person who buys and cooks the food may make dietary change more likely. The diet needs to be perceived as lifelong rather than a short-term response to an acute event. The social significance of food should not be ignored – the individual does not want to perceive themselves as a social outcast at the meal table. The nurse needs to be sensitive to the meaning of food in the patient's life and should be aware of the cultural and social significance of eating.

Cigarette smoking The World Health Organization estimates that tobacco use was responsible for the deaths of 4.9 million people worldwide in 2002 (WHO 2006b). 250 million teenagers and children in the world today will be killed by tobacco use unless smoking behaviour trends change dramatically (WHO 2006b). In the UK, approximately 28% of men and 24% of women smoke cigarettes (British Heart Foundation 2004) whereas it is estimated that in the Western Pacific Region of the world 62% of men and only 6% of women are reported to engage in tobacco consumption (WHO 2006). The proportion is highest in the 16–24 age group and declines with age (DOH 1999). Within the various ethnic groups, males from the Bangladeshi and Caribbean communities show particularly high smoking rates: 42% and 34% respectively (British Heart Foundation 2004).

For both men and women, cigarette smoking is one of the major risk factors for cardiovascular disease. The risk of morbidity and mortality is dramatically greater for smokers than for non-smokers, particularly in people under the age of 50 years and those who have other risk factors.

There are a number of compounds in cigarette smoke that are harmful: nicotine stimulates catecholamine secretion which, in turn, promotes platelet aggregation, increased heart rate, blood pressure and oxygen consumption. Carbon monoxide also appears to increase platelet adhesiveness and reduce oxygen supply which, in the presence of coronary lesions, may increase the incidence of angina pectoris.

Every opportunity should be taken to discuss smoking cessation with the patient. The nurse should assess whether the patient is ready to make a change and whether they might be receptive to help at a particular time (see p. 000 for the cycle of change). If the patient is in the pre-contemplation stage, simply reminding them that they could consider stopping smoking might help move them into the contemplation stage and eventually on to action to stop smoking.

It is worthwhile considering the complex behaviour that surrounds smoking. There is the addiction to nicotine and the routine of social behaviours. Patients may therefore need pharmacological interventions to help address the addiction and subsequent cravings on cessation of smoking and they may also need to consider behaviour modification. There are a number of strategies to facilitate smoking cessation:

● Pharmacological strategies include the use of nicotine replacement therapy and, for some patients, the use of bupropion. Nicotine replacement therapy is available in a variety of products including lozenges, chewing gum and patches. These products can be used to help the patient who has set a definite quit date and they are recommended for use over a period of 8–9 weeks. After this time some patients will be able to remain off cigarettes for the long term
● Providing information that is tailored to the individual's needs (Box 12.1). A patient who has already experienced a recent cardiac condition may be more receptive to messages on the impact of smoking on the heart and health
● Eliciting social support can be beneficial. Family members and friends can discuss their roles in helping the person to stop smoking. There can be great benefit in partners deciding to stop smoking at the same time. This can be a source of support and encouragement
● Self-help and discussing with the individual, behaviours that are associated with the activity and how to avoid these situations, at least initially when attempting to stop, can be helpful. Social and psychological reinforcers that contribute to smoking behaviours can be very powerful in preventing successful cessation
● A gradual reduction of the number of cigarettes smoked can be a successful strategy, but current advice focuses upon choosing a particular day or date to stop as the most successful approach. The person is then advised to keep busy, to alter usual routines that may be linked to smoking, to drink plenty of fluids, to become more active and to treat themselves with the money saved
● Cessation programmes are often available in the individual's community. The nurse should be aware of these programmes and facilitate the patient's referral as appropriate.

Diabetes mellitus People with diabetes have such a high risk of coronary heart disease that the management of their condition is considered to be secondary prevention rather than primary prevention (Williams et al 2004). It is therefore

Box 12.1   Advice for smokers

1   It is best to choose a day or a date to stop smoking. Most people are more successful with this method, rather than cutting down slowly.

2   Tell patients that they are making a major decision: i.e. a 65-year-old who smokes two packets of cigarettes a day may forfeit 6 years of life but can regain 4 of those years by stopping smoking.

3   If a patient resumes smoking, provide reassurance that stopping smoking is like any other new skill: several tries may be necessary.

4   If the patient has one cigarette, inform the patient that this does not mean immediate dependence; however, emphasize that it should not become habitual.

5   Inform patients that withdrawal symptoms are generally most severe 2–4 days after stopping and symptoms slowly subside during the following week, but reach a second peak about 10 days after stopping, before slowly tapering off permanently. Emphasize that symptoms will be short lived and can often be countered by planning for them.

6   Advise patients that any weight gain is unlikely to exceed 2.5–3 kg (5–10 lbs), and that very few ex-smokers maintain the added weight for more than 1 year. Suggest an exercise programme.

essential to discover people with diabetes, impaired fasting glucose or impaired glucose tolerance at an early stage. This allows for the early implementation of interventions including pharmacological and dietary management. In addition to the detection of glucose intolerance it is important to identify patients who might be at risk of diabetes in the future, those who are obese, who have a family history of diabetes or have had gestational diabetes. These patients can be provided with advice about diet and exercise and in some it will prevent the progression to diabetes mellitus (see Ch. 18).

Obesity   Obesity is a major risk factor for CVD (WHO 1998) and is also a major indicator for hypertension, hyperlipidaemia and diabetes mellitus. The current prevalence of obesity in the UK is 22% which compares with 36% in the USA, 24% in Canada, 1% in India and 7% in South Africa (WHO 2006c). Surveys demonstrate that obesity is increasing in the UK (British Heart Foundation 2004, DoH 1999). Across the world, figures are expected to rise to 24% in the UK, 44% in the USA, 25% in Canada, 2% in India and 8% in South Africa by 2010 (WHO 2006c). In addition to being overweight, body shape is important. People who have an 'apple' shape have a higher risk of developing CHD than those who have a 'pear' shape (Daniels 2002). Excess fat around the abdomen has been associated with high blood pressure, diabetes and dyslipidaemias. It can therefore be useful to measure the patient's waist and hips and to include this information when assessing their risk for CVD.

Physical activity   Physical inactivity is estimated to cause 2 million deaths worldwide each year (WHO 2006d). Estimates of physical inactivity across countries range from 31% to 51% with a global average of 41% (WHO 2006d) (the WHO define physical inactivity as less than 2.5 hours of exercise per week). In the UK the government has recommended that each person should engage in 30 minutes of moderate intensity exercise on five or more days of the week (British Heart Foundation 2004). Exercise can include activities such as such as brisk walking, cycling or climbing stairs and should be enough to produce breathlessness. Most importantly, exercise should be enjoyable. Using the UK government guidelines, levels of physical activity are low in the UK, with only 37% of men and 24% of women meeting the activity guidelines suggested by government (i.e. a level of physical inactivity rate of 63% in men and 76% in women). There is evidence that physical activity is important in the prevention of obesity and high blood pressure (Williams et al 2004). Those who have had a heart attack or those with heart failure are now being encouraged to participate in supervised exercise programmes to improve their exercise tolerance. People who have uncontrolled blood pressure should delay embarking upon an exercise programme until the blood pressure is sufficiently treated.

High alcohol intake   A regular high intake of alcohol causes hypertension and is associated with excess IHD. Binge drinking is associated with an increased risk of stroke. Patients should not be discouraged from having a moderate intake of alcohol up to the recommended limits of 21 units for men and 14 units for women spread evenly over the week with 2 days off alcohol, particularly of red wine as it is thought to have a beneficial affect on the lipid profile and to protect against IHD.

Factors influencing high-risk behaviour

High-risk behaviours such as smoking, lack of exercise, excessive alcohol consumption and unhealthy diet are often seen as voluntary elements of lifestyle. There is, however, some debate as to the extent to which this is so. Diet may be determined at least in part by income and the availability of different foods. Smoking and alcohol consumption, in particular, may be regarded as being determined by social and peer pressures. Certain individuals or groups of individuals may not have the time, money or necessary transport to enable them to engage in leisure or sporting activities.

The environmental, political, economic and social forces that act on individuals and groups to influence behaviour need to be understood before change interventions can be identified and implemented. It is important for nurses to understand how they might be able to assist each individual in their personal and particular situation. A broad understanding of the influences on the individual and the best ways to work with the patient, given their personal strengths and constraints, is essential to lay the groundwork for sensitive and empathic nursing practice.

THE PERSON WITH A CARDIOVASCULAR DISORDER

ASSESSMENT

Assessment of the individual's cardiovascular function provides data needed to identify actual and potential health problems, guide nursing intervention and evaluate care. A cardiovascular assessment includes:

- health history
- physical examination
- diagnostic procedures
- knowledge of manifestations of cardiovascular disorders.

The nurse collects and analyses the assessment data, formulates patient-centred problems and develops a goal-oriented plan of care with the patient and family, which is then implemented and evaluated.

Health history

The health history will assist the nurse in defining the patient's health problems. The depth and manner in which this information is collected will depend on the patient's clinical status and availability of family or significant others.

If the patient is acutely ill, then brief, direct questions should be used to identify essential information during admission procedures. If the patient's status is stable, the nurse may conduct a formal interview using more open-ended questions. Other information can be obtained through less formal conversation throughout interaction with the patient. The nature of the nurse–patient relationship is important in establishing the significance of the problem for the patient and family.

The health history includes data concerning the patient's primary health problems, history of present illness, current medication, past health history, family history, and social and personal history.

Primary health problem

The patient identifies the chief concern or reason for contact with the healthcare system. Common cardiovascular health problems include chest pain, dyspnoea, syncope, palpitations and intermittent claudication.

History of present illness

This is a detailed investigation of the patient's presenting problem, primary health problem and previously prescribed treatment plan. It is important to use a systematic approach when gathering these data to ensure the information is comprehensive. One method of organizing this data collection is use of the PQRST mnemonic (see Ch. 128).

Current medication

The patient's current medication regimen including over the counter medications and alternative and complementary therapies should be reviewed.

Past health history

Assessment includes the patient's general state of health, major health problems and treatment plans, hospital admissions, surgical procedures and injuries. The patient's response to these events provides data concerning coping strategies. Allergies to food, medication and environmental agents are identified and allergic reactions described.

Family history

Information concerning the patient's blood relatives may suggest a specific cardiac problem or the potential to develop a specific problem. The patient may be questioned about whether any family member has ever had hypertension, diabetes mellitus, ischaemic heart disease, stroke, vascular disease or hyperlipidaemia.

Social and personal history

These data facilitate an understanding of the person's uniqueness as an individual and suggest needs for health teaching and discharge planning. Data are gathered in the following areas:

- *Personal characteristics*. These include the patient's age, marital status, education, occupational experiences, socio-economic status and religious beliefs
- *Lifestyle*. Information concerning the individual's daily activities is collected, including dietary, bowel and sleep habits. Usual activities, and data concerning use of tobacco, alcohol, caffeine and social drugs is useful. Identification of these factors can help to facilitate planning in health promotion activities
- *The patient's perception of the illness and ability to cope*. What does this illness mean to the patient? This provides information as to the patient's level of understanding about the condition and the impact on his or her life. How the patient has coped with other problems may identify coping strategies that the nurse can facilitate when planning care with the individual
- *Relationships with others*. The patient is questioned about the network of family and friends to assess social support systems available. The family and significant others' perceptions of the patient's condition and coping will provide information as to their level of understanding and their ability to handle the situation
- *Home environment*. Who is living with the patient? Describing the physical characteristics of the home including stairs, location of bathroom (toilet facilities), etc., will help to start discharge planning. This is particularly important for the individual with reduced activity resulting from cardiac dysfunction as daily routines will need to be modified to accommodate changes in function
- *Knowledge of cardiovascular function*. The patient's understanding of the condition and the treatment plan is important for planning health education. Does the patient know the current medical diagnosis and what this means in terms of treatment and lifestyle? For example, does the patient who has had a myocardial infarction understand activity limitations and medication schedules?
- *Quality of life*. There is a wide individual variation in response to physical illness. Some individuals are able to

continue to lead full and satisfying lives despite major symptoms and disability, whereas others with much less serious medical problems become gravely handicapped (Mayou and Bryant 1993). This issue needs to be explored so that a knowledge of the reality of illness for each individual can be used in subsequent care planning. Kleinman et al (1978) give the following questions designed to elicit culturally sensitive important patient information:

a) What brings you here?

b) What do you think has caused your illness?

c) Why do you think it started when it did?

d) What do you think this illness does to you?

e) How severe is your illness?

f) What kind of treatment do you think you should receive?

g) What are the most important results you hope to receive from treatment?

h) What are the chief problems your illness has caused for you?

i) What do you fear most about your illness?

Basic physical examination of the cardiovascular system

In this section, basic physical examination techniques for assessing the person's cardiovascular system are described. Certain of the techniques described are often carried out by the doctor. However, increasingly, nurse practitioners are undertaking these skills as part of nurse-led practice. It is also necessary for nurses to understand the principles of these techniques in order to gain a wider appreciation of the patient's experience and to be equipped to explain the nature of the techniques to patients.

Basic physical examination is a cornerstone of the nurse's methods of data collection. Performing a physical examination facilitates gathering the objective data on the person's cardiovascular system, which is necessary to establish a baseline of the person's condition and to assess ongoing changes in health status.

General appearance

1 *Facial expressions*

Does the patient appear alert, anxious, distressed, exhausted? Grimacing or biting of lips are noted as they may be signs of pain.

2 *Posture*

Does the patient appear comfortable, restless, agitated? Is he or she sitting or lying supine?

3 Skin and mucous membranes:

a) *Colour*: examine skin in symmetrical areas, noting any increase or loss of pigmentation, redness, pallor, cyanosis and jaundice. Ask the patient whether there have been any recent changes in the colour of the skin. Observe for signs of bleeding such as petechiae, bruising or haematomas.

b) *Moisture*: inspect skin for dryness, oiliness or sweating (diaphoresis).

c) *Hair pattern*: note hair distribution on limbs or the glossy, shiny appearance of the skin surface.

4 *Observations*

Observe the patient for respiratory rate noting any respiratory distress or cough.

Palpation

This method of examination is used to assess **skin**, peripheral pulses and the chest.

Skin

1 *Capillary refill*. This is noted by applying pressure to the nail-bed and releasing quickly. A normal response is for the nail-bed to blanch on pressure and quickly to reperfuse and become pink when pressure is released. An abnormal response is a delay of more than 2 seconds in the return to pink.

2 *Temperature*. The skin is palpated symmetrically to establish the temperature of the skin using the back of the hand and noting generalized warmth or coolness of any localized areas.

3 *Turgor*. A fold of skin is lifted and the speed with which it returns into place is noted.

4 *Oedema*. Assessment is made for oedema in symmetrical locations, including feet, ankles, lower arms and sacrum. Three fingers are pressed firmly over symmetrical bony surfaces for 5 seconds, and released. Pitting oedema, which is continued depression of the skin and underlying tissue after pressure is released, is noted.

5 *Chest*. The chest is palpated anteriorly in a methodical systematic way. Feel for the beat of the apical pulse which should be gentle and brief. If it is more vigorous than normal this is called a 'heave' or a 'lift'.

Peripheral arterial pulses   Arterial pulses are assessed for rate, rhythm and amplitude (volume) at symmetrical locations on the body. The carotid, brachial, radial, femoral, popliteal, dorsalis pedis and posterior tibial pulses can be included.

The heart rate can be assessed by counting the pulse rate. The radial or carotid pulse rate can be palpated and counted for 60 seconds to establish heart rate.

The heart rhythm can be initially assessed using the pulse. The radial or carotid pulse is palpated to identify whether the rhythm of pulses is regular. If it is irregular, any pattern present is noted.

The pulse amplitude may be described and recorded as follows:

- not palpable
- barely palpable, weak, thready
- decreased, moderate impairment
- full
- bounding.

Auscultation

Arterial blood pressure Arterial **blood pressure** is an important predictor of morbidity and mortality, and is therefore one of the most important clinical observations. Recording a blood pressure appears simple, but it is a skill that must be performed carefully. There is clear evidence that care is not always taken in doing this (Hatchett 2001). Importantly, treatment for high blood pressure (hypertension) will be initiated on the results of these readings and they therefore need to be accurate and reliable. Unless the reading is very high, several recordings will be taken over a short period of time to provide a more accurate assessment (Hatchett 2001).

Arterial blood pressure is measured in millimetres of mercury (mmHg). This is by means of a blood pressure monitoring device and a stethoscope, using the brachial artery. Increasingly, electronic digital devices are being used instead of the mercury sphygmomanometer. Mercury is known to be a toxic substance and its use is slowly being banned worldwide in medical devices because of the dangers of accidental spillage. The general technique of recording a blood pressure is described here using either an electronic device or an auscultatory device.

The patient should be sitting comfortably with the arm supported at heart level. Tight clothing should be removed from the arm and the patient should be discouraged from talking during the procedure. The cuff of the blood pressure apparatus is applied to the upper arm just above the elbow. The appropriate sized cuff should be used ensuring that it encircles at least 80% of the upper arm. A cuff that is too large will underestimate the blood pressure and one that is too small will overestimate. The cuff is inflated with air, which compresses the brachial artery. If the auscultatory method is being used, the stethoscope is applied over the brachial artery just below the cuff. When the cuff pressure becomes greater than the blood pressure, no pulse is heard or sensed by the machine. The air in the cuff should be pumped 30 mmHg above this point and then is slowly released and the height of the mercury on the manometer is noted when the pulse is first heard (this is known as Korotkoff phase 1). This corresponds to the systolic blood pressure.

With further slow deflation of the cuff, the pulse gradually becomes softer. The level of the mercury is again noted just before the pulse becomes inaudible (Korktkoff phase 5) or when there is a pronounced change in the sound heard, known as muffling (Korktkoff phase 4). This represents the diastolic blood pressure. The result should be recorded to the nearest 2 mmHg. The electronic device will note the changes in these sounds and provide a digital figure. The blood pressure should be assessed in both arms on the first occasion and at least twice on each occasion thereafter and if there are marked differences between the two recordings it should be repeated again (Williams et al 2004).

If the blood pressure is recorded as 100 mmHg, this simply means that the pressure of the blood on the walls of the vessel is sufficient to raise a column of mercury to a height of 100 mm. The normal blood pressure in a healthy young adult in a sitting position is below 120/80 mmHg.

In older patients or patients with diabetes, or when the person has a history of fainting or dizziness when changing position, the blood pressure should be taken in two positions if possible: sitting and after standing for 2 minutes. Under normal conditions, the systolic pressure will either drop slightly or stay the same when the person rises, while the diastolic pressure rises slightly.

Heart sounds Auscultation of the heart involves listening to the heart with a good stethoscope using a systematic approach. **Heart sounds** are assessed considering the following characteristics: frequency, intensity, duration and location.

Two loud sounds are produced in quick succession in each cardiac cycle and two other very soft sounds can be heard which only the experienced ear will normally detect. These are followed by a brief pause before being repeated in the next cycle. Through a stethoscope, the heart sounds will be heard as a lubb-dubb and are produced by closure of the heart valves.

The first heart sound, S_1, is a prolonged low-pitched sound (lubb). It is produced by the closing of both atrio-ventricular valves, the mitral and the tricuspid, just before ventricular systole. Although closure of the two valves occurs almost simultaneously, the mitral valve closes slightly before the tricuspid valve. Therefore, the mitral component is heard slightly before the tricuspid and is the main component of the first heart sound. S_1 is heard best over the apex (fifth left intercostal space) of the tricuspid and mitral areas using the diaphragm of the stethoscope.

The second sound, S_2, is briefer and higher pitched (dubb). It is produced by the closing of both semilunar valves, the aortic and the pulmonary, just before diastole. As the aortic valve closes slightly before the pulmonary valve, the aortic component of S_2 will be heard slightly before the pulmonary. The components of the second sound are normally affected by respiration. During inspiration, closure of the pulmonary valve is delayed because of the increased venous return to the right heart. The difference in the two components of S_2 is therefore more apparent. This is referred to as *physiological splitting* and disappears during expiration. S_2 is best heard in the second intercostal space, either side of the sternum using the diaphragm of the stethoscope.

The remaining faint sounds are known as S_3 and S_4, and are connected with atrial emptying. They follow S_2.

Clinical characteristics of impaired cardiac function

Any impairment in circulation due to an abnormal heart condition is reflected in signs and symptoms, which are produced by various factors: (1) a reduced blood supply to the heart and tissues throughout the body, causing a reduced nutrient and oxygen supply and an accumulation of metabolic wastes; (2) malfunctioning of the conduction system; and (3) the inability of the heart to eject the blood it receives. The last factor results in an excessive volume in the venous system, creating congestion and increased pressure that interfere with the function of tissues and organs.

The signs and symptoms of cardiac conditions vary with the degree to which circulation is impaired and with the form and location of the heart condition. Those that are discussed here do not necessarily all occur in every patient, nor are they all inclusive; they are the more common problems presented by cardiac patients.

Abnormal pulse

The pulse rate may be abnormally fast or slow and the intervals between the heart beat may be unequal. The volume may vary. Some specific abnormalities of the arterial pulse are described below.

Pulsus alternans With pulsus alternans, the heart beats are regular but vary in amplitude. This condition is produced by changes in the left ventricular contractile force and is often precipitated by a premature ventricular beat. It is frequently associated with left ventricular failure resulting from hypertension, cardiomyopathy or aortic valve disease.

Pulsus bigeminus Premature contractions alternating with normal heart beats result in variation in the strength of the heart beats. This alteration in pulse volume from beat to beat is called the bigeminal pulse. It differs from pulsus alternans in that the weaker beat occurs regularly after a stronger, normally conducted, beat.

Pulsus paradoxus Normally, the strength of the arterial pulse falls during inspiration because of pooling of blood in the pulmonary vascular system. This occurs because of the more negative intrathoracic pressure and expansion of the lungs causing a reduced left ventricular stroke volume. If the blood pressure falls more than 10 mmHg (the normal fall during inspiration), the pulse is called pulsus paradoxus. Causes include cardiac tamponade, chronic constrictive pericarditis, emphysema and bronchial asthma.

Blood pressure

Arterial blood pressure is an important indicator of the patient's circulatory status. The systolic pressure depends on the cardiac output and, obviously, will fall with a reduced output by the left side of the heart.

Dyspnoea

The patient may experience shortness of breath or laboured breathing only on exertion, or it may be present even at rest. This can be due to pulmonary congestion. The left side of the heart may not be forwarding all the blood it receives, and the blood is dammed back in the pulmonary veins. This can result in pulmonary oedema, a sign of which is dyspnoea which occurs when the patient is recumbent and which is referred to as *orthopnoea*. It may be relieved when the patient sits upright. Dyspnoea can also be due to IHD, and particularly, angina. The patient tends to complain of breathlessness that occurs with exercise and improves with rest, although in severe cases, patients may be dyspnoeic at rest.

Cough

In pulmonary oedema, fluid escapes into the alveoli from the capillaries in the congested pulmonary system and this acts as a cough stimulus. The fluid may be expectorated as a frothy sputum and in severe heart failure may contain blood. Cough might also be significant in patients who have a history of chronic obstructive airways disease. Long-term problems with breathing can lead to cor-pulmonale, the heart condition associated with respiratory disease.

Hypoxia

Any impairment in circulation will create an oxygen deficiency in tissues. The cardiac output may be reduced, or a disturbance in pulmonary circulation may reduce the exchange of gases in the lung. Symptoms of an oxygen deficiency are many and varied, because the function of all structures is affected. The brain quickly reflects oxygen deprivation and reduced mental efficiency, restlessness, apathy and disorientation are manifested. If the deficiency is severe, consciousness is lost and, unless the supply to the brain is promptly re-established, there is likely to be permanent brain damage.

Severe pain (angina) occurs when muscle tissue, such as the myocardium, is deprived of adequate oxygen. Hypoxia may also cause cyanosis, a bluish colour, which is usually seen first in the peripheries such as the nail-beds and then in the lips.

Oedema

Excess fluid accumulates in the interstitial spaces of the tissues in cardiac disease when the heart cannot forward the blood it receives. The blood backs up in the veins and venules, raising the venous blood pressure. Normally, at the venous end of the capillaries, the colloidal osmotic pressure exceeds the hydrostatic pressure of the blood, and interstitial fluid moves into the capillary. However, if the hydrostatic pressure of the blood in the distal portion of the capillaries exceeds the osmotic pressure in the tissues, interstitial fluid will not be moved into the capillaries.

The retention of sodium ions also contributes to the formation of oedema in the cardiac patient. The decreased sodium excretion is promoted by the reduced blood flow through the kidneys, which results from the impaired circulation and impaired functioning of the kidney. An increased secretion of aldosterone by the adrenal cortices of an adenoma can also result in the retention of sodium.

Oedema is a very characteristic sign of some weakening in heart function. Considerable fluid accumulates before the oedema becomes apparent; a person may retain 4.5–7.0 kg of excess fluid before the oedema becomes evident. It appears first in the dependent parts of the body where gravity most hinders venous return. If the patient is ambulant, it becomes evident first in the ankles and feet but, if in bed, it appears initially in the sacral region.

Pain

Chest **pain** may result from a variety of conditions. Non-cardiac causes include musculoskeletal disorders such as cervical arthritis, gastrointestinal disorders such as reflux oesophagitis and gallbladder disease, pulmonary conditions such as pulmonary embolus, and psychological states such as severe anxiety.

Pain of non-cardiac origin may mimic that of cardiac origin. For example, the pain of oesophageal spasm is usually burning in nature, located substernally and may be relieved by glyceryl trinitrate (GTN). Non-cardiac disease is ruled out by a careful history, physical examination and specific diagnostic tests such as gastric or gallbladder investigations. The chest pain that cardiac patients experience is usually due to the deficiency of oxygen in the myocardium. It is important to determine the location, nature and precipitating or contributing factors of chest pain in order to distinguish the specific cause. The pain may be described as sharp, aching, squeezing, a feeling of heaviness or weight on the chest or a sensation of pressure within the chest. It may be mild or excruciating. It may be localized to one area or may radiate across the chest, and into the back, neck, jaw, shoulders and/or arms. It may be precipitated or aggravated by activity, breathing cold air or certain bodily positions, and may be relieved by resting or a change of position. Table 12.1 describes some causes of chest pain.

Palpitations

Palpitations are experienced by people who become conscious of their beating heart. This may be due to the apex of the enlarged heart striking the chest wall with each contraction, or it may occur with an increased stroke volume in extrasystole, or with ectopic beats or arrhythmias (see p. 295). Palpitations may also be experienced by patients who are having an acute anxiety attack and this contributes to their sense of impending doom.

General debilitation, loss of strength, and decreased mental and physical efficiency

Weakness, loss of appetite and weight, general apathy and reduced efficiency occur as the result of the reduced nutrient and oxygen supply, venous congestion and the accumulation of metabolic wastes.

Abnormal heart sounds

Cardiac murmurs are abnormal heart sounds caused by abnormalities within the heart. The most frequent causes of heart murmurs are stenosed and incompetent valves and openings between the right and left sides of the heart. Murmurs may also occur in an aneurysm – a localized saccular dilatation of an artery.

In determining the significance of a murmur, the doctor considers when it occurs in the cardiac cycle, its intensity, quality of sound, duration, factors that alter the sound (such as respiration and change of position) and the patient's history. It is also important to note where the murmur is most audible during the chest examination. For example, those that are heard in the apex area of the heart can tend to be related to the mitral valve and those that are heard over the right sternal border are related to the aortic valve. Murmurs in some people may have no great significance.

Occasionally the S_3 or S_4 heart sound becomes pronounced, producing a gallop rhythm. This may be associated with

Table 12.1	Differential diagnosis: causes of chest pain			
	Angina	**Gastrointestinal**	**Musculoskeletal**	**Respiratory**
Provocation	Exercise Emotional upset	Related to food consumption	Related to trauma, physical effort	Increases with inspiration or trunk movement
Palliation	Rest Glyceryl trinitrate	Antacids	Mild analgesics, heat, rest	Little relief
Quality	Tightness	Burning, discomfort, wind	Ache	Sharp, grabbing (pleurisy, pneumothorax or pulmonary embolism) or dull, aching in pneumonia
	Stops patient activity	Patient carries on activity	Patient carries on activity	Lower chest, sometimes bilateral
Region	Retrosternal	Epigastric/retrosternal	Intercostal	Pneumothorax on entire side of chest
Radiation	Arm, wrist, hand, jaw	Unlikely, but possibly through to back	Back, shoulder, chest	Pneumothorax radiates to back
Severity	Moderate/severe	Variable	Moderate, but variable	Moderate to severe
Timing	Tends to be related to exercise	Vague onset, but may waken patient from sleep	Shortly after physical effort	Sudden onset and then continual pain

From Walsh et al (1999). Reprinted by permission of Butterworth-Heinemann.

significant pathology such as hypertension, CHD or thyrotoxicosis, or may be heard in pregnancy.

Clinical diagnostic studies

The cardiac patient may require a number of diagnostic studies to evaluate disease processes and treatments. The nurse requires an understanding of these procedures and their implications to manage patient care effectively and to teach patients who wish to be more knowledgeable about their own care. Blood tests, non-invasive and invasive diagnostic procedures are discussed below.

Blood tests

A number of blood tests are conducted when investigating heart disease, including biochemical markers for myocardial damage (such as troponin levels), full blood counts, blood cholesterol levels, glucose levels and urea and electrolyte levels. These are discussed elsewhere in this book.

Non-invasive diagnostic procedures

Non-invasive diagnostic procedures include electrocardiography, echocardiography, nuclear magnetic resonance imaging and chest radiography.

Electrocardiography Electrocardiography (ECG) is the study of the electrical activity associated with heart contractions. The **electrocardiogram**, which produces a graphic recording of heart activity, provides one of the most dependable aids in assessing heart function and in diagnosing heart disease. It is also non-invasive and painless to the patient.

Each heart contraction results from electrical currents that spread from the heart and can be monitored from the surface of the body. These currents are detected when electrodes are placed on the external surface of the body and make up the ECG recording.

The electrical complexes are recorded on graph paper (see Fig. 12.5). The horizontal axis of the graph paper represents time. Each small horizontal square indicates 0.04 second. Each large square is composed of five small squares and is therefore equal to 0.20 second.

The vertical axis of the graph indicates voltage. Each small vertical square represents 0.1 millivolt (mV), whereas a large square composed of five small squares equals 0.5 mV. The electrical activity over each cycle is divided into the P, Q, R, S and T sections.

The baseline of the graph paper represents zero electrical potential. Deflections above the baseline are considered positive, and deflections below the baseline are considered negative. When a wave form has both a positive and negative component, it is considered biphasic.

The *P wave* represents atrial depolarization. It begins when the electrical impulse leaves the SA node and initiates atrial depolarization. The P wave may be positive, negative or biphasic, depending on the monitoring lead, and should be no more than 2–3 mm high.

The *P–R interval* is the time interval from the beginning of the P wave to the beginning of the QRS complex. The normal P–R interval is 0.12–0.20 seconds. The P–R interval represents the time for an impulse to travel from the SA node to the ventricular Purkinje fibres.

The *QRS complex* represents ventricular depolarization. The Q wave is the initial downward (negative) deflection following the P wave, the R wave is the initial upward (positive) deflection following the Q wave, and the S wave is the downward deflection following the R wave. The QRS complex should not exceed 0.10 second in duration and the normal amplitude varies significantly depending on the monitoring lead.

The *ST segment* is an interval of zero potential, the period between completion of depolarization and the beginning of repolarization (recovery) of the ventricles. Usually it is isoelectric, but it may normally deviate 2.0 mm above or below the baseline.

The *T wave* represents the recovery phase after contraction or return of the ventricular muscular fibres to their resting state. Normally, the T wave is slightly rounded, asymmetrical and not more than 5–10 mm in height, depending on the lead.

A *standard 12-lead ECG* records electrical conduction events from 12 different angles or leads, six recordings from the limb leads, and six recordings from the chest leads. The ECG tracing is studied for deviations by understanding the tracing made by a normal heart, including the direction, contour and timing of the waves and segments. Information is obtained that is related to impulse formation and conduction, and to the condition and response of the myocardium. As the 12-lead ECG can provide a variety of angles of the conduction waveform, this enables a far easier diagnosis of an arrhythmia than can be offered by a bedside monitor alone. It also indicates whether any specific area of the heart is damaged, because each lead examines a particular area of the heart (Walsh and Kent 2001).

The patient should be given a brief explanation of the procedure and told that it takes approximately 5 minutes and that it is important to lie still during the procedure to produce a good tracing. The patient should be aware that the electrical recording will not cause any discomfort and

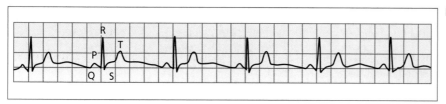

Figure 12.5 A normal electrocardiogram.

there is no danger of electrocution. It is important to make sure that the patient is relaxed and warm during the procedure to reduce any non-cardiac electrical interference with the recording.

In most coronary care units the nurse is responsible for obtaining the ECG. Nurses working in these specialty areas interpret ECG patterns and changes in the ECG tracings of patients connected to cardiac monitors. Nurses are becoming increasingly responsible for ECG interpretation and should always be aware of the results and their significance for the individual patient. Nurses who are trained to administer thrombolytic (clot busting) agents will have to act upon ECG interpretation, as will nurses trained in the skills of advanced life support (ALS).

Bedside monitoring   While on a specialized cardiac unit, the patient's cardiac functioning may be monitored by bedside equipment. This equipment allows continued surveillance of the patient's ECG tracing, with rapid identification of abnormal or changing rhythms and prompt treatment.

Telemetry monitoring   A telemetry monitoring system can be used in hospital to monitor an ambulant patient's cardiac activity. This method incorporates a transmitter (a small battery-powered unit), which can fit into a pocket, and a receiver and monitor, which are commonly housed in the coronary care unit. The patient, attached to the transmitter by means of chest electrodes, can be in a ward in another part of the hospital as long as he or she is within the working radius of the transmitter and receiver. The cardiac rhythm can therefore be monitored in the coronary care unit by nurses who are able to recognize cardiac arrhythmias. This system is important because it allows patients to begin the process of appropriate mobilization without feeling imprisoned by the monitoring system.

Ambulatory electrocardiography   The Holter technique of electrocardiography is a means of studying, over a prolonged period of time, the electrical activity of the heart during a person's normal daily activities. The ECG is recorded continuously on a magnetic tape while the patient performs normal activity, usually for 24 hours. The patient keeps a diary of activities and symptoms over the recorded period. The tape is then analysed by computer for arrhythmias, which can be correlated with activities (such as sleep and exercise) and symptoms.

This technique can be used to detect and document suspected or known cardiac rhythm disturbances and to assess cardiac function during symptoms such as syncope, palpitations or chest pain.

The nurse should explain the procedure to the patient. As the machinery cannot be immersed in water, the patient will not be able to have a bath or shower during the test. It is very important that the patient maintains a normal level of activity during the test and records all symptoms and activities in the diary.

Exercise electrocardiography   An exercise ECG, also known as a stress test, graded exercise test or exercise tolerance test, is used to detect and evaluate ischaemic heart disease while the individual exercises. Exercising increases myocardial oxygen demand and this test assesses the ability of the coronary arteries successfully to meet the increased demand. Thus it is useful in the evaluation of chest pain and the assessment of cardiac reserve or presence of IHD following myocardial infarction or cardiac surgery. Electrodes are attached to the patient, who is monitored continuously during the procedure. Periodically, recordings are printed.

The patient exercises on a treadmill or rides a bicycle at gradually increasing speeds against a regulated amount of resistance, according to an established protocol. The exercise continues until the patient reaches a pre-determined maximal heart rate according to age and sex. The test is discontinued earlier if the patient develops chest pain, hypotension, severe ventricular arrhythmias, marked ST depression, undue dyspnoea or fatigue. The exercise ECG is considered positive for ischaemia if the ECG shows an ST segment depression of 1 mm or more.

On the day of the test, the patient should have a light meal and should not smoke for 2 hours before the procedure. The patient should come to the test prepared to exercise, wearing loose-fitting trousers or shorts and lace-up walking shoes, with socks to prevent blisters. It is important that the patient knows that she or he can stop the test at any time and that any symptoms, including chest discomfort, light-headedness, leg cramping and weakness, must be reported to the staff. After the test, the patient should be encouraged to rest and not to take a hot shower within 2 hours of completing the test.

Patients are likely to want to know the outcome of the test and any implications for their future. Many patients feel reassured as their performance gives them some indication of their exercise capabilities, which they can then translate into activities of daily living.

Echocardiography   This is a non-invasive test used to detect ventricular dysfunction, valvular abnormalities, pericardial effusions, intracardiac masses and congenital defects.

High-frequency sound waves are aimed at the heart from a transducer held against the skin. Sound waves reflect or 'echo' off thoracic structures, are picked up by the transducer, visualized on a screen, and recorded on videotape or on a strip chart recorder for analysis.

Doppler echocardiography   This is a valuable adjunct to the conventional echo examination. Using ultrasound, it provides information concerning blood flow patterns by assessing blood velocity at multiple locations of the heart or great vessels. Doppler colour flow mapping provides information concerning direction of blood flow. Doppler imaging is especially useful in evaluating valvular heart disease and the presence of septal defects.

Patients should be aware that they will need to lie quietly in a dimly lit room for 20–30 minutes while the technician performs the echocardiogram. They will also be asked to change position several times during the procedure.

Oesophageal echocardiography Minute transducers mounted at the end of a gastroscope have been developed to image the heart anteriorly. This procedure is useful for visualizing the aortic and mitral valves, the aorta and the left ventricle in patients for whom the traditional echocardiography procedure has not produced the required information. It is useful because it reduces the impedance of skin, muscle and bone in gaining a clear picture. The patient is asked to fast for 6 hours before the procedure and is likely to be given lidocaine (lignocaine) spray to anaesthetize the throat.

Nuclear magnetic resonance imaging Magnetic resonance imaging (MRI) is a non-invasive diagnostic technique used to obtain high-resolution, tomographic, three-dimensional images of body structures. It allows visualization of cardiac chambers and blood vessels to determine structure, function and tissue characteristics.

Contraindications for MRI include the presence of pacemakers or implantable cardioverter defibrillators (ICDs) because the magnetic field can interfere with their operation. The presence of surgical clips and mechanical valves may produce considerable image artefact. The patient who suffers from claustrophobia or those who are acutely ill and unstable are not good candidates for this investigation.

Patients should be aware that they will be enclosed in the MRI scanner for about 30 minutes. No discomfort is felt during the procedure. The development of magnetic resonance contrast media to enhance images is creating a greater interest in this technique in cardiac patients. These require a much smaller injected volume and are less toxic than the more usual X-ray contrast media.

Chest radiography A radiograph of the chest can provide valuable information about the heart and lungs. Heart size may be assessed relatively accurately; the normal heart should be less than 50% of the width of the thoracic cavity and not exceed 16 cm. Cardiac enlargement is an early sign of cardiac failure, but an enlarged cardiac shadow may be seen in other conditions, such as valvular disease, cardiomyopathy, cardiac aneurysm and pericardial effusion. The location of invasive catheters, such as pacemaker or pulmonary artery catheters, can also be identified. There have been several advances in chest X-ray techniques in recent years. Of note are computed and digital radiography. Computed radiography uses a phosphor plate instead of conventional film. Following exposure the phosphor plate is scanned by a laser, and the image is digitized and stored electronically. In both computed and digital radiography, images can be manipulated electronically from one exposure, without increasing the radiation dose to the patient, by taking a further radiograph (Halstead et al 2001).

A brief explanation by the nurse may help allay any apprehension on the part of the patient.

Invasive diagnostic procedures

Radionuclide imaging techniques Nuclear cardiology includes a group of diagnostic tests in which tracer substances called radionuclides are injected into the bloodstream and their distribution in cardiac chambers is measured using a computer and a gamma camera. Tracer substances are composed of two components: the radionuclide and the substance to be tagged.

Tracers are characterized by their chemical behaviour, their physiological and biological half-life, and by the type of radiation emitted. For example, tracers that emit gamma radiation are used to make most of the measurements in nuclear cardiology.

Gamma rays emitted from the patient are detected with a gamma camera, and an image of the distribution of radioactive isotope in the area of interest is obtained. This information on isotope distribution and the relative amounts of isotope present can be obtained in fractions of a second and stored in a computer for subsequent analysis.

Nuclear cardiology techniques are relatively non-invasive, requiring only peripheral intravenous injections, and are considered safer than invasive techniques. Some measures are carried out while the patient is at rest and others during exercise.

Information provided varies with the test performed. Some tests estimate myocardial blood flow; others show cardiac haemodynamics such as cardiac output, stroke volume or ventricular performance. Radionuclide techniques may be divided into two general types: (1) first-pass techniques, in which only the first transit of a radionuclide bolus through the circulation is analysed; and (2) equilibrium studies in which serial studies can be obtained over time.

Two nuclear myocardial imaging techniques will be described: the thallium and technetium scans.

Thallium myocardial imaging Thallium-201 is an element with properties similar to potassium and is the radiopharmaceutical of choice for myocardial perfusion scintigraphy. Myocardial perfusion scintigraphy is recommended by NICE where the exercise tolerance test has not given accurate results (NICE 2003a). This may occur more commonly with women, people with diabetes or in people who are unable to exercise adequately for the exercise tolerance test. Clearance of the thallium-201 from the blood is rapid and extraction by the myocardium is high.

Thallium-201 scanning provides an assessment of myocardial tissue perfusion. Normally, coronary blood perfusion is equal throughout the myocardium, and thallium-201 would be distributed evenly in the tissue. In areas of myocardial ischaemia or necrosis, little or no thallium would be picked up. These areas of no perfusion would be seen as dark or 'cold' spots on the composite computerized image. In some patients, myocardial perfusion may be normal at rest, even with severe coronary disease. With exercise, however, the blood supply in the area supplied by the diseased vessels will differ from that supplied by normal vessels. Thus thallium imaging may be paired with exercise stress testing to evaluate myocardial perfusion at rest and when stressed.

After the heart has been stressed, exercise-induced ischaemia or previous myocardial infarction with a non-viable scar will produce a perfusion defect or cold spot. A second myocardial scan (or reperfusion image) is usually done 3 hours later. During the rest period, the exercise-induced ischaemic tissue will be reperfused and will no longer show as cold spots. This is called the redistribution pattern.

Technetium myocardial imaging   The radioactive substance in this procedure is ^{99m}Tc-labelled pyrophosphate. This test detects the size, location and approximate age of myocardial damage within 7–10 days of damage. The technetium-99m is absorbed by injured myocardial cells and images obtained of the heart will show these areas as 'hot' spots or bright areas. The scanning to obtain images takes approximately 30 minutes to perform.

Cardiopulmonary angiography   There are various techniques whereby the pulmonary and cardiac circulation can be assessed. The most widely used method involves the selective placement of a suitable catheter in the vessel or cardiac chamber proximal to the region being investigated. Injected radio-opaque contrast medium flows away from the catheter tip, and its path may be recorded and stored electronically on a compact disk.

Cardiopulmonary angiography may be used to investigate and diagnose a number of abnormalities, including valvular lesions, such as stenosis or regurgitation, pulmonary emboli, cardiac tumours, myocardial dysfunction, coronary artery stenosis or occlusion.

Cardiac and pulmonary angiography is invasive and not without complications; these may include a haematoma at the catheter insertion site, an allergic reaction to the contrast media, and chest pain during the procedure. As with all investigations, the potential benefit from making a correct diagnosis must exceed the risk from the diagnostic procedure. The indications for the test must be clear and the patient fully informed of what to expect. It is the doctor's duty to discuss the procedure with the patient and to gain consent, but the nurse must have sufficient understanding to respond to additional questions to help to reduce anxiety. High levels of anxiety may exist amongst patients before the procedure, particularly if invasive, because of a fear of the unknown (Halstead et al 2001). Peterson (1991) found that patients had concerns over a variety of issues, including the waiting time on the day of the procedure, the actual test, lying flat on a hard table, insertion of the catheter and possible complications. Teaching the patient relaxation techniques prior to the procedure reduces stress. Patients are likely to be less anxious if they are told what sensations to expect (Peterson 1991), although some respond better if they are not told in too much detail what the procedure is like.

It is the policy of most hospitals that informed, written consent be obtained before angiography. Food and fluids are withheld for the preceding 4 hours and opiate pre-medication is advisable. There are few contraindications to the administration of radio-opaque contrast media. Although most patients experience a sensation of warmth with the injection, major side-effects, which include respiratory dis-tress, hypotension, urticaria, nausea and vomiting, are fortunately rare. Treatment will depend on the severity of the reaction, but intravenous fluids, antihistamines, steroids, adrenaline (epinephrine) and oxygen should be available. Full resuscitation equipment needs to be on hand in case of problems resulting from ischaemia.

Right heart and pulmonary catheterization   This investigation provides information about the right side of the heart and the pulmonary circulation. Under local anaesthesia and sterile technique, the common femoral vein (usually the right) is punctured using a stiletted needle. The stilette is withdrawn and, once venous backflow occurs, a guidewire is threaded through the needle into the vein as far as the inferior vena cava. The needle is removed and an appropriate catheter is passed over the wire until it is in a satisfactory position, as judged by fluoroscopy. A small injection of contrast medium will confirm the position of the catheter tip.

If a pulmonary angiogram is required for suspected pulmonary emboli, the catheter is guided through the tricuspid and pulmonary valves. In the assessment of right ventricular function, valvular disease or congenital defects, the catheter will be placed in the appropriate cardiac chamber.

Left heart and coronary artery catheterization   The femoral or brachial artery is used for evaluation of the left heart and coronary arteries. The technique of catheter introduction is similar for arterial studies, but more care is required because the pressures are higher. The catheter is passed retrogradely up the aorta. Crossing the aortic valve usually causes very little disturbance to cardiac or valve function; however, arrhythmias may be induced, so continuous cardiac monitoring is mandatory.

Cardiac catheterization also allows haemodynamic measurements and other parameters, such as the degree of oxygenation of blood within the various chambers, to be recorded (Table 12.2). This may be valuable in the investigation of congenital heart disease. For example, with an

Table 12.2   Range of normal resting haemodynamic values

| | | Pressure (mmHg) | |
	Mean	Systolic	End diastolic
Right atrium	0–8		
Right ventricle	9–16	15–30	0–8
Pulmonary artery		15–30	3–12
Pulmonary artery 'wedge' and left atrium	1–10		
Left ventricle		100–140	3–12
Systemic arteries	70–105	100–140	60–90

atrial septal defect, increased oxygen tension may be found in the right side of the heart.

The role of the nurse The nurse has a major role in preparing the patient for cardiopulmonary angiography. As indicated above, informed written consent is required. The patient is informed of the equipment that may be seen during the procedure, the sterile precautions that will be taken, and some of the physical sensations that will be experienced, such as a feeling of pressure when the catheter is introduced and the warm flush that immediately follows injection of the contrast medium. Although each step is usually explained during the procedure, the patient's anxiety is often decreased when given this information beforehand. Some institutions may provide leaflets describing the experience.

The patient's reaction must be observed closely during the procedure. The ECG is monitored constantly. Irritation of the myocardium by the catheter may rarely precipitate ventricular fibrillation, so a defibrillator is close at hand. The patient experiences little discomfort but may complain of a fluttering or irritation in the chest, especially during movement of the catheter. The patient is advised that this is a temporary sensation.

The sheaths, which introduced the catheter, are often removed by the doctor in the angiography laboratory. However, the nurse may perform this when the patient returns to the unit. Pressure is then applied over the groin area, which can be for a minimum of 10 minutes to stop bleeding from the artery. Special manual compression devices and collagen seals into the vessel have all been designed to reduce the length of time for which the nurse has to press on the groin. There has been controversy over how long the patient should then stay on bedrest to reduce damage to the artery and to prevent haematoma formation. It is likely that patients will lie flat for an hour and gradually be sat upright. The patient needs to be able to drink in order to clear the radio-opaque dye from the system. Searle and Hoff (2000) found that bedrest of 2–3 hours, followed by gentle mobilization, produced few side-effects such as haematoma formation. In addition, the pulse below the catheter insertion site is checked every 15 minutes for the first hour and then at gradually increased intervals if it remains normal. An irregular, rapid or weak pulse is promptly reported to the doctor. The wound is observed for redness and tenderness, which may indicate irritation or phlebitis.

Despite the above measures, there may still be an area of bruising and skin discoloration as a result of bleeding into the tissues around the puncture site. This will fade over a week or so. Patients discharged straight home need to be given advice and a contact telephone number in case of any problems. Patients frequently wish to discuss their feelings following the procedure. Although one probable reaction is relief that the procedure has been completed, anxiety about the findings and their implications is often evident.

Electrophysiology studies An electrophysiology study (EPS) is an invasive procedure used to assess and facilitate management of recurrent symptomatic arrhythmias. The heart is deliberately provoked in an attempt to identify the existence, type and severity of the rhythm disturbance. The heart is stimulated using pacing catheters. The catheter electrodes are usually introduced via the right femoral vein (it is rare to use an artery), and are positioned with radiographic (fluoroscopic) guidance in the right side of the heart, which will receive the stimuli. Once the pacing catheter(s) are in place (Fig. 12.6), programmed stimulation is used to induce the rhythm disturbance. Figure 12.6 illustrates the three catheter positions, but a fourth may be placed in the coronary sinus, enabling recording and pacing from the left atrium (Bygrave 2001).

If the arrhythmia is induced, medications and various manoeuvres may be attempted to prevent or treat it. A long-term treatment regimen can thus be established.

Preparation and post-procedure management of the patient undergoing EPS by the percutaneous route are similar to those described for cardiopulmonary angiography. However, the patient will also have to be in a 'drug-free state' to prevent their usual medication suppressing the arrhythmias that are being induced. After the procedure it may be necessary to monitor the heart rhythm, depending on the diagnosis (Bygrave 2001). The patient with significant arrhythmic disturbances may require ongoing evaluation using EPS.

Measurement of venous blood pressure Venous **blood pressure** is an important parameter in the care of seriously ill patients. It reflects the intravascular volume and the ability of the heart to cope with the blood it receives via the venous system. Measurement of the venous pressure may be made in a peripheral vein, such as the median basilic, or in a large central vein, such as the superior vena cava.

Central venous pressure Central venous pressure (CVP) is more reliable than the peripheral. It may be used as a guide for fluid replacement in the dehydrated or post-operative patient, or for a critically ill patient.

An intravenous catheter is passed into the superior vena cava via the subclavian or internal jugular vein, or occasionally into the inferior vena cava via a femoral vein. The catheter is attached to a three-way stopcock which is also connected to a water manometer and intravenous infusion. An alternative, and more frequently used, method employs a pressure transducer in the CVP cannula and electronic monitoring of the CVP reading. In setting up the CVP line, the zero level of the manometer is positioned at the level of the right atrium, which is approximately in line with the mid-axillary and suprasternal notch. The most important factor is that the equipment is at the same level for each recording, so the initial level is usually marked on the patient's skin. In most instances the changes in the venous pressure or the trend of recordings are more significant than the actual level.

To take a CVP reading, patients should be lying on their back, although they can sit up; however, they must be in the same position for each recording. The pressure is generally

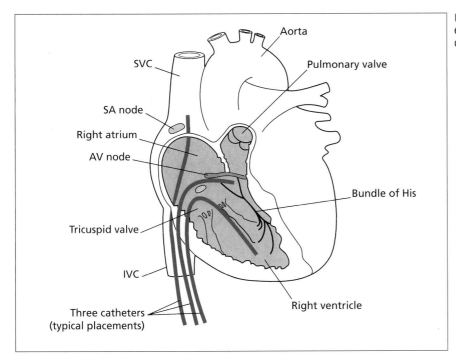

Figure 12.6 Placement of catheters in electrophysiology studies. SVC, superior vena cava; IVC, inferior vena cava.

recorded hourly. When the catheter is introduced, the stopcock is adjusted to allow fluid to flow to the patient. Then, to determine the venous pressure, the stopcock is turned to direct the fluid up into the manometer to a level of approximately 30–35 cm. The valve is then adjusted to close off the flow from the intravenous bag and to establish a flow between the manometer and the catheter. When the back pressure fluid from the venous system balances the downward pressure of the column of fluid, the fluid level remains relatively stationary, rhythmically rising and falling 1–2 cm with respirations. The height of the fluid column above the base line is the CVP. After recording this, the stopcock is readjusted to allow the intravenous solution to flow to the patient.

The normal CVP is approximately 3–12 cmH$_2$O when recorded with a water manometer set on an infusion (drip) stand. When an electronic transducer is used to measure CVP, the normal range is recorded in millimetres of mercury, and is approximately 0–8 mmHg. This varies with the patient's size, position and state of hydration. As the normal range is quite wide, it is important to note the recorded trends in CVP readings to detect changes in the patient's condition. The significance of CVP is determined in conjunction with the arterial blood pressure, the hourly output of urine, pulse rate and volume, and ECG. The nurse needs to know the levels at which the doctor is to be informed, and the type, volume and rate of flow of the infusion must be prescribed.

Other nursing responsibilities include observation for complications such as inflammation at the insertion site. This may be prevented by the use of aseptic technique during catheter insertion and during the application of dressings. Interference with flow may be minimized by periodic

flushing with a solution of heparinized saline to prevent clotting, and loosely coiling the tubing to prevent it from kinking.

Measurement of pulmonary artery pressure (wedge pressure) To obtain more specific information about the functioning of the left side of the heart, pulmonary artery and pulmonary capillary pressures are measured. This procedure is used for critically ill patients in whom early detection of left ventricular dysfunction is important.

A flow-directed pulmonary artery catheter (sometimes called a Swan-Ganz catheter) (Fig. 12.7) is inserted under sterile conditions into a central vein, such as the internal jugular or subclavian vein. A tiny balloon at the tip of the catheter is inflated and the catheter floats into the right atrium, right ventricle and pulmonary artery, at which time the pulmonary artery pressure may be measured. The catheter is then advanced into a branch of the pulmonary artery until it becomes wedged in a pulmonary capillary. The changing monitored pressure tracings allow the doctor to know where in the heart the catheter is as it is advanced. The balloon is inflated and 'wedged' in the pulmonary artery, hence the term 'wedge pressure'. It may then monitor pressure in the lungs and the left heart chambers. Thus, the catheter offers a reflection of the functioning of the left side of the heart, without directly entering these high-pressure chambers. The balloon must always be deflated until the next pressure reading, to allow blood to flow through to the lungs.

The nurse is responsible for monitoring pressures, reporting abnormalities and preventing complications. The normal pulmonary artery pressure is 25/10 mmHg, and the normal pulmonary capillary 'wedge' pressure is 4–12 mmHg. An

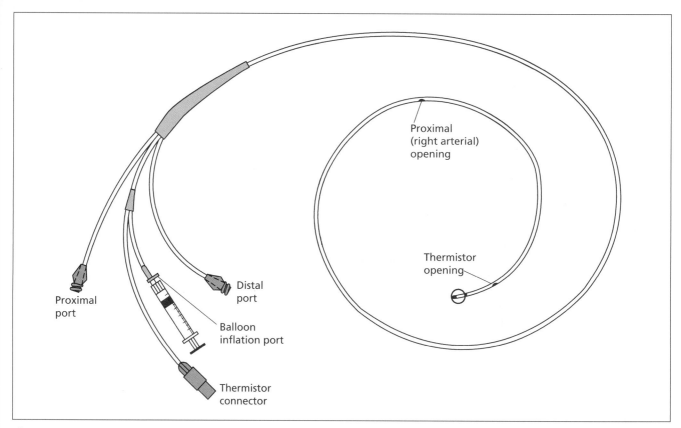

Figure 12.7 Thermodilution pulmonary artery catheter.

increase in this latter reading can indicate left ventricular failure.

NATURE OF PATIENTS WITH A CARDIAC CONDITION

Patients with cardiovascular problems are a diverse group. There are varying degrees of impairment and a wide range of psychological responses. Individuals will display different ways of coping with and adapting to unique situations. The heart is frequently perceived as symbolizing life and health. Not being able to see the heart and related structures means that those with problems need to rely on information from healthcare professionals before they can conceptualize the extent of their disorder. Misconceptions and unfounded fears are common. Most people will know someone who has had a cardiac condition, and it is easy for information to become distorted. Significant others will also be greatly affected, as will the dynamics of family life. The ability to plan ahead and to retain a sense of control over the future may be lost.

Some individuals may have a slight physical abnormality or a condition that has been cured. The heart may carry some structural change or a scar (e.g. after myocardial infarction) but cardiac efficiency is such that no long-term restrictions on activities are necessary. Some such people may have unwarranted fears and, despite advice to the contrary, restrict their activities unnecessarily. There may be a fear of extending the damage or triggering off an old problem. Some people worry about dying. There is often a feeling that a first event, such as a myocardial infarction, is a warning and a subsequent second attack is inevitable and will be fatal. Alternatively people may experience benefits as a result of their diagnosis and continue to display activities associated with the sick role in order to guarantee themselves continuing attention and support from others. Families are frequently uncertain how to respond to individuals with cardiac problems. They may have similar perceptions to the patient or their views may contrast significantly. A tightrope is often walked, balancing between overprotection and apparent indifference. Wives of coronary patients, for example, have been shown to engage in secret surveillance activities, monitoring their partner's every move, during the first few weeks at home (Thompson et al 1995). The role of the nurse with these patients is to try to dispel any unfounded fears and encourage an active and fulfilling lifestyle. Talking through unresolved fears and offering positive reassurance may be of benefit.

Some people are left with limited cardiac function, and some restrictions on activity are necessary. The disorder may have resulted in adaptive changes to the heart (dilation, hypertrophy and/or acceleration) in order to avoid heart failure. Energy expenditure needs to match functional capability and therefore limitations will be individual. Some may only have to give up strenuous competitive sports. Feelings of anger and a reduced sense of self-worth may accompany enforced changes in lifestyle. Frustration is a common response. Relationships may suffer as partners have to take on new roles and accept limitation in their own lives. Other relationships may be enhanced through caring and the increased openness that illness sometimes brings. The aim is to help each individual to live a useful and satisfying life within their own limitations. Individuals and their families may need support in accepting and adjusting to changes in lifestyle. Advice about appropriate activities – work, leisure, etc., and the importance of rest – may help in regaining a sense of direction and control. Ongoing medical treatment may be necessary to control symptoms. Concordance can be achieved when the individual understands the reasoning behind treatment regimens and can be further enhanced if there is a good relationship with the healthcare team. Realistic expectations are important.

Some patients may have a functional capacity that means they experience symptoms such as shortness of breath and chest pain on minimal exertion. They may be limited to self-care activities or be completely dependent on others. Such individuals are likely to be dependent on the care and support of their families, with resulting consequences for family dynamics. There may be a regression to child-like status with associated feelings of inadequacy, powerlessness and low self-esteem. Individuals may resent their situation and become angry and uncooperative in the eyes of their carers. They may become depressed and withdraw from life as they once knew it. Such individuals need to be helped to retain some sense of self-value and purposefulness. The family needs to be involved in care planning and decision making. Physical care can be demanding and demoralizing, and carers need a forum to express their feelings in confidence. Family members may suffer physical exhaustion and experience feelings of guilt at possible negative feelings towards their situation.

If the patient is at a terminal stage in their disease process, they need care geared towards supporting them and their families through this difficult time. Deciding when the condition has become terminal can be a problem for some healthcare professionals geared to preserving life. End-stage heart failure, although irreversible, has often not been given the same priority as other conditions such as cancer or acquired immune deficiency syndrome (AIDS). Respite care in a hospital or hospice may be a way of relieving pressure on the family. The primary healthcare team will also have input at this stage.

COMMON PROBLEMS RELATED TO CARDIOVASCULAR FUNCTION

Analysis of data gathered during assessment may identify a number of problems related to the individual's cardiovascular status, emotional response to disease and alterations in lifestyle. The most common problems occur as a result of:

- decreased cardiac output
- activity intolerance
- chest discomfort
- effects on family/carers
- anxiety and other psychological responses
- alterations in lifestyle and self-care.

See Table 12.3.

Decreased cardiac output

The individual may experience shortness of breath, lethargy, weakness, palpitations, swollen ankles, weight gain, changes in elimination pattern and/or changes in appetite. Management *goals* include:

1 reducing the workload of the heart
2 improving contractility of the heart
3 identifying and treating associated patient problems
4 monitoring effects of interventions.

Nursing intervention
Reducing the workload of the heart

Rest   Rest is important in the treatment of the patient with reduced cardiac output because it reduces the demand on the heart by reducing body requirements for oxygen. The decrease in muscular activity leads to a reduction in venous return. Filling pressure (preload) is decreased and there is greater efficiency of ventricular emptying at systole. Thus, the heart works more effectively and cardiac output increases. Renal blood flow increases as less blood is needed to supply the muscles. Recumbency-induced diuresis also decreases intravascular volume, increases urine volume and reduces oedema.

The benefits of rest need to be weighed against the severity of the problem and possible consequences of inactivity. The patient could be advised to be on *complete bedrest*, which tends to mean absolute minimal activity with help with most activities of living, or *bedrest*, which refers to the patient being able to participate in some degree of personal care. Care plans need to be specific in the amount of activity the patient is performing. The patient may react negatively to restrictions on activity and they need to know the rationale behind such restrictions and the length of time they are likely to last. Strategies need to be worked out with the patient which allow activity that induces minimal symptoms. The effect of any activity on or by the patient needs to be monitored. Intervention by the various health professionals needs to be coordinated to allow time for rest. Activity needs to be spaced out. Creating an environment conducive to rest is important.

Once an acute episode has passed, the patient is likely to be able gradually to increase activities. Intermittent rest periods throughout the day and after activities should be encouraged.

Positioning   The position that the patient with decreased cardiac output finds most comfortable in bed may be determined by his or her breathing. If the patient is experiencing

Table 12.3 Common problems related to cardiovascular disorders

Problem	Related factors	Defining characteristics
Decreased cardiac output	Cardiac arrhythmias Impaired contractility of myocardium Changes in preload Altered afterload Coronary vasospasm Changes in myocardial automaticity	Altered level of consciousness Changes in blood pressure Changes in cardiac output, pulmonary capillary wedge pressure Arrhythmias Jugular venous distension Decreased or absent peripheral pulses Increased bodyweight Altered rate and depth of respirations Crackles in lungs Changes in skin colour Decreased or absent urine output Fatigue
Activity intolerance	Immobility Imbalance between oxygen supply and demand Generalized weakness Sedentary lifestyle Impaired myocardial contractility Impaired nutritional status Limited cardiac reserve Arrhythmias Lack of knowledge about energy conservation	Statement of fatigue, weakness Inactivity Dyspnoea on exertion Chest pain on exertion Expression of decreased energy Significant changes in heart rate, blood pressure on exertion
Chest discomfort	Decreased myocardial perfusion Increased myocardial oxygen requirements	Statement of chest pain Facial grimacing Clenched fist on chest Changes in rate and depth of respirations Altered blood pressure Changes in heart rate, rhythm Sweating
Effects on family	Disruption of family functioning due to patient's illness, hospitalization, treatment Lack of knowledge of cardiovascular disease process, management plan Altered sexual feelings and behaviour	Decreased family involvement in social and community affairs Failure to participate in usual family activities Lack of family participation in patient's care
Anxiety and other psychological responses	Prognosis Diagnosis Treatment plan	Complaints of anxiety, anger, denial, guilt, depression Sleeplessness Restlessness Abnormal rate or rhythm of pulse Abnormal rate of respirations Increased blood pressure Lethargy, withdrawal, hostility, non-compliance

a profound decrease in cardiac output and little dyspnoea, the supine position is preferable. This position facilitates venous return to the heart and reduces the heart's workload. The patient who is experiencing dyspnoea will be more comfortable with the head of the bed elevated, but the height of elevation should only be that at which the dyspnoea is minimal.

Patients may manifest orthopnoea, that is, less difficulty in breathing with the trunk in the upright position. This position increases the vital capacity and tends to reduce the volume of blood returned to the heart and to the pulmonary system. Pressure of abdominal viscera on the diaphragm is reduced. Some patients may be still more comfortable in a true sitting position – with the lower limbs down. A special cardiac bed on which the foot of the bed can be lowered to provide a chair-like support is available. Alternatively the patient may find comfort from sitting in a chair. The sitting position promotes the formation of peripheral oedema in the dependent parts but relieves the pulmonary congestion to some extent; peripheral oedema is much less serious than pulmonary oedema.

In the sitting position a pillow placed longitudinally at the patient's back may help to provide some comfort. Pillows should be used at the sides to support the arms and relieve the fatiguing pull on the shoulders. A change may be effected by arranging a table and pillow over the bed, upon which the patient may rest the head and arms. Cot sides may be kept up on the bed to safeguard the patient when in the upright position, as the patient may become drowsy and fall to the side, or may experience cerebral hypoxia which causes disorientation. The sides are also useful when a change of position is made because they may be grasped by the patient and used for added support. Patients in the upright position are encouraged to assume the recumbent position for periods to help reduce circulatory stasis and oedema in the lower parts of the body. However, patients should not be forced to do this if they are suffering from severe dyspnoea.

In patients with heart conditions, as with all patients, the general principles of positioning apply. Good body alignment is respected to prevent contractures, hyper-extension and circulatory stasis. *Even a slight change in position* every 1–2 hours is helpful. A footboard is used to prevent foot drop.

Constipation should be prevented and the patient cautioned against straining at stool because of the stress it places on the heart. A mild laxative or stool softener may be given as necessary.

Drug therapy   Nursing responsibilities towards patients receiving drug therapy include:

- administering the drug
- explaining its purpose
- monitoring the effect – changes in fluid balance, weight, oedema and breathing pattern
- observing for side-effects – dehydration, hypokalaemia, muscle weakness, arrhythmias, etc.

Vasodilator drugs reduce the workload of the heart by producing either venous dilatation (relaxing smooth muscle in the veins, thereby reducing venous return) or arterial dilatation (reducing myocardial work by decreasing peripheral vascular resistance). This lowers the heart's demand for oxygen, because less blood is returned to be pumped through the chambers due to the vessel dilatation. *Diuretics* reduce preload, blood volume and ventricular filling pressure, and resolve pulmonary and systemic congestion. *Angiotensin-converting enzyme (ACE) inhibitors* inhibit the conversion of angiotensin I to angiotensin II and are therefore very effective in lowering blood pressure. *Thrombolytics* are drugs that dissolve thrombi, which may be occluding a vessel. They are of major value when a patient is suffering a myocardial infarction (MI). *Beta-blockers* (beta-adrenergic blockers) block the β-adrenergic receptors in areas such as the heart. They can be used to treat the pain of angina by reducing the heart rate and thus the demand for oxygen. It is the mismatch between the supply and demand of oxygen by the myocardium that causes anginal pain.

Myocardial contractility can be enhanced with the use of inotropes, which increase ventricular activity. They tend to be given by intravenous infusion and are commonly seen in the coronary and intensive care environment. Examples are *dobutamine* and *dopamine*. *Digoxin* is a mild oral inotrope. Unfortunately, inotropes can overstimulate the heart, leading to myocardial hypoxia with the possibility of ventricular arrhythmias.

Identifying and treating associated patient problems
Shortness of breath   Appropriate positioning of the patient, spacing out activities, encouraging rest and administering drug therapy may help ease shortness of breath. In addition, oxygen therapy may be beneficial because it helps correct the ventilation–perfusion imbalance that leads to hypoxia. Sometimes opiates in the form of diamorphine prove helpful as they reduce anxiety, leading to systemic vasodilatation, which improves cardiac efficiency.

Palpitations   The patient in hospital may require frequent ECGs or constant cardiac monitoring. Individuals, particularly those at home, need to be aware of the importance of reporting any abnormal heart sensations. Changes in heart rate and rhythm need to be assessed for their nature and frequency, and for the effect they have on the individual concerned.

Oedema and weight gain   The patient with fluid retention and oedema is at increased risk of pressure sore development and problems associated with reduced mobility. They may also have negative feelings about their body image and become depressed and withdrawn. Drug therapy needs to be given as prescribed and its effects monitored. Elevating swollen limbs may also help. Individuals need to have realistic expectations about the effects of treatment and to be aware of the importance of frequent pressure relief for affected areas.

Changes in elimination pattern   Prolonged immobility and gastrointestinal stasis may lead to constipation requiring a mild apperient. Diuretic therapy is likely to lead to an increase in the volume and frequency of urine output. The timing of administration of these drugs should be planned around the patient's day to avoid disruption, particularly at night. Despite possibly feeling lethargic, it is usually easier to use the bedside commode than a bedpan.

Changes in appetite   Gastrointestinal congestion, ascites and/or lethargy may lead to a reduction in appetite. An easily digestible diet should be available and encouraged. A high salt intake needs to be discouraged because it attracts excess water and has been linked to factors such as high blood pressure, which can lead to further complications (e.g. heart failure). Those who are overweight need to be advised of the benefits of weight reduction as this reduces myocardial workload and enables exercise to be taken more easily, thus improving cardiac function.

Monitoring effects of interventions   The effect of interventions designed to improve cardiac output can be evaluated through monitoring:

- fluid balance
- daily weight
- blood pressure, heart rate
- subjective feelings
- level of exercise tolerance
- associated clinical features.

Activity intolerance

Patient goals

1 The patient will be able to perform planned activities without increased dyspnoea and fatigue.
2 The patient will understand and participate in a planned physical activity programme.

Nursing intervention

Activity progression   An acute episode of cardiovascular dysfunction will often confine the patient to bed until symptoms abate. This means that the patient is dependent on the nurse to facilitate care. It is important to discuss this necessary dependence with the patient so that its purpose, importance and temporary nature are understood.

The patient is encouraged to perform mild activities such as cleaning teeth, washing face and hands, and feeding, as long as reaching is avoided. Exercising the lower limbs to prevent venous stasis is commenced. Most patients are helped to use a bedside commode, as this demands less energy than using a bedpan. Undisturbed rest periods are provided following short periods of activity, for instance after eating or bathing.

As the patient's condition improves, activities and ambulation are gradually increased. An important principle in gradual ambulation is pacing activities. Rest periods are alternated with activity, and certain activities may be avoided for a period of time. These may include pushing, pulling, lifting or straining.

When patients learn that they have a heart condition or are recovering from an acute cardiac illness, they are advised as to whether former activities may be resumed or whether it will be necessary to curtail some activities. On the basis of the functional capacity of the heart, some individuals may consider themselves doomed to complete invalidism and an early death. They may have an unjustified fear of another attack or of participating in any activity, creating unnecessary problems and hardships for themselves and their families or carers. Maximum independence should, however, be the ultimate goal. Some may find that a few simple adjustments in their pattern of living are necessary, while others are more restricted.

There are several ways of assessing the patient's capacity for activity and any limitations. The patient's response to a gradual increase in energy expenditure is a key indicator of progress. This will probably begin with self-care activities which are progressively extended to include more strenuous efforts. The assessment programme may go on over several weeks or months, and the patient may require considerable encouragement to persevere. An exercise tolerance test may give the patient positive encouragement as to how far they can push themselves.

The nurse may assist in the assessment of the patient by observing and recording responses to various activities. Any complaint of shortness of breath, palpitations, fatigue or an undue increase in the pulse rate are noted, and the effort is discontinued.

It is helpful to have patients list their regular pattern of activity. It may then be apparent what changes, if any, are necessary. This is useful in getting patients to think and talk about how much they will be able to do. It encourages patients to plan independently and to reach a compromise between activity and restriction. Ideally, patients should be given the information, advice and support, and encouraged to decide for themselves what they can or cannot do. Individuals need to have the confidence to listen to their own body's response to activity and exercise, and to interpret what they find and modify their activity levels accordingly. Those with cardiovascular disorders will be of a variety of ages and previous levels of fitness. They will have varying expectations of and needs for future activity levels. Standardized activity programmes are likely to be inhibitive for some and overambitious for others. Individually setting short- and long-term objectives will give a sense of direction and encourage motivation. Practical information regarding daily activities such as gardening is more useful than simply suggesting a gradual return to normal.

Once the patient is free of pain and other early symptoms and feels quite well, activities may still be restricted. Time may drag, so some effort should be made to provide suitable diversions in which the patient is interested. Reading or radio and television programmes may occupy the patient. Some hobby may be pursued without overtaxing the heart. Visitors are restricted at first, but later they help to relieve the patient's boredom. Visitor selection should be made by the family to avoid those who might excite or distress the patient. Visitors should be made aware of time limitations as it may be difficult for patients to ask them to leave if they become tired.

Planned physical activity programme   *Physical activity* refers to any body movement that uses energy, for example housework, gardening, etc. *Exercise* refers to structured body movement that is performed with the purpose of enhancing health and fitness.

Following an acute cardiac event, or the diagnostic label of some form of heart disorder, there is a temptation for many consciously to avoid physical activity and exercise. The symptoms brought on by exercise may mimic those of a cardiac problem (e.g. breathlessness and sweating), and therefore cause anxiety. Loss of confidence may prevent participation in the simplest of activities. A vicious circle ensues: the less active the individual becomes, the more likely they are to experience symptoms of breathlessness and fatigue.

The benefits of physical activity include:

- enhancement of physical working capacity, enabling individuals to work harder for longer with less effort
- improvement in the efficiency of the cardiovascular system
- improvement in posture
- helping in weight management, thus improving self-esteem
- improvement in sense of well-being and stress reduction
- reduction in the risk of further disorders such as further episodes of IHD, hypertension, intermittent claudication and diabetes.

The benefits of aerobic exercise for cardiac patients include:

- improvement of collateral circulation
- decreased resting heart rate
- increased maximal exercise capacity
- improved peripheral circulation and blood pressure reduction
- increased levels of HDL.

Structured exercise is now generally viewed as beneficial to the majority of patients with heart failure, to increase their functional capacity (Gould 2001).

Individuals who experience angina need gradually to increase their exercise levels. The threshold at which they experience pain is likely to increase. Following myocardial infarction or heart surgery, activity levels should again be built up gradually and regular exercises introduced as soon as surgical wounds have healed (4–6 weeks).

In hospital   Many hospitals have structured activity programmes beginning as soon as the acute stage is over. The more active the patient is in hospital, the more likely they are to have the confidence to build up activity at home. A typical plan of activity progression in hospital would involve the following:

1 Rest in bed, chair, carrying out own toilet/hygiene activities at the bedside. Perform gentle neck, arm and leg exercises.
2 Walk around the bed area, sit in the bathroom for wash at the sink, be wheeled to bathroom, gradually increase gentle exercises.
3 Walk around ward area, walk to bathroom and toilet, increase exercises.

4 Walk around more frequently. Use the shower, then rest.
5 Build on the above plus monitored use of the stairs.

First weeks at home   Day-to-day activities should be gradually increased over the first few weeks at home. The distance walked each day should gradually be increased to build up stamina. Small amounts of activity need to be followed by rest. Individuals should be encouraged to monitor their own body's response and recognize appropriate and inappropriate signs. Gently warming up before exercise is important to loosen the joints, as is cooling down once the activity is over.

Exercise should be avoided until at least 2 hours after a heavy meal as blood and hence oxygen is diverted to the gut to aid digestion. Extremes of temperature should also be avoided. If chest pain, nausea, excessive shortness of breath, faintness, palpitations and/or excessive sweating is experienced, the activity should be stopped.

Activity that is moderate, rhythmic, continuous and aerobic such as walking, cycling and swimming should be encouraged initially. Heavy lifting, pulling, pushing, impact activity or anything that involves a sudden burst of activity should be avoided at first.

Chest pain
Patient goals
Management goals include:

1 early recognition of chest discomfort
2 elimination of chest discomfort
3 prevention of further chest discomfort.

Nursing intervention
Early recognition of chest pain   This requires that: (1) the individual is able to acknowledge and report chest pain as appropriate; and (2) healthcare professionals are aware of chest pain.

Each patient needs to be taught the significance of chest pain and to be made aware of the importance of acknowledging the signs and symptoms, and of reporting them to others when appropriate. Some patients may not realize that the sensation they are experiencing is anything to do with the cardiovascular system. The pain can be similar to that of indigestion. Others may have been told that their pain is cardiac, but choose to ignore or deny it. People sometimes try to work through their pain, continuing with activity as a method of distraction. The response to pain is likely to depend on an individual's perception of the significance of the pain and other factors, such as health perception and the need to be seen by others as being well.

Some studies have shown that nurses' assessments of patients' pain are not always reliable (Watt-Watson et al 2000), although others have demonstrated that assessments are more accurate if nurses have been taught about the significance of symptoms (Thompson et al 1994). Nurses need to be aware of typical words used to describe cardiac pain, the site and radiation of such pain, and likely associated symptoms, bearing in mind that individual experiences can differ widely. In hospital there will be access to other means of assessment including ECG, cardiac monitoring, blood pressure recording and blood tests. Totally painless cardiac ischaemia is possible resulting in patients having what is described as a 'silent myocardial infarction'; nurses therefore need to be aware of changes in the ECG pattern associated with ischaemia.

Elimination of chest pain

Administration of nitrates   Nitrates act by relaxing vascular smooth muscle. This results in decreased peripheral vascular resistance and venous return, with a subsequent decrease in stroke, volume and cardiac output. The net effect is a decrease in the oxygen consumption of the heart.

Glyceryl trinitrate (GTN) is a short-acting vasodilator administered in tablet, skin patch or spray form. The tablet is placed under the tongue where it is absorbed very quickly (sublingual). The patient may experience a tingling feeling on the tongue at first and should obtain relief in 1–2 minutes. Patients should not take multiple doses to obtain quick relief of pain. If relief is not apparent after three tablets taken at 5-minute intervals and the patient is outside the hospital, he or she should come to the hospital as soon as possible and/or call for emergency assistance. If the patient is in hospital, the nurse will initiate therapy as prescribed. The initial dosage of GTN should be 0.3 mg. This reduces the likelihood of severe headaches, which often occur in the initial stage of treatment. People who suffer attacks of angina are advised to carry the drug at all times. It should be replaced periodically so that a fresh supply is available when required. Tablets should be kept in a dark glass container and those not being carried should be stored in a cool, dark place, because GTN is affected by both light and heat. The patient is advised that there may be a mild fullness, warmth or throbbing in the head. When patients need to take nitrates regularly (see below) these side effects usually diminish. In emergency situations GTN may be administered intravenously.

Administration of analgesics   An analgesic such as diamorphine is usually given to relieve severe pain not relieved by nitrates. The drug may be administered intravenously in small doses in pre-hospital care, the A&E department and in the coronary care unit. Intramuscular injections raise creatine phosphokinase readings, as this enzyme is also present in skeletal muscle, and diagnosis of a myocardial infarction may be obscured. However, the majority of units are now using biochemical markers such as the troponins, with levels recorded a set number of hours apart to determine the presence of myocardial damage. The effect of diamorphine on the respirations should be noted, as depression of the respiratory centre may occur. This drug will reduce preload, afterload, sympathetic tone and the patient's anxiety.

Administration of oxygen   Oxygen is usually administered in order to increase arterial oxygen tension, which may help to relieve the myocardial pain caused by hypoxia and prevent extension of the infarction. Observations are made of the patient's response to oxygen. Its effectiveness will be indicated by reduced pulse rate, less dyspnoea, improvement in colour, less restlessness and improved oxygen saturation levels as monitored by pulse oximetry.

Prevention of further chest pain

Administration of nitrates   Long-acting nitrates, such as the buccal tablets that are placed in the buccal cavity (between upper lip and gum) and left to dissolve, can be used if regular attacks of angina are being experienced. Other nitrate tablets used to control angina include *isosorbide dinitrate* and *isosorbide mononitrate*. Modified-release preparations prolong the effects. In hospital, intravenous nitrate therapy may be prescribed. The dose is usually low initially and increased in response to pain. Some people may experience hypotension and feel light-headed on standing. A headache is common, and paracetamol may help. GTN tablets may be taken prophylactically before an activity known to produce angina, although there is a danger of psychological dependence and not being able to get an accurate picture of the level of activity needed to produce pain.

Reduction of workload on the heart   The reduction of workload on the heart is important so that there is sufficient oxygen available to the myocardium to meet the demands placed upon it. Pacing of activities to ensure adequate periods of rest between periods of activity can facilitate balanced supply and demand on the heart.

Anxiety reduction   Increased anxiety levels increase the likelihood of chest pain as the stress response stimulates the sympathetic nervous system. Biofeedback or relaxation techniques such as background music may help. Distraction, such as watching the television, may also help. The nurse should ensure a calm relaxing environment for the patient at all times.

Anxiety and other psychological responses

Goals

Goals will be individual and centred around the response of each person concerned. They may include the person being able to talk about feelings of anxiety or to show signs of a reduction in anxiety.

Nursing intervention

People with heart disease are frequently anxious. Serial measurements of the anxiety levels of coronary patients have shown that anxiety is highest on admission to the coronary care unit and immediately after transfer to the ward, falling rapidly over the following week and rising just before discharge (Thompson et al 1987).

The common knowledge that the heart is a most vital organ and that heart disease is a frequent cause of death produces a great emotional reaction in the person advised of a diagnosis of a heart disorder. This response is likely to be very individual and depends on factors such as age, perception of the significance of the diagnosis, and expectations for the future. The complex range of emotions produced can be described in terms of response to loss: loss of health, loss of status, loss of income, loss of confidence, and loss of any notion of invincibility. The individual is likely to go through the stages described in models of grieving, including numbness, denial, disbelief, grief, guilt, anger, despair, depression and disorganization (see Ch. 4). Anxiety is the most common initial response. All the above responses are normal, although they may become prolonged and then lead to serious distress. There is no set pattern to coping, and responses will depend on individual personality and experience. Reorganization and acceptance are the final stages of adaptation, although not all will work through to this response.

The aim is to encourage individuals to accept the reality of their situation and adjust accordingly. The emotional energy invested in grief and anger needs to be reinvested in positive coping for the future. The individual needs to:

● accept the reality of the situation
● work through negative emotions
● adjust emotionally to changed circumstances
● make necessary changes in lifestyle, employment, etc., in order to move with confidence to an acceptable quality of life.

The nurse who understands the patient's condition, and who knows what to look for and what to do, usually displays calm and composure which contribute to the patient's confidence and security. Brief and precise explanations of all equipment, routines, tests and procedures usually prove helpful. A quiet, controlled atmosphere may do more toward allaying fear than verbal reassurance.

Patients may pose direct questions about their condition, such as: 'Is it serious?' or 'Will I recover?' Answers should be honest and supportive. Each patient must be helped to find a coping strategy appropriate to his or her personal situation and own strengths and weaknesses. This is done through effective communication with the patient. Effective communication includes listening to the patient and responding to any cues, introducing statements to which the patient might respond, and allowing the patient to discuss feelings. Considerable help and peace of mind may be derived from a priest or other religious leader.

If the patient is very upset, the nurse remains until the patient is less apprehensive, and confirms that someone is close by and will be in and out frequently. The presence of a close member of the family who will not disturb the patient may provide additional comfort. Occasionally, diazepam or another anti-anxiety drug may be prescribed.

There may be a problem at home that contributes to the patient's unrest, which should be discussed if appropriate or arrangements made for assistance from the social services or primary healthcare team.

Effects on family or carers
Patient's family or carer's goals
1 The family/carer(s) will express feelings of support and awareness of available resources.

2 The family/carer(s) will be able to participate in the patient's treatment as appropriate.

It is important to understand that the family may not necessarily be a close or blood relative of the patient. A detailed nursing assessment will ascertain who the patient regards as closest emotionally to them and who can offer support.

Nursing intervention
Members of the patient's family often experience shock and anxiety in response to the patient's diagnosis. Seeing someone close to us in pain and seriously ill is a very frightening experience. Relatives of patients have described their initial reaction as 'feeling numbed and dazed'. As reality sets in, anxiety about the patient's survival and future increases.

Good relationships between family members and healthcare professionals need to be fostered early on. Soon after admission the family needs to be advised about suspected diagnosis and initial treatment. Family members may be uncomfortable in approaching nursing staff to ask questions and so should be invited to discuss their feelings and concerns. Relatives as well as patients are reassured by simple explanations of equipment, procedures and routines. In talking to the family, the nurse may elicit information about the patient's habits, likes and dislikes, and emotional reactions, which are helpful in planning care.

Alleviating the anxieties of relatives and/or close family friends allows them to be more supportive of the patient. As with the patient, concern may prevent the members of the family from absorbing all that they are told. Explanations and instructions may have to be repeated. The family should be included in teaching programmes provided for the patient or in programmes specifically designed for them to ensure they understand the patient's condition. Visiting times need to be viewed as an important contribution to recovery. Open visiting is encouraged in many areas with thought to individual patient needs.

Dynamics within the family may take a while to reestablish themselves. They may never return to how they were before the event. Relationships may be perceived as stronger or weaker. The anxiety created from having cardiac disease can have a clear detrimental effect on resuming sexual activities (Friedman 2000). Couples are often open about discussing sexual matters once the subject has been mentioned, and nurses need to examine their own feelings towards the issue. Partners may have unresolved feelings of guilt at having contributed in some way to the problem. It is not always relevant for nurses to become involved in complex family issues but they need to be aware of the important part they play in recovery and offer support and advice as appropriate.

Patients in the community will need the support of their general practitioner, nurse practitioner and practice or district nurse. More practices are establishing support groups for individuals with similar problems. Self-help groups may help to foster positive attitudes and provide a means of social support.

There is evidence that spouses experience significant distress when a partner is experiencing a cardiac disease (Kettunen et al 1999, O'Farrell et al 2000), yet professional support, particularly of the spouse, is often inappropriate or inadequate. A simple programme of in-hospital counseling for coronary patients and spouses has a number of benefits, including a reduction in anxiety and depression (Thompson 1990). Patients in early recovery from myocardial infarction or cardiac surgery have been found to want information on the side-effects of treatment and knowledge of their disorder (Jaarsma et al 1995).

Alterations in lifestyle and self-care

Patient goals

1 The patient will show knowledge of the disease process.
2 The patient will engage in lifestyle modification to reduce risk.

Nursing intervention

Patient's knowledge of the disease process To make the best possible adjustment to illness and recovery, the patient must have some understanding of the illness and how he or she can assist in recovery. Provision of this information helps to give the patient realistic expectations and some control over the situation. Teaching programmes are adjusted to specific patient needs and capabilities, as learning capacity varies among individuals. Patients experiencing cardiovascular conditions often have many misconceptions of their condition and how it will affect their future. It is useful for the nurse to find out what the patient already knows and to obtain information about lifestyle. The nurse has many opportunities to reinforce and elaborate on explanations given by the doctor and to respond to further questions.

During the acute stage, the patient is often too anxious to absorb much information. *Simple* explanations of equipment being used and procedures common to coronary care units are usually adequate. Following transfer to the general ward, the patient is usually better able to participate in a planned programme. Written as well as verbal instruction may be provided. Visual aids such as heart models or diagrams help to enhance learning.

Short teaching sessions are necessary, as many patients with cardiovascular conditions tire easily. It is helpful if one of the family can be present during the teaching session. Acknowledgement is made of the feelings that the patient has in response to the illness. The patient may wish to express verbally the feelings being experienced, such as discouragement, fear, anger and/or depression; the nurse should provide opportunities for free expression and should be a willing listener.

Use should be made of the many useful pamphlets and booklets available from the British Heart Foundation (the web address for the BHF can be found at the end of this chapter). Many of these deal with rehabilitation, and appropriate copies may be given to the patient to read, backed up with individual information and advice.

Lifestyle modification The harmful effects of smoking are so severe that the patient is advised to discontinue.

Clarification of the prescribed diet is made. The nurse should be sensitive to individual patient needs, particularly in relation to social and cultural issues. Many patients are advised to continue with a low sodium (salt) intake and a limited number of calories. Meal planning should be discussed and the importance of keeping weight within the normal range and avoiding large meals is explained. Preferably, the discussion of the diet should be with the family as well as the patient. Directions and suggestions are given to the patient in writing, and an appropriate diet booklet can be obtained from the British Heart Foundation, the Health Education Authority or the dietetic department.

The medications that are to be continued are discussed, and written instructions are provided. Early signs of untoward reactions are cited; included with these are directions about what to do if they develop. For example, if an anticoagulant such as warfarin is to be continued, the patient and a family member are advised of the action of the drug and the necessary observations to recognize bleeding. They are told that bleeding from body orifices, discoloured areas of the skin (bruises and petechiae), bleeding gums, and persistent bleeding from minor cuts or injuries are to be reported immediately to the doctor or clinic. If there is dental work to be done, the patient should advise the dentist that he or she is receiving warfarin. The patient is given an identification card to carry which states that he or she is receiving warfarin. Regular visits to a clinic for INR testing will be arranged.

Many patients with heart conditions are required to take digoxin continuously and should understand that loss of appetite, nausea or diarrhoea may indicate the need for some adjustment in the dosage of the drug. If the patient is an elderly person who lives alone and perhaps has some difficulty with their memory, they may require the use of medication containers such as Dosette packs to help them to take their medications at the right time.

Progressively increased activity is encouraged to condition the patient to the level of activity that corresponds to the heart's ability.

Changes may be necessary at home if the patient is not able to use stairs. It may be helpful to have a member of the primary healthcare team or an occupational therapist or social worker to assess the home situation before the patient is discharged. For example, a bedroom and bathroom may have to be provided on the ground floor.

It should be pointed out to the patient and family that moderation in everything is a good rule for persons who have had a heart illness. Some work, exercise, rest and recreation are important for everyone. Situations that are likely to add undue strain should be anticipated and avoided. Enough time should be allowed to prevent rushing. For example, rather than having to run for a bus, the patient should plan to leave earlier. Climbing, walking against a strong wind, lifting, pushing and fatigue are to be avoided. Constipation, infections and emotional upsets also tend to increase the demands on the heart. Suitable recreational activities, which meet both interests and cardiac functional capacity, may be suggested. Exercise is beneficial and walking is a particularly good exercise. Regular hours of rest at night and, if necessary, a rest period during the day are recommended.

The doctor, a social worker or the nurse may discuss necessary adjustments in the person's work situation with the employer or occupational health nurse. Assistance might be given to find suitable employment or to obtain retraining if a change in occupation is indicated.

Some follow-up service is important. The patient and family are advised of the resources outside the hospital, and a referral may be made to the cardiac rehabilitation programme, general practitioner or district nurse. Home visits by a nurse can be very helpful; they provide an opportunity for the patient and family to ask questions and receive counseling on the various aspects of care. At the same time the patient's condition and progress can be observed.

An individual may choose not to follow advice given but may still gain support from the nurse–patient interaction. Understanding what has happened and what to expect during recovery may enable the patient and family to cope, without necessarily influencing subsequent behaviour patterns.

CAUSES AND TYPES OF HEART DISORDER

Heart disorders may be classified as *congenital* or *acquired*. Various sub-classifications may be used in acquired heart disease. Some authors concentrate on structure, such as pericardium, myocardium and endocardium. Others highlight the causes of heart disease, such as trauma, infections, degenerative processes, and hypermetabolic and hypometabolic processes. This text classifies heart disorders as:

● congenital cardiovascular defects
● disorders of cardiac muscle
● disorders of myocardial blood supply
● disorders of electroconduction
● disorders of myocardial pumping capacity
● disorders of the vascular system.

CONGENITAL CARDIOVASCULAR DEFECTS

Congenital cardiovascular defect implies a structural abnormality that was present at birth in the heart or the large proximal blood vessels. It has been only within the past two or three decades that many of the congenital cardiovascular defects have been identified and successfully treated by surgery. Many are recognized shortly after birth if the infant survives. Others may go undiscovered for months or years because the heart maintains an adequate circulation by compensation. As in so many congenital deformities, the cause remains obscure.

An individual's response to a congenital condition is likely to alter with time. The significance of the problem may not become apparent until the person gets older and starts to want to plan ahead, for example starting a family. Uncertainty as to how symptoms of the disorder will increase with time may produce feelings of fear, uncertainty and loss of control. To meet such needs there has been an emergence in recent years of Grown Up Congenital Heart Teams, known as GUCH teams. They aim to meet the needs of adolescents and young people with congenital cardiovascular defects who are making the transition to independent adulthood.

Many types of heart malformation occur. They may be classified into three main groups: (1) those that produce a left-to-right shunt of blood; (2) those that offer resistance to the blood flow; and (3) those that cause a right-to-left shunt (Fig. 12.8).

ANOMALIES THAT CAUSE A LEFT-TO-RIGHT SHUNT

Several malformations occur that produce an abnormal pathway that permits a direct flow of blood from the left side of the heart or aorta to the right heart or pulmonary artery, creating a bypass of the systemic circulation and an overloading of the pulmonary circulation. These anomalies include patent ductus arteriosus and septal defects.

Atrial septal defect

An opening between the two atria (Fig. 12.8c) may be due to failure of the foramen ovale to close after birth or to a gap in the septum, either above or below the foramen ovale. There are three types. The most common is termed an *ostium secundum* defect and is found in the middle of the atrial septum. The other two are *ostium primum* and *sinus venosus* (Farrelly 2000). Blood in the left atrium will flow through the opening into the right atrium, increasing the volume of blood in the pulmonary system. The right atrium, right ventricle and pulmonary artery enlarge. Pulmonary hypertension develops and causes dyspnoea, particularly on exertion. The reduced systemic circulatory volume retards physical and mental development and efficiency. The size of the opening may be so small that it goes undiscovered, and the patient may not experience any respiratory or circulatory difficulty.

Surgical repair of an atrial septal defect is usually accomplished by open heart surgery. Some defects may be closed simply by suturing, whereas others may require a patch of Teflon.

Ventricular septal defect

An opening in the ventricular septum results in a left-to-right shunt and produces problems similar to those cited in atrial septal defect: pulmonary hypertension, enlargement of the right ventricle and pulmonary arteries, and a deficient systemic circulation. If the defect is small and the patient is

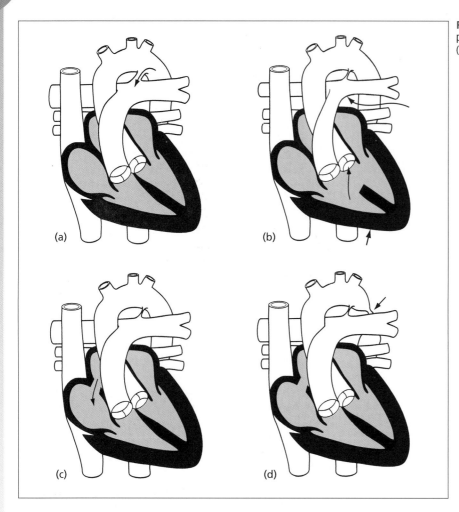

Figure 12.8 Congenital cardiac defects: (a) patent ductus arteriosus; (b) tetralogy of Fallot; (c) atrial septal defect; (d) coarctation of aorta.

asymptomatic, surgery is not indicated. Moderate to severe defects may be closed by patching with either pericardial tissue or Teflon. Occasionally the defect closes spontaneously in the young child.

Patent ductus arteriosus

Normally, after birth, a gradual spontaneous constriction and atrophy of the ductus takes place. If it remains open, the blood in the aorta, under a pressure approximately five to six times that in the pulmonary artery, is shunted into the pulmonary artery (Fig. 12.8a). This increases the volume of blood entering the lungs, resulting in a high pulmonary blood pressure and dilatation of the pulmonary vessels. The patient experiences dyspnoea, particularly on exertion. There is a corresponding increase in the venous flow into the left atrium and left ventricle, causing dilatation and hypertrophy of the left side of the heart. The volume of blood in the systemic circulatory system is less than normal, and the resulting oxygen and nutritional deficiencies delay normal mental and physical development.

The patent ductus arteriosus is corrected by surgical division and suturing of the two ends of the vessels.

ANOMALIES THAT CAUSE RESISTANCE TO BLOOD FLOW WITHIN THE CIRCULATION

The severity of the problem is determined by the degree of constriction or stenosis found in the pulmonary artery or aorta.

Pulmonary stenosis

A stenosis of the pulmonary valve or artery offers resistance to the outflow of blood from the right side of the heart. The right ventricle enlarges and the pressure in both the right ventricle and atrium is above normal. Blood may be backed up in the venous system, while the blood volume entering the pulmonary system is below normal. The latter creates an oxygen deficiency throughout the body which is manifested by fatigue, shortness of breath and, less frequently, cyanosis. Symptoms may not be present for several years.

This malformation may be treated surgically by incision of the constricted ring.

Aortic stenosis

A defect comparable to pulmonary stenosis may occur in the aorta and offer resistance to left ventricular outflow. The left side of the heart enlarges and the pressure in both left chambers is greater than normal; this may be reflected in an increased pulmonary pressure if the restriction is severe. The cardiac output is lower and reduces arterial blood pressure and the systemic circulation as well as the blood supply into the coronary arteries. The defect may be treated by operation, using an extracorporeal pump oxygenator (cardiopulmonary bypass) during the procedure.

Coarctation of the aorta

Coarctation is a stricture in a segment of the aorta (Fig. 12.8d). *Post-ductal coarctation* occurs just beyond the obliterated ductus arteriosus and distal to the origin of the left subclavian artery. The second type, *pre-ductal coarctation*, develops in the segment of aorta before the entrance of the ductus arteriosus. With this latter type the ductus usually remains patent.

Blood volume and pressure are increased behind the stricture, and the work of the left side of the heart is increased greatly. The blood volume and pressure are high in the upper extremities and head, but are abnormally low in the body parts that derive their blood supply from below the stricture. A difference in growth and development may be seen between the areas supplied from behind the stricture and those supplied from the aortic flow distal to the stricture. The patient may experience headaches, epistaxis, dyspnoea on exertion, leg cramps and fatigue.

Surgical treatment of the condition involves resection of the constricted area and an end-to-end anastomosis, or in some instances, the area is excised and a graft of inert material introduced.

ANOMALIES THAT CAUSE A RIGHT-TO-LEFT SHUNT

A shunting of blood from the right side of the heart to the left involves a combination of two or more anomalies. Normally, the pressure is much higher in the left side of the heart than in the right. A stenosis that offers resistance to flow from the right ventricle may increase the pressure in the right side to a level exceeding that in the left side. If a septal defect coexists with this increased pressure, blood is shunted from the right to the left side of the heart.

One of the most frequently seen combinations of anomalies that produces a right-to-left shunt is the *tetralogy of Fallot* (Fig. 12.8b). Tetralogy denotes a set of four conditions: pulmonary stenosis, ventricular septal defect, dextraposition of the aorta which causes it to override the septal defect, and right ventricular hypertrophy. The pulmonary stenosis produces an increased pressure in the right ventricle, causing a right-to-left shunt. The volume of blood flowing through the pulmonary system for oxygenation is reduced. Unoxygenated blood escapes into the aorta and a general systemic hypoxia occurs, manifested by cyanosis and dyspnoea, especially on physical exertion, and by clubbing of the fingers. Compensatory responses to the oxygen deficiency develop in the form of polycythaemia, high haemoglobin level, and increased pulse and respiratory rates.

Correction of these defects is possible by means of open heart surgery and the use of the cardiopulmonary bypass machine. The septal opening is patched, and the pulmonary stenosis is relieved. Occasionally the surgeon may decide not to perform corrective surgery but will proceed with a palliative surgical procedure, referred to as a 'shunt'. This consists of an anastomosis between the subclavian and pulmonary arteries (Blalock-Taussig shunt) to divert a larger volume of blood through the lungs for oxygenation.

MISCELLANEOUS CONGENITAL CARDIAC ANOMALIES

A wide variety of anomalies can occur; many are not yet amenable to treatment, and others may be so severe that the infant cannot survive. *Transposition of the great vessels* is relatively common and may be treated surgically. In this anomaly, the pulmonary artery originates from the left side of the heart and conducts the oxygenated blood back to the lungs, and the aorta rises from the right ventricle, carrying unoxygenated blood into the systemic circulation.

Valvular atresia (absence of an opening) is another form of anomaly that occurs most frequently with the tricuspid valve, but may also develop with the aortic valve. Tricuspid atresia raises the pressure within the right atrium to a level exceeding that in the left atrium, and blood flows through the foramen ovale. This anomaly is frequently accompanied by a ventricular septal defect and is corrected surgically.

DISORDERS OF CARDIAC MUSCLE

In this section, discussion will focus on cardiomyopathies and inflammatory disorders of the heart, including rheumatic fever, infective endocarditis and pericarditis, as well as the nurse's role in caring for people with these disorders.

CARDIOMYOPATHY

Cardiomyopathy is a term used to describe diseases that affect the myocardium and have no obvious cause.

Three types of cardiomyopathy have been identified, based on their pathophysiological abnormalities: (1) dilated cardiomyopathy, where enlargement of the cavity of the ventricle is seen; (2) hypertrophic cardiomyopathy, where there is a thickening of the ventricular wall, associated with a small cavity; and (3) restrictive cardiomyopathy, where the ventricle becomes stiff and resistant to filling.

Dilated cardiomyopathy

This is the most common of the three types. It is characterized by dilated, usually thin-walled, ventricles which produce poor systolic function and low cardiac output. A variety of conditions has been associated with this disorder, including viral infections (poliovirus, coxsackie B virus), immunological disorders, systemic hypertension and exposure to toxic agents (particularly alcohol).

Symptoms of this disorder include congestive heart failure, particularly left-sided failure, fatigue, activity intolerance, chest pain and tachyarrhythmias. As a result of relative stagnation of blood in the ventricles, patients may experience systemic or pulmonary emboli.

The patient will be supported with a range of drugs, such as digoxin and furosemide (frusemide), for as long as possible. End-state dilated cardiomyopathy may be treated surgically with cardiac transplantation. More recently the use of mechanical left ventricular assist devices, such as the Jarvik 2000 Impeller Pump, have been used to reduce the workload of the ventricle and facilitate some improvement in cardiac function.

Hypertrophic cardiomyopathy

This is characterized by a hypertrophied left ventricle, particularly the septum, with no dilatation of the chamber. Thus the left ventricle has thickened walls but there is no enlargement of the chamber size. Symptoms of hypertrophic cardiomyopathy include dyspnoea, palpitations, syncope, angina pectoris and activity intolerance. The first sign of this disorder may be sudden death.

Medical management of hypertrophic cardiomyopathy focuses on improving cardiac output by enhancing diastolic function, reducing contractility and preventing ventricular arrhythmias.

Surgical management may be indicated, with a septal myotomy being performed. This procedure involves the removal of a portion of the hypertrophied septum, thus widening the outflow track from the left ventricle to the aorta. However, the patient is usually very sick at this stage and the surgical risk is high. A specific form of cardiac pacing, which depolarizes the septum at a slightly earlier stage of the cardiac cycle, may be used to encourage a particular movement in the cardiac muscle to reduce the obstruction to the outflow of blood. An implantable cardioverter defibrillator (ICD) (see p. 301) may be used for those who have survived cardiopulmonary arrest.

Several medications are generally contraindicated in the treatment of hypertrophic cardiomyopathy, although they may be used with careful supervision. Digitalis is contraindicated because it increases contractility and increases outflow obstruction. Nitrates and diuretic therapy are avoided because they cause decreased venous return to the heart.

Restrictive cardiomyopathy

This is the least common of the three types of cardiomyopathy. It is characterized by rigid, hypertrophied ventricular walls and impaired diastolic filling, leading to decreased cardiac output. This loss of compliance may be a result of myocardial infiltration and/or fibrosis.

This disorder may manifest as pulmonary congestion, activity intolerance and chest pain. Atrial arrhythmias, particularly atrial fibrillation, are common.

Medical management of this disorder is also palliative in nature and involves managing the symptoms of heart failure by diuretic therapy, and fluid and sodium restriction.

INFLAMMATORY DISORDERS OF THE HEART

The inflammatory process may result in destruction of normal functional tissue followed by its replacement with scar tissue, which is fibrous in nature and less specialized.

Diseases that produce inflammatory heart lesions and impaired function include rheumatic fever, infective endocarditis and pericarditis.

Rheumatic fever

Rheumatic fever causes inflammation of heart structures and can still be cited as a factor linked to valve replacement in later life. However, the incidence of the disease has declined significantly over the past 50 years in Western Europe and the USA. In industrialized countries the annual incidence is around 0.5 cases per 100 000 children of school age. In developing countries rheumatic fever remains an endemic disease, with an annual incidence ranging from 100 to 200 per 100 000 school-aged children (Olivier 2000). Although any or all parts may be affected by rheumatic fever, the valves and the myocardium are the most frequent sites and tend to sustain greater permanent damage. The disease is a complication of a group A streptococcal infection, which is usually respiratory. A period of 1–5 weeks may lapse between the infection and the onset of rheumatic fever, during which time the patient may have recovered completely from the infection.

The inflammatory response, which may occur in the joints as well as the heart, is thought to be due to a sensitivity of the affected individuals to the antibodies that were formed in response to the invading bacteria. This sensitivity is present only in certain individuals – not all those with streptococcal infection develop rheumatic fever. The symptoms of the acute stage vary in intensity and may be so mild that they go unrecognized. In some, joint involvement and fever may be predominant with no evident symptoms referable to the heart, and it is not until much later that it becomes known that cardiac tissue was involved and sustained permanent damage.

Rheumatic fever may cause acute myocarditis with subsequent scarred areas that reduce myocardial efficiency and impair the conduction system. The valves are the most common area of the heart to be affected, and the mitral and aortic valves are the most susceptible. They frequently become scarred, distorted and functionally impaired. Both the valve ring at the opening and the valve cusps may be affected. Following the acute inflammation, scarring occurs, the orifice is diminished and the edges of the cusps may fuse. These changes result in resistance to the forward movement of the blood, thus increasing the work of the heart chamber behind the obstruction. Damage of this type is referred to as a *stenosis*. Normally, the mitral opening in an adult is large enough to admit three fingers; in severe stenosis it can become so restricted that only one finger may be introduced.

In some instances, the scarring of the valvular cusps produces a thickening and loss of tissue which prevents them from coming together to close off the opening completely. This incomplete closure allows a regurgitation or backflow of blood through the valve, and is called *valvular incompetence* or *regurgitation*. An added strain is placed on the heart chamber behind the incompetent valve. Many patients with rheumatic heart disease have combined stenosis and incompetence in the affected valve. If the mitral valve is involved, the left atrium develops dilatation and hypertrophy to compensate for the resistance of stenosis and the backflow of valvular incompetence (i.e. the leaking of the blood back through the valve). In the case of aortic valvular damage, the left ventricle dilates and hypertrophies. Prolonged strain created by a damaged valve, increased demands on the already weakened heart, or further progress of the initial rheumatic disease process may result in decompensation or heart failure.

Treatment of rheumatic fever includes drug therapy (antimicrobial preparations, salicylates, corticosteroids), rest and possible surgery.

In the acute stage of rheumatic heart disease the patient may receive large doses of penicillin to destroy any haemolytic streptococci that may still be active in the body. Reactivation of the disease occurs very readily with any subsequent streptococcal infection. Patients with rheumatic fever, particularly children, continue on prophylactic doses of oral penicillin or on a monthly intramuscular injection of a large dose which is slowly absorbed. Antiinflammatory drugs may be used to decrease inflammation.

Nursing management of patients with rheumatic fever may focus on:

● lack of knowledge about prophylactic antibiotic use
● activity intolerance related to fatigue
● ineffective coping related to managing the disease process.

Infective endocarditis

Infective endocarditis is inflammation of the endocardium, primarily the heart valves. Factors predisposing to infective endocarditis include parenteral drug use (of note is prolonged intravenous drug abuse, with poor skin preparation), valvular abnormalities (either congenital or acquired in origin), rheumatic fever, minor infections, dental procedures and cardiac surgery. The term subacute bacterial endocarditis (SBE) is slightly dated now, as the disease can be caused by organisms that are not bacterial in origin (Mason 2001). Presentation can vary between patients, but tends to include fever, sweats, chills, anorexia, fatigue, weight loss, arthralgia (pain in the joints), myalgia (pain in the muscles) and back pain (Mason 2001). The fever is usually low grade unless an organism such as S*taphylococcus aureus* is involved. The onset of symptoms may be insidious and more commonly affects previously damaged heart valves.

In infective endocarditis, the organisms implant on areas of the endocardium, and clusters of vegetative structures form consisting of inflammatory exudate, fibrin, platelets and bacteria. As the infection subsides, the affected areas become scarred; if a valve was involved, incompetence is likely to develop, and the patient then has the same problems as mentioned in relation to rheumatic fever.

Symptoms may include signs of infection such as fever, malaise, chills, joint tenderness and petechiae. Valvular destruction usually produces a cardiac murmur, heard on auscultation, and signs of embolism, caused when fragments of vegetative lesions break away and lodge downstream in an artery. Diagnosis is confirmed by blood cultures which identify the causative organism. Echocardiography may be useful in visualizing vegetations on heart valves.

Treatment of infective endocarditis includes eradicating the infecting organism by long-term antimicrobial therapy. Surgical repair of damaged valves may be required.

Nursing management of the patient with infective endocarditis may focus on the following problems:

● lack of knowledge about the disease process, need for antibiotic prophylaxis and treatment
● activity intolerance related to fatigue
● anxiety related to the disease process and length of the recovery period.

To assist in reducing issues related to the last point, some hospitals have been using home intravenous antibiotic therapy (HIVAT). This is generally used with patients who understand the illness and the importance of the antibiotic treatment, and is usually reserved for specific bacterial infections such as penicillin-sensitive streptococcal infections. Importantly, these tend to have a reduced risk of disease-related complications (Mason 2001).

Pericarditis

Pericarditis is an inflammation of the pericardium and is most commonly caused by bacterial and viral infections, cardiac injury or an autoimmune reaction. Fluid accumulates in the pericardium as part of the inflammatory response, causing a pericardial effusion. The pressure exerted on the heart by this fluid may prevent its normal filling, creating a condition referred to as *cardiac tamponade*. In some instances, extensive scarring of the visceral pericardium may prevent normal stretching and filling of the heart chambers.

Symptoms of pericarditis may include chest pain, which is exacerbated by movement, pyrexia and dyspnoea. A pericardial friction rub may be heard on auscultation. A paradoxical pulse may be present if cardiac tamponade has occurred. ECG changes characteristic of pericarditis include elevation of ST segments, followed several days later by T-wave inversions. Chest radiography and echocardiography may be used to identify a pericardial effusion.

Treatment goals for the patient with pericarditis include relieving pain, controlling the underlying cause and preventing complications. Explaining the cause of pain is important because there may be fears that it is due to a myocardial infarction.

Medical treatment includes non-steroidal anti-inflammatory agents, such as salicylates and indometacin, and occasionally corticosteroids to combat inflammation. Antibiotics are prescribed for bacterial pericarditis. The patient must be observed carefully for complications such as cardiac tamponade.

Nursing management of the patient with pericarditis may focus on the following problems:

- chest pain related to pericardial inflammation
- anxiety related to illness
- lack of knowledge about the disease process and management.

DISORDERS OF MYOCARDIAL BLOOD SUPPLY

CORONARY ATHEROSCLEROSIS

A narrowing or obstruction in the coronary arteries reduces the blood supply to the myocardium, and causes what is called *ischaemic heart disease*. It results in a deficiency of oxygen and nutrients to the muscle. The reduced oxygen supply is most significant and is quickly reflected in reduced myocardial efficiency. The heart muscle can withstand only a very small oxygen debt, as it is much more susceptible to a reduced oxygen supply than skeletal muscle. In most instances the decreased blood supply to the myocardium is due to degenerative changes in the arteries that produce a narrowing of the lumen of the vessels. Fatty substances, which include cholesterol, are deposited within the intima of the arteries to cause *atherosclerosis*. These fatty plaques interfere with the nutrition of the cells in the intima, leading to necrosis, scarring and calcification, which leave the surface rough and the lumen reduced. These roughened constricted areas allow less blood through and predispose to thrombus formation and occlusion of the vessel (Fig. 12.9).

Atherosclerosis usually develops gradually. While the blood supply through the artery is being reduced, a collateral circulation develops in an effort to increase the supply to the myocardium, but this supplementary circulation is rarely sufficient to provide enough oxygen to the heart muscle during strenuous physical exertion. *Acute coronary syndromes* (ACS) is a term used to define patients with ischaemic cardiac chest pain of recent origin, with one of the following: unstable angina, non-Q-wave myocardial infarction (no Q waves seen on the 12-lead ECG), acute myocardial infarction with ECG changes of ST segment elevation and Q-wave development (NICE 2002).

ANGINA PECTORIS

The term angina pectoris describes a clinical syndrome characterized by chest pain. 'Pectoris' indicates the general location (chest) and '**angina**' refers to the choking, suffocating nature of the pain. This condition arises because of an imbalance between the oxygen being supplied to the myocardium and the energy being expended. The pain, arising from heart muscle fibres that are deficient in oxygen, is usually precipitated by physical exertion or emotional stress, which increases the workload of the heart. There is a need for a greater blood supply than is being delivered by the coronary circulation. It is estimated that just under 1.2 million people in the UK live with or have experienced angina, with 341 000 new cases being diagnosed each year (British Heart Foundation 2004).

Chest discomfort often develops suddenly and is retrosternal, and frequently may radiate to the left or both shoulders and arms, and occasionally up the neck to the jaw. The pain may, however, be atypical and arise only in the arms, jaw or neck, and not in the chest. It is usually relieved within a few minutes by resting and/or by glyceryl trinitrate (GTN) but may last as long as 30 minutes. The patient may become short of breath.

Angina may remain a stable condition brought about by predictable precipitating factors with no change in the severity or frequency of the attacks. *Stable angina* is usually associated with fixed obstructive coronary artery disease (Fig. 12.10a). It is then controlled by limiting those activities or situations known to cause pain and by medication. However, the pain may progress in frequency and intensity if the atherosclerotic process in the coronary arteries proceeds more rapidly than the development of collateral circulation. This condition is known as *unstable angina*. Activities may then need to be curtailed greatly. Pain may be experienced at rest.

Unstable angina is distinguished from stable angina by four characteristics:

1 The syndrome has developed within the previous month.
2 A pattern of stable, exertion-related angina pain becomes less predictable, more prolonged, frequent or severe.
3 The syndrome occurs at rest.
4 The pain is not relieved as promptly with GTN as it is with stable angina.

Unstable angina frequently precedes myocardial infarction and is the reason why it is treated promptly. The pathology of unstable angina involves varying amounts of fixed obstructive coronary disease and dynamic obstruction caused by platelet activation and thrombosis (Fig. 12.10c).

Prinzmetal angina refers to a type of unstable angina in which the pain occurs at rest and often at the same time each day. It is not precipitated by exertion. The underlying cause is spasm of the coronary arteries, and obstructive coronary artery disease may or may not be present.

Diagnosis of angina pectoris is made by means of a thorough history, resting electrocardiography, exercise stress test and/or radionuclide imaging. Cardiac angiography is used to assess the degree of narrowing and occlusion within the coronary arteries.

Figure 12.9 Development and progression of atherosclerosis. From Crumbie and Lawrence (2001).

Development of atherosclerosis

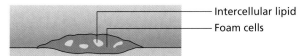

- Intercellular lipid
- Foam cells

Early lesion or fatty streak

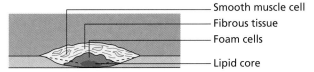

- Smooth muscle cell
- Fibrous tissue
- Foam cells
- Lipid core

Advanced lesion or fibrous plaque

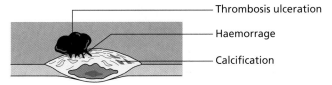

- Thrombosis ulceration
- Haemorrage
- Calcification

Complicated lesion, with ulceration, calcification or haemorrhage

The progression of atherosclerosis

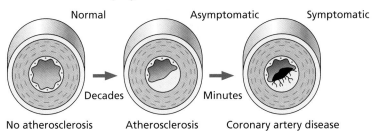

Normal   Asymptomatic   Symptomatic

Decades   Minutes

No atherosclerosis   Atherosclerosis   Coronary artery disease

Injury hypothesis of atherogenesis

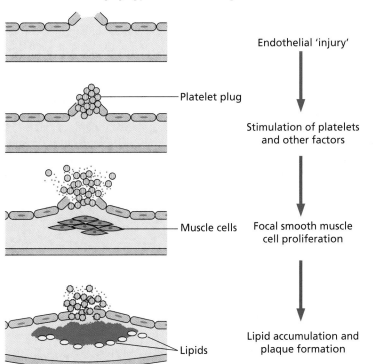

- Platelet plug
- Muscle cells
- Lipids

Endothelial 'injury'

↓

Stimulation of platelets and other factors

↓

Focal smooth muscle cell proliferation

↓

Lipid accumulation and plaque formation

The initiating stimuli could be mechanical, chemical, toxic, viral or immunological (e.g. hypertension, smoking)

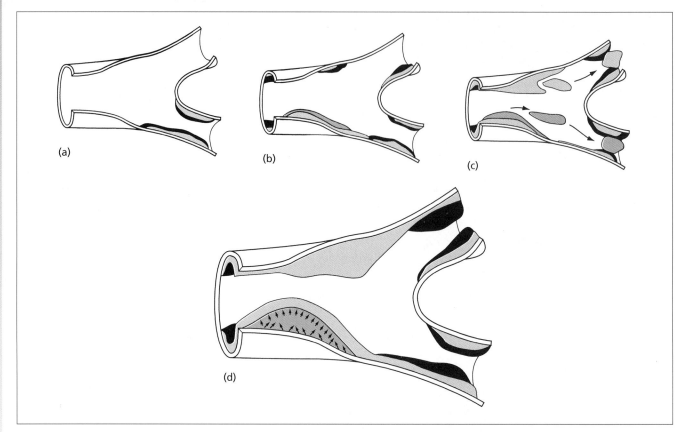

Figure 12.10 Coronary artery obstruction by (a) plaque formation, (b) clot formation around plaque, (c) thrombi on top of fixed plaque formation and (d) vessel haemorrhage.

Medical management

Management of angina pectoris is focused on balancing myocardial oxygen supply and demand to ensure the supply is greater than or equal to the demand. Interventions focus on immediate care, reducing or eliminating risk factors, activity management, medications, percutaneous transluminal coronary angioplasty (PTCA) and the intra-aortic balloon pump.

Immediate care

At the start of an angina attack, patients should be advised to stop whatever they are doing, sit down and take a sublingual glyceryl trinitrate (GTN) tablet or a squirt of their GTN spray. If this does not relieve the pain in 5 minutes, a further dose of GTN should be taken. Once the pain is resolved, any remaining tablet can be spat out or swallowed. Tablets can be bitten to increase the surface area and speed up the action of the drug if the pain is particularly severe.

In hospital, it is useful to monitor how often pain is occurring and to identify any precipitating factors. A 12-lead ECG recorded during pain can highlight the area of heart muscle involved and record any abnormal heart rate or rhythm associated with ischaemia.

Risk factor modification

Altering lifestyle to reduce the progression of coronary artery disease is highly desirable (see p. 252).

Activity management

The patient is advised that strenuous physical activity and emotional outbursts should be avoided. Moderate exercise below the point of producing pain is encouraged. Walking is excellent exercise and should be done on a regular basis. The individual should begin with short walks on level ground, gradually increasing the distance over a period of weeks. Regular, medically supervised, exercise programmes are recommended for some patients. Regular exercise improves muscle tone and general well-being and stimulates the development of collateral circulation in the myocardium. With exercise, normal weight is more easily maintained. The psychological benefit of exercise to the patient cannot be overestimated.

Medications

One of the cornerstones of the management of angina is pharmacological therapy. The medications commonly used are presented in Table 12.4.

Percutaneous transluminal coronary angioplasty

Percutaneous transluminal coronary angioplasty (PTCA) provides an alternative for some patients who might otherwise require coronary artery bypass surgery. It can also be used as an alternative to thrombolysis in acute myocardial infarction (MI). PTCA is a non-surgical method of dilating stenotic or occlusive lesions in the coronary arterial system.

Table 12.4   Drugs used in the management of angina

Medication	Example	General action in angina
Nitrates		
Short-acting	Glyceryl trinitrate	Vasodilate vascular smooth muscle Decrease preload, decrease afterload Vasodilate coronary arteries
Long-acting	Isosorbide dinitrate modified release	As above
Beta-blockers		
	Propranolol Atenolol	Decrease heart rate, automaticity Decrease force of contraction Decrease myocardial oxygen consumption
Calcium channel blockers		
	Nifedipine Diltiazem	Dilate coronary and peripheral vessels
Anteplatelet therapy		
	Aspirin and Clopidogrel	Decrease platelet aggregation
Potassium channel openers		
	Nicorandil	Sustained dilatation of arterial resistance and conduction vessels Little haemodynamic effect on heart rate, blood pressure or cardiac contractility

Patients are generally prepared as for cardiac catheterization. Approximately 2–3% of patients may require subsequent coronary graft surgery due to complications such as *acute coronary occlusion* (closure of the vessel during the procedure), and therefore PTCA is carried out on sites with a cardiothoracic surgical capability or rapid accessibility.

Criteria for selection of patients include:

1 Acute MI, where:
   a) thrombolysis is inappropriate
   b) there is cardiogenic shock, or
   c) large anterior infarct – known as primary angioplasty – is present.
2 Recent onset of angina pectoris.
3 Angina resistant to medical treatment.
4 Angina symptoms of sufficient severity to compromise the quality of life of the patient.
5 Single-vessel disease, which technically makes the procedure easier, although those with multi-vessel disease can be treated, the risk of complications is higher in this group.
6 Anyone being considered for coronary artery bypass grafts.

Diagnostic testing before this procedure is similar to that for coronary bypass surgery and includes coronary angiography. Nursing care includes giving both physical and emotional support to the patient, as the procedure is often frightening. The patient should be given an explanation of ischaemic heart disease and of all the tests carried out before the procedure, the risks involved, the possible need for bypass surgery and the expected results of this treatment.

PTCA is performed using local anaesthesia in the cardiac catheterization laboratory. A guide catheter is introduced into the right or left femoral or brachial artery. This catheter is advanced under fluoroscopy to the affected coronary artery. Once through the stenotic narrowing in the coronary artery, a dilating catheter is slipped through the guide catheter. When positioned within the atherosclerotic lesion, the dilating balloon is inflated. The resultant stretching of the coronary arterial muscle wall widens the lumen of the artery, allowing blood to flow more freely.

Possible complications include bleeding or thrombosis of the affected artery due to injury of the vascular endothelium, acute coronary occlusion, coronary artery spasm and rupture of the artery, causing cardiac tamponade. These complications may result in acute myocardial infarction (1–2% of cases).

Medications such as nifedipine and beta-blockers may be given either before or during the procedure to prevent coronary artery spasm. Intravenous GTN may be administered to promote vasodilatation. Generally patients receive an anticoagulant such as heparin, which may be followed by treatment with warfarin or antiplatelet drugs (NICE 2000).

After the procedure the patient is returned to the acute cardiac unit. Cardiac monitoring is initiated and a 12-lead ECG is recorded to assess for signs of ischaemia or infarction related to the vessel that has been treated. Heparin will have been administered during the procedure. It is important for the nurse not to remove the introducer sheaths until the recorded activated clotting time (ACT) is reduced to the desired protocol range. This is normally between 130 and

175 seconds, and indicates that excessive bleeding will not occur on sheath removal. Pressure is applied to the groin during sheath removal to reduce the risk of bleeding. Biochemical markers such as troponin T are recorded to assess whether any myocardial damage has occurred because of the procedure. Time spent on bedrest following sheath removal varies, but will be at least 2–3 hours. It is likely that a *stent* (a tiny circular wire mesh used to hold open the coronary artery) will be inserted during the PTCA procedure to offer greater patency to the vessel wall. Some units perform a PTCA in the morning and discharge that evening, but many will stay in hospital for 24 hours. Patients will be discharged home on aspirin for long-term use, and with a short course of an oral antiplatelet drug such as *clopidogrel* or *ticlopidine* to prevent vessel occlusion.

Intra-aortic balloon pump   Occasionally counter-pulsation with the intra-aortic balloon pump is utilized for the patient with unstable angina prior to coronary artery surgery. The intra-aortic balloon is inserted into the aorta from one of the femoral arteries; it is inflated during diastole and deflated as the heart ejects its contents during systole. In this way it reduces afterload and myocardial oxygen demand, decreases myocardial ischaemia and relieves angina. The intra-aortic balloon pump is an invasive method of treatment; consequently, the patient and family require a great deal of support from nursing and medical staff. See Hatchett (1998) for further discussion of this intervention.

Nursing management

The nursing management of a patient with angina focuses on the following health problems:

- lack of knowledge
- activity intolerance
- potential for chest discomfort
- anxiety and other psychological problems.

CASE   Ann Carter was a 70-year-old woman diagnosed with stable angina 6 months before. She had been referred to the community nurse to be monitored for her ability to manage her angina. Mrs Carter lived with her daughter and son-in-law in a bungalow. When visited in her home, Mrs Carter expressed anxiety related to her inability to cope with chest pain when it occurred. She was concerned that she would not do the 'right things'.

Mrs Carter's primary health problem was identified as a knowledge deficit related to her disease process and management. The *goals* of care for Mrs Carter were that she could:

1 recognize symptoms of myocardial ischaemia
2 undertake appropriate interventions to reduce and eliminate myocardial ischaemia if it occurred
3 engage in activities to prevent myocardial ischaemia.

Nursing intervention
- Mrs Carter was asked to describe the signs and symptoms of myocardial ischaemia which she had

experienced. Descriptors that described myocardial ischaemia were reinforced and other possible symptoms were discussed
- The patient was questioned as to her understanding of the cause of her angina. The concept of myocardial ischaemia was clarified. The heart's need for enough oxygen to meet its demands was emphasized and the impact of ischaemic heart disease was discussed. This was achieved using straightforward language and was reinforced with diagrams
- Mrs Carter was prompted to discuss what she did when she experienced chest pain. The use of rest and correct administration of glyceryl trinitrate were reinforced. She was encouraged to tell whomever she was with that she was experiencing chest discomfort, so that they could assist her as needed. If the chest pain was not relieved by rest and glyceryl trinitrate in the prescribed time, Mrs Carter was advised to ask to be taken to the nearest hospital where she could be assessed by healthcare professionals
- Preventive strategies to avoid angina were also discussed. Mrs Carter indicated that she did not get overtired. The need to alternate activity and rest was reinforced. Use of glyceryl trinitrate prophylactically when Mrs Carter engaged in activities that caused angina was encouraged
- An educational booklet was given to Mrs Carter to read. This provided her with a reference so she could review any concerns.

Evaluation
At the end of the visit, Mrs Carter could describe signs and symptoms of myocardial ischaemia, actions she would take if she developed chest pain, and how she planned to pace herself. On a follow-up visit, 2 weeks later, Mrs Carter described how she had successfully managed an episode of chest discomfort. She had also paced her activities, incorporating more quiet periods into her life. Mrs Carter expressed feelings of increased confidence in her ability to manage further episodes. She was also referred for assessment of further treatment that would reduce the symptoms of angina, such as PTCA or coronary artery bypass grafting.

ACUTE MYOCARDIAL INFARCTION

Acute **myocardial infarction** (MI) or 'heart attack' is the most serious and acute form of ischaemic heart disease. A coronary artery becomes blocked and the myocardial area which it supplies suffers oxygen deficiency and cell necrosis. The blockage may be due to the rupture of an atheromatous plaque, with associated thrombus formation as blood clots around the area. This can occur suddenly, and compensation through collateral channels is inadequate to maintain the myocardial cells. The resulting area of necrotic tissue is referred to as an *infarction*.

The extent of the infarction varies from patches of 1–2 cm in diameter to widespread areas of necrosis. One or more layers of the heart may be involved. The area of infarction becomes soft and then eventually fills in with firm, fibrous, scar tissue. Survival and the extent of subsequent restrictions depend upon the amount of myocardial damage and the area of the heart affected. Death may occur immediately or within a few hours. Obviously, the remaining viable heart tissue must compensate for the loss of functional tissue.

Occlusion may be preceded by some manifestations of coronary insufficiency such as angina, or it may occur suddenly without any previous warning. Although the condition can clearly be fatal, about half of all people who suffer a heart attack will survive beyond 28 days and the survival rate is improving by approximately 1.5% each year (British Heart Foundation 2004). Survival will depend critically on prompt diagnosis and instigation of appropriate treatments such as early thrombolysis (see below).

Types of myocardial infarction

It is difficult to delineate the precise area of the myocardium that is affected, but general areas can be identified from the 12-lead ECG. This is important to know because damage to each area can produce different complications. Although other areas of the heart may be involved, most infarctions occur in the left ventricle.

Anterior wall infarction

The anterior wall of the left ventricle is infarcted due to an occlusion of the left anterior descending artery. The interventricular septum may also be involved, in which case it is called an *anteroseptal* infarct.

Lateral wall infarction

An infarction in the lateral wall of the left ventricle is associated with an occlusion of the lateral branch of the left circumflex artery. Occasionally both the anterior descending and the left circumflex branches are obstructed, and the infarction is designated *anterolateral*.

Inferior wall infarction

This term implies an infarction of the part of the left ventricle that rests on the diaphragm. It is usually due to occlusion of the right coronary artery.

Posterior wall infarction

This type is usually due to occlusion of the posterior branch of either the right coronary or left circumflex artery. It is sometimes called a true posterior infarction to distinguish it from an inferior infarction.

Right ventricular infarction

The right ventricle may infarct in conjunction with an inferior or posterior left ventricular infarction. It is usually caused by occlusion of the artery that perfuses the posterior ventricular wall, either the right coronary artery or, less commonly, the left circumflex artery.

Symptoms

Pain

The most common presenting complaint of patients with myocardial infarction is severe chest pain. The pain may last for several hours or until relieved by analgesics. It should not persist for days; prolonged pain may be an indication of pericarditis or an extending infarction. Up to 25% of patients do not experience any pain (*silent MI*). Time of onset of pain has been shown to peak at around midnight and 6 a.m. – times when individuals are likely to be awoken from sleep with pain rather than engaging in vigorous physical activity (Thompson et al 1991).

Dyspnoea

Dyspnoea may be due to pulmonary congestion or pain. It may also occur as activity is increased. Relief of pain and congestion may relieve the dyspnoea. It is important to note whether shortness of breath is present at all times or, if intermittent, how it is precipitated and what measures relieve it.

Skin

The skin may be cool and moist, and have a greyish colour in response to the decreased cardiac output.

Nausea and vomiting

Nausea and vomiting may be experienced at the time of the attack, lasting from several hours to 2–3 days. Occasionally, nausea and vomiting occur in response to the opiates being administered.

Weakness and tiredness

Extreme weakness may be experienced and may persist for many days. Many patients complain of tiredness for weeks after an infarction; the exact cause of this is not clearly defined. Some suggest it results from decreased oxygen perfusion of the tissues due to a lowered cardiac output. It has also been attributed to weakened skeletal muscles as a result of even a brief period of immobilization. The patient may have been in a state of physical exhaustion before the attack or may be emotionally exhausted from the experience.

Heart rate

The pulse becomes rapid and weak, and may be imperceptible at the time of the attack. Initially, a few patients may exhibit bradycardia, followed by tachycardia.

Blood pressure

Owing to the decreased pumping efficiency of the heart, the blood pressure can fall, but initially following an MI it may be raised due to an augmented sympathetic response.

Temperature

Myocardial necrosis causes an increase in body temperature ranging from 37.7 to 39°C. The temperature usually rises within 24–48 hours and returns to normal by the sixth or seventh day. If the increased temperature persists for longer, it may be due to complications.

Psychological reactions

An MI carries the threat of death or long-term disability of the patient. The sudden change in well-being may lead to feelings of vulnerability and helplessness. The patient is required to make very rapid adjustments to both the illness and change in environment.

Anxiety is the most common psychological response. It is manifested by various overt and covert behaviours, such as tenseness, restlessness, short attention span, inability to concentrate, crying, constant talking and expression of feelings of anxiety. The patient may appear generally relaxed but may exhibit more subtle manifestations of anxiety such as darting eye movements. There are various instruments available for measuring anxiety. Three of them, the Stait-Trait Anxiety Inventory (STAI), the Hospital Anxiety and Depression scale (HAD scale) and a linear analogue anxiety scale, have been shown to give effective measurements for coronary patients (Elliot 1993). Patients may also show denial, refusing to acknowledge the seriousness or even the presence of symptoms, and may be angry and/or depressed. These emotional responses may appear in varying degrees and at any time during hospitalization or may not become evident until after discharge from the hospital. The individual's interpretation of the experience and personal coping pattern influence responses.

Diagnosis

Medical diagnosis of an acute MI is made using the clinical history, changes in the 12-lead ECG, and via biochemical markers and serum enzymes.

Changes in the electrocardiogram

Theoretically, three types of changes are present in the myocardium when an infarction develops. These define three concentric areas, referred to clinically as the *area of infarction*, the *area of injury* and the *zone of ischaemia*, resulting in a distinctive ECG pattern. In the central infarcted area, irreversible structural changes occur with resulting necrosis of tissue. As electrical impulses cannot be conducted through this tissue, the normal ECG pattern is altered resulting in a pronounced pathological Q wave (see Fig. 12.11).

Surrounding the zone of infarction is an area of injury that suffers a decreased blood supply, but the damage is not permanent. Although specific abnormal ECG changes are produced, these may revert to normal if the blood supply is restored. Electrodes placed over the injured area will record a ST segment elevation due to leakage of positively charged ions from damaged cells.

The zone of ischaemia surrounds the area of injury and may also return to normal once the blood supply is restored. Inverted T waves indicate ischaemia.

ST elevations appear within several hours following an infarction and disappear in a few days. In the early stages T waves become taller and appear as an extension of the elevated ST segment. They later become inverted. Q waves appear within 1–2 days and persist (Fig. 12.11). The area of infarction will be reflected in leads that view that portion of the heart. Thus, *inferior* infarctions can be identified in leads II, III and AVF, *anterior* infarctions can be identified in the anterior leads V_1 to V_4, and *lateral wall* infarction in leads I, AVL, V_5 and V_6. Under normal conditions no leads face the posterior wall of the heart, so diagnosis is based upon reciprocal changes in leads facing the opposite wall; that is, increased R waves in leads V_1 and V_2.

Changes in biochemical markers and serum enzyme levels

Certain intracellular biochemical markers and enzymes known to be persistent in myocardial cells are released into the blood when the cells are damaged or destroyed. Serial determinations of the serum concentrations of these enzymes can provide information concerning the presence and degree of cardiac damage. The normal values of serum enzymes vary depending on laboratory techniques and sampling methods.

In the coronary care unit, the most commonly ordered biochemical markers and enzyme level estimations are those for troponin T or I, creatine phosphokinase (CPK), aspartate aminotransferase (AST) and lactic dehydrogenase (LDH) (see Table 12.5). Diagnosis of a myocardial infarction can be confirmed by elevations of these biochemical and enzyme levels.

Creatine phosphokinase (CPK)   CPK is present in cardiac and skeletal muscle and in brain tissue. CPK levels begin to rise in the serum 4–8 hours following MI, peak at 12–24 hours, and return to normal in 3–4 days.

A rise in CPK levels may also be caused by pericarditis, severe congestive heart failure, electrical cardioversion and

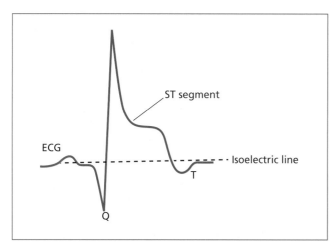

Figure 12.11   Electrocardiographic changes indicating acute myocardial infarction: Q wave, ST elevation and T-wave inversion.

Table 12.5   Increases in serum enzyme levels (units/litre) following myocardial infarction

Enzyme	Day of admission	Day 2	Day 3	Day 7
CPK	6	162	5	5
AST	14	177	201	23
LDH	151	513	789	419

A troponin T value should be less than 0.1 mg/L. There are several Troponin I assays available and values will vary depending on the system used to record the level. It is advisable to consult the manufacturer's literature. Myoglobin concentration should be less than 100 mg/L.

intramuscular injections. Thus, to determine the source of raised CPK levels, electrophoresis or radio-immunoassay can be used to separate CPK into three fractions or isoenzymes. The *MB isoenzyme* has been found predominantly in the myocardium. Studies have shown that CK-MB (or MB-CPK) is very sensitive and specific for the diagnosis of acute MI, provided that it is determined between 6 and 36 hours after the suspected infarction.

Thus, in assessing the presence of an acute MI by means of CPK levels, it is important to ensure that blood samples are drawn on admission and every 6–8 hours for 24 hours after the onset of chest pain.

Aspartate aminotransferase The concentration of AST rises within 8–12 hours after an MI, reaching a peak at 18–36 hours and usually returning to normal within 3–4 days. Raised aspartate aminotransferase (AST) levels are also seen in patients with hepatic and skeletal muscle disease, pulmonary embolism and pericarditis. This is a problem for the diagnosis of MI because there are no cardiac-specific isoenzymes of AST. Thus, the routine use of AST in diagnosis of acute MI is debatable.

Lactic dehydrogenase Lactic dehydrogenase (LDH) is present in most body organs including the heart, kidneys, lungs, liver and skeletal muscle. After an acute MI, the LDH level becomes raised in 8–24 hours, peaks at 3–6 days and returns to normal in 8–14 days.

A rise in total LDH concentration may also occur in patients with pulmonary embolism, neoplastic disorders, hepatic disease and shock. Thus, it is important to assess LDH isoenzyme levels to assess whether cardiac damage is causing increased enzyme levels. LDH has five isoenzymes and cardiac muscle contains primarily LDH_1. A rise in the proportion of LDH_1 exceeding 40% of the total LDH value and an increase in the ratio of $LDH_1 : LDH_2$ is considered a sensitive indicator of MI. Thus, when a patient has a suspected MI that occurred more than 2 days previously, LDH isoenzyme analysis can be more revealing than CPK analysis.

The troponins and myoglobin

The troponins are known to be highly sensitive markers of myocardial damage, and are beginning to supersede cardiac enzyme testing. The blood levels do take several hours to rise, and it is usual to record a troponin level on admission and again in approximately 8 hours. The other advantage is that, together with another biochemical marker called myoglobin, their presence can be measured as a bedside test. Treatment for myocardial damage can therefore be given quickly with the assurance of a positive test result. Myoglobin rises at an earlier stage compared with other markers, owing to its small molecular size, allowing it to escape more easily from damaged myocardium into the bloodstream.

Other diagnostic procedures

Other procedures that may be used to assess the extent of MI include echocardiography, radionuclide imaging and thallium stress electrocardiography.

Medical management

Patients with acute MI are best managed on a coronary care unit, although some are cared for on medical wards and some at home. Coronary care units have essentially been designed to serve three purposes:

1 The provision of a separate area within the hospital for the care and monitoring of patients with acute MI or other cardiac disorders.
2 The provision of high-quality specialized care.
3 The provision of personnel and equipment immediately available for resuscitation.

Ideally, this service should be available for all, with no exclusion criteria such as advanced age.

The most important area of management must be the attempt to re-establish blood flow to the myocardium through the blocked coronary artery. Management will also focus on areas of control of symptoms, reducing the workload of the heart, and the recognition and treatment of complications. It is also important to have a strategy to identify patients at high risk, to reduce subsequent development of heart failure, and to have effective measures for secondary prevention to reduce the incidence of reinfarction as well as to promote rehabilitation.

Control of symptoms

Pain relief See page 272.

Reducing myocardial workload Reducing the myocardial oxygen demand may limit the size of the infarcted area. Beta-blocking agents are used to reduce heart rate, myocardial contractility, blood pressure and cardiac output. They are used with extreme caution or may be contraindicated in patients with hypotension, chronic airway disease or peripheral vascular disease.

Prevention of arrhythmias During the convalescent phase of MI, ventricular extrasystoles and supraventricular and ventricular arrhythmias are associated with a poor prognosis. However, treatment with prophylactic antiarrhythmia drugs is no longer popular because of adverse side-effects.

Acute myocardial reperfusion

Thrombolytic therapy Evidence that coronary thrombosis is a very early event in acute MI, recognition of the prognostic importance of infarction size, and evidence that infarction size might be reduced by early intervention have resulted in thrombolytic therapy becoming the most significant recent development in the management of the patient with acute MI. Several intravenous agents that lyse (break down) clots are currently being used in patients who have sustained an acute MI; these agents include streptokinase and tissue plasminogen activator (tPA). Research to evaluate the impact of these agents on morbidity and mortality, as well as to establish the most effective management protocols, is ongoing. Nonetheless, the benefit of this form of treatment is clear, together with the need to initiate therapy as soon as the diagnosis has been confirmed. In addition, it has been known for some time that all patients who are experiencing an MI should be given 300 mg aspirin to chew as soon as possible (ISIS-2 1988). This is not for its analgesic effect, but its antiplatelet properties. Aspirin appears to augment the effects of thrombolysis and increase the chance of survival. Patients who are allergic to aspirin or who have a history of problematic bleeding, such as those with a peptic ulcer, are generally not offered aspirin.

Thrombolytic therapy is used to break down clots in the affected artery, restore the blood flow, save the myocardium from damage, preserve the function of the left ventricle and reduce mortality (Tough 2005). Therapy needs to be initiated as soon as possible after the onset of MI to give maximum benefit. Thus, enabling patients who are experiencing chest pain to attend units that can promptly administer these agents has become increasingly important. Contraindications are related to issues of bleeding problems. These will vary between units but generally include active bleeding, CVA within the previous 3 months (in some units this may extend to periods of up to 1 year), severe systemic arterial hypertension, bleeding disorders, and major surgery or traumatic injury in the last 6 months.

Nurses need to be aware of the possible complications of bleeding, arrhythmias, allergic reaction, drop in blood pressure, as well as anxiety and lack of knowledge, which might accompany the administration of thrombolytics. There is evidence that individuals who have received streptokinase develop antibodies that reduce the effectiveness of subsequent administration of the drug. Those having this form of thrombolytic therapy need to be issued with a card detailing the date and dose of drug given so that an alternative can be offered if necessary. To speed the administration of thrombolytic agents, specially trained nurses are now instigating treatment to agreed protocols before the medical team has arrived (Quinn et al 2001).

CASE Mr Abdulla is a 65-year-old man with a known history of stable angina. Following his evening meal, he experienced chest pain which, although not intense, increased with discomfort throughout the evening. It was central, retrosternal, and radiated down his left arm. He took little notice, presuming it was indigestion from his rich evening meal. He awoke at 5 a.m., sweating, feeling nauseous and with an increased intensity of pain. His wife called the GP, but he was at another call and, after eventually being contacted, arrived some 20 minutes later. The GP noted Mr Abdulla's ashen complexion and sweaty skin. He took the blood pressure, recorded as 110/70 mmHg, and assessed the presenting chest pain. He immediately called an ambulance and gave Mr Abdulla 2.5 mg diamorphine intravenously. In addition 300 mg aspirin was given. Oxygen was administered, together with a tablet of sublingual glyceryl trinitrate (GTN). Mr Abdulla was admitted via ambulance to hospital where a nurse-led thrombolysis programme was in operation. This allowed a rapid clinical assessment and the speedy administration of a thrombolytic agent.

Patients like Mr Abdulla can sometimes mistake pain that occurs after an evening meal as indigestion and therefore delay seeking help. The GP in the critical incident described quickly identified the symptoms as cardiac in nature. It was important that the diamorphone was administered intravenously as intramuscular injections prior to possible management with thrombolytic agents can result in haematoma formation at the injection site. It is worthwhile reflecting on the possible consequences of this incident for Mr Abdulla and his wife. It is also worthwhile considering how nurses could contribute to the rapid management of Mr Abdulla's condition and what support could be offered to the patient and his wife at this worrying time.

Anticoagulants Heparin therapy is used routinely by some cardiologists when there is evidence on ECG of left ventricular thrombus, active deep vein thrombosis or anterior wall MI. Heparin may also be used prophylactically for a patient with an inferior wall MI experiencing atrial arrhythmias, and also those having congestive heart failure. Heparin may also be administered after thrombolytic therapy. Low-dose heparin may be used for patients with a high risk of venous thromboembolism.

Antiplatelet drugs Multiple trials with aspirin have shown that daily low-dose aspirin (75–150 mg) significantly reduces the risk of reinfarction and death following MI. In addition NICE (2004) recommend that clopidogrel should be used in addition to aspirin in patients with non-ST-segment-elevation acute coronary syndrome. Treatment with the combination of aspirin and clopidogrel should be continued for 12 months after the patient's most recent attack and aspirin should be continued thereafter.

Percutaneous transluminal coronary angioplasty and coronary artery bypass surgery These procedures may be indicated for the acutely unstable individual who requires aggressive therapy to prevent death after coronary angiography is conducted. Discussion can be found on page 282.

Stents Some centres are increasingly using stents inserted during a procedure similar to angioplasty to increase and maintain myocardial perfusion.

Medications There is much evidence that certain drugs and therapies when administered to the patient with angina, unstable angina and MI do improve survival and clinical outcome. The National Service Framework for Coronary Heart Disease (DoH 2000b) is a government-initiated document that has highlighted specific standards to achieve in the treatment of these and other cardiac conditions. These standards include, unless contraindicated, the use of thrombolytic agents, aspirin, beta-blockers, angiotensin-converting enzyme (ACE) inhibitors and lipid-lowering drugs such as the statins in the treatment of MI. Much work is in place and ongoing in the hospital and community to improve service delivery to meet such standards, and includes collaborative practice between all members of the healthcare team.

Recognition of complications

Doctors and nurses share responsibility for assessing and recognizing complications of an acute MI. It is important for the nurse to have a sound understanding of the possible complications so that rapid identification and initiation of treatment, as required, is conducted. Complications following MI include arrhythmias, congestive heart failure, pericarditis, mitral regurgitation, myocardial rupture, aneurysm, and systemic or pulmonary emboli.

Arrhythmias   Arrhythmias usually occur early following a myocardial infarction. The most serious arrhythmia that may be seen is *ventricular fibrillation*; this is treated by cardiac defibrillation. *Bradyarrhythmias* are unusually slow heart rates (e.g. Wenckebach heart block), and are most often associated with inferior wall infarctions. As the SA node and the AV junctional tissue are most often supplied by the right coronary artery, occlusion of this vessel will lead to their decreased functioning. Anterior MIs are more likely to lead to failure and arrhythmias, such as *sinus tachycardia* and rapid *atrial arrhythmias*, and to interventricular conduction disturbances, such as *Mobitz type II block*. *Complete AV block* (third-degree or complete heart block) may follow either inferior or anterior wall infarction.

Heart failure   Mild congestive heart failure occurs in many patients due to the decreased efficiency with which the heart contracts. Gross left ventricular failure is more common following an anterior infarction. Heart failure is suspected if there are crackles on chest auscultation, complaints of shortness of breath, orthopnea, peripheral oedema and reduction in activity tolerance. See below for a further discussion relating to heart failure (p. 304).

Pericarditis   Pericarditis following an MI is thought to be due to an autoimmune reaction in which antigens originate from the injured myocardial tissue and cause inflammation of the pericardium. It is known as Dressler's syndrome, and may occur as early as 24 hours after the infarction. The pain that accompanies pericarditis is similar to that of MI, but is sometimes more excruciating. It is alarming to the patient, who may think that he or she is having another MI. A friction rub may be heard on auscultation, but is not always present in the early stages. The patient's temperature may remain raised for more than 1 week. Treatment is usually with non-steroidal antiinflammatory drugs such as indometacin or soluble aspirin. A corticosteroid preparation may be used.

Mitral regurgitation   This complication may occur when a papillary muscle dysfunctions or ruptures, causing the valve to become incompetent. This is a grave complication which may be corrected by surgery. Less severe mitral insufficiency may be due to infarction of the papillary muscle.

Myocardial rupture   Myocardial rupture, when present, usually occurs within 7 days. It is more often seen in patients with transmural infarctions. Rupture of the inter-ventricular septum usually occurs within the first 2 weeks and is a very grave prognostic sign. Instead of flowing normally from the left ventricle into the aorta, blood is re-routed to the right ventricle, increasing the demands on it and flooding the lungs.

Aneurysm   An aneurysm is a ballooning out of the infarcted myocardial tissue, causing the heart to contract in a disruptive fashion. If large, it seriously impedes the maintenance of normal cardiac output. The extent of the aneurysm may be determined by a myocardial scan, and in some instances may be corrected by surgery.

Emboli   Emboli occur because clots formed in the healing area of the myocardium break loose and escape into the circulation. Pulmonary emboli may arise in the leg veins due to circulatory stasis, and may be prevented by exercising the limbs. The treatment for emboli includes anticoagulant drugs.

Risk stratification

Assessment of left ventricular dysfunction, residual ischaemia and the tendency to arrhythmias is important for identifying patients at high risk of complications so that treatment can be targeted appropriately. Clinical features, ECG, chest radiography, echocardiography, exercise testing and radionuclide studies are important assessment tools.

Rehabilitation

Cardiac rehabilitation is the process by which patients with ischaemic heart disease (IHD) are enabled to achieve their optimal physical, emotional, social, vocational and economic state (World Health Organization 1993). Cardiac rehabilitation services for the patient and partner need to include the following (Stokes and Thompson 2001):

- a tailored exercise programme
- risk factor modification, including specific advice on smoking cessation, activity, work, changes in lifestyle, relaxation and stress management
- attention to the psychological sequelae of IHD for both the patient and family, especially the partner.

Numerous studies have shown that comprehensive rehabilitation programmes can produce worthwhile improvements in quality of life and it is recommended that they be routinely offered to all patients with IHD (DoH 2000b, Thompson et al 1996). Ideally, programmes should be individually targeted and cater for groups such as the elderly, women and those from minority ethnic groups. Routine care needs to be accompanied by a means of identifying those who need additional support.

Rehabilitation can be seen as a process that begins in hospital from the time of admission and extends out into the community.

Community support needs to follow on as soon as possible from that provided in hospital. Ideally, the patient and partner should have some support during the first 2 weeks at home – even if this is only a telephone link with the hospital or practice nurse. Some programmes incorporate home visits in the first few days at home. Later support can involve individual and group sessions linked with exercise, either in hospital or a community-based setting. Home-based rehabilitation may be more appropriate for some individuals. The 'Heart Manual', a home-based programme, has been shown to increase confidence in recovery and produce a positive perception of progress (Linden 1995).

After 3 or 4 months, some programmes offer a long-term community-based support group which encourages self-help and peer support for long-term health maintenance.

Nursing management

The nursing management in the acute phase of a patient who has sustained an MI is illustrated using a clinical example (Case 12.3).

CASE   Robert MacGregor was a 57-year-old man, who was married with two grown-up children. He was admitted to hospital via ambulance with the diagnosis of acute anterior wall myocardial infarction. On the day of admission, he awoke from sleep at 12.15 a.m. with 'crushing' chest discomfort, which radiated down his left arm. He felt nauseated and sweaty, and was short of breath. He felt something was seriously wrong and woke his wife. She telephoned the ambulance service and Mr MacGregor arrived at the hospital approximately 1 hour after his chest pain started.

Mr MacGregor's past medical history did not include any cardiovascular disorders or bleeding problems. He had sustained several injuries to his left knee which had required surgical correction. Mr MacGregor had several risk factors for ischaemic heart disease, including his age, sex and habit of smoking a pack of cigarettes a day for 40 years. He did not know his cholesterol levels and did not have hypertension. Mr MacGregor considered his position as a taxi driver to be stressful. His father had died from a myocardial infarction in his seventies.

Care in the coronary care unit

Mr MacGregor's initial assessment indicated that he was medically stable. His vital signs were stable and he was in normal sinus rhythm. Interventions included:

- Oxygen via nasal cannulae at 4 L per minute was commenced
- An intravenous line was set up
- A 12-lead electrocardiogram showing changes consistent with an anterior wall myocardial infarction was recorded
- A troponin T level was obtained and was repeated again in 8 hours to assess for myocardial damage
- Diamorphine hydrochloride 5 mg i.v. was given with good relief of chest pain
- Aspirin 300 mg was administered, and thrombolytic therapy was commenced to reduce the size of the myocardial infarct, as there were no contraindications. Streptokinase was administered via intravenous infusion
- The doctor and nurse met with Mrs MacGregor to discuss her husband's condition and to provide reassurance.

Mr MacGregor was somewhat restless and fully conscious. He indicated that he had no discomfort in his chest and that he was worried about his wife. Mr MacGregor knew that he had had a myocardial infarction. His respiratory rate was 14 breaths per minute and he remained on oxygen 4 L per minute via nasal cannulae. His blood pressure was equal in both arms and was 120/60 mmHg. The cardiac monitor showed that Mr MacGregor remained in normal sinus rhythm, 72 beats per minute with ventricular ectopic beats (VEBs) approximately 5–10 per minute.

After 1 hour the streptokinase infusion was complete and a heparin infusion was started.

Four priority health problems were identified in the provision of nursing care for Mr MacGregor:

1. potential for chest pain
2. potential decrease in cardiac output
3. anxiety
4. potential for haemorrhage.

Potential for chest pain

Mr MacGregor was encouraged to report any episodes of chest pain. A visual analogue scale was used to quantify any pain experienced, a score of 10 meaning the worst possible pain and a score of 0 no pain. Intravenous diamorphine was given for pain during the acute period, a total of 12.5 mg being required over the first 12 hours. Glyceryl trinitrate was placed at the bedside on the second day so that Mr MacGregor could have control over his pain management and rapid pain relief. He kept nursing staff informed when he used this so that they could assess the effectiveness of pain management and the degree of ischaemic pain.

Evaluation

Mr MacGregor experienced only one episode of pain after the first day. He felt confident at using GTN tablets and in managing any episodes of pain experienced after discharge.

Potential decrease in cardiac output

This was related to damaged myocardium, as evidenced by 12-lead ECG changes, presence of ventricular arrhythmias, clinical history and biochemical markers/cardiac enzymes.

The *goals* in caring for Mr MacGregor were that:

1. Mr MacGregor would be pain free.
2. He would reduce the workload on his heart.
3. No further ventricular arrhythmias causing haemodynamic instability would be experienced.
4. Mr MacGregor would report any episodes of myocardial ischaemia (experienced through chest pain, and assessed by nursing staff via the 12-lead ECG).

Nursing intervention

- Mr MacGregor's vital signs were monitored every 4 hours for any changes in blood pressure. His heart rate and rhythm were monitored continuously for any changes. Close attention was paid to ventricular arrhythmias as the patient had had VEBs. Initial damaged ventricular muscle predisposed him to fatal ventricular arrhythmias

- Mr MacGregor was initially advised to remain on bed/chair rest to limit cardiac workload. His activity level was gradually increased over several days to allow the heart time to recover and to facilitate assessment of his activity tolerance
- The importance of avoiding straining and of performing isometric exercises was stressed. A laxative was given, as necessary, to avoid constipation
- A quiet environment was provided to facilitate rest. Mr MacGregor was encouraged to rest for an hour after each meal to reduce myocardial workload
- Supplemental oxygen via nasal cannulae was administered continuously for the first 24 hours and if he had chest pain. This ensured additional oxygen was available to improve myocardial oxygen supply if required.

Evaluation

Mr MacGregor experienced no further arrhythmias. He reduced his cardiac workload by resting quietly in bed and performing gentle exercises. He reported that he experienced no episodes of chest discomfort.

Anxiety

Anxiety was related to diagnosis and admission to hospital, as evidenced by inability to concentrate, apprehension and difficulty in sleeping.

The *goals* in treating this problem were that:
1 Early signs of anxiety would be detected.
2 Mr MacGregor would participate in activities that would reduce or eliminate his anxiety.

Nursing intervention

- Reassurance and comfort were provided for Mr MacGregor. The nurse stayed with him frequently, speaking calmly and providing competent, efficient care
- A quiet environment was provided and sensory stimulation was reduced. The door was partly closed and the lights were dimmed during rest periods to facilitate sleep
- Mr MacGregor was informed of the procedures and treatments he could expect. He was kept up to date, with the use of language he could understand. The patient was encouraged to ask questions about his environment and condition. Honest, concise information was provided to clarify his understanding of heart disease. As Mr MacGregor liked to read, he was given a pamphlet to reinforce the information provided. He was informed that many patients find it difficult to concentrate while in hospital, so he should not be alarmed by his poor concentration span
- Visitors were limited to the immediate family. Mrs MacGregor was encouraged to visit her husband and was kept informed of his condition. She was encouraged to attend the cardiac family support group to meet other partners and receive support from them
- Mr MacGregor took a mild sedative in the evening to encourage sleep
- Mr MacGregor was informed about the cardiac rehabilitation programme, and he and his wife were invited to attend.

Evaluation

Mr MacGregor indicated that he felt less anxious and more in control of his environment when he was well informed. He eagerly asked questions about his condition and prognosis. The booklet was helpful as he recorded questions he wanted to ask the doctor in it, so that he would not forget them. Mrs MacGregor enjoyed the family support group and found it helpful. Both Mr and Mrs MacGregor were keen to join the rehabilitation group which started 3 weeks after discharge. The rehabilitation coordinator would visit them at home during the first week to offer support, answer questions and assess their progress.

Potential for haemorrhage

There was a potential for haemorrhage related to the thrombolytic agent and concurrent administration of anticoagulant.

The *goals* were that there would be:
1 Absence of all subjective and objective signs of gastrointestinal, vascular and soft tissue haemorrhage
2 Early detection of bleeding, within 15 minutes of commencement.

Nursing intervention

- Vascular punctures were kept to a minimum
- All intravenous and puncture sites were observed frequently for bleeding. Any bruising was outlined and assessed more frequently for increasing size
- All bodily excretions were inspected for signs of blood
- Mr MacGregor was informed of the risk of bleeding and was encouraged to report immediately any signs of bleeding to the nurse
- Mr MacGregor used his own electric razor and soft toothbrush.

Evaluation

Mr MacGregor showed no signs of haemorrhage during his stay in the coronary care unit.

When Mr MacGregor improved and was transferred from the coronary care unit to the general medical ward, several other health problems became more important. These included activity intolerance, potential for chest pain and alteration in lifestyle and self-care. The cardiologist requested further investigations of his cardiac functioning and the condition of his coronary circulation, to determine further care. Medical treatments such as beta-blocking therapy were commenced and the cardiac rehabilitation team became involved prior to an uneventful discharge.

DISORDERS OF ELECTROCONDUCTION

Normally, the rate and rhythm of heart contractions are established by impulses generated in the sinoatrial (SA) node at a rate between 60 and 100 beats per minute (Fig. 12.12). A disorder of rate or rhythm is referred to as a *cardiac arrhythmia*, and is due to some disturbance in the formation or conduction of impulses. The **arrhythmia** may be of short duration or persistent, and may be functional in origin, result from organic heart disease or be associated with an electrolyte imbalance, such as hypokalaemia.

An arrhythmia may have significant haemodynamic consequences. For example, an excessively slow or fast heart rate may decrease the cardiac output and blood pressure, thus compromising the perfusion of vital organs such as the brain, kidneys, liver and the heart itself. Arrhythmias may also predispose the patient to thrombus formation. It is important for nurses to have a sound knowledge of arrhythmias and their management in order to plan and provide care for patients with these health problems. Arrhythmias can also act as a pre-warning to further, more life-threatening, rhythm disturbances, and a knowledge of certain arrhythmias is imperative for the employment of skills where nurses are trained to provide prompt definitive treatment, such as in the use of defibrillation in cardiopulmonary arrest.

Common irregularities include tachycardia (fast heart rate), bradycardia (slow heart rate), ectopic beats (extrasystoles), flutter, fibrillation and heart block. The arrhythmia is further defined by the site of its origin: *sinus* arrhythmia originates in the SA node, *atrial* originates in an atrium, *junctional* originates in the AV junctional area, and *ventricular* originates in a ventricle. Importantly, tachycardia needs to be treated promptly to slow and steady the heart, producing a good cardiac output. Bradycardias are treated cautiously to avoid inadvertently stopping the heart altogether. Cardiac pacing may be used to speed up the rate in a longer-term bradycardic problem.

TACHYCARDIAS

Sinus tachycardia

In this rhythm the heart rate is greater than 100 beats per minute, and the impulse originates in the SA node. It is not always an abnormal rhythm, because it occurs during and after exercise and in response to emotional stress. It may be

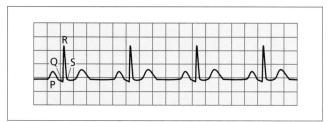

Figure 12.12 Sinus rhythm.

a normal response to an abnormal state, such as pain, severe anxiety, fever, anaemia, infection, hyperthyroidism, myocardial infarction and heart failure. It may also result from medications, for example atropine, adrenaline (epinephrine), isoprenaline hydrochloride and thyroid extract, or other drugs such as alcohol and nicotine (Fig. 12.13).

Tachycardia is significant for two reasons: coronary blood flow occurs predominantly during diastole. With tachycardia, the diastolic time is shortened, reducing the time for perfusion of the myocardium. Also, an increased heart rate increases the need of the myocardium for oxygen. In someone with narrowed coronary arteries, tachycardia may precipitate myocardial ischaemia.

Primarily, treatment is directed at correcting the underlying cause, but it may be necessary to reduce the rate by giving a drug such as a digitalis preparation or a beta-blocker.

Paroxysmal atrial tachycardia/narrow complex tachycardia

This is an abrupt onset of a very rapid heart rate, usually 150–250 beats per minute, initiated in the atria. It has several names and may be called a supra (meaning above) ventricular tachycardia (SVT). It may last a few seconds or longer. Such attacks cannot be explained in some persons; in others they may be related to organic heart disease or digitalis toxicity (Fig. 12.14). The narrow QRS complex indicates that the fast arrhythmia is originating in the atria, not in the ventricles, as this part of the ECG (the QRS segment) is normal.

A rapid heart rate of this type is serious if imposed on a diseased heart. When this arrhythmia occurs, the patient is advised to rest and the doctor is notified. If the patient is subject to recurring attacks, he or she is encouraged to recognize and avoid possible precipitating factors such as fatigue, emotional stress, or excessive smoking or coffee drinking. In some instances an attack may be relieved by measures that increase parasympathetic (vagal) innervation to the heart. Among those suggested is pressure on the carotid sinus. *Caution must be used in relation to the manoeuvre.* Carotid sinus massage applied injudiciously may result in asystole. It should be performed only by a doctor. The Valsalva manoeuvre, which involves an inspiration followed by voluntary closure of the glottis and an effort to exhale, may prove helpful. This reduces the venous return from the extremities and head, thus reducing the volume of blood entering the heart, which in turn decreases the cardiac output and the arterial blood pressure. An antiarrhythmic agent such as adenosine (which blocks the electrical

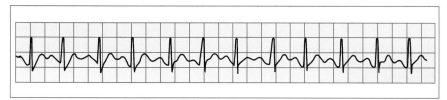

Figure 12.13 Sinus tachycardia: rate over 100 per minute; P wave and QRS are normal in 1 : 1 relationship.

impulses reaching the ventricles for a few seconds, breaking the tachycardic cycle), verapamil, a beta-blocker or digoxin may be used. Disopyramide or amiodarone may be useful. Long-acting quinidine preparations are sometimes prescribed.

Ventricular tachycardia/broad complex tachycardia

The term ventricular tachycardia (VT) usually refers to a run of rapidly repeated ventricular beats, essentially regular in rhythm, at a rate of 100–210 per minute. The impulses actually occur in the ventricles themselves and dominate as the fast pacemaker of the heart. Any rate above 60 per minute that is initiated in the ventricles might be considered tachycardia because the ventricles normally do not initiate impulses at more than 25–40 beats per minute. However, rates between 60 and 100 per minute are usually distinguished from the faster rates. They are usually referred to as *accelerated idioventricular rhythms* but are also called *slow ventricular tachycardia* (Fig. 12.15). The broad QRS complex indicates that the abnormal impulse originates in the ventricles themselves.

Ventricular tachycardia is a serious arrhythmia as there is always the danger that it will lead to ventricular fibrillation. It is usually due to ischaemic heart disease and is frequently present following myocardial infarction.

Treatment includes defibrillation, cardioversion (if a pulse is present) and/or antiarrhythmic drugs such as intravenous lidocaine (lignocaine). Other drugs that may be used include intravenous procainamide or flecanide.

BRADYCARDIAS

Sinus bradycardia

Sinus bradycardia is discharge of the SA node at a rate less than 60 beats per minute (Fig. 12.16).

Circulation may be adequately maintained by an increased stroke volume in a person with sinus bradycardia. With fewer contractions, more blood collects in the heart chambers to produce greater stretching of the myocardial fibres, resulting in a stronger contraction and increased output. Obviously this can occur only if the myocardium is in good condition. If the heart rate is less than 30–40 per minute, circulatory insufficiency is likely to occur, especially with physical activity.

The most common causes of sinus bradycardia are a decreased blood supply to the SA node or increased vagal tone. Circulatory reflexes may initiate a compensatory increase in the heart rate but, if the cause persists and becomes progressively severe, the heart muscle will gradually become weaker and less responsive, producing fewer contractions. Any disturbance that initiates an increase in the number of vagal nerve impulses to the heart will produce a decrease in the heart rate. An example of this would be bradycardia produced by carotid sinus massage or, in some people, by vomiting. Other examples of conditions in which slowing of the heart rate may be secondary are increased intracranial pressure (see p. 683) and myxoedema (a deficiency of thyroid secretion; see p. 577).

The pulse rate may normally be slower in those with well-developed cardiac reserve, such as well-trained athletes. In such people, the venous return is of greater strength, producing an increased stroke volume with each contraction.

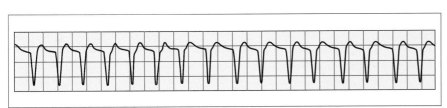

Figure 12.14 Paroxysmal atrial tachycardia.

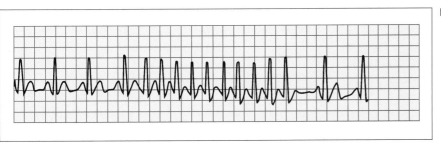

Figure 12.15 Ventricular tachycardia.

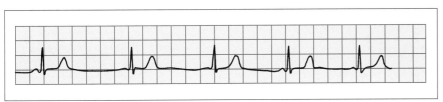

Figure 12.16 Sinus bradycardia.

Sinus bradycardia does not require treatment unless the individual is symptomatic. Atropine sulfate may be administered to decrease vagal tone. If the arrhythmia is due to the administration of medication, this should be withheld and re-evaluated.

ECTOPIC BEATS (EXTRASYSTOLES)

When impulses that influence the heart rate and rhythm are generated elsewhere than in the SA node, the contractions are called *ectopic*, *premature beats* or *extrasystoles*. The beats tend to be individual, but may occur in a small sequence or increase in frequency. The ectopic or premature beat occurs when the myocardial fibres are in the relative refractory period following a normal contraction. The impulse from the SA node for the succeeding normal contraction is ineffective, because it arrives when the muscle fibres are in the absolute refractory period following the premature beat, and no contraction takes place. This causes a longer than normal pause before the next normal contraction, and the heart 'misses' a beat. The next normal contraction may be stronger because of the prolonged filling period. The time between the normal heart contraction, which precedes the extrasystole, and the one that follows is equal to two normal cardiac cycles. The subject usually describes the experience as the heart 'missing a beat'.

Ectopic, or premature beats, may be due to ischaemic areas or to inflammation in the heart muscle. The fibres may also become irritated and hypersensitive as a result of certain toxic conditions, such as may occur with the excessive use of tobacco, coffee, tea or alcohol. The ectopics may occur irregularly, with varying lengths of time between them. The incidence may be so rare as to have no clinical significance but they should be investigated if persistent. Ectopic beats may arise regularly and at a rate in excess of that of the normal SA pacemaker, resulting in tachycardia.

Atrial ectopic beats

The ectopic focus is in the atria and the complex occurs earlier than expected. Atrial ectopic beats are significant because, if they occur during the vulnerable period of the atria, they may precipitate more serious atrial arrhythmias, such as atrial flutter or atrial fibrillation. They may or may not be conducted to the ventricles, depending upon the state of conduction through the AV node and the refractory period at which they occur. Treatment is not usually required unless they occur with great frequency or unless progression to more serious arrhythmias is feared, as may occur following myocardial infarction. If a precipitating cause is recognized, it should be eliminated (Fig. 12.17).

Ventricular ectopic beats

The ectopic focus is in the ventricle, and therefore there will be no related P wave on the ECG. Occasional ventricular ectopic beats may be innocuous, but they may also precipitate ventricular tachycardia and/or fibrillation. If they occur in a diseased heart, in groups of three or more, more frequently than 5 per minute, arise from more than one focus (multifocal) or are on the T wave of the preceding complex, they are considered serious and require treatment. The usual immediate treatment is lidocaine (lignocaine), given by bolus i.v. injection followed by a continuous i.v. drip. An oral drug such as disopyramide might be given when the lidocaine (lignocaine) infusion is gradually tapered off; however, many patients do not require this (see Fig. 12.18).

FLUTTER

Atrial flutter

As with atrial tachycardia, atrial flutter is due to a rapidly firing ectopic focus in the atria. The atrial rate usually falls between 250 and 350 beats per minute and a characteristic sawtooth pattern is seen on the ECG. AV block is usually present, so that the ventricular response may vary from 150 to 175 beats per minute (Fig. 12.19). Atrial flutter may occur with mitral stenosis, ischaemic heart disease and chronic obstructive pulmonary disease. The usual treatment is electrical cardioversion (see below) when the patient is haemodynamically unstable. Digoxin is the drug of choice to slow the ventricular rate by blocking impulses at the AV node. It may convert the flutter to atrial fibrillation, which is easier to manage.

FIBRILLATION

This is an arrhythmia in which the normal rhythmic contractions of the myocardium of either the atria or ventricles are replaced by extremely rapid (250–500 per minute), ineffective contractions, irregular in force and rhythm. As a result the heart does not achieve the contraction and relaxation that permit normal emptying and filling of the chambers.

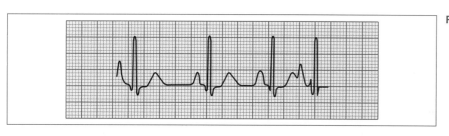

Figure 12.17   Atrial ectopic beat (arrowed).

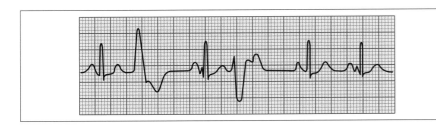

Figure 12.18 Ventricular ectopic beat (arrowed).

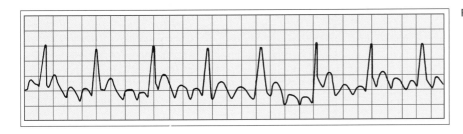

Figure 12.19 Atrial flutter.

Atrial fibrillation

Atrial fibrillation (AF) is a fairly common arrhythmia in which electrical activity in the atria is totally disorganized. It is due to myocardial disease which may be the result of coronary insufficiency, valvular heart disease, congestive heart failure or acute infection. The atria are never completely empty, and normal filling cannot occur. Since little pressure is created by the atrial contractions themselves, the flow of blood into the ventricles is due mainly to drainage under the influence of gravity. This aspect may not adversely affect the cardiac output. Only a proportion of the impulses arising in the atria are conducted through the AV node to the ventricles. However, those that do pass through may far exceed the normal in frequency, and are irregular, although the QRS complex is normal (Fig. 12.20). Cardiovascular problems may therefore occur, owing to the high heart rate experienced. Cardiac output falls as a result of decreased ventricular diastolic filling time, and the pulse may be weak and irregular.

To control the ventricular response, digoxin, verapamil and beta-blockers such as propranolol may be used. To decrease atrial tissue irritability, quinidine can be used. Procainamide and amiodarone may be used in more resistant cases. Cardioversion may be used with the patient who is haemodynamically unstable.

A complication that may follow atrial fibrillation is embolism. The blood that was not forwarded into the ventricles during fibrillation may have formed a thrombus in an atrial chamber and then, when normal heart action is re-established, the thrombus may be moved out into the circulation. Therefore, for those who have been in atrial fibrillation for some time, anticoagulation will be given for several weeks with warfarin, in addition to a drug such as digoxin to slow the heart rate, before cardioversion is attempted. In the elderly, treatment may fail to revert them to sinus rhythm and a drug such as digoxin is used on a long-term basis to slow and steady the heart rate.

Ventricular fibrillation

In ventricular fibrillation (VF), very rapid, asynchronous quivering arises in the ventricular myocardium because the electrical activity occurs in a totally disorganized sequence (Fig. 12.21). The contractions are so ineffective in pumping that the condition very quickly proves fatal. The pulse and blood pressure become unobtainable within a few seconds, the patient quickly loses consciousness, pupils dilate, reflexes are lost and cyanosis is likely to develop. Prompt emergency treatment may re-establish circulation. If the patient is being moni-tored in a coronary care unit, the arrhythmia may be identified immediately at onset, and treatment would consist of immediate defibrillation. Defibrillation is an expanding part of the nurse's role but hospital policy on who may defibrillate should be followed at all times. An important guideline is that it must be initiated very quickly to increase the chance of survival.

Ventricular fibrillation may occur with irritation of the heart during heart catheterization, because of coronary occlusion by the catheter or when conditions such as myocardial infarction, hypothermia, hypoxia, hypokalaemia and electrical shock exist. Very frequently ventricular fibrillation is preceded by ventricular ectopic beats. Prompt administration of an antiarrhythmic drug may prevent serious ventricular tachycardia and fibrillation.

HEART BLOCK

This is a condition in which impulse formation is depressed or impulse conduction is blocked. Although conduction may be interrupted between the SA node and the atria, the term 'heart block' usually refers to a disorder of conduction at the junctional tissues, which are the AV node and the common bundle (bundle of His). The SA node or the conduction pathway may be damaged by inflammatory disease such as rheumatic fever, coronary insufficiency, pressure from scarred

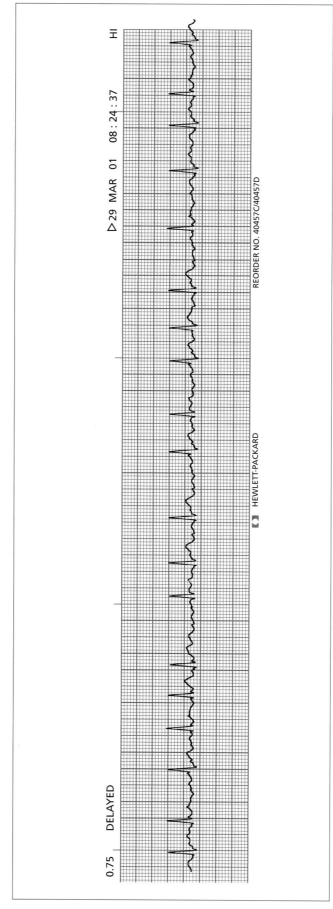

Figure 12.20   Atrial fibrillation with varying ventricular responses.

or calcified tissue, or surgical trauma. In the latter, this is notably following cardiac valve surgery.

Sinoatrial block

In sinoatrial block, impulses either are not formed in the SA node, fail to be conducted from it, or emerge very slowly (Fig. 12.22). If sinoatrial impulses are not received by the atria, occasional beats may be dropped, cardiac standstill may occur, or the ventricles may respond to impulses arising from a lower pacemaker, such as the junctional tissue. In the latter instance a junctional rhythm will result.

The seriousness of a SA block depends on the extent to which the heart rate is slowed and cardiac output is decreased. A slow rate may precipitate other arrhythmias. Specific precipitating causes include drugs such as digoxin and some antiarrhythmic drugs, salicylates, ischaemic heart disease, myocardial infarction and increased vagal tone.

Treatment is directed at removing the cause, when possible, and improving conduction between the SA node and the atria by drugs such as atropine and isoprenaline. If drug therapy is not effective, artificial pacing may be required.

Heart block at junctional tissues occurs in varying degrees of severity and may be categorized as first degree, second degree (types I and II) and third degree, or complete AV block. Conduction may be impaired in the bundle branches, referred to as *right* or *left bundle branch block*.

First-degree atrioventricular block

First-degree heart block is usually due to delayed conduction through the AV node, and the interval between atrial and ventricular contractions is lengthened. This is exhibited on the ECG by a prolonged P-R interval (greater than 0.20 seconds) (Fig. 12.23). It may be caused by increased vagal tone, digoxin toxicity, inflammatory heart disease or coronary artery disease. First-degree AV block may progress to second- and third-degree block, but in the absence of evidence of disease requires no treatment. Digoxin may be discontinued or the dosage reduced.

Second-degree atrioventricular block

Second-degree or partial block refers to a more advanced disturbance in which some of the sinus impulses fail to get through and activate the ventricles. It may be divided into Mobitz type I or Wenckebach, and Mobitz type II.

In *Wenckebach block* the period of time between atrial and ventricular conduction becomes progressively longer, until finally an atrial impulse is completely blocked. The ECG shows progressively longer P–R intervals, until finally a P wave is not followed by a QRS complex. The P–R interval

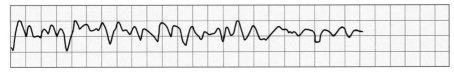

Figure 12.21 Ventricular fibrillation: chaotic ventricular activity.

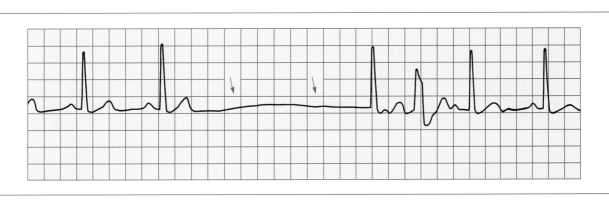

Figure 12.22 Sinoatrial block (the arrows indicate where a sinoatrial impulse (P wave) should have occurred).

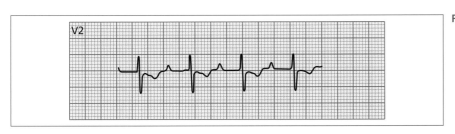

Figure 12.23 First-degree heart block.

following this dropped ventricular beat is close to the normal range, but with each successive beat it lengthens and the cycle repeats itself. The patient may be conscious of a decreased ventricular rate if the change occurs suddenly, but may exhibit no physical symptoms (Fig. 12.24).

Type II second-degree block is more serious than type I. At specific intervals impulses are blocked at the AV node and an atrial beat fails to be followed by a ventricular beat. The ratio of atrial to ventricular beats may vary, for example 2 : 1, 3 : 1, 4 : 3, or 3 : 2. The P–R interval is constant. The patient may experience syncopal (fainting) attacks (Fig. 12.25).

Both second-degree blocks may be due to inflammatory or fibrotic processes, ischaemic heart disease, infarction, or drugs such as digoxin, beta-blockers or verapamil. Atropine sulfate may be required to increase the heart rate, and temporary cardiac pacing may be needed if the ventricular rate is slow.

Complete atrioventricular block

In this arrhythmia, conduction is so disturbed that no impulses reach the ventricles, and the atria and ventricles beat independently at their own inherent rhythms. The block may occur at the AV node, or the bundle of His. It is a more advanced block and may be caused by any of the disorders responsible for type II partial blocks. As atrial impulses are unable to penetrate the AV node, a lower pacemaker takes over and controls the ventricles. If this 'rescuing' pacemaker is initiated in the junctional tissue, the ECG will show a QRS complex that is normal in appearance and is not wide unless there is an associated bundle branch block. If the pacemaker is in the ventricles, the QRS complexes will be wide and abnormal in shape (Fig. 12.26).

This condition may be managed with an infusion of isoprenaline if the patient shows signs of a decreased cardiac output. A temporary cardiac pacemaker may be required and evaluation of the need for permanent cardiac pacing conducted to manage this arrhythmia. A permanent pacemaker is rarely used in the first instance, because the condition may be temporary, for example following cardiac surgery.

TREATMENT OF CARDIAC ARRHYTHMIAS

Treatment of heart arrhythmias includes the use of a pacemaker, implantable cardioverter defibrillator (ICD), medications and/or defibrillation.

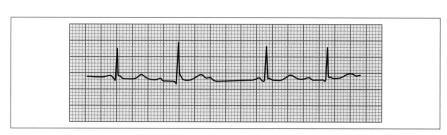

Figure 12.24 Wenckebach block.

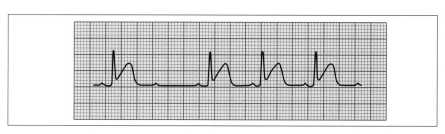

Figure 12.25 Type II second-degree block.

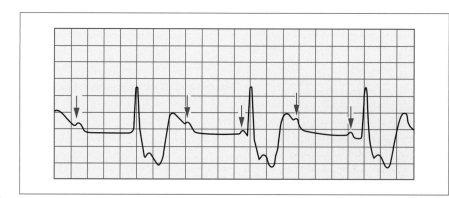

Figure 12.26 Complete heart block (the arrows indicate sinoatrial impulses (P waves) occurring regularly but independently of ventricular activity).

Artificial cardiac pacemakers

In serious conduction defects, and sometimes in the treatment of tachyarrhythmias, electrical stimulation may be provided by an electronic battery-operated pacemaker to stimulate or control cardiac contractions.

An artificial pacemaker generates an electrical stimulus which is used to send a specific electrical current to the myocardium to control or maintain a minimum heart rate. Every pacemaker consists of a pulse generator, which emits and senses electrical impulses, and a wire catheter with one or more electrodes that conduct the impulses to the heart. This electrode or lead system may transmit impulses by contact with the endocardium established through the venous route into the right atrium and/or ventricle, or by contact with the epicardium established by thoracotomy (e.g. after cardiac surgery). Contact may also be made by the transthoracic approach when the pacing stimulus is delivered through electrodes applied on the external anterior and posterior chest wall in an emergency. This latter method is quite painful to the patient.

If the conduction defect is transient, a *temporary* pacemaker is used. A pacing electrode is introduced through the external jugular, subclavian, antecubital or femoral vein, and advanced into the right ventricle under fluoroscopy or via a special flotation catheter with a little balloon on the end. The electrode wire is connected to an external battery-operated pacemaker. The site of insertion of the electrode is secured with a sterile dressing.

When the conduction defect is irreversible, a *permanent* pacemaker is implanted within the body. The electrode is introduced transvenously, usually through the right cephalic or right external jugular vein, and the battery unit is implanted subcutaneously in a supermammary pouch on the chest wall. Alternatively, it is implanted beneath the muscle of the upper abdominal wall. This requires a small incision. Pacemaker functioning can be described based on: (1) the heart chamber paced, (2) the chamber in which the heart's intrinsic electrical impulse is sensed, (3) the mode of pacemaker response, (4) its programmable characteristics,

and (5) the antitachy-arrhythmic features. Often, only the first three positions are used to describe a particular pacemaker's functioning (Table 12.6).

Essentially all pacing systems must have two wires to complete the electrical circuit. The *bipolar* system uses two wires placed against the myocardium (Fig. 12.27b). A temporary system will invariably use a bipolar system (with an external pacing box). If one of the wires is believed not to be working, perhaps because pacing spikes cannot be seen on the ECG with a good electrical output, either wire can be 'bypassed' by pushing a needle under the skin and connecting this to the temporary pacing box to complete the electrical circuit.

There are several modes of pacemaker, categorized according to their pattern of activity. The pacemaker may be preset to discharge at a fixed rate, by demand or at a rate that corresponds to cardiac activity. *Fixed rate pacing* is asynchronous, meaning that it does not sense the heart's own impulses. The pacemaker therefore delivers a predetermined rate of impulses, even if the heart is generating its own spontaneous rhythm. A second mode of pacing is the *demand mode*. In this mode, the pacemaker is programmed to sense the heart's intrinsic electrical activity and to fire only when the intrinsic rhythm falls below a preset rate. This

Table 12.6 Positions describing pacemaker functioning

	Position		
	I	**II**	**III**
Category	Chamber(s) paced	Chamber(s) sensed	Mode of response
Letters used	V – ventricle A – atrium D – dual (atrium and ventricle)	V – ventricle A – atrium D – dual (atrium and ventricle) O – none	T – triggered I – inhibited D – dual O – none

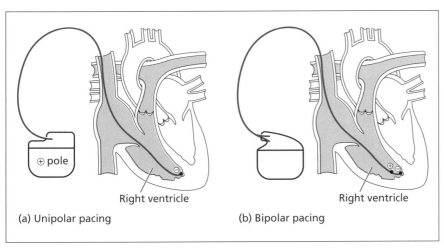

Figure 12.27 VVI pacing systems. From Barnett (2001), with permission.

(a) Unipolar pacing (b) Bipolar pacing

Right ventricle

Right ventricle

⊕ pole

avoids dangerous competition between the heart and the pacemaker, as well as the risk of two differing messages being sent to the myocardium, for example a stimulus to depolarize during repolarization. This would run the risk of inducing a life-threatening cardiac arrhythmia.

Nurses caring for patients with cardiac pacemakers learn how to recognize that the device is working from the characteristic ECG patterns. Generally, when working, a small vertical horizontal *pacing spike* occurs before a P wave in atrial pacing and before a slightly abnormal QRS complex in ventricular pacing. In the latter, if the wire is quite high in the ventricle, the QRS complex may appear fairly normal. Also, P waves may be seen to wander through the rhythm strip, because atrial activity may still be functioning while the ventricle is paced, but there is no association between the two chambers. In dual-chamber pacing, a spike appears before the P wave *and* before the corresponding QRS complex. Pacing spikes with no complexes indicate a lack of electrical *capture*, or depolarization of the myocardium.

Nursing care of the patient with a pacemaker

Nursing care involves assisting in the preparation of the patient for implantation of the pacemaker. The patient may be apprehensive because of the symptoms of bradycardia such as dizziness and fainting, and may also be fearful of the procedure and being dependent on an electrical device for their heart beat. When explaining the need for a pacemaker, the doctor reviews the procedure with the patient. The nurse reinforces this explanation and answers any further questions before the patient signs the consent form. Explanations are also given to the family and carers.

Temporary pacemakers are usually implanted under local anaesthesia in the angiography department, in the radiology department or occasionally, in an emergency, at the bedside. Permanent pacemakers are inserted in the operating theatre or the angiography department.

Following the implantation of a permanent pacemaker, the patient is monitored continuously until it has been established that the pacemaker is functioning properly. Rest is indicated for the remainder of the day. If a temporary pacemaker has been inserted, mobility is restricted, depending upon the site of insertion as well as the patient's general condition. Cardiac monitoring may be continued as long as the temporary pacemaker is being used.

The nurse is responsible for monitoring and reporting the patient's rhythm, for checking the operation site and cleansing the wound as necessary, for assessing and reporting any complications, and for supporting the patient and providing any information needed.

Complications that could occur include malfunction of the pacemaker, perforation of the myocardial wall by an electrode, breakage or dislodgement of the electrodes, thrombus formation, and infection, such as phlebitis, endocarditis or septicaemia. Malfunction may occur because the pacemaker fails to fire, fires too rapidly, or fires erratically. Malfunctioning may be detected by cardiac monitoring or

by ECG, as well as by the presence of signs and symptoms, such as decreased pulse rate, dizziness and/or fainting.

Following perforation of the myocardium, blood can seep into the pericardium, causing cardiac tamponade. The resulting compression of the heart causes low blood pressure, tachycardia, increased central venous pressure and distended neck veins. The electrode may also stimulate innervation to the upper abdominal or lower chest muscles, resulting in spasm. This is uncomfortable for the patient and more common with a large and thinned right ventricle. The doctor should reposition the wire in such cases. Breakage or dislodgement of the electrode will result in a change in the shape of the QRS complex and in the heart rate.

The nurse should be alert to electrical hazards in the environment. Electrical equipment must be properly earthed and the external pulse generator of temporary pacemakers must be kept dry. If epicardial wires are used, which emerge through the chest wall, following cardiac surgery, the ends should be wrapped in gauze or the fingers of rubber or latex gloves. This prevents static from clothes sending an electrical impulse along the wire to the heart.

Caution regarding electrical hazards includes avoiding close contact with large electrical motors; for example, in a machine shop the patient may develop arrhythmias as a result of the electrical interference. Microwave ovens may cause similar interference with some pacemakers if the oven is faulty with an inadequate door seal. Small home appliances, if properly grounded, produce no untoward effects. Contact sports might be allowed on the doctor's advice. The patient's dentist should be advised that the patient is wearing a pacemaker before any electrical equipment is used. It is advisable for the patient to notify airport security of their cardiac pacemaker to avoid triggering the alarms.

The patient should carry an identification card indicating the type of pacemaker in place and the doctor to be notified in case of difficulty. Before travelling, the patient should obtain the name of a local doctor or hospital in case of an emergency.

The implantable cardioverter defibrillator (ICD)

This is a small internal device which looks rather like a pacemaker. It is designed to track the heart rhythm and deliver a series of small direct current (DC) shocks to the myocardium when a life-threatening arrhythmia is detected. This aims to terminate the arrhythmia. It is designed for patients who are known to be prone to this sort of event, perhaps due to cardiac disease, and where other treatments alone are not effective. Although the use of these devices has saved many lives, it has emerged that there is a need for psychological support for patients receiving the ICD (James 2001). This is because patients are often discharged home within a few days of implantation and may have concerns over a variety of issues. These include how the shock will feel (although many units now administer a test shock before discharge), whether they can be touched during the shock, whether an ambulance will need to be called after a shock is delivered, through to the dangers to partners during sexual activity. In fact, the shock is small enough not to affect those touching the patient. However, a structured programme for patients receiving the device is needed to allay fears in both the patient and loved ones, and to prevent the device from having an adverse effect on quality of life.

Drugs used to manage arrhythmias
Drugs commonly used to manage cardiac arrhythmias are described in Table 12.7.

Defibrillation and cardioversion
In *defibrillation* two electrodes ('paddles') are placed on the chest wall. The standard technique is to place one paddle to the right (the patient's right) of the upper part of the sternum, below the clavicle and the other paddle over the fifth left intercostal space in the mid-clavicular line. The technique will vary according to the type of defibrillator being used and many areas now use automated devices that require electrode pads to be placed on the patient's chest. Whichever device is used a strong electrical discharge is passed through the electrodes for a brief period once the defibrillator is discharged. When this happens all the muscle fibres of the myocardium are thrown into contraction together and then enter a refractory period simultaneously. This quiescent period may give the normal pacemaker, the

SA node, an opportunity to take over. It is important to make sure that no one is touching the bed or the patient during the electrical discharge to prevent them from receiving a shock. Shocks are delivered in a set sequence with rest periods of 2 minutes between each shock to reassess the rhythm and review the strength of shock that is needed (Resuscitation Council UK 2005a). An overview of the current resuscitation guidelines can be found in Appendix 1.

Cardioversion differs from defibrillation in only one important aspect. It is a synchronized procedure designed to deliver smaller amounts of electrical energy to the heart at a set time in the cardiac cycle. The same equipment is used to perform cardioversion as defibrillation but a synchronization circuit is activated to allow for timing of the cardiac cycle. After the machine is discharged, the shock is held until the next QRS complex is tracked and then it is discharged. This prevents the shock from being delivered during ventricular depolarization and causing ventricular fibrillation. Cardioversion is used to treat ventricular tachycardia and rapid atrial arrhythmias, such as atrial fibrillation and flutter, when the patient is haemodynamically unstable.

Some patients are admitted for electrical cardioversion as day cases, such as those in atrial fibrillation. They will have been fully anticoagulated on warfarin to avoid the formation of any clots that might be forced into the circulation on restoration of normal sinus rhythm. Patients need to be

Table 12.7	Drugs commonly used to manage cardiac arrhythmias	
Drug	**General actions**	**Clinical uses**
Cardiac glycosides e.g. Digoxin	Increase force of contraction without significantly increasing oxygen utilization Decrease conduction through AV node	Atrial arrhythmias, notably atrial fibrillation
Sodium channel suppressors e.g. A. Quinidine sulfate Procainamide	Depress automaticity Slow conduction Decrease myocardial contractility	Atrial arrhythmias Ventricular arrhythmias
B. Lidocaine (lignocaine)	Depress ventricular ectopic foci	Ventricular arrhythmias, ventricular ectopic beats
β-Adrenergic blockers e.g. Sotalol	Decrease ventricular ectopy Decrease heart rate Increase PR interval Decrease myocardial contractility Decrease myocardial oxygen demand	Ventricular arrhythmias Supraventricular arrhythmias
Prolong repolarization e.g. Amiodarone	Decrease ventricular conduction Increase duration of the action potential	Atrial arrhythmias Recurrent ventricular tachycardia/ fibrillation
Calcium channel blockers e.g. Verapamil	Prolong refractory period of AV node	Atrial arrhythmias

advised not to eat or drink for at least 5 hours before the procedure as they will be having a general anaesthetic. Cardioversion is normally performed on a coronary care unit or a day-case ward. The procedure takes about 15 minutes. After-effects tend to be related to the anaesthetic, and the patient may have a sore chest. Cardioversion is not always successful as it does nothing to remove the underlying cause of the arrhythmia. The potential outcome therefore needs to be fully explained.

CARDIOPULMONARY ARREST

Cardiopulmonary arrest means the sudden cessation of effective ventricular contraction *and* respirations. Cardiac arrest essentially means the cessation of effective ventricular function, but the terms may be used interchangeably. The condition includes ventricular tachycardia (VT) when there is no pulse, ventricular fibrillation (VF) and asystole. Possible causes are myocardial ischaemia, respiratory insufficiency, heart block, electric shock, metabolic acidosis and adverse reactions to medications.

Cardiac arrest must be recognized as a critical emergency. This condition is diagnosed when the individual is assessed as unconscious, not breathing and having no pulse. It is imperative that oxygen supply be re-established to the brain within 3–4 minutes of cardiac arrest to prevent irreversible anoxic brain damage.

Basic cardiopulmonary resuscitation (CPR) must be commenced as soon as cardiac arrest is diagnosed. The ABC steps are Airway, Breathing and Circulation (Fig. 12.28). It is every nurse's responsibility to be prepared and well versed in conducting basic life support. Regular practical updates, usually 6 monthly to yearly, allow the skill to be reassessed and competence maintained.

A: Airway After unresponsiveness has been determined, help is summoned, the airway is opened using the head-tilt/chin-lift or jaw manoeuvre. A Guedal airway may be used to maintain patency of the airway until such time as endotracheal intubation occurs.

B: Breathing After the airway is opened, assessment for respiration is conducted. Once absence of breathing is determined, definitive assistance such as an ambulance or the cardiac arrest team is called. Artificial resuscitation is started. To deliver respirations the rescuer gives two breaths, ensuring the patient's nose is pinched closed. In a hospital or clinic, resuscitation should be performed using a pocket mask with oxygen attachment, or a self-refilling bag-mask device, again attached to an oxygen source. This offers a greater percentage of oxygen to the patient. The bag-mask device is hard to use by one person, as there is a need to keep the airway open, hold the mask in place and inflate the bag. It is much more effective if one person holds the mask over the face with two hands while tilting the chin, and another squeezes the bag to ventilate the lungs. Laryngeal mask airways (LMAs) are being used by nurses in hospital to offer an even higher oxygen percentage. These consist of a tube with a rubber flange on the end. This is inserted into the mouth and inflated over the larynx, then connected to the bag-valve device (Simons 1999). The use of these devices is known as basic life support with adjunct therapy.

C: Circulation Circulation is achieved by delivering, external chest compression is started immediately. This consists of the regular application of vertical pressure at a point one-third up the sternum from the xiphoid process. Both hands should be used, with the fingers interlocked, applying pressure with the heels of the hands and maintaining the elbows locked in an extended position so that the arms are straight. The increase in intrathoracic pressure produces a limited circulation of blood which, if it is to be effective, must force sufficient blood into the arteries to produce pulsation in the carotid and femoral arteries. The sternum should be depressed 4–5 cm in an adult. The thoracic cage is quite flexible in an unconscious person and the possibility of injury to the ribs is therefore reduced. This technique of resuscitation is simple, requires no special equipment, and may be done anywhere. Finding the carotid pulse can be difficult in a collapsed patient, and current guidance suggest this wastes time.

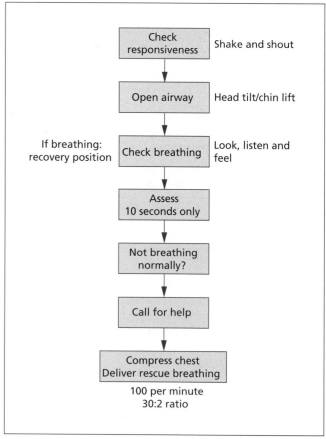

Figure 12.28 In-hospital resuscitation. From Resuscitation Council UK (2005b). See appendix 1

After every 30 compressions the lungs are ventilated twice, hence the ratio of compressions to respirations is 30 : 2 (Resuscitation Council 2005a). The aim should be to deliver at least 100 compressions per minute.

Basic CPR is enhanced by the provision of advanced cardiac life support by trained personnel who are prepared to diagnose and provide definitive therapy. One member of the team attaches electrodes to the patient and continuous cardiac monitoring is begun to determine the underlying cardiac rhythm. Another member of the team inserts an intravenous line for the infusion of medications. If ventricular fibrillation or pulseless ventricular tachycardia has caused the arrest, a defibrillator is used to deliver an electric shock through electrodes onto the chest wall. Emergency drugs are given as required. To be optimally effective, advanced life support follows a particular algorithm guideline from the Resuscitation Council (2005a) (see Appendix 1).

Care following resuscitation

The patient who has been resuscitated requires constant observation of the vital signs. If possible, the patient is transferred to an intensive care unit and continuous monitoring of heart action is established. An intensive care unit will be used if mechanical ventilation is required. An X-ray is usually ordered to assess for any damage to the chest following CPR, the position of any central lines or an endotracheal tube if in place. A variety of blood tests will be taken to assess electrolyte and blood gas levels (e.g. oxygen and carbon dioxide levels). What has happened will be discussed with relatives and loved ones, and if there are any specific problems encountered such as cerebral oedema due to hypoxia of the brain these will be assessed and treated. Peripheral pulses are checked for volume, rhythm and rate, together with regular recordings of the blood pressure and oxygen saturation levels via a pulse oximetry probe. The defibrillator and mechanical ventilator are kept nearby and ready for immediate use.

The patient may be very apprehensive and should be advised of the improvement in condition and of the importance of rest and minimal emotional stress, and is assured that someone will either be present or close by so that treatment may be quickly instituted should it be needed.

Ethical issues: decisions to withhold cardiopulmonary resuscitation

Although decisions to withhold CPR have been debated extensively during the past two decades, such decisions remain a common and difficult ethical problem for most healthcare providers. The usual presumption in any instance of cardiac arrest is that CPR will be attempted. However, there are situations in which CPR does not appear to be appropriate. The main difficulties in trying to determine whether or not CPR is appropriate can be reduced to three: determining in *which* situations CPR should be withheld, determining *who* should make that kind of decision, and determining *how* the decision should be made and implemented. A typical situation is described in Case 12.4.

CASE **The decision to withhold CPR**

Mrs Zabranska is an 86-year-old woman who has been admitted to hospital with increasing shortness of breath. Tests show that she has lung cancer that has metastasized throughout her chest. She has been an active woman until recently and agrees to a trial of radiotherapy to control the malignancy to a certain extent. After a week she starts to deteriorate.

If Mrs Zabranska has a cardiac arrest, should she be resuscitated? How should such a decision be made?

Background

Deciding not to resuscitate is, of course, a controversial issue. Like many technological advances, CPR raises ethical issues that previous generations of healthcare providers did not have to face. The imperative to extend life-sustaining technology to an ever wider range of patients brings eventually with it the need to set limits to the use of the technology. When CPR was introduced in 1960 its goal was to prevent sudden and unexpected death from cardiac arrest. Before long it was applied to almost anyone who suffered cardiac arrest (i.e. anyone who died). Now, in most hospital practice, and in most hospital policies, it is presumed that in the event of cardiac arrest CPR will be performed unless a specific decision not to resuscitate is made. In the 1960s, any decisions not to resuscitate were made by doctors verbally at the time of making rounds.

As practitioners were confronted with increasing and sometimes inappropriate use of CPR, and as nurses became more uncomfortable at being left with only verbal orders, attempts were made to establish guidelines for making decisions about CPR. The nurse has an obligation to determine whether there are such advance directives.

Although limitation of treatment decisions is usually couched in terms of the principle of autonomy, or 'patient wishes', other principles are involved in actually coming to the decision. A decision to forego CPR is usually guided by balancing the benefits and the burdens of the treatment for a patient. When the burdens of a treatment such as CPR appear to be disproportionate to the benefits that may be obtained, it is important for the caregivers to initiate a discussion of the appropriateness of CPR for the individual. In evaluating a decision, the benefits and the burdens are both considered from the point of view of the patient. At present, most policies require that decision-making on this issue include the patient or relatives, and that decisions be made only after discussion with the patient or relative.

A further issue that might be considered is balancing the benefit to the patient with the burdens that the treatment will place on family members or society in general. Certain types of underlying disease and other characteristics of the patient are associated with reduced survival, and for some associated complications (e.g. pneumonia) the chances are practically zero. It may be possible, with further study, to define the circumstances in which CPR would be definitely futile, and would therefore not even have to be offered.

Until then, the patient or patient's family should be involved in the decision-making. Jevon (1999) states that there are several possible consequences of deciding not to carry out a resuscitation and these include:

- denial of a peaceful and dignified death
- distress for the relatives
- denial of care for other patients while the crash team are attending to the patient
- repeated failures for the crash team leading to demoralization and
- inappropriate use of valuable resources.

To aid decision-making and the support of everyone involved in such a decision, the British Medical Association, the UK Resuscitation Council and the Royal College of Nursing have produced guidelines (BMA/RCN 2002). The term *do not attempt resuscitation* (DNAR) is used, and the overall responsibility lies with the consultant or general practitioner in charge of the patient's care. He or she should discuss the decision with other healthcare professionals involved in the patient's care. The decision must always be on an individual basis, be clearly documented in the medical and nursing notes, and should be conveyed to all those who need to know it. Unless the patient refuses, decisions on resuscitation should be communicated to those close to the patient, who should be a part of the decision-making process.

Since the early 1990s there has been an increased awareness of the need to allow relatives and loved ones to witness the resuscitation of the patient. Traditionally, staff have considered that loved ones would get in the way, or be unable to cope with seeing events. However, there is little evidence to support this and many are grateful to see all that was done (Kidby 2003), as opposed to sitting for prolonged periods in a waiting room. We do also need to question whether we have the right and whether it is ethically correct to stop a loved one being with the patient at what may be the end of their life. There is, however, a need for someone to stay with the person, explain proceedings and support them (Quinn and Hatchett 2001).

Communication

While there has been increased awareness of the ethical aspects of decisions regarding CPR, actual practice does not seem to have kept pace with our understanding. Thus, although it is common for institutions to have policies on the subject, the level of communication on this subject between patient and doctor is still disappointing. Decisions need to be communicated both verbally and in writing.

Although it is still considered to be the role of the doctor to carry out the discussions and make the decisions regarding CPR with patients and families, it is often the nurse who makes the initial assessment that the appropriateness of CPR should be questioned and who assumes the role of facilitator of the decision-making process. It is important, therefore, that the nurse has a clear understanding of the principles on which decisions regarding the withholding of CPR should be made.

HEART FAILURE

Heart failure can be defined as an insufficient cardiac output to meet the metabolic demands or needs of the body. It may be acute or chronic. In the acute situation there is a sudden and severe failure of cardiac function, perhaps due to myocardial infarction or a condition such as cardiomyopathy. In the chronic situation, failure occurs over many months or years, primarily due to ischaemic heart disease, or a condition such as hypertension or a valvular disorder. In this case the body will implement a variety of compensatory mechanisms to maintain cardiac function, for example enlargement of the heart (hypertrophy). The person may be admitted to hospital many times with a worsening of their condition, when it is known as *decompensated* heart failure, i.e. they can no longer compensate for the deterioration in their heart's function. Chronic heart failure is a debilitating condition, with the person becoming increasingly breathless, tired and severely restricted in activities. Lozano et al (2001) state that heart failure is a condition which is ill-defined and therefore it is difficult to compare prevalence rates between countries. However, figures from the British Heart Foundation (2004) indicate that approximately 660 000 people are living with chronic heart failure, with 65 000 new cases appearing each year.

Although the mortality rate from CHD is slowly declining, admissions for chronic heart failure appear to be rising (Sharpe and Doughty 1998). This is due to an ageing population, but also because treatments are allowing patients with the condition to survive for longer periods. It is now clear, however, that mortality figures for chronic heart failure are comparable to those for many malignant diseases. In fact, those with the condition often fair much worse (Millane et al 2000). This has led to the increased involvement of palliative care teams in managing this condition, as well as the use of specific treatments to improve the quality of life.

Heart failure may involve either side of the heart. However, as both sides of the heart work in series, one side does not usually fail for long before the other is affected.

In *left-sided heart failure*, the left side of the heart cannot forward all of the blood it receives to the systemic circulation. As a result, blood backs up in the pulmonary circulation (Fig. 12.29). The pulmonary vessels become congested and the alveoli gradually fill with serous fluid.

A serious consequence of left-sided heart failure may be acute pulmonary oedema. This condition occurs when the alveoli fill up with serous fluid and the exchange of respiratory gases is impaired. A patient in acute pulmonary oedema will manifest symptoms of acute respiratory distress including dyspnoea and cough. Rapid treatment is necessary to prevent further deterioration of respiratory function. This will include the use of a diuretic, often intravenously, and nitrates. The diuretic reduces oedema and therefore helps breathing, while nitrates dilate the venous system to reduce blood returning to the heart (reducing the preload). To a lesser extent, nitrates also reduce the resistance in front of the heart (the afterload) through arterial dilatation. These actions reduce the workload on the heart and enable it to pump more effectively. Augmentation of contractility will be achieved with the use of a drug such as digoxin.

Right-sided heart failure may be secondary to failure of the left side, or it may occur independently. When the right side of the heart fails, it cannot effectively forward blood to the pulmonary arteries and lungs. As a result, increased pressure is placed on the venous system. This leads to venous congestion and oedema developing in tissues and organs (Fig. 12.30).

Symptoms of heart failure

Respirations Dyspnoea is the most common symptom of heart failure. Pulmonary oedema impairs gas exchange and may induce hypoxia. In mild or early failure, dyspnoea may be experienced only with exertion. With severe heart failure, it is present at rest. With acute pulmonary oedema, it is severe. Patients will commonly complain of breathlessness on lying down (orthopnea) and will often compensate by using several pillows to prop themselves up in bed at night.

Cough Due to congestion and fluid in the alveoli and bronchial tubes, cough may be present. The frequency, characteristics and amount of sputum are noted. Frothy, colourless sputum occurs in pulmonary oedema, and blood may appear from the rupture of capillaries and arterioles in severe congestion.

Pulse The pulse may be rapid, weak and irregular, as tachycardia frequently accompanies severe heart failure. The strength, rate and rhythm of the pulse should be noted frequently.

Blood pressure It is important to assess the blood pressure because uncontrolled hypertension can be a contributory factor in heart failure. Some of the treatments used once heart failure has been diagnosed will have an antihypertensive effect (e.g. ACE inhibitors) and therefore it is valuable to check the patient's blood pressure to avoid the adverse consequences of hypotension.

Body temperature Many patients with cardiac insufficiency register a subnormal temperature as their heat production is reduced because of inadequate circulation, deficiency in oxygen and resulting decrease in metabolism.

Colour The colour of the lips, nail-beds and skin may show pallor due to generalized vasoconstriction. There may be cyanosis of lips and nail-beds.

Generalized oedema Failure of the right side of the heart causes fluid to accumulate in the systemic venous circulation. The

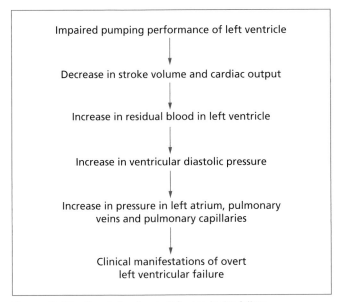

Figure 12.29 Events leading to left ventricular failure.

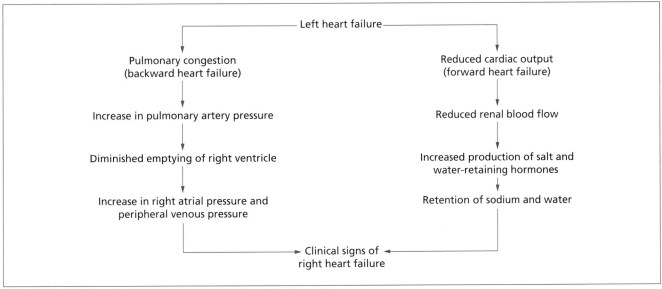

Figure 12.30 Sequence of events leading to right heart failure.

reduced venous return to the heart leads to a reduction in left ventricular output, and compensatory mechanisms occur in an attempt to maintain adequate perfusion of vital organs. This causes further retention of fluid. Systemic venous and capillary pressures are raised due to back pressure from the failing heart. As a result of abnormal pressure gradients, fluid escapes from the vascular system into the interstitial tissues, resulting in oedema.

Oedema is usually found in the dependent areas of the body. If the person is mobile, swelling first appears in the feet and ankles, but if the person is confined to bed oedema may first become apparent in the back and sacral region. As it becomes more severe, all body tissues become affected and ascites may develop.

The most accurate method of observing the patient for oedema is by daily weighing, which should be at the same time each day wearing similar clothes. Up to 7 kg (7 L) of water may be retained before oedema becomes visibly obvious.

Fluid balance

An accurate record is kept of the patient's fluid intake and output. A positive balance is brought to the attention of the doctor, particularly if the urinary output is decreased to less than 0.5 mL per kg per hour. The amount of sweating is noted as a large amount of fluid may be lost in this manner. In the patient whose cardiac function is severely deteriorated, a urinary catheter allows an hourly assessment of urine output. Urinary output provides a useful guide to general tissue perfusion, because the kidneys are one of the last organs to be served with blood when there is disruption to cardiac function. If the person is passing at least 0.5 mL/kg of urine per hour, then the vital organs of heart, brain and lungs are receiving an adequate blood and oxygen supply.

Chest or abdominal pain

Chest pain and any apparent precipitating causes are observed and reported immediately. Abdominal pain may be due to the congestion and poor perfusion of internal organs. Abdominal distension may be associated with reduced peristalsis as a result of congestion and reduced blood supply to the intestines.

Anorexia

The patient may not eat because of lack of strength or because of dietary restrictions that make meals unpalatable. Congestion of internal organs due to oedema may contribute to loss of appetite. Anorexia may also result from drug toxicity (e.g. digoxin). The amount and type of food the patient eats should be observed at every meal.

Fatigue

Feeling tired all the time is a common concern of people with heart failure; the degree of fatigue should be noted at rest as well as in relationship to specific activities.

Orientation and level of consciousness

When circulation and/or the oxygen content of the blood perfusing the brain are inadequate, the patient's cerebral functioning may decrease. Observations are made regarding the patient's level of consciousness; orientation to person, time and surroundings; and response to stimuli such as questioning.

Anxiety

It is very important to observe the patient for fear and apprehension. Anxiety may initiate the release of adrenaline, which stimulates the heart at a time when the aim is to reduce cardiac workload. The patient's apprehension may indicate a need for information, explanations or sedation.

Diagnosis

Diagnosis of heart failure can be made using the history, physical examination and a number of other investigations. A 12-lead ECG should be performed and in some areas the blood can be tested for natriuretic peptides. If either of these tests show abnormal findings the patient should have an echocardiogram and this will provide information relating to the underlying functional abnormality of the heart. Other tests are carried out mainly to exclude other causes of the patient's symptoms including; chest radiography, thyroid function tests, urea and electrolytes, creatinine, blood glucose, lipids, full blood count, urinalysis and spirometry.

Medical management

Management of a patient with heart failure focuses on two areas. The cause of heart failure must be determined and corrected if possible. Often the underlying cause is a myocardium that is so severely damaged after myocardial infarction(s) that it cannot function effectively and the condition cannot be cured without a heart transplant. The second focus of treatment is improving the functional ability of the heart. The National Institute of Clinical Excellence have developed an algorithm for the treatment of heart failure (NICE 2003b). This can be summarized as follows:

- *Lifestyle modifications.* Patients who smoke should be encouraged to stop and those who drink excessive amounts of alcohol should be advised to reduce their intake and in some cases stop drinking alcohol altogether. Patients should be encouraged to engage with regular aerobic exercise as part of a planned rehabilitation programme
- *Reduce fluid accumulation.* A diet restricted in sodium may be useful in decreasing fluid retention. Diuretics are essential in the treatment of heart failure. In severe heart failure a fluid restriction may be advocated of 1–1.5 L in 24 hours. It is important to explain this to the patient and to devise an acceptable distribution of fluid intake over each 24-hour period
- *ACE inhibitor treatment.* All patients who have heart failure due to left ventricular failure should be treated with ACE inhibitors titrated up to the highest possible dose. If an ACE inhibitor is contraindicated or is causing intolerable side-effects, angiotensin II receptor agonists can be used instead
- *Beta-blocker treatment.* Once the patient has reached the highest tolerable dose of ACE inhibitor, beta blockers

should be introduced at the lowest possible dose and again should be titrated upwards to the highest possible dose. Bisoprolol and carvedilol are the two beta-blockers that are licensed for use in heart failure

- *Spironolactone*. If the patient remains symptomatic the aldosterone antagonist spironolactone can be introduced. Patients should be regularly monitored for their renal function as hyperkalaemia and deteriorating renal function can be a problem with this treatment
- *Digoxin*. In patients who remain symptomatic in spite of treatment with diuretics, ACE inhibitors and beta-blockers, or in patients who are experiencing atrial fibrillation, digoxin, may be required. Digoxin improves myocardial efficiency by improving contractility with only a moderate increase in oxygen consumption by the myocardium.

Nursing management

Nursing management of the person with congestive heart failure focuses on several specific problems. These include:

1 decreased cardiac output
2 fluid volume excess
3 anxiety
4 alteration in lifestyle and self-care.

Decreased cardiac output
Goals

1 The patient will demonstrate signs of improved cardiac contractility.
2 The patient will show signs of improved oxygenation.
3 The workload of the heart will be reduced.

Nursing intervention   Nursing intervention with patients who have heart failure will vary according to the severity of the symptoms. Some patients will be admitted to hospital with acute symptoms and others will be managed with mild symptoms in the community setting. In the acute situation inotropic agents such as digoxin, dobutamine and dopamine may be administered and will require close monitoring and specialist care. Nursing staff are responsible for the administration of these medications and monitoring for adverse reactions. Patients in the community may require, with the support of the nurse, to engage with structured exercise programmes to increase their functional capacity and they will need monitoring, support and advice as they work towards maximizing their treatment with ACE inhibitors and beta-blockers. The following considers a range of nursing interventions with patients who have heart failure, whether they are in the hospital setting with an acute exacerbation of their condition or they are in the community in a more stable situation.

Oxygenation of the tissues   Oxygen may be administered by mask or nasal cannulae to increase arterial oxygen concentration. It will be effective only if delivery to the tissues is improved.

The nurse should explain the procedure to the patient briefly and remain until the patient is accustomed to the mask or nasal cannulae. Observations are made of the patient's response to the oxygen. Its effectiveness will be indicated by reduced pulse rate, less dyspnoea, improvement in colour and less restlessness.

In severe pulmonary oedema, oxygen may be given under positive pressure (i.e. greater than atmosphere pressure) to counteract the movement of fluid from the capillaries into the alveoli.

Patients may require oxygen in the acute situation but may also need long-term treatment with oxygen in the home as they reach the terminal stages of their condition.

Administration of medication   Drugs that are used to treat heart failure are summarized in Table 12.8. The nurse will monitor the effectiveness of these medications and needs to ensure that each patient understands their medication. ACE inhibitors and beta-blockers, when given in small doses and gradually increased over several weeks, have a beneficial effect on the morbidity and mortality of patients with chronic heart failure (Clark et al 2000). Spironolactone has also proved beneficial in this respect. The nurse may note that these drugs have been added to the patient's medication regimen.

Promotion of rest   Rest is important in the treatment of the patient with heart failure because it reduces the demand on the heart by reducing body requirements for oxygen. For the patient in failure, rest in bed is necessary until the oedema has decreased.

Once the acute episode has passed, the patient is able to get out of bed for gradually increasing intervals. Intermittent rest periods during the day and after activities are arranged, and the patient rests before and after meals and between procedures.

Physical comfort will contribute to the patient's rest and may be promoted by change of position, bathing, warmth, etc. Anticipation of need and the planning and provision of undisturbed rest periods are important. Cooperation is sought from the laboratory, dietary and house-keeping staffs to minimize interruptions to rest periods. In the home the family should be informed of the need to rest properly and to avoid unnecessary stress for the patient.

Activity   Rest has been emphasized as an important phase of the treatment of cardiac patients, but it is well known that there are certain disadvantages inherent in bedrest. The limbs should be put through passive movements to promote venous drainage and prevent phlebo-thrombosis. Gentle massage is also helpful. If the patient's condition permits, it may be suggested that he or she gradually commences foot, leg and arm exercises. The patient is also encouraged to take 5–10 deep breaths every 1–2 hours to expand the lungs fully. As soon as possible, the patient is encouraged to get out of bed to use a commode, because the use of a bedpan for defaecation places considerable strain on the patient.

Observations are made of reactions to any activity so that undue stress on the heart may be avoided. These will also assist in defining the patient's future activities and the amount of rest and restriction that will be necessary. In the community the patient may engage with a rehabilitation programme in order to try to build up their physical fitness and their tolerance of exercise.

Positioning The patient should be positioned in such a way as to facilitate ease of breathing. The person who is experiencing dyspnoea will be more comfortable with the head of the bed elevated, but only by a sufficient amount to be effective.

Patients with congestive failure manifest orthopnoea, that is, less difficulty in breathing with the trunk in the upright position. A semi-upright or upright position increases the vital capacity and tends to reduce the volume of blood returned to the heart and the pulmonary system. Pressure of abdominal viscera on the diaphragm is reduced. Some patients may be still more comfortable in a true sitting position (i.e. with the lower limbs down). A special cardiac bed on which the foot of the bed can be lowered to provide a chair-like support is available. Alternatively the patient may find comfort from sitting in a chair. The sitting position promotes the formation of peripheral oedema in the dependent parts but relieves the pulmonary congestion to some extent; peripheral oedema is much less serious than pulmonary oedema.

In the sitting position, a pillow placed longitudinally at the patient's back may help to provide some comfort. Pillows should be used at the sides to support the arms and relieve the fatiguing pull on the shoulders. A change may be effected by arranging a table and pillow over the bed, upon which the head and arms may rest. Cot-sides may be kept up on the bed to safeguard the patient when in the upright position, as the patient may become drowsy and fall to the side, or may experience cerebral hypoxia which causes disorientation. The sides are also useful when a change of position is made because they may be grasped by the patient and used for added support. Patients in the upright position are encouraged to assume the recumbent position for brief periods to help reduce circulatory stasis and oedema in the lower parts of the body. However, patients should not be asked to do this if they are suffering from severe dyspnoea.

Good body alignment is essential to prevent contractures, hyperextension and circulatory stasis. *Even a slight change in position* every 1–2 hours is helpful. A footboard is used to prevent foot drop.

Elimination Constipation and straining at defaecation are to be avoided because of the undue strain placed on the heart. A mild laxative may have to be given to keep the stool soft. Abdominal distension is also to be avoided, because it raises the diaphragm and further inhibits the patient's breathing. Use of the bedpan requires more energy than getting out of bed and using a commode. Therefore it is preferable for the patient to use a bedside commode. When a patient receives a diuretic it will mean frequent use of the urinal, bedpan or commode, which can be very exhausting.

Fluid volume excess Some patients may be experiencing the symptoms of fluid overload. The nurse will need to administer medications to produce diuresis (Table 12.8) and will need to monitor the effectiveness and any adverse reactions of these. Low-sodium diets may be prescribed to reduce oedema and prevent further accumulation of fluid in the tissues. Sodium restriction varies with patients, depending upon their cardiac function and amount of oedema. Normally the average daily salt intake is 10 g daily.

Table 12.8 Medications used in the treatment of heart failure

Medication	Example	Comments
Diuretics	Furosemide, bendroflumethiazide, amiloride	For the relief of congestive symptoms and fluid retention, titrated up and down according to need
Angiotensin-converting enzyme (ACE) inhibitors	Enalapril, lisinopril, captopril, perindopril, ramipril	All patients with heart failure due to left ventricular dysfunction should be treated with ACEI; therapy should be titrated up to the optimal tolerated dose
Beta-blockers	Bisoprolol, cavedilol	Initiated in patients with heart failure due to left ventricular dysfunction after treatment with an ACE inhibitor and diuretic has been initiated
Aldosterone agonists	Spironolactone	Patients who remain symptomatic despite optimal therapy (specialist advice should be sought)
Digoxin	Digoxin	Patients with worsening or severe heart failure
Angiotensin II receptor agonists	Losartan, candesartan, irbesartan	May provide an alternative for patients who cannot tolerate ACE inhibitors but at the time of publication, angiotensin II receptor agonists are not licensed for the treatment of heart failure

NICE (2003b)

This is approximately double what is recommended for any person's needs. If no salt is added to food either at the table or in cooking, and no salted foods are used, the intake may be reduced to approximately 3 g. With the advent of the newer and more potent diuretic drugs, severe dietary sodium restriction is not mandatory, as it was previously for most patients with heart failure. A great deal of salt is found in ready-made meals, processed meats, soups and snacks. Food may initially appear tasteless without adding salt, but taste receptors do adjust over a few weeks, so that salted food is then difficult to take. A sodium content of less than 0.2 g per 100 g of food label is generally recommended (Hatchett 2001). The nurse should explain the purpose of the diet and relate it to symptoms the patient is experiencing. There are many spices and foods allowed that help to make a low-sodium diet more palatable.

If the patient with heart failure is overweight, the calorie intake is reduced in an effort to reduce weight. The lower-calorie diet should contain less fat but enough of the other foods to meet nutritional requirements.

Anxiety Patients who have been diagnosed with heart failure may become extremely fearful and anxious about the future. Their close relatives and friends may also be concerned and they will need a great deal of support and sensitive nursing care to deal with their fears and psychological distress. In addition to the activities listed above the nurse can help by providing information, listening to the worries of the patient and their family and simply by acting as a resource and support at times of distress. It is important to think ahead and anticipate the needs of the patient both in the hospital setting and at home. The patient may need to be introduced to the multidisciplinary team and may need the support of occupational therapists, physiotherapists and others to achieve the highest possible level of quality of life as they learn to live with their heart failure.

THE PERSON HAVING CARDIAC SURGERY

Correction of acquired heart disease includes surgery for coronary artery disease and for stenosed or incompetent cardiac valves. The fact that the heart must function immediately after operation presents a problem different from that in many areas of the body. The heart must heal while continuing to maintain adequate circulation. This creates the need for greater support and for minimizing physiological demands.

Progress in this area was delayed until the introduction of the pump-oxygenator (bypass machine). This machine permits extracorporeal (outside the body) oxygenation of blood and maintenance of circulation while the heart is arrested and opened to provide a direct surgical approach. During operation the heart is exposed by median sternotomy; the aorta is clamped off and cardiopulmonary bypass maintained via cannulae in the atria and descending aorta. Circulation thus bypasses the heart and lungs. The body temperature is lowered to 32°C in order to reduce the metabolic activity of the heart so that the cells can survive the interruption of the coronary circulation. In addition, to reduce metabolic demand further, cardiac arrest is induced by a variety of methods. This may be the use of electric paddles, which causes the heart to fibrillate (the muscle twitches rather than contracts), or through the use of high doses of potassium in a solution known as *cardioplegia* injected around the heart. The blood is heparinized in order to prevent coagulation and thrombus formation. On completion of the cardiopulmonary bypass, the heparin is neutralized by the administration of protamine sulfate.

After the procedure, the aorta is unclamped, the patient re-warmed and normal cardiac rhythm restored by internal defibrillation. Cardiopulmonary bypass is stopped, the cannulae removed and the chest closed. As a general rule the whole operation takes 3–4 hours.

The bypass machine is not without complications and these have been noted for several years. Those of particular note include the potential for neurological, renal and pulmonary damage. Neurological damage is the most significant. This can range from temporary memory loss and changes in personality, through to disorientation, agitation and inappropriate behaviour. The latter is known as *post-pump psychosis* or *delirium*, and the exact cause is unknown. The nurse can assist by orienting the patient to time and place, reducing noise levels and sensory overload, such as maintaining night and day patterns, and the use of familiar people such as family and friends. Ultimately, sedation may be required until recovery occurs over the following few days. At worse the patient may suffer a cerebrovascular accident (CVA), perhaps through emboli entering the cerebral circulation. Because of these effects, *off-pump* cardiac surgery has emerged. This form of surgery is performed on the beating heart, and may use a variety of mechanical devices to stabilize the area of the heart that the surgeon is working upon (Glenville 1999, Openshaw and Durbridge 2001).

Surgery for ischaemic heart disease

Both direct and indirect methods are used to revascularize the myocardium. The indirect method involves implanting the internal mammary artery into the myocardium, but is rarely used because revascularization is not immediate.

The most popular procedure is the *aortocoronary bypass surgery*, in which one end of a resected saphenous vein is anastomosed to the aorta and the other to the coronary artery beyond the point of obstruction. The right or left internal mammary artery may also be used as a grafting vessel. The blood supply to the myocardium is immediately improved.

The British Heart Foundation estimate that there are approximately 30 000 bypass operations carried out in the UK annually (British Heart Foundation 2005). This figure has undergone a six-fold increase since 1980. The overall mortality rate is approximately 3–4%. A strategy of early operation significantly reduces the mortality rate (Yusuf et al 1994). Coronary artery bypass grafts do not last indefinitely, and may require replacement in approximately 10 years. The mortality rate is higher for patients having a repeat procedure.

General indications for bypass surgery include:

- symptoms despite maximum medical therapy
- triple coronary vessel disease
- left mainstem coronary artery stenosis
- unstable angina.

The overall physical and psychological condition of the patient is generally taken into account. Patients who show a positive attitude toward risk factor modification (for example stopping smoking) may be more likely to have their case viewed favourably. Nurses may find themselves drawn into debates over issues such as whether smokers should be offered surgery. Patients who feel they have been unfairly treated may need specific support and advice.

Angioplasty (PTCA) may also be used in coronary artery disease (see p. 282).

Surgery for diseased valves

The surgeon can significantly enlarge the size of the orifice of stenosed valves in some individuals by dilating the valve. Others, however, may require valve replacement.

Certain patients with regurgitation of the aortic, mitral and/or tricuspid valves, who no longer respond to medical treatment, require total replacement. This is accomplished with an artificial valve prosthesis or the use of tissue homografts. Artificial valves require anticoagulation for life with warfarin to prevent thrombus formation on the valve. Tissue valves do not require this, but do not last as long. Tissue valves are usually advocated for patients such as women of childbearing age, for whom taking warfarin would be dangerous to the fetus, or the elderly.

PREOPERATIVE NURSING CARE

Most patients have tests such as cardiac catheterization carried out several weeks in advance and then return to the hospital 1–2 days before the operation. Time is needed before surgery to gather baseline information such as weight, fluid balance and vital signs. A range of blood tests including cross-matching and blood-clotting measurements will be necessary. Nurses are ideally placed to provide cardiac surgery patients with advice, information and support before surgery. Patients and their families need to be clear about the operation itself and likely effects for the future.

Informed written consent will need to be obtained and any worries or misconceptions addressed. Anxiety is a normal response to impending surgery. The individual needs to appreciate the risks of surgery balanced against the risks of continuing untreated. Some patients will need support to help them arrive at a decision regarding surgery. There is evidence of a positive association between the length of time patients have to wait for surgery and levels of anxiety, depression, and disturbed family relationships, irrespective of the severity of illness (Underwood et al 1993).

POSTOPERATIVE NURSING CARE

Nursing objectives for the patient include:

- monitoring and maintaining adequate respiratory and haemodynamic function
- pain relief
- assistance with activities of living
- psychological support
- evaluation of the recovery process
- preparation for discharge home.

Complications

Complications of bypass grafting include:

- angina
- pain at both chest incision and graft sites
- leakage at the incision site producing discomfort and shock
- hypertension as a result of increased sympathetic activity produced by lack of blood flow during operation
- shortness of breath due to heart failure or chest infection
- hyperglycaemia as a result of increased sympathetic response
- confusion or disorientation due to the effects of the bypass machine, cerebral hypoxia, medication and/or sepsis.

The patient is mechanically ventilated until normal body temperature has been regained. Prolonged ventilation increases the risk of complications such as chest infection and pulmonary damage. Therefore, in many units, nurse-led extubation occurs. The nurse will assess the patient and follow a set plan, integrated care pathway or algorithm. When the nurse considers that all parameters have been met, including satisfactory blood gases, respiratory pattern and body temperature, the endotracheal tube is removed and an oxygen mask is put in place. Arterial and central venous pressure (CVP) lines are used to monitor cardiac pressures for the first 18–24 hours. Any cardiac arrhythmia or change in heart rate is detected with a cardiac monitor. Blood pressure, pulse and respirations need to be monitored closely. Fluid input and output are recorded to detect possible fluid retention. One of the major roles of the nurse is to administer intravenous fluids and possibly an inotrope (a drug that stimulates cardiac contractility) depending upon the patient's haemodynamic status.

Level of consciousness, orientation and restlessness need to be observed as they may be linked to a fall in cardiac output/blood pressure or occur as a result of hypoxia, as well as inadequate pain relief. Any weakness or loss of function, possibly a result of a thrombus or embolus, needs to be reported. The chest drainage system needs to be observed at regular intervals to check that it is functioning correctly and the drainage observed for possible bleeding around the heart. One of the dangers of cardiac surgery is *cardiac tamponade* (bleeding below the pericardium). This is indicated by rising CVP, falling blood pressure and tachycardia.

This is an emergency situation and the surgeon will have to reopen the chest, stop the bleeding and evacuate the accumulated blood.

Dressings on the chest and graft sites need to be checked regularly for excessive bleeding and haematoma formation. Compression stockings may be used to reduce venous stasis and the risk of thromboembolic complications. The patient will usually be able to eat a solid diet on the first or second post-operative day. Intravenous fluids will be given before this. Mouth care may ease the discomfort of a dry mouth and help to prevent infection. Activity is increased as tolerated over the first 2 days and early mobilization is encouraged. The patient's way of coping needs to be assessed so that appropriate support can be given. Patients are usually ready for discharge after about a week.

Pain and discomfort

Pain from median sternotomy may cause discomfort for a few weeks; there may also be discomfort from incision sites. Leg pain and swelling may still be present for up to 1 year after operation. Delayed wound healing may also be a problem. Activities such as sneezing, coughing, bending over, raising the hand above the head and twisting to the side may cause difficulty. Helping the patient to hug a cushion when coughing supports the sternum and aids more effective expectoration. Patients may need help with washing and dressing for the first few weeks. Angina is likely to return in about 25% of patients within 5 years of bypass surgery, although the symptoms are not necessarily as severe as before operation.

Information for recovery

The increasing trend for shorter hospital stays minimizes the time available for information giving and support for discharge. It is therefore important that the time available is used effectively to establish a relationship with the patient and family on which to build individualized care. Finally, staff members need support and guidance concerning the patient's likely recovery pattern (Knoll and Johnson 2000). Patients need realistic expectations. A positive outcome for surgery does not have to mean a complete reversion to a pre-symptomatic lifestyle. Alternative goals may be more appropriate. Knowing how each individual perceives their situation may assist in helping them to identify realistic outcomes. Many patients find their early progress disappointing. Exercise tolerance may be less than expected. Pain may be more severe than anticipated. Appropriately supervised and progressive exercise programmes can be helpful in identifying problems, increasing activity levels, boosting confidence and providing support. Outpatient support via telephone links has been found to be associated with positive feelings about recovery, although there is evidence that, although helpful, such support does not necessarily reduce levels of anxiety and depression in the early period following discharge (Roebuck 1999). Those who have been severely restricted by angina for many years may find the return to normality difficult to cope with. The potential for a change in lifestyle is not always welcome.

Families need to be aware of the possibility of mood swings and signs of anxiety and/or depression. Short-term memory loss and difficulties with concentration are not uncommon. Some individuals experience feelings of poor self-esteem and of anticlimax.

DISORDERS OF THE VASCULAR SYSTEM

Disorders may involve arteries or veins. Arterial disorder commonly leads to a reduction in blood supply to peripheral tissue resulting in ischaemic pain and possibly gangrene. Alternatively the patient may experience continuously raised arterial blood pressure, known as hypertension. Venous problems lead to interference with the normal drainage of venous blood back to the heart causing congestion and oedema within the tissues. Vascular conditions may be chronic, developing slowly over a considerable period of time, or they may be sudden and acute.

HYPERTENSION

Hypertension is a condition in which there is a sustained increase in arterial blood pressure. Defining hypertension is problematic, because the normal range does vary – creating a blurring between normotensive and hypertensive people. A blood pressure of 135/85 mmHg may be seen as acceptable, but if the patient has a condition such as diabetes or renal disease this blood pressure recording may be considered to be too high.

It is absolutely essential that the blood pressure is measured accurately. Figure 12.31 outlines the steps that are important to measure a patient's blood pressure. Treatment decisions are made on the results of blood pressure recordings and therefore it is the responsibility of the nurse to make sure that the results are an accurate reflection of the patient's condition.

Antihypertensive drug treatment is recommended for those with a sustained systolic blood pressure reading of 160 mmHg or greater, or a diastolic pressure of 100 mmHg or more (Williams et al 2004). In the presence of target organ damage or a cardiovascular disease risk of 20% or greater the threshold for treatment is lower (see Fig. 12.31). Cardiovascular risk can be calculated using the risk prediction charts which can be found in the British National Formulary (2006).

Sustained hypertension is a serious condition and is sometimes termed 'the silent killer', because few if any symptoms may be encountered until organ damage has occurred. A sustained increase in blood pressure results in vascular disease. The changes in the arterial walls involve thickening and sclerosis, which alter the blood supply to tissues and ultimately may reduce their functional ability. The arterial wall may develop necrotic areas that may

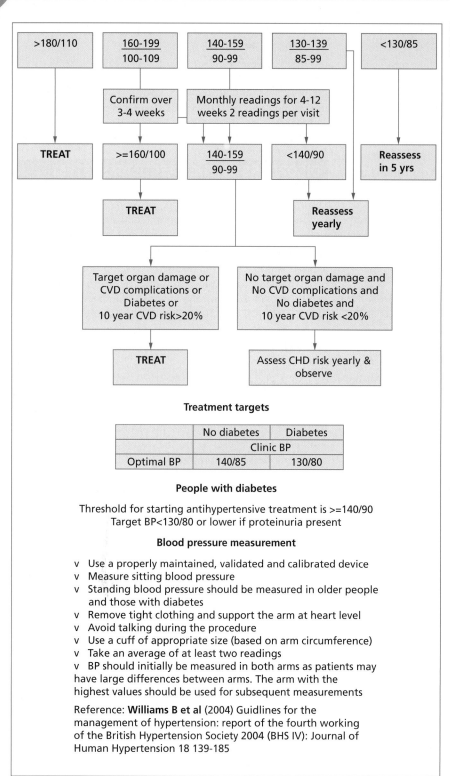

Figure 12.31 Thresholds for intervention in patients with hypertension. (British Hypertensive Society 2004).

weaken or rupture under high pressure. The wall may also thicken and so narrow the lumen of the artery. Thrombosis is likely with such diseased arterial walls.

Four organs that are the most frequent targets for damage are the heart, kidneys, brain and eyes. The sustained increase in arterial blood pressure greatly increases the workload of the heart. The myocardium hypertrophies in response to the increased demands, but there is not an adequate increase in the coronary blood supply and eventually some pump failure develops. Hypertension is a major risk factor for developing coronary disease. Thickening and sclerosis of the coronary arteries may cause ischaemic heart disease, the

patient may experience angina pectoris or suffer a myocardial infarction. Kidney function becomes impaired as the result of sclerosing haemorrhage or thrombosis of the renal arteries, which destroys functional tissue. Retinal haemorrhages and oedema of the optic disc can occur, resulting in degenerative changes in the eyes.

Types of hypertension

Hypertension may be classified by aetiology as *primary* (essential) or *secondary*. Approximately 90% of people with hypertensive disease are said to have essential hypertension; the remaining 10% have secondary hypertension.

Primary or essential hypertension

Primary hypertension is most frequently referred to as *essential* or *idiopathic hypertension*. The cause of this type of hypertensive disease is not known; no initial disturbance in the areas commonly associated with secondary hypertension has been established. It may cause cardiac or kidney disease but is not preceded by either. Heredity is thought to be a factor, because most persons with the condition have a history of a parent or grandparent having had it.

Secondary hypertension

Secondary hypertension is distinguished from essential hypertension by having an identifiable cause. Common causes include renal disease, endocrine disorders and medications.

Renal disease Any condition that reduces blood flow through the kidneys or destroys renal functional tissue causes hypertension. Examples of such conditions are sclerotic changes or stenosis of a renal artery, nephritis and polycystic disease. The ischaemic kidney reacts by secreting a proteolytic enzyme called renin. In the bloodstream, renin acts upon a plasma protein to produce angiotensin I, which is then converted to angiotensin II by another enzyme, primarily in the lining of the lungs. Angiotensin II causes widespread vasoconstriction of the arterioles and increased peripheral resistance, leading to an increase in arterial blood pressure. Angiotensin II also inhibits the secretion of aldosterone by the adrenal glands, which increases the blood pressure through its influence on sodium and water retention.

Endocrine disorders A phaeochromocytoma is a tumour of the adrenal medulla. Tumours may be single or multiple. The tumour cells secrete adrenaline, in the same way as normal medullary cells; this produces vasoconstriction and an increased cardiac output with a corresponding increase in arterial blood pressure. Removal of the tumour restores a normal blood pressure.

An increased output of aldosterone by the cortex of the adrenal glands may also be responsible for hypertension. The increased secretion may be idiopathic or may be due to a tumour. Aldosterone increases the reabsorption of sodium by the kidney, leading to water retention and an expansion of the intravascular volume, increasing the arterial blood pressure. Aldosterone may also have a direct vasocon-

stricting effect. A general increase in the secretion of all of the adrenocorticoids causes Cushing's disease, which is also accompanied by hypertension.

Medications Some women taking oral contraceptives may develop hypertension. It is thought that the oestrogen component of the pills may be responsible by stimulating hepatic synthesis of angiotensinogen, which leads to increased amounts of angiotensin. If the contraceptive agent is discontinued for 6 months, blood pressure usually returns to normal.

Symptoms

A person may have an abnormally high arterial blood pressure for a long period without symptoms. The condition is often discovered on a routine physical examination. Those who do experience symptoms may complain of a throbbing occipital headache or migraine. The headache may be accompanied by weakness, dizziness, visual disturbances, epistaxis, palpitations, angina pectoris and dyspnoea. Symptoms of emotional instability, memory lapses and personality changes may indicate cerebrovascular damage. Later, other manifestations appear as the heart, kidneys, brain or eyes become damaged by the persisting hypertension. The person who manifests even a slight increase above the normal in both systolic and diastolic blood pressures should undergo careful investigation to determine a possible primary cause. Several systems may be investigated in an attempt to identify the cause of hypertension; tests include, ECG, urinalysis, urea and electrolytes and lipid levels as a minimum.

Medical treatment

If the hypertension is secondary, treatment is directed toward correcting the primary condition. In essential hypertension, treatment is directed at: (1) lowering the blood pressure in an effort to prevent serious complications; and (2) having the patient adjust life to reduce the demands on the cardiovascular system and kidneys. The treatment depends on the blood pressure and the signs and symptoms of impaired function in vulnerable organs. The patient with borderline hypertension may simply be advised to reduce weight, stop smoking, decrease salt intake, increase exercise and engage with stress reduction techniques. People with more severe hypertension will receive drug therapy to lower the blood pressure (Table 12.9).

Nursing care

Goals

1 The patient's blood pressure is within normal limits.
2 The patient can describe the disease process and the factors contributing to disease management.
3 The patient can describe health behaviours needed to manage the hypertension.
4 The patient actively participates in a disease management programme.

Table 12.9 Examples of oral medications used in management of hypertension

Group	Example	General action
Angiotensin-converting enzyme (ACE) inhibitors	Captopril, ramipril, enalapril	Inhibit the conversion of angiotensin I to angiotensin II
Alpha-adrenoceptor blocking drugs	Prazosin, doxazosin	Peripheral arteriolar vasodilator
Beta-adrenoceptor blocking drugs	Propranolol, atenolol, bisoprolol, carvedilol	Block β-adrenergic receptors of sympathetic nervous system
Calcium-channel blockers	Nifedipine, amlodipine, felodipine	Interfere with the inward displacement of calcium ions
Angiotensin-II receptor antagonists	Losartan, eprosartan, irbesartan	Similar to ACE inhibitors and have their effect on the renin angiotensin system
Diuretics Thiazides	Bendroflumethiazide	Inhibit sodium reabsorption in the kidney
Loop	Furosemide	Powerful diuretics that inhibit reabsorption in the loop of Henlé
Potassium sparing	Amiloride	Causes retention of potassium

Nursing intervention

Diet

- Discuss with patient and family the need to achieve and maintain a normal bodyweight as this may facilitate lowering of blood pressure
- Reduction of sodium intake is likely because excess sodium expands intravascular volume and aggravates hypertension. The degree of restriction depends on the severity of disease. A 'no added salt' diet may be recommended. If adequate sodium reduction is achieved by diet, drug therapy is likely to be reduced. Patients should generally aim for foods with less than 0.2 g per 100 g, and be informed to avoid those with a high sodium content (e.g. processed meats, soups, ready-made meals and certain snack foods)
- Reduction of alcohol intake is recommended because alcohol increases the risk of obesity and may cause a rise in blood pressure. The recommended intake is 3–4 units of alcohol per day for men and 2–3 units for women with 2 days break during the week. Binge drinking, for example saving up the daily units, is an unhealthy practice.

Exercise   Discuss with the patient a plan of regular exercise to be undertaken once the hypertension is under control. Regular physical activity is a beneficial strategy to achieve and maintain a satisfactory weight.

Stopping smoking   Great emphasis should be placed on encouraging patients to stop smoking as the coexistence of smoking as an additional risk factor in hypertensive patients confers a greatly increased risk of subsequent cardiovascular events.

Stress management   The relationship between stress and hypertension has not been clearly defined. However, stress reduction is advocated as a health promotion activity:

- Encourage the person to express feelings of stress and to identify stressors in the environment that are both avoidable and unavoidable. Facilitate the patient's planning of strategies that can be used to reduce or eliminate the available stressors in a defined time
- Teach the patient relaxation techniques that can be used to reduce stress in a variety of settings. There are a number of resources available in the community to teach relaxation techniques, as well as books, cassette tapes and compact discs which can be purchased.

Medications

- Medications required to control hypertension need to be taken regularly for long periods of time. This may be difficult for the patient to understand if they feel asymptomatic. Ensure that the patient and family have accurate perceptions of the use and need for these drugs and their possible side-effects
- Assist the patient in developing a simple, convenient schedule to take medications that is tailored to fit personal habits
- Discuss side-effects of the patient's medication and encourage the patient to seek advice if side-effects occur. One important and reasonably common side-effect of antihypertensive treatment is erectile dysfunction. It is important to ask the patient if this side-effect has occurred because it could be a difficult subject for the patient to approach. A non-threatening questioning technique can help to address these concerns, for example: 'There are a number of side-effects from most blood pressure tablets and these include skin rashes, dizziness, lethargy and problems with getting an erection; have you experienced any of these problems?'

Evaluation

Evaluate the effectiveness of care by assessing whether the patient:

1 has blood pressure within normal limits identified for him or her
2 can describe hypertension and the factors contributing to disease management
3 can discuss behaviours being followed to promote health.

ARTERIAL DISORDERS

Aortic aneurysm

An aneurysm is a saccular dilatation of the wall of an artery and develops as a result of weakness in the wall of the vessel in that area. The weakness in the majority of cases is due to atherosclerosis but may also be caused by an infectious disease (e.g. syphilis), congenital defect, trauma or a condition of the connective tissue such as Marfan syndrome. The aorta and cerebral arteries are the most common sites of aneurysms.

The aneurysm that does not extend completely around the artery is referred to as a *saccular aneurysm*. If it involves the complete circumference, it is classified as a *fusiform aneurysm* (Fig. 12.32).

Separation of the layers of the aorta is referred to as a *dissecting* aortic aneurysm, even though no dilatation may be present. The tear is often in the intima and may be due to bleeding in the medial layer from the vasa vasorum. The dissection may extend lengthwise for a considerable distance and may involve branches of the aorta. The aortic aneurysm may also be classified according to the section of the artery in which the defect is located; for example, it may be designated as a thoracic or abdominal aortic aneurysm.

A serious threat to any patient with an aneurysm is rupture of the weakened vascular area: the rapid loss of blood almost always proves fatal.

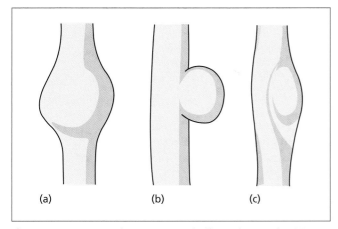

Figure 12.32 Types of aneurysm: (a) fusiform; (b) saccular; (c) dissecting.

Manifestations

Signs and symptoms may be absent until the aneurysm is large enough to compress adjacent structures. The majority of aortic aneurysms are abdominal. The patient may complain of mid-abdominal, lumbar or pelvic pain, often severe. Physical examination may reveal an expansile, abdominal mass. Femoral pulses may be reduced. The patient with a thoracic aneurysm may experience chest pain, dyspnoea, hoarseness due to vocal cord paralysis and/or congestion of the veins in the neck because of pressure on the superior vena cava. With an abdominal aneurysm, careful physical examination, radiography, echocardiography and/or aortography are means of confirming the diagnosis. Scanning techniques such as computed tomography, which may be performed with contrast dye to enhance results, and magnetic resonance imaging (MRI) are also used to provide images of the aneurysm.

Symptoms of a dissecting aortic aneurysm include pain, often described as ripping or tearing in nature, which may involve the chest, back and/or abdomen. There may be a discrepancy in pulses at various locations in the body. This is a serious situation with a need to control the pain, which may be severe, and to lower and stabilize the blood pressure with intravenous drugs such as a beta-blocker. This reduces the haemodynamic stress on the aortic wall. Controlling the blood pressure is very important to reduce the risk of the aneurysm rupturing. Occasionally hypotension may present, but hypertension is more common.

Treatment

In recent years, encouraging advances have been made in the surgical treatment of aneurysms. If a small blood vessel is affected, it may be tied off and the flow of blood diverted to another artery. In treating an aortic aneurysm, the area is resected and replaced with a graft of inert synthetic material such as Teflon or Dacron, which does not cause tissue reaction.

Arterial occlusion

Acute occlusion occurs suddenly as a result of external compression, thrombosis or embolism. It is serious because there is a lack of collateral circulation to the tissues supplied by this artery.

Arterial thrombosis occurs with the formation of an abnormal blood clot (*thrombus*) within an artery, usually as the result of narrowing of the lumen of the artery by atherosclerotic changes. The stasis in the blood flow predisposes to the formation of the clot, partially or completely blocking the vessel. If the vessel is not completely blocked, treatment is directed towards preventing the clot from enlarging to occlude the vessel and towards keeping it at the site of formation to prevent an embolism.

Arterial embolism is the blocking of an artery by a foreign mass that has been carried by the bloodstream until it reaches an artery too small for it to pass through. The foreign mass is referred to as an *embolus*.

Most frequently an embolus consists of a thrombus that breaks loose from its site of origin, but it may consist of air, fragments of vegetations from diseased cardiac valves, fat, atherosclerotic plaques or small masses of tissue or cancerous cells. The effects of an embolism are determined by the localization of the embolus. Obviously, if it is an end-artery, the tissue entirely dependent upon that artery becomes necrotic. An embolus originating in a vein or the right side of the heart is likely to cause a pulmonary embolism blocking the arterial supply to an area of lung tissue. One arising from the left side of the heart or a large systemic artery may produce a cerebral embolism or may plug a smaller artery. The site of arterial occlusion by an embolus may also be a lower extremity.

Chronic arterial occlusion can develop as a result of gradual changes in the walls of the vessels, causing narrowing of the lumen. It may also be of functional origin due to hyperactivity of the sympathetic nervous system, causing excessive vasoconstriction. Gradual occlusion of an artery allows for collateral circulation to be established, which ensures a supply of oxygenated blood to peripheral tissue, for at least a while.

The most common causes of chronic occlusion are atherosclerosis and arteriosclerosis. The arteries in any area of the body may be affected, but the coronary, cerebral and renal arteries are frequent sites. When the abdominal aorta and/or medium- and large-sized arteries are involved, the condition may be referred to as *arteriosclerosis obliterans*. The arteries of the extremities are also a relatively frequent site of chronic occlusion which may be referred to as *peripheral vascular disease*. In this condition there is progressive loss of the blood supply to the legs, leading to intermittent claudication and the appearance of necrotic tissue, usually on the toes and feet. Patients are typically of late middle age to elderly, have a history of smoking, and are often diabetic. Amputation may be necessary; this is discussed in detail in Chapter 24.

Two other forms of peripheral vascular disease are Raynaud's disease and thromboangiitis obliterans.

Raynaud's disease is a condition in which episodes of excessive vasoconstriction occur in the digits of the hands and/or feet. The cause is obscure, but the episodes are most frequently precipitated by cold or emotional stress. The disease is more common in women, usually develops before the age of 40–45 years and is bilateral.

Thromboangiitis obliterans (Buerger's disease) is a chronic occlusive disease in which there is an inflammation and thickening of the walls of limb arteries, predisposing to thrombosis. It has a higher incidence in young men and in Jewish people. The parts are very tender and painful, and necrotic areas develop in the distal portions of the digits. The condition is seriously aggravated if the person smokes. The cause of this disease is unknown.

Signs and symptoms of arterial insufficiency in the extremities

Gradual reduction in the arterial blood supply to the extremities produces the following signs and symptoms.

Intermittent claudication   This is leg pain that occurs with exercise and is relieved by rest. The blood supply is sufficient to meet the tissue needs when the part is at rest. However, with exercise, oxygen demands cannot be met and metabolic wastes are not readily removed from the muscle tissue. The result is ischaemic muscle pain. Rest allows increased supply of oxygen to tissues and removal of metabolic waste, thus relieving the discomfort. This symptom usually worsens progressively and increasingly limits the distance a patient may walk before the pain occurs.

Rest pain   Muscle leg pain at rest indicates advanced peripheral vascular disease. This pain may be described as burning or numbing and may become more prominent at night.

Peripheral pulses   Peripheral pulses may be absent or weakened. A Doppler flowmeter may be used to listen to the pulsation of arteries in an area where the vessels are deeper and cannot be palpated by the fingers. A comparison is made of the pulses in both legs and may reveal that one is weaker than the other, indicating partial occlusion in that leg. Complete occlusion could be indicated by an absence of the pulse.

Colour   A difference in the colour of the two extremities or an abnormal change in both extremities, if both are involved, will probably be present. In Caucasians the skin may become white and blanched, or it may become dusky red or mottled, depending on the amount of blood in the capillaries and the amount of reduced haemoglobin in the blood. On being raised, the limb becomes even paler as the venous drainage increases but, on being lowered, it fails to increase its colour quickly as the normal limb would do with the rush of arterial blood into it. The superficial veins are slow in filling when the limb is lowered; normally, they fill in approximately 5 seconds.

Skin changes   The skin temperature and moisture may be different in the two limbs. The affected one exhibits a coldness to the touch and may be unusually moist. Limb tissues may atrophy, causing the affected limb to become smaller than the other. The skin becomes dry and shiny, and loses its hair. Nails thicken and become brittle and ridged.

Necrosis   Ulcerated or gangrenous areas may develop, denoting areas of tissue completely deprived of blood supply. Ulceration is a superficial area of devitalized tissue; gangrene is a more massive area of dead tissue.

Diagnosis

In most instances, a thorough history and an adequate vascular physical examination result in an accurate diagnosis of occlusive arterial disease. Various tests may be used to diagnose and assess vascular disease.

Exercise tolerance   The patient is required to walk or perform some form of exercise until intermittent claudication occurs. The length of time from the start of activity until the occurrence of pain is noted.

Ankle brachial pressure index The systolic blood pressure in the legs should be equal to or slightly higher than the systolic pressure in the upper limbs. When arterial narrowing occurs, a reduction in pressure occurs distal to the lesion. The ankle brachial pressure index is calculated from the ratio of ankle to brachial systolic pressure (Donnelly et al 2000). It is a sensitive marker of arterial insufficiency.

A Doppler probe will assist in detecting blood flow at the ankle which occurs as the sphygmomanometer cuff is deflated, indicating the lower limb systolic pressure. When the brachial systolic pressure is divided by ankle systolic pressure, the result should be greater than 1. A ratio of less than 0.9 indicates the presence of arterial disease, and if the ratio is less than 0.5 severe ischaemia is present (Vowden 2001).

Doppler ultrasonography Doppler ultrasonography is based on the principle that the frequency of reflected sound waves from moving objects (such as red blood cells) shifts in proportion to the velocity of the object and the direction of movement. Continuous-wave Doppler ultrasonographic equipment produces an audible signal when the probe is held over the artery, indicating movement of blood in the vessel (Donnelly et al 2000).

Duplex ultrasonography The combination of real-time ultrasonography and Doppler studies is being used increasingly in the evaluation of patients with arterial disease. A two-dimensional picture of the reflected ultrasound waves is provided. Characteristic changes can be seen near areas of stenosis. The great advantage is that it is non-invasive and in some parts of the body (e.g. carotid vessels) its accuracy in assessing the degree of stenosis is comparable to that of arteriography. Furthermore, the Doppler aspect of the study yields valuable information about the haemodynamic significance of any stenosis identified.

Angiography A radio-opaque contrast medium containing iodine is introduced into the arteries, and radiographs are taken. Arterial narrowing or obstruction may be located in this way, and some information regarding the amount of collateral circulation present may also be obtained.

Magnetic resonance angiography This technique has developed rapidly over recent years. It can image a moving column of blood, but does not require ionizing radiation or iodinated contrast dye (Donnelly et al 2000). It is limited by both cost issues and accessibility to the scanning equipment.

Medical management
Vasodilating and anticoagulant drugs have been used to treat patients with arterial occlusive disease.

Although many drugs are promoted as agents capable of increasing peripheral blood flow, many are universally ineffective. Any α-adrenergic blocking drug will increase the flow through the skin, but no drug can increase flow to muscles when the underlying disease is atherosclerosis of a major artery.

Anticoagulant drugs may be prescribed to prevent and treat thrombosis. The most widely used anticoagulants are heparin and warfarin. Aspirin may be used to prevent platelet aggre-gation. Heparin is given parenterally because it has no effect orally. It is thought to block the effect of thrombin on fibrinogen, thereby preventing clot formation. Heparin therapy is usually extended over several days and then gradually replaced by a warfarin preparation given orally. Warfarin takes effect in approximately 48 hours, so it is started before the heparin is withdrawn.

The dosage and frequency of warfarin administration is dependent upon the prothrombin time, which indicates the effectiveness of the extrinsic system in producing clotting. It is reported as the international normalized ratio (INR). The dosage of heparin is decided by the partial thromboplastin time (PTT), which is another measure of clotting time. A therapeutic level is generally considered to be 1.5 times to twice the normal values for PTT although the therapeutic target will vary according to the patient's medical condition.

Warfarin carries the risk of producing haemorrhage as a side-effect, especially as it is prone to interaction with other drugs that potentiate its effects. Broad-spectrum antibiotics, such as erythromycin and metronidazole, are one such group of drugs. These drugs produce the risk of bleeding but their therapeutic value may be considered to outweigh this risk.

The nurse's responsibilities include close observation for signs of haemorrhage. The patient should be taught to monitor this potential problem for themselves before discharge. Profuse bleeding from minor cuts, bleeding gums, haematuria, haematemesis, blood in the stool, petechiae and abnormal vaginal bleeding indicate problems and should be reported promptly. In the event of bleeding, the drug is discontinued, and vitamin K (for those taking warfarin) and a blood transfusion may be given to counteract the reduced coagulation. Protamine sulfate, a heparin antagonist, is given if severe bleeding occurs as a result of heparin administration.

The prothrombin or partial thromboplastin time is determined before the anticoagulant drug is administered. Patients outside the hospital taking anticoagulants are usually required to report to the clinic, initially weekly, for an international normalized ratio (INR) level check.

Surgical management of arterial disease
A direct surgical approach may be employed in which the surgeon chooses to perform an endarterectomy, bypass or graft. An endarterectomy is the removal of the thickened intima and atheromatous plaques from the artery, and is used when the disease is localized to a relatively small area. The establishment of a bypass channel in order to reduce the arterial insufficiency may be achieved by transplanting one end of another artery into the occluded artery below the site of obstruction or by an autogenous venous graft. The latter consists of the removal of a section of vein (usually the saphenous), reversing it (because of the valves) to ensure flow in the right direction and attaching it to the affected artery above and below the occlusion. The surgeon often elects to resect the affected segment of the artery and replace it with an inert synthetic (Teflon or Dacron) graft. This type of graft is relatively porous and is eventually incorporated

into host tissues. An intima develops within it fairly quickly as cells proliferate through the interstices and from the host intima of the artery at each end of the graft. A layer of fibrous tissue also develops on the exterior surface, reinforcing the tube.

The most common site of major vascular surgery for occlusive disease is the aorta and the iliac and femoral arteries. Failure of surgical intervention may lead to amputation of the affected limb as ischaemic pain becomes continuous and gangrene may develop.

Nursing care

Arterial occlusive disease (peripheral vascular disease) is a chronic condition, and the patient will probably have to continue with the prescribed care and precautions indefinitely. This may create considerable hardship for the patient and family, depending on the severity of the disease and the limitations it imposes. Adjustments may have to be made in occupational and social life; the patient may become partially or completely dependent financially and for personal care, and will certainly find it difficult to accept the situation. The nurse must be alert to the possible implications for the patient and family, and should provide the necessary assistance and guidance.

Impaired skin integrity related to ischaemia

Goals
1 The patient will have intact skin.
2 The patient will inspect the skin daily.

Nursing intervention The patient is taught to inspect the skin daily for signs of irritation or injury. The presence of neuropathy may reduce the person's awareness or perception of pain, thus daily inspection may be the only reliable indicator of skin integrity.

Daily bathing in comfortably warm (not hot) water using a mild soap is recommended. Gentle and thorough drying is important, and special attention is given to the areas between the digits. If the skin is dry, the limbs may be gently massaged with a light emollient. Nails are cut straight across but not right down to the soft tissue. Corns should be removed by a chiropodist; the patient should not undertake to 'pare' them with sharp instruments.

The patient is advised of the importance of well-fitting shoes and socks or stockings. Socks should be loose and are changed daily. The patient is instructed to avoid walking about in bare feet: a cut, abrasion or infection could be serious because resistance to infection is lowered and healing is poor as a result of the impaired blood supply. If injury does occur, even of a minor nature, it should receive prompt medical attention as the potential for sepsis and gangrene is great.

Good general nutrition is essential to promote tissue healing and prevent tissue breakdown.

Decreased tissue perfusion related to reduced blood flow

Goals The patient will have:

1 extremities warmer to touch
2 improved colour of skin
3 reduced oedema of extremities.

Nursing intervention

Positioning The horizontal position is used when the patient rests. Occasionally, raising the head of the bed may be used to encourage the flow of blood into the lower limbs by gravity. Position should be changed at frequent intervals throughout the day, and long periods of standing must be avoided. The patient is advised not to cross the legs and, when sitting, pressure on the popliteal region should be avoided. If ambulatory, the patient sits or lies down every 2–3 hours and elevates the feet for 10–15 minutes.

Exercise Many authorities indicate the most effective treatment for intermittent claudication is physical exercise, especially walking. It is suggested that the patient should walk for 20–30 minutes each day at a slow to moderate pace on a level surface. The patient may do this by walking to the point of intermittent claudication, stopping until the discomfort disappears, and then continuing to walk until the distress develops again. The underlying theory is that exercise increases collateral circulation.

Passive and active exercises may also be prescribed: flexion and extension of the legs, feet and toes may be used for lower limbs, and similar exercises may be employed for the arms and fingers if these are the sites of the arterial insufficiency. Exercises promote emptying and filling of the vessels and stimulate the development of collateral circulation.

Protection from cold Exposure to cold with lowering of normal body temperature produces undesirable responses: peripheral vasoconstriction and increased metabolism. Special precautions are necessary in cold weather. Extra, warm clothing should be worn. If exposure to cold precipitates an episode, the patient is advised to take a warm drink and seek a warm environment. Local heat applications to the affected parts are discouraged because there is a reduced nerve sensitivity leading to the risk of localized tissue damage. The patient is advised to wear warm socks or to wrap the feet in a warm blanket rather than applying a hot-water bottle.

Smoking The use of tobacco should be discontinued, because it promotes vasoconstriction and aggravates the disease. The patient should be given advice and an explanation relating to the effects of smoking and should be given all the necessary support to engage with smoking cessation.

VENOUS DISORDERS

Reduction in venous return leads to congestion and oedema, which interfere with normal cell function and eventually prevent a normal arterial volume from reaching tissue cells. Common venous conditions are varicose veins, deep vein thrombosis (DVT), thrombophlebitis and phlebothrombosis.

Varicose veins

When venous blood meets with increased resistance to its forward flow, the walls of the veins become dilated and tortuous, the valves become damaged and incompetent, and the blood tends to pool and stagnate. The condition may be referred to as varicosities, or as varicose veins. Trunk varices are varicosities in the line of the long or short saphenous vein, or one of its branches in the legs. Reticular veins are dilated, tortuous subcutaneous veins, not belonging to the main branches of the long or short saphenous vein. Telangiectasia are intradermal and are often called thread or spider veins (London and Nash 2000). The superficial veins of the lower extremities are most susceptible. Because of our upright position, the venous pressure in the lower limbs is increased by gravity. Other common sites of varicosities are the veins of the anal canal (haemorrhoids), spermatic veins (varicocele), oesophageal veins (oesophageal varices) and the vulvar veins in pregnant women due to pressure from the enlarging uterus. Although resistance to the flow of blood is the main cause of varicosities, it is now believed that they are caused by inherently weak vein walls, which leads to dilatation and separation of the valve cusps in the vein (London and Nash 2000). Long periods of standing, obesity and increasing age can all predispose to the development of varicose veins in the lower extremities.

Manifestations

Varicose veins cause local oedema of the tissues, crampy pains or aching, and a full, heavy feeling in the affected area. The congestion and oedema in the tissues interfere with the normal supply of oxygen and nutrients reaching the cells, leading to fibrosing of subcutaneous tissues and, in some instances, necrosis of superficial tissue, producing what is referred to as a varicose ulcer. The affected area appears swollen and discoloured, and the veins are seen as tortuous, bulbous protrusions. These veins readily become inflamed (phlebitis), and occasionally the vessel wall ruptures, causing haemorrhage.

Diagnosis

The test most frequently performed for varicosities in the lower limbs is the *Trendelenburg test*. While the patient is in the horizontal position, the leg is elevated above the level of the pelvis until the superficial veins appear to be empty. The patient then stands, and the veins are observed as they fill. Normally they fill relatively slowly from below; with varicosities, the incompetent valves allow them to fill from above as well. Hand-held Doppler or colour duplex scanning is used to assess the structure and functioning of the veins.

Conservative management

The patient is instructed to avoid situations and factors that tend to increase the resistance to venous flow, to provide support to the veins and tissues by elastic compression stockings, and to assist drainage by elevation of the limb at intervals.

Surgical treatment

With more severe varicosities in the lower limbs, surgical treatment in the form of ligation and stripping of the veins may be employed in some people. The affected vein is ligated above the varicosity, its connecting branches are severed and tied. The venous blood then returns via the deep veins. The great saphenous vein is the one most frequently ligated. This necessitates several small horizontal incisions along the course of the vein. Compression bandages are applied from the foot to the groin after the operation, and the foot of the bed is elevated. The nurse observes the feet for colour and warmth to assess for an adequate circulation, and the incision sites are inspected for signs of bleeding. Mobilization is encouraged at an early stage, often on the day of operation if the patient is able, and certainly the next day. This facilitates good venous return. Standing is avoided. Compression stockings are provided for several weeks at home. The patient can return to work within 1–3 weeks depending on the occupation and its association with risk factors such as heavy lifting. Weight reduction is advised and support offered, straining at stool is discouraged, while regular walking is actively encouraged, increasing the distance each day.

Deep vein thrombosis

A **deep vein thrombosis** (DVT) is a blood clot occurring in the deep veins of the leg. It is usually due to venous stasis or slow flowing blood around the venous valve sinuses (Gorman et al 2000). Box 12.2 highlights the main factors predisposing to this condition.

Manifestations

Deep vein thrombosis may be asymptomatic and is notoriously difficult to diagnose by physical examination alone. It is confirmed in only one of every three cases suspected clinically (Gorman et al 2000). Further investigations are always required. Signs and symptoms may include pain in the calf area (particularly on walking) and localized tenderness. Swelling around the area of thrombosis may occur with pitting oedema, together with a raised skin temperature. It is important when performing a nursing assessment to consider whether the patient falls into one of the 'at risk' categories (Box 12.2), and to consider educating vulnerable patients with regard to identifying possible signs of DVT.

Diagnosis

A full medical history is always taken and a physical examination performed.

D-Dimer testing   D-Dimer is a circulating degradation product of fibrin production. Fibrin is involved in the clotting process. D-Dimer concentrations are raised in conditions such as DVT and pulmonary embolism. Levels can be increased in other conditions, but this remains a valuable test.

Contrast venography   Contrast venography utilizes X-ray imaging with an injected contrast medium to see blockages in the vein. An alternative form is radionuclide (radioactive)

Box 12.2   Risk factors for the development of deep vein thrombosis (DVT)

- Varicose veins

- Age above 40 years

- Clinical history in the patient or family of DVT or pulmonary embolism

- Immobility, for example as a result of prolonged bedrest, paralysis or stroke

- Surgical procedures lasting for more than 30 minutes. These are notably orthopaedic, neurosurgical, urological or gynaecological surgery (Gorman et al 2000). Surgery reduces venous return because of lack of mobility in the legs, preventing the muscles in the calves from squeezing blood back towards the heart. The clotting cascade can also be triggered by surgical intervention

- Pregnancy. This can raise intra-abdominal pressure and hinder venous return of blood

- Serious illnesses such as myocardial infarction, heart failure, sepsis; these can interfere with blood flow through the main and microcirculation

- Disorders that encourage abnormal blood clotting

- Obesity. This may cause pressure and obstruction to the venous return

- Underlying malignancy. This may affect both clotting and venous return

- The term *thrombophilia* may be used, and refers to a tendency of the blood towards clotting

- Recent controversy over the adverse effects of prolonged air travel has led to ongoing research into the so-called 'economy class syndrome' associated with the risk of DVT to passengers

---

venography, which uses the injection of radiopharmaceuticals to produce images of the occlusion.

Compression ultrasonography This has emerged in recent years as a valuable diagnostic tool in DVT. Pressure is applied to the vein with an ultrasound probe. This compresses the walls of the vessel, but will not occur if a thrombus is present. The lack of vessel collapse can be visualized on a screen. As a technique it is known to be less effective in the veins of the calves.

Duplex scanning Colour duplex scanning utilizes ultrasound and may be used to image the venous system in certain areas, such as with more proximal DVTs.

Complications

Part or all of the DVT may break free and travel within the circulation. This may lead to emboli blocking the blood flow to organs, particularly in the lungs (pulmonary embolism). The patient becomes breathless and experiences chest pain. An area of lung may infarct – at worse, this may prove fatal.

Prophylaxis

Nursing staff should be aware of the factors predisposing to DVT. Patients should be encouraged to mobilize when able in order to encourage venous return. A good fluid intake is encouraged unless contraindicated, for example in severe heart failure. Subcutaneous heparin (an anti-coagulant) and graded compression stockings, which encourage venous return, may be necessary in high-risk groups.

Treatment

Nursing care should aim to reduce the presenting symptoms, prevent complications and reduce the size of the thrombus. The affected leg is elevated when resting. This will help to reduce swelling and compression around the area. Early mobilization is now seen as beneficial (Gorman et al 2000). Graded compression stockings will be prescribed. An accurate measurement of the limb is needed to ensure that the correct size of stockings are used. These should not be rolled down or have wrinkles in them. A spare pair is usually given to allow one pair to be washed. Anticoagulation is given as soon as a diagnosis has been made. This is usually a bolus dose of heparin (5000 units) and either a constant heparin infusion or subcutaneous low molecular weight heparin.

Monitoring the activated partial thromboplastin time (APTT) occurs at approximately 6-hour intervals to ensure that adequate anticoagulation has been achieved. A therapeutic range of 1.5–2 times the laboratory value of a normal PTT (the control) is usually recommended. Heparin will not break down the clot, but will prevent it from enlarging as it dissolves naturally. An oral anticoagulant, usually warfarin, is started immediately, but takes about 3 days to prolong the prothrombin time adequately, measured as the international normalized ratio (INR). The target range is approximately 2–3, or slightly higher for a recurrent DVT. Heparin is not available as an oral drug and is stopped when the INR has reached the target range for 24 hours with the oral anticoagulant.

The INR will be measured several times over the subsequent few days, then weekly as an outpatient assessment or in the patient's general practice. The time is then lengthened as the INR target range stabilizes. Patients are advised of the risks of bleeding such as the occurrence of bruising or blood in the urine or stools. These should be reported to the healthcare team. A small booklet is kept by the patient with the result of the INR and the prescribed dose of warfarin, which alters depending on the result. Activities known to be a risk to bleeding, such as gardening, contact sports and handling pets that may scratch, should be avoided. The oral anticoagulant will be prescribed for a number of months.

Approximately 35% of patients with a DVT are cared for in the community (Gorman et al 2000). Subcutaneous heparin is administered by the patient or community healthcare team. If the patient with a DVT is pregnant, heparin is administered by subcutaneous injection as warfarin is contraindicated in pregnancy. It is stopped before delivery and then restarted following the birth for several weeks to approximately 3 months.

THROMBOPHLEBITIS AND PHLEBOTHROMBOSIS

Phlebitis is an inflammation of the walls of a vein and may be caused by injury, prolonged pressure or infection. The endothelial lining is damaged and a thrombus develops at the site of inflammation, producing a secondary condition known as thrombophlebitis.

Phlebothrombosis is the formation of a blood clot within a vein with no associated inflammation, and for this reason may be referred to as a *bland* or *silent thrombosis*. It is nearly always due to slowness or stasis of the circulation, such as occurs with prolonged bedrest, inactivity or pressure causing resistance to the venous blood flow. The serious factor in both phlebothrombosis and thrombophlebitis is the blood clot, which becomes a potential embolus. The silent thrombus or that associated with inflammation may be carried along in the bloodstream and may eventually lodge in an artery to cause an embolism. Phlebitis and venous thrombosis may occur in any vein, but the most frequent site is the saphenous veins of the legs.

Manifestations

Thrombophlebitis in superficial veins produces local pain, tenderness and swelling. The pain may vary from moderate discomfort on touching the limb to severe cramping. If the leg is involved, there may be calf pain during dorsiflexion of the foot. Systemic symptoms such as fever, headache and general malaise develop. If the vein is superficial, the overlying skin becomes red and hot. It may be taut and shiny.

With deep vein thrombosis, the process may be silent. No symptoms may be present until the thrombus is swept along and causes an embolism. In either phlebothrombosis or thrombophlebitis, the thrombus may become large enough to block the vein, causing severe congestion, oedema and pain.

SUMMARY

Cardiovascular disease is one of the most important single causes of death in the UK and contributes to a significant level of morbidity. It is of multifactorial origin, so there is no one single preventive measure that would reduce its incidence dramatically. A combination of strategies is therefore needed to reduce the morbidity and mortality associated with cardiovascular disease. Nurses have a major role in preventing cardiovascular disorder and in improving the quality of life for patients, and their loved ones, living with heart disease. However, the government also has an important role in health promotion, and considerable interest has been shown by the government in targeting heart disease through national standards, manifest in documents such as the National Service Framework for Coronary Heart Disease (DoH 2000b). This may go some way to addressing the issue of Britain's mortality statistics from cardiovascular disease which are amongst the worst in Europe.

ACKNOWLEDGEMENT

The author would like to acknowledge the work of Richard Hatchett in his original work on this chapter in the previous edition of *Watson's Clinical Nursing and Related Science*.

REFERENCES

Balarajan R (1991) Ethnic differences in mortality from ischaemic heart disease and cerebrovascular disease in England and Wales. British Medical Journal 302: 560–564.

Barnett M (2001) Cardiac pacing. In: Hatchett R, Thompson DR, eds. Cardiac nursing: a comprehensive guide. Edinburgh: Churchill Livingstone, p 391–425.

British Heart Foundation (2004) Coronary heart disease statistics. Online. Available: http://www.heartstats.org/ 17 March 2006.

British Heart Foundation (2005) Coronary heart disease statistics Online. Available: http://www.heartstats.org/ 17 March 2006.

British Hypertension Society (2004) Guidelines for the management of hypertension: report of the fourth working party of the British Hypertension Society 2004 (BHS IV). Journal of Human Hypertension 18: 139–185.

British Medical Association/Royal College of Nursing (2002) Decisions relating to cardiopulmonary resuscitation: a joint statement from the British Medical Association, the Resuscitation Council (UK) and the Royal College of Nursing. London: BMA/RCN.

British National Formulary (2006) British national formulary London: BMA/Royal Pharmaceutical Society of Great Britain.

Bygrave A (2001) Electrophysiology studies. In: Hatchett R, Thompson DR, eds. Cardiac nursing: a comprehensive guide. Edinburgh: Churchill Livingstone, p 369–390.

Clark J, Queener S, Burke V (2000) Pharmacological basis for nursing practice. St Louis: CV Mosby.

Crumbie A, Lawrence J (2001) Living with a chronic condition: a practitioner's guide to providing care. Oxford: Butterworth Heinemann.

Daniels L (2002) Diet and coronary heart disease. Nursing Standard 16(43): 47–52.

Department of Health (1999) Health survey for England. Cardiovascular disease 1998. London: DoH.

Department of Health (2000a) Saving lives: our healthier nation. London: DoH.

Department of Health (2000b) The national service framework for coronary heart disease. London: DoH.

Donnelly R, Hinwood D, London NJM (2000) ABC of arterial and vascular disease: non-invasive methods of arterial and venous assessment. British Medical Journal 320: 698–701.

Elliot D (1993) Comparison of three instruments for measuring patient anxiety in a coronary care unit. Intensive and Critical Care Nursing 9: 193–200.

Farrelly R (2000) Congenital heart disease 1. Nursing Times 96(24): 47–50.

Friedman S (2000) Cardiac disease, anxiety, and sexual functioning. American Journal of Cardiology 86(2A): 46–50F.

Glenville B (1999) Minimally invasive cardiac surgery (editorial). British Medical Journal 319: 135–136.

Gorman WP, Davis KR, Donnelly R (2000) ABC of arterial and venous disease: swollen lower limb 1. General assessment and deep vein thrombosis. British Medical Journal 320: 1453–1456.

Gould M (2001) Chronic heart failure. In: Hatchett R, Thompson DR, eds. Cardiac nursing: a comprehensive guide. Edinburgh: Churchill Livingstone, p 187–217.

Halstead F, Turner B, Wilson S (2001) Diagnostic procedures. In: Hatchett R, Thompson DR, eds. Cardiac nursing: a comprehensive guide. Edinburgh: Churchill Livingstone, p 125–147.

Hatchett R (2001) Clinical observation and monitoring devices. In: Hatchett R, Thompson DR, eds. Cardiac nursing: a comprehensive guide. Edinburgh: Churchill Livingstone, p 69–95.

ISIS-2 (Second International Study of Infarct Survival) Collaborative Group (1988) Randomised trial of intravenous streptokinase, oral aspirin, both, or neither among 17187 cases of suspected acute myocardial infarction: ISIS-2. Lancet ii: 349–360.

Jaarsma T, Kastermans M, Dassen T et al (1995) Problems of cardiac patients in early recovery. Journal of Advanced Nursing 21: 21–27.

James J (2001) The management and support of patients with internal cardioverter defibrillators. In: Hatchett R, Thompson DR, eds. Cardiac nursing: a comprehensive guide. Edinburgh: Churchill Livingstone, p 495–505.

Jevon P (1999) Do not resuscitate orders: the issues. Nursing Standard 13(40): 45–46.

Kettunen S, Solovieva S, Laamanen R et al (1999) Myocardial infarction, spouses' reactions and their need of support. Journal of Advanced Nursing 30(2): 479–488.

Kidby J (2003) Family-witnessed cardiopulmonary resuscitation. Nursing Standard 17(51): 33–36.

Kleinman A, Eisenberg L, Good B (1978) Culture, illness and care. Annals of Internal Medicine 88: 251–258.

Knoll SM, Johnson JL (2000) Uncertainty and expectations: taking care of a cardiac surgery patient at home. Journal of Cardiovascular Nursing 14(3): 64–75.

Linden B (1995) Evaluation of a home based rehabilitation programme for patients recovering from acute myocardial infarction. Intensive and Critical Care Nursing 11: 10–19.

London NJM, Nash R (2000) ABC of arterial and venous disease: varicose veins. British Medical Journal 320: 1391–1394.

Lozano R, Murray C, Lopez A et al (2002) Miscoding and misclassification of ischaemic heart disease mortality. Geneva: WHO.

Mason S (2001) Infective endocarditis. In: Hatchett R, Thompson DR, eds. Cardiac nursing: a comprehensive guide. Edinburgh: Churchill Livingstone, p 287–298.

Mayou R, Bryant B (1993) Quality of life in cardiovascular disease. British Heart Journal 69: 460–466.

Millane T, Jackson G, Gibbs CR et al (2000) ABC of heart failure: acute and chronic management strategies. British Medical Journal 320: 559–562.

Munro J, Edwards C (1995) Macleod's clinical examination. Edinburgh: Churchill Livingstone.

National Institute for Clinical Excellence (2000) Appraisal guidance on technologies for specialist cardiac services. London: NICE.

National Institute for Clinical Excellence (2002) Guidance on the use of glycoprotein IIb/IIIa protein inhibitors in the treatment of acute coronary syndromes. Technology appraisal guidance No. 47. London: NICE.

National Institute for Clinical Excellence (2003a) Angina and myocardial infarction – myocardial perfusion scintigraphy (no.73) Online. Available: http://www.nice.org.uk 17 March 2006.

National Institute for Clinical Excellence (2003b) Chronic heart failure. Management of chronic heart failure in adults in primary and secondary care. NICE: London

National Institute for Clinical Excellence (2004) Acute coronary syndromes – clopidogrel (No. 80) Online. Available: http://www.nice.org.uk 17 March 2006.

O'Farrell P, Murray J, Hotz SB (2000) Psychologic distress among spouses of patients undergoing cardiac rehabilitation. Heart and Lung 29(2): 97–104.

Olivier C (2000) Rheumatic fever: is it still a problem? Journal of Antimicrobial Chemotherapy 45: 13–21.

Openshaw A, Durbridge M (2001) Early extubation protocols, the emergence of high dependency units and the newer revascularisation techniques. In: Hatchett R, Thompson DR, eds. Cardiac nursing: a comprehensive guide. Edinburgh: Churchill Livingstone, p 544–563.

Peterson M (1991) Patient anxiety before cardiac catheterisation. Heart and Lung 20: 643–647.

Quinn T, Hatchett R (2001) Cardiopulmonary resuscitation. In: Hatchett R, Thompson DR, eds. Cardiac nursing: a comprehensive guide. Edinburgh: Churchill Livingstone, p 481–494.

Quinn T, Webster R, Hatchett R (2001) Coronary artery disease: angina and unstable angina. In: Hatchett R, Thompson DR, eds. Cardiac nursing: a comprehensive guide. Edinburgh: Churchill Livingstone, p 151–188.

Resuscitation Council UK (2005a) Resuscitation guidelines 2005. London: Resuscitation Council.

Resuscitation Council UK (2005b) In house hospital resuscitation. Online. Available: http://www.resus.org.uk/pages/inhralgo.pdf 30 Jul 2006.

Roebuck A (1999) Telephone support in the early post-discharge period following elective cardiac surgery: does it reduce anxiety and depression levels? Intensive and Critical Care Nursing 15(3): 142–146.

Scandinavian Simvastatin Survival Study Group (1994) Randomised controlled trial of cholesterol lowering in 4444 patients with coronary heart disease: the Scandinavian Simvastsatin Survival Study. Lancet 344: 1383–1389.

Searle M, Hoff L (2000) Bedrest after elective cardiac catheterisation. Professional Nurse 15(9): 588–591.

Sever PS et al (2003) Prevention of coronary and stroke events with atorvastatin in hypertensive patients who have average or lower than average cholesterol concentrations in the Anglo Scandinavian Cardiac Outcomes Trial Lipid Lowering Arm (ASCOT-LLA): a multi centre randomized controlled trail. Lancet 361: 1149–1158.

Sharpe N, Doughty R (1998) Epidemiology of heart failure and ventricular dysfunction. Lancet 352 (Suppl 1): S13–S17.

Simons R (1999) The airway at risk. In: Colquhoun MC, Handley AJ, Evans TR, eds. ABC of resuscitation. London: BMJ Books, p 19–24.

Stokes H, Thompson DR (2001) Cardiac rehabilitation. In: Hatchett R, Thompson DR, eds. Cardiac nursing: a comprehensive guide. Edinburgh: Churchill Livingstone, p 29–39.

Thompson DR (1990) Counselling the coronary patient and partner. London: Scutari.

Thompson DR, Webster RA, Cordle CJ et al (1987) Specific sources and patterns of anxiety in male patients with first myocardial infarction. British Journal of Medical Psychology 60: 343–348.

Thompson DR, Sutton TW, Jowett NI et al (1991) Circardian variation in the frequency of onset of chest pain in acute myocardial infarction. British Heart Journal 65: 177–178.

Thompson DR, Webster RA, Sutton TW (1994) Coronary care unit patients' and nurses' ratings of intensity of ischaemic chest pain. Intensive and Critical Care Nursing 10: 81–88.

Thompson DR, Ersser S, Webster RA (1995) The experiences of patients and their partners 1 month after a heart attack. Journal of Advanced Nursing 22: 707–714.

Thompson DR, Bowman GS, Kitson A et al (1996) Cardiac rehabilitation in the United Kingdom: guidelines and audit standards. Heart 75: 89–93.

Tortora G, Grabowski S (2000) Principles of anatomy and physiology, 9th edn. New York: John Wiley.

Tough J (2005) Thrombolytic therapy in acute myocardial infarction. Nursing Standard 19(37): 55–64.

Underwood MJ, Firmin RK, Jehu D (1993) Aspects of psychological and social morbidity in patients awaiting coronary artery bypass grafting. British Heart Journal 69: 382–384.

Vowden P (2001) Doppler assessment and ABPI: interpretation in the management of leg ulceration. Online. Available: http://www.worldwidewounds.com/2001/march/Vowden/Doppler-assessment-and-ABPI.html#whats-in-a-number 30 Jul 2006.

Walsh M, Kent A (2001) A & E nursing, 4th edn. Oxford: Butterworth-Heinemann.

Walsh M, Crumbie A, Reveley S (1999) Nurse practitioners; clinical skills and professional issues. Oxford: Butterworth Heinemann.

Watt-Watson J, Garfinkel P, Gallop R et al (2000) The impact of nurses' empathic responses on patients' pain management in acute care. Nursing Research 49(4): 191–200.

Williams B, Poulter NR, Brown MJ et al (2004) Guidelines for the management of hypertension: report of the fourth working party of the British Hypertension Society 2004 (BHS IV): Journal of Human Hypertension 18: 139–185.

World Health Organization (1993) Needs and action priorities in cardiac rehabilitation and secondary prevention in patients with coronary heart disease. Copenhagen: WHO.

World Health Organization (1998) Obesity: preventing and managing the global epidemic. Report of WHO Consultation on obesity. Geneva, WHO.

World Health Organization (2005) Ten statistical highlights in global public health. Online. Available: http://www.who.int/whosis/2006highlights/en/index.html 30 Jul 2006.

World Health Organization (2006a) World health statistics 2006. Online. Available: http://www.who.int/healthinfo/statistics/en/ 30 Jul 2006.

World Health Organization (2006b) Basic health information on tobacco use. Online. Available: http://www.wpro.who.int/NR/exeres/61805311-B034-45C1-AFE8-7756D2487268.htm 30 Jul 2006.

World Health Organization (2006c) WHO Global InfoBase. Online. Available: http://www.who.int/ncd_surveillance/infobase/web/InfoBaseCommon/ 30 Jul 2006.

World Health Organization (2006d) Global strategy on diet, physical activity and health: physical activity http://www.who.int/dietphysicalactivity/publications/facts/pa/en/index.html 30 Jul 2006.

Yusuf S, Zucker D, Peduzzi P et al (1994) Effect of coronary artery by-pass graft surgery on survival: overview of 10 year results from randomised trials by the Coronary Artery Bypass Graft Surgery Trialists Collaboration. Lancet 344: 563–570.

FURTHER READING

Cooke F, Metcalfe H (2000) Cardiac monitoring 1. Nursing Times 96(23): 45–46.

Cooke F, Metcalfe H (2000) Cardiac monitoring 2. Nursing Times 96(25): 45–46.

A well illustrated and brief guide to attaching a patient to bedside cardiac monitoring.

Farrelly R (2000) Congenital heart disease 1. Nursing Times 96(24): 47–50.

Farrelly R (2000) Congenital heart disease 2. Nursing Times 96(28): 43–46.

A well illustrated and briefly explained overview of the more common congenital heart defects in children, with a guide to current treatments.

Hampton JR (2003) The ECG made easy, 6th edn. Edinburgh: Churchill Livingstone.

A popular and valuable handbook from the basics to the more advanced practice of ECG interpretation.

McGhie AI, ed. (2001) Handbook of non-invasive cardiac testing. London: Arnold.

There is an array of non-invasive cardiac investigations the patient may undergo from exercise electrocardiography, to echocardiography and nuclear cardiology tests. This useful handbook dedicates specific chapters to all of these tests, allowing the healthcare professional to allay fears and explain the procedures to patients and loved ones.

Swanton RH (2003) Cardiology pocket handbook, 5th edn. Oxford: Blackwell Science.

A very useful but detailed handbook, from the well respected cardiologist, which provides a quick reference to the many presenting cardiac conditions.

USEFUL WEB SITES

British Heart Foundation
http://www.bhf.org.uk

Coronary Heart Disease Statistics
http://www.heartstats.org
British Hypertension Society
http://www.bhsoc.org
Resuscitation Council UK
http://www.resus.org.uk
National Service Framework for Coronary Heart Disease
http://www.dh.gov.uk/PolicyAndGuidance/HealthAndSocialCareTo
    pics/CoronaryHeartDisease

Vowden P (2001) Doppler assessment and ABPI: interpretation in
    the management of leg ulceration. Online. Available:
    http://www.worldwidewounds.com/2001/march/Vowden/
    Doppler-assessment-and-ABPI.html#whats-in-a-number
    30 Jul 2006.
An excellent resource for guidance on the measurement of ABPI.

Caring for the patient with a respiratory disorder

Wendy Fairhurst-Winstanley

INTRODUCTION

Health problems affecting breathing and the respiratory system strike at the very root of human well-being and are common in a wide range of patients. Illness affecting the respiratory system ranges from acute life-threatening episodes (e.g. an acute asthmatic attack) to long-term debilitating conditions such as chronic bronchitis. Other systems of the body, particularly the cardiovascular system, are often involved. The consequences of such health problems are not only physical: severe psychological distress can also occur and be accompanied by major social disruption. After a brief overview of relevant anatomy and physiology, this chapter examines the assessment of patients with respiratory disorders before looking at some of the more specific issues relating to the care and treatment of patients with certain disorders.

RESPIRATORY STRUCTURES

The structures concerned with **ventilation** are the upper and lower respiratory tracts, respiratory muscles, thorax and portions of the nervous system (Fig. 13.1).

UPPER RESPIRATORY TRACT

The upper airway is formed by the nose, mouth, pharynx and larynx. It serves as a passageway for air being inspired and expired; filters, warms and moistens the inhaled air; and provides the protective reflexes of sneezing and the closing off of the larynx to prevent aspiration of fluid and solids. Irritation of the pharynx and larynx may also initiate the cough reflex.

LOWER RESPIRATORY TRACT

The lower tract consists of the trachea, bronchi and two lungs. The trachea continues to warm and filter the inspired air. It divides into the two *primary bronchi* known as the right main bronchus and the left bronchus. The right bronchus is wider and shorter than the left and any foreign object that is inhaled tends to lodge in the right bronchus (Hinchliff et al 1996). The bronchi subdivide into the *bronchioles*, which in turn lead to the respiratory bronchioles. At the terminal end of each respiratory bronchiole is a thin-walled sac known as an *alveolus*. The alveoli are covered by networks of capillaries and it is in this part of the respiratory tract that gaseous exchange takes place.

ASSESSMENT

NURSING ASSESSMENT OF A PATIENT WITH A RESPIRATORY DISORDER

When making an initial assessment of a patient, nurses need to use their skills of observation, measurement and interpersonal communication. Information may be gathered from the patient, their relatives or significant others, and other members of the multidisciplinary team. Depending upon the patient's condition, the nurse will need to prioritize the information required to plan immediate care, adding to this at a later time when necessary and possible.

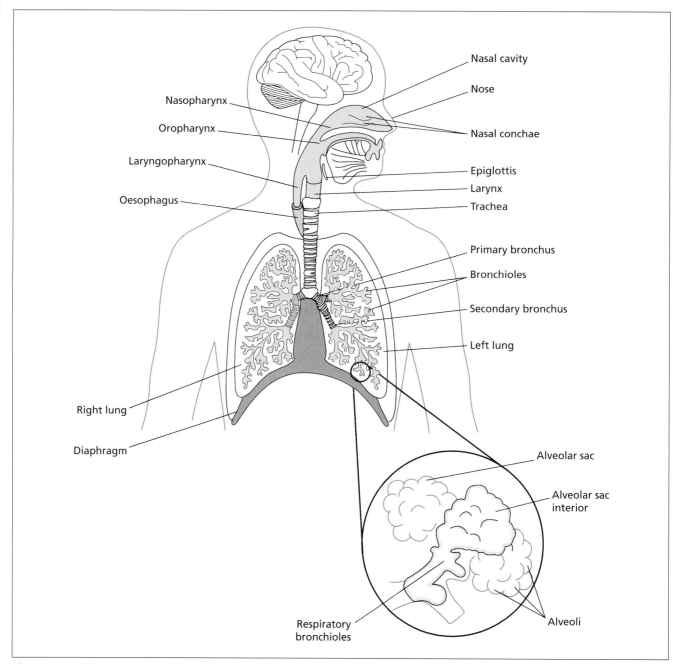

Figure 13.1 The respiratory system.

On first meeting the patient, the nurse should take an overview of his or her general appearance in order to gain a feeling for the overall health status of the patient. The facial expression might give clues as to mood; colouring should be noted to check for signs of a flushed, red appearance that might indicate pyrexia. Cyanosis (a bluish discoloration around the lips that is a late sign of severe respiratory failure) may be noted. The patient's posture should be observed to note whether it indicates a sense of ease and relaxation or the anxiety and tenseness, associated with difficulty in breathing.

The nurse seeks to obtain information about the person's respiratory function, past history related to respiratory disorders and treatment programme, in order to identify factors that contribute to the promotion as well as any impairment of airway clearance. The information the nurse obtains from the patient and/or others should include:

- the symptoms that prompted the patient to seek health care
- a description of the precipitating events
- duration of the symptoms
- the person's perception of the causes and implications of the symptoms
- the patient's past medical history
- the patient's family medical history
- current medication

- lifestyle and social factors such as occupation and housing conditions
- smoking status
- immunization status (influenza and pneumococcal).

Possible symptoms manifested by the patient include cough, wheeze, sputum production, breathlessness, fever and pain:

Cough The presence, frequency and depth of the **cough** are noted as well as the nature and sound. The PQRST symptom analysis tool (see p. 128) should be used for an accurate description of the cough:

P *Provocation/palliation*: Does anything in particular bring on the cough (e.g. smoking) or relieve it?
Q *Quality*: Is it hard and racking, croup-like, hacking, shallow, deep and rattling, or does it have a whooping sound? Is the cough productive and if so, what colour is this?
R *Region/radiation*: Does coughing produce any symptoms elsewhere?
S *Severity*: Does the cough disrupt everyday life or prevent sleeping? Is it associated with pain? Is the cough getting worse or better? How does this compare to previous episodes of cough?
T *Time*: How long has the cough been present? Is it worse at any particular time such as at night? Is it worse at any particular time of the week (e.g. worse during the week when at work) or at any particular time of year (e.g. worse in the winter)?

Wheeze Wheeze is a high-pitched musical sound which is often audible to the patient and others even without the assistance of a stethoscope. Wheeze is classically heard in patients who have asthma and may be constant during an acute exacerbation or may be intermittent. Patients may find that the wheeze is triggered by exercise or by walking into a smoky atmosphere or they may find that a weekend at home with the cat might bring it on. Wheeze is an important indicator of restriction to air flow and should be noted as a significant respiratory symptom.

Sputum It is necessary to determine the consistency (mucoid, watery, purulent, tenacious, frothy or blood streaked), colour, smell and amount, and whether the amount has increased recently.

Breathlessness The patient may complain of breathlessness and the history should reveal whether it occurs with usual activity, increased effort or when at rest, and whether it interferes with daily activities and sleep pattern. It is useful to find out if the patient needs to be propped up in bed at night in order to breathe. Orthopnea relates to breathlessness that comes on when the patient is lying flat and this can point to a cardiovascular source of the breathlessness rather than primarily a respiratory cause. It should be noted whether the patient's speech is audible, clear and effortless, or whether the responses are weak, short and jerky phrases with apparent effort. The patient is questioned as to what was done to pre-vent or modify the breathlessness and whether the suggested actions were effective in preventing or alleviating it.

Fever/pyrexia The patient may have a **fever** and give a history of having night sweats. The recording of the patient's temperature should therefore form part of a baseline assessment against which changes can be monitored.

Pain and discomfort This may be associated with the chest, breathing activities or coughing; the nature of the **pain**, its severity, duration and precipitating factors should be noted alongside any strategies that the patient has found useful in relieving or lessening the discomfort.

In addition to exploring the presenting symptoms associated with the respiratory system it is important to enquire about the patient's smoking status. Past smoking history is as important as current smoking history and so it is useful to explore with the patient how many cigarettes they used to smoke before quitting and for how many years they smoked them. Smoking is significantly related to the development of some respiratory problems such as chronic obstructive pulmonary disease (COPD) and lung cancer (British Thoracic Society 2004) and knowledge of whether a person smokes can aid in prioritizing differential diagnoses.

The patient's understanding of the respiratory problems should be explored carefully. If the patient is severely distressed, questions should be kept to a minimum and if possible asked in such a way that they may be answered by a nod or shake of the head. More detailed discussions should be saved until the patient's breathing is easier.

Observation of whether the airway is patent, followed by assessment of respiratory rate, depth and rhythm, may identify serious problems immediately, and in all patients provides a vital basic record that can be used as a baseline to monitor subsequent progress. The tongue of an unconscious patient may, for example, block the airway. If the brain is deprived of oxygen, serious damage occurs within 3 minutes. Any obstruction to the upper airway is potentially fatal within minutes, hence the importance of always beginning an assessment by checking that the upper airway is clear.

Assessment of respiration

To avoid the patient being conscious of having the breathing monitored, which may affect the rate, it is suggested that the respiratory rate is taken immediately after the pulse, while still holding the patient's wrist. The healthy adult breathes 12–18 times per minute at rest, although this rate is much quicker in infants – 40 breaths per minute is typical of a newborn baby. A rapid respiratory rate (*tachypnoea*) in an adult may indicate anxiety, pain, pyrexia, metabolic disorders (e.g. acidosis) or may be the result of the body attempting to compensate for inadequate oxygenation due to a wide range of cardiovascular and respiratory disorders (e.g. heart failure or shock). Slower breathing rates are associated with sleep or with disorders and drugs that depress the respiratory centre (e.g. opioids).

Observation of the thorax should also be carried out to note its shape, size and symmetry, in addition to forming an impression about the amount of effort involved in breathing. Long-standing respiratory disease leads to a characteristic barrel shaped chest. The chest may also be described as pigeon chest (pectus carinatum) or funnel chest (pectus excavatum). Paradoxical chest movements (i.e. one part of the chest wall appears to move in the opposite direction from the rest of the chest wall) indicate ribs fractured in two places, known as a *flail segment*. This is potentially fatal as the ensuing lung collapse may make it impossible for the patient to achieve sufficient ventilation to be compatible with life.

Unequal participation of the two sides of the chest in respiratory movements may be evident, or unusual retraction or ballooning of the intercostal spaces may occur. For example, in patients with atelectasis or pneumothorax, in which a part or all of the lung is not being inflated, there is diminished movement of the chest wall on the affected side. Similarly, this may occur if a large section of alveoli is consolidated with fluid or secretions. Excessive retraction or ballooning is associated with extreme difficulty in getting air in or out of the air passages.

Breathing pattern

Normal respirations are regular, effortless and quiet. Irregularities in breathing may relate to rate, volume, rhythm or the ease with which the person breathes. The following terms are used to indicate characteristic breathing patterns:

- *Eupnoea* is quiet, normal breathing at the rate of about 12–18 times per minute in the adult. Respirations are more rapid and shallow in the infant and pre-school child, gradually reaching adult levels by the age of 10–12 years
- *Dyspnoea* refers to a subjective awareness of a disturbance or difficulty in breathing
- *Tachypnoea* is rapid breathing, usually with reduced tidal volume
- *Bradypnoea* is an abnormally slow rate of respiration
- *Hyperpnoea* is an increase in the volume of air breathed per minute due to an increase in either the rate or depth of respirations, or to both
- *Orthopnoea* is dyspnoea which is present when the patient is lying down but is relieved to some extent by sitting up
- *Cheyne–Stokes* respiration is characterized by a few seconds of apnoea followed by respirations that gradually increase in frequency and volume to a peak intensity and then gradually subside to a period of apnoea. This pattern is cyclical
- *Biot's pattern* of breathing is characterized by a few respirations varying in volume, followed by a prolonged period of apnoea
- *Kussmaul's* respirations are rapid and very deep.

In dyspnoea the patient experiences discomfort and the need for increased effort or work in ventilation. The individual's perception of difficult breathing or shortness of breath may be due to physiological or psychological stress. The experience of **dyspnoea** is anxiety provoking because the person knows that breathing is essential to life; the emotional reaction tends to aggravate and perpetuate the problem further. The individual may describe it as tightness in the chest, shortness of breath, unable to get enough air, or suffocating. The dyspnoeic patient frequently has a distressed appearance, is restless and may be perspiring. The difficulty may be present only on exertion and may be episodic. The frequency of the episodes and whether their occurrence is related to a particular time of day, activity or certain situations or factors are noted.

Other factors

When completing an initial assessment or as part of the ongoing assessment the nurse would also seek to gather information on the following factors:

Past history of respiratory disorders and treatment programme   The person is asked whether there has been any trauma or surgery to the chest or respiratory passages, or any respiratory infections. The existence of any associated health problems such as asthma or COPD is also determined. Information is obtained about all prescription and non-prescription drugs the person has been taking regularly or intermittently. The name, dosage, frequency, purpose and perceived effectiveness of each drug is noted (if the patient is able to supply this information).

Health-promoting behaviours and risk factors   Assessment includes data about factors in the person's lifestyle and health habits that are likely to increase the risk for problems. Smoking status, exercise, diet, weight and utilization of the health service should be assessed. The patient's occupation and possible exposure to irritants should be noted in addition to housing conditions, the presence of pets and exposure to infectious diseases such as TB in the community. Recent travel is an important risk factor and it is also necessary to enquire about known allergies and the patient's personal reaction to allergens.

The person's perceptions of altered respiratory status   The person's perception of their current health and attitude towards known risk factors such as smoking should be determined. It is important also to recognize which factors are beyond the control of the patient, such as working conditions, air pollution or poverty, and consider ways in which their effects may be reduced. Giving up work or moving away from a city may not be feasible or acceptable to the patient.

The nurse also assesses the individual's understanding of previously prescribed treatment. It is important to determine why the person sought health care and what his or her goals are for care. What does the individual state as the priority for care? Many respiratory problems are chronic in nature and it is therefore important that the person recognizes the long-term nature of the illness and the implications of this. Family support should be discussed to discover something of the social setting the patient has come from and will return to, as that setting may have significant influence over his or her health.

Family medical history It is important to enquire whether the patient has any family members who have experienced respiratory problems. Many respiratory conditions, such as asthma, show familial tendencies and others may be directly inherited such as alpha-1-antitrypsin deficiency. Alpha-1-antitrypsin deficiency is the only proven genetic link to COPD and people with this deficiency may demonstrate signs of respiratory dysfunction in their 20s or 30s (Holt 2001).

Pulse oximetry

Pulse oximetry is a non-invasive measurement of arterial oxygen saturation. Some 97% of the oxygen transported in the bloodstream is attached to haemoglobin (Hb) within red blood cells. The other 3% is dissolved in the plasma. When haemoglobin is carrying its maximum amount of oxygen (four molecules per Hb molecule) it is considered saturated; the extent to which this occurs is referred to as oxygen saturation or 'sats' for short.

To interpret oxygen saturation readings, Hb levels must be known. If the patient is anaemic (low Hb level), less oxygen is required to provide a high oxygen saturation. However, the total amount of oxygen in the bloodstream could be inadequate for metabolic requirements and the patient may be hypoxic despite an apparently satisfactory oxygen saturation reading on the pulse oximeter.

Pulse oximetry works by measuring the transmission of red and infrared light across a pulsatile arterial bed, such as a finger or earlobe. As these beams of light are transmitted, oxygenated haemoglobin absorbs more infrared light. De-oxygenated blood absorbs more red light. The pulse oximeter processor then determines how much of each type of light has been absorbed to calculate the saturated oxygen value.

Normal Hb levels and tissue perfusion are essential if pulse oximetry readings are to provide an accurate picture of the amount of oxygen in the bloodstream. Abnormal Hb concentration, very low levels of normal Hb or severe tissue underperfusion (shock) can undermine the accuracy of pulse oximetry readings. Temperature and blood pH also affect the relationship between saturation levels measured by pulse oximetry and the actual amount of oxygen in the bloodstream as measured by the partial oxygen pressure (PO_2). Therefore, whilst the oxygen saturation is a useful measure of respiratory function, it should be combined with other measures of blood chemistry to obtain an accurate picture of patient progress.

Patient movement may cause interference with the oximeter reading, introducing inaccuracy. If blood pressure is being measured on the same arm, inflation of the cuff will affect saturation readings as arterial blood flow is temporarily impeded. Nail polish should be removed as this will interfere with the transmission of light through the nailbed and hence the pulse oximeter reading, if the probe is attached to a finger. Finally, limb oedema may impede absorption of red and infrared light. If the patient has peripheral oedema, extra care should be taken not to cause pressure damage with the finger probe. When nursing the patient, the nurse should observe the probe site for pressure tissue damage. Frequently moving the probe to other digits will prevent this.

Peak flow rate measurement

One further method of assessment that the nurse may use is to measure peak flow rates for the patient. This is a test of the maximum rate of exhalation (**peak expiratory flow rate**) a patient can achieve (in litres per minute) by the patient blowing as hard as possible into a simple instrument. This assesses the degree of impairment in respiratory function due to airway narrowing in diseases such as asthma.

The nurse needs to instruct the patient on how to use the peak flow meter and should ensure that the patient adopts a position that is both comfortable and facilitates the greatest lung expansion. It is advised that the patient should be sitting for safety reasons even though greater lung expansion can be achieved when standing. After taking a deep breath in, the patient should try to ensure that the mouth is closed around the mouthpiece, and should then exhale as deeply and rapidly as possible. It is usual practice to ask the patient to do this three times, with the best result being recorded. In addition to recording the result, the type of peak flow meter used should also be recorded as different instruments have been shown to give varying results (Sharp 1993). Peak flow meters are available on prescription and many patients monitor their own respiratory function at home.

MEDICAL ASSESSMENT AND RELATED INVESTIGATIONS

A range of techniques is employed to assess respiratory function. Although formerly the sole preserve of the medical profession, other health staff such as nurse practitioners and physiotherapists are now incorporating these techniques into their practice in order that they may expand their role. A fuller account of these techniques can be found in Walsh (2005).

PHYSICAL EXAMINATION OF THE CHEST AND BREATHING PATTERN

Inspection

General Inspection

Inspection of the respiratory system begins by generally observing the patient's hands and facial expression. The hands should be observed for finger clubbing, a clinical sign of chronic respiratory problems and for capillary refill. Capillary refill is assessed by pressing on the patient's finger end and watching how quickly the colour of the finger turns from a blanched white to a well-perfused pink colour. In addition the colour of the fingers and hands can be noted for signs of peripheral cyanosis and also the nicotine staining associated with smoking. The patient's face may also give clues of chronic respiratory distress as there may be vertical lines around the mouth which result from the long-term effects of pursed lip breathing or they may simply look anxious and fearful as they are struggling to get the next breath.

Thorax

Normally, the thorax is symmetrical. It is important to note any difference on either side and any apparent abnormality in the shape or bony framework of the thorax. Scoliosis or kyphosis may interfere with normal breathing. If the chest is barrel shaped, this may indicate chronic airflow limitation. A funnel-shaped chest is characterized by depression of the sternum, whereas a pigeon chest involves an outward location of the sternum and inward depression of the first few ribs with minimal impairment of breathing.

Chest movements associated with respirations

The frequency, rhythm and depth of respirations are noted by observing the chest. The thorax is normally symmetrical. On inspiration, as the diaphragm descends, the lower rib cage moves slightly outward and upward. The upper rib cage simultaneously expands slightly. Expiration is a passive process of elastic recoil and of slightly longer duration than inspiration. A short pause occurs before the next inspiration.

Accessory muscles

Rhythmic movement of the diaphragm is observed with normal respiration. Use of the accessory muscles indicates some degree of respiratory distress and is characterized by retraction of the supraclavicular and suprasternal areas and elevation of the shoulders during inspiration. Enlargement of the accessory muscles, particularly the sternocleidomastoid muscles, occurs with chronic airflow limitation.

Palpation

This method of examination is used to assess chest excursion, symmetry, structural abnormalities and tenderness. The chest should be palpated to ascertain the shape of the thoracic cage, its elasticity and to note any crepitations or coarse vibrations associated with respiratory movement. Chest excursion on inspiration may be assessed by placing the hands on the chest with the fingers slightly outspread and the thumbs just meeting at the midline (Fig. 13.2). This reflects the extent of expansion and depth of respiration. As the patient breathes in, the hands are normally separated by the chest expansion. Whether the range of the chest excursion is the same on both sides is also noted; if it is equal, the thumbs are moved an equal distance from the midline on each side. Normally the movements of the two sides are symmetrical.

The chest is also palpated to note the quality of tactile fremitus. The hands are placed on the chest bilaterally and as the patient speaks the palpable vibrations on the chest are evaluated for their presence and symmetry. Decreased or absent vibrations when assessing fremitus may indicate an effusion or excessive air in the lungs; increased fremitus occurs in the presence of a solid mass or consolidation (Seidel et al 1999). Finally the significant lymph nodes around the chest (such as the supraclavicular nodes) should be palpated to determine their size.

Percussion

The chest can be percussed to assess the percussion tones heard throughout the thoracic cage. Areas of hyper-

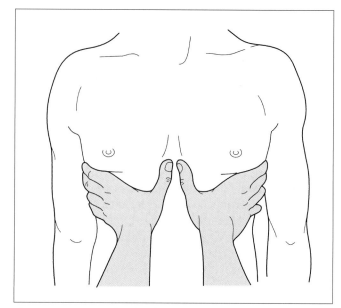

Figure 13.2   Assessing the chest excursion on inspiration.

resonance are associated with the hyperinflation found in emphysema or pneumothorax and areas of dullness are associated with pleural effusion (Seidel et al 1999). The important finding to note is lack of symmetry and therefore percussion notes are compared bilaterally using each lung as a control for the other.

Auscultation

The diaphragm of the stethoscope is best used to listen to breath sounds (auscultation). Normal respirations present characteristic sounds as air enters and leaves the lower respiratory tract. Absence of such sounds or the accompaniment of other sounds may indicate excessive secretions in an area or constriction or blockage of an airway in a section of the lung:

- *Vesicular breath sounds* are heard in normal respirations. They are a soft, low-pitched sound and are heard over all the lung areas except over the main bronchi. The inspiratory phase of a vesicular sound is longer and louder than the expiratory phase. The differences may be attributed to the movement of inspiratory air into progressively smaller air passages (and vice versa in the case of the air being exhaled). Normal breath sounds can also be described as *tracheal or bronchial* (heard over the trachea) and *broncho-vesicular* (heard over the bronchi)
- *Adventitious sounds* are abnormal sounds superimposed on breath sounds as a result of a disease process within the tracheobronchial tree and/or lungs. These include crackles, wheezes, stridor and pleural friction rub:
  - *Crackles* (*rales* or *crepitations*) are described as fizzing or popping sounds created by the equalization of airway pressures during the explosive reopening of previously collapsed airways closed on inspiration, or by air bubbling through pulmonary oedema

– *Wheezes* (rhonchi) are whistling, musical sounds associated with spasm of the bronchial walls; they tend to occur on expiration, although inspiratory wheezes can also be heard

– *Stridor* is a distinctive sound heard on inspiration when there is partial airway obstruction; a totally obstructed airway is usually silent as there is no air movement to produce any sound

– *Pleural friction rub* is a characteristic rough, grating sound produced when inflamed roughened pleurae rub against each other on inspiration. It becomes audible during the latter part of the inspiratory phase.

Functional assessment

Functional assessment and investigations of the patient's tolerance of physical effort are carried out to determine how energy expenditure in performing various activities may be reduced and how the environment may be modified to facilitate functioning:

1 The patient's level of daily activity should be assessed, especially the ability to:
   a) feed self
   b) dress, shave or shower without assistance
   c) climb stairs unaided
   d) perform household activities such as vacuuming, making beds, preparing food
   e) carry out strenuous activity at work.

2 Factors that bring on breathlessness should be assessed:
   a) simple daily tasks such as shaving, dressing, tying shoelaces
   b) extra effort such as climbing stairs
   c) during the night
   d) getting up in the morning?

3 Steps that the person takes to relieve breathlessness should be noted such as using a bronchodilator before activity.

4 Effort tolerance may be assessed with the use of a treadmill. A chair should be available in case the patient needs to stop and rest. The resting heart rate is recorded as well as the pulse rate on completion of the test. A pulse oximeter is used to determine changes in arterial oxygen saturation associated with the exercise. The test estimates the patient's horizontal walking capacity. This information assists in planning an acceptable daily routine and an exercise programme to increase effort tolerance.

The patient's perception of their condition

Further data are obtained to identify how the patient perceives the respiratory dysfunction. Questions that could be asked include:

a) What does it mean to the patient?
b) What losses in functioning are most relevant to the patient?
c) What losses is he or she able to accept?
d) How does he or she feel about it?

e) Is the attitude one of hopeless resignation or unrealistic denial?
f) Is the patient motivated to pursue a self-care programme?

Pulmonary function tests (Table 13.1)

An objective measurement of lung volumes may be determined by spirometry at the bedside, in the clinic, health centre or patient's home. (Spirometry is the measurement of air taken into and expelled from the lungs and the speed at which this process takes place.) Changes in lung volumes provide the best objective measurement of airflow limitation. The normal values for the different lung volumes have been established from studies made on normal subjects. They vary with height, age, sex and ethnicity. Lung volume determinations can be used to identify potential risks of respiratory complications in preoperative patients and to monitor changes in the postoperative period. They may also be used to differentiate between diagnoses of asthma or COPD. Vital capacity (VC) and timed forced expiratory volume (FEV) are used most frequently:

● *Vital capacity* (VC) is represented by the volume of air exhaled following a maximal inspiration. To determine the VC, the individual breathes through a mouthpiece that is connected to a tube leading to a spirometer. The normal VC ranges from 3500 to 5000 mL. The VC provides information about compliance, which is the effort required to stretch the lung. Diseased lung requires more effort to achieve expansion and hence is said to have less compliance

● *Forced vital capacity* (FVC) is the maximum volume of air that can be forcibly and rapidly exhaled following a maximal inspiration

● *Peak expiratory flow rate* (PEFR) measures the maximum rate at which air can be exhaled

● *Timed forced expiratory volume* (FEV_t) records the percentage of vital capacity that can be expelled in 1 second (FEV_1). Normally about 80% of the vital capacity is expired in 1 second. FEV_t provides information about the resistance to expiratory airflow.

The FVC, FEV1 and PEFR provide the most useful information that is routinely used in the measurement of lung function. In addition to these clinically relevant readings the residual volume (RV), functional residual capacity (FRC) and tidal volume (V_T) are measurements of lung function that may be altered in the respiratory distressed patient:

● *Residual volume* (RV) is the volume of gas remaining in the lungs at the end of a maximal expiration

● *Functional residual capacity* (FRC) is the air remaining in the lung after passive exhalation in normal breathing; no forceful or increased effort is used

● *Tidal volume* (V_T) is the volume of air exhaled following a normal breath. The normal is usually stated as being 450–500 mL with the individual at rest, but varies with individuals and their activities. *Minute ventilation* (or

Table 13.1 Summary of pulmonary function measurement

Test	Description	Comments
Vital capacity (VC)	The maximal volume of air exhaled following a maximal inspiration (normal: 3500–5000 mL)	Reduced in restrictive airway disease because of limited lung expansion. In obstructive airway disease, the total lung capacity is increased but VC may be reduced due to air trapping with increased residual volume
Tidal volume (V_T)	The volume of air exhaled following a normal breath (normal: 450–500 mL)	
Forced vital capacity (FVC)	The maximum volume of air that can be forcibly and rapidly exhaled following a maximal inspiration	Reduced in obstructive airway disease due to air trapping
Timed vital capacity (FEV_t)	The percentage of vital capacity that can be expelled in 1 second (FEV_1), 2 seconds (FEV_2) and 3 seconds (FEV_3) (normal ranges: FEV_1, 80%; FEV_2, 90%; FEV_3, 95%)	Reduced in obstructive airway disease because of increased airway resistance; usually normal in restrictive airway disease
Residual volume (RV)	The volume of gas remaining in the lungs at the end of a maximal expiration (normal: 25–40% of total lung capacity, e.g. 1500 mL)	Increased in obstructive airway disease
Functional residual capacity (FRC)	The volume of air remaining in the lung after a passive exhalation in normal breathing (normal: about 3000 mL)	Increased in obstructive airway disease

minute respiratory volume) is determined by multiplying the tidal volume by the number of respirations per minute.

Spirometry readings can be helpful in providing an objective measurement of the patient's lung function. The results, however, do not always correlate with the patient's subject report of their symptoms. The results of spirometry should therefore only be used to provide some useful information and should be considered in context with the patient's history.

RADIOLOGICAL EXAMINATION

Chest radiography

The most common X-ray examination of the respiratory system is the chest X-ray. This may reveal the location and size of lesions in the lungs or surrounding bony cage. In addition the nature of the lesion can be gauged from its radiological appearance, e.g. metastases are generally seen as white shadows. Trauma to the lungs, for example caused by damage to the ribs resulting in a pneumothorax, can also be assessed as the collapsed lung will appear as an area devoid of lung markings. The mediastinum can also be assessed and should be centrally positioned. Misplacement of the mediastinum generally indicates pathology, e.g. consolidation of a lung. The heart size can be assessed. If the

cardiothoracic ratio (the maximum diameter of the heart divided by the maximum diameter of the chest) exceeds a third to a half, this indicates pathology. The major blood vessels in the chest, such as the aorta, can also be visualized, for example for widening, which in the aorta could indicate tearing after a deceleration injury, typically resulting from a road traffic accident. Also the position of the diaphragm can be assessed, for example elevation of the diaphragm may indicate pathology such as a sub-phrenic abscess.

A chest X-ray is ideally undertaken with the patient standing to allow the diaphragm to descend maximally, when the patient takes a deep breath in. The X-ray film is placed in front of the patient to allow the heart to be brought as close to the film as possible and the patient to bring their shoulders forward thus clearing their scapulae from their lung fields. In sick patients the film can be taken at the bedside if necessary. In all cases the patient must be cleared of all radio-opaque objects above the waist. A gown should be provided. The exposure will be taken after the patient has been instructed to breathe in and hold their breath, to allow full expansion of the lungs and no blurring on the resulting film.

Computed tomography is a further examination commonly performed in the chest, which gives diagnostically superior images, e.g. to establish the relationship of lung metastases to the airways; to diagnose chest wall disease; to categorize

mediastinal lesions; to guide biopsies of chest lesions. This is a cross-sectional imaging technique, which uses a pencil beam of X-rays on a rotating gantry to build up the image. This provides detail of the lungs and mediastinum and can be 'windowed' to show either area optimally.

Magnetic resonance imaging provides similar information to computed tomography but uses radio-waves in a magnetic field. Whilst it is less commonly performed than CT, it has advantages in some cases. This is because it can obtain images in any plane, which may be valuable to distinguish small lesions from blood vessels, e.g. in the hilar region of the lungs.

The detection of pulmonary embolism, a life-threatening condition which can occur in patients with normal chest X-rays, has been traditionally performed using *radionuclide perfusion and ventilation scans*. These provide images of the blood flow to the lungs, and a mismatch between the perfusion and ventilation scans, typically an area of the lung that is not perfused, is suggestive of a pulmonary embolus.

Computed tomography pulmonary arteriography is a technique that is overtaking radionuclide scanning in the detection of pulmonary embolus. Intravenous, iodine-containing, contrast agent is injected to opacify the pulmonary arterial tree and a series of CT scans are obtained in one breath hold. Emboli which are significant will show up as filling defects in this arterial tree. A similar technique can be performed with MRI but is less common.

BIOCHEMICAL AND HAEMATOLOGICAL MEASUREMENTS

Blood gas analysis

Impairment of respiratory ventilation and gas exchange are reflected in changes in the levels of **blood gases**. Normal values are shown in Table 13.2. A blood specimen for gas analysis is withdrawn using an heparinized syringe, and any air is expelled from the syringe before it is covered with a cap to prevent atmospheric gas exchange (Szaflarski 1996). If the sample remains at room temperature it must be analysed within 10 minutes; otherwise the syringe is placed on ice in a special labelled container and sent promptly to the laboratory (samples stored on ice should be analysed within 1 hour) (Clutton-Brock 1997). The samples used to be taken from the femoral artery when firm pressure had to be applied to the arterial puncture site for at least 7 minutes, or until bleeding has ceased and the site was then protected with a sterile covering. More commonly now arterial blood gases are determined by taking a sample of blood from the ear lobe. This is less invasive for the patient and it is a procedure that can be carried out in the outpatient setting.

Electrolyte concentrations

Determination of electrolyte values, particularly hydrogen carbonate ions (2428 mmol/L) is necessary to interpret changes in acid–base balance.

Erythrocyte count, haemoglobin and haematocrit determination

It is important to know whether the erythrocyte count is normal because erythrocytes contain the haemoglobin that carries the oxygen. Obviously, a deficiency of red blood cells or haemoglobin may produce an oxygen deficiency. The haematocrit represents the percentage of erythrocytes by volume. Normal values are shown in Table 13.3.

Leucocyte count A total and differential count of the white blood cells may be ordered since this information may be useful in confirming infection and distinguishing between an acute disease, such as pneumonia, and a chronic one, such as tuberculosis (see p. 344).

BACTERIOLOGICAL AND CYTOLOGICAL STUDIES

Specimens of sputum, throat secretions, pleural fluid or tissue may be examined for pathogenic organisms and/or malignant cells.

Sputum is examined microscopically in a smear or by culture for organisms, bronchial casts, eosinophils and cancer cells. Tests are also done to identify the antimicrobial drug(s) (usually antibiotics) to which the infecting organisms present in the sputum are sensitive. This can help to guide treatment decisions for the patient. Ideally the sputum specimen should be collected first thing in the morning, because the secretions that accumulate during the night

Table 13.2 Normal values of blood gases

	Normal value
Pao_2	11–13.3 kPa (80–100 mmHg)
$Paco_2$	4.8–6.0 kPa (35–45 mmHg)
pH	7.35–7.45
[H⁺]	35–45 nmol/L
Plasma carbon dioxide level	20–32 mmol/L (20–32 mEq/L)
Arterial oxyhaemoglobin saturation	95–97%

Table 13.3 Normal values for erythrocyte count, haemoglobin and haematocrit

	Normal value
Erythrocyte count	
Men	$4.5–6.53 10^{12}$/L
Women	$3.8–5.83 10^{12}$/L
Haemoglobin concentration	
Men	13–19 g/dL
Women	12–15 g/dL
Haematocrit	
Men	40–50%
Women	37–47%

may have a higher concentration of organisms. The mouth should be clean and free of residual food particles. The patient is given a small sputum container and is instructed to cough deeply to raise the sputum from the lungs. When the specimen is obtained, the container is labelled and delivered to the laboratory. Sputum specimens may be collected during or after postural drainage. They may also be obtained by tracheal aspiration if the patient is unconscious or too weak to cough. The sputum specimen container is attached to the suction catheter, which allows the sputum to flow directly into the container.

Bacteriological studies may also be made of secretions from the *throat* and *pleura*.

Skin tests for tuberculosis

A tuberculin skin test is used in the diagnosis of tuberculosis and to identify those who have been exposed. The test involves an intradermal injection of tuberculin bacillus extract using a syringe and needle (Mantoux test) or a multiple puncture apparatus (Heaf, Tine or Mono-Vac). Tuberculin extract preparations include purified protein derivative (PPD) and old tuberculin (OT), which are available in several strengths. The forearm is the usual site of inoculation. Results are interpreted in 48–72 hours. A positive reaction is characterized by an area of induration of 10 mm or greater.

HISTOLOGICAL EXAMINATIONS

When a malignancy is suspected a biopsy of the tumour is usually taken:

Bronchial biopsy Bronchial tissue can be examined visually by means of a bronchoscope, and samples of tissue and cells may be obtained by brushing or aspirating secretions from the involved areas.

Lung biopsy A lung biopsy may be necessary to confirm the diagnosis when radiological studies reveal pulmonary infiltration or lesions. Lung tissue can be obtained for examination by open thoracotomy, bronchoscopy or percutaneous needle biopsy. Transbronchial biopsy involves the introduction of a bronchoscope and the insertion of long flexible forceps into the involved area. Small samples of tissue may be obtained in this manner. Percutaneous needle biopsy involves the insertion of a needle into the diseased area to obtain a small sample of tissue. The procedure is useful when the lesion is localized.

Lymph node biopsy The scalene lymph nodes (or the supraclavicular nodes) are situated in a pad of fat anterior to the scalenus anterior muscle in the neck and can be found by palpating just above the clavicle. These nodes drain the lungs and mediastinum. The nodes can be examined histologically to help determine the spread of bronchogenic carcinoma and the indications for surgical resection or the prognosis in diseases such as sarcoidosis, tuberculosis or lymphomas such as Hodgkin's disease.

Pleural biopsy Pleural fluid and tissue may be obtained during open thoracotomy but are usually obtained by thoracocentesis. A specially designed needle is inserted into the pleura and samples are taken. Tissue from several sites may be required to confirm a diagnosis of tuberculosis or a malignancy.

SPECIFIC DISORDERS

DISORDERS OF THE LOWER RESPIRATORY TRACT

Pneumonia

Pneumonia is the term generally used to indicate infection and inflammation of lung tissue. Haslett et al (1999) define pneumonia as an acute respiratory illness with shadowing on the chest radiograph. It is an inflammatory condition of the lung in which the alveoli are usually filled with fluid and blood cells. Pneumonia is classified as community or hospital acquired due to the significance of potentially resistant bacterial strains in the treatment of the illness. This is a particular problem in hospital-acquired pneumonia. It is obviously imperative that the patient be treated with the correct antibiotic regimen to be effective against the causative organism. A further important category of patients who may develop pneumonia are immunocompromised persons, such as those with acquired immune deficiency syndrome (AIDS).

Pneumonia caused by pneumococci is a common type of pneumonia, but other bacteria or viruses may be the cause. Non-bacterial and non-viral causes include: aspiration of gastric secretions, food, fluids (*aspiration pneumonia*), and retention of secretions, which occurs frequently in the immobilized elderly or debilitated individual (*hypostatic pneumonia*).

It should be remembered that the most common respiratory complication faced by individuals with human immunodeficiency virus (HIV) infection is *Pneumocystis carinii pneumonia* (PCP). The individual with PCP may be critically ill and is likely to present with a dry, non-productive cough, shortness of breath, high fever and night sweats. PCP may be difficult to diagnose as the individual may have a normal chest radiograph and breath sounds. Bilateral infiltrates are likely to be present in an abnormal chest radiograph. Diagnosis is usually made by cultures obtained by bronchoscopy.

PCP is readily treated with antibiotic regimens. Combinations of drugs such as trimethoprim-sulfamethoxazole (TMP/SMX) and dapsone or pentamidine may be used to treat the infection. These drugs must be used with caution because of their side-effects. For example, TMP/SMX may cause severe rash. Pentamidine given intravenously can cause nausea, orthostatic hypotension and hypoglycaemia.

Prophylactic regimens are also effective in preventing PCP. Prophylaxis is available to patients using a decreased amount of the above medications. Pentamidine when used

for prophylaxis is given in aerosol form, generally with a hand-held nebulizer. Prophylactic regimens are usually initiated when the patient's T4 count drops below 200 000 cells/L. The patient is taught to assess for signs of infection and learns to monitor respiratory rate and function. Nursing care is similar to that for other patients experiencing respiratory impairment.

Manifestations

The onset, symptoms and course of disease vary with different types of pneumonia. Infection of the alveoli results in their filling with inflammatory exudate (plasma, blood cells, pathological organisms and cellular debris) that readily overflows into other alveoli, extending the infection. A whole lobe of lung tissue may become consolidated or the consolidation may be patchy; pulmonary ventilation and diffusion are impaired, and the oxygen tension of the blood is reduced to below normal. The PCO_2 level generally remains normal or may be decreased. The increased respiratory rate caused by the initial increase in the PCO_2 results in increased amounts of carbon dioxide being excreted by the normal areas of the lung. Within a few days the exudate becomes more liquid and may be gradually eliminated from the alveoli by expectoration and absorption. This process is referred to as *resolution*. The disease may clear up with dramatic rapidity when specific antibacterial drugs are administered. It may run a course of 5–10 days; if untreated, it may rapidly prove to be fatal.

The onset of some infective pneumonias may be very sudden; they frequently begin with a chill, followed by fever (e.g. pneumococcal). Hypostatic, staphylococcal and atypical (viral) pneumonias have a gradual onset (less abrupt than the pneumococcal type). The last two may be associated at the onset with upper respiratory infection.

The pulse rate and respirations increase. The latter may be shallow and accompanied by an audible grunt characteristic of pleuritic pain. The nostrils flare on inspiration and the face may be flushed. Cyanosis of the lips, tongue and nailbeds may develop. The patient's cough may be hacking, painful and unproductive at first; later, it becomes less painful and is productive. In bronchopneumonia the sputum is tenacious, blood streaked and mucopurulent. In pneumococcal pneumonia, the sputum is usually rust coloured and becomes purulent as resolution takes place.

The patient experiences general malaise, weakness, headache and aching pains. The leucocyte count is raised in some types of pneumonia (e.g. pneumococcal, staphylococcal) and normal or below normal in others (e.g. atypical). Sputum examination and culture, blood culture and serology are used to identify the causative organism. Specific antimicrobial therapy is determined by culture and sensitivity tests.

An example of a clinical situation is described in Case 13.1.

CASE George Fleming was an emergency admission to the medical unit with a diagnosis of right lower lobe pneumonia. Upon admission, a thorough nursing history and assessment were completed. Further data were obtained from his

daughter and from the results of diagnostic tests and additional assessments as they became available on his health record. Relevant findings included:

- *General appearance*. George was a well-nourished man in his mid-seventies, with obvious respiratory distress and diaphoresis
- *Vital signs*. Respirations were rapid at 32 per minute; pulse was 110 per minute; and oral temperature was raised to 38.2°C
- *Respirations* were laboured with moderate retraction of the intercostal spaces. Crackles and wheezes were heard over the right middle and lower chest on auscultation. No abnormal breath sounds were heard over the left lung
- *Cough* was dry and hacking, producing a small amount of blood-streaked sputum
- *Pain and discomfort*. The patient experienced occasional episodes of stabbing chest pain that increased with respirations and travelled to his right shoulder
- *Cognitive and perceptual status*. The patient was oriented to the person but was confused as to time and place
- *Chest radiography* demonstrated consolidation in the right lower lobe
- *Sputum analysis* showed a positive Gram stain for bacterial pneumococci
- *White blood cell count* was increased to 17 000 per mL
- *Arterial blood gas* analysis showed a raised $PaCO_2$ of 52 mmHg, a decreased PaO_2 of 70 mmHg, and a decreased oxygen saturation level of 86%
- *Psychosocial history*. George is retired. He lives alone in the home that he and his wife occupied until her death 3 years ago. His only daughter lives nearby.

The patient's daughter stated that her father was normally bright, alert and oriented. He was an active participant in planning and organizing events for the local pensioner's group. He had complained of a cold and flu-like symptoms a few weeks before, but seemed to be improving. His present illness had come on suddenly.

Based upon an analysis of available data, the following major patient problems were identified:

1 The patient is unable to achieve normal lung ventilation due to the retention of respiratory secretions secondary to infection (i.e. ineffective airway clearance).
2 The patient is confused and disoriented in time and space, probably because of cerebral hypoxia as a result of the first problem.
3 The patient has severely limited activity owing to shortness of breath.
4 The patient is lacking in knowledge about how to improve airway clearance.

Box 13.1 illustrates the plan of care devised to deal with each of these problems. In this plan, where there are two goals for each problem, the interventions apply to both.

After 7 days the patient was able to feed, wash and dress himself, walk to the bathroom independently and describe plans for his discharge. He was alert and oriented. Owing to pressure on beds he was discharged a day earlier than planned; this caused considerable inconvenience for his

Box 13.1 Patient care plan for George Fleming, an elderly man with pneumonia

Goals	Nursing intervention	Rationale
Patient problem 1: Ineffective airway clearance related to retention of respiratory secretions secondary to inflammation of respiratory passages as a result of infection		
1 Respiratory rate will be 20–24 per minute within 3 days (date …)	Assess respiratory rate and depth, breathing pattern and breath sounds 2 hourly	Ongoing objective data provide a basis for planning further nursing interventions and identification of signs of respiratory failure
2 Breathing pattern will be regular, requiring minimal effort, and breath sounds normal within 3 days (date …)	Monitor body temperature 4 hourly	Provides objective data on disease progress and response to therapy
	Obtain a sputum specimen for culture and sensitivity as ordered	Antibiotic therapy alters sensitivity of organisms
	Administer i.v. antibiotics 6 hourly as prescribed	Treatment of infection
	Administer oxygen at 24% by mask as prescribed	To promote gas exchange and decrease respiratory effort
	Ensure patient is sitting upright	To facilitate lung expansion
	Demonstrate and supervise deep breathing and coughing techniques 2 hourly during day and when awake at night	To improve breathing pattern; promote removal of secretion
	Provide anti-inflammatory analgesic preparation 4 hourly as prescribed until temperature within normal range	To reduce body temperature and promote comfort to facilitate lung expansion
	Offer juice, warm tea or water 2 hourly or more often. Leave fluids within reach. Monitor fluid intake and maintain at 2 L daily or greater	Adequate hydration facilitates movement of secretions
	Cleanse mouth with diluted mouthwash after coughing (2–4 hourly) more	With increased expectoration of secretions, frequent mouth care is required
Patient problem 2: Confusion and disorientation in time and space due to cerebral hypoxia		
1 Mr Fleming will be oriented to time and place as well as person within 4 days (date …)	Assess cognitive status 4 hourly	To evaluate changes in hypoxic state
	Call Mr Fleming by name and introduce yourself on each encounter	To promote orientation and decrease confusion and anxiety
2 Mr Fleming will participate in interactions with nurses, family and other visitors	Provide repeated explanations of all care activities before and during the procedures	
	Engage Mr Fleming in conversations during all activities	
	Encourage daughter to talk to him during visits	

continued

Box 13.1 *Cont'd*		
Goals	**Nursing intervention**	**Rationale**
Patient problem 3: Severely limited activity due to dyspnoea		
Mr Fleming will gradually resume self-care and other activities of daily living, becoming independent in 7 days (date …)	Plan care activities to allow for uninterrupted rest periods. Adjust assessment and care to be completed when he is awake	To promote maximum rest
	Assist Mr Fleming with all aspects of self-care initially. Increase his participation gradually as tolerated	To prevent exhaustion
	Assess daily for bowel function. Obtain order for stool softener if straining occurs	Constipation is a side-effect of analgesic medications and dehydration. Straining at stool increases energy expenditure
	Sit Mr Fleming upright	To depress diaphragm and decrease effort of breathing
Patient problem 4: Lack of knowledge concerning care after discharge		
Mr Fleming and his daughter will state a plan for home care and maintenance of respiratory function	To teach Mr Fleming and his daughter to observe for signs and symptoms of respiratory distress	Mr Fleming and his daughter will recognize complications quickly and seek help
	Assist them to develop a plan for Mr Fleming to obtain regular and adequate nutrition and fluids and adequate rest when he returns home	Mr Fleming and his daughter will be informed about his needs
	Make a referral to the community nurse for follow-up care	Resources should be available within the community to ensure continuity of care

daughter who had to take him home at very short notice. A community nurse visit was arranged as part of the follow-up but this was later than planned because of the premature discharge. Local social services promised that a home help would be able to visit once a week, but owing to staff shortages no-one came in the first week after discharge. Despite these problems, the patient recovered fully.

Chronic obstructive pulmonary disease and asthma

Disease of the airway may be broadly categorized as either reversible or irreversible, dependent upon whether the airways respond to treatment (Brewin 1997). The diagnosis of particular disorders is not, however, so simple as there is often overlap and what started as a reversible condition may over a period of time lead to irreversible damage to the airways.

Chronic obstructive pulmonary disease (COPD) has been defined by the British Thoracic Society (BTS) as 'A chronic slowly progressive disorder characterized by airways obstruction … which does not change markedly over several months. Most of the lung function impairment is fixed, although some reversibility can be produced by bronchodilator (or other) therapy' (BTS 1997, p. 2). As airway

obstruction gradually increases, breathing patterns change and become less efficient until eventually they are unable to meet the ventilatory needs of the body. COPD is a general term that covers many conditions (e.g. chronic bronchitis, emphysema and bronchiectasis) which share the same underlying lung conditions (Haughney 1998). The term COPD acknowledges the fact that chronic respiratory disease may be caused by a number of simultaneously occurring pathological processes. COPD affects mainly older patients and most cases are linked to a history of tobacco smoking. Asthma may contribute to the development of COPD.

The nursing care required by patients with COPD is discussed after an overview of the various disorders.

Chronic bronchitis

The disease is characterized by hyperactivity of the mucus-secreting glands of the bronchial mucosa in response to prolonged or frequently recurring irritation. As with all forms of COPD, tobacco smoke is the principal cause, although atmospheric pollutants such as dust, industrial fumes and smoke also contribute to the problem.

The bronchial mucosa undergoes a chronic inflammatory process, together with hypertrophy and an increase in the number of mucus-secreting glands. Airway obstruction results from the narrowing of the bronchial lumen as a result of hyperplasia of the mucus-secreting glands and the increased production of sputum. Initially the patient usually experiences a cough in the morning (often referred to as smoker's cough) but it progressively becomes more frequent and is accompanied by dyspnoea, and the production of sputum. Although chronic bronchitis and emphysema are classified as separate disorders, they commonly coexist. A frequent complication of chronic bronchitis is chest infection as secretions are not expectorated and become infected. Individuals with chronic bronchitis are usually well aware of the further debilitation and lethargy that results from a chest infection and need to be vigilant for the first signs of an exacerbation in order to obtain prompt treatment. Infective bronchitis is the most common cause of an acute exacerbation of chronic bronchitis, which may in turn lead to respiratory failure and death (Bloom 1995).

Pulmonary emphysema

Pulmonary **emphysema** is a chronic disorder characterized by destruction of alveoli walls and a loss of lung surface area for gas exchange together with a loss of elasticity due to damage to the connective tissue (Springhouse Corporation 2000). Smoking is the principal cause. Destruction of the pulmonary lung units occurs with ageing in all lungs but is accelerated in some, leading to clinical emphysema. The damage is not uniform. It may affect only the central portion of the pulmonary lobules (centralobular emphysema) or it may result in destruction of most of the structures within a terminal unit, including the alveolar ducts and alveoli (panlobular emphysema). The onset is insidious but, once initiated, is progressive and non-reversible. The disease is more common in men than in women. The lung damage cannot be repaired but the patient may be helped to breathe more effectively and live with less disability. Patients who smoke may be helped to delay the progression of the disease by being encouraged to stop smoking.

Medical approaches to treatment of COPD   The British Thoracic Society (BTS) and the Global Initiative for Chronic Obstructive Lung Disease (GOLD) categorize COPD as mild, moderate, severe and very severe according to spirometry readings and symptoms. FEV_1/FVC is expressed as a ratio of the forced expiratory volume expired in 1 second compared with the forced vital capacity, and the FEV_1 is expressed as a percentage of the predicted FEV_1 for the individual patient:

- Mild ($FEV_1/FVC < 70$, $FEV_1 < 80\%$, with or without symptoms)
- Moderate ($FEV_1/FVC < 70$, $FEV_1 > 50\% < 70\%$, with or without symptoms)
- Severe ($FEV_1/FVC < 70$, $FEV_1 > 30\% < 50\%$, with or without symptoms)
- Very severe $FEV_1/FVC < 70$, $FEV_1, < 30\%$ or presence of chronic respiratory failure or right heart failure (GOLD 2004).

Both GOLD and the BTS recommend treatment guidelines for each group (BTS 1997, GOLD 2004).

Drug treatment   The National Institute for Clinical Excellence (2004) have produced guidance which emphasizes that clinicians should, in planning drug therapy, respond to patients' reporting of symptoms and experience rather than simply look at objective measures of lung function. Simple questions about changes in symptoms, exercise tolerance and quality of life should be used (Halpin 2004). The MRC dyspnoea scale may be useful for this (NICE 2004). While lung function tests may be useful in initial diagnosis and as a guide to severity, it is now established that lung function measurements (spirometry) do not fully relate to levels of dyspnoea and disability in COPD (MacNee and Calverley 2003). Regular therapy with short-term bronchodilators (e.g. salbutamol) is the first line of treatment, moving onto the use of long-acting B2 agonists (e.g. salmeterol) and anti-cholinergic agents (e.g. ipratropium) if patients remain symptomatic. Use of inhaled steroids remains controversial but currently, NICE recommend that inhaled corticosteroids should be used in patients with an FEV_1 less than 50% predicted and a history of two or more exacerbations in the previous year (NICE 2004). Some patients may experience such severe symptoms that they ultimately need oxygen therapy to help them cope with their activities of daily living. Non-drug measures applicable to all groups include smoking cessation, exercise, vaccination against influenza and pneumonia and pulmonary rehabilitation where appropriate.

Asthma

The prevalence of **asthma** in the UK has increased significantly in recent decades. It has been estimated by Asthma UK that 5.5 million people in the UK live with asthma; 1.1 million are children and there are over 1400 deaths per year (Asthma UK 2004). The increased incidence may partly reflect an increased awareness of, rather than a real increase in, the disease. Asthma can be described as a syndrome comprising bronchial inflammation, airway hyper-responsivseness and usually reversible airway obstruction (Rees and Kanabar 2000). It is characterized by variable airway obstruction, bronchial hyper-reactivity and often persistent inflammation (Kilgarriff 2000).

Stimuli that may precipitate the asthmatic response include: allergens (especially the housedust mite), viral respiratory infections, irritating inhalants (smoke, chemicals, air pollutants), cold dry air, emotional stress and physical exercise. An asthma attack may also be triggered by a response to drugs such as acetylsalicylic acid (aspirin), beta-blockers and non-steroidal antiinflammatory drugs. Asthma often begins in childhood but may develop at any age. Childhood asthma may gradually resolve with growth into adulthood, but adult-onset asthma tends to be a more permanent problem with which the person has to learn to live. Frequently there is a personal and/or family history of one or more allergies.

Medical approaches to the treatment of asthma   Most patients with asthma have their condition controlled and monitored by the primary healthcare team. There are, however, occasions when an individual's asthma may become so severe that hospital admission is required. Regardless of the location of care, the British asthma guidelines produced by the British Thoracic Society and Scottish Intercollegiate Guidelines Network (2003) provide comprehensive, multi-disciplinary guidance on best practice. A key feature of the current approach to the treatment of asthma is the early use of preventive anti-inflammatory therapy, usually in the form of inhaled corticosteroids. The dose of inhaled corticosteroid should be titrated according to symptoms, peak flow recordings and other drug therapy with the goal of administering the lowest effective dose for long-term control and optimal quality of life (Lipworth 1999). The use of preventive corticosteroid should reduce the need for symptomatic relief with short-acting inhaled bronchodilators (β_2 agonists).

If β_2 agonists such as salbutamol are required to relieve shortness of breath more than once daily, the emphasis must be placed on prevention of attacks. Frequent use of these short-acting drugs in mild to moderate asthma is a cause for concern. The long-acting β_2 agonists such as salmeterol play a role in the long-term management of asthma and are usually administered at the same time as inhaled steroids.

Additionally, a group of drugs known as leucotriene receptor agonists (LTRAs) have an anti-inflammatory effect. They are used as 'add on' drugs and may be prescribed for people with mild to moderate asthma and are particularly useful for those with exercise-induced asthma if inhaled corticosteroids and an inhaled β_2 agonists are insufficient (British National Formulary 2006).

The main emphasis within asthma care is prophylaxis – the prevention of an asthma attack or exacerbation. Prophylactic treatments such as inhaled steroids are, however, effective only when used correctly. For most patients with asthma, inhaled medication needs to be taken daily even when they are free of symptoms. From a review of the literature, Ward and Reynolds (2000) estimated that approximately half of all patients with asthma do not comply with their prescribed treatment regimen, emphasizing a very important role for nurses in working with patients to help them understand their condition and its recommended management.

The effects upon families or patients with asthma can be devastating, with the disease causing major practical and emotional problems for everyone, not just the sufferer. Nurses are ideally placed to help patients manage their asthma with the least disruption to their life. Patients should be taught that lack of response to a bronchodilator is a vital warning sign of an impending serious attack. This is a sign that is often missed. Patients can also be taught routine peak flow monitoring at home, in the same way that patients with diabetes monitor blood glucose levels. Deterioration in peak flow is a warning sign that, if acted upon, could avert a major medical emergency.

The monitoring of peak expiratory flow rates (PEFRs) at home in addition to early recognition of deterioration in symptoms can facilitate the early detection of decreased respiratory function and gives the individual with asthma the potential for greater control. The BTS/SIGN (2003) guidance highlights a number of evidence-based points which may help people with asthma adhere to suggested management regimens. These include interventions that are designed to meet the needs of individuals with asthma and are focused on improved communication between healthcare professionals and patients. Simple written instructions can increase patient concordance and presenting important information in a repetitive fashion can improve patient recall. BTS and SIGN offer the following practical guidance:

- Use open-ended questions like: 'If we could make one thing better for your asthma what would it be?'
- Make it clear you are listening and responding to the patient's concerns and goals
- Reinforce practical information and negotiated treatment plans with written instruction
- Consider reminder strategies
- Recall patients who miss appointments.

More recent approaches to asthma care have included the use of written action plans focused on individual needs. Patients monitor their respiratory function (usually by recording PEFR and noting any symptoms such as sleep disturbance, etc.) and the clinician provides them with guidelines on appropriate action to take based upon their observations (BTS/SIGN 2003).

For patients to take control of their asthma it is vital that they are able to identify the signs of an impending attack and understand what actions they should take. Patients also need to learn the skills of measuring (and recording) their PEFR and of taking their inhaled medication. Nurses need to be able to teach patients about their condition and provide correct instruction on the use of inhaler devices and peak flow meters.

The acute asthma attack   Warning signs of increasing bronchial reactivity include frequent awakening at night, decreased physical effort tolerance, shortness of breath on getting up in the morning, cough and (if the patient is measuring it, a decreased peak expiratory flow rate).

The reaction of the over-responsive airway to stimuli is oedema and thickening of the mucosa, hypersecretion by the mucous glands and spasmodic contraction of bronchial and bronchiolar muscle tissue. This causes diffuse narrowing of the tracheobronchial tree and obstruction to airflow. Expiration is impeded and the lungs become hyperinflated, resulting in severe dyspnoea and wheezing.

During an acute asthmatic attack the patient experiences tightness in the chest, wheezing and dyspnoea. The accessory muscles of respiration are used and expiration is prolonged. The patient usually appears distraught and may assume an upright sitting position. The sputum is scant and thick, and the pulse and respiratory rates are rapid. In some cases the patient may not be able to speak and physical examination of the chest will show that there is little air entry into the lower lobes of the lungs. Often patients can be treated with inhaled short acting beta 2 agonists, however, patients suffering a severe asthmatic attack may require intubation and artificial ventilation for a period if they do not respond to nebulized and intravenously administered bronchodilator therapy. Repeated peak flow measurements and arterial blood gas values are good guides to progress, together with vital sign monitoring. The importance of psychological support during acute episodes of respiratory distress cannot be overemphasized.

Management of a severe asthmatic attack   As the onset of an asthmatic attack may be sudden and without warning, treatment has to be immediate and appropriate to the severity of the attack. This can be categorized into four types: mild, moderate, severe and life-threatening (see Box 13.2).

Key factors in the history that should be ascertained at assessment include whether the patient:

- is a known asthmatic and what medication he or she takes
- has any known allergies and may have been exposed to allergens
- has a cough and whether it is productive
- has any nocturnal symptoms
- is wheezing
- is a smoker.

The flow charts depicted in Figures 13.3 and 13.4 summarize treatment and care for a serious attack in hospital and in the community respectively.

If the patient has been admitted, the nurse should ensure before discharge that:

1 The basic pathophysiology of asthma has been explained to the patient and is supported by leaflets.
2 The patient knows about all his or her asthma medicines and their actions.

Box 13.2   Characteristics of various types of asthma attack

Mild or moderate
The speech is normal
Pulse < 110 per min
Respiratory rate ≤ 25 per min
Peak expiratory flow rate (PEFR) greater than 50% of the normal for that person

Severe
Unable to complete sentences
Pulse > 110 per min
Respiratory rate > 25 per min
PEFR less than 50% of the normal for that person

Life-threatening
The patient is unable to speak
Bradycardia and hypotension
Signs of exhaustion
PEFR less than 33% of the normal for that person
Silent chest on auscultation
The patient is cyanosed

---

3 The patient's PEFR has been monitored throughout his or her hospital stay, not just during the acute exacerbation; it must be greater than 70% of the patient's predicted or best recent value.
4 Inhaled corticosteroid therapy has been maintained throughout the admission and the patient is taking both inhaled and oral corticosteroids.
5 The patient has adequate inhaler technique and has been taking inhaled drugs for at least 24 hours.
6 In conjunction with the patient, the identification of trigger factors has begun and avoidance strategies are being considered, and an individualized written action plan has been provided.
7 Follow-up appointment arrangements have been made.
8 The patient has been instructed on how to monitor PEFR and has been supplied with a PEFR meter and diary card.
9 A detailed written discharge summary has been prepared for the general practice.
10 The patient knows what to do if his or her condition deteriorates soon after discharge.

It is clear that nurses and other health professionals need to work in partnership with patients to ensure optimum control of asthma and least disruption to daily life.

Problems common to patients with COPD

Altered breathing pattern   The most frequent symptom of COPD is a prolonged expiratory phase, as demonstrated by an increase in the forced expiratory time. Other characteristics of the breathing pattern of a person with COPD are rapid shallow respirations and use of the intercostal and accessory muscles. Shortness of breath is experienced by many, but not all patients, despite severe airflow limitation. Dyspnoea varies daily with changes in activity, increased effort and during sleep.

Poor activity tolerance   Respiratory muscle fatigue develops in persons with COPD in response to the increased airway resistance, which in turn increases the work of breathing. The inspiratory muscles have to generate greater negative pressures to ventilate the lungs. Muscle fatigue occurs when the inspiratory muscles are no longer able to maintain the force required for ventilation.

Activity intolerance increases with exercise and stress and impairs the individual's ability to perform usual activities. Eventually, the effort of breathing consumes all the individual's energy. In addition to spirometry it is important to take into account markers of deterioration such as nutritional status, body mass index and self-reported accounts of breathlessness.

Inadequate nutrition   Weight loss and muscle wasting are recognized problems in persons with chronic lung disease. Dyspnoea increases with eating and yet an increased caloric intake is needed because of the increased energy expended with breathing. Associated problems include a loss of appetite and decreased senses of taste and smell.

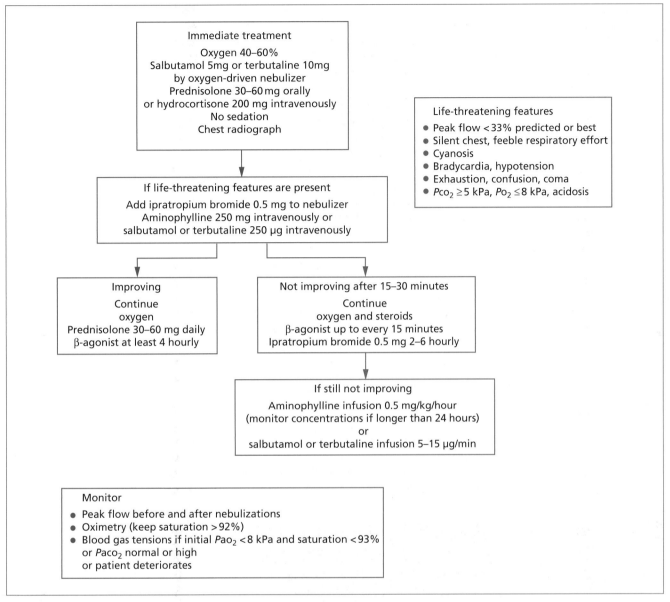

Immediate treatment

Oxygen 40–60%
Salbutamol 5mg or terbutaline 10mg
by oxygen-driven nebulizer
Prednisolone 30–60 mg orally
or hydrocortisone 200 mg intravenously
No sedation
Chest radiograph

Life-threatening features

- Peak flow <33% predicted or best
- Silent chest, feeble respiratory effort
- Cyanosis
- Bradycardia, hypotension
- Exhaustion, confusion, coma
- $P\text{co}_2 \geq 5$ kPa, $P\text{o}_2 \leq 8$ kPa, acidosis

If life-threatening features are present

Add ipratropium bromide 0.5 mg to nebulizer
Aminophylline 250 mg intravenously or
salbutamol or terbutaline 250 µg intravenously

Improving

Continue
oxygen
Prednisolone 30–60 mg daily
β-agonist at least 4 hourly

Not improving after 15–30 minutes

Continue
oxygen and steroids
β-agonist up to every 15 minutes
Ipratropium bromide 0.5 mg 2–6 hourly

If still not improving

Aminophylline infusion 0.5 mg/kg/hour
(monitor concentrations if longer than 24 hours)
or
salbutamol or terbutaline infusion 5–15 µg/min

Monitor

- Peak flow before and after nebulizations
- Oximetry (keep saturation >92%)
- Blood gas tensions if initial $P\text{ao}_2 <8$ kPa and saturation <93%
  or $P\text{aco}_2$ normal or high
  or patient deteriorates

Figure 13.3   Treatment of acute severe asthma in hospital.

Inadequate knowledge   Long-term management of COPD requires the patient to be an active participant in the care process. The individual requires knowledge of the disorder; an understanding of the use, actions, administration and side-effects of the medications; the ability to perform breathing retraining techniques; information on factors influencing respiratory function; and information about community resources.

Nursing intervention
Although COPD is irreversible, patient care has improved sufficiently over the past few decades to enable patients to live useful and satisfying lives. The patient's *goal* is to achieve an effective breathing pattern so that greater levels of activity can be tolerated. This can be shown by the patient being able to:

1 demonstrate a decreased respiratory rate and increased depth of respirations
2 demonstrate improvements in objective measurements of lung function (spirometry)
3 report decreased episodes and severity of dyspnoea
4 tolerate increased levels of activity.

Smoking cessation   For patients who have COPD and continue to smoke, smoking cessation is the cornerstone of their management. Stopping smoking can prevent the progression of the disease. The nurse can assist patients by emphasizing the importance of stopping smoking and directing them to smoking cessation services either in hospitals, community or general practice. The greatest success can be achieved by offering nicotine replacement therapy or bupropion in addition to counseling.

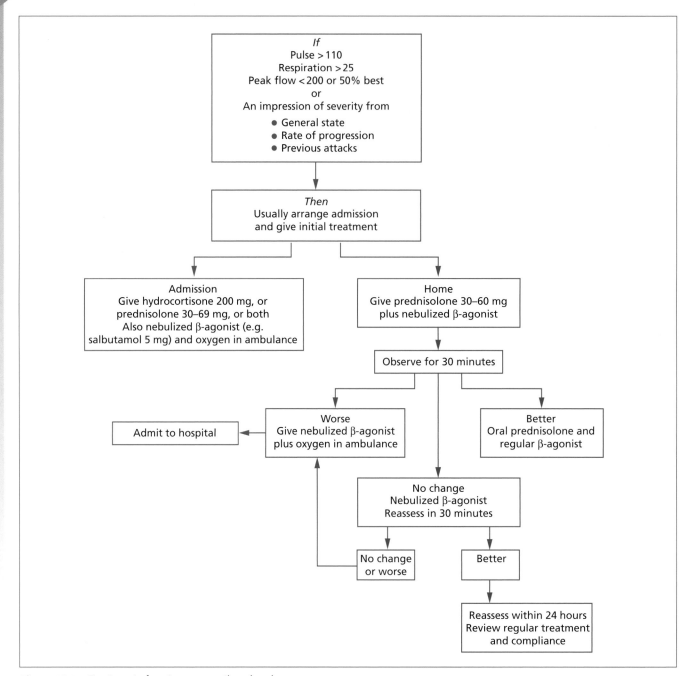

Figure 13.4   Treatment of acute severe asthma in primary care.

Breathing   Assessment of the individual's respiratory status is ongoing and focuses on the relationship of the deterioration in respiratory function to the person's ability to function in daily living activities. Interventions to improve dyspnoea are limited. The person's home and work environments are assessed for possible respiratory irritants and the individual is directed to appropriate resources for help (such as occupational therapists) in altering the environment where this is possible.

The nurse can assist the individual to gain control over the respiratory pattern. During an acute episode, the nurse can provide emotional support and at the same time teach the person to relax and control breathing. The nurse should stay with the person and may place his or her hands on the patient's shoulder and abdomen while quietly repeating instructions and encouragement to breathe slowly and deeply, gradually altering the breathing pattern and decreasing fear. Patients are taught the techniques of breathing retraining and relaxation. Nurses need to educate patients about their medication and ensure that the patients are able to administer it correctly themselves.

During an acute episode of breathlessness the patient should be discouraged from talking unnecessarily and helped to find a comfortable position (usually sitting up with arms supported). The nurse works in collaboration with the patient, general practitioner, physiotherapist, occupational therapist and pharmacist to teach the patient and family to monitor and manage the respiratory care programme.

Activity Once respiratory muscles become fatigued, they must be rested. Interventions are directed toward decreasing the work of breathing and increasing the individual's tolerance. Patients are helped to plan their daily activities to include periods of rest before and after activity, and to learn more effective ways of performing daily living activities. Inhaled medications are administered to dilate the bronchial airways and to decrease inflammation, thus decreasing the effort of breathing. Postural changes such as sitting in the forward leaning position may also facilitate breathing. The use of general body exercises and respiratory muscle training can help to improve respiratory muscle strength and to develop a more effective breathing pattern. Pulmonary rehabilitation programmes tend to focus on these exercises and many patients find that these programmes transform their lives.

In his study of people with COPD, Williams (1993) made extensive use of extracts from interviews conducted with sufferers. These graphically illustrate the tremendous difficulties that some people have to manage in order to continue with some semblance of everyday life. For example, one woman within the study described how it would take her more than 2 hours to vacuum her living room because of the need to take frequent rests. The study also highlights the extent to which some people go to disguise their reduced exercise tolerance, perhaps by pretending to be waiting for someone when they need a rest when walking. Nurses need to discover how an individual already copes in order to give effective advice and help.

Nutrition Although no randomized controlled longitudinal studies have been carried out to date to show that nutritional support alters the outcome for persons with chronic respiratory disease, malnutrition is a recognized patient health problem.

A nutritional assessment should be carried out on all patients with COPD and, if necessary, a referral made to the dietician. Nurses can help by carefully timing the administration of nebulizers so that they are not administered immediately before meals, unless the patient requires the medication in order to have sufficient breath to eat. Oxygen can be administered via nasal cannulae (see Fig. 13.5) to enable the patient to benefit from the oxygen whilst eating. The presentation of small appetizing meals interspersed with nutritious snacks can be very helpful as many patients with respiratory problems feel unable to eat a large quantity of food at any one time. Fresh chilled water should always be available and the patient should be encouraged to take frequent small sips to counteract the drying effect of tachypnoea (and oxygen therapy). Regular mouth care can also enhance a patient's appetite and make the mouth feel more pleasant.

Teaching Self-monitoring and self-care are essential components of the management programme. The patient needs to learn to cope with the limitations imposed by the disease, prevent complications and comply with the negotiated

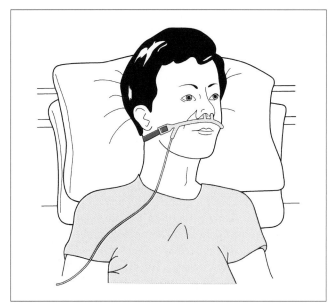

Figure 13.5 Plastic cannulae or prongs inserted into the nostrils to deliver oxygen.

treatment plan if a satisfactory lifestyle is to be achieved. As with any chronic disorder, the individual ultimately has to learn to live with the disease process and to manage his or her daily routine accordingly. In recent years the use of guided self-management of asthma has gained in popularity and emphasizes the need for partnership between the patient and health practitioner. In simple terms, self-management involves the patient keeping well and adjusting treatment according to a treatment plan developed in advance with the doctor or appropriate health professional (Partridge 1996). Changes in treatment are usually in response to changes in peak flow recordings and other symptoms. Patients therefore need to be educated about how to measure and record peak flow and how to use the treatment plan to adjust their medication.

Drugs to promote ventilation and improve airflow
Patient teaching related to drug therapy As there are no cures for many chronic respiratory disorders, treatment programmes and drug therapy are planned for each individual according to personal goals, lifestyle situation, respiratory status, response to drugs and other therapeutic measures. The patient usually assumes responsibility for self-management of the therapeutic regimen and therefore requires the knowledge and skill necessary not only to administer the drugs but also to make decisions regarding the plan. The individual learns to monitor responses to medications, determine when adjustments are desirable and when to seek further professional assistance.

The teaching plan should include:

● Information about the action, duration of effect, method of administration and side-effects of prescribed medications
● Instruction and practice in the proper use of metered-dose inhalers for optimal delivery of the medication into the bronchial tree (Fig. 13.6). For individuals who have

difficulty manipulating the metered-dose inhaler, a spacer device may be used which reduces the need for the patient to coordinate inhalation with the activation of the metered-dose inhaler

● Patient participation in the development of the medication schedule to meet the individual's needs.

The BTS/SIGN guidelines state that successful educational interventions that have resulted in clinical benefit have been delivered by trained asthma healthcare professionals (BTS/SIGN 2003) and the effectiveness of nurses teaching patients with chronic respiratory disease has been demonstrated by a number of studies. An early study by Howard (1987) showed that a structured teaching programme had the effect of reducing hospital admissions and the lengths of such admissions when necessary, in a sample of 115 patients (predominantly white males). The effect was a reduction of between 15% and 25% in the number of days this group would have been expected to spend in hospital. Nursing time spent on such activities is cost effective when consideration is given to the substantial savings that could be made by hospitals, and clearly the improvements in health status are very beneficial to patients.

Pulmonary tuberculosis

Tuberculosis is an infectious disease caused by the tubercle bacillus. The organism may attack other tissues in the body, but in Europe and North America the lungs are most frequently the primary site of invasion – although most organs in the body can be attacked. Infection is usually by inhalation of droplets bearing tubercle bacilli. The droplets have been expelled into the air by the sneezing or coughing of a person with active disease.

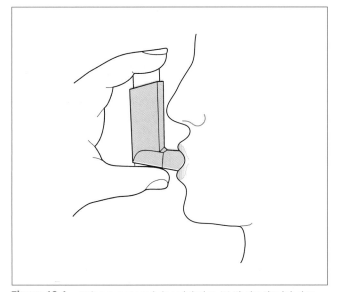

Figure 13.6   Using a metered-dose inhaler. (1) Shake the inhaler. (2) Exhale fully. (3) Spray once into wide open mouth as you inhale fully. (4) Hold breath for 5 seconds before exhaling. (5) Repeat for each puff ordered.

Tuberculosis is a disease of poverty, readily taking advantage of those with weakened resistance due to poor nutrition and general health. Social conditions, therefore, play a large part in determining susceptibility to the disease. Homeless persons and the elderly, together with members of ethnic communities originating from the Indian subcontinent, are perhaps most at risk in the UK. People who live with HIV are more susceptible to tuberculosis and the HIV epidemic has contributed to the resurgence of tuberculosis in recent years (Chief Medical Officer 2002). Children and adolescents are at greater risk than adults. Tuberculosis is responsible for 2 million deaths per year, the majority being in sub-Sahara Africa. The incidence of tuberculosis in the UK has increased in recent years: there were 5778 new cases in 1988, 6564 new cases in 1993 (Central Statistical Office 1995) and 7835 new cases in 2003 (TB Alert 2004).

Disease process

Small rounded nodules, with a tendency toward central necrosis, develop at the site of tissue invasion by the bacilli. These are referred to as *tubercles* and are composed of lung tissue cells, leucocytes, other phagocytic cells, fibroblasts and tubercle bacilli. If the body defences are strong enough to destroy the organisms, the lesion heals and may calcify.

In some instances, the reproduction of the tubercle bacilli may be minimal; a few continue to survive within the tubercle but remain confined and dormant. This person, having been infected and still harbouring live bacilli, will show a positive tuberculin test approximately 2–10 weeks after the initial infection; defensive cells have become sensitized and tend to inhibit or slow up the growth of tubercle bacilli. At a later date, if resistance is lowered, the reproduction of the tubercle bacilli may be accelerated and active disease develops. When the bacilli continue to multiply, the tubercle necroses centrally, producing soft caseous material that may eventually be discharged from the tubercle, leaving a cavity. This caseous discharge is highly infective.

The initial infection does not affect pulmonary function. The later stages of tuberculosis, which are becoming again more common in Britain and Europe, produce systemic and local symptoms. The constitutional symptoms are vague and non-specific; they include lassitude, fatigue, malaise, loss of appetite and weight, fever (usually low grade) in the latter part of the day, tachycardia and night sweats. Symptoms produced by the local disease process at the site of the lesion in the lungs are cough, sputum, haemoptysis, dyspnoea and chest pain if the pleura is involved.

Diagnostic investigation

The investigation of a patient for pulmonary tuberculosis involves tuberculin testing, chest radiography and bacteriological examination of sputum.

Treatment

Patients remain at home and continue to work during the course of their treatment. The principal factors in the plan of patient care are prolonged chemotherapy, rest and patient and family education.

The administration of specific antimicrobial drugs over a long period of time has proved very successful in the prevention and treatment of tuberculosis. Preventive therapy for susceptible contacts involves the administration of isoniazid 300 mg daily for 6 months (Haslett et al 1999). The recommended treatment for infected patients commences with an initial phase of 2 months' treatment with isoniazid, rifampicin and pyrazinamide together to kill as many bacteria as possible, as quickly as possible (British National Formulary 2006). After 2 months of treatment this may be decreased to isoniazid and rifampicin only for a further 4 months. Longer periods of treatment or other drugs may be needed if there is evidence of resistance to these antibiotics. The nurse should be familiar with the treatment plan and with the actions and possible side-effects of the drugs so that adverse reactions can be recognized early and the patient can be taught what to look for and what to do if side-effects occur. The following drugs are used:

Isoniazid This is taken orally. This drug is usually well tolerated. Liver function should be checked before use as the drug can be toxic to the liver. Peripheral neuropathy is the main side-effect, and is usually associated with pre-existing risk factors such as malnourishment, alcoholism or diabetes.

Ethambutol This is used if resistance to first-choice drugs is likely. Patients receiving ethambutol should be assessed for visual acuity before treatment and monitored for changes, as the main side-effect is loss of visual acuity and colour blindness.

Rifampicin This is taken orally 1 hour before or 2 hours after the ingestion of food to promote maximum absorption. Adverse gastrointestinal effects such as heartburn, epigastric distress, nausea and diarrhoea may occur and can be minimized by administering the drug with food. Patients should be helped to establish a routine that best suits their responses. Patients should be aware that rifampicin may impart a red-orange colour to the urine, faeces, sputum, sweat and tears. Soft contact lenses may become permanently discoloured. The patient's liver function is monitored regularly.

Streptomycin This antibiotic is rarely used and only if resistance is a problem. It is given intramuscularly and serious side-effects are damage of the auditory nerves and consequent loss of hearing.

Pyrazinamide This drug is often added during the first 2 months of therapy. It occasionally causes hepatitis, hyperuricaemia, gastrointestinal disturbances or arthralgia.

In view of the lengthy courses of chemotherapy required to treat tuberculosis, there is a significant risk of patients failing to take their medication correctly or simply stopping altogether. This contributes to the problem of emerging resistance to current medication. Close supervision and reinforcement of teaching about the importance of completing the full course are therefore required in the community care setting.

Lung cancer

Lung cancer is the most common cancer in men and the primary cause of cancer deaths in both men and women. The incidence of lung cancer has been rising over the last 50 years. Cigarette smoking is a major risk factor for the development of lung cancer, with more than 85% of lung cancers being directly attributable to smoking (Mera 1997). Most patients present with symptoms late in the course of the disease and it has been estimated that approximately 70% of patients presenting with symptoms already have metastases (Mera 1997). In view of the high mortality rate for the disease and the strong links to smoking, the most important issue in relation to lung cancer is prevention and the use of health promotion strategies aimed at a reduction in smoking.

Characteristics of cancer of the lung

Early symptoms are usually absent or vague. The person may have a persistent non-productive cough. Later, the sputum may be blood streaked. Dyspnoea, localized chest pain and wheezing may develop. General symptoms include fever, chills, sweating (especially night sweats), anorexia, weakness, fatigue and weight loss. Symptoms are often insidious. Confirmation of the presence of lung cancer requires further diagnostic investigations.

Treatment of lung cancer

Treatment of lung cancer usually involves a combination of chemotherapy, radiation and surgical resection. Small cell lung cancers, which are characterized by rapid cell growth and metastases, are usually sensitive to chemotherapy and radiation. The non-small-cell variety are usually removed surgically. Most patients show some response to treatment but the 5-year survival rate remains poor.

Chemotherapy Combinations of various chemotherapeutic agents may be prescribed for patients who have metastatic disease on diagnosis and for those with recurrent disease. No effective drug regimen for cancer of the lung has been proven; the use of chemotherapy is therefore limited primarily to individuals with small cell lung tumours.

Radiotherapy Radiation is used as a primary treatment, in combination with surgery, or for palliation. The total dose of and the schedule for radiation depends on the treatment goal.

Surgical treatment Surgical resection is the treatment of choice for persons with non-small-cell lung cancer with no evidence of extrathoracic metastases. Surgical treatment consists of a thoracotomy and resection of the involved lung tissue and regional lymph nodes.

Pneumonectomy, in which an entire lung is removed, involves the ligation of a large pulmonary artery, two large pulmonary veins and a bronchus. The phrenic nerve on the operative side is crushed or severed to permit the diaphragm to rise to reduce the size of the cavity that remains. Pneumonectomy is used when extensive tissue must be excised.

A *lobectomy* is the removal of a lobe of a lung and is used when the disease is confined to that particular lobe.

Segmental resection is used when the person's disease is localized to a segment of a lung, making it possible to conserve functional tissue and lessen the degree of overdistension in the other lung by removing only the affected segment.

Wedge resection is used when the disease is localized and small, or when conservative treatment is indicated because of a poor prognosis.

Nursing care of the person having chest surgery

Preoperative nursing care Before operation the patient and family may be anxious and frightened. They may be denying the diagnosis of lung cancer and the severity of the prognosis, while at the same time they may be struggling to make decisions regarding treatment.

The patient is usually fatigued and restless, and may appear thin and emaciated from recent weight loss and poor appetite. Chest pain and discomfort may not develop in the early stages. Respiratory function is usually impaired as a result of a history of heavy smoking and resulting chronic airflow disease as well as the lung cancer. The patient may experience a persistent non-productive cough and shortness of breath.

The patient's day is occupied with numerous diagnostic studies, including chest radiography, cytological studies of sputum, bronchoscopy and pulmonary function studies.

The goals for nursing intervention during the preoperative period are: (1) to improve respiratory function before surgery; (2) to alleviate the anxiety of the patient and family by providing support during the decision-making process and in coping with the diagnosis and prognosis; and (3) to provide information about the operative procedure and expectations for the patient and family before and after the operation.

Postoperative nursing care The arterial blood pressure, pulse and respirations are noted every 15 minutes for the first 2–3 hours and then the interval is increased to 0.5–1 hour for the succeeding 8–10 hours if the vital signs are stabilized.

The rise and fall of both sides of the chest in respiration should be noted. Dyspnoea, decreased movement of one side of the chest on inspiration (except in pneumonectomy), cyanosis or chest pain may manifest a pneumothorax and should be reported promptly to the doctor. This may develop as a result of air or fluid collecting in the pleural cavity and compressing the lung. It must be treated quickly by chest aspiration (thoracocentesis), or the patient may die from respiratory insufficiency. Respirations are also observed for audible moist sounds. Portable chest radiography may be done daily for 2–3 days to determine lung expansion and detect the presence of fluid and air in the pleural cavity.

The wound area and chest drainage are examined frequently for any indications of bleeding. The sealed drainage system is checked frequently for functioning and the tubing connections are examined for security. The volume of drainage is measured at regular intervals. The intake and output are recorded and the fluid balance is estimated.

Arterial blood specimens may be necessary for blood gas determinations which indicate possible respiratory insufficiency and the need for mechanical assistance and/or increased oxygen inhalation.

In the case of a pneumonectomy, turning is from the back to the affected side only. With partial resection, the patient usually may be turned from back to left side, to back to right side, and so on. If a sternum-splitting incision is used, the patient is generally most comfortable on the back, but is encouraged to assume a lateral position for at least brief periods.

Disorders of the pleurae

Pleural effusion   Pleural effusion is an accumulation of an abnormal quantity of fluid in the interpleural space and is a symptom associated with a variety of conditions. The fluid may be a transudate or an exudate. A transudate may collect in the pleural space as a result of increased venous pressure incurred by congestive heart failure or an intrathoracic tumour which interferes with venous drainage in the area. Cirrhosis of the liver may cause a pleural effusion, as well as ascites. An accumulation of exudate in the pleural space indicates irritation and inflammation of the pleura associated with infection.

The patient with an effusion may experience some pleuritic pain, which is stabbing and is worse on inspiration before the excess fluid collects. The condition may develop insidiously and may go unrecognized until the increasing volume of fluid compresses the lung, causing dyspnoea and impaired pulmonary ventilation.

A chest aspiration (thoracocentesis) is done to relieve the pressure on the lung and to obtain a specimen of fluid for examination. Treatment is directed toward the disease causing the effusion. A culture is made of the aspirated fluid for identification of the causative organisms and their antibiotic sensitivity. The patient receives antibiotics parenterally or orally, and the drug may also be injected into the thoracic cavity following aspiration. Surgical drainage may be necessary, especially if the pus is thick. A collection of pus in the pleural cavity is known as *empyema*. Early breathing exercises to promote re-expansion of the lung are important, because the visceral pleura tends to become thick, fibrous and resistant to stretching, reducing lung compliance and the vital capacity.

Pneumothorax   Pneumothorax is a term used to describe a situation where a rupture in the visceral and/or parietal pleura allows air to accumulate in the pleural space, leading to collapse of part of the lung. This may occur after trauma or spontaneously. In *tension pneumothorax* the rupture acts as a one-way valve so that air enters the pleural space on each respiration but cannot escape. This leads to a progressive build-up of air in the pleural space, collapse of the whole lung and displacement of the trachea away from the affected side. Major blood vessels become kinked and blood flow to the brain may be seriously impaired. Unlike a *simple pneumothorax*, which often resolves itself with the air in the pleural space being gradually reabsorbed, a *tension pneumothorax* is a life-threatening emergency. An accumulation of blood acts in the same way to compress the lung and is known as a *haemothorax*.

In order to expand the collapsed lung it is necessary to remove any blood or air from the pleura. This is done by introducing a drainage tube which is sutured in place and secured via an underwater seal drain to prevent air re-entering the pleural space. If the patient has a pneumothorax, the chest drain is inserted high in the lateral chest wall, while to drain fluid and blood a site low down the lateral chest wall is selected. Drains may be inserted in both sites if blood and air need to be drained from the pleura (*haemopneumothorax*).

Assessment

Nursing assessment focuses on the person's respiratory status and breathing pattern. The breathing pattern of an individual with decreased lung expansion resulting from a pleural effusion or pneumothorax is characterized by: decreased lung volumes, dyspnoea, use of the accessory muscles of respiration, and rapid shallow breathing. In non-emergency situations the nurse should ascertain the effect of the respiratory impairment on the patient's lifestyle and ability to carry out usual daily activities. Physiological measurements of pulmonary function are obtained, when possible, and the results used to validate the analysis of the nursing history and physical examination completed by the nurse. Additional data are collected from the patient, family and the health record.

The patient's *goal* is to achieve a functionally effective breathing pattern with adequate gas exchange. The patient should demonstrate:

1 a normalizing respiratory pattern
2 increased lung volumes
3 blood gases within the normal range.

Measures to restore normal intrathoracic pressure
The intrathoracic space lies between the visceral and parietal pleurae; the membranes are normally separated only by a thin film of fluid. Disruption of the pleura by disease, trauma or chest surgery results in air or fluid entering this space; the normal negative intrapleural pressure is lost. The increased pressure restricts lung expansion on inspiration and may cause collapse of the lung. Closed chest drainage is usually established. A thoracocentesis (pleural aspiration) may be performed to remove fluid from the pleural cavity, as well as for diagnostic tests.

Closed chest drainage   A closed or water-seal drainage system is established to allow the escape of air and fluid from the pleural cavity and re-establish the normal negative pressure, while preventing any reflux.

Methods   Various methods are used to achieve closed drainage, but the principle is the same with all: to allow air

and fluid to pass in one direction only. The difference in the methods is generally in the number of compartments or containers used, whether or not suction is applied, and whether or not a flutter valve is introduced into the system. The compartments of the disposable chest drainage systems are comparable to the bottles or containers described in Figure 13.7.

Water-seal drainage may be established with one container fitted with a two-holed stopper through which two glass or plastic tubes pass (Fig. 13.7a). The chest tubes are connected to a fairly long tube leading to the drainage container. This drainage tube is connected to a tube that has its distal end submerged at all times in sterile water or sterile normal saline to a designated depth. The depth of tube submersion determines the pressure exerted by the water – hence the term water-seal drainage. A small, short tube, serving as an air vent, passes through the second hole of the tight-fitting two-holed stopper. The water level must be marked clearly on the container (or recorded in the care plan) so that the amount of drainage can be determined accurately.

With each expiration, the respiratory muscles relax, the intrapleural space is diminished and the pressure within the space is increased; this pressure exceeds that exerted by the water at the end of the tube, so fluid and air are forced from the cavity into the water in the container. The air may be seen bubbling through the water, from which it passes, escaping from the container through the vent. With inspiration the pleural space enlarges and the pressure within it decreases, causing water to rise several centimetres in the distal end of the tube. The evacuation of fluid and air from the intrapleural space results in greater space and less pressure. As a result, lung expansion is increased.

The alternating changes in pressure in the pleural cavity result in repeated fluctuations in the water level in the distal end of the drainage tube; these fluctuations correspond to the patient's breathing in and out, and indicate a patent system. If the water level does not oscillate, the tube may be blocked by a blood clot or fibrin. If this occurs the doctor should be notified at once as blocked tubing may cause a tension pneumothorax or surgical emphysema. The tube should not be milked by hand or by using mechanical rollers in an effort to relieve the blockage as even a small amount of negative pressure may result in lung tissue being sucked into the drainage system (Welch 1993). Fluctuation of the fluid level in the tube ceases when the lung has fully re-expanded. The doctor confirms this by chest radiography before removal of the drainage tube.

Coughing and deep abdominal breathing alter the intrapleural space and pressure to a greater degree than normal respirations and, as a result, are important in promoting drainage of the cavity, removal of air and fluid, and the re-expansion of remaining lung tissue.

To prevent water from being sucked into the chest, the drainage container must be kept well below the level of the patient (0.5–1 metre below the patient's chest). The negative chest pressure is equivalent to 10–20 cm H_2O and sucks

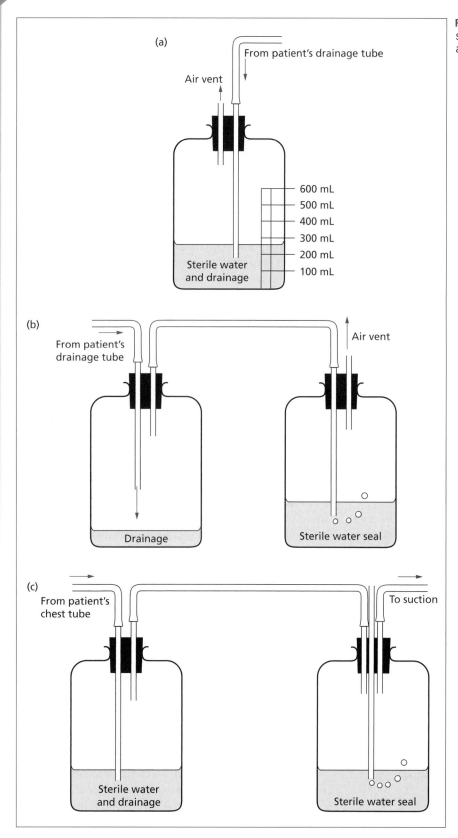

(a)

From patient's drainage tube

Air vent

600 mL
500 mL
400 mL
300 mL
200 mL
100 mL

Sterile water and drainage

(b)

From patient's drainage tube

Air vent

Drainage

Sterile water seal

(c)

From patient's chest tube

To suction

Sterile water and drainage

Sterile water seal

Figure 13.7 Underwater-seal chest drainage system using (a) one bottle, (b) two bottles, and (c) two bottles and suction.

the water up into the tube only to that level. If the container is lifted or moved, caution is observed to prevent traction on the tube, which might result in its dislodgement.

A safer method for preventing the possibility of water accidentally entering the chest cavity, and which also keeps the drainage separated from the water, is to use two containers. The second one contains the water, leaving the drainage container dry (Fig. 13.7b). When only one container is used, fluid drainage from the chest raises the level of the fluid, increasing the pressure at the distal end of the tube. More pressure is then required to force the fluid down on expiration and allow the escape of air and fluid. Blood and serum are more likely to collect and clot in the tube. In the two-container system, the first container is sealed and does not contain water. The second tube in container 2 is short and acts as an air vent. A disadvantage of the two-container system is its bulk, which makes it difficult for the patient to mobilize without assistance.

If there is a considerable amount of air leaking into the pleural cavity from the intrapulmonary space, or if the patient's cough and respirations are not sufficiently strong to facilitate the clearance of fluid and air from the chest cavity, *continuous gentle suction* may be applied. This necessitates a two-container system; the first container serves as a drainage container and water seal. The short air-vent tube in container 1 is connected to the second container, which has a three-holed stopper through which two short tubes and one longer tube pass (see Fig. 13.7c). The lower end of the longer tube is submerged in water to a designated depth. The upper end is open to the air. This tube controls the degree of suction applied to the pleural cavity. One short tube is connected to container 1; the second short tube is connected to a suction apparatus. The usual suction machine creates too strong a negative pressure to be applied directly to the pleural cavity. This may be reduced by a valve and meter (such as is used in wall suction) inserted between the suction and the water-seal container. If the portable suction machine is used, the negative pressure is controlled by the depth of submersion of the lower end of the open glass tube in container 2. A continuous bubbling in the control container (container 2) indicates that the suction is being maintained.

Disposable closed drainage receptacles with two compartments comparable to the two-container system are available. The receptacle is attached to suction and is suspended from the side of the bed, eliminating the danger of containers being knocked over and broken.

The water-seal system is cumbersome and also restricts patient mobility. The nurse and patient are continuously apprehensive of such things as tubes becoming disconnected and containers being broken. As a safety measure and to permit greater freedom in turning and earlier ambulation, some surgeons prefer to introduce a plastic flutter valve into the system. It is placed between the chest drainage tube and the drainage container. Suction may still be applied. The system may be placed on a small cart or pole with wheels to allow the patient to move around the unit.

Responsibilities and precautions   When any method of water-seal drainage is used, it is important that the nurse understands the purpose and operating principles of the system. The nurse must be familiar with the precautions to be observed to prevent air and fluid from entering the chest cavity, as this could cause a collapse of the lung and life-threatening respiratory insufficiency.

If the container system is used, the container should be calibrated so that the volume of water used is known and the drainage may be measured.

The system must be checked at frequent intervals for patency. This is determined by noting the oscillating water level in the submerged tube; this rises with inspiration and falls with expiration. When suction is employed, fluctuations of the water level do not occur because the continuous suction holds the water level in the tube at a fixed level. The suction may be interrupted briefly and the column of water observed for fluctuations. If the water level does not fluctuate in a closed system, the tube should be examined for possible kinks or compression caused by the patient lying on it. If the system remains non-functional, the doctor is informed at once.

As a precaution, connections may be taped with adhesive to prevent their separation and to keep air from entering the system. The taping of connections is controversial (Godden and Hiley 1998), but there is currently no firm evidence to support either taping or not taping and it is therefore up to the practitioner to decide on the most appropriate approach in a given situation. The containers may be placed in a rack to prevent accidental moving or knocking over. Visitors and ward personnel are warned not to disturb them.

To prevent dragging, the chest drain tubing may be loosely fastened to the patient's clothing using tape and a safety pin. This is better than securing it to the bedding as it allows the patient greater mobility, although care must be taken by the patient and staff to remember its presence when clothing is changed.

The characteristics and volume of the drainage are noted and recorded frequently, especially during the first 24–48 hours. The drainage may be coloured by blood at first, but gradually clears and decreases in amount.

The drainage container must be changed only by someone who fully understands closed drainage. Each drainage tube is clamped close to the chest wall with two chest drain clamps, and the container is quickly replaced by a clean, calibrated, sterile container.

If an interruption or break in the closed system should occur as a result of the disconnection of a tube or a broken container, a closed drainage system should be re-established as soon as possible. There has been debate as to whether or not clamps should be applied in this situation (Williams 1992), as the application of clamps could lead to the development of a tension pneumothorax and possibly death. In view of the potentially serious consequences resulting from clamping the drain for more than a few moments, it is safer to leave the drain open to the air as this will result in no more than a simple pneumothorax. As a precaution, an extra set of sterile containers and connections should always be available. As soon as the underwater-seal drainage system has been re-established, the doctor should be informed of the incident and the patient closely observed for signs of impaired breathing or other distress. It is important to remain calm and inform the patient of what you are doing, and why, as they will be understandably anxious.

Regular frequent staged coughing and deep breathing are important because they increase the intrapulmonary and intrapleural pressures, forcing air and fluid out of the cavity and promoting lung expansion. The patient should be ambulatory as soon as possible.

Patients should be instructed to inform the nurse if they experience any pain so that analgesia can be given or the prescription reviewed if it is ineffective. A patient experiencing pain will be reluctant to move about, cough or breathe deeply and this in turn will hamper lung expansion (Avery 2000).

When turning the patient, or when giving any care, precautions are taken not to dislodge or disconnect the drainage tubes. A final check is made to make sure the patient is not lying on a portion of the tube and that there are no loops or kinks present to interfere with drainage.

Even if the system appears to be functioning satisfactorily, any patient complaint of pressure or pain in the chest, dyspnoea, cyanosis or a rapid, weak pulse is reported promptly.

When the lung is fully expanded and no fluid remains in the pleural cavity, the tubes are removed. The water in the closed drainage container will have stopped fluctuating, and the lung expansion is confirmed by percussion, auscultation and chest radiography.

When the tube is withdrawn from the chest cavity, the wound is covered with a dry, secure dressing. In most cases a purse-string suture has been inserted around the tube and this is tightened off when the tube is removed and covered with a dry, secure dressing. A chest radiograph should be taken following removal of the drain, and the respiratory rate recorded. The patient continues to be observed closely for the next 24 hours for possible leakage of air into the chest and ensuing pneumothorax.

Evaluation   If the person's breathing is more effective and dyspnoea, hypoxaemia and hypercapnia are absent or sufficiently modified to permit optimal daily functioning, care may be judged to be successful. Respiration should be regular, with symmetrical chest expansion, and of normal rate and depth for that individual. There should be evidence that the causative and contributing factors are modified: if pain was present, the person will state absence of pain; injuries to the chest will demonstrate healing; and repair and expansion of any impaired lung tissue will be shown by radiography.

Clamping of underwater-seal drainage systems   As mentioned above, some confusion exists among nurses and other healthcare workers regarding the indications for clamping underwater-seal drains. Following a review of the relevant literature, Williams (1992) identified only three valid reasons for clamping:

1 Following a pneumonectomy to maintain the central position of the mediastinum and its contents
2 When changing the drainage bottles
3 In patients with spontaneous pneumothorax, when re-inflation of the affected lung is confirmed by chest radiography, thus allowing observation for recurrent pneumothorax before the intercostal drain is removed.

When clamps are applied they should both be placed on the drain itself (i.e. above the first connection), not on the tubing connecting the drain to the drainage bottle.

Thoracocentesis (pleural aspiration)   A thoracocentesis is the withdrawal of fluid or air from the pleural cavity. Normally pleural fluid serves to lubricate the pleura. Excessive fluid and air interfere with lung expansion. Chest expansion will be asymmetrical, with distension and decreased movement present on the affected side. A thoracocentesis is performed to remove excessive pleural fluid to facilitate lung expansion, for diagnostic purposes or to instil medication into the pleural cavity. After preparation of the skin and injection of a local anaesthetic, the doctor inserts a needle through an intercostal space into the pleural cavity. A three-way adaptor (stopcock) is attached to the needle to enable withdrawal of fluid through attached tubing or a syringe, and closing of the system when fluid is not being aspirated. Care must be taken to maintain a closed system and prevent air from entering the pleural space.

Nursing interventions for the patient having a thoracocentesis are summarized in Box 13.3.

Restricted lung expansion

Ventilation may be restricted if bony structure is abnormal or there is rigidity of the wall. *Scoliosis* (a deformity in which the spine is S shaped with one shoulder higher than the other) causes stiffness of the chest wall, as well as limiting the size. Surgical removal of ribs (*thoracoplasty*) results primarily in a reduction in the size of the thoracic cavity. Restriction to thoracic expansion may also occur following chest surgery when the patient tends to immobilize the chest and take shallow respirations to minimize the pain.

Blunt trauma to the chest wall may produce fractures of one or more ribs. The pain caused by such an injury may be severe and, as a result, the patient is reluctant to breathe deeply. When ribs are fractured in two places (a flail segment), that section of the chest wall becomes unstable and, when negative pressure is created within the thoracic cavity for inhalation to occur, collapse of the chest wall inwards occurs (Fig. 13.8). This is known as *paradoxical respiration*. The result is that the lung is not adequately ventilated and life-threatening respiratory failure may ensue, particularly if the injury is associated with a haemopneumothorax. Early

Box 13.3 Nursing intervention in the management of the patient having a thoracocentesis

Goals	Nursing intervention	Rationale
Patient problem: Ineffective breathing due to excess fluid in the pleural space		
1 The patient will state he or she understands the procedure and what to expect during the procedure	The patient is informed of the procedure, and what to expect during the procedure	Knowledge of what to expect can reduce anxiety and opportunity is provided to answer the patients concerns
2 The patient's breathing will be regular, rhythmical and not laboured	The nurse checks that the consent form has been signed following the doctor's explanation to the patient of the purpose of the test and expected and other outcomes, and that chest radiography has been carried out	Radiographs provide information as to the exact anatomical location of the fluid and air in the pleural cativity
3 Chest expansion will be symmetrical, with a usual degree of excursion	The prescribed sedation is administered prior to the start of the procedure	Sedation may be required to promote relaxation and decrease discomfort and anticipatory pain
	The patient is placed in a sitting position, leaning forward, with head and arms resting on a table or several pillows	Fluid is dependent and therefore accumulates in the lower portions of the pleural cavity when the patient is upright, making it easier to remove
	During the procedure the nurse provides physical support for the patient and instructs him or her to remain still while the needle is being inserted and while it is in place	To prevent spontaneous movement by the patient which may result in trauma to the pleura and lung
	During the procedure the nurse provides ongoing explanations as to what is occurring. As the antiseptic solution is applied, the patient is told to expect a feeling of cold; injection of the local anaesthetic will be felt and a pressure will be experienced as the thoracocentesis needle is inserted	Patient cooperation increases and anxiety is decreased when he or she is aware of what is happening
	A sterile transparent dressing or a gauze dressing sealed with tape is applied as the doctor withdraws the thoracocentesis needle	To prevent air from entering the pleural cavity To protect the site from micro-organisms
	The patient is assisted to a comfortable position in bed and assessed at least every 15 minutes for the first 2 hours. Observations include respiratory rate, depth and rhythm, pulse rate, presence of blood, frothy sputum, uncontrolled cough, dyspnoea, cyanosis, chest pain or tightness, and feelings of dizziness or faintness. The site is inspected and the surrounding tissue palpated for puffiness or crackling	If a large amount of fluid is removed, lung expansion occurs suddenly and pulmonary and cardiac distress may occur. Spontaneous pneumothorax and subcutaneous emphysema may occur following thoracocentesis. A portable chest radiograph is usually ordered to verify that a pneumothorax is not present
	The volume, colour and consistency of the pleural fluid is determined and recorded. The specimen containers are labelled and sent promptly to the laboratory	Accurate, prompt documentation is a legal requirement. Prompt labelling and discharge of specimens ensures identification of the specimen and that contamination of the specimen does not occur

death after chest trauma is usually due to hypoxia or hypovolaemia. Such injuries often require urgent positive pressure artificial ventilation, for which the patient needs intubation.

Restricted lung expansion may be the result of impaired nerve supply to the respiratory muscles, as occurs in the Guillain-Barré syndrome and poliomyelitis, or it may be due to muscular weakness incurred by a chemical deficit at the myoneural junction (myasthenia gravis). The impaired muscle contraction causes dyspnoea and, if severe enough, respiratory failure. Involvement of the diaphragm increases symptoms and assisted ventilation is usually necessary. Severe obesity alters the mechanics of breathing by decreasing lung inflation, chest wall compliance and lung volumes.

RESPIRATORY FAILURE

Respiratory failure is a disorder of respiratory function that is present when a person is unable to maintain adequate arterial blood levels of oxygen and carbon dioxide.

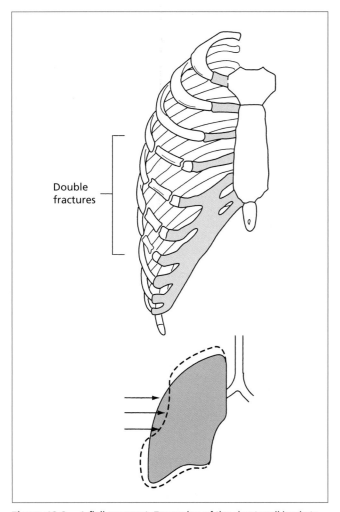

Figure 13.8 A flail segment. Expansion of the chest wall leads to the pressure inside the chest being lower than atmospheric pressure. Therefore the flail segment collapses in on the lung, preventing proper expansion and ventilation.

A PaO_2 of less than 8.0 kPa (60 mmHg) or a $PaCO_2$ of more than 6.2 kPa (45 mmHg) is the parameter used to define respiratory failure.

Causes

Respiratory failure may be encountered in any clinical area and may be associated with a variety of disorders, including:

- trauma or surgery that lead to shock
- intrapulmonary disorders, such as acute and chronic airway obstruction, resistive disorders and pulmonary vascular disorders
- central nervous system disorders, such as drug overdose, brain tumour, cerebral injury or haemorrhage
- neuromuscular disease that involves respiratory muscle innovation (e.g. myasthenia gravis and Guillain-Barré syndrome)
- sepsis, especially if the organisms are Gram negative
- obstructive and central sleep apnoea.

Patients with a history of chronic obstructive pulmonary disease (asthma, chronic bronchitis) and cardiac or kidney disease, and those who are obese or debilitated, are predisposed to develop respiratory failure.

Respiratory failure may be the result of alveolar hypoventilation, inadequate oxygenation of the blood (as occurs in ventilation perfusion imbalance) or right-to-left shunt. In some instances more than one problem is present. Ventilation perfusion inequality is the most frequent cause and is largely responsible for the low PO_2 in respiratory failure that results as a complication of obstructive and restrictive diseases and adult respiratory distress syndrome (ARDS). Alveolar hypoventilation is characterized by the retention of an excessive volume of carbon dioxide, accompanied by hypoxaemia. The patient develops respiratory acidosis because of the raised $PaCO_2$. It is frequently associated with general hypoventilation due to neuromuscular disturbances and chest wall injury. When diffusion is impaired the carbon dioxide retention is initially slight and hypoxia is usually minimal.

Failure to oxygenate the blood adequately may be due to abnormal distribution of the inspired gas, ventilation perfusion inequality or shunting of the blood through unventilated areas of the lung. The alveoli may be filled with fluid, or the alveoli are not ventilated because of an airway obstruction or atelectasis. As a result, the blood may flow through the capillaries around the alveoli without gas exchange taking place. When blood enters the arterial system without going through ventilated areas of the lung, it is referred to as a shunt, such as occurs with a heart defect when the blood moves directly from the right side of the heart to the left. In other instances the alveoli may be ventilated but the respective capillaries do not receive an adequate blood supply or are occluded (*ventilation perfusion mismatching*).

When respiratory failure is severe, pulmonary capillary epithelium is damaged, which leads to haemorrhage and interstitial oedema. The oedema decreases diffusion because fluid lies between the alveoli and capillaries. Fluid infiltrates the alveoli; surfactant is destroyed by proteins that leak through the permeable capillaries; and functional terminal respiratory units collapse. The capillaries dilate, the alveolar walls hypertrophy and the lungs become fibrotic. Defective gas diffusion becomes extensive and very serious. This severe form of acute respiratory failure may be referred to as *adult respiratory distress syndrome* (ARDS) or *shock lung*. There is increased resistance to air entry in the airways and alveoli.

Characteristics

The person may manifest the effects of hypoxaemia. Dyspnoea or tachypnoea may be present, or in ventilatory failure, respirations may be depressed and are slow, irregular and shallow. The pulse rate increases and arrhythmias may develop. The patient may be restless and complain of headache or dizziness. Disorientation, apathy and slow responses develop as a result of the cerebral hypoxia, and may progress to unconsciousness. Periodic sustained contraction of a group of skeletal muscles (asterixis), slurred speech and mood fluctuations may occur if there is marked retention of carbon dioxide. The tidal and minute volumes are usually reduced.

Respiratory failure may develop quickly in a few hours after the initial insult, or the onset may be insidious over a few days or weeks. Serial monitoring of the patient's blood gases and tidal volume, and close observation of the characteristics of the respirations in circumstances where respiratory insufficiency may occur, are important in early recognition of the problem.

Treatment

The underlying disorder that initiated the respiratory failure is treated and therapy is immediately directed toward improving ventilation and oxygenation of the blood. Airway obstruction is alleviated by removing retained secretions, through coughing, postural drainage and suctioning. A bronchodilator (e.g. salbutamol) is administered and respiratory stimulants may be given. Respiratory depressants are avoided. Corticosteroids are useful for some patients to improve their airflow.

Infections are treated promptly as they may produce respiratory failure in patients with chronic airflow limitation.

The aspiration of acid from the stomach into the lungs (acid reflux) occurs in many people with chronic respiratory failure, particularly when they are lying down. Measures to correct or modify the problem are developed in collaboration with the patient. Dietary measures include the avoidance of caffeine and eliminating evening snacks. The head of the bed is elevated on blocks. Antacid medications and histamine (H₂) antagonists such as ranitidine may be used to minimize the effects of the stomach acid.

Diuretics are prescribed to decrease fluid overload in persons with cardiac complications. Changes in bodyweight are monitored and the person's ankles are observed for swelling.

Oxygen may be administered by Venturi mask (see Fig. 13.9) at a concentration of 24–28%. Caution must be exercised in administering oxygen to individuals whose main respiratory stimulus is hypoxaemia as the delivery of uncontrolled oxygen via nasal prongs or a simple mask may depress respiration and increase the likelihood of respiratory failure. The number of hours of oxygen therapy per day is individually prescribed and will vary at different times for the same patient as the requirements fluctuate. A person who requires home oxygen for 14 hours a day when well may require continuous oxygen therapy during a respiratory infection that has increased the respiratory failure.

Additional nursing measures include exercise programmes to strengthen respiratory muscles and the use of breathing techniques. Patients with chronic respiratory failure are encouraged to remain active, eat a well-balanced diet, maintain their desired body weight and get adequate rest and sleep. Individuals and their families are taught to monitor their respiratory status, to adjust the therapeutic regimen to prevent complications, and to treat them early when they do occur.

PATIENTS REQUIRING RESPIRATORY ASSISTANCE

CARE OF THE PATIENT WITH AN ARTIFICIAL AIRWAY

When there is an actual or potential obstruction of the upper airway, intervention is needed to secure efficient and reliable ventilation of the lungs.

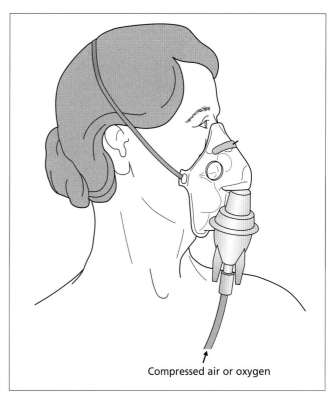

Compressed air or oxygen

Figure 13.9   Venturi mask (entrainment mask).

Endotracheal intubation

An oropharyngeal airway is useful in emergency and following anaesthesia to safeguard the airway against blockage by the tongue, should the patient be unconscious and have therefore lost the gag reflex and the ability to cough. The airway should be introduced inverted and then rotated into the correct position over the back of the tongue. Once in situ, it should be left until the patient recovers consciousness sufficiently for the gag reflex to return; at this stage the patient will cough the airway out spontaneously.

The site of the obstruction may be lower than the oropharynx; there may be severe facial trauma threatening the airway; or the patient may require artificial ventilation. In cases such as these a different solution is required and the patient will either have an endotracheal tube introduced as a temporary measure, or a tracheostomy may be performed, which could be temporary or permanent.

Common clinical situations in which an endotracheal tube is passed include emergency airway management (e.g. trauma, cardiac arrest), before operation to facilitate artificial ventilation and anaesthesia, and to allow efficient airway management for artificially ventilated patients in intensive care units.

The tube is usually passed (this is called *intubation*) through the mouth into the trachea, although the nasal route may also be used. If the patient is conscious, a quick-acting anaesthetic drug and a muscle relaxant (e.g. suxamethonium) are usually administered intravenously to permit intubation. The patient's airway is totally dependent upon the endotracheal tube thereafter; if muscle relaxant drugs have been used, the patient will be unable to breathe spontaneously as all muscles in the body will be paralysed. Maintaining ventilation, and hence the life of the patient, is therefore totally in the hands of the medical and nursing staff.

The endotracheal tube bypasses the upper airway where warming, humidification and filtration occurs; it also bypasses the vocal chords, so the patient cannot speak. If the tube is to be in situ for any length of time, it is important that the artificial ventilation system in use permits air to be warmed and humidified. The patient cannot drink, which means regular oral toilet is needed, otherwise the patient's mouth will become dry and *Candida* infection is possible.

If the patient is conscious, communication will be a major problem and aids such as a pencil and paper are vital. Ashworth (1980), in a now classical piece of nursing research, showed that nurses failed to communicate with intensive care patients if they could not talk back. Every effort should therefore be made to communicate with ventilated or unconscious patients. If possible patients should be informed beforehand that they will not be able to speak after intubation, and the temporary nature of the condition explained.

For intubation, any dentures should be removed and the patient should be positioned on the back, with the head extended and slightly supported to ensure correct alignment of the mouth, pharynx and larnyx. Using a laryngoscope the endotracheal tube is introduced and the proximal portion is secured to the patient's face. The tube is made from soft plastic and is pliable (Fig. 13.10). The tube is equipped with an inflatable cuff a short distance above the distal end. The cuff remains soft when inflated, thereby exerting only a low pressure on the tracheal walls and thus minimizing the risk of tissue damage through trauma or ischaemia. When inflated, the tube prevents the aspiration of vomitus and oral secretions. It also permits more effective ventilation by preventing the escape of gases being delivered under pressure.

When the tube is in position, the cuff is inflated with air if the patient is to receive mechanical ventilatory assistance. Near the proximal end of the fine tube leading to the cuff, and through which the air is introduced, there is a small balloon-like dilatation that remains inflated when the tube is clamped. This dilatation is observed frequently and, as long as it remains inflated, the cuff is also inflated.

Immediately after insertion of the tube, and then at regular intervals, the chest is auscultated to determine whether air is entering both lungs. If the tube is too low, the inflated cuff could completely block off a bronchus and cause atelectasis of the respective lung. A radiograph may be taken to check the position of the tube.

The endotracheal tube is distressing and a source of discomfort to the conscious patient. Prolonged use may cause damage to the vocal chords and ulceration in the trachea. If an artificial airway is necessary for a prolonged period, a tracheostomy is performed and the endotracheal tube removed.

Periodic deflation of the cuff should not be necessary if a large-volume low-pressure cuff is used. The inspired gas is humidified before entering the endotracheal tube to liquefy secretions and prevent encrusting within the tract and tube. Frequent deep suction through the endotracheal tube is necessary.

Suctioning may deplete the amount of oxygen reaching the alveoli. The patient may be given oxygen prior to suction, and again following suction. The patient's pulse is monitored for possible cardiac dysfunction and arrhythmias (due to hypoxia) during and after the suctioning. If any irregularity occurs, suctioning is immediately discontinued and oxygen is administered with the self-inflating bag and mask.

Using sterile gloves, the nurse passes a sterile catheter through the tube into the trachea. Suction is not applied while the catheter is being introduced. When in position, suction is applied intermittently and the catheter is rotated and withdrawn. If the airway is not clear of secretions, the catheter is not allowed to become contaminated and may be reintroduced into the trachea. It will probably be necessary to ventilate the patient with the self-inflating bag before passing the catheter again. If the secretions are tenacious, 5–10 mL of a sterile saline solution may be introduced into the tube, followed by immediate suction. After suction the patient is hyperoxygenated.

Frequent mouth care is necessary, and suctioning of the oropharyngeal area at frequent intervals is done to remove the secretions that may form in response to the presence of

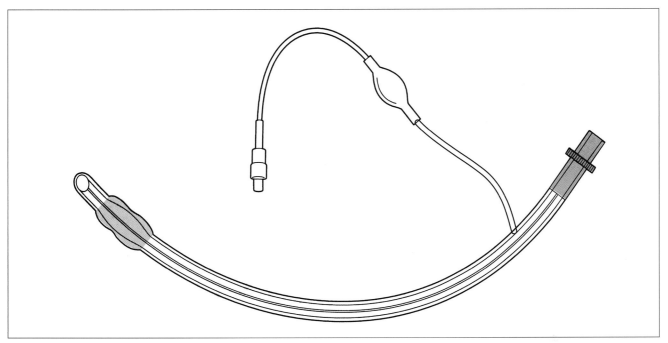

Figure 13.10   An endotracheal tube with inflatable cuff which provides a seal between the trachea and tube. After the tube is inserted, the cuff is inflated by introducing a specified volume of air through the fine attached tube, which is then clamped.

the tube. When the patient is to be *extubated*, the emergency (resuscitation) trolley should be accessible so the patient can be quickly reintubated if necessary.

Before the cuff is deflated and the tube is removed, secretions are suctioned from the oropharynx to prevent aspiration. After removal of the tube, the patient is observed for respiratory distress and insufficiency. A nurse remains in attendance, constantly monitoring the patient's respirations, pulse and colour. The patient is usually apprehensive and needs the nurse's presence and reassurance.

Tracheostomy

Tracheostomy tubes are similar to endotracheal tubes but are inserted through an incision in the neck, directly into the trachea; they are therefore much shorter. The artificial airway bypasses the larynx and air passages above.

Indications for a tracheostomy include:

1 An upper airway obstruction (e.g. laryngeal tumour).
2 Prolonged, mechanically assisted, ventilation where a seal is necessary to prevent loss of ventilatory gas that is under pressure.
3 The need for more efficient access to retained pulmonary secretions which, unless removed, may cause serious respiratory problems such as atelectasis and pneumonia.
4 The prevention of recurrent aspiration of oral secretions and vomitus.

Since endotracheal intubation has been more commonly used and may be performed very quickly, tracheostomy is rarely used in an emergency situation. The procedure is generally elective, and is performed with an endotracheal tube in

position and under aseptic conditions in an operating room. It may be necessary as an emergency measure if the patient cannot be intubated because of facial injuries or burns, laryngeal oedema or severe upper airway infection. If the tracheostomy is performed because the patient has had a laryngectomy, the tracheostomy becomes permanent for that patient.

The operative procedure is undertaken with the patient in the dorsal position, with the head and neck hyperextended. A pillow or folded sheet is placed under the shoulders. A vertical or horizontal incision is made about 2 cm above the suprasternal notch to expose the upper part of the trachea. This is then opened, usually at the level of the second and third cartilaginous rings, and a tracheostomy tube is introduced. The tube is held in position by laterally attached tapes which are tied securely around the neck.

Tracheostomy tubes are available in various sizes. The diameter and length of the tube selected depends upon the size of the trachea, and is slightly smaller in diameter than the trachea. The tubes may be made from plastic, silver or nylon, and may be single or consist of two parts – an inner and outer cannula (Fig. 13.11). When a double-lumen tube is used, the outer cannula is fitted with an obturator that extends beyond the distal end of the tube. Its end is blunt and smooth, which facilitates the introduction of the tube. As soon as the tube is in position, the obturator is removed and the inner tube is inserted and secured.

The tube with an inner cannula provides a more efficient means of clearing the airway of secretions, because the inner tube can be removed and readily cleansed without the risk of compromising the airway. The single tube (without

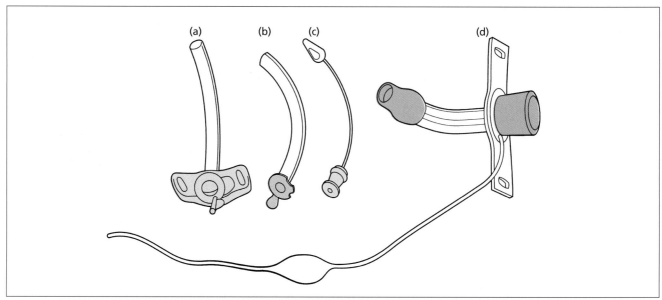

Figure 13.11 Tracheostomy tubes. (a) Outer part of metal tracheostomy tube. (b) Inner part of metal tracheostomy tube. (c) Obturator used during insertion of the outer metal tube. (d) Polyethylene cuffed tube.

an inner cannula) must be changed about every 3 days or more often if secretions accumulate within the tube. The tube with an inner cannula may be left for a longer period.

Most synthetic tubes now in use have a high-volume low-pressure cuff which encircles the lower part of the outer tube. After the tube is in position, the cuff is inflated by introducing a small amount of air via a fine tube that leads into it. The cuff creates a seal between the trachea and the tube, and prevents air from entering or escaping around the tube, in addition to preventing the aspiration of secretions or fluid into the tract below. This type of tube is used most frequently for patients who require mechanical assistance in breathing.

The amount of air required to produce a seal without unnecessary pressure on tracheal tissue varies from 2 to 10 mL. While introducing the air, the nurse listens and tests for the escape of air from around the tube. The tracheostomy tube may be blocked off momentarily while testing for leakage around the tube. When the inflation is completed, the end of the fine tube is clamped. The amount of air used in inflating the cuff is recorded each time; any significant change observed from one time to another is reported. A decreased amount of air used may indicate swelling and oedema in the air passage tissues.

Near the proximal end of the fine inflating tube is a small balloon-like dilatation. This is inflated and, because it is visible, may be checked frequently to determine whether the tube and the cuff below remain inflated. Obviously, if the small pilot balloon becomes deflated, a leak in the system is indicated and the cuff will be deflated, thus losing the intratracheal seal.

A variety of tubes are available that facilitate upper respiratory breathing or speaking and are used when weaning patients from mechanical ventilation.

Tracheostomy care

The nurse should appreciate that the patient is dependent upon the patency of the tracheostomy tube for breathing. Constant attention and meticulous care are necessary to prevent serious complications and to reduce the patient's fear of choking. Sensitivity to the patient's fears and needs is important, because the patient cannot communicate verbally.

Preparation for tracheostomy The doctor explains the procedure to the patient and family and informed consent is obtained. The nurse assesses the patient's understanding of the procedure. The patient is assured that someone will be in constant, close attendance and that provision will be made for communication by writing. A similar explanation is given to the family. Opportunities are provided for the patient and family members to ask questions and to receive further clarification.

Preparation to receive the patient This includes assembling sterile suction equipment, ventilator if indicated, adaptor to fit the tracheostomy tube, oxygen administration equipment and a tray with various sizes of sterile tracheostomy tubes in case the one inserted becomes dislodged. Sterile tape for securing the tube in place, gauze squares, tracheal dilator, artery forceps and a sterile syringe to inflate the cuff are required. A catheter mount, which can be used to connect an Ambu bag (see Fig. 13.12) to the tracheostomy tube should emergency resuscitation be required, is essential. A humidifier should also be switched on and ready for use; the type will depend on whether the patient is to receive mechanical ventilatory assistance; if not, a nebulizer may be available that fits over the opening of the tube. Equipment for frequent mouth cleansing should be available, and a pencil and pad for written communication.

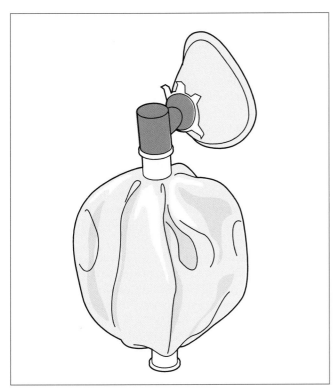

Figure 13.12 Ambu resuscitator: a self-inflating hand-compressible breathing bag and mask.

Position The head of the bed is usually elevated to approximately a 45° angle if the patient is conscious and the blood pressure and pulse are stable.

Assessment Frequent monitoring of blood pressure, respiratory rate and sounds, pulse and colour is necessary. An increase in the respiratory rate, crackles and wheezes, and an increased pulse rate may indicate the need for suction. The patient may still experience respiratory insufficiency due to obstruction in the tract below the tracheostomy. This could be evidenced by marked respiratory effort, unequal movement of the sides of the chest and retraction of the soft tissues in the intercostal and supraclavicular spaces. Cyanosis and distress not relieved by suctioning are reported promptly. Increasing restlessness, especially if accompanied by a rapid pulse rate, may indicate hypoxia or bleeding.

The neck and area around the incision are inspected for possible interstitial emphysema due to air leaking into the subcutaneous tissue. The wound is observed for bleeding in the immediate postoperative period and then checked daily for signs of infection and sloughing.

The tube is checked frequently for patency and the characteristics (consistency, colour, amount) of the tracheobronchial secretions are noted. Increased secretion occurs in response to the tracheal trauma and is usually coloured by blood at first, but the blood content should gradually diminish and disappear.

Suction Frequency of suctioning is determined by assessment of the patient's breathing and the rate of production of secretions. It is possible that an apparent decrease in secretions actually means they have just become thicker and more readily retained. Sterile saline may be instilled into the tube and followed immediately by suctioning to help loosen tenacious secretions.

If the patient is receiving mechanical ventilatory assistance or oxygen, he or she may be hyperoxygenated before suction (100% oxygen for 35 minutes). Suctioning removes air and oxygen from the respiratory tract, as well as removing secretions, and may cause hypoxaemia and ensuing cardiac arrhythmia. The development of hypoxaemia is related to the duration of suctioning and the frequency of passing the suction catheter.

The trachea is suctioned using a sterile glove and a sterile suction catheter moistened in sterile water or normal saline. The negative pressure is not applied during the insertion of the catheter but is applied when it is in position and during withdrawal. Suctioning must be brief and not longer than 10–15 seconds. If it must be repeated, the patient is allowed several breaths or is given oxygen again.

Secretions and suction may initiate coughing. Secretions escaping from the tracheostomy tube are gently wiped away with sterile gauze. The mucus and exudate must be cleaned away quickly before being drawn back into the tube with a breath.

Tube and wound care The wound and surrounding skin are kept as free of secretions as possible. The wound and area under the tube are protected with a dressing; a number of dressings are now available that have been developed for this specific purpose, many of which contain foam, thus increasing their absorbency and patient comfort. If the tapes securing the tube become soiled, they are replaced with fresh sterile tapes. It is advisable to have two nurses (or the help of a relative) when changing the tapes so that one person can gently but firmly hold the tracheostomy tube in place while the other changes the tapes. This reduces the risk of the tube becoming displaced during the procedure (e.g. as a result of the patient coughing). The tapes should always be tied in a double bow or knot as a single bow can easily become undone if the tapes are inadvertently caught on something.

The inner cannula of the tracheostomy tube is carefully removed and cleansed as often as necessary (perhaps even hourly). Hydrogen peroxide or sodium bicarbonate solution may be used to soak the tube to loosen crusts of mucus, and the cannula is then cleansed using a small tube brush or applicator. It is then rinsed in water. The outer cannula is suctioned if necessary before the inner cannula is reinserted. Precautions must be taken not to displace the outer tube; the tapes that secure it are checked frequently.

Single tubes are usually changed by the surgeon or an experienced trained nurse, as often as necessary to ensure patency. The tube with an inner cannula may be changed weekly. A tray with sterile replacement tubes and the necessary equipment is kept at the bedside.

Should the tube come out of the trachea because of vigorous coughing or carelessly tied tapes, the tracheal opening closes and the patient is threatened with asphyxia. Prompt action is necessary. The tracheal wound may be quickly reopened with the sterile tracheal dilator or artery forceps, which are always kept at the bedside in the event of such an emergency. The opening is held open until the doctor (or experienced nurse) arrives and inserts the sterile tracheostomy tube.

An alternative course of action if you witness the displacement of a tracheostomy tube would be quickly to open one of the sterile tracheostomy tubes which should be by the patient and insert this into the stoma. This may be less traumatic than the use of tracheal dilators, particularly if the surgical wound is fresh.

Humidification Humidification of the inspired gas is very important to prevent encrustations forming within the trachea and the tube, as these will increase airway resistance.

Fluids and nutrition A minimum fluid intake of 3000 mL is recommended to help liquefy pulmonary secretions, unless contraindicated by cardiac insufficiency and oedema. An accurate record is kept of the intake and output. The patient is not usually permitted any fluids or food by mouth; they are administered intravenously. Some patients are fed via a nasogastric tube.

If the tracheostomy is to be permanent, or the patient is not on a ventilator, oral fluids are introduced gradually; if tolerated, a soft diet is given and increased gradually to a regular diet. The nurse remains with the patient until sufficient confidence is gained.

Mouth care Oral hygiene is important for comfort and to reduce the risk of infection. The mouth is cleansed and rinsed every 2 hours until the patient is taking normal meals, at which time regular cleansing of the teeth and rinsing of the mouth after each meal and at bedtime suffice.

Communication The patient is likely to be fearful of choking and concerned about his or her inability to cough up the secretions and to communicate. When the nurse leaves the bedside, the patient is advised of the errand and how long it will take. A call-bell is given to the patient, who will be more secure knowing that someone can be called if necessary.

The nurse talks to the patient, informing him or her of progress and what is to happen next. It is very helpful to try to anticipate information the patient might want but cannot ask for. A pad and pencil are kept readily within reach, and the patient is encouraged to communicate feelings and needs. Hand signals are developed to enable the patient to communicate yes or no, or to make routine requests by raising one or more fingers. Family members are encouraged to talk to the patient.

Extubation If the patient has been receiving mechanical ventilatory assistance, removal of the tracheostomy tube is not considered until he or she is breathing successfully without the ventilator. When the tracheostomy is a temporary measure, the patient is gradually returned to breathing through the upper tract. In order to lessen tracheal injury and scarring, the tube is removed as soon as possible, but without compromising adequate ventilation. The protective reflexes should be responsive; the epiglottis and glottis should be closed to prevent aspiration, the gag reflex should be present and the patient should be able to swallow fluids and food without risk of aspiration.

If a cuffed tube has been used, the cuff may be deflated for 24–48 hours before the tube is removed and the patient's ability to keep upper tract secretions out of the lower tract is observed. A sterile tracheostomy tray with tubes of several sizes is kept at the bedside in case a tube has to be reinserted after extubation. Sterile suction equipment should also be available.

When the tracheostomy tube is removed, the wound is cleansed, the wound edges are approximated and taped, and a firm dressing is applied. Healing occurs spontaneously; sutures are not considered necessary. The patient is advised to place a hand over the area and exert some pressure when coughing. He or she may be fearful of not being able to breathe when the tube is removed, so is assured beforehand that breathing is adequate via the normal route. A nurse remains following removal to be certain that no difficulty is experienced. After discharge, the patient needs to be monitored to check for possible scarring and tracheal stricture resulting from irritation and trauma.

Home tracheostomy care If the tracheostomy is permanent, the patient is instructed about the care of the tube and the stoma. This is done as soon as the patient is well enough to undertake the care in the hospital, so confidence will be developed. If possible, and with the patient's consent, a member of the family also receives instructions about the necessary care and precautions.

The patient and family are referred to the district nurse who is able to obtain the necessary suction equipment and dressing supplies, and also give instruction in the use and care of the equipment. The patient and family are advised how to conceal the site of the tracheostomy using collared shirts, a scarf or high-necked garments.

An explanation is made of the danger of aspirating water through the tracheostomy tube. In the past, a person with a tracheostomy was not allowed to swim, but there are now several devices available that make swimming a safe form of recreation. These devices need to be fitted professionally and care must be taken when first entering the water. Precautions must also be used when taking a shower.

The patient is advised to return to the outpatient department or to the general practitioner at regular intervals, for changing the tube and examination of the stoma. Eventually, when the stoma is firmly healed and the tracheal opening remains patent, the patient or a member of the family may be taught to change the outer cannula, or the tube may be removed permanently for patients in whom a laryngectomy has been performed. Precautions should be used to avoid close contact with those in the environment with respiratory infection.

PATIENTS REQUIRING MECHANICAL VENTILATION

Mechanical ventilation supports respiration automatically by delivering air with an enhanced concentration of oxygen and in the process fully expanding the lungs. It is indicated when respiratory failure occurs and the patient is unable to maintain their own adequate arterial blood gases. However, only those patients who can benefit from respiratory support and have a realistic chance of survival should be established on mechanical ventilation.

INDICATIONS OF THE NEED FOR MECHANICAL VENTILATION

The decision to ventilate a patient mechanically is usually taken by an anaesthetist. However, when appropriate, this may be discussed with the patient and family. Mechanical ventilation may be indicated in a number of different circumstances including:

- post-surgery (e.g. following elective or emergency major abdominal, gastric, cardiac or neurological surgery)
- post-trauma (e.g. for a flail chest, multiple fractures, massive blood loss or spinal injury)
- acute ventilatory or respiratory failure (e.g. respiratory arrest, adult respiratory distress syndrome, infection or sepsis, or cerebral haemorrhage, multiple organ failure)
- impending acute respiratory failure (e.g. respiratory muscle weakness due to Guillain-Barré syndrome, self-poisoning)
- chronic conditions (e.g. chronic pulmonary disease).

Clinical investigations that may help to identify the need for mechanical ventilation include blood gas analysis, chest radiography and lung function tests. Mechanical ventilation is usually carried out via a positive-pressure ventilator which actively administers gas into the patient's lungs via a series of tubes and an artificial airway (commonly an endotracheal or tracheostomy tube). These ventilators are either volume or pressure controlled, which mimics the mechanism that normally terminates the patient's inspiratory phase.

VOLUME-CONTROLLED VENTILATORS

The inspiratory phase ends after a pre-set tidal volume or minute volume has been delivered. The machine will deliver this volume to the patient. However, lung compliance is reduced in most patients who require ventilation. This means that, to deliver a satisfactory volume to the patient, the pressure in the lungs may be high. This high airway pressure may cause further damage to the lungs. To prevent this, pressure-controlled ventilation may be used.

Pressure-controlled ventilators

This mode of ventilation delivers the inspiratory gas until a pre-set pressure is reached. This then determines the volume of gas the patient receives. The greater the compliance of the lungs, the lower the inflation pressures required to obtain a satisfactory minute and tidal volume. By controlling the airway pressure in this way, further lung damage may be avoided (*barotrauma*). Pressure-controlled ventilation also provides a greater distribution of gas around the lung.

Positive-pressure ventilation, regardless of the type of ventilator used, may be divided into controlled or assisted ventilation. In *controlled* ventilation the patient is making no respiratory effort and respiration is entirely dependent on the ventilator. An *assisted* ventilation mode may be used when patients are capable of making some respiratory effort themselves: the ventilator is literally assisting the patient to breathe. Recent advances in positive-pressure ventilator therapy have included development of the biphasic intermittent positive airway pressure (BIPAP) mode. In this mode, pressure alternates between two adjustable pressure levels. These levels are positive end-expiratory pressure (PEEP) and inspired pressure. Between these two pressures the patient can be ventilated manually or allowed to breathe spontaneously. This mode benefits the patient as it allows one mode to be used from the instigation of ventilation all the way through the ventilation episode. It allows much greater patient comfort whilst reducing the need for sedation. By having the airway pressure controlled, the patient is at much less risk of barotrauma. The extent of the assistance provided by the ventilator is variable and is determined by the mode selected by the anaesthetist.

The use of positive-pressure ventilators is largely limited to intensive care settings where nurses and other staff are skilled in the care of ventilated patients and the staffing levels allow close observation. Patients in intensive care environments who are mechanically ventilated are frequently sedated and in some instances will receive muscle relaxant drugs to enable them to tolerate the artificial airway and mechanical ventilation. These patients are totally reliant upon nursing staff for their personal safety and the fulfilment of their needs.

LOCALIZED AIRWAY OBSTRUCTION

Localized obstruction of airflow is less common than chronic airflow limitation and causes less residual impairment.

OBSTRUCTION OF THE NASAL PASSAGES

The narrow nasal passages are particularly susceptible to obstruction. Obstruction may be the result of:

- trauma causing deviation of the septum and nasal fractures

- foreign bodies in the nose, which are common in childhood
- growths and polyps
- inflammation of the nasal mucosa as a result of irritation from pollution, allergies, smoking or infection.

Signs and symptoms include asymmetry of the nose from trauma, bleeding, and thin to thick purulent drainage. The person breathes through one nostril or the mouth when obstruction is present.

OBSTRUCTION OF THE PHARYNX

Inflammation and enlargement of the adenoids in the nasopharynx and of the tonsils in the oropharynx interfere with breathing and swallowing. Foreign bodies that are of sufficient size to lodge in the oropharynx are usually relatively easy to remove. Smaller objects that pass on to the larynx and bronchi pose a greater hazard.

OBSTRUCTION OF THE LARYNX

Oedema, laryngeal spasm or aspiration of a foreign body may cause obstruction in the larynx. Any constriction or obstruction in the larynx is manifested quickly by hoarseness, dyspnoea, stridor, cyanosis, and increased but ineffective inspiratory effort, evidenced by the retraction of the intercostal spaces. Prompt emergency measures are necessary or death may ensue as a result of asphyxia.

OBSTRUCTION OF THE TRACHEA

Aspiration of a foreign body, scarring following trauma or surgery, or pressure from an aortic aneurysm or neoplasm of a neighbouring structure may narrow the trachea and offer resistance to the flow of air. Inspiratory and expiratory stridor result and hypoventilation leads to hypercapnoea and hypoxaemia.

Obstruction of the airway by an aspirated foreign body presents an acute emergency. The patient should be slapped vigorously between the scapulae. Alternatively, someone standing behind the individual places the arms around the victim's trunk just below the diaphragm, clasping the hands in front. Pressure is applied with the arms and hands (Fig. 13.13). The compression (*Heimlich hug or manoeuvre*) forces air under pressure through the airway and may dislodge the aspirated mass. If this procedure does not dislodge the object, a laryngoscope may be quickly introduced through which the offending object may be retrieved. If the patient's breathing is completely obstructed, an emergency tracheostomy may have to be performed to establish an airway before the foreign body can be removed.

For *oedema* or *spasm*, intubation may be performed in which a tube is passed beyond the obstruction into the trachea to establish an airway, or the doctor may do a tracheostomy. If oedema of the larynx is due to an allergic response, the patient is given adrenaline 1:1000 intramuscularly. An adrenal corticosteroid preparation such as prednisolone may be prescribed for a brief period to reduce tissue sensitivity. Local applications of ice to the neck may also be suggested.

OBSTRUCTION OF A BRONCHUS

If a foreign body is inhaled, it may pass into either bronchus, but most often the right bronchus is blocked. Localized obstruction may also be caused by enlarged lymph nodes surrounding the bronchus. Complete obstruction leads to atelectasis (collapse of the lung) beyond the obstruction.

SUMMARY

The constant exchange of oxygen and carbon dioxide between an individual and the environment is essential to life. Impairment of respiratory function threatens the

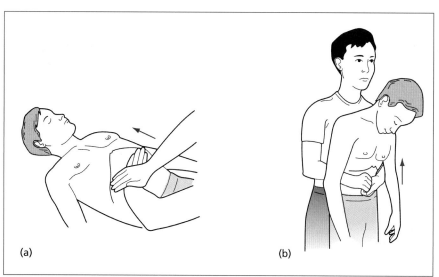

Figure 13.13 The Heimlich method of dislodging a foreign body from the larynx or trachea. If the patient has collapsed or is unable to stand, crossed hands can be placed just below the ribcage and a firm upward thrust exerted (a). Alternatively, if the patient can stand, the thrust may be performed by someone standing behind the patient and clasping their hands below the ribcage (b).

(a)　　　　　　(b)

individual's survival and either temporarily or permanently disrupts health and the quality of life. Respiratory disorders are common and familiar occurrences. Each of us has experienced the difficulties with airway clearance that result from acute respiratory infections. We can relate to the fear and apprehension demonstrated by persons with acute respiratory distress. It is much more difficult to appreciate fully the enormous personal impact that chronic respiratory disorders have on the patient and family, their daily functioning and lifestyles. Medical advances have been made in the management of acute and chronic respiratory disorders, but medical cures do not exist for most respiratory diseases. Patients and their families must learn to live with the resulting health problems.

The nursing care of people with respiratory problems includes the negotiation of long-term patient goals and outcomes as well as goals and outcomes for the current clinical situation. Nurses are assuming an increased role in helping patients with respiratory conditions and their families to acquire self-management skills and to achieve productive lives. Advances in nursing research related to respiratory function are providing scientific rationales for the selection of specific nursing strategies and are helping nurses to evaluate the effectiveness of therapeutic measures. Nurses are becoming better prepared and able to assume greater responsibility for providing nursing solutions to patients' respiratory health problems. Nurses need to be working collaboratively with other health professionals, patients and carers to optimize respiratory function and quality of life for those with respiratory disorders.

ACKNOWLEDGEMENT

We would like to thank Gillian Marshall, Principle Lecturer in Rdiography and Imaging Science at St Martins College, Lancaster, for her contribution to this chapter.

REFERENCES

Ashworth P (1980) Care to communicate. London: Royal College of Nursing.

Asthma UK (2004) Where do we stand Asthma in the UK today. London: Asthma UK.

Avery S (2000) Insertion and management of chest drains. NT Plus – Respiratory Care 3–6, published with Nursing Times 96(37).

Bloom SR (ed.) (1995) Tooheys medicine, 15th edn. Edinburgh: Churchill Livingstone.

Brewin A (1997) Comparing asthma and chronic obstructive airways disease (COPD). Nursing Standard 12(4): 49–53.

British National Formulary (2006) British National Formulary. London: British Medical Association/Royal Pharmaceutical Society of Great Britain.

British Thoracic Society (1997) Guidelines for the management of chronic obstructive pulmonary disease. Thorax 52(5): S1–S32.

British Thoracic Society (2004) Position statement on tobacco. Online. Available: http://www.brit-thoracic.org.uk 25 Aug 2005.

British Thoracic Society, Scottish Intercollegiate Guidelines Network (SIGN) (2003) British guideline on the management of asthma. Thorax; 58(Suppl).

British Thoracic Society, Scottish intecollegiate Guidelines Network (SIGN) (2005) British guideline on the management of asthma. A national clinical guideline. Available: http://www.bit-thoracic.org.uk January 2007

Central Statistical Office (1995) Annual abstract of statistics. London: HMSO.

Chief Medical Officer (2002) Joint tuberculosis committee of the British Thoracic Society guidelines. Online. Available: http://www.dhsspsni.gov.uk/publications/2002/HSS(MD) 8-2002.pdf 21 Jan 2006.

Clutton-Brock TH (1997) The assessment and monitoring of respiratory function. In: Goldhill DR, Withington PS, eds. Textbook of intensive care. London: Chapman and Hall, p 345–355.

Godden J, Hiley C (1998) Managing the patient with a chest drain, a review. Nursing Standard 12(32): 35–39.

Global Initiative for Chronic Obstructive Lung Disease (GOLD) (2004) Global strategy for the diagnosis, management and prevention of Chronic Obstructive Lung Disease. Online. Available: http://www.goldcopd.com 2 Aug 2005.

Halpin D (2004) NICE guidance for COPD (editorial). Thorax 59: 181–182.

Haslett C, Chivers E, Hunter J et al (1999) Davidson's principles and practice of medicine, 18th edn. Edinburgh: Churchill Livingstone.

Haughney J (1998) The role of inhaled steroids in COPD: the search for evidence. Asthma in General Practice 6(1): 5–7.

Hinchliff SM, Montagne SE, Watson R (1996) Physiology for nursing practice, 2nd edn. London: Baillière Tindall.

Holt K (2001) Chronic obstructive airways disease In: Crumbie A, Lawrence J, eds. Living with a chronic condition. Oxford: Butterworth Heinemann, p 101–120.

Howard J (1987) Respiratory teaching of patients, how effective is it? Journal of Advanced Nursing 12(2): 207–214.

Kilgarriff J (2000) A practical guide to treating asthma. Nursing Times 96(31): 43–44.

Lipworth BJ (1999) Modern drug treatment of chronic asthma. British Medical Journal 318: 380–384.

MacNee W, Calverley PMA (2003) Chronic obstructive pulmonary disease 7: Management of COPD. Thorax 58:261–265.

Mera S (1997) Understanding disease: pathology and prevention. Cheltenham: Stanley Thornes.

National Institute for Clinical Excellence (2004) Management of chronic obstructive pulmonary disease in adults in primary and secondary care. Clinical guideline 12. Online. Available: http://www.nice.org.uk 1 Aug 2005.

Partridge MR (1996) Self-management plans: uses and limitations. British Journal of Hospital Medicine 55(3): 120–121.

Rees J, Kananbar D (2000) ABC of asthma, 4th edn. London: BMJ, Publishing.

Seidel HM, Ball JW, Dains JE et al (1999) Mosby;s guide to physical examination, 4th edn. St Louis: Mosby.

Sharp J (1993) Which peak flow meter? Nursing Times 89(3): 61–63.

Springhouse Corporation (2000) Handbook of pathophysiology. Springhouse, PA: Springhouse Corporation.

Szaflarski NL (1996) Preanalytic error associated with blood gas/pH measurement. Critical Care Nurse 16(3): 89–100.

TB Alert (2004) TB in the UK. Online. Available: http://www.tbalert.org/projects/uk/uk.php 21 Jan 2006.

Walsh M (2005) Nurse practitioners; clinical skills and professional issues, 2nd edn. Oxford: Butterworth Heinemann.

Ward M, Reynolds C (2000) Patient empowerment: the key to compliance in asthma. Nursing Times Plus 96(37): 8–9.

Welch J (1993) Chest drains and pleural drainage. Surgical Nurse 6(5): 7–12.

Williams S (1993) Chronic respiratory illness. (Experience of illness series.) London: Routledge.

Williams T (1992) To clamp or not to clamp? Nursing Times 88(18): 33.

FURTHER READING

Williams S (1993) Chronic respiratory illness (Experience of Illness series). London: Routledge.

This book provides a useful insight into the real life experiences of people living with a respiratory illness, and the problems they experience.

NT Plus (2000) Respiratory care (produced in conjunction with the Association of Respiratory Nurse Specialists). Published with Nursing Times 96(37).

This supplement to Nursing Times *contains a number of useful articles relating to the care of patients with respiratory problems. The articles include: insertion and management of chest drains; patient empowerment – the key of compliance in asthma; asthma and women; identifying and treatment* Pneumocystis carinii *pneumonia.*

Wooddrow P (2000) Intensive care nursing – a framework for practice. London: Routledge.

This British book on intensive care nursing contains sections throughout on the respiratory problems encountered by critically ill patients and related nursing care. As well as being a resource for nurses in intensive care units, the book is also a useful source of information for nurses caring for highly dependent patients outside specialist units.

14 Caring for the patient with a haematological disorder

Audrey Yandle

INTRODUCTION

Blood has been recognized as an important symbol of life throughout history. Folklore and religion have contributed to beliefs that blood has many attributes. These include not only its physiological functions but also its sacred and fantastic properties. Titmuss (1970) in his book *The Gift Relationship*, suggested that attitudes to blood and values associated with its possession, inheritance and loss are a distinctive feature of many different cultures. Bathing in blood, anointing with blood and drinking blood have been practised either in reality or symbolically since ancient times. Historically, blood was identified as one of the four chief fluids or humours of the body along with phlegm, yellow bile (choler) and black bile (melancholy); the balance of which was believed to determine a person's physical and mental attributes. The sanguine temperament described the person in whom the blood predominates over other humours, giving rise to a person with a ruddy complexion, and a courageous, hopeful and amorous disposition. Blood-letting was practised as a treatment for many ailments in the belief that it would help to restore the balance of the body's humours.

Fears about blood also abound, and it is often the unexpected loss of blood that prompts individuals to seek medical advice without delay. Thus, blood may simultaneously be perceived as a life-giving substance and a symbol of disease and death. Beliefs about so-called 'bad blood' have re-surfaced in recent years, initially in connection with fears related to infection with the human immunodeficiency virus. More recently, concerns have focused on risks related to transmission of the hepatitis C virus and Creutzfeldt–Jakob disease as a result of blood transfusion. Anxieties about blood transfusion are not new. Solzhenitsyn (1968) described the blood transfusion procedure and wrote of the fears and suspicions of the recipient of a transfusion in a Russian cancer unit in the 1950s.

Blood is one of the most familiar tissues of the body because it is frequently seen as a result of minor injuries. It is also readily sampled and examination of its constituents provides information about the function of other body tissues and organs. A specimen of blood is frequently taken and analysed as an aid to the diagnosis of a wide variety of conditions and to monitor the effects of treatment. Thus, blood can be seen as a window into our bodies as well a source of strength and vitality.

PHYSIOLOGY

Blood is a red, fluid connective tissue that is pumped throughout the vascular system by the heart and is composed of two compartments: the **plasma** and **cellular components**. Blood constitutes around 6–8% of body weight and an adult has between 4 and 6 L of blood.

Blood has a number of important functions:

- It is a medium for the transportation and distribution of cellular requirements and metabolic products between cells in different parts of the body and the external environment
- It is vital to the maintenance of homeostasis. Continuous exchange of constituents across capillary walls between the blood and the fluid surrounding the cells (interstitial fluid) keeps the cellular environment relatively constant
- It plays an important role in defending the body against infection, injury and blood loss

● Blood regulates body temperature and heat loss by distributing heat energy produced by metabolic reactions throughout the body and between the body and the external environment. This helps to keep the body's core temperature within narrow limits.

PLASMA

Plasma is a straw-coloured fluid composed of water, proteins and a wide variety of solutes and makes up approximately 55% of blood. The formed elements (red and white blood cells and platelets) are suspended in the plasma (Fig. 14.1) and make up approximately 45% of blood.

The plasma proteins

Serum albumin, serum globulin and serum fibrinogen are the main **plasma proteins**. Their large molecular size prevents these proteins from diffusing easily through the capillary walls. The resulting concentration of these relatively non-diffusible substances within the capillaries is responsible for what is referred to as the colloid osmotic pressure or oncotic pressure of the plasma (about 25–28 mmHg or 3.3–3.7 kPa). Excessive loss or diminished production of these proteins, albumin in particular, results

in the reduction in the oncotic pressure and the subsequent accumulation of fluid in the tissues, known as oedema. These proteins also contribute to the viscosity (or thickness) of blood, which is 3–5 times that of water.

Serum albumin, fibrinogen and α and β globulins are formed in the liver from amino acids derived from ingested foods. In situations of protein starvation they can be synthesized from tissue protein. Gamma (γ) globulins (also known as immunoglobulins) are produced by plasma cells derived from B lymphocytes. Plasma also contains a number of specialized proteins.

The functions of the plasma proteins may be summarized as follows.

Albumin
● Albumin exerts an intravascular oncotic pressure that influences fluid exchange between the interstitial and intravascular compartments
● Albumin increases blood viscosity.

γ-Globulin
● γ-Globulin contributes to the immune response. It is the antibody fraction of the blood that binds to antigenic material and in doing so helps to inactivate or destroy pathogens and toxins.

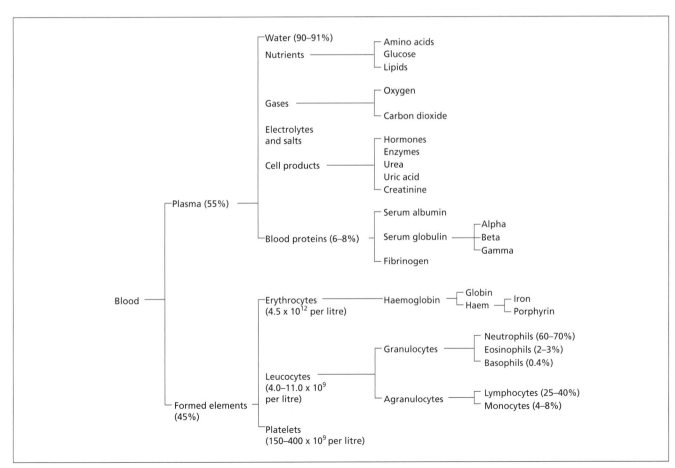

Figure 14.1 Composition of blood.

Fibrinogen

- Fibrinogen plays a key role in blood coagulation, protecting the individual from excessive blood loss
- At the site of inflammation or injury, the coagulation cascade turns fibrinogen into an insoluble fibrin mesh, thereby forming a stable clot (thrombus) and allowing tissue repair and healing to take place.

General functions of plasma

- Plasma proteins combine with both alkalis and acids, and can act as a buffer to maintain a normal blood pH between 7.35 and 7.45
- The proteins bind substances such as hormones, enzymes, lipids, fat-soluble vitamins and essential ions during their transport in the blood. This prevents too rapid an escape of these substances by filtration in the renal glomeruli
- Many exogenous substances are also bound to plasma proteins. Drugs bound in this way (e.g. warfarin) may be biologically inactive until the protein reservoir is saturated or until they are displaced by a more strongly bound substance
- Among the plasma proteins is a group known collectively as the complement system. These proteins enhance the inflammatory and immune responses.

Formed elements of the blood

The formed elements are the **erythrocytes** (red blood cells), the **leucocytes** (white blood cells) and the **thrombocytes** (platelets).

Blood cell production (**haematopoiesis**) starts at an early stage of fetal development, and by 6–7 months of fetal life, the production of new blood cells is located in the bone marrow. After birth and during childhood, most of the bones contain red bone marrow and participate in haematopoiesis. When growth is complete, only the red bone marrow in the cancellous (spongy) tissue of the skull bones, vertebrae, sternum, pelvis and proximal ends of the femur and humerus continue to produce blood cells.

The formed elements of the blood all develop from common **pluripotent stem cells**. When stimulated, these stem cells may differentiate into one of two types of committed stem cell: the lymphoid stem cell and the myeloid progenitor cell. The development of a stem cell through the acquisition of particular cell characteristics and functions is termed differentiation. Cells also undergo amplification or multiple cell divisions leading to colonies of cells in the bone marrow that continue to amplify and differentiate into the various types of blood cells. The cells respond to various haematopoietic growth factors; these are involved in the orchestration of the two key processes of amplification and differentiation. Figure 14.2 summarizes how the different blood cells develop.

Erythrocytes

The normal red blood cell is a flexible, elastic, biconcave disc. During the process of maturation, the cell loses its nucleus and so the circulating erythrocyte has no nucleus and is incapable of division and repair.

The function of the red blood cells is the transportation of oxygen and carbon dioxide between the tissue cells and the lungs. The major constituent of the cell is haemoglobin, a complex protein made from the protein globin and an iron-containing pigment, haem. Each haemoglobin molecule is composed of four globin chains (two α and two β chains) attached to four haem molecules. Each red cell contains about 640 million haemoglobin molecules. Oxygen has an affinity for this compound: four molecules of oxygen combine with one molecule of haemoglobin to form oxyhaemoglobin. This combination is loose and reversible so when there is little or no free oxygen in the red cell's environment, oxygen is freed from the red blood cell and diffuses into the plasma.

It is the red pigment in the haemoglobin of red blood cells that gives blood its colour. The colour varies according to the amount of oxygen combined with the haemoglobin. A high concentration of oxygen produces a brighter red coloration. This difference can be seen when comparing arterial blood, which is oxygenated and therefore a bright red colour, and venous blood, which is deoxygenated and a darker duller colour.

Some of the carbon dioxide carried in the blood (approximately 27%) is transported in the red blood cells in the form of carbaminohaemoglobin. When the haemoglobin takes on oxygen in the lungs, the carbon dioxide is released into the plasma and then diffuses into the alveoli. Most of the remainder of the carbon dioxide is converted to carbonic acid and then to bicarbonate. Only a small percentage of carbon dioxide is not taken up by the red cell and remains dissolved in the plasma.

Erythropoiesis   In **erythropoiesis** a committed myeloid stem cell is stimulated to begin a series of cell divisions that result in an amplification of cell numbers. During these cell divisions, changes occur that result in the appearance of haemoglobin in the cell: the loss of the nucleus, a reduction in cell size, and finally loss of the reticular network. **Reticulocytes** are nucleated red cells at the last stages of development; normally only a small percentage can be found in peripheral blood. An elevated or decreased reticulocyte count can be a useful indicator in the investigation of anaemia.

In health, the rate of production and maturation of the red blood cells normally approximates the rate at which old cells are removed from the circulation and destroyed in a process called haemolysis. This results in the red cell count and the amount of haemoglobin remaining relatively constant. Tissue hypoxia is the essential factor in the regulation of erythropoiesis. The red bone marrow does not respond directly to hypoxaemia (lowered concentration of oxygen in the blood) but the resulting tissue hypoxia stimulates the production of a hormone, **erythropoietin**, mainly by the kidneys. Erythropoietin acts by increasing the rate of production of red cells from stem cells and shortening the period of maturation. As more red cells are released, delivery

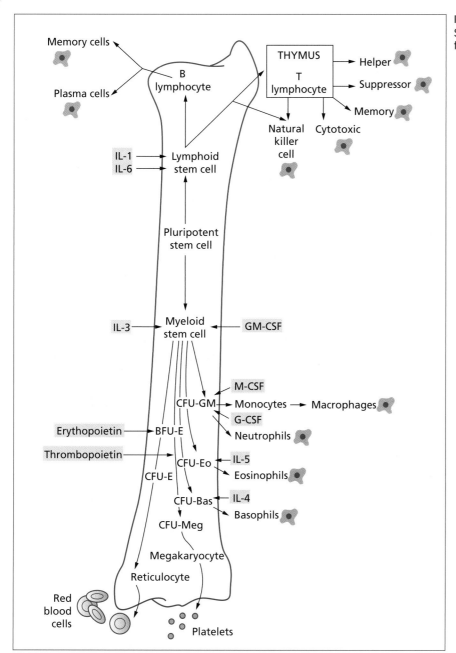

Figure 14.2 Development of blood cells. Sites of action of some haematological growth factors are indicated.

of oxygen to the tissues increases and erythropoietin production declines. This negative feedback mechanism acts to increase the number of red cells produced if the rate of red cell destruction is increased or if there is increased need: for example, if there is a loss of red cells as a result of haemorrhage and at high altitudes, where the oxygen tension of the air is low.

Essential for an adequate production of normal erythrocytes by the bone marrow is a supply of protein, iron, vitamin B_{12}, folic acid and vitamin C. Iron is essential for the formation of haemoglobin. Only limited amounts are absorbed from the small intestine; this is then loosely bound with **transferrin** to be transported in the plasma. Excess iron is stored in the liver and other cells as **ferritin** and

haemosiderin, and can be released as iron when needed by the bone marrow. The majority of iron used in the formation of haemoglobin is derived from breakdown of worn out erythrocytes. Only a small amount of dietary iron is required under normal circumstances and its absorption from the small intestine is inhibited when transferrin and ferritin are saturated. Extra dietary iron and medicinal iron preparations are not absorbed but simply eliminated in the faeces. If erythropoiesis is increased, as it is in pregnancy, or in conditions causing hypoxia, the iron stores are utilized and intestinal absorption increases accordingly.

Vitamin B_{12} and folic acid are required for production of nucleic acids in all cells, and erythrocytes with their rapid rate of turnover are no exception. Vitamin B_{12} can be

absorbed only in the presence of a glycoprotein known as intrinsic factor, which is secreted by the parietal glands in the gastric mucosa (see Ch. 15). Together they form a complex, which is absorbed in the distal ileum. The vitamin B_{12} is released into the portal circulation to be carried to the liver, where it is stored until required. Stores are usually sufficient to last for up to 3 years even if the ability to absorb the vitamin is lost. Folic acid is absorbed in the small intestine and also stored in the liver, but stores are normally sufficient to last for only 3–4 months if intake ceases. Vitamin C promotes iron absorption and also helps to preserve folic acid, which is very quickly destroyed during food preparation. It is also an important factor for red blood cell production.

Red blood cells survive in the circulation for approximately 120 days. The cell membrane becomes fragile and less flexible as the cell ages, and eventually it ruptures as it is squeezed through small capillaries. The phagocytic macrophages destroy damaged cells and haemoglobin is broken down. Iron is recycled along with the constituent amino acids of globin, and the remainder of the haem molecule is eventually excreted in the bile. This cycle is illustrated in Figure 14.3. Red cell destruction (**haemolysis**) mainly takes place in the spleen but can also occur in the liver.

Leucocytes

White blood cells are less numerous, larger than erythrocytes and have nuclei. Healthy people have at least five types of white cells or **leucocytes** in the circulating blood (Fig. 14.2):

- **Granulocytes** are formed in the red bone marrow. Three types are recognizable by the staining characteristic of their cytoplasm: *neutrophils* (stain with a neutral dye),

eosinophils (stain with and acid dye) and *basophils* (stain with basic dyes)

- **Lymphocytes** are smaller than granulocytes and also originate from the bone marrow. Some immature lymphocytes migrate to the thymus gland where they are processed and activated to become *T lymphocytes* (**T cells**). Several subsets of T cells exist, including **memory, helper** and **suppressor** or **regulatory** T cells. *Natural killer cells* (**NK cells**) are another type of lymphocyte, and appear to be a further subset of T lymphocytes. A second type of lymphocyte, *B lymphocyte (***B cells***)* travel from the bone marrow to lymphatic tissue, primarily lymph nodes, where they fully mature. When activated, these eventually develop into **plasma cells** and **memory B cells**. Mature lymphocytes circulate in the blood and between the blood and the lymphatic tissues, where they spend most of their life

- **Monocytes** are the largest white blood cells. After their formation in the red bone marrow they circulate in the blood for only a short time (10–20 hours) before migrating into the tissues where they become **macrophages**. These cells form the **reticuloendothelial** system in bone marrow, liver spleen and lymph nodes.

Leucopoiesis Stem cells in the blood-forming organs are stimulated to produce precursors of the white cells, *myeloblasts, monoblasts* and *lymphoblasts* (Fig. 14.4). The physiological stimuli responsible are not fully understood, but increased leucopoiesis is associated with infection, haemorrhage and tissue destruction, whereas drugs such as sulfonamides, gold and most cytotoxic drugs result in a reduced white cell count. Numerous haematopoietic growth factors are involved in the process of differentiation and

Figure 14.3 Life cycle of erythrocytes.

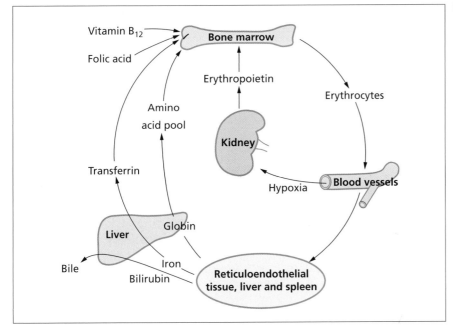

proliferation of the leucocytes. Some of these are normally found in plasma, others are detected only when there is an inflammatory response or in response to a stimulus such as an antigen or endotoxin. They include interleukins and colony stimulating factors. Figure 14.2 illustrates the site of action of some of these growth factors.

Functions of the leucocytes Leucocytes serve as an important body defence, destroying many injurious substances such as micro-organisms and the products of degenerating tissues. Neutrophils and monocytes are chemically attracted to areas of bacterial invasion and tissue damage. This process is known as **chemotaxis**. Neutrophils then ingest and digest foreign particles by a process known as **phagocytosis** and, when worn out, are themselves phagocytosed by macrophages. Monocytes and macrophages respond more slowly but have a greater capacity for ingesting foreign particles and debris. Macrophages have a number of other functions concerned with the inflammatory and immune responses.

Eosinophils participate in allergic reactions, in defence against parasitic invasion and in the resolution of the inflammatory response. Basophils contain heparin and histamine, and are very similar to tissue **mast cells**. They are involved in hypersensitivity, anaphylactic and inflammatory reactions.

T lymphocytes are responsible for cell-mediated immunity, and B lymphocytes for humoral immunity involving the production of antibodies.

The lifespan of the white blood cells varies enormously depending on the type of cell and the body's need for protection. A neutrophil may survive for only a few hours in the presence of an infection, whereas lymphocytes can survive for years in the spleen and lymph nodes. Leucocytes that are destroyed or die are disposed of through phagocytosis by the macrophages of the reticuloendothelial tissues.

Blood platelets
Platelets are the smallest of the formed elements of the blood. They are oval, non-nucleated, granular structures containing important substances, including calcium, potassium, several clotting factors, serotonin, adrenaline, adenosine diphosphate (ADP) and enzymes.

Stem cells in the red bone marrow develop into giant cells called *megakaryocytes* under the influence of a cytokine called thrombopoietin. The megakaryocytes disintegrate, releasing platelets; each megakaryocyte is capable of producing about 4000 platelets. Platelets have a lifespan of 8–12 days and production is increased following tissue trauma and destruction and in hypoxaemia. At any one time about one-third of the platelets are to be found in the spleen, which acts as a reservoir.

The major function of platelets relates to **haemostasis** (arrest of bleeding) following injury to a blood vessel. This is achieved through:

1 Adhesion – platelets stick to the injured area, especially if collagen is exposed.
2 Release of cytoplasmic contents as a result of cellular deformation.
3 Aggregation – an increase in platelet stickiness caused by the release of cellular contents results in nearby platelets adhering to the original clump. This produces a platelet plug that prevents further blood loss.
4 The provision of a surface on which the coagulation cascade takes place, ensuring the construction of a strong fibrin plug, fully sealing the damaged area.

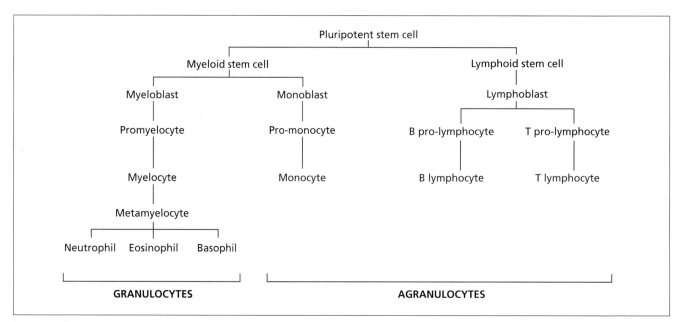

Figure 14.4 Formation of white blood cells (leucopoiesis).

Haemostasis and blood coagulation

The formation of a primary haemostatic plug by the clumping together of platelets is one of the mechanisms for restricting blood loss following the rupture of a blood vessel. The others are:

- *Local vasoconstriction* – chemicals released by platelets stimulate a contraction of smooth muscle in the wall of the injured blood vessel which lasts for about 20 minutes
- *Clot formation* – this process involves the formation of a jelly-like mass in the blood by the conversion of the soluble plasma protein fibrinogen to an insoluble mesh of thin threads called fibrin in which are entangled blood cells forming the mass or clot. Clot formation is triggered either by contact of the blood with a foreign surface or by the release of tissue factor (thromboplastin) from damaged cells, and results in a series of amplification reactions between the numerous clotting factors (Table 14.1). The extrinsic pathway is first to act, producing a short burst of thrombin. This first pathway is soon curtailed by inhibitors. The slower intrinsic pathway then ensures the continued production of thrombin which, in turn, produces insoluble fibrin from fibrinogen. The intrinsic and extrinsic pathways are now known to complement each other and are seen as two interrelated parts of a single process. Figure 14.5 illustrates the coagulation cascade. The process of clot formation takes about 3–6 minutes. The clot then shrinks in size as a result of contraction of contractile proteins, and serum (plasma minus the clotting factors and fibrinogen) is extruded. The fibrin mesh pulls together the edges of the break and further checks the loss of blood

- *Fibrinolysis* – as the healing process begins, fibroblasts proliferate, filling the area with fibrous tissue. Fibrin is degraded into waste debris by the action of the enzyme plasmin (an active product of the plasma protein plasminogen) and the debris is cleared by the macrophages. The waste debris of fibrin consists of various sized pieces of the protein and is termed fibrin degradation products (FDPs).

These coagulation mechanisms operate during normal day-to-day activities when tiny blood vessels sustain injury and in minor trauma. If a major blood vessel, especially an artery, is interrupted, these physiological responses may not be adequate to control blood loss and pressure; ligation or cautery may be required.

Uncontrolled systemic coagulation is potentially dangerous, as is uncontrolled fibrinolysis. The body therefore produces various inhibitory substances such as anticoagulants and fibrinolytic inhibitors to counteract these processes.

BLOOD GROUPS

In 1900 Karl Landstiener discovered that human blood differs from one individual to another. This difference arises from the presence or absence of specific antigens (agglutinogens) on the surface of red blood cells and on the presence or absence of specific antibodies (agglutinins) in plasma. This explains why blood cannot be taken at random

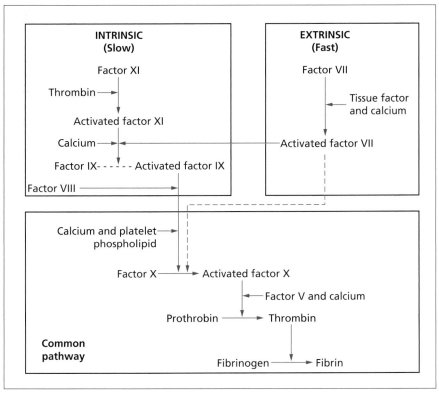

Figure 14.5 The process of blood coagulation. (Modified from Hoffbrand and Pettit 1993.)

from one person and transfused into another. The blood, when of a different type to that of the recipient, may cause a serious reaction and can sometimes be fatal. Many different blood group systems are now known, but the ABO and Rhesus systems are of the most clinical importance.

The ABO blood group

Blood type is determined genetically, with the genes for A and B agglutinogens being co-dominant. An individual's blood is typed as A, B or AB if it has those agglutinogens present on the red blood cells. If no agglutinogens are present, then the blood is termed type O.

The blood plasma does not contain agglutinins that will agglutinate the red cells; therefore, plasma of an individual with blood type AB will contain no antibody, whereas plasma of an individual with blood type O will contain both. An individual whose red cells express either A or B agglutinogens will have plasma containing anti-B or anti-A antibodies, respectively (Table 14.2). These antibodies are termed *naturally occurring* as, unlike most other antibodies, there is no need for exposure to the specific antigen for their formation.

Blood is grouped by adding specially prepared serum containing either anti-A or anti-B serum to a sample of the blood to be typed and observing for clumping of the red cells. The relative incidence of blood group antigens varies from race to race but, worldwide, types O and A are more common than B and AB.

The Rhesus (Rh) blood group

Several antigens (agglutinogens) are involved in this system but the D factor is of greatest clinical significance:

- Approximately 85% of Caucasians possess the D factor and are classified as being Rh positive. Those without the D factor are said to be Rh negative
- The gene for the D agglutinogen is always dominant, so an Rh(D)-positive individual may have inherited the gene from only one or from both parents (Fig. 14.6)
- Antibodies against the D factor do not occur naturally: they develop in the plasma of Rh(D)-negative blood when the D factor is introduced on red blood cells of Rh(D)-positive blood. Anti-D antibodies develop slowly and, after an initial exposure, do not usually reach a sufficient concentration to cause a reaction before the red blood cells are destroyed naturally
- A second exposure to Rh(D)-positive blood will, however, result in a reaction causing agglutination of the donor cells.

When an Rh-positive fetus develops within an Rh-negative mother, some of the fetal red blood cells or D antigen released by worn-out erythrocytes may pass through the placenta into the maternal circulation. This usually occurs at delivery. The mother then forms antibodies that diffuse into the fetal circulation in subsequent pregnancies causing agglutination of the fetal erythrocytes. This causes a severe haemolytic disease of the newborn. It is rare for this to occur in a first pregnancy. There is a chance that maternal sen-

Table 14.1	Blood clotting factors
Factor number	**Name**
I	Fibrinogen
II	Prothrombin
III	Tissue factor (thromboplastin)
V	Labile factor
VII	Proconvertin
VIII	Antihaemophilic factor
IX	Christmas factor
X	Stuart–Prower factor
XI	Plasma thromboplastin antecedent
XII	Hageman factor
XIII	Fibrin stabilizing factor
Pre-K	Prekallikrein
HMWK	High molecular weight kininogen

The sequence of roman numerals indicates the order in which the clotting factors were identified and is not related to the sequence of their participation in the clotting process.

Table 14.2	The ABO blood group system			
Phenotype (blood group)	**Genotype**	**Red cell antigens present (agglutinogens)**	**Naturally occurring plasma antibodies (agglutinins)**	**Plasma agglutinates red blood cells of blood type**
A	AA or AO	A	Anti-B	B and AB
B	BB or BO	B	Anti-A	A and AB
AB	AB	A and B	None	None
O	OO	None	Anti-A and anti-B	A, AB and B

Subgroups of the A antigen exist but are of little clinical importance.

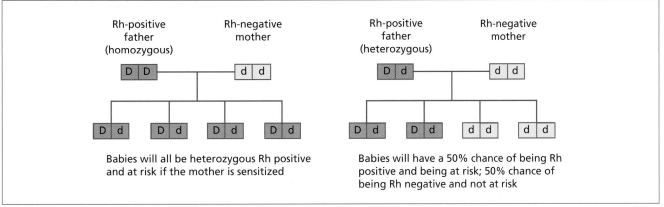

Figure 14.6   Inheritance patterns of Rh blood group factors. The gene for agglutinogen D is always dominant. If the mother is Rh negative and her baby is Rh positive, the mother will form anti-Rh antibodies.

sitization may occur following spontaneous or induced abortion, amniocentesis, chorionic villus sampling, ectopic pregnancy, antepartum haemorrhage and abdominal trauma. This can be prevented by administering anti-D immuno-globulin to agglutinate Rh-positive antigen before the mother can produce her own antibodies. It is usual practice to administer anti-D after any of the potentially sensitizing episodes detailed above, at 28 and 34 weeks of pregnancy and within 72 hours of delivery (BNF 2005) in order to protect any subsequent child from being affected.

When the fetus is Rh negative and the mother is Rh positive there is no problem, because there is no agglutinogen to stimulate antibody production.

BLOOD DISORDERS

Blood disorders (dyscrasias) may affect erythrocytes, leucocytes, platelets or the coagulation process. The problem may be due to a defect originating in the blood-forming red bone marrow, or it may involve the lymphoid and reticuloendothelial tissues. Disorders may be inherited or acquired; they may represent a primary condition or occur secondary to some other pathological process or its treatment. A haematological malignancy such as leukaemia, an inherited haemoglobinopathy such as thalassaemia, and infection with the malaria parasite are examples of primary disorders. A condition such as renal failure that produces a secondary anaemia, and cytotoxic chemotherapy given for a non-haematological malignancy that causes bone marrow depression with anaemia, neutropenia and thrombocytopenia, are examples of problems caused by other disease states or by treatment. Deficiency of an essential requirement may also result in a blood disorder. Blood cells that are defective, whatever the cause, are likely to function abnormally and may be rendered susceptible to premature or excessive destruction.

Blood disorders may develop at any point during a person's lifespan, although the incidence of some blood disorders predominates at the extremes of life. Women of reproductive age are subject to the particular demands of menstrua-

tion and pregnancy, and as such experience a greater risk of anaemia.

Like disorders affecting other body systems, disorders of the blood may be acute or chronic. Whatever the cause, dysfunction has an effect on many other body systems because of the numerous and essential functions of blood. The physical manifestations of blood disorders are therefore many, varied and frequently non-specific.

HEALTH ASSESSMENT

Assessment of an individual's normal and altered haematological status involves knowledge of the person's health history, physical examination and observation, medical diagnostic procedures and knowledge of the haematological system. Collection and analysis of these data form the basis for the identification of an individual's problems and the development of a care plan with specific nursing interventions.

HISTORY

In taking a patient history, information that may be of significance includes any family history of haematological disorders, a drug history (any cytotoxic drug, immunosuppressive drugs including antibiotics, gastric irritants such as non-steroidal anti-inflammatories and drugs affecting blood coagulation are of particular interest), an occupational history (providing clues about any exposure to toxic chemicals) and a nutritional history. The nurse should enquire about the nature of the patient's stools as chronic bleeding from the gastrointestinal tract, as occurs for example in cancer, will lead to melaena (see p. 15) and anaemia.

Common presenting symptoms are often non-specific and include fatigue, lethargy, weakness, breathlessness, pain and weight loss. People with blood disorders can also report fevers, night sweats and repeated infections, and may have indications of unusual bleeding such as a tendency to bruise easily or prolonged or excessive bleeding from a cut. These factors should all be explored when taking a health history.

PHYSICAL ASSESSMENT

Physical assessment should include observation of the person's general appearance and behaviour. Pallor and lethargy may suggest a decrease in the number of red blood cells and oxygen-carrying capacity. The colour of the mucous membranes is inspected, and may be abnormally pale in the case of the conjunctiva, or the tongue may be a beefy red with glossitis (indicating classic iron deficiency anemia). Other unusual features such as stomatitis should be noted. On examination, the skin may be pale and dry; with some conditions jaundice may be present. This can result in itching and excoriation of the skin from scratching. The presence or absence of bruises and petechiae are noted when examining the skin, as this may indicate that the person has an increased tendency to bleed.

Blood pressure and pulse rate and volume are recorded and compared, if possible, with normal values for the particular patient. Respiratory rate and rhythm are also assessed at rest and after exercise, as a reduction in the ability of the blood to transport oxygen places a greater demand on the respiratory and cardiovascular systems which will be more obvious after activity. The person's cognitive status should also be assessed for evidence of confusion or a decreased level of consciousness.

INVESTIGATIONS

A variety of investigations are used to assist in the diagnosis of blood disorders. Some of these are described in Tables 14.3–14.5. Microscopic examination of a stained blood film is used to assess the shape, size and appearance of blood cells and to detect abnormal cells and parasites such as those causing malaria. A variety of radiological investigations may also be helpful in determining the cause and extent of the haematological disorder, including radiography, ultrasonography, computed tomography, magnetic resonance imaging and nuclear medicine studies.

BONE MARROW EXAMINATION

This is a useful test for establishing haematological function. It involves examining a small sample of the bone marrow obtained from inside the bone (bone marrow aspiration) and a small piece of the bone itself (bone marrow trephine biopsy). Blood smears are made of the aspirated bone marrow and the bone specimen is cut into thin sections. Microscopic examination of these specimens provides information about the structure of the bone marrow cavity, the number and different types of cells and their stages of development and maturity. It may also show the presence of cells foreign to the bone marrow, as in secondary carcinoma.

The site chosen requires red bone marrow to be easily accessible; in adults, the posterior iliac crest is usually preferred. An alternative site is the anterior iliac crest, and if only an aspirate is required the sternum may occasionally be used. In children, bone marrow may be sampled from the tibia and a general anaesthetic is given.

The individual is positioned prone or on their side when aspirating from the iliac crests; supine for a sternal aspiration. The skin is cleansed and the area infiltrated with local anaesthetic. When the anaesthetic has taken effect, the specialized aspiration needle is inserted. The individual

Table 14.3	Laboratory tests for assessing erythrocytes (normal values vary slightly between laboratories)	
Test	**Normal values**	**Description**
Red blood cell count (RCC)	Males: $4.5–6.3 \times 10^{12}$/L Females: $4.2–5.5 \times 10^{12}$/L	The normal red cell blood count varies with sex, age, altitude and exercise. It increases with hypovolaemia and decreases with hypervolaemia.
Haemoglobin concentration (Hb)	Males: 14–18 g/dL (8.1–11.2 mmol/L) Females: 12–16 g/dL (7.4–9.9 mmol/L) Children (3 months to puberty): 10–14 g/dL	The normal values for haemoglobin vary with age, sex, altitude and exercise. Hypovolaemia leads to increased levels and hypervolaemia to decreased levels.
Packed cell volume (PCV) or haematocrit Erythrocyte indices	Males: 40–50% Females: 37–47%	The volume of red blood cells in blood is expressed as a percentage of the total blood volume.
Mean corpuscular volume (MCV)	76–96 fL (femolitres)	This is the average size of individual red cells (normocytic). A raised MCV indicates a macrocytic anaemia. A lower MCV indicates a microcytic anaemia.
Mean corpuscular haemoglobin (MCH)	27–32 pg (picograms)	This is the average amount of haemoglobin per red cell (normochromic).

continued

Table 14.3 *Cont'd*

Test	Normal values	Description
Mean corpuscular haemoglobin concentration (MCHC)	30–35 g/dL	This is the average weight in grams of haemoglobin in 1 decilitre (dL) of red blood cells.
Reticulocyte count	0.5–1.5%	The percentage of circulating non-mature, non-nucleated red blood cells. Results are indicative of bone marrow activity.
Serum vitamin B_{12}	160–925 ng/L	B_{12} is necessary for red blood cell production. It requires intrinsic factor for its absorption from the gastrointestinal tract. Its level is determined to diagnose macrocytic anaemia.
Serum folate	3.0–15 mg/L	Folic acid is required for the normal production of red and white blood cells and DNA. Its absorption depends on a normally functioning intestinal mucosa. Its level is determined to diagnose macrocytic anaemia.
Serum ferritin Red cell mass (RCM)	10–250 mg/L Males: 20–33 mL/kg Females: 20–27 mL/kg	Indicates the total body iron stores. Determined by labelling the red blood cells with chromium-51 (^{51}Cr). This is used in the diagnosis of polycythaemia.
Erythrocyte sedimentation rate (ESR)	Up to 12 mm/h	Measures how rapidly red blood cells settle out of unclotted blood. Alteration in the blood proteins results in aggregation of the red cells and they fall faster. This is a non-specific test, but raised values are indicative of active inflammatory processes.
Sickle-cell test	Negative	Demonstrates the presence of haemoglobin S. A reducing agent is used to deoxygenate the erythrocytes and the cells are examined microscopically for evidence of sickling. Red blood cells that contain haemoglobin S are distorted and sickle- or crescent-shaped when deprived of oxygen.
Haemoglobin electrophoresis	Adult: (% of total) HbA 95–98%, HbA_2 1.5–3.5%, HbF_1 2%, HbC 0%, HbS 0% Newborn: HbF 40–70% Infant: HbF 2–10% Child (> 6 months) HbF 1–3%	Used to identify the different types of haemoglobin present in the red blood cells when investigating haemoglobinopathies and thalassaemia. Haemoglobin S is the most common of the abnormal haemoglobins.
Coombs' test Direct Indirect	Negative (no agglutination) Negative (no agglutination)	Erythrocytes are mixed with Coombs' reagent to test for agglutinins that lead to clumping and haemolysis. The direct test detects antibody or complement bound to the red cells as found in immune haemolytic anaemias. The indirect test is used in routine cross-matching before transfusion and during pregnancy. It detects antibody in the serum.

Table 14.4 Laboratory tests for assessing leucocytes (normal values may vary slightly between laboratories)

Test	Normal values	Description
White blood cell count (WCC)	$3.7–11.0 \times 10^9$/L	
Differential count Neutrophils Eosinophils Basophils Monocytes Lymphocytes	$1.7–7.5 \times 10^9$/L (40–75%) $0.03–0.44 \times 10^9$/L (1–6%) $0.015–0.1 \times 10^9$/L (<1%) $0.2–0.8 \times 10^9$/L (2–10%) $1.5–3.5 \times 10^9$/L (20–50%)	In certain disease conditions, the percentages of the various types on leucocyte are increased relative to others.

Normal values may be lower for West Indian, African and Middle Eastern people.

Table 14.5 Laboratory tests for assessing platelets and clotting functions of the blood

Test	Normal values	Description
Blood platelet (thrombocyte) count	$150-400 \times 10^9$/L	
Bleeding time	2–5 minutes (varies with method used)	This is the time it takes bleeding to stop naturally – that is, the period of time blood continues to escape from an 'open' area.
Prothrombin (PT) or International normalized ratio (INR)	11–15 seconds 2–4	This is the time it takes for coagulation following addition of thromboplastin and calcium to the specimen. The INR is designed to produce consistent results in all laboratories regardless of reagents used and it the ratio of the PT of the patient to that of a person not taking anticoagulants.
Partial thromboplastin time (PTT) Activated partial thromboplastin time (APTT)	PTT 40–100 seconds APTT 30–45 seconds	The partial thromboplastin time is a general test of coagulation used for screening and to monitor anticoagulant therapy. Clotting deficiencies other than factor VII, XIII and platelets can be detected. The activated partial thromboplastin time (APTT) involves the addition of activators to the regular test reagent to shorten the clotting time.
Plasma fibrinogen	2–4 g/L	This indicates the fibrinogen concentration.

should be warned that discomfort occurs from the pressure needed to pass the needle through the cortex of the bone into the marrow and from the aspiration of the marrow fluid. On removal of the needle, pressure is applied until bleeding stops and the site is covered with a plaster or dry dressing and should be kept dry for 24 hours. If an outpatient, the individual is observed for at least 1 hour to ensure bleeding has ceased.

ERYTHROCYTE DISORDERS

A deficiency or excess may occur in the number of circulating red blood cells, or the red blood cells may function abnormally. Variations in the size, shape and haemoglobin content may be present. Certain descriptive terms are used to denote some of the characteristics that are noted when blood is examined microscopically:

- Macrocytes are erythrocytes that are larger than normal
- Microcytes are erythrocytes that are smaller than normal
- Normochromic describes cells that possess a normal amount of haemoglobin
- Hypochromic describes cells that are deficient in haemoglobin
- Hyperchromic describes cells with a haemoglobin content that is greater than normal
- Poikilocytic cells are cells with an abnormal shape.

ANAEMIA (ERYTHROCYTE AND HAEMOGLOBIN DEFICIENCY)

The term **anaemia** denotes a reduction in the oxygen-carrying capacity of the blood. This occurs as a result of fewer circulating erythrocytes than is needed or a decrease

in the concentration of haemoglobin. Anaemia is normally defined as a haemoglobin level in the blood of less than 13.5 g/dl in men and 11.5 g/dl in women. It is sometimes also classified according to the size of the red cell and amount of haemoglobin in the erythrocytes. For example, iron deficiency causes an anaemia where the cells are hypochromic and microcytic, and the disease may be referred to as a hypochromic microcytic anaemia.

Causes

Anaemia may be caused by decreased production of red blood cells (erythropoiesis) or by excessive destruction or loss. Anaemia that is due to decreased erythropoiesis may result from a deficiency of factors essential for normal production or by depressed bone marrow activity. It may also occur secondary to some other disorder such as renal disease, and because of this, the patient may undergo extensive investigation to determine the cause of the anaemia. Excessive destruction of red blood cells leading to anaemia may be caused by problems within the red blood cells (intracorpuscular defects) or result from factors outside the red blood cells (extracorpuscular factors).

General effects and characteristics

Whatever the cause or type of anaemia, it presents a common problem: a decrease in the capacity of the blood to transport oxygen. This is manifested in a variety of signs and symptoms attributable to tissue and organ hypoxia and the ensuing reduced metabolism. These are shown in Figure 14.7.

The occurrence and severity of these manifestations depend on three factors:

1 *Speed of onset* – a gradually developing anaemia may be tolerated without any significant incapacity, whereas a relatively small but rapid blood loss may produce marked symptoms.

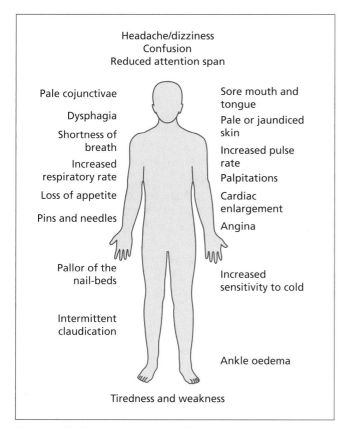

Headache/dizziness
Confusion
Reduced attention span

Pale cojunctivae

Dysphagia

Shortness of breath

Increased respiratory rate

Loss of appetite

Pins and needles

Pallor of the nail-beds

Intermittent claudication

Sore mouth and tongue

Pale or jaundiced skin

Increased pulse rate

Palpitations

Cardiac enlargement

Angina

Increased sensitivity to cold

Ankle oedema

Tiredness and weakness

Figure 14.7 Symptoms and signs of anaemia.

2 *Severity* – mild anaemia often causes no problems, and even severe anaemia may result in relatively few symptoms in a young and otherwise healthy person.

3 *Age* – anaemia tends to be tolerated less well by the elderly because cardiac compensatory mechanisms may also be impaired.

4 *Health status of the person* – anaemia in the context of other health problems may be less well tolerated by the individual.

Anaemia due to abnormalities of erythropoiesis

Anaemia may result from a lack of an essential nutrient in the diet, defective absorption or an increased demand which cannot be met by the normal supply of factors essential for red cell production. The nutritional deficiency anaemias seen most often are those resulting from a lack of iron, vitamin B₁₂ or folic acid. A healthy diet is very important in preventing such deficiencies occurring.

Nurses should be proactive in the primary prevention of such problems by promoting healthy eating guidelines at every opportunity, as a normal varied diet supplies essential nutrients in excess of the body's usual requirements. A wide variety of community, workplace and institutional settings offer opportunities for nurses to interact with individuals, either on a one-to-one basis or in groups, to promote healthy eating. Those who should be particularly targeted include pregnant women, mothers with babies and toddlers, schoolchildren and adolescents, the elderly and those in hospital or residential care. It is obviously important to take into account each individual's dietary preferences and circumstances, such as the special needs of vegetarians and vegans, and to be sensitive to cultural influences in diets and food preparation.

Dietary sources of iron are liver, red meat, some green vegetables, fish and cereals (which are often supplemented with iron during processing). Vitamin B₁₂ is found in liver, red meat, eggs, shellfish and dairy produce. Sources of food rich in folate includes liver, eggs, vegetables such as broccoli, peas, spinach, brussel sprouts and potatoes, cereals and yeast, but cooking may reduce the folate content of food by up to 95%.

The ability of a person to afford or to access a healthy diet takes the problem to a different level. It is society's responsibility to ensure that its members can afford and obtain foodstuffs that will prevent any individual from developing diseases such as deficiency anaemia. This is a professional responsibility that may involve nurses in campaigning for client groups at risk, such as schoolchildren who need healthier and affordable school meals, or the elderly who face cuts in community care and the closure of local food stores, or for rights of refugees and asylum seekers. The elderly form an especially vulnerable group because, even if they are able to afford a healthy diet, they often have physical disabilities and other health problems that make acquiring, preparing and eating food difficult.

Iron deficiency anaemia

Iron deficiency is common worldwide (Nowak and Handford 2004). It is characterized by small red blood cells with less than the normal content of haemoglobin (microcytic hypochromic). There is usually a slight reduction in the total number of red blood cells. Iron deficiency may be due to chronic blood loss, an insufficient nutritional intake of iron, impaired intestinal absorption or an increased requirement for iron. Pregnant and lactating women and pre-school children are those most at risk of iron deficiency because of an increased need for iron to meet the needs of the fetus and for growth during infancy. In adults, the most common cause is chronic blood loss, especially from the gastrointestinal tract or genitourinary tract. Women of reproductive age are at risk because of menstrual blood loss, increased demands during pregnancy and lactation and blood loss at delivery. Iron deficiency anaemia is uncommon in men unless there has been a loss of blood, development of hypochlorhydria secondary to gastric disease, atrophy of the gastric mucosa or gastrectomy. Other causes of blood loss include cancer, peptic ulcer and haemorrhoids, and in tropical climates infestation with hookworms which may be responsible for chronic blood loss. In addition to the general symptoms of anaemia identified in Figure 14.7, the person with iron deficiency anaemia may experience soreness and inflammation of the mouth and tongue. Iron is essential for the production of enzymes which play a key role in maintaining healthy epithelium (cytochromes), consequently iron deficiency results in disorder of the epithelial lining of the mouth and tongue. The tongue may be very red and may have a smooth, glazed appearance due to atrophy of the papillae. Inflammation of the gastric mucosa may develop from the same mechanism (gastritis) leading on to achlorhydria (Walsh 2006). Rarely the patient with a severe anaemia complains of dysphagia (difficulty in swallowing). The combination of dysphagia, stomatitis (inflammation of the mouth) and atrophic glossitis (inflammation of the tongue with atrophy of papillae) in anaemia may be referred to as the Plummer–Vinson syndrome. Changes in the fingernails are common in those with prolonged iron deficiency. The nails become brittle and concave or spoon shaped.

Investigations Serum ferritin concentration is the most reliable guide to iron deficiency; it is likely to be less than 12 mg/L. When gastrointestinal bleeding is suspected as a cause of chronic blood loss, other investigations such as faecal occult bloods and endoscopy may be required.

Treatment If a source of blood loss (such as a peptic ulcer, colonic cancer or uterine fibroids) is identified as the cause of the anaemia, steps should be taken to treat this and stop the blood loss. When iron supplementation is required, medicinal iron is usually given in the form of an oral ferrous salt such as ferrous sulfate 200 mg taken three times a day, or ferrous gluconate 600 mg three times daily. Both preparations are normally continued for at least 4 months in order to raise the haemoglobin to normal levels and replenish the iron stores. Gastrointestinal irritation and constipation or diarrhoea are not uncommon side-effects of iron therapy and may be reduced by taking iron preparations after food. Stools are darkened by iron, and older patients in particular may find that iron has a constipating effect. Parenteral iron is rarely indicated.

Preventive strategies at an individual level include promoting dietary changes that will increase the intake of haem iron (iron from animal products); increase the intake of vitamin C and other acidic or fermented foods that promote iron absorption; and reduce intake of iron absorption inhibitors such as coffee, tea and some cereals. Other foodstuffs may be fortified, for example cereals and weaning foods and follow-on baby milks. Control of parasites such as hookworms are important strategies in some parts of the world for reducing iron deficiency. Iron supplementation is recommended for pregnant and lactating women in areas where iron deficiency anaemia is prevalent.

Vitamin B$_{12}$ deficiency (pernicious anaemia)

When there is a deficiency of vitamin B$_{12}$, red blood cells are produced that are larger than normal but fewer in number. The cells show considerable variation in both shape and size. Although the red cells have a haemoglobin content that is greater than normal, the deficiency in the total number of erythrocytes results in an insufficient oxygen-carrying capacity of blood. The condition is sometimes referred to as megaloblastic anaemia, in reference to the larger erythrocyte produced in this type of deficiency.

The cause of vitamin B$_{12}$ deficiency is usually non-absorption of the vitamin. Inadequate dietary intake is rare and associated with starvation or in individuals who are vegans (eat no animal or dairy products). Malabsorption of the vitamin is the most common cause of deficiency and results from failure of the gastric parietal cells to produce intrinsic factor, the glycoprotein that binds vitamin B$_{12}$ and facilitates its transfer across the intestinal wall. This condition, characterized by atrophy of the parietal cells, is known as pernicious anaemia. It is an autoimmune disorder that has a tendency to occur in families and is associated with those whose blood is group A. It is more common in females, and has an insidious onset and a peak occurrence around the age of 60 years.

Malabsorption of vitamin B$_{12}$ may also occur as a result of partial or total gastrectomy, which removes the source of intrinsic factor. Any gastrointestinal condition or operation that results in the formation of blind or stagnant loops of small intestine (e.g. diverticular disease, Crohn's disease, ileal resection) may predispose the individual to vitamin B$_{12}$ deficiency because bacterial growth proliferates in conditions of stasis, using up available B$_{12}$ before it can be absorbed.

Clinical characteristics In addition to the general symptoms of anaemia, the patient may experience gastrointestinal and nervous system changes. The tongue is often sore and smooth, and a beefy red colour. There is loss of appetite but the person does not necessarily lose weight. The lack of vitamin B$_{12}$ may cause degeneration of myelin and nerve fibres in the spinal cord and peripheral nerves. The patient may present with neurological symptoms such as a symmetrical tingling or 'pins and needles', or coldness and numbness in the extremities. Unless the deficiency is corrected, serious motor disturbances may develop in the form of muscular weakness, ataxia (loss of coordination and staggering) and paralysis. If the deficiency is prolonged and severe, degeneration of the optic nerves may occur, causing serious impairment of vision. When degenerative changes occur in the spinal cord, the condition is known as subacute combined degeneration of the cord. In severe pernicious anaemia the skin may show some jaundice, a result of increased haemolysis or erythrocyte breakdown.

Investigations Laboratory examination of the blood reveals a deficiency in the number of erythrocytes and macrocytic hyperchromic cells. Bone marrow examination shows hyperplasia of the bone marrow but a failure in erythropoiesis, as evidenced by a large proportion of immature cells. A lack of intrinsic factor is often associated with a lack of gastric acid (achlorhydria), which is also produced by the parietal cells, and thus in investigation of pernicious anaemia there may be an attempt to test and stimulate gastric acid secretion after administering histamine or pentagastrin. The Schilling test or a variant of it may also be used to evaluate the absorption of vitamin B_{12}. This involves measuring the concentration of radioactively labelled B_{12} excreted in a 24-hour collection of urine. The radioactive dose is administered orally and is followed by a dose of unlabelled vitamin B_{12} administered subcutaneously, which flushes the radioactive vitamin, which has been absorbed, out into the urine. Serum cobalamin (B_{12}) levels can be used as a measure of the body's cobalamin status.

Treatment Vitamin B_{12} deficiency is treated by intramuscular injection of hydroxocobalamin to overcome the problem of malabsorption. Up to 1 mg of hydroxocobalamin is administered three times a week for 2 weeks. Thereafter, an injection of the drug is required at 3-month intervals for life to maintain normal haemoglobin and erythrocyte levels (BNF 2005).

The haematological response to treatment is rapid and may result in temporary depletion of iron stores and insufficient haemoglobin production. For this reason, ferrous sulfate is sometimes administered concurrently when treatment is initiated. Potassium levels should also be monitored to detect potential hypokalaemia. Neurological symptoms improve only slowly and may never disappear completely.

In contrast to pernicious anaemia, the anaemia associated with a dietary deficiency of vitamin B_{12} or intestinal disease does not manifest as hypochlorhydria or lead to degenerative changes in the nervous system. Individuals who are strict vegans may take oral vitamin B_{12}. When the anaemia is secondary to intestinal disease and malabsorption has been demonstrated, parenteral vitamin B_{12} is given. Following total or partial gastrectomy or ileal resection, vitamin B_{12} should be given prophylactically.

Folic acid deficiency anaemia

Like vitamin B_{12}, folic acid (folate) is an essential requirement for DNA synthesis. Its lack results in a form of anaemia very similar to that of vitamin B_{12} deficiency. The cause of folate deficiency may be:

- an inadequate diet (alcoholics and those with anorexia are at particular risk)
- malabsorption (such as in coeliac disease, Crohn's disease and tropical sprue)
- increased requirements, particularly during pregnancy
- drug induced (e.g. by the cytotoxic drug methotrexate or anticonvulsants such as phenytoin).

Investigations Haematological changes are the same as those found with vitamin B_{12} deficiency (macrocytic hyperchromic cells are seen microscopically); however, the person does not manifest achlorhydria, decreased vitamin B_{12} absorption or have nervous system involvement.

Treatment Folic acid 5 mg orally daily for 4 months is usually sufficient to restore normal haematological findings and to replenish body stores. In malabsorption states, a higher dose may be needed. A person with severe megaloblastic anaemia needing urgent treatment should not be given folic acid alone until vitamin B_{12} deficiency has been definitely excluded. This is because there is a risk of precipitating neurological symptoms in a person with B_{12} deficiency. Until the underlying cause of the anaemia has been determined, it is therefore necessary to give vitamin B_{12} concurrently.

Folic acid is sometimes given prophylactically to women during pregnancy and to patients with severe haemolytic anaemias. It is recommended that all women who are planning to become pregnant take folic acid supplements at a dose of 400 mg daily before conception and for the first 12 weeks of pregnancy. This has been shown to reduce the incidence of babies born with neural tube defects and also helps to prevent maternal anaemia (Lumley et al 2001).

Vitamin C deficiency

This results in scurvy and is associated with a diet lacking in fresh fruit, potatoes and green vegetables. People eating a very restricted diet such as infants and the elderly sometimes develop anaemia and are deficient in vitamin C as well as iron and folate. Vitamin C improves iron absorption by reducing ferric iron to ferrous iron, which is more readily absorbed. It also enhances the catalytic action of folic acid in erythropoiesis.

Anaemia secondary to blood loss

Blood loss may be either acute or chronic. Common causes for chronic blood loss include gastrointestinal lesions and menorrhagia. In chronic blood loss, the result is often iron deficiency anaemia, which was discussed above. Acute blood loss may be the result of trauma, surgery, haematemesis, haemoptysis or obstetric haemorrhage.

The sudden loss of blood removes erythrocytes from the circulation, reducing the oxygen-carrying capacity of the blood. Initially, the blood count may remain within normal parameters, as there is an equivalent loss of plasma during a bleeding episode. As the plasma volume generally returns to normal within 1–3 days after the initial blood loss, the remaining pool of red cells is then dispersed into this increased circulatory volume. It is at this time that the severity of anaemia can be more accurately measured.

Under normal circumstances, the bone marrow responds quickly to increased tissue hypoxia and the red cell count returns to normal within 4–5 weeks. As a considerable amount of iron may be lost as a result of the bleeding episode, haemoglobin production may be impaired, necessitating the administration of iron supplements to replenish iron stores and increase the level of haemoglobin production.

If the blood loss is 20% or more of the total blood volume, or if bleeding cannot be arrested quickly, rapid replacement by means of a blood transfusion may be necessary. This will help to prevent acute renal failure (p. xxx) and minimize the normal physiological responses to acute blood loss that may lead to cardiac, renal, respiratory or gastrointestinal problems. Rapid transfusion quickly increases the total circulating volume as well as the number of red cells available to carry oxygen. In severe blood loss, the replacement of plasma, platelets and clotting factors may also be required. Specific protocols for the management of massive blood loss and transfusion exist as this represents a medical emergency associated with a high morbidity and mortality rate. Management of severe blood loss includes the surgical control of bleeding, management of the circulatory volume and maintenance of adequate blood oxygen-carrying capacity (UK Blood Transfusion Services 2001).

Anaemia due to abnormal red cell destruction (haemolytic anaemias)

A reduced red cell lifespan with abnormal or increased destruction is characteristic of the haemolytic anaemias. This abnormality may be either inherited or acquired. Destruction related to a defective red cell reflects the inherited haemolytic anaemias, whereas, for the most part, the acquired haemolytic anaemias are due to increased destruction of normal red cells. One exception to this is paroxysmal nocturnal haemoglobinurea, where an acquired red cell defect is the primary cause of the haemolysis. Destruction of the red cell may take place within the bloodstream (intravascular haemolysis) or in the spleen and liver (extravascular haemolysis).

Acquired haemolytic anaemias

Autoimmune haemolytic anaemia (AIHA) is caused by the production of an antibody that is targeted against one or more of the person's own red cell surface antigens. AIHA is divided into warm or cold types, depending on the temperature at which there is maximum antibody activity (37°C or 4°C). Both types may either be primary (idiopathic) or secondary to another disorder. Examples include SLE or other autoimmune diseases, lymphoproliferative diseases such as lymphoma or CLL, some drugs including methyldopa and infections such as mycoplasma pneumonia and infectious mononucleosis (Hoffbrand et al 2001). Warm AIHA can be treated with immunosuppressive therapy such as steroid treatment or other immunosuppressive drugs, and a splenectomy may be considered if steroid treatment fails. Management of cold AIHA involves immunosuppression and includes keeping the patient warm.

Alloimmune haemolytic anaemia is caused by the reaction between the antibodies of one individual and the red cells of another. This may occur as a result of a mismatched blood transfusion, following transplantation or in haemolytic disease of the newborn, where a Rhesus-negative mother with Rh antibodies reacts to a Rhesus-positive fetus causing intravascular haemolysis in the child. Alloimmune haemolytic anaemia is a potentially life-threatening condition. *Transfusion-related haemolytic anaemia* is discussed later in this chapter.

Other extrinsic causes for abnormal haemolysis include drug-induced haemolytic anaemia and infections through either direct damage, toxins or autoantibody formation. Microangiopathic haemolytic anaemia may occur in disseminated intravascular coagulation, in patients with artificial heart valves, in thrombotic thrombocytopenic purpura (TTP), malignant hypertension, pre-eclampsia and meningococcal septicaemia (Mehta and Hoffbrand 2000). In these haemolytic anaemias, treatment of the underlying cause of the red cell destruction is a clinical priority, as well as managing the haemolysis itself.

Anaemia of chronic disorders

Chronic inflammatory disorders such as chronic infections, connective tissue disorders and malignant disease can result in a mild and often stable anaemia. This anaemia appears to arise out of a number of processes such as reduced release of iron, reduced red cell lifespan and a reduced erythropoietin response, secondary to the production of cytokines such as interleukin-1 (IL-1) and tumour necrosis factor (TNF). This anaemia is often exacerbated by other factors.

The anaemia of cancer is one example of the multifactorial process of some anaemias:

- Iron deficiency (and folate deficiency):
  1 Inability to eat because of:
     - the location of the cancer (e.g. oropharyngeal, GI)
     - treatment of the cancer by radiotherapy or chemotherapy producing side-effects such as mucositis and GI disturbances, loss of appetite, nausea and vomiting, taste changes, pain
     - length of treatment
     - fatigue
     - psychological factors.
  2 Reduced absorption:
     - vitamin C
     - gastric ulcer prophylaxis.
  3 Blood loss:
     - G-U, gynaecological, G-I cancers
     - oesophageal varices secondary to metastatic disease of the liver and Mallory–Weiss tears due to retching
     - multiple phlebotomies
     - aggravated by quantitative and qualitative platelet defects and abnormalities of the coagulation cascade.
- Impaired erythropoiesis:
  - reticuloendothelial blockade of iron utilization
  - reduced erythropoietin production
  - resistance of bone marrow to erythropoietin
  - bone marrow failure due to treatment or infiltration.
- Immune haemolytic:
  - Chronic lymphocytic leukaemia, non-Hodgkin's lymphoma, Hodgkin's disease, multiple myeloma, teratomas of the ovary, seminoma, thymoma, hypernephroma, breast, lung, renal cell, G-I adenocarcinoma.
- Microangiopathic:
  - G-I adenocarcinoma, breast, lung
  - Factors from tumour or direct effects of tumour cells on vasculature
  - tumour emboli.

Inherited haemolytic anaemias

Defects of the red cell can be related to:

- an abnormality of the cell membrane
- abnormal metabolism
- abnormal haemoglobin.

Much of the pathology associated with these chronic anaemias can be described in terms of the process of red cell destruction. The anaemia itself may, in some disorders, be relatively mild and is often reasonably well tolerated. However, at times of stress, such as during a period of infection or extra need, the anaemia may become more pronounced. In these anaemias folate deficiency is fairly common; therefore folic acid supplements may be needed. The increased bilirubin concentration may predispose individuals to gallstones, particularly those with relatively high rates of haemolysis. There is also increased urobilinogen in the urine and faeces, making both darker in colour. Itching, either persistent or intermittent, may also be present. Splenomegaly may feature in disorders where the spleen is the major site of destruction.

Hereditary spherocytosis and hereditary elliptocytosis

Haemolytic anaemias resulting from an abnormal red cell membrane include *hereditary spherocytosis* and *hereditary elliptocytosis*. The haemolytic anaemia is classified according to the shape of the abnormal red cell, as the names imply. Most are inherited, although there is some evidence of spontaneous mutations in individuals with spherocytosis. In general the anaemia tends to be mild to moderate, depending on the rate of haemolysis. Folate deficiency is common, and infection (particularly some viral infections) can cause an acute haemolysis. A palpable spleen is relatively common. Nevertheless, many individuals remain only mildly symptomatic. For those whose symptoms are not easily tolerated, splenectomy may be helpful.

Glucose-6-phosphate dehydrogenase (G6PD) deficiency

An important example of haemolysis resulting from abnormal metabolism of the red cell is glucose-6-phosphate dehydrogenase (G6PD) deficiency. The genetic deficiency is on an X-linked gene, which means that by and large it affects males. The majority of women are only carriers, but a small population of women is affected, although usually only mildly. Heterozygote women are afforded a degree of protection from falciparum malaria (Hoffbrand et al 2001). The incidence varies greatly throughout the world, from very rarely amongst northern Europeans to over 20% in southern Europe, parts of Africa and Asia. The highest frequency appears to be in south-east Asia and parts of the Middle East (Luzzatto and Gordon-Smith 1999).

In most, the haemolysis is acute and manifests itself only in the presence of a specific trigger. Certain medications, fava beans and infections are known triggers. Medications that act as triggers include some antimalarials, antibiotics, analgesics and antihelminths (Hoffbrand et al 2001). Care should be taken to avoid these as far as possible. For healthcare workers, this is particularly relevant in relation to medications that may unknowingly be prescribed and administered to susceptible individuals. In acute attacks, the intravascular haemolysis can greatly vary in severity, as can the symptoms. Renal failure is associated with G6PD haemolysis.

In severe anemia, therapy includes supportive care such as maintaining a high urine output, blood transfusions, the treatment of any underlying infection and the immediate removal of any other specific trigger. In some individuals, the haemolysis may be chronic.

Haemoglobinopathies

The complex haemoglobin (Hb) molecule occurs normally in three forms. The type is determined by slight variations in the globin portions of the four subunits. HbA is the principal haemoglobin of adults, HbA_2 is approximately 2% of adult haemoglobin and HbF (fetal haemoglobin) is usually less than 1% Hb in adults (Arif and Mufti 1998). Adult haemoglobin contains two α- and two β-globin chains with a haem pocket within each chain.

The term haemoglobinopathy indicates the presence of red blood cells containing an inherited abnormality of haemoglobin, the result of a genetic mutation that causes a disorder in synthesis of the haemoglobin molecule. This may result in a structural variation in one or more of the globin chains causing a decreased production of structurally normal haemoglobin and premature haemolysis of the erythrocyte. The most common haemoglobinopathies are thalassaemia and sickle-cell anaemia.

Thalassaemia

The thalassaemias are a group of autosomal recessive inherited disorders affecting the synthesis of the globin part of the haemoglobin molecule in the red cell. Either the α- or the β-chain of the globin molecule can be affected, leading to an imbalance in the production of α- and β-chains and a fundamental instability of the globin molecule. This leads to a range of syndromes, the clinical characteristics of which are related to the degree of α- and β-chain imbalance (Haslett et al 2002).

The thalassaemias occur predominantly in the Mediterranean, parts of Africa, the Middle East, the Indian subcontinent and south-east Asia (Nowak and Handford 2004). They are among the most common inherited disorders and are thought to have evolved because they can confer partial resistance to the malaria parasite. The thalassaemias are classified according to their severity. Thalassaemia major is a severe transfusion-dependent form; thalassaemia minor is a carrier state with few, if any, clinical implications. Thalassaemia intermedia is a less severe form, with a degree of anaemia and splenomegaly (Nowak and Handford 2004).

β-*Thalassaemia major* is a severe form of the disease, with red cell destruction both within the bone marrow and in the spleen. Children born with this disorder have severe anaemia, fail to thrive and have a myriad of problems. The spleen and liver enlarge and the chronic anaemia causes extramedullary haemopoiesis, causing bony deformities. These children are transfusion dependent: without treatment they seldom survive into adolescence. The need for frequent transfusions creates its own problems, including iron overload and organ damage.

Apart from regular transfusions, regular iron chelation therapy, such as subcutaneous desferrioxamine, is required to reduce iron overload. A splenectomy may be required to reduce transfusion requirements. Bone marrow transplantation may be an option for some individuals. Long-term cardiac, liver and endocrine problems require management as they arise.

Thalassaemia intermedia is less severe: individuals exhibit a moderate anaemia, sometimes requiring transfusion support. Many of the clinical symptoms of β-thalassaemia major are absent.

β-*Thalassaemia minor* (or trait) is least severe, with mild anaemia. Individuals often remain completely asymptomatic, except perhaps at times of stress, such as in pregnancy.

In α-thalassaemia, the clinical picture is related to the number of functioning α genes present. In parents who are carrying the α thalassaemia trait there is a one in four chance that a child could have the complete absence of α-globin production which is incompatible with life and results in intrauterine or neonatal death and the syndrome *hydrops fetalis* and there is a one in four chance that the child could inherit *Haemoglobin H disease*, which is a consequence of only one functioning gene and results in anaemia and splenomegaly. One or two α-gene deletions result in thalassaemia trait. This is often asymptomatic, although some individuals may have mild anaemia.

Genetic counselling should be offered to those individuals found to be carriers. Partners of carriers should also be tested. Appropriate and unbiased information and support should be offered to couples who are both carriers, alongside the option of antenatal testing so that informed choices can be made about pregnancy.

Sickle-cell disease   This is a group of hereditary recessive blood disorders characterized by red cells that contain an abnormal form of haemoglobin called HbS. The globin chain structure is changed by the substitution of the amino acid glutamic acid by valine, effectively changing the behaviour of the whole protein molecule. As this is a recessive disorder, individuals who inherit HbS from only one parent have what is termed a sickle-cell trait (HbAS), whereas individuals who inherit HbS from both parents have sickle-cell anaemia (HbSS). Figure 14.8 shows examples of inheritance of HbS. Other variants of sickle-cell disease include HbSC and HbS β-thal.

It is predominantly a disease of the African-Caribbean population, but also affects individuals with Mediterranean, Middle Eastern and Asian Indian ancestry. Sickle-cell trait seems to offer some protection from a common type of malaria, falciparum malaria, so there is a higher incidence

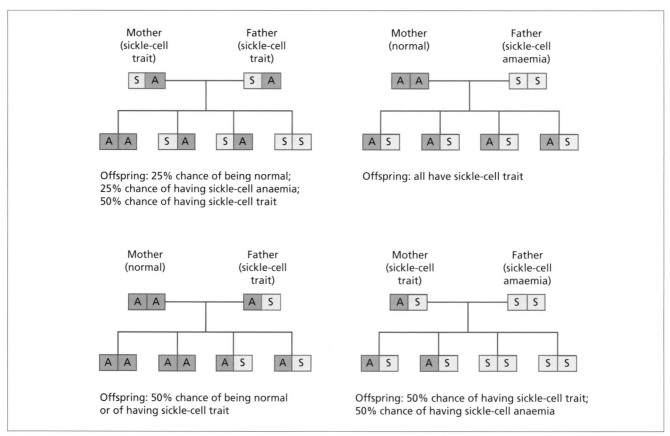

Offspring: 25% chance of being normal; 25% chance of having sickle-cell anaemia; 50% chance of having sickle-cell trait

Offspring: all have sickle-cell trait

Offspring: 50% chance of being normal or of having sickle-cell trait

Offspring: 50% chance of having sickle-cell trait; 50% chance of having sickle-cell anaemia

Figure 14.8   Examples of inheritance of sickle-cell disease. S, gene for Hbs; A, gene for normal haemoglobin.

of HbS inheritance in regions where malaria is prevalent. Diagnosis is often made within the first 2 years of life; young babies are often protected from symptoms of the disease because of the high levels of HbF (fetal haemoglobin) produced in early life.

The exact mechanisms by which changes in the properties of deoxygenated haemoglobin molecules cause the red cells to sickle (change shape from a biconcave disc to a crescent or sickle shape) is not yet fully understood but appear to be complex. Red cells with high levels of HbS dehydrate abnormally, making the red cell dense and encouraging the abnormal linking of neighbouring globin chains. It is thought that these denser red cells deform through this process of linking as they release oxygen molecules in the capillaries. The red cells undergo repeated cycles of 'sickling' and 'de-sickling' and are soon no longer able to return to their normal shape. These distorted crescent-shaped red cells become trapped in the microcirculation, causing blockages and producing the range of clinical manifestations of sickle-cell disease. Another consequence of this 'sickling' process is that the red cell lifespan is shortened from a normal 120 days to as little as 25–35 days, resulting in a haemolytic anaemia.

The course of sickle-cell anaemia is very variable. Some affected individuals are able to live almost normal lives, whereas others experience repeated crises with great incapacity and disability. The reason for this variation is not yet known. The clinical manifestations of sickle-cell disease are varied but include:

- severe episodes of acute pain, a consequence of vaso-occlusion
- acute chest syndrome
- splenic sequestration crisis
- avascular necrosis of bone and joints
- osteomyelitis
- chronic skin ulceration – frequently on lower limbs
- renal dysfunction
- stroke
- retinopathy
- anaemia
- priapism
- infections
- cardiomegaly
- bone marrow necrosis
- aplastic crisis.

Exacerbation of this sickling process, with vascular occlusion and severe pain, is termed a sickle-cell crisis or vaso-occlusive crisis. Precipitating factors of a crisis include physiological stresses such as exposure to cold or heat, dehydration, infection, physical exertion or any situation where the person experiences hypoxia or stress. Often, it is a combination of factors that induces a crisis. At times there are warning signs, but often the crisis is unpredictable and quite sudden.

Pain is a key feature of a vaso-occlusive crisis, often requiring strong opiate analgesics to control it. Although some mild sickle-cell crises can be managed effectively at home with oral analgesics, often the person is unwell and requires hospital admission for management and pain control. Initially patients require strong opiate analgesics to control the pain. This can be given as intramuscular injections, subcutaneous infusion or intravenous infusion, including patient-controlled analgesia (PCA) systems, depending on the clinical situation (see Ch. 8). Prompt, effective pain relief is imperative as pain is a potent physiological and psychological stressor, and may contribute to an increasing cycle of sickling and to other serious complications, as well as being very distressing for the person in pain. Often the pain is intense, engendering fear and anxiety and rendering the patient immobile. Appropriate pain assessments must be undertaken to identify the location and nature of the pain and to permit ongoing evaluation of the pain management strategy. Pain management with medication should be either continuous or given by the clock to ensure sustained pain relief. Non-steroidal anti-inflammatory agents can be added, if suitable. Comfort measures such as the use of pillows, positioning, warmth and reassurance are other important elements of the pain management strategy. The British Committee for Standards in Haematology has published guidelines for the management of pain in sickle cell anaemia (Rees et al 2003).

If the precipitating cause is a suspected infection, antimicrobials are prescribed. This is important as a large proportion of patients with sickle-cell disease are functionally asplenic (the spleen does not function) from an early age as a consequence of splenic infarctions from repeated crises. In the initial stages, rest and careful monitoring are essential. Sustained hydration is also essential, orally if tolerated, or as an intravenous infusion. Oxygen therapy is given to prevent any further hypoxia and the oxygen saturation levels are carefully monitored. Falling oxygen saturations may indicate a chest crisis or be a side-effect of the opiate analgesia. A chest crisis is a serious complication of sickle-cell disease and often leads to death from multiple fat emboli in the lungs leading to ventilatory failure. Urgent and effective medical management must be instituted promptly. Another serious complication is splenic sequestration; a rapidly falling haemoglobin level and abdominal discomfort or pain and distension are indicators of possible sequestration. Again, prompt medical intervention is essential. Transfusions of red cells or red cell exchange procedures may be required to reduce the proportion of sickle cells in the circulation and to help stabilize the seriously ill patient.

Once the person's condition has been stabilized and the pain is satisfactorily under control, gentle mobilization and rehabilitation can begin. This may be a rapid or slow process, depending on a number of factors. Regaining independence and a sense of control is a priority for patients. Pain relief can be titrated according to need, but a sudden increase in pain may signal the onset of another crisis and should be monitored carefully. A sample critical pathway that highlights some of the care interventions can be found in Box 14.1.

Chronic pain is often a consequence of bone and joint necrosis, and may be difficult to control effectively. Joint damage may reduce mobility, as can chronic skin ulcers. Strokes can occur at any age but are more frequent in childhood and can be devastating, leaving the person seriously disabled. Priapism (a persistent erection in the male) is another serious complication that may be difficult to treat and may induce impotence. The chronic anaemia and red cell breakdown may result in cardiomegaly and the development of gallstones. Patients with sickle-cell disease are often slightly jaundiced, a result of the continual red cell turnover. Damage to the renal capillaries may cause chronic renal failure; the individual typically passes large amounts of dilute urine, predisposing them to dehydration (see p. 615). Repeated transfusions may lead to iron overload.

Prevention of crises and complications includes:

- good nutrition and hydration (3 L of fluid per day)
- managing changes in the weather by keeping warm or cool as appropriate
- good housing with effective heating
- managing stress and stressful situations
- appropriate vaccinations including protection against pneumococcal infection (Davies et al 2002)

Box 14.1 Critical pathway for sickle-cell crisis

On arrival assessment	Days 1–3 assessment	Days 4–10 assessment
• Pain assessment	• Pain assessment – quantitative and qualitative – regular and consistent	• Pain assessment – quantitative and qualitative – regular and consistent

• Baseline:
  – O$_2$ saturations
  – vital signs
  – level of consciousness
  – hydration status
	• Clinical examination including abdomen, chest and CNS	• Clinical examination including abdomen, chest and CNS

• Clinical examination including abdomen, chest and CNS	• Anaemia	• Anaemia
	• Respiratory function	• Respiratory function
• Full blood count, U&E, blood cultures, group and save	• Level of consciousness	• Level of consciousness
	• Hydration	• Hydration
• Chest X-ray	• Renal function	• Renal function
• Assess need for vascular access	• Self-caring activities	• Self-caring activities
• Assess ability to drink	• Psychological status/mood	• Psychological status/mood
	• Support needs	• Support needs
		• Preliminary discharge assessment
Intervention	**Intervention**	**Intervention**

• Analgesia:
  – institute promptly and at a dosage that relieves pain effectively
  – repeat regularly and titrate to pain levels
  – maintain a regular analgesia schedule
	• Analgesia:
	  – titrate to pain levels
	  – maintain a regular analgesia schedule
	  – institute an appropriate drug delivery system (e.g. patient controlled analgesia (PCA) device)
		• Analgesia:
		  – titrate to pain levels
		  – maintain a regular analgesia schedule
		  – discuss changing needs with the patient
		  – implement analgesia strategy to meet needs

• Oxygenation:
  – maintain O$_2$ saturations > 90%
  – O$_2$ via humidified mask
  – mechanical ventilation, if required
	• Oxygenation:
	  – maintain O$_2$ saturations > 90 %
	  – O$_2$ via humidified mask
	  – mechanical ventilation, if required
		• Oxygenation:
		  – maintain O$_2$ saturations > 90 %
		  – O$_2$ via humidified mask if required

• Monitor hourly:
  – pain levels
  – O$_2$ saturations
  – vital signs
  – level of consciousness/CNS
  – renal function
	• Monitor hourly initially – increase or reduce according to assessment findings (see above):
	  – pain
	  – vital signs and O$_2$ saturations
	  – level of consciousness
		• Monitor 2–4 hourly – increase or reduce according to assessment findings (see above):
		  – pain
		  – vital signs and O$_2$ saturations
		  – level of consciousness
		  – fluid input and output

continued

- prophylactic penicillin during childhood, adolescence and for some adults
- prompt management of infections
- folic acid supplements
- a home analgesia strategy including anti-inflammatory drugs and opiates

- access to effective medical and nursing care both in the community and in the acute sector.

Treatment strategies to prevent veno-occlusive crises can include a regular programme of prophylactic red cell transfusions with concomitant iron chelating agents to reduce

Box 14.1 *Cont'd*		
On arrival assessment	**Days 1–3 assessment**	**Days 4–10 assessment**
• Hydration: – oral/i.v. – maintain input of 3 litres in 24 hours unless contraindicated • Intravenous antibiotics if infection is suspected • Vascular access, if required • Provide comfort and reassurance: – orientate the person as necessary – offer explanations for interventions – help with positioning/movement as required – provide a restful environment	– nausea and vomiting – fluid input and output • FBC, U&E – if there are signs of anaemia, liver or renal dysfunction • Hydration: – oral/i.v. – maintain input of 3 L in 24 hours unless contraindicated • Start or continue i.v. antibiotics in the presence of fever • Nutrition • Ensure the provision of nutritious and easily digestible foods • Provide comfort and reassurance: – help with hygiene needs – provide items such as fresh sheets – provide a restful environment – discuss care needs	• FBC, U&E – if there are signs of anaemia, liver or renal dysfunction • Hydration: – oral/i.v. – maintain input of 3 L in 24 hours unless contraindicated – consider an oral hydration schedule, if tolerated • Start, continue or change i.v. antibiotics in the presence of fever • Start a rehabilitation/mobilization programme titrated to energy levels and pain levels • Review venous access – consider oral therapy in place of i.v. if client is stable • Formulate a preliminary discharge strategy but only when client is physically and psychologically ready to start dialogue with the clinical team • Provide comfort and reassurance: – help with hygiene needs – provide a restful environment – discuss changing care needs
Notes • Prioritize prompt and effective analgesia and assessment • Ensure adequate pain relief is maintained to minimize physiological stress and further sickling of red cells and deoxygenation • Keep client warm and comfortable • Consider possible complications: – chest crisis – splenic sequestration – cerebral vascular accident or other CNS involvement – sepsis • Monitor client closely	**Notes** • Prioritize regular or continuous effective analgesia and assessment • Consider possible complications: – chest crisis – splenic sequestration – cerebral vascular accident or other CNS involvement – sepsis • At this early stage avoid reducing analgesia unless warranted by the clinical situation, i.e. respirations < 10–12/minute or impaired level of consciousness	**Notes** • Prioritize regular or continuous, effective analgesia and assessment • Consider possible complications: – chest crisis – splenic sequestration – cerebral vascular accident or other CNS involvement – sepsis • Avoid early withdrawal of analgesia • Remain alert for increasing levels of pain that may signal the onset of complications or a new crisis
U&E, urea and electrolytes; FBC, full blood count.		

the iron overload associated with regular transfusions. For selected individuals, hydroxyurea, a cytotoxic agent, can be used to increase the level of fetal haemoglobin in red cells. This treatment does have some potentially significant side-effects, which must be weighed against the benefit of reduced crises. Stem cell transplantation is a potential cure for sickle cell anaemia. However, due to the significant morbidity and mortality and the requirement of an HLA matched donor, this strategy may only be appropriate for selected individuals with severe disease or poor quality of life.

Sickle-cell disease: nursing management issues

Sickle-cell disease presents a challenge for nurses working in both hospital and community settings. The establishment of sickle-cell centres has greatly enhanced knowledge, promoted understanding of the condition and promoted a multidisciplinary and culturally sensitive approach to care. This is important because the disorder affects ethnic and racial groups that may have been disadvantaged in relation to health care. Coordinated services with specialist medical and nursing teams as well as access to general practitioner services and sickle-cell specialist community nurses are important features of good care.

Although most individuals with sickle-cell disease have infrequent hospital admissions, a proportion will have repeated severe painful crises requiring regular admission to hospital. Unfortunately, because of their frequent and regular presentation in A&E departments, many of these patients may become labelled as manipulative and addiction prone, and analgesia is restricted at the very time it is most needed. Morphine is the drug of choice to relieve the pain, such is its severity (Black and Hawkes 2005). The impact of a poor client–carer relationship that arises from a lack of communication, lack of mutual understanding and a clinical situation that offers the potential for conflict is an important issue in the care of patients with sickle-cell anaemia.

Physical care during a crisis is only part of the nurse's role. The ability of the nurse to help individuals and families to adjust their lifestyle and develop strategies for overcoming health difficulties is equally important. Like other chronic illnesses, sickle-cell disease has many psychological and practical implications. Genetic counselling and support should be offered to individuals and couples when considering pregnancy and parenthood, so that they are better able to make informed decisions. This counselling should provide an honest appraisal of risk but be unbiased so that couples can feel free to make personal informed decisions about their future and that of their children (Atkin et al 1998).

Social support is extremely important to the well-being of families; local parent support groups and the Sickle Cell Society are helpful in meeting this need. The financial implications of raising a child with sickle-cell disease also need to be addressed, because maintaining an optimal environment may be very expensive in terms of heating, bills, etc. Teachers also need to be briefed on how the condition may interfere with a child's daily routines and school performance, as it is very easy for a cycle of disadvantage to be set up. Adolescents with sickle-cell disease, like those with any chronic illness, can generate particular challenges for families and carers. Illness can have a negative impact on a young person's increasing need for independence and self-determination, leading to a potential conflict between the need to sustain health promoting behaviour and the need for freedom and experimentation. Concordance with medications can be a particular challenge (While and Mullen 2004). In adult life, individuals may be disadvantaged in terms of employment as a result of their need for a relatively constant environment, and as a consequence of the chronic manifestations of the disease, such as leg ulcers, the need for hip replacement following bone necrosis and visual loss from retinal damage. This complex disease with its many manifestations requires a multidisciplinary approach to care and nurses are ideally placed to coordinate care and resources so that the disabling effects on individuals and their families are minimized.

Nursing management of the person with anaemia

Anaemia is a symptom of an underlying disorder and the care required by an anaemic patient varies with the cause and the severity of the anaemia. Many individuals with anaemia are treated as outpatients, especially if the anaemia is chronic as in pernicious anaemia. Others may need regular supervision, intermittent treatment and may need to substantially modify their way of life, as in the example of sickle cell anaemia. For some people, anaemia may be cured entirely by treatment of the underlying cause, such as a bleeding ulcer. Depending on the underlying cause, there may be other symptoms and problems in addition to those attributable to anaemia. An example would be the problem of jaundice in haemolytic anaemia, or vascular occlusion in sickle-cell disease. Whatever the cause of the anaemia, the patients have one common difficulty: a decreased capacity of the blood to transport oxygen.

Assessment

History It is important to begin by establishing to what degree the patient is incapacitated by the anaemia. This will vary from very mild to extensive disruption of their normal daily activities. Knowledge of the clinical characteristics of anaemia should lead the nurse to be alert to any indication of their presence from the history given by the patient. The patient is also asked about gradual or sudden changes in daily activities, changes experienced with exertion, and any increased need for rest and sleep.

The history should include information about the sequence of events leading up to the present situation, such as recent surgery or trauma or unusual bleeding. Occupational and social circumstances should be determined together with past health history and medication history. It may also be relevant to enquire about any history of anaemia in other family members. For women of reproductive age it is important to enquire about any menstrual problems, such as heavy, prolonged or frequent periods.

It may be relevant to obtain a nutritional history assessing the intake of essential nutrients and focusing especially on the adequacy of iron and vitamin B_{12} intake.

Taking a health history also provides an opportunity to assess the patient's knowledge and understanding of their anaemia, its cause and any prescribed therapeutic measures.

Physical examination This begins with a general observation of the person's appearance and behaviour, noting indications of anaemia such as pallor and signs of fatigue or pain. The skin and mucous membranes, especially the conjunctivae, are examined for pallor and in the case of haemolytic anaemia for initial or increasing jaundice. The tongue is inspected, as vitamin B_{12} deficiency produces a red, smooth, sore tongue. Nails are observed for brittleness and any abnormalities of shape such as spooning or clubbing, which can occur with anaemia. Neurological disorder may also develop, such as sensory disturbance, depression or memory loss. Respiratory and heart rates are recorded and any changes on exertion noted.

The person diagnosed or suspected of having pernicious anaemia may demonstrate signs of degenerative changes in the nervous system. Therefore, any complaint of tingling, numbness and paraesthesia (pins and needles) in the extremities, loss of fine movement, difficulty in holding small objects, limb weakness, ataxia or impaired vision should be noted.

If the person has sickle-cell anaemia, they are regularly observed for swollen, tender and painful areas, changes in body function or their mental and physical abilities that may be indicative of areas of vascular occlusion.

Laboratory test results should be consulted and nursing measures adapted according to abnormalities and changes. For example, a fall in the haemoglobin level, packed cell volume or erythrocyte count may suggest that the patient's activity level should be restricted to reduce oxygen requirements until treatment takes effect.

Patient problems related to anaemia
The reduced capacity of the blood to carry oxygen may give rise to some or all of the following problems:

- inability to sustain the usual level of activity
- potential reduced quality of life as an outcome of fatigue
- potential risk of tissue damage and injury
- pain due to tissue ischaemia or hyperplasia of the bone marrow
- impaired thought processes.

The person may also experience problems such as:

- inability to maintain an adequate dietary intake of nutrients essential for red blood cell production
- lack of knowledge concerning the disease process, treatment and measures to promote health.

Nursing interventions
The goals of intervention for the person with anaemia are that:

1 The person will achieve an acceptable level of activity while maintaining vital signs within the normal range.
2 The person will be able to maintain their normal roles and responsibilities.
3 The person will state that they have a strategy to effectively manage fatigue.
4 The person's skin and mucosal tissues will remain intact and no accidental injury will be experienced.
5 The person will state that he or she is pain free.
6 The person and their family will report improvement in thought processes.
7 The person will be able to select appropriate foodstuffs and maintain an adequate dietary intake, as indicated by improvement in laboratory blood results.
8 The person will be able to describe the cause and characteristics of the anaemia, the treatment plan and discuss plans to modify lifestyle and to minimize the risk of complications.

Activity Individuals are assisted to modify their level of activity in order to decrease the demand for oxygen, and nursing care is planned to achieve this. An explanation of the basis of the fatigue and weakness experienced, and emphasis on the importance of balancing rest and activity, may help the person to understand what is happening and to accept limitations on activity. Activity is encouraged but the importance of resting before becoming fatigued and breathless is explained. Assistance may be required to enable the person to perform essential activities, such as maintaining personal hygiene and dressing, with the minimum of effort.

Severe anaemia may cause shortness of breath or dyspnoea, even at rest, and the person may be less distressed with the head of the bed raised or in a sitting position, and with good ventilation. Oxygen administration may be necessary during the acute period. Prolonged use is inadvisable as increasing the concentration of oxygen in the blood suppresses erythropoiesis (development of new red blood cells). A blood transfusion of packed cells may be administered. Individuals may have questions about the safety of blood transfusions and wish to explore problems associated with this treatment, especially if they are required regularly and on a long-term basis.

In the long term, if the person is active and employed it may be necessary to encourage adjustments to their normal lifestyle. The nurse should help the individual and family to evaluate the usual daily routines and identify activities that are priorities so that a plan may be developed that aims at avoiding sudden strenuous activity and schedules rest periods. The person's activity tolerance is reviewed regularly and, taking the clinical condition into account, activity is increased or decreased accordingly.

Skin and mucosal tissues   The reduced oxygen supply to the tissues increases the risk of pressure sore development, especially if activity is limited. The person with anaemia should be carefully assessed, using a risk assessment scale such as that of Norton or Waterlow, and the appropriate precautionary measures instituted. This may range from 2-hourly changes of position to the use of special pressure-relieving systems (see p. 837). People with haemolytic anaemia who are jaundiced often experience *pruritus* (itching). Warm or tepid water is used for bathing and use of soap is avoided. Calamine lotion may be applied to relieve itching; the fingernails should be kept short and clean to prevent excoriation and infection, should the person scratch the irritated areas. Skin creams and emollients are useful in keeping skin hydrated and supple, and in preventing dry, cracked skin.

In pernicious and iron deficiency anaemias, ulcerative lesions of the oral mucosa and a sore raw tongue may occur. Regular cool, mild mouthwashes may be soothing. A soft toothbrush is advised for cleaning the teeth. Hot spicy foods are best avoided and the mouth should be cleaned regularly.

The person who is very weak and dizzy as a result of anaemia may be at risk from falls. It is important to assess this risk and to manage the person's environment to minimize the possibility of accidental injury. The person who has a sensory loss as a result of anaemia may demonstrate poor coordination and be at risk of injury from dropping objects. They will also be less sensitive to heat and may therefore be susceptible to burns. If the person with anaemia is also susceptible to infection, additional safety precautions may be required. These are discussed later.

Pain   The person with anaemia may experience angina-like pain, headache, pain due to marrow hyperplasia or splenic enlargement or pain due to vascular occlusion and ischaemia as a result of a sickle-cell crisis. Whatever the cause, the pain should be fully assessed, using a pain chart, and analgesia administered as required to achieve effective pain relief.

Thought processes   Confusion and slow cognitive responses may become apparent. The individual should be reassured that mental disturbance and a reduced concentration span are associated with the condition and should improve. This is because treatment, generally aimed at increasing the oxygen-carrying capacity of the blood, will also improve cerebral oxygenation.

Diet   When nutrition has been identified as a problem, the nurse and dietician should discuss with the person and family the importance of diet. Food preferences are identified and help given to plan menus that will provide the necessary nutrients in an acceptable form. Foods should be light,

easily digested and provide protein, iron, vitamins B_{12} and C and folic acid. Dietary sources of iron include red meats, liver, eggs, fish, green leafy vegetables, enriched whole-grain cereals, and bread and dried fruits. The absorption of iron is reduced by the presence of tea, coffee, milk and antacids but is promoted in the presence of vitamin C. Sources of vitamin B_{12} include red meats, liver, eggs and dairy produce. Folic acid is present in meat (especially liver), whole-grain cereals, leafy vegetables, beans, brewer's yeast and dairy products. Citrus fruits particularly, and other fruits and vegetables, are good sources of vitamin C. These vitamins are heat sensitive and therefore destroyed by prolonged cooking.

Anorexia may be an accompanying problem and may be exacerbated if the person has a sore mouth. Small, frequent meals and avoidance of certain foods may help. Oral care is important and food should be presented attractively. Help with eating and social contact at mealtimes should be provided as necessary. Older people at home may require a carer or meals-on-wheels, arranged through their community care manager. Voluntary agencies such as Age Concern and local authorities provide daycare and luncheon clubs, which provide a nutritious meal and social contacts. Dietary intake may be supplemented by prescriptions of iron and vitamins.

Extra fluids are very important for the person with a haemolytic anaemia, especially sickle-cell anaemia. The person who is hospitalized during a sickle-cell crisis should have fluid intake recorded and may require intravenous hydration if unable to maintain a good oral intake (2–3 L per 24 hours for an adult).

Knowledge and lifestyle   A full explanation of the nature of the disorder and reasons for symptoms experienced should be made to the individual and family members. The person is advised of changes that might indicate a recurrence of the disorder and the need to seek medical help.

Information should be provided about the prescribed treatment and plan of care, and the person's understanding evaluated by having him or her carry out procedures such as medication administration and the planning and preparation of food. Explanations should be provided about any prescribed drugs and possible adverse effects. For example, the person prescribed iron should be warned to expect dark stools and possible gastrointestinal irritation. Long-term iron therapy has a tendency to cause constipation and thus the importance of a high-fibre diet should be stressed. The necessity of getting regular maintenance doses of vitamin B_{12} should be stressed to the person with pernicious anaemia, and a district nurse referral made to facilitate this if attendance at the clinic for the injections is not possible.

In the case of sickle-cell anaemia, parents should receive an explanation of the disease and factors that predispose to crises. Children and parents can be advised of the importance of prophylactic care during remission. This involves living as normally as possible but avoiding chilling, contact with people with infections, high altitudes, over-fatigue and stressful situations. A well-balanced diet, plenty of fluids and adequate rest are important. Proper dental care and immunization against infectious diseases are stressed, as well as attendance at clinics for regular physical and haematological assessment.

Individuals with hereditary forms of anaemia may wish to be advised of genetic counselling opportunities for themselves. It is important that they feel able to make informed choices about their chances of having affected children (see Case Study 14.1).

CASE Claudia is a 19-year-old girl whose parents are Ghanaian. She came to a family planning clinic for advice regarding contraception. She and her boyfriend were having regular sex and she wanted a reliable method of contraception in addition to using sheaths to protect herself from sexually transmitted infection.

In taking a history it emerged that Claudia had sickle-cell anaemia and had experienced numerous crises throughout her childhood. She was currently well. She was well informed about her condition, as was her boyfriend, and was very aware of the implications of pregnancy for her health.

Claudia's contraceptive choices were limited by her condition, as an intrauterine device would be unsuitable because of the risk of exacerbating anaemia and increased risk of infection, and the combined oral contraceptive pill was unsuitable because of the potential risk of thromboembolism. This left a progestogen-only form of contraception as her main option. Claudia was willing to try the progestogen-only pill; the possibility of irregular periods did not concern her as these were already irregular. She was in the habit of taking folic acid supplements and prophylactic antibiotics and therefore felt quite confident of her ability to take the pill on time. Following consultation with the doctor, Claudia left the clinic with condoms and a 3 months' supply of Carazette to start on the first day of her next period.

The issues facing Claudia should be reflected upon, including her immediate needs for contraception and her needs for the future relating to potential pregnancy and the need for genetic counselling.

Persons with haemolytic spherocytosis who have had a splenectomy, and those with sickle-cell anaemia or thalassaemia who have impairment of splenic function, require teaching regarding the potential for post-splenectomy sepsis. Pneumococcal vaccine may be administered as a preventive measure.

Evaluation Objective measurement of the effectiveness of nursing intervention for the person with anaemia is provided by ongoing laboratory results which show that the haemoglobin, red blood cell counts, haematocrit, vitamin B_{12} and folate levels are within the normal ranges for the individual. Care has been effective if the patient reports a decrease or absence of the clinical symptoms previously identified.

Evaluation of patient and family teaching is based on assessment of their knowledge of dietary and treatment measures and their verbalization of strategies to control symptoms and resume usual daily activities. Questions regarding the therapeutic plan should be answered and the person should be aware of community resources for ongoing health care.

POLYCYTHAEMIA (ERYTHROCYTE EXCESS)

Polycythaemia refers to an excessive number of erythrocytes and a corresponding increase in haemoglobin concentration. *Secondary polycythaemia* occurs when there is a physiological compensatory increase in the number of erythrocytes by the red bone marrow in response to a low concentration of oxygen in the blood and an increase in erythropoietin. It normally occurs at high altitudes where the atmospheric oxygen tension is low, and in pathological conditions in which there is tissue hypoxia. Examples of the latter are chronic obstructive pulmonary disease and certain congenital malformations of the heart. It can occur in individuals who are heavy smokers, and in people with renal disease when there is inappropriate secretion of erythropoietin. A relative polycythaemia also occurs as a result of excessive plasma loss, for example following extensive burns or excessive vomiting and diarrhoea.

Primary polycythaemia is also known as *polycythaemia rubra vera* (PRV). It is a very rare, malignant, myeloproliferative disorder of the red bone marrow in which there is uncontrolled production of an excessive number of red blood cells. It may be accompanied by some overproduction of granulocytes and platelets. The cause of this malignant disorder is unknown, although it would appear to result from some mutation in a pluripotent stem cell which gives it a proliferative advantage in comparison to normal stem cells. Onset usually occurs between 50 and 70 years of age and its rarity can be gauged by its prevalence of about one case per million population in the USA (Black and Hawkes 2005).

Clinical characteristics

Primary polycythaemia increases the total red cell volume and viscosity of the blood. The blood pressure is raised and the workload of the heart is increased. Heart failure may develop insidiously as a result of increased cardiac demands. The rate of flow through the blood vessels is reduced, which, together with the increased number of erythrocytes and blood viscosity, predisposes to the development of thrombi. Occlusion of arterial or venous vessels may occur, causing a cerebrovascular accident, transient ischaemic attacks, coronary thrombosis, intermittent claudication, deep vein thrombosis, etc. The spleen enlarges in many cases because of the increase in red cell destruction. Bleeding, as a result of qualitatively poor platelets, can also be a potential problem.

Symptoms vary greatly: an individual may not experience any discomfort and be unaware of any problem until the condition is discovered during a routine blood test; others may experience symptoms such as headache, dizziness, blurred vision, or complain of a full feeling in the head. Pruritus (itching), especially after a hot bath, is an unpleasant, although not dangerous, symptom associated with this condition, as is gout due to uric acid derived from the increased breakdown of red blood cells. A person with primary polycythaemia often appears plethoric (with a very ruddy complexion), while the distal parts of limbs, especially the lower limbs, may be cyanotic owing to sluggish circulation. Peptic ulceration occurs in up to 10% of patients and is apparently attributable to an increase in gastric acid secretion.

The person with a secondary polycythaemia is usually cyanosed due to the underlying cardiac or respiratory disease. Diagnosis is based on a number of blood tests including increased haematocrit and red cell mass, and a bone marrow aspiration. Exclusion of respiratory and renal disease is indicative of PRV.

Treatment and care

The aim of treatment is to reduce the risk of thrombosis and alleviate the symptoms. How this is achieved varies and also depends on the duration and severity of the condition and on the age of the patient. A phlebotomy (venesection) is the simplest way of producing a temporary reduction in symptoms.

Initially, up to 500 ml blood may be removed once or twice a week until the packed cell volume (PCV) is down to about 45%. Red cell and platelet apheresis is a rapid way of achieving this (Box 14.2). Repeating this at regular intervals may be the only treatment needed, although iron and folate supplements may be prescribed to prevent deficiencies occurring. In patients with PRV, if phlebotomy is required very frequently, or the platelet count is too high, the risk of thrombosis is high and treatment with a myelosuppressive drug such as hydroxyurea may be used to suppress erythropoiesis. Radioactive phosphorus (^{32}P) is of value in treating older patients with severe disease. These agents are avoided in younger persons if possible, because of concerns about their carcinogenic potential. The value of other treatment strategies such as recombinant interferon-α therapy is still under evaluation.

Unless a complication such as thrombosis, peptic ulcer or cardiac insufficiency occurs, a person with polycythaemia is not usually treated as an inpatient. Pain should be alleviated and a reasonable amount of activity encouraged with the aim of preventing circulatory stasis. When pruritus is a significant problem, medication with antihistamines may be helpful in alleviating the itching. Close supervision by the haematology team and the patient's general practitioner is important, and the patient and family are alerted to early indications of potential complications such as thrombosis and advised of the importance of prompt action. Frequently PRV can be managed for long periods with relatively little disturbance to the individual's daily life. In the long term

---

Box 14.2 Apheresis

The term apheresis is derived from a Greek word meaning to take away or withdraw, and describes the process of removing one circulating blood component, usually through the use of automated blood cell separators, while returning the other components to a donor or patient. This procedure can be used for therapeutic purposes or as a method of collecting blood components for transfusion. Either cells (cytapheresis) or plasma solutes (apheresis) may be withdrawn.

The process involves the use of a closed system whereby an amount of blood is drawn from the person and mixed with anticoagulant to prevent clotting. It is then processed through a centrifuge or filter to remove the desired component. The remaining components are recombined and returned to the patient or donor. If required, the component being removed can also be replaced.

For example:

- In polycythaemia, red cells and platelets can be removed from a symptomatic patient

- In sickle-cell disease, a large volume of abnormal red cells can be removed and these are then replaced through a simultaneous blood transfusion in order to maintain the patient's red cell count within normal limits (this is called red cell exchange)

- In myeloma, plasma containing large amounts of abnormal paraproteins can be removed to reduce the symptoms of hyperviscosity, and normal plasma can then be transfused

- In acute leukaemia, large numbers of white cells can be removed from the circulation to relieve the symptoms of a high white cell count or to reduce the tumour load prior to chemotherapy

- In stem cell transplantation, stem cells can be collected from the donor using cytapheresis

- In transfusion practice, platelets can be collected from volunteer donors at specific blood donor sessions.

Therapeutic apheresis can be used for a range of indications other than those cited above; these have simply been selected as examples.

(10–15 years), about 20% of patients go on to develop acute leukaemia or myelofibrosis.

LEUCOCYTE DISORDERS

Alterations in the number of leucocytes may involve increased or decreased production of cells as a result of a variety of benign and malignant processes.

LEUCOCYTOSIS

The number of leucocytes in the circulation increases to a level in excess of the normal ($4.0–11 \times 10^9$/L) in a variety of situations. These include infection, inflammatory diseases, pregnancy, after trauma or surgery, in malignancy, after acute haemorrhage or as a side-effect of drugs. This increase is referred to as a leucocytosis and is usually predominant in one type of white cell.

LEUCOPENIA

Leucopenia may be defined as a reduction in the number of leucocytes below the normal lower limit of 4×10^9/L. This may be due to a decreased production or an increased destruction of white cells. The deficiency is most commonly seen in the granulocyte cell line, particularly the neutrophils. Lymphopenia, a deficiency of lymphocytes is relatively uncommon but may be a consequence of corticosteroid therapy, trauma or surgery, Hodgkin lymphoma, systemic lupus erythematosus (SLE) and acquired immune deficiency syndrome (Arif and Mufti 1998).

NEUTROPENIA

The primary function of neutrophils is one essential part of the body's defence against infection. This requires the ability to migrate to the site of infection or injury and to destroy bacteria. A normal neutrophil count is generally between 2.5 and 7.5×10^9/L, although a lower threshold of 1.5×10^9/L is normal for some groups. Neutropenia may be defined as a peripheral count below 1.5×10^9/L. However, serious infections are not generally seen until the neutrophil count is less than 0.5×10^9/L (Howard and Hamilton 1997).

Neutropenia may be the result of a reduced production of neutrophils, as in bone marrow failure, increased destruction, as in immune neutropenia, or pooling into the spleen. *Benign idiopathic neutropenia* is a familial disorder that is not associated with an increased risk of infection. The production of neutrophils is normal but there is an increased proportion of neutrophils out of the circulation, with a resulting lower number in the peripheral blood. *Cyclical neutropenia* is a genetic disorder where the neutrophil count falls every 14–21 days and is associated with an increased risk of infection. Certain chemicals, drugs and infections may produce an *immune neutropenia* through a direct toxic effect on the bone marrow or through an immune process. Bone marrow infiltration with carcinoma, cytotoxic chemotherapy, irradiation, hypersplenism and some autoimmune disorders can also cause neutropenia, sometimes with an associated pancytopenia.

Management and care

The cause of neutropenia should be identified and, if possible, eliminated. Infections should be treated promptly with broad-spectrum antibiotics, as septicaemia is a serious and potentially fatal complication of neutropenia. Prophylactic antibiotics may have a role to play in some patients, as does the use of haemopoietic growth factors. In a small group of patients with immune neutropenia, splenectomy may be considered (Roberts et al 1999). Nursing care of the patient with neutropenia includes a careful assessment of the current infection status and the risk of infection (including the client's environment, personal hygiene and dietary infection risk) and client education and support in the management of risk, and in identifying the early warning signs of infection or sepsis. A more detailed discussion of these issues can be found in the section on management of patients with white cell disorders.

LEUKAEMIA

Leukaemia is a heterogeneous group of malignant disorders characterized by the uncontrolled proliferation of immature haematopoietic cells. It is thought that these malignancies arise from a single, mutated, early progenitor or stem cell. The malignant cells are characterized by uncontrolled cell growth, arrested development and resistance to normal cell death, and they also lack the expected mature cell functions. The cells rapidly overwhelm the bone marrow, preventing the production of normal red cells, white cells and platelets; they eventually spill over into the peripheral blood and may invade other organs such as the spleen.

Classification

Classification is important because it has a bearing on disease course, treatment choice and outcomes. The classification of leukaemia is, in the first instance, according to the general course of the disease, termed either acute or chronic. In general, acute leukaemias involve the more immature cells (blasts) whereas chronic leukaemias tend to involve more mature cells. The next classification is according to the originating cell line, either myeloid or lymphoid.

These broad categories can then be further subdivided into subtypes based on other morphological, cytogenetic or molecular characteristics such as surface markers. So, for example, AML M3 refers to (A) acute (M) myeloid (L) leukaemia and M3 describes the cell as having stopped at the promyelocytic stage of development. CML Ph+ refers to (C) chronic (M) myeloid (L) leukaemia that is positive for the Philadelphia chromosome, denoting a particular genetic translocation. An important classification involves the type of chromosomal damage seen in the malignancy. This has implications for the treatment strategies selected and outcomes as some abnormalities have a more favourable prognosis and demonstrate a better response to treatment. In acute myeloid leukaemia, the inversion of chromosome 16 has a favourable prognosis, whereas the deletion of chromosome 5 or 7 has a less favourable prognosis (Hoffbrand et al 2001). This may need to be taken into account when making decisions about treatment options.

Incidence and aetiology

Leukaemia is one of the less common types of cancer. Although leukaemia occurs in all age groups, it has a higher incidence in the older age groups and, overall, there is a higher incidence in males. There are also geographical variations in the incidence of particular types of leukaemia; for example, chronic lymphocytic leukaemia is common in countries such as the USA, Canada and the UK but much less so in Japan, India or South America (Cartwright 1998).

Certain predisposing factors have been linked to the leukaemias. Particular genetic predispositions, such as in Down's syndrome, Fanconi anaemia, Bloom's syndrome and ataxia telangiectasia, are associated with leukaemia. There are also slightly higher rates of leukaemia in certain families, which also points to the possibility of a genetic predisposition. Pre-existing bone marrow dysfunction, such as in aplastic anaemia or myelodysplasia, is also associated with a higher incidence of leukaemia.

Environmental factors associated with leukaemia include ionizing radiation, chemicals such as benzene, exposure to agrochemicals and previous treatment with particular cytotoxic agents (Cartwright 1998). Occupational exposure to benzene and agrochemicals has been associated with leukaemia. Although there are reports of other possible occupational links with haematological malignancy, these are always difficult to demonstrate clearly owing to the inherent difficulties of epidemiological studies. The relationship between ionizing radiation and leukaemia was initially demonstrated by the high incidence of leukaemia in survivors of the Japanese atomic bombs and, subsequently, in follow-up studies with workers on atomic test sites. Long-term low-dose exposure, such as in the early days of the development of X-ray technology, also demonstrates an increased rate of haematological malignancies, including leukaemia. Treatment with cytotoxic chemotherapy, particularly alkylating agents, can lead to the subsequent development of leukaemia, termed secondary leukaemia. There is also a reported increase in the risk of secondary leukaemia in solid organ transplant recipients as well as bone marrow transplant recipients, particularly in those who received total body irradiation.

Despite a continued search for possible infective agents, only one to date has been strongly associated with the development of leukaemia. The human T-lymphocytic virus (HTLV-I) has been demonstrated to induce a T-cell leukaemia in susceptible individuals. This virus, although uncommon in Europe, is a common infective agent in the Caribbean, where its relationship with leukaemia has been demonstrated. Although there is some indirect evidence that infection may be one possible factor in childhood leukaemia, no clear evidence has yet come to light.

In the majority of *de novo* cases of leukaemia, however, the answer to the question of 'Why me?' must remain unanswered. The development of a malignancy is a complex, multistep process involving factors in the person, in the environment and at a cellular level. For the individual facing an unwelcome diagnosis, this may seem a rather unsatisfactory response to an important question. One of the roles of the healthcare worker is to help the client look forward and to adjust to their situation, while also trying to make sense of what has happened.

Acute leukaemia

Acute leukaemia may be either myeloid or lymphoblastic. Acute myeloid leukaemia (AML) is most commonly seen in adults, whereas acute lymphoblastic leukaemia (ALL) is predominantly, although not exclusively, a disease of childhood. Presenting features vary from general non-specific symptoms at diagnosis to the disease manifesting itself as an acute illness. The presenting problems are, in the main, associated with ineffective bone marrow function. With the expanding pool of leukaemic cells in the bone marrow, the production of normal red cells, white cells and platelets decreases rapidly, resulting in signs and symptoms of anaemia, neutropenia and thrombocytopenia. The person often complains of feeling more tired than usual and may be short of breath on exertion or at rest. They may have persistent or repeated infections, such as a sore throat or chest infection. The patient may also present with an overt septicaemia and be acutely ill. Often there is evidence of increased bruising or the client may describe a history of nosebleeds or abnormal gum bleeding. Women may complain of heavy menstrual loss. The more acute presentations of thrombocytopenia include retinal haemorrhage resulting in loss of vision, gastrointestinal bleeding or cerebral haemorrhage. Symptoms associated with a high peripheral white cell count include blurred vision, speech changes, memory changes and a fluctuating level of consciousness.

Diagnosis is made from examination of a bone marrow aspirate and trephine. Cytochemistry, immunophenotyping and cytogenetic tests permit identification of the leukaemia type, help to identify some important prognostic factors and aid in deciding the optimal treatment strategies. Other tests include: baseline blood counts to determine the degree of anaemia and thrombocytopenia, a clotting screen to detect abnormal clotting, biochemical investigations to assess renal, cardiac and liver function, microbiological cultures, chest radiography and physical assessment. A lumbar puncture to assess any central nervous system (CNS) involvement will be performed if ALL is suspected because CNS involvement is a feature of this condition. Other tests will be requested according to clinical need.

Priority of care at the time of presentation includes supportive treatment in the form of appropriate blood product administration, antibiotic treatment if required, and appropriate venous access, often through the insertion of a central venous catheter. Prevention of infection and haemorrhage are two important goals of care. Any clotting abnormalities require prompt treatment. If the white cell count is raised and the patient is symptomatic leukapheresis, a procedure involving the selective removal of the white cells from the client's circulation, may be considered.

Rapid confirmation of diagnosis is imperative to allow for the prompt institution of treatment. As fertility is an important issue in the care of patients with acute leukaemia, it may be possible to consider sperm banking before starting chemotherapy. For women, collecting eggs is not currently possible at diagnosis because of the time factor and technical difficulties. Even for men, the option of sperm banking depends on their clinical status at the time of diagnosis and on the services available. However, every effort should be made to address this important need, if possible.

The initial aim of treatment for acute leukaemia is to induce a rapid remission of the disease. This requires the use of an intensive schedule of combination cytotoxic agents appropriate to the type of leukaemia. These combinations are different for AML and ALL. Other factors, such as the patient's age and some specific prognostic factors, may alter the regimen chosen. The aim of combination chemotherapy is to increase cell death by combining drugs with different modes of action or ones that work synergistically. Box 14.3 lists common cytotoxic drugs used in the treatment of acute myeloid leukaemia and examples of combination chemotherapy for AML. In addition to cytotoxic and cytokine therapy, new agents, targeting cell surface markers for example, are being assessed for potential efficacy.

As the aim of treatment is to attack the abnormal blood cells developing in the bone marrow, the doses of cytotoxic chemotherapy used will induce profound bone marrow failure with neutropenia. The patient will therefore be at high risk of developing life-threatening infections and septicaemia. Careful monitoring of the patient's condition is fundamental to effective clinical care. A prompt response to any sign of infection is important. Any pyrexia should be immediately investigated and the appropriate blood cultures and microbiological specimens sent. Patients will be started immediately on broad-spectrum intravenous antibiotics. Most units have specific protocols that provide clinical guidance on antibiotic use in neutropenic patients. As the risk of infection-related morbidity and mortality is high in this population of patients, the prompt use of appropriate antibiotic therapy is a cornerstone of good practice. Good assessment skills are also vital as the inflammatory processes, such as swelling, redness, heat and pain, that normally help to signpost infection are often greatly diminished or absent. Getting to know the person, their usual routine and being able to recognize when they are feeling 'off-colour' is also useful in helping to identify the early signs of infection or some other problem.

Infection control measures such as effective handwashing by all members of the clinical team, a clean and dust free environment, the systematic use of aseptic technique when

Box 14.3 Some cytotoxic drugs commonly used in the treatment of acute myeloid leukaemia				
Antimetabolites	**Alkylating agents**	**Anthracycline antibiotics/DNA binding agents**	**Mitotic inhibitors**	**Miscellaneous**
Cytosine arabinoside (Ara-C, cytarabine)	Cyclophosphamide	Daunorubicin Doxorubicin Idarubicin Mitoxantrone	Vincristine Etoposide	Amsacrine
Sample induction chemotherapy for AML:				
ADE Cytarabine (Ara-C) Daunorubicin Etoposide (VP16)	FLAG-Ida Fludarabine Cytarabine (Ara-C) GCSF (growth factor) Idarubicin	DA Daunorubicin Cytarabine (Ara-C)		
Sample consolidation chemotherapy for AML:				
MACE Amsacrine (Amsa) Cytarabine (Ara-C) Etoposide (VP16)	MiDAC Mitoxantrone Cytarabine (Ara-C)	Ara-C High-dose Cytarabine as a single agent		
Source: Medical Research Council Working Parties on Leukaemia in Adults and Children (2002)				

managing the central venous catheter and during any invasive procedure, and ensuring the patient's personal hygiene are important elements in a strategy to minimize the infection risk for the patient. The provision of a low microbial diet and the use of prophylactic antibiotics and antifungal agents may also be used to protect neutropenic patients from infection. Finally, minimizing the microbial load of the patient's immediate environment through the use of single rooms, controlled air-delivery systems and limiting visitors may also be used as part of the infection control strategy.

Blood product support at this time will be required to manage the anaemia and thrombocytopenia that follows intensive chemotherapy. The safe management of transfusions is an important element in the care of haematology patients. The patient's haemoglobin level will be maintained with the use of packed red cells. Often patients require a blood transfusion every 3–5 days. The need for more frequent transfusions should alert the team to the possibility of internal bleeding. Platelet transfusions will be required every 2–3 days, sometimes more frequently if there is evidence of bleeding or infection. Any signs of bleeding such as bruising and petechiae, gum bleeding, epistaxis, or gastrointestinal bleeding will need to be promptly reported. Spontaneous and potentially life-threatening bleeding including haematemesis, haemoptysis and cerebral haemorrhage can occur, particularly in the context of very low platelet counts ($<10 \times 10^9$/L). Daily platelet counts and vigilance are therefore imperative.

Nutritional and fluid support may also be required at this time. Mucositis and its associated pain, oral candida infection, nausea and vomiting, and anorexia may all prevent the patient from eating and drinking sufficiently. Nutritional deficiencies, weight loss and muscle loss are all frequent consequences of this rigorous treatment. Ensuring a fluid and nutritional intake that maintains renal function and meets the body's increased metabolic requirements may require intravenous hydration and total parenteral nutrition at this time (see Ch. 17). A nutritious diet with supplements is important for those who are still able to eat and drink. A multidisciplinary approach to nutrition, including the expert support of a dietitian and regular nutritional assessments, will prove valuable in preventing excessive weight loss and nutritional deficiencies.

Minimizing the inevitable consequences of the higher doses of cytotoxic chemotherapy used in the treatment of leukaemia invariably proves a challenge for the clinical team. Nausea and vomiting, diarrhoea, mucositis, pain, anorexia and pyrexia will all require prompt assessment and treatment. Renal failure as well as cardiac and liver problems may complicate the clinical picture. The patient will need intensive support for up to 21–28 days. Once bone marrow function is restored, the risk of infection and bleeding decreases markedly and the patient generally feels better. Problems with other organs, such as the kidneys, may persist in particular individuals. Loss of appetite and weight loss may also become long-standing problems for some patients.

Remission induction chemotherapy usually comprises one or two cycles of treatment. Remission is defined as a specific reduction in the number of leukaemic cells or the absence of detectable disease, rather than the complete absence of disease. For this reason, consolidation and intensification chemotherapy are given as a prolonged attack on the leukaemia cells that are known to be present, even though they may be undetectable. In the case of ALL, CNS therapy will be added to treatment, as in this disease the CNS provides a particular sanctuary site for malignant cells. Consolidation chemotherapy involves giving repeated courses of the same drugs at similar doses as were given to induce remission, whereas intensification involves giving higher doses or different drug combinations. The specific drugs used for consolidation or intensification cycles may vary to some extent, but the treatment-related problems remain the same.

After the appropriate cycles of consolidation-intensification chemotherapy, patients with ALL will start a maintenance programme of chemotherapy. Maintenance chemotherapy usually involves lower doses of drugs and is given on an outpatient basis. At this point, also, particular subgroups of patients will be considered for other treatment strategies such as allogeneic bone marrow transplantation or autologous stem cell transplantation.

It is important to remember that with each cycle of treatment, the patient may have accumulating problems such as weight loss and anorexia. The body's ability to heal itself will be seriously tested. The patient's own personal and psychological resources will also have been greatly challenged. Loss of weight and hair loss may engender issues of altered body image. The treatment-induced fatigue and loss of physical strength may be difficult for patients, particularly for those who had previously led active lives. The possible loss of fertility may need to be addressed sensitively. Extended periods of hospitalization may often lead to a feeling of loss and isolation from family life, friends and work. There may be concerns over financial matters or loss of income, affecting both the patient and their family. Changes in family members' roles may require personal adjustment. Fear and anxiety is a natural response to the threat of a serious illness and treatment; effective personal coping strategies and an effective support system will be helpful for the client at this time.

A therapeutic relationship between the clinical team and the patient and their family is a key aspect of care. Clients need to feel free to raise their concerns and personal worries; therefore, the development of trust and confidence between staff and client is vital. This element of trust needs to be in relation to the quality of clinical care offered and the personal and team approach to the client. The individual's response to illness, its meaning for them and the worries they may have all need to be acknowledged, respected and explored in a sustained effort by the clinical team to support the person at this critical time in their lives (see Case Study 14.2).

CASE Helen, a 26-year-old woman, attended her GP's surgery complaining of a persistently sore throat and a productive cough following a viral infection. On examination, Helen appeared rather pale and slightly short of breath. A blood sample was sent to ascertain Helen's full blood count. That same day, the GP rang Helen at home, requesting that she and her husband come to the evening surgery for the results. The doctor confirmed that Helen was anaemic, with a haemoglobin level of 9.1 g/dl, but also mentioned a low platelet count (25×10^9/L) and high white cell count (30×10^9/L) that were suggestive of leukaemia.

Helen was referred to her local hospital for immediate admission. That evening, Helen had a bone marrow aspiration and trephine performed to confirm the preliminary diagnosis, and a central venous catheter inserted. She was started on intravenous antibiotics to treat the chest infection and was given a 2-unit blood transfusion. The diagnosis of acute myeloid leukaemia was confirmed by the haematologist later that evening. Helen was told that treatment would have to start as soon as possible, probably the next day.

Initial treatment included a combination regimen of cytarabine, doxorubicin and etoposide that lasted for 8 days. Helen was placed in a single room and remained in protective isolation until her white cell count returned to 0.5×10^9/L – in Helen's case, this took 24 days. Her main problems during this induction cycle of chemotherapy were mucositis, which prevented her from eating and resulting weight loss (3 kg in total). She did have one episode of fever and remained on intravenous antibiotics throughout most of this initial admission. Once her bone marrow function had returned, Helen was allowed home for a few days. After 1 week at home, Helen returned for a second course of chemotherapy, identical to the first. Again, mucositis and weight loss were two important problems and again she required intravenous antibiotics.

Following recovery of her bone marrow function, Helen had a bone marrow biopsy to determine her remission status. After another week at home Helen returned to the good news that she was in complete remission. The third course of chemotherapy included mitoxantrone, cytarabine and etoposide. This resulted in a prolonged stay in hospital for Helen as the return of her bone marrow function was delayed following this cycle of chemotherapy. By this time, Helen was becoming rather withdrawn and had lost a considerable amount of weight, so it was agreed that a longer stay at home with the aim of putting on weight and spending time with her family and friends would be beneficial.

Some 2 weeks later, Helen returned feeling generally better in herself and ready to face her final course of chemotherapy. At this point, the possibility of a bone marrow transplant was addressed with Helen and her husband, as Helen had a sister who was an identical match. After careful consideration of the risks and benefits, Helen opted not to have a stem cell transplant as she did not want to face permanent infertility at this time in her life. She described her sister's bone marrow as her insurance policy for the future in case of relapse. Her final course of chemotherapy went reasonably well, and Helen went home after 27 days in hospital. Helen is still in remission after 18 months and attends the outpatient clinic regularly for check-ups.

The issues facing Helen and her partner both at diagnosis and later as the treatment progressed should be considered. Reflect upon the issues raised for the future and what implications this illness might have upon their relationship and their plans.

Chronic leukaemias
Chronic myeloid leukaemia

This is a haematological malignancy characterized by the overproduction of neutrophils and their precursors. It is thought to arise from a genetic change in a pluripotent stem cell. The vast majority of persons with chronic myeloid leukaemia (CML) have a specific translocation of genetic material between chromosome 9 and 22, termed the Philadelphia (Ph) chromosome. This translocation results in the production of an altered protein (fusion protein) with abnormal functions. This protein has enhanced activity of tyrosine kinase, an enzyme that helps to send proliferation signals through the cell. The abnormal protein sends excessive cell growth and division signals leading to a clonal proliferation of the abnormal cell. The possible causes of CML are unknown, although there is an association with ionizing radiation (Cartwright 1998). The median age for its development is 40 years, and men and women are affected equally.

The disease appears to have two or three distinct phases; most patients present in the first phase, a relatively stable and chronic phase. After a period of months or, often, years, the disease frequently progresses to an accelerated phase, where the signs and symptoms of increasing bone marrow failure are in evidence. The final phase is one of transformation to acute leukaemia.

Presenting symptoms vary and the disease is sometimes found on routine blood testing. The patient may complain of left hypochondrial pain and may give a history of weight loss and night sweats. The spleen is often enlarged and there may be associated anaemia, with its accompanying fatigue, exercise intolerance and shortness of breath. The patient may occasionally have signs of hyperviscosity from the high white cell count and the often accompanying raised platelet count. These include disturbed vision, headaches and, rarely, priapism. High uric acid levels may predispose the occasional individual to gout. The presenting clinical picture is often related to the stage at which the disease is discovered. A relatively normal spleen and no anaemia probably indicate early disease. As the disease advances, an increasing proportion of blast (early precursors) cells can be seen in the bone marrow and peripheral blood. There are often increased signs of bone marrow failure leading to anaemia and a deterioration in general health. The final stage of the disease usually presents as acute leukaemia. The prognosis at this stage is often poor.

The choice of treatment for CML depends on a number of factors including the age of the patient at diagnosis and the availability of a suitable human lymphocyte antigen (HLA)-matched donor for allogeneic transplant. Although volunteer unrelated donors may be considered, sibling donors are preferred as the outcome is much more favourable with a sibling transplant. Although transplantation is the treatment of choice in CML, only a minority of patients will have this as an option.

Alternative treatment choices include cytotoxic chemotherapy (hydroxyurea or busulphan) and α-interferon. These may be given singly or in combination and can extend the chronic phase of the disease by months or years. A new therapy that has been developed as a result of the advances in molecular science is imatinib (Gleevec). This is a tyrosine kinase inhibitor and therefore limits the activity of the fusion protein that drives clonal proliferation. All of these treatments have potentially severe side-effects; interferon-α and imatinib in particular may not be tolerated by all patients. It is only after careful consideration of all of the patient-related factors that the most suitable treatment regimen can be selected. Patients in blast crisis can be treated with the combination cytotoxic regimens available for the treatment of acute leukaemia with the aim of inducing an often short-lived remission.

Chronic lymphocytic leukaemia is a B-cell malignancy and is considered a disease of the elderly; it is rare before the age of 50 years. It is also the most common type of leukaemia in Europe and North America. Its cause is unknown. Many cases are discovered following routine blood tests. Symptoms, if present, may include those related to anaemia, weight loss and night sweats. An enlarged spleen is common and the patient may complain of a feeling of fullness after a light meal. Some 10–20% of patients develop an immune haemolytic anaemia (Hamblin and Oscier 1998). There may be urinary symptoms from kidney or prostatic involvement. Enlarged lymph nodes are present and are useful for disease staging. The presence of an enlarged spleen, liver and anaemia are other staging markers (Mehta and Hoffbrand 2000). The disease may remain stable for a period of years or may progress to more aggressive disease. A major cause of death in patients with CLL is infection (Hamblin and Oscier 1998).

Treatment is not necessary for a proportion of patients. For those whose disease or symptoms require treatment, chlorambucil, an alkylating agent, is commonly used. Corticosteroids, usually prednisolone, may be given alongside chlorambucil or if there is an associated haemolytic anaemia. Fludarabine, a nucleoside analogue, is another effective cytotoxic agent in CLL. Combination chemotherapy is another possible approach for patients with progressive disease. More recently, monoclonal antibodies such as Campath-1H (anti CD52) and rituximab (anti CD20) have been used with some success (Greer et al 2004). Monoclonal antibodies target specific antigens on a cell's surface and then enlist the body's own immune response to

effect cytotoxicity or programmed cell death (apoptosis). Splenic irradiation, splenectomy or stem cell transplantation can also be useful in selected individuals (Greer et al 2004). As this can be a slowly progressive disease, maintaining a good quality of life is an important objective in patients with CLL. Supportive measures, such as the prompt treatment of infection, minimizing possible treatment-related side-effects, and supporting the person to lead a normal life are therefore important care elements.

Myelodysplastic syndrome

Myelodysplastic syndrome (MDS) is a disease of the older adult and is characterized by abnormalities of the various myeloid cells with ineffective haematopoiesis. This results in cytopenias in the context of an active bone marrow. The abnormalities are both quantitative and qualitative, so there are both reduced numbers of cells and the cells do not function optimally. The cells also undergo apoptosis (programmed cell death) more readily than expected. It is a disease of the haematopoietic progenitor cell, leading to a clonal expansion of the abnormal stem cell population and abnormalities in multiple cell lines. Chromosomal abnormalities are often present. It can be a primary condition or develop as a consequence of treatment with chemotherapy or radiotherapy. Myelodysplasia can also evolve into acute leukaemia.

MDS is an often slowly progressive disease and is sometimes diagnosed by chance following a blood test for an unrelated problem. The symptoms of MDS are related to the lack of functioning blood cells and are those of anaemia, thrombocytopenia and neutropenia. Shortness of breath on exertion, fatigue, unexplained bleeding, easy bruising and repeated infections are common symptoms.

Treatment selection depends on a number of factors such as the person's age and the severity of the symptoms. An important factor is the number of blasts (abnormal immature white cells) in the bone marrow. For some individuals, supportive measures such as transfusions and antibiotics may be the only interventions. Individuals may be transfusion dependent for long periods of time and may therefore also require iron chelating therapy to avoid excessive iron overload. Cytokines such as erythropoietin or growth factors may be used to reduce or manage symptoms. Immunosuppression may be useful for selected individuals with bone marrow failure. Low dose or intensive cytotoxic chemotherapy or stem cell transplantation can be used for younger patients and for those with higher blast counts. Newer therapies, such as differentiating agents, monoclonal antibodies and signal inhibitors, are being investigated for their usefulness in MDS (Erba 2003).

Aplastic anaemia

Partial or complete failure of bone marrow activity is an anticipated result of the toxic action of certain drugs or chemicals such as cytotoxics, excessive exposure to radiation, or invasion of the bone marrow by malignant cells. However, in susceptible individuals, an idiosyncratic response to particular pharmacological agents (e.g. chloramphenicol, gold salts), industrial chemicals (e.g. benzene) or certain viral infections (e.g. viral hepatitis) are thought to be capable of inducing bone marrow failure. Others may have an inherited predisposition such as in Fanconi anaemia, where a progressive deterioration of bone marrow function may be observed in affected individuals. However, the majority cases of bone marrow failure are idiopathic and the cause remains unknown.

Aplastic anaemia is an uncommon disease, affecting all age groups with an approximately equal male to female ratio. There is a greater incidence of aplastic anaemia in the Far East; this has led to suggestions of possible environmental factors in some cases. It is generally thought to be a consequence of multiple underlying factors including a reduced or damaged stem cell population, a damaged marrow microenvironment, and a complex and poorly understood immune process, resulting in either a sudden or insidious reduction in bone marrow production and eventual pancytopenia.

Presenting clinical features will be commensurate with the degree of marrow failure present. Many patients will manifest signs and symptoms of anaemia, neutropenia and thrombocytopenia. Infection, including life-threatening bacterial infections, bleeding and general weakness and lethargy with minimal exercise tolerance are common presenting features. Diagnosis is one of exclusion and is made from examination of the patient's bone marrow, peripheral blood count and a careful history. It is important to rule out other possible causes of bone marrow failure, such as malignancy or an inherited disorder, as this would have a great bearing on the appropriate choice of treatment. Initial treatment includes supportive care in the form of red cell and platelet transfusions and prophylactic or therapeutic antibiotics until the diagnosis is confirmed. Subsequent choice of treatment will be dependent on the severity of the bone marrow failure, any predisposing factors such as drug-induced aplasia, and the presence of a matched sibling donor for possible transplantation. Other factors involved in the decision-making process include the age of the patient, their general state of health and any concomitant health problems.

The current treatment of choice for patients under 55 years with severe bone marrow failure is allogeneic stem cell transplantation with a suitable matched donor (Marsh et al 2003). Currently this is the only potentially curative treatment for aplastic anaemia. Immunosuppression with anti-lymphocyte globulin (ALG) or antithymocyte globulin (ATG) is an alternative treatment, offering overall success rates of about 50–70% (Mehta and Hoffbrand 2000). With immunosuppressive therapy, treatment success is often defined as transfusion independence rather than a return to a normally functioning bone marrow. Treatment with ALG or ATG may be supplemented by the administration of cytokines or cyclosporin. For some patients with non-severe aplastic anaemia, immunosuppression with cyclosporin alone or support with transfusions may also be options. Patients treated with immunosuppression may well relapse after months or years, and can subsequently be offered further immunosuppressive treatment. For those individuals where treatment fails, supportive care in the form of transfusions and measures to prevent infection can be offered.

Skilled nursing care in the management of the side-effects and complications of the disease and treatments is vital to the success of therapy. A therapeutic environment where supportive care, information giving and education facilitate the development of effective coping skills for living with a chronic and life-threatening illness is also paramount. A more detailed discussion of some of the nursing care issues can be found later in this chapter.

STEM CELL TRANSPLANTATION

Stem cell transplantation (SCT) has become an increasingly useful treatment for a range of haematological conditions. The main purpose of SCT is to eradicate the patient's own faulty stem cell population and replace it with healthy haemopoietic stem cells. These healthy stem cells can be from another person (*allogeneic transplant*) or they can be the patient's own cells, which have been previously collected and stored (*autologous transplant*). SCT can also be used to replace or manipulate an abnormal immune system, as in autoimmune disease or immunodeficiency syndromes, for example.

Autologous transplant

The term transplant in the context of autologous transplantation is commonly used but is a little misleading, as the cells returned to patients are their own. Another term for this is stem cell rescue, which reflects an important aspect of autologous SCT: one main objective of autologous SCT is to re-populate the patient's marrow after high-dose chemotherapy and/or radiotherapy. The bone marrow is very sensitive to the effects of cytotoxic chemotherapy and radiotherapy, and this has been an important dose-limiting factor in their therapeutic use. By collecting and storing the patient's stem cells before treatment with chemotherapy and/or radiotherapy, these therapies can now be given at a much higher dose. The stem cells are then returned to the patient and these re-populate the bone marrow, effectively rescuing the patient from treatment-related bone marrow failure. This technique is commonly used in the treatment of haematological malignancies when a donor is not available, or in older patients where allogeneic transplant would pose too great a risk. It is now also being used as part of the treatment strategy for some solid cancers, such as high-risk breast cancer. It may also have a place in the treatment of autoimmune diseases; all these strategies are currently being evaluated for their effectiveness.

Allogeneic transplant

Allogeneic transplantation requires a donor whose own genetic make-up closely resembles that of the patient. This type of 'matching' relates to the human lymphocyte antigen (HLA) complex that allows the immune system to recognize self and non-self. It is important that the donor and recipient's HLA complex closely match so that the donor stem cells are accepted and then tolerated by the recipient's immune system. Successful matching most often involves siblings as they have the best chance of inheriting similar antigen combinations from their parents. A volunteer unrelated donor transplant from either national or international donor registries is possible, but the chances of finding a match is often small and the immune problems associated with this type of donor transplant make it a less favourable option. A third type of allogeneic transplant is from an identical twin and is referred to as a syngeneic transplant.

The transplant process

Stem cells can either be collected directly from the bone marrow using a general anaesthetic, or can be obtained from peripheral blood (PBSCs). For a bone marrow harvest, no specific preparation is required, whereas PBSCs have to be coaxed out of the bone marrow with the use of growth factors, chemotherapy or both; this is termed mobilisation. The cells are then harvested using a number of apheresis procedures. There are benefits and limitations with each method of collection so that the choice of method depends, in part, on the clinical circumstances. Broadly speaking, PBSC is now a very common collection method for both autologous and allogeneic transplantation, however a bone marrow harvest is still a method used for some allogeneic donors or if insufficient numbers of cells are collected using peripheral stem cell mobilisation and harvest procedures. One important benefit of the PBSC method is that the recipient's bone marrow function is restored more quickly compared with a transplant procedure using a bone marrow harvest. However, the use of growth factors in healthy donors prior to a PBSC collection may pose as yet unknown risks to the donor (Gluckman 1998), whereas the risks of anaesthesia are now well established.

SCT involves three distinct stages. The first stage is referred to as *conditioning* and often involves high-dose (myeloablative) cytotoxic chemotherapy and may also include total body irradiation. Reduced intensity regimens are now also being used that do not involve myeloablative doses of chemotherapy but require manipulation of the immune system to ensure graft survival and disease eradication. The exact type of conditioning used will depend on many factors including the nature of the disease and the degree of immunosuppression needed for a successful transplant. Once conditioning is complete the transplant stem cells are re-infused into the patient; this process is not unlike a blood transfusion.

Bone marrow failure is a feature of the next stage of transplant. This may last anywhere from 14 to 25 days or longer, depending on the type of stem cells and the conditioning used. At this time the patient is very vulnerable to infection, bleeding and anaemia, and requires intensive support. As mentioned above, autologous stem cells and those collected from a peripheral stem cell harvest tend to recover more speedily than those from a donor or those collected directly from the bone marrow. In lower intensity regimen transplants, the intense pancytopaenia is avoided.

The final stage of transplant is again variable in length and involves the reconstitution of the patient's *immune system*. The patient remains susceptible to bacterial, viral and fungal infections and may still require support including antibiotics and transfusions at this time. For allogeneic transplant recipients, this final stage is generally longer than in autologous transplantation as suppression of the immune system is greater and longer lasting to allow the graft to establish itself. At this time, some of the long-term complications of conditioning and transplantation may begin to manifest themselves.

The list of possible complications associated with stem cell transplantation is extensive. Many complications arise as a consequence of the high-dose chemotherapy and radiotherapy used, the bone marrow failure, the immune dysfunction and the metabolic problems related to the prophylactic and therapeutic treatments needed during the acute transplant phase. Allogeneic transplant recipients are also at risk of graft-vs-host disease and graft rejection, and often require extended immunosuppressive therapy. Other transplant-related complications include pulmonary, endocrine and neurological problems or may involve other organs such as the kidneys or liver. Endocrine problems often include premature menopause for women. Infertility in both men and women is often a very distressing but often inevitable side-effect of the treatment.

Undergoing such an arduous procedure and coping and living with its complications and side-effects is a challenge for patients and their families. A degree of psychological distress and anxiety is an inevitable consequence of the stress of transplantation and the subsequent disruption to normal life. Healthcare workers involved in caring for these patients require many skills to be able to minimize the physiological and psychological effects of the procedure effectively. Knowledgeable nurses with the skills to encourage and support patients are vital to the success of transplantation. As transplantation involves a number of complex events and processes, and these cannot be discussed in detail in a brief overview, a Further Reading list has been given at the end of this chapter.

BIOTHERAPY – IMMUNOTHERAPY

Cytotoxic chemotherapy and radiotherapy currently remain the mainstay of treatment for haematological malignancies. An important drawback to these therapies is that they do not target cancer cells specifically and therefore damage healthy cells and tissues alongside cancer cells. They also have serious side-effects and are therefore not suitable for all patients. Despite developments in the supportive care of patients and refinements in the therapeutic strategies used, cure rates for a number of these cancers still remain disappointing. Developments in the understanding of the molecular biology of the cell, cancer biology and the body's immune processes have opened the door to new approaches in the treatment of cancer.

Cytokines are important chemical messengers. One such cytokine is the growth factor granulocyte colony stimulating factor (GCSF). This has been used successfully for over 10 years to support patients with treatment-induced neutropenia as well as to mobilize stem cells prior to stem cell transplantation. It is currently also being assessed for its usefulness as part of first line chemotherapy schedules to make leukaemia cells more sensitive to chemotherapy. Another cytokine, α-interferon, has cytostatic and other effects and is routinely used as single therapy or as adjuvant or maintenance therapy for some haematological malignancies.

Monoclonal antibodies to cell surface antigens permits the targeting of tumour cell and makes use of the body's immune system to destroy malignant cells. These antibodies can be used as either monotherapy or in combination with other therapies. Rituximab, used in the treatment of lymphoid malignancies, is one example. Antibodies can also be linked to radioactive particles or other anti-tumour agents, providing targeted radiotherapy or chemotherapy for tumour cells, while sparing normal cells and potentially reducing toxicity. Allogeneic stem cell transplantation can also be used as immunotherapy by exploiting the tumour vs malignancy effect. This is where the transplanted immune cells attack the remaining tumour cells and destroy them. Other immunotherapeutic strategies are also currently being developed and refined for clinical use.

These various biotherapies are welcome additions to the range of treatment available to cancer patients. They are not, however, without their side-effects and toxicities. Side-effects can include flu-like symptoms and patients may also experience a degree of pain or discomfort as well as fatigue. Nausea and vomiting and anorexia may also be experienced. Monoclonal antibodies can generate tumour lysis syndrome, a consequence of rapid cell death and the release of chemicals predisposing the person to renal failure and metabolic problems. A hypersensitivity reaction is a possible complication; this is treated as a potential medical emergency. The side-effects of these therapies can have a negative impact on the person's quality of life; for some patients the side-effects will be severe enough to warrant discontinuation of the therapy. One of the roles of the nurse caring for patients receiving biotherapy is to be aware of the side-effects of individual treatments and to minimize and manage these appropriately.

LYMPHATIC DISORDERS

INFECTIOUS MONONUCLEOSIS (GLANDULAR FEVER)

This is a benign infectious disease involving the lymphatic system and is seen most commonly in adolescents and young adults. The causative organism is the Epstein–Barr virus (EBV). The disease is not highly contagious but is transmitted by the oropharyngeal route, via saliva, often through kissing. It has an incubation period of 4–6 weeks.

Clinical characteristics

Symptoms vary from one person to another and are often non-specific. Common complaints include sore throat, headache, neck stiffness, fatigue, anorexia, nausea and vomiting and general malaise. The person has a fever, which may be intermittent, and there is usually enlargement and tenderness of the superficial lymph nodes (cervical, axillary and inguinal). The spleen is often enlarged and tender, and palpation may also reveal abdominal tenderness due to involvement of the mesenteric lymph nodes. An erythematous or maculopapular rash is developed by some individuals with glandular fever and occasionally the person is jaundiced.

Investigations

The total leucocyte count is raised and may range from 10 to 20×10^9/L. A differential count reveals an increase in lymphocytes and monocytes, and many of the lymphocytes are atypical. The number of granulocytes may be below normal. A mild to moderate anaemia may exist together with thrombocytopenia. Diagnosis is confirmed by a positive Paul–Bunnell test. Increased levels of heterophile antibodies appear in the serum of patients with infectious mononucleosis: these antibodies cause the agglutination of sheep red blood cells, which is the basis of the Paul–Bunnell test. The Paul–Bunnell reaction does not become positive until the second week of infection because it depends on production of immunoglobulin M (IgM). A rapid slide test (the Monospot test) using horse red blood cells is easier to carry out and is considered to be more specific.

Treatment and care The disease usually runs a self-limited course of 2–4 weeks and is managed at home with symptomatic care. Goals for the person with infectious mononucleosis are to:

- obtain adequate rest until the temperature returns to normal
- obtain a satisfactory degree of relief from distressing symptoms
- avoid spread of the disease to others
- avoid secondary infections.

Paracetamol may be prescribed to relieve the headache, fever and general body discomfort. Non-steroidal anti-inflammatory agents can also be used in the absence of hepatic pathology. Warm saline gargles may help to soothe a sore throat. Rest is advisable until the temperature returns to normal. If there is evidence of a concomitant bacterial infection, antibiotics can be prescribed but some penicillin-based antibiotics should be avoided as they can cause a rash in infectious mononucleosis (IM).

Convalescence may take some weeks and occasionally a relapse can occur. The prolonged fatigue experienced may result in the person feeling discouraged and depressed. Nurses can convey understanding and reassurance that these reactions are normal and that fatigue will resolve over time. It may be helpful to set realistic goals for the resumption of normal activities whilst stressing the importance of adequate rest. When the spleen is enlarged, the individual should be advised to avoid contact sports because there is a danger that an abdominal injury could lead to rupture of the spleen. Any moderate to severe abdominal pain in the context of an enlarged spleen should be closely monitored as this could indicate a ruptured spleen. This is a rare but serious complication of IM. Occasionally, the person will have a moderate haemolytic anaemia and rarely will develop bone marrow failure.

MALIGNANT LYMPHOMAS

This term is applied to a group of neoplastic diseases that primarily affect lymphoid tissue rather than bone marrow. They are characterized by painless, progressive enlargement of the lymph nodes and the spleen. In some conditions, the proliferating cells invade extralymphatic tissues and organs. This group of diseases is divided into Hodgkin's disease (HD), which is the most common form of lymphoma, and non-Hodgkin's lymphomas (NHL).

Hodgkin's disease

Hodgkin's disease is a disease of unknown aetiology. Although there is some evidence of a viral connection, with traces of Epstein–Barr virus being detected in 30–50% of cases, it is not likely to be the sole cause. Hodgkin's disease may develop at any age but incidence peaks between the age of 20–30 years and after 50 years of age. There is a higher incidence of the disorder in males. The 5-year survival rate has improved dramatically, from only 20% in the 1960s, and is currently approaching 90%. This is mainly due to the introduction of interdisciplinary care and advances in chemotherapy and radiotherapy techniques.

Hodgkin's disease is classified histologically into four subtypes. This is known as the Rye classification:

1 lymphocytic predominant
2 nodular sclerosing
3 mixed cellularity
4 lymphocyte depleted.

Large atypical cells known as Reed–Sternberg cells seen in the affected lymph nodes are characteristic of Hodgkin's disease and are present in different numbers in the various subtypes. The lymphocyte-predominant form of the disease tends to be associated with a more favourable prognosis than the other subtypes.

Clinical characteristics
The disease often has an insidious onset and most patients present with a painless enlargement of one group of lymph nodes. In two-thirds of patients it is the cervical nodes that enlarge. The disease spreads progressively to other lymphoid and non-lymphoid tissue throughout the body, producing a variety of symptoms. The enlarging nodes may cause pressure on nerves, resulting in pain, or may impose on neighbouring organs causing dysfunction. Enlarged axillary and inguinal nodes frequently interfere with venous and lymphatic drainage, leading to oedema in the arms or legs. Enlarged mediastinal nodes may cause a distressing cough, dyspnoea or difficulty swallowing (dysphagia). The spleen becomes enlarged causing abdominal discomfort.

Constitutional problems do not usually present until the later stages. The patient gradually develops fatigue, weakness, fever, anorexia, loss of weight and pruritus. Drenching night sweats and alcohol-induced pain are sometimes reported.

Diagnosis is made by histological examination of an affected lymph node and observation of the Reed–Sternberg cell.

Non-Hodgkin's lymphomas

Non-Hodgkin's lymphomas (NHLs) are proliferative disorders of B and T lymphocytes, with about 80% being of B-cell origin. The NHLs usually originate in the peripheral lymphoid tissues and are often widespread at diagnosis. They are less predictable in terms of pattern of spread than Hodgkin's disease and have a very variable prognosis. Some of the NHLs are relatively benign, whereas others are aggressive and rapidly fatal. The diverse nature of these disorders makes their classification very complex and various classification systems exist.

Although the cause is unknown, NHLs are associated with a variety of factors, including damage to the immune system caused by radiation, immunosuppressive drugs and environmental chemical hazards. Viral infections are also believed to contribute to the complex aetiological process and there is an increased incidence of NHL in individuals with AIDS. As a group, NHLs are the most common type of haematological malignancy, with an incidence of around 1 in 10 000. Although forms of NHL affect all ages, the incidence increases with increasing age and men tend to be affected more often than women.

Clinical characteristics
Painless enlargement of peripheral lymph nodes may be the first indication of a problem, although generalized disease is not uncommon. Sometimes large masses are detected in the chest and abdomen, and the gastrointestinal tract is the most commonly involved extranodal site after the bone marrow because it contains a lot of lymphoid tissue. Many other tissues may be involved including tonsils, bone, skin, testicles, central nervous system, liver and spleen, giving rise to a wide variety of symptoms, including respiratory difficulty, superior vena cava obstruction, abdominal swelling and ascites, lower limb oedema and intestinal obstruction. Recurrent fever, night sweats, weight loss and fatigue are other general symptoms that may occur. Diagnosis is confirmed by histological examination of an excised lymph node or tumour biopsy.

Investigation and staging of malignant lymphomas

When a diagnosis of Hodgkin's disease or NHL has been confirmed, a series of investigations is organized to determine the extent of the disease. These include: a full blood count, bone marrow aspiration and biopsy, blood chemistry, liver function tests, chest radiography and immunoglobulin estimations. Computed tomography, magnetic resonance imaging, lymphangiography (occasionally), isotope scans, ultrasonography and lumbar puncture may also be indicated. For the person with Hodgkin's disease, accurate staging is crucial in determining the best treatment option. Surgical assessment with a staging laparotomy, liver biopsy and splenectomy used to be routine, but advances in radiological techniques have virtually eliminated the need for such surgery with all its inherent risks.

Malignant lymphomas are staged according to the spread of the disease using the Ann Arbor classification, revised in 1989 to take account of specific nodal involvement in stage III and the importance of tumour bulk as a prognostic indicator (Fig. 14.9). NHLs are also classified according to histological appearance and immunological tests into different subtypes using the Revised European American Lymphoma (REAL) system. The use of techniques such as cell morphology, immunophenotyping and chromosomal changes in combination with clinical features assists the medical team in making treatment decisions and in identifying prognosis and the likely response to treatment. Disease progression of the different types of NHL can be classified ranging from indolent to highly aggressive.

Treatment and nursing care

Treatment may consist of radiation therapy, chemotherapy, immunotherapy, bone marrow transplantation or a combination of these. Care is aimed at helping the person with a malignant lymphoma to understand the disease and the side-effects of treatment and to cope with both the physical and psychological sequelae of diagnosis and treatment.

Treatment of Hodgkin's disease

Radiotherapy Radiotherapy is used to treat early-stage disease, either alone or in combination with chemotherapy. Involved nodes and those in adjacent areas are irradiated in very early cases. When treating all lymph node groups above the diaphragm, an extended 'mantle' field is irradiated. The equivalent field used to treat lymph nodes below the diaphragm is known as an 'inverted Y' field (Fig. 14.10). A combination of the two given 3–4 weeks apart may be used for stage III disease and involves total nodal irradiation. Localized radiotherapy is also used to treat bulky or painful tumour masses in patients with advanced disease who are receiving chemotherapy as the primary treatment. Side-effects of the radiotherapy vary according to the field of treatment and all patients need information and opportunities to discuss treatment, potential side-effects and how these may be minimized.

A person having mantle irradiation may experience a dry mouth, altered taste, dysphagia, vocal changes, skin soreness and hair loss in the treatment area. These effects are temporary and usually completely reversible. A person having inverted Y irradiation is likely to experience gastrointestinal disturbances, colic, flatulence and diarrhoea, and will need dietary advice to control these problems. Young women who wish to remain fertile can be offered oophoropexy (repositioning of the ovaries) via laparoscopy to allow the ovaries to be shielded during treatment. Men normally have their testes shielded to protect testicular function. Blood counts and haemoglobin concentrations are determined frequently as bone marrow depression may occur. The general effects of radiotherapy are discussed in Chapter 11.

Chemotherapy Chemotherapy with or without radiotherapy is used to treat stage III or IV disease, and anyone with adverse prognostic factors such as weight loss greater than 10% in 6 months, fever and night sweats (referred to as B symptoms), multiple sites and/or bulky disease. A number of cytotoxic agents are used, including chlormethine (mustine), vincristine, vinblastine, prednisolone, procarbazine, cyclophosphamide, chlorambucil, dacarbazine and bleomycin. These are usually given in combinations at 4-week intervals for up to six cycles. Some combinations (those containing alkylating agents) are more likely than others to cause infertility, which is an important consideration for many patients when selecting a treatment plan. They are also associated with an increased risk of developing a secondary malignancy at some later date. Six to eight cycles of chemotherapy are normally administered (see Case Study 14.3).

Chemotherapy is also used for patients whose disease relapses, and developments in the use of growth factors and stem cell rescue have offered opportunities for administering high doses of chemotherapy to this group and to younger patients with poor prognostic factors as primary treatment.

CASE Paul is 26 years of age. He has been married to Jane for 4 years and they have no children. Paul works in the computer department of a large bank. Two years ago he noticed a swollen gland on the right of his neck. His general practitioner treated this as an infected lymph gland for several weeks before referring Paul for a biopsy, which revealed that he had Hodgkin's disease. He was diagnosed as having stage Ia disease and a course of local radiotherapy was given to the neck and axillary area.

As the course of radiotherapy progressed, Paul started to complain of low back pain, which got progressively worse. Shooting leg pains inhibited walking and the pain woke him at night. Various analgesics were prescribed but failed to control the pain adequately. Paul was reassured that the pain was unrelated to the Hodgkin's disease because investigations over several months failed to reveal a cause for the pain. Eventually, Paul alerted medical staff to the fact that his back pain became much worse after drinking beer. A MRI scan was then performed and a shadow was detected

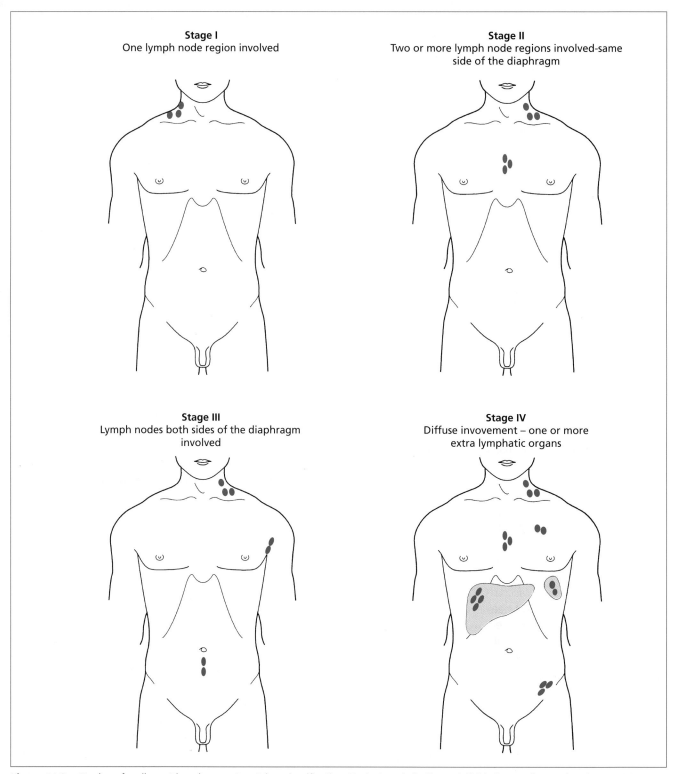

Figure 14.9 Staging of malignant lymphomas: Ann Arbor classification. Each stage is further subdivided according to the absence (A) or presence (B) of any of the following symptoms: weight loss >10% of body weight in 6 months; fever >38°C; night sweats. A suffix E indicates localized extranodal involvement in stages I, II and III. A suffix S indicates involvement of the spleen in stage III.

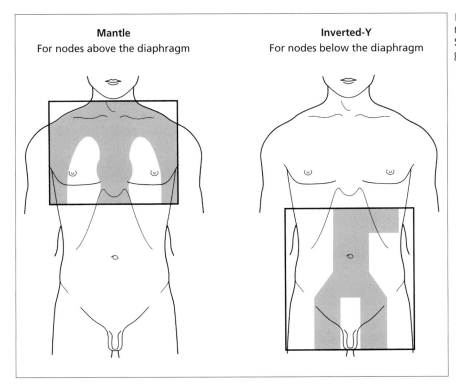

Mantle
For nodes above the diaphragm

Inverted-Y
For nodes below the diaphragm

Figure 14.10 Mantle and inverted-Y radiotherapy fields for Hodgkin's disease. Shaded areas are irradiated with 35–40 Gy given over 4–5 weeks.

on the lumbar vertebrae. Biopsy of the vertebra confirmed Hodgkin's disease and a bone marrow biopsy revealed extensive infiltration of the marrow.

At this point chemotherapy was planned and an opportunity to discuss sperm banking was offered. Paul was advised that only healthy sperm could be preserved successfully. As his disease was widespread and involved the bone marrow, it was felt that the quality of his sperm would be too poor to preserve and Paul and his wife decided not to proceed with sperm banking.

Paul then commenced six cycles of chemotherapy. The first course of treatment was accompanied by severe nausea and vomiting but in subsequent treatments this was controlled with ondansetron. Paul experienced some bone marrow depression between courses of treatment and had to be admitted for intravenous antibiotics for a suspected infection. Deep mouth ulcers causing severe facial swelling, pain and an inability to eat were the side-effects of treatment that Paul identified as causing him the most distress. Eventually Paul had his wisdom teeth removed, as it was believed that these were the source of the infection. Paul also recalled the repeated venipunctures by different members of staff as being the 'ultimate torture for someone with a bit of a needle phobia'.

After completion of the chemotherapy Paul returned to work and has been promoted. His response to treatment has been followed by 3-monthly bone marrow biopsies in outpatients, and these have remained clear to date.

Consider the issues facing Paul and his wife both at diagnosis and later as the treatment progressed. Reflect upon the issues raised for the future and what implications this illness might have upon their relationship and their plans.

Treatment for non-Hodgkin's lymphoma The treatment chosen depends on the person's medical history and the classification and characteristics of the disease. Radiation therapy and chemotherapy are used singly or in combination. For low-grade tumours, radiotherapy alone or single-agent chemotherapy may be adequate treatment. For persons with intermediate-grade disease, combination chemotherapy with or without local radiotherapy is used to produce remission rates of up to 75% and a significant improvement in survival rates. Aggressive high-grade NHLs are managed with intensive combination chemotherapy.

A typical chemotherapy combination used is called CHOP, which is a combination of cyclophosphamide, Adriamycin (doxorubicin), vincristine and prednisolone. Response is often rapid but there is a high relapse rate. Intrathecal methotrexate may be given to prevent CNS relapse. High-dose chemotherapy and autologous stem cell rescue may be recommended for patients who relapse. The role of α-interferon and other biological response-modifying agents are also being evaluated in the management of NHL. Rituximab, an anti CD20 antibody is now being successfully used as a treatment strategy. Other antibodies are also being assessed for efficacy. Radioimmunotherapy, such as radio-isotopes attached to anti CD 20 are also being assessed in the context of relapsed disease. In future, other targeted therapies could also help to enhance or even perhaps replace the more conventional treatment strategies such as chemotherapy or radiotherapy for specific types of lymphomas.

Nursing intervention The potential patient problems, goals and nursing interventions for the patient with a malignant lymphoma are similar to those for patients with leukaemia. Following the investigational procedures, initial therapy aimed at achieving remission may be given as an inpatient or on an outpatient basis depending on the drugs and doses used. During this period the patient will need careful surveillance and may need supportive measures such as blood transfusion and intravenous antibiotics and symptomatic care, for example analgesia for pain relief. Following remission the patient can usually return to a normal lifestyle.

Nurses should be closely involved with the patient and family members in discussions about treatment plans, care and prevention of side-effects (especially infection). The need for rest, information about medication and follow-up are important, as is support in coping with the therapy and its side-effects, such as fatigue and nausea. Risks of future infertility should be explained. Opportunities for sperm banking exist and it is becoming increasingly possible to freeze and store eggs or ovarian tissue for future use. However, in lymphoma for example, some concerns have been expressed over the theoretical risk of re-introducing the cancer with the tissue implantation (Simon et al 2005). Women treated with chemotherapy are less likely to become sterile than men, but periods usually become irregular or stop during chemotherapy. The re-establishment of menstruation after chemotherapy tends to be age-related. Contraceptive advice therefore needs to be available and women who experience an early menopause may need hormone replacement therapy to control their symptoms.

With much treatment being given to outpatients, it is essential that patients have an out-of-hours contact number should problems arise at home and that details of the most recent blood counts are easily available. Information for patients is available from a number of sources including The Hodgkin's Disease Association, Leukaemia Research Fund and Cancer BACUP and may be accessed via a telephone helpline, information booklets or the internet.

MULTIPLE MYELOMA

Multiple myeloma is a malignant disease characterized by a proliferation of abnormal plasma cells in the bone marrow. Plasma cells develop from B lymphocytes after they have been stimulated by an antigen, and they secrete antigen-specific immunoglobulins. These plasma cells exist in lymphoid and connective tissue throughout the body. In multiple myeloma a malignant clone (a group of identical cells derived from a single cell) of plasma cells produces one of the immunoglobulins in excess and in a form that is not capable of maintaining normal humoral immunity. The abnormal protein produced is known as paraprotein and may be found in the plasma and urine. It is a malignancy that accounts for about 1% of all malignant disease but remains an incurable condition affecting mainly those in late middle to old age.

Clinical characteristics

The disease tends to have an insidious onset, with early symptoms being pain and general malaise. The malignant plasma (B) cells produce cytokines which unfortunately encourage bone destruction by stimulating osteoclasts (p. 821). Multiple, diffuse areas of bone destruction develop; these areas are seen as well circumscribed or 'punched out' lytic bone lesions on radiography and typically affect the skull, ribs and axial skeleton (Haslett et al 2002). The breakdown in bone structure frequently results in pathological fractures, especially in weight-bearing bones such as the vertebrae. Changes in posture and stature may be evident. The patient often experiences pain in the area of the bone lesions, which worsens with movement, jarring and pressure. As the disease progresses, the patient experiences more and more pain and may become increasingly incapacitated. The vertebrae are a common site of involvement and pressure on the nerve roots by the tumours and/or collapsing vertebrae causes severe back and/or lower limb pain. In extreme cases, this may progress to spinal cord compression and, if treatment is delayed, interruption of nerve impulses may result in paraplegia.

The excessive production of abnormal paraprotein occurs at the expense of normal immunoglobulin synthesis. This reduction in the synthesis of normal antibodies predisposes the patient to infections, which are usually respiratory in origin, although bladder infections and skin lesions are not uncommon. Abnormal quantities of immunoglobulins in the blood occasionally cause a hyperviscosity syndrome which may result in bleeding problems, visual disturbance, neurological problems and heart failure.

As the bone marrow becomes crowded with plasma cells, red cell production falls and the person with multiple myeloma is frequently anaemic. In advanced disease white blood cell and platelet production are also reduced, further predisposing the individual to infection and a bleeding tendency.

Breakdown of bone tissue gives rise to the release of calcium, and hypercalcaemia (normal calcium level 2.33–2.6 mmol/L) develops in about 30% of patients. Excretion of the increased serum calcium by the kidneys entails an increased loss of water. If the fluid intake is not correspondingly increased, the patient becomes dehydrated, the serum calcium is retained and urinary output falls. Nausea, thirst, loss of appetite, cardiac dysrhythmias, constipation and disorientation and confusion may all be symptoms of hypercalcaemia.

Urinalysis may record proteinuria, and electrophoresis of urine may demonstrate the presence of an abnormal protein known as Bence Jones protein, which is excreted by the kidneys. In high concentration this protein may be precipitated in the renal tubules, forming casts that damage the tubules and may cause renal insufficiency. A combination of factors such as proteinuria, hypercalcaemia and raised serum urate caused by rapid breakdown of cells contributes to the high incidence of renal impairment with this condition.

Investigations

These include blood tests, which may reveal an increased erythrocyte sedimentation rate, erythrocyte, leucocyte and platelet counts below normal, and raised serum calcium and urea levels. Examination of a specimen of bone marrow shows the presence of large numbers of plasma cells, often with abnormal forms. Serum electrophoresis and urine electrophoresis demonstrate the presence of an abnormal paraprotein in the serum, urine or both.

Treatment

Care of the patient with malignant myeloma involves the administration of chemotherapy, radiotherapy and supportive care to relieve symptoms. Often the person with multiple myeloma remains stable and symptom free for several years, but overall the prognosis of patients with this malignancy remains poor. Alkylating agents such as melphalan or cyclophosphamide are given with or without prednisolone. Combination chemotherapy is also used, particularly for younger patients and when high-dose chemotherapy and stem cell rescue is an option, α-interferon may be given as maintenance treatment. All of these treatments have recognized toxicities and these have to be factored in when considering treatment options. Unfortunately, current treatments do not offer a clear survival benefit and options must be considered carefully in terms of the potential benefits and inevitable side-effects of intensive treatment.

For individuals with advanced disease, palliative chemotherapy or radiotherapy can be used to relieve symptoms. Supportive care is crucial. Allopurinol may be prescribed to decrease uric acid production and prevent impaired renal function. Patients with hypercalcaemia are hydrated with intravenous fluids and given a diuretic and steroids to reduce serum calcium levels. Administration of a bisphosphonate drug is an effective way of both reducing hypercalcaemia and managing bone pain. Analgesics are likely to be needed to control the pain of bone lesions until chemotherapy or radiotherapy produces a response.

Radiotherapy, in particular, is very useful in the treatment of bony deposits as it alleviates pain and reduces the likelihood of pathological fractures or spinal cord compression. Multiple bone lesions may be treated effectively with hemi-body irradiation. Plasmapheresis is used to treat hyperviscosity syndrome. This involves the removal of plasma containing the paraproteins and replacement with plasma protein fraction. Surgery may be required to treat pathological fractures. Blood transfusion and platelets may be needed to manage anaemia and thrombocytopenia.

Nursing care

The person with multiple myeloma requires regular medical and nursing assessment as significant changes can occur in a short space of time (e.g. vertebral collapse leading to spinal cord compression). Posture, the degree and difficulty of movement, and amount of incapacity and pain require regular assessment. Laboratory data relating to blood counts and blood chemistry need to be evaluated to indicate whether the patient's condition is improving or worsening. For example, rising serum calcium levels or increasing uraemia may indicate the need for hydration and detailed fluid balance recording.

Some of the goals for the patient with multiple myeloma include:

- achieving adequate pain control
- maintaining mobility to prevent further demineralization of bone
- preventing injury related to pathological fractures and/or vertebral collapse (any numbness or increasing loss of sensation; weakness and loss of movement; urine retention and constipation; and back pain of increasing severity should be reported urgently)
- preserving independence and the ability to maintain expected roles and responsibilities.

Involvement of a multidisciplinary palliative care team is vital at an early stage to ensure good symptom control, preserve independence and provide ongoing emotional support for the individual with a myeloma.

NURSING MANAGEMENT OF THE PERSON WITH A LEUCOCYTE OR LYMPHATIC DISORDER

White blood cells (WBCs) or leucocytes are composed of populations of granulocytes (neutrophils, eosinophils and basophils), lymphocytes (T and B cells) and monocytes. Their primary function is the protection of the body against foreign invasion. When there is either a quantitative or qualitative (i.e. numerical or functional) decrease in leucocytes, the body's natural defences are impaired, the person becomes immunocompromised and is susceptible to infection from bacteria, fungi or viruses. Bacterial infections are often caused by the spread of commensal bacteria to a new and previously sterile site; for example, intestinal flora may enter the bloodstream. Infection may arise from either Gram-positive or Gram-negative bacteria and quickly develop into sepsis; in the immunocompromised individual life-threatening sepsis is a common problem. Virus infections are often a result of reactivation of a latent organism but may also be a new infection. Fungi such as candida or aspergillus can be a major threat to an immunocompromised patient. Candida is frequently found in small numbers in healthy individuals; simple colonization can quickly turn into a life-threatening systemic infection in the immunocompromised person. Aspergillus is a common air-borne spore that can invade the lungs of a susceptible individual, with serious consequences.

Susceptibility to particular infections is related both to the degree of immunosuppression and to the predominant type of white cell dysfunction. Frequently, however, immunosuppression is complicated by a variety of other factors such as the nature of the disease, treatment, overall bone marrow function, reduced mucosal barriers (as with the use of central venous catheters) and the person's overall state of health.

Assessment

Systematic and continuous assessment of the person with a white cell disorder is important during the acute phases of illness and treatment. Changes in health status that may be indicative of infection, need to be identified promptly, as infection may rapidly become generalized and life-threatening.

Health history

During the initial assessment, it is important to establish the possible factors that may have contributed to the person's current situation. Particularly in circumstances where the cause of the white cell disorder is unknown and malignancy is not suspected, previous or recent exposure to chemicals, radiation, toxins or drugs may cast some light on the possible causes of the disorder. The previous medical history may also provide some clues to the origin of the problem.

Specific questions aimed at identifying possible signs of infection may provide useful assessment information. These may include the presence or absence of:

● redness, swelling, warmth, abnormal discharge
● fever, chills, shivering, unexplained sweating
● general malaise or weakness
● sore mouth, throat, eyes or ears
● skin lesions or rashes
● pain and discomfort in the abdomen, joints, rectal or perineal areas
● changes in the character or colour of stools, diarrhoea
● nausea or vomiting.

The presence of one of these symptoms could be explained by many pathologies, however it is the combination of signs and symptoms that points towards a possible white cell disorder. This is true of many diseases of course and the advanced nurse practitioner learns to combine a comprehensive medical and nursing history with their physical assessment to arrive at a working hypothesis of what may be wrong with the patient (see Ch. 1). Another major component of the health history is identification of the person's and their family's response to the illness, diagnosis and treatment. This is particularly relevant when the diagnosis may be malignancy or another life-threatening illness such as bone marrow failure. Anxiety and fear are common reactions, as may be denial and anger. In many instances, the treatment regimens as well as the disease process itself places the patient at risk of infection. The infections and their debilitating side-effects are often very distressing to patients and their families and, even if expected, may engender fear and anxiety. It is not surprising that the emotional responses of the patient and the family are likely to fluctuate as the person's clinical situation and health status alter.

Physical assessments

1 Baseline observations of the person's blood pressure, pulse, temperature and respirations are taken.
2 Skin and all body sites with high potential for infection are examined. These include the skinfold areas (buttocks, axillae, perineum, breasts), insertion sites of intravenous cannulae or central venous catheters, and wound sites for signs of redness, warmth, swelling or discharge.
3 The mouth is inspected for candida infection or ulceration. Dental hygiene is assessed.
4 The person's respiratory status is assessed. The presence and nature of any cough and sputum is noted as well as any dyspnoea, pain or discomfort or alteration in breathing pattern.
5 Patterns of bowel elimination and the colour and consistency of stools are noted. Any history or presence of diarrhoea is established.
6 Urine is examined for any signs of infection such as cloudiness or odour. Any report of frequency or dysuria is noted.
7 The person's state of hydration is assessed and fluid intake and output are monitored.
8 Any signs of anaemia are noted.

Tests

The person's white cell count and differential are monitored regularly. Throat, wound, perineal or other swabs are sent for microbiological culture and sensitivity, as required. Urine, stool or sputum samples are also sent for culture and sensitivity testing, as required. Blood cultures are also sent to be cultured for an infective agent, if the person has a raised temperature. Some may be sent to establish a baseline; subsequent samples may then be sent if infection is suspected.

Patient problems

A key health problem is the potential risk of local or systemic infection due to immunosuppression or bone marrow failure. Other problems may include:

● risk of bleeding from thrombocytopenia in the presence of bone marrow failure
● fatigue in the presence of infection or bone marrow failure-associated anaemia
● anxiety related to the diagnosis, treatment and potential outcomes; lack of knowledge of the disease process and treatment; fear of the unknown; loss of control over life events and uncertainty over the future
● pain due to the disease process, infection (e.g. oral candida) and treatment (e.g. stomatitis)
● nutritional deficiencies, weight loss and inadequate fluid intake from a multitude of factors including treatment side-effects, nausea, pain, infection, diarrhoea, anorexia and others
● body image issues associated with treatment side-effects such as hair loss, weight loss, long-term central venous catheters, pallor, loss of muscle mass
● lack of effective coping strategies related to altered roles and relationships, prolonged treatment and hospitalization, body image and loss of control.

In addition, treatment-related toxicity may frequently generate a range of specific problems.

Nursing interventions
Prevention of infection

Environment The decision to isolate the person with a white cell disorder depends on the level of risk assessed, the facilities available, the anticipated length of isolation required, the anticipated degree and length of neutropenia, and other factors such as the potential risk presented by other patients. In general terms, however, scrupulous cleaning, staff education and supervision, and the removal of items likely to introduce infection into the client's immediate environment (e.g. flowers) will help to reduce the risk of infection.

While in hospital, the person who is severely neutropenic (a neutrophil count of 0.5×10^9/L or less) is often nursed in a single room or, if facilities are available, in a room designed with positive air pressure to facilitate the provision of a clean environment. Again, it is assessment of the client's associated risk factors (e.g. the use of intensive chemotherapy, radiation, immunosuppressive drug therapy, bone marrow transplantation, the overall degree of bone marrow failure and the client's general state of health) that will ensure the risk is minimized. Protective isolation can then be used effectively for those patients who are at high risk of infection, while not necessarily restricting those at lower risk. An assessment process is also useful when facilities are limited. In this environment, limiting the number of individuals in the room at any one time, maintaining equipment and supplies for the client's sole use, and maintaining a high standard of cleaning services are other important measures.

Personal hygiene An important nursing responsibility involves the promotion of meticulous personal hygiene in order to reduce the potential for infection. The person is encouraged to shower daily, establish an oral hygiene routine and practice good perineal care. Particular attention is given to the perineum, groin, axillae and skinfolds when showering or bathing. The person is taught to note any redness, tenderness, swelling, unusual skin lesions or discharge and report these to the clinical team. Antiperspirants are avoided as they can lead to blockage of the sweat glands and subsequent infection. Men should be advised to use an electric razor to decrease the potential for causing breaks in the skin while shaving. Women are also advised to take precautions if wishing to shave areas such as the legs.

Oral hygiene Effective oral care is central to the prevention of infection, the maintenance of nutritional status and patient comfort and well-being. Treatment for haematological malignancies often causes significant destruction of the oral mucosa, may induce a severe reduction in salivary secretion and increase the risk of infection. Infection originating in the mouth can easily lead to a systemic infection with its associated risks. Appropriate oral care is, therefore, an important part of health-promoting care. Regular and consistent assessment of oral status with an appropriate tool can provide useful baseline data, monitor the response to nursing interventions and help to identify new problems as they arise. Assessment may include both the physical assessment of the status of the oral cavity and a functional assessment of the client's ability to swallow, speak, eat and drink. A pain assessment may also be useful when damage to the oral cavity is a possibility.

The prevention of trauma to the oral mucosa is necessary in the prevention of infection. Dentures should be checked to ensure that they fit properly and ill-fitting dentures should not be worn. Dentures should regularly be cleaned thoroughly and, if prophylactic mouthwashes or suspensions are prescribed, the dentures should be removed before using the treatment. Oral hygiene should be practised regularly using a soft toothbrush, taking care to avoid gum trauma or bleeding. If the mouth is painful, soft swabs can be used in place of the toothbrush. Mouthwashes can be used to remove debris or thick mucus. Dental floss should be avoided when the white cell count or platelet counts are low or when there is damage to the mucosa. A dental referral may be required if the patient has not been having regular checks or there is evidence of dental caries or gum disease. This is often required before intensive treatments that predispose the patient to mucositis and opportunistic infections. The person should also be warned that any dental treatment may need antibiotic cover and that this should be discussed with their doctor.

Bowel care As infections originating from the intestinal tract are common in neutropenia, it is important that the patient understands the importance of avoiding constipation and rectal straining that may damage the rectal mucosa and provide entry for organisms found in the gastrointestinal tract. Maintenance of regular bowel habits is promoted and a bowel routine using stool softening or other mild non-irritating laxatives can be established and implemented with each patient when needed. Careful assessment of regular patterns and risk factors, such as the use of opioid analgesia, can encourage the implementation of preventive measures. Suppositories, enemas and rectal tubes should not be used as they may cause damage to the mucosa. If constipation or diarrhoea is a problem, the person's diet and fluids are reviewed accordingly. Women should also be advised to wipe from front to back when performing perineal cleansing after each bowel motion to reduce the risk of introducing infection to the urinary tract. Careful handwashing is also encouraged. Abnormal pain, tenderness, discharge or itching should be reported promptly to the healthcare team.

Food and fluids The patient may need support and encouragement to maintain a nutritionally balanced diet containing sufficient calories, protein and vitamins to meet physiological needs. The person at risk of infection may need to follow a low pathogen diet as it is recognized that food can be a major source of pathogenic bacteria. At a minimum, they may be advised to avoid high-risk foods such as, lightly cooked eggs and pâtés, as well as unpasteurized milk and milk products such as ice cream; soft, ripened and blue cheeses; foodstuffs containing raw egg, raw fish and meat products; and other high-risk foods such as salads. Soft fruits and bananas may also be avoided. Other diets may recommend cooked food only and, for those in sterile environments, food may even be irradiated before eating (Buchsel and Whedon 1995). It is recommended that water should be boiled (Bouchier 1998). Ice cubes can be a source of bacteria, so are not recommended for use by at-risk patients.

A range of diets with a variety of different recommendations has been developed over the years by teams with the primary responsibility of providing care for immunocompromised patients, and this continues to be a source of ambiguity in terms of best practice. However, it is important to note that, as in other aspects of care, a range of factors can affect the overall infection risk from food. For example, the individual who is neutropenic but living at home will not have the same level of risk as a client taking prophylactic antibiotics to sterilize the gastrointestinal tract or the bone marrow transplant recipient. Assessment and effective teamwork, including the dietitian and the infection control team as well as the nursing and medical team caring for the person, can help to overcome some of these inevitable ambiguities.

Patient and family teaching   The person with a white cell disorder often wishes to be kept informed of their blood counts and needs to be taught the normal ranges for white cell and neutrophil counts and the significance of variations from normal. An understanding of the functions of white cells and the causes for a decrease in counts can also help the patient to understand the significance of changes. Inclusion of the patient's family in these discussions, if appropriate, is important.

Meticulous handwashing is an essential infection control measure for staff, patients and visitors. Good handwashing technique can be demonstrated to the person and to families and visitors, and this is encouraged before any direct contact between the patient and others. The person and family are also advised to caution anyone with a recent infection, such as respiratory infections, shingles or chickenpox, not to visit the patient in hospital or at home while their count is low. Crowds, particularly in poorly ventilated environments, should also be avoided. Other work-related or recreational activities with a possible infection risk can be discussed by the client and the team on an individual basis.

The early identification of infection when at home is also important and patients and their families can be taught how to recognize early signs of infection. A raised temperature above 37.5°C or chills, even without a fever, should alert the family to contact the hospital team.

Delivery of nursing care   The nurse and other caregivers should take precautionary measures to prevent the transfer of potentially infectious organisms from themselves to the patient. The need for regular and meticulous handwashing cannot be overstressed. Clean uniforms or clothing and the removal of outer garments such as white coats before entering the room is also important, as is the effective use of aprons and gloves. It is also best if the least number of caregivers is used to provide care. Similarly, if there is an indication that the caregiver has a potential or actual infection, a change of allocation should be provided. Strict aseptic technique should be maintained in the management of wounds and intravenous sites and lines. Equipment should be cleaned regularly and disposables such as infusion lines changed at regular intervals, usually every 24–48 hours.

The nurse has the overall responsibility to maintain a safe environment for the patient at risk; this includes the supervision of domestic staff and the provision of safe food as well as ensuring that all team members maintain consistent and high-quality infection control measures. Effective management of the clinical environment is an essential part of the nursing role in the care of this group of patients.

Early identification of infection
Specific assessment for infection takes place at least every 4 hours, but as often as the clinical situation warrants. A member of the medical team is alerted if:

- the oral temperature rises above 37.5°C
- the person experiences chills, rigor, tachycardia, cyanosis, cold clammy extremities, unexplained abdominal or rectal pain
- the person becomes irritable, restless, complains of a headache or shows an alteration in level of consciousness.

A blood sample is taken for aerobic and anaerobic cultures and a specimen of urine, sputum, stool, wound swabs, throat swabs or swabs from any lesion are sent for microbiological analysis and culture, as appropriate. Intravenous antibiotic therapy is then initiated as quickly as possible if there is any suspicion of infection. It is usually continued for at least 5 days, or for 48 hours after any fever has resolved, depending on clinical circumstances. Further antibiotic therapy may be prescribed. As mentioned previously, antibiotic protocols that have been designed specifically for the particular needs of neutropenic patients are usually in place.

Management of central venous access
Many patients, particularly those requiring intensive or prolonged cytotoxic chemotherapy regimens, long-term transfusion support, bone marrow transplantation or other procedures requiring frequent and reliable venous access will have a central venous catheter (CVC). Although a variety of CVC devices are commonly used in practice, for patients requiring intensive treatments a skin-tunnelled single or multi-lumen catheter such as the Hickman catheter is a frequent choice (Fig. 14.11). This CVC is tunnelled under the skin before entering the vessel. A Dacron cuff located under the skin permits the tissue to seal tightly around the catheter. Once healed, this can provide a natural barrier to microbes, potentially reducing the risk of infection. The material used for the catheter is relatively inert, allowing the catheter to remain in place for extended

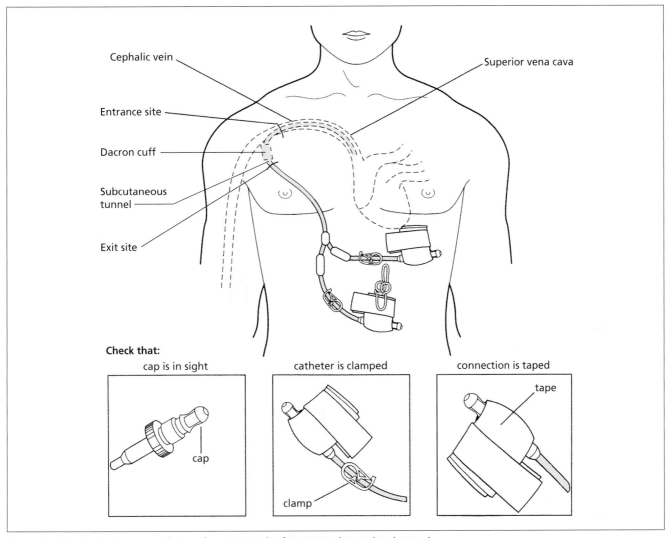

Figure 14.11   Central venous catheter: placement and safety precautions to be observed.

periods of time – often months or even years. Other CVCs in common use include peripherally inserted central venous catheters (PICCS) which, as the name suggests, are inserted via the antecubital vein.

The benefits of long-term CVCs include:

- reduced need for repeated venepuncture for blood sampling, so preserving the integrity of veins
- multiple access allowing for simultaneous administration of multiple therapies including intravenous drugs, fluids or total parenteral nutrition
- the administration of large volumes or continuous therapies
- safer administration of cytotoxic drugs, reducing the risks of extravasation
- reliable access for the administration of blood and blood products
- rapid intravenous access in the event of an emergency.

Despite the many clear advantages of CVCs in the care and treatment of patients with haematological conditions, there are a number of potentially serious complications that healthcare professionals must manage effectively. Microbial contamination of the catheter lumen is a serious problem that can often lead to life-threatening infections and sepsis. Strict asepsis in the management of CVCs, particularly when accessing the catheter lumen, changing equipment such as giving sets or caps, or when changing the exit site dressing is imperative.

The risk of air embolus or serious blood loss from an open lumen (as well as the potential to introduce infection) can be minimized through the use of luer lock connections, the systematic use of the integral clamp on each lumen (Fig. 14.11) and the use of closed system caps and access devices. Artery forceps or sharp-edged clamps should never be used as these may damage the catheter.

Patency of the catheter can be maintained by regular flushing with an appropriate solution at least once a week when the catheter is not in use or after each use. Local clinical practices vary in relation to line flushing, with regard to both frequency and the solutions used. The British Committee for Standards in Haematology issued guidelines for the management of central venous lines in 1997, which remain the latest guidance to date and these include some catheter-flushing protocols that may support decision-making in this area (BCSH 1997).

Although clinical practices may well vary, this is nevertheless an important aspect of catheter care, as a thrombus within the lumen can reduce the lumen size, limiting flow and predisposing the patient to a catheter infection. It can also cause a catheter to break with the pressure exerted during flushing or bolus administration, it may cause a clot to enter the circulation or may require the removal of the catheter if all patency is lost. Occasionally, a thrombus may develop external to the lumen, causing partial or complete obstruction of the vessel. A patient complaining of discomfort in the shoulder region should be investigated promptly for the possibility of infection, a catheter break or the presence of a thrombus.

The patient will need time and support to become familiar with and accept the catheter. The nurse should be sensitive to issues of body image and help the client to feel confident and skilful in catheter management, particularly before discharge. Education of both the client and family members in the effective management of long-term CVCs is an important nursing role; addressing anxieties and concerns is also important for the long-term success of this intervention. Some of the possible goals of a teaching programme to facilitate client independence in catheter management are outlined in the care plan shown in Box 14.4.

Evaluation

Review of care should demonstrate that assessment for signs of infection has been continuous and that the patient and family have been taught and understand measures for decreasing potential sources of infection, can identify signs of infection and know what to do if an infection develops. Persons with disorders of white cells should be supported in altering their behaviours sufficiently to decrease the risks of infection while still enjoying a balanced lifestyle and social activities.

RESPONSES OF INDIVIDUALS TO MALIGNANT DISORDERS OF WHITE BLOOD CELLS

The diagnosis of a malignant disorder of white blood cells such as leukaemia or lymphoma has a dramatic impact on the person and his or her family. The emotional and psychological impact of the diagnosis is only the beginning of a long and very challenging road to acceptance and adjustment. Their lives are altered forever.

The dialogue in Case Study 14.4, condensed from an actual nurse–patient interaction (the names have been altered), helps to highlight some of the issues from an individual perspective.

CASE James Adams is a 22-year-old man who was in his second year of college when he was diagnosed as having leukaemia. During the interview he recalled many of his experiences from the time of his diagnosis to his 2-year interview. He shared his perceptions of the impact his diagnosis had on himself, his parents and his younger brother, and how his family and health professionals had helped him to cope.

James: 'When I was first diagnosed I felt that I was the only one who had this disease. I thought once you had it, it was the end. Slowly I began to realize there was a chance that this thing could be beaten through chemotherapy. I went through the stages of anger, denial and acceptance. I let the stages take their course, but it was very hard to accept and took a long time. I remember people coming up to me and saying, "You have cancer", and I would say, "No, I don't, I have leukaemia. There is a difference". That was just another way of denying it, even though cancer and leukaemia are the same thing. I could not believe it was happening to me. I was the healthiest person in the world'.

Cheryl (nurse): 'You have told me about the support and encouragement you have received during this time. How have your family, friends and the healthcare workers helped you in coping and adapting to your diagnosis of leukaemia?'

James: 'My family and friends were always very supportive. There were times when I was very irritable and told them that I did not want anything to do with them. They always managed to give me a "sort of shake" and put things back into perspective. When I was at my lowest point, they would drag me out of the house, even though I did not want to go, and take me for a drive. They made me look at things in a different perspective – to open my eyes – and say, "What am I doing sitting here feeling sorry for myself?".

The nurses taught me how to deal with all the different things I was exposed to like needles, hospitals, and dealing with things mentally and emotionally. The nurses could provide more support if they had more time for each patient – the time they have sometimes is not quite enough.

The chaplain made me look at things in a different light. The doctor, of course, helps with the treatments and all the side-effects. I think it takes a very caring and special individual to work on a haematology ward because you develop close relationships with the patients. I have known some of the nurses for 2 years. The nurses are aware of everything the patients are going through and know what each patient likes and dislikes. When you spend as much time in hospital as I do, you like to have a sense of independence. That is something the nurses on haematology allow me to have. It does a lot for me psychologically'.

Cheryl: 'How has your leukaemia altered your life?'

James: 'There are many restrictions. At certain times I cannot drink alcohol. I have to be in hospital a lot. I am in for 1 week each month, and if there are complications I am in longer. Following treatments, you do not feel well and therefore are not up to doing what you would like to do. I have a Hickman [central venous] catheter and therefore

Box 14.4 Care plan for central venous catheters

Goal	Intervention
● The catheter will remain in place and intact for the duration of clinical need	**1** The CVC will be stitched in place and stitches will remain until the tunnel and exit site are fully healed (approx. 21 days) (or until the catheter is removed if not intended as long-term vascular access).
	2 Appropriate dressings and support are used to reduce the weight of the catheter on the exit site and the tail(s) are fixed to the chest.
	3 Strategies are developed to support and protect the CVC during normal activities such as sleeping, exercise and work.
	4 Strategies will be implemented to maintain patency and prevent thrombus formation, including a regular flushing schedule and the use of a lock technique when flushing.
● The catheter will remain infection free	**5** Strict aseptic practice will be maintained at all times when handling or using the line.
	6 The number of individuals accessing the line is kept to a minimum.
	7 Strategies are developed to minimize line accessing (e.g. blood tests are timed with drug administration, etc.).
	8 An occlusive dressing is used to protect the exit site when bathing, showering, etc.
	9 The dead space is removed prior to using or flushing the CVC.
	10 The integrity of the CVC is maintained whenever possible.
	11 Microbiological cultures are sent whenever infection is suspected and antibiotic therapy is instigated at the earliest opportunity.
● The client and key individuals will demonstrate skilled, confident and knowledgeable practice in the care, maintenance and use of the catheter	**12** An educational strategy is designed to facilitate the client or family members to: a) explain the purpose, use and care of the CVC b) demonstrate the ability to hand-wash to a high standard and to apply basic principles of asepsis to catheter management c) demonstrate the ability to prepare a syringe with a flushing solution, flush the catheter and dispose of the equipment safely d) change the cap on the catheter safely e) identify safety precautions and action to be taken in case of problems arising f) identify how they will obtain further supplies of equipment g) identify likely activities that may need to be curtailed or restricted and modified.
● The potentially negative impact of the catheter on the client's body image, sense of self-mastery and personal freedom will be minimized	**13** Support will be offered to the client before and after catheter placement and their personal concerns will be identified.
	14 Partners and family are included in the preparation and education process, as appropriate.
	15 The client is facilitated to take responsibility for catheter management as quickly as is appropriate in the individual clinical and personal circumstances.
	16 Help and support in catheter management is offered until the client feels confident.
	17 Access to other clients with long-term catheters may be appropriate.

cannot be as athletic as I would like to be. I cannot play contact sports. If I was injured it would cause a lot of problems for me. But the goal is to get through therapy and hopefully get back to a normal lifestyle'.

Cheryl: 'Do you have any comments you would like to make to a newly diagnosed leukaemic patient?'

James:
1 Try to lead as normal a life as possible.
2 Your attitude is important. If you let it beat you mentally, then you have not got a hope.
3 It is good to talk to people – that has been my experience. I speak to the nurses, the chaplain, the doctors – as many

people as possible. They help you put things in perspective when you are really upset and you cannot look at things logically.

4 Speak to someone who has gone through a similar experience. When I spoke with a volunteer from the Cancer Society, I thought, "How come you are okay? People with this disease do not have a chance". Seeing this young man and realizing that he had gone through some hard times and was okay now I thought, "Well, if he can do it, I can do it too". As a result of my experience, I appreciate little things more and take advantage of every minute. The time I spend with family, friends and nurses, I appreciate a lot more. I take things one day at a time'.

HAEMORRHAGIC DISORDERS

Effective blood coagulation is the result of a complex interaction between vascular, platelet and plasma factors. A defect or abnormality in any of these may predispose an individual to excessive or prolonged bleeding. The cause may be primary, either inherited or acquired, or secondary to other diseases or pathological processes. Abnormal bleeding is commonly the result of a deficiency in clotting factors, excess anticoagulant, or may arise from a reduced number of platelets (thrombocytopenia) or, less commonly, dysfunctional platelets or vessel wall abnormalities. Secondary causes of abnormal coagulation include liver disease, malignancy, obstetric complications, trauma and burns. A bleeding disorder is often characterized by one or more of the following features: (1) prolonged bleeding following tissue damage, (2) spontaneous bleeding into mucous membranes, tissue, joints, skin and/or organs, and (3) bleeding in multiple sites.

DISORDERS OF PLATELETS

Thrombocytopenia

Thrombocytopenia can be very broadly defined as a platelet count below 125×10^9/L. In practice, however, clinical manifestations of thrombocytopenia often reflect a much lower platelet count, certainly below 100×10^9/L, although often the count may drop much lower. As a slight drop in the platelet count may have a straightforward explanation, mild thrombocytopenia may not necessarily be a cause for clinical concern.

Thrombocytopenia can, however, also be the result of a number of different pathological processes. These include failure of production, a reduced platelet lifespan, removal of platelets from the circulation or dilution of platelets in the circulation. Bone marrow failure in diseases such as leukaemia, myeloma or aplastic anaemia, is a frequent cause of thrombocytopenia. It can also be the result of bone marrow toxicity following treatment with cytotoxic chemotherapy or radiotherapy. Other causes for a reduced production of platelets by the bone marrow include infections as well as drugs known selectively to suppress platelet production.

A reduced platelet lifespan may be the result of an immune process involving platelet antibodies, drugs or infections. Platelet destruction within the blood vessels is one result of disseminated intravascular coagulation. Sequestration by the spleen may reduce the platelet count through pooling into the spleen. A dilution effect may be a result of massive blood transfusion. It is also important to remember this dilution effect when transfusing an individual with a low platelet count.

Bleeding from the mucous membranes is characteristic of thrombocytopenia. Conjunctival haemorrhages, nose bleeds, bleeding gums as well as skin bruising are all common sites of bleeding. Heavy menstrual blood loss or gastrointestinal bleeding may also be a feature. Intracranial bleeding is a less common but very serious complication of a low platelet count.

Immune thrombocytopenia

Drugs (e.g. quinine, heparin), infections (e.g. malaria, Epstein–Barr virus), connective tissue diseases (e.g. systemic lupus erythematosus) and some malignancies (e.g. chronic lymphocytic leukaemia) are associated with immune thrombocytopenias.

Idiopathic thrombocytopenia purpura (ITP), as the name implies, is a spontaneous event involving the systematic destruction of platelets by the reticuloendothelial system. These platelets have previously been coated with antibody through an autoimmune process. Acute ITP is predominantly a disease of childhood and often follows a viral illness. The platelet count often falls to below 20×10^9/L and may lead to spontaneous bleeding. The problem may resolve spontaneously or may require steroid therapy or intravenous immunoglobulin.

Chronic ITP is a disease of adulthood and is more insidious in nature. It rarely resolves spontaneously and may become a lifelong illness. The platelet count varies in chronic ITP, and very mild cases may not initially require treatment. For those whose platelet count puts them at risk of spontaneous bleeding or who have signs of active bleeding, therapy in the form of oral corticosteroids or intravenous immunoglobulin (IVIg) may be required. A splenectomy may be considered for patients who fail to maintain satisfactory platelet counts despite therapy with corticosteroids or IVIg. Other treatments for those who remain refractory to conventional therapy include other immunosuppressant drugs such as cyclophosphamide or azathioprine. Other immunomodulating agents such as IFN-α, Anti CD20 antibody (Rituximab) or Campath 1H have been used with some success (BSH Guidelines 2003, see Further Reading).

Platelet function disorders

Defects of platelet function may either be hereditary or acquired. Aspirin therapy, for example, is a common cause of an acquired platelet function defect. Platelet function can be assessed in a variety of ways. A bleeding time is a direct assessment of the formation of a **platelet plug** in a wound. This is done by making a small incision in the patient's forearm and recording the time to the cessation of bleeding. Platelet aggregation studies can also be used to assess platelet response to the common agonists (e.g. adenosine diphosphate (ADP), collagen) involved in the formation of an effective platelet plug. More specialist tests may also be required to diagnose the more obscure causes of platelet dysfunction.

Impairment may result from a failure of any of the stages of platelet plug formation; however, the majority of the syndromes associated with these defects are relatively rare.

COAGULATION FACTOR DEFICIENCIES

Deficiencies in blood **clotting** factors may be inherited or, less frequently, acquired. Failure of coagulation may be result of a deficiency in factor production, clotting factors that are either structurally or functionally abnormal, presence of antibodies to clotting factors, or excessive consumption of clotting factors. The next section describes the most common disorders of clotting factors, including haemophilia A and B and von Willebrand disease.

Haemophilia

Haemophilia is an X-linked recessive inherited disorder that leads to a deficiency in either factor VIII (haemophilia A) or factor IX (haemophilia B or Christmas disease). As the genetic defect is carried on an X chromosome, it is transmitted from mother to son. Men inherit an X chromosome from their mother and a Y chromosome from their father. Women inherit two X chromosomes, one from each parent. As this abnormality is carried on the X chromosome, men who inherit the abnormal gene are automatically affected as they have only one X chromosome. Women who inherit the abnormal gene also inherit a normal gene on the second X chromosome and therefore only become carriers of the disease. For this reason, haemophilia is a disease that almost exclusively affects men (Fig. 14.12). It is interesting to note, however, that occasionally women have been born with haemophilia. This could occur if a female carrier and a male haemophiliac were to have children. In practice, this is a very rare occurrence but there have been documented cases

(Tuddenham and Laffan 1999). It is also thought that a proportion of new cases of haemophilia, as in families with no known history of the disease, may be due to spontaneous mutations.

Clinical characteristics

Haemophilia is usually recognized in the first year of life, often once the child begins to crawl. Transplacental transfer of clotting factors from the mother to the fetus prevents excessive bleeding at birth but in some cases, there may be persistent bleeding from the umbilical cord. Persistent bleeding when the infant is circumcised or injured can also lead to early diagnosis of the disorder. Some babies present with large bruises, leading to the suspicion of non-accidental injury. This may be a source of great stress and trauma for parents and families until an accurate diagnosis is made. A sensitive approach to assessment and diagnosis in these circumstances is vital.

The severity of bleeding is closely related to the individual's factor VIII level. Severe haemophiliacs (about 50% of cases) will have frequent spontaneous bleeding into joints, muscles and organs. Moderately severe haemophiliacs (about 30% of cases) will bleed after minor trauma and have some spontaneous bleeding episodes. Mild haemophilia (about 20% of cases) is characterized by severe bleeding after trauma or surgery (Tuddenham and Laffan 1999). The severity of the disease appears to be linked with the type of mutation found in the gene.

A key feature of the bleeding pattern is its persistence. Bleeding may be a continuous slow ooze or intermittent and continue for days. Joints, frequently but not exclusively the weight-bearing ones, are typical sites of bleeding. Some joints are more frequent 'targets' for bleeding; this leads to repeated irritation, inflammation and destruction of these target joints. Muscle bleeding is common and can cause pain and local neuropathy, as well as long-term ischaemic damage and contractures. Bleeding into soft tissues, such as the oropharynx, is less common but may cause problems such as obstruction. Gastrointestinal bleeding as in haematemesis or malaena requires investigation to exclude other possible causes for bleeding, such as malignancy. As blood is a potent irritant, repeated assaults on the integrity of joints and muscle tissue can lead to permanent and severe damage, resulting in a marked decrease in functional ability and long-term disability.

Treatment and care

The key to successful treatment of a bleeding episode is the prompt administration of clotting factors to limit the amount of blood leaking into joints, muscle or tissue. Clients frequently become adept at recognizing the onset of a bleeding episode, even before clinical signs appear. The availability of clotting factors in the home and skill in their self-administration offers the potential to minimize damage caused by frequent bleeding episodes. Although clotting factors are frequently administered as a response to bleeding, prophylactic administration of clotting factors is seen as the

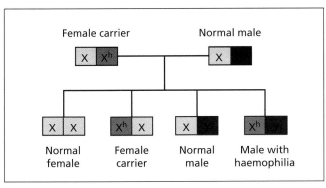

Figure 14.12 Inheritance of haemophilia. X^h, haemophilia gene; X, normal X chromosome; Y, normal Y chromosome.

most effective strategy for minimizing the often crippling long-term damage of severe haemophilia.

Two limiting factors in the provision of prophylaxis have been availability of supply and cost. Increased plasma supplies and the development of recombinant factor VIII production have increased the overall availability of clotting factors, but cost continues to be a very real problem. In the long term, however, the cost implications need to be balanced against the benefits, including reduced need for orthopaedic surgery, hospital admissions and long-term disability as well as a myriad of other important quality-of-life issues.

Complications of treatment A proportion of patients with severe haemophilia will develop antibodies to factor VIII. These are known as inhibitors. Inhibitors often develop in childhood but may occur at any point. The treatment options for a patient with inhibitors are dependent on the level of antibody and its response to factor VIII administration. In those whose antibody response is mild or whose antibody level is low, increased doses of factor VIII may be sufficient. In those whose response is high, porcine factor VIII may be an option. Others may require alternative factor infusions, in an attempt to bypass some of the clotting cascade. In refractory patients, the use of immunosuppression and immunoglobulin infusions and other complex therapies have been tried with varying degrees of success (Tuddenham and Laffan 1999).

A devastating complication of the use of factor concentrates has been the transmission of infections, of which two of the most important are hepatitis and human immunodeficiency virus (HIV). Screening for hepatitis B has been in place since the 1970s. Nevertheless, for years an unknown infective agent was causing liver disease in individuals with haemophilia. This is now known to be the hepatitis C virus (HCV). HIV infection in haemophilia was first documented in the early 1980s, and a proportion of patients now live with one or other, or both, of these viruses. The physical, psychological and emotional impact of chronic liver disease and HIV on clients and their families cannot be underestimated. Care strategies that are able to meet the multiple and complex health needs of this client group pose many important challenges for healthcare providers. Careful screening of blood products and treatment with solvents has now eliminated new transmission of HIV, HCV and other known viral agents, but it must be remembered that as yet unknown infections may pose a health threat in the future to those dependent on blood product derivatives.

Care Following a bleeding episode, local supportive measures can be instituted. An inflamed joint may require support and a period of rest, but activity and movement should be resumed as soon as possible to promote mobility. Appropriate pain relief measures must also be instituted at this time. Physiotherapy plays an important part in maintaining function and mobility in damaged joints or muscles and should be offered as part of a comprehensive care package.

The complex nature of this disease combined with the multiple problems associated with severe haemophilia have led to the development of a strategy for the provision of care and services to this client group. Designated haemophilia centres, where there is both expertise and access to a range of services, information and support, are considered key to the provision of quality care. Dedicated teams of doctors, nurses, physiotherapists and social workers combined with the availability of orthopaedic, dental, haematology, rehabilitation and other services within one locality can provide prompt, informed, appropriate services and a coordinated approach to care provision.

In the initial stages after diagnosis, one of the main functions of the nurse is to implement an effective teaching programme for the person and their family, enabling them to manage the disease and its consequences effectively. This can also promote a sense of personal control in the face of a lifelong condition with the very real risk of disability and ill health. This programme may include information about the nature of the disorder and its possible consequences, management of home factor administration, risk assessment and essential precautions, management of a bleeding episode, effective self-care measures, and effective use of services available, including emergency access and long-term support. It is also important for parents of a child with haemophilia to be given the opportunity to reflect on the implications of the disease for the child during the various stages of development and to address their anxieties. This can help them develop a more realistic view of both limitations and possibilities. An important goal is to maintain a home environment and lifestyle which is as normal as possible and to minimize the risk of overprotection and the promotion of dependency. For this, parents may require personal support and encouragement, as well as practical support.

Managing the child at school can be a concern for parents, and problems may arise from a lack of knowledge and understanding on the part of the authorities. The expertise of haemophilia centres can be used successfully to facilitate this through the provision of information and education enabling children, their parents, teachers and the education authorities to develop effective strategies that meet the child's needs in the school environment.

Self-care measures such as the management of venous access, the management of childhood illness, the use of over-the-counter medications, dental hygiene and the home management of bleeding and rehabilitation can promote a sense of independence for the client and the family. As the child gets older, parents may need support in handing over the responsibility of health management to the child.

The adult with haemophilia will have gained considerable expertise in managing the condition but may still require support in areas such as employment and the management of increasing disability. The aim in any intervention should be the facilitation of independence and personal decision-making. The Haemophilia Society, with its extensive support network, information, publications, events and campaigning, can be an effective resource for individuals with haemophilia, their families and professionals involved in their care.

Caring for the individual with haemophilia and HIV or HCV can be particularly challenging for the healthcare professional, who may share some of the great emotional strain experienced by the client, their partners and their family. Effective teamwork and a commitment to the provision of comprehensive care can help to support this particular client group.

Von Willebrand's disease (VWD) Von Willebrand factor (VWF) is a protein synthesized by endothelial cells and megakaryocytes. Its primary purpose is to bind platelets to the endothelium and it also carries factor VIII in plasma. In VWD, the factor defect may be either quantitative or qualitative, so that either the factor is in short supply or there may be sufficient amounts but it functions ineffectively. The quantitative deficiency is by far the more common. A rarer type involves a defect of the actual platelet receptor sites for VWF, causing abnormal use of VWF.

Clinical symptoms vary depending on the severity of deficiency. A minority of patients have a severe form of the disease; this is characterized by a very limited production of VWF and a marked decrease in factor VIII levels. These patients are susceptible to spontaneous bleeding, which may at times be life-threatening. This less common type more closely resembles the clinical picture of haemophilia A. Treatment of severe VWD involves the administration of factor VIII.

Milder forms of the disease reflect the reduced platelet function, with gum bleeding, epistaxis, prolonged bleeding after injury and increased bruising. Women may experience menorrhagia. Others may have noticeably increased bleeding only after surgical interventions, such as dental extractions or major surgery. Those with milder disease may require little or no intervention, except before operation. If bleeding is a problem and treatment is required, desmopressin (DDAVP) infusions can be used to stimulate the release of VWF from the body's stores. Some subtypes of VWD do not respond to DDAVP. Before a surgical intervention, DDAVP, cryoprecipitate or mixed purity factor VIII may be required. For those with a platelet receptor site defect, platelet concentrates would be a treatment option.

VASCULAR PURPURA

An abnormality of blood vessels may be a cause of abnormal bleeding. A common cause for extensive bruising in older persons is senile purpura. This results from a loss of subcutaneous tissue and collagen, leading to inadequate support of the vessels and increased vessel rupture following mild trauma. Purpuric lesions may also follow infections and certain types of septicaemia. Allergic purpura may be caused by inflammation of the vessel wall; this is precipitated by an allergic response to chemicals, toxins or other stimuli. Vitamin C deficiency (scurvy) may also cause bleeding from multiple sites. Vitamin C supplements quickly resolve the problem.

Long-term administration of steroid therapy may cause atrophy of collagen fibres, leading to a loss of support of blood vessels. Some rare collagen disorders may cause bleeding as a result of the failure of platelets to adhere to abnormal collagen after injury. Hereditary haemorrhagic telangiectasia is a rare disorder characterized by the development of angiomatous malformations in the nose, mouth, gastrointestinal tract, skin and urinary tract, which bleed easily with minor trauma. Iron deficiency anaemia is a common problem in persons with this rare condition.

VITAMIN K DEFICIENCY

Vitamin K is essential in the production of prothrombin and factors VII, IX and X by the liver. Vitamin K is derived from vegetables in the diet and from intestinal flora. A deficiency may result from a dietary deficiency, impaired absorption or defective utilization of vitamin K. Dietary deficiency is most often seen in patients requiring intensive medical care and those on high or prolonged doses of antibiotics, as these can seriously diminish the number of intestinal bacteria. Malabsorption may be the result of conditions such as coeliac disease or chronic biliary obstruction. Haemorrhagic disease of the newborn may be the result of lack of synthesis in an intestinal tract still free of organisms or low placental transfer of vitamin K, or even a low level of the vitamin in breast milk. Liver disease may also result in reduced synthesis of clotting factors, including prothrombin. Vitamin K deficiency may be treated with parenteral or oral administration of vitamin K (phytomenadione). Haemorrhage or deficiency secondary to liver disease may also require the administration of fresh frozen plasma or clotting factors.

EXCESS OF ANTICOAGULANT: HEPARIN OR WARFARIN TOXICITY

Excessive bleeding may be a result of anticoagulant drug therapy such as heparin and warfarin. Anticoagulant agents are commonly used to treat acute venous thrombosis (e.g. deep vein thrombosis) and pulmonary embolus or as prophylaxis for individuals at risk of thrombosis. Patients with prosthetic valves, arterial grafts and those with an inherited or acquired predisposition to thrombus formation are often on long-term or lifelong anticoagulant therapy. In all individuals on anticoagulant therapy, excessive bleeding following trauma or bleeding in the absence of vascular trauma may be an indication of an increased anticoagulant effect. This could be due to an excess of the drug or be the result of a drug interaction.

Unfractionated heparin disrupts the clotting process by potentiating the activity of antithrombin which, in turn, deactivates prothrombin Xa, IXa and XIa. In addition, it has an effect on thrombin and impairs platelet function. Low molecular weight heparin has a more specific activity, and is longer lasting than heparin with a lesser effect on thrombin and platelets and a lower risk of bleeding (Black and Hawkes 2005). Warfarin inhibits vitamin K action on factors II, VII, IX and X, producing an overall decrease in these circulating factors over a period of 2–3 days. As warfarin does not offer an immediate anticoagulant effect, patients may commonly need alternative anticoagulant therapy such as heparin at the outset and will need to maintain multiple anticoagulant therapy until the optimum therapeutic level of warfarin-based anticoagulation has been achieved. The anticoagulant effect of continuous heparin infusion is monitored by measuring the activated partial thromboplastin time (APPT).

Warfarin requires regular monitoring for as long as the patient is on therapy. The prothrombin time is measured and expressed as an international normalized ratio, commonly referred to as the INR. This is the ratio of the patient's prothrombin time to an international standard. Oral anticoagulant dosages can be altered to maintain the patient within a specified INR range to ensure maximum therapeutic effect and to minimize the risk of excessive anticoagulation with its increased risk of haemorrhage.

If bleeding does occur, or the INR is excessively raised, anticoagulant therapy is withheld and, if necessary, fresh frozen plasma or factor concentrates can be administered. Vitamin K may also be given but this results in a prolonged resistance to warfarin. Protamine sulfate inactivates heparin and may be used for serious bleeding however, as heparin has a short half-life, stopping the infusion or reducing the dose is often sufficient to correct an increased APTT.

Nursing responsibilities related to clients on anticoagulant therapy include assessment and education regarding:

- the aim of therapy and its possible side-effects and complications
- the importance of medication compliance and regular monitoring
- the warning signs of possible over-coagulation requiring prompt intervention
- the importance of informing relevant individuals (e.g. dentists) of drug therapy
- the importance of maintaining adequate supplies of the drug to ensure continued therapeutic levels. This includes taking sufficient supplies on holiday, etc. and obtaining further supplies in good time to avoid running out of the drug
- the potential for drug interactions, including prescription and over-the-counter medications such as aspirin-based compounds, and alcohol
- the risks associated with injury and the immediate management of bleeding.

DISSEMINATED INTRAVASCULAR COAGULATION

Disseminated intravascular coagulation (DIC) is a potentially fatal condition that is often a secondary development to a serious primary illness. It is characterized by inappro-

priate and excessive stimulation of the clotting mechanisms resulting in the simultaneous formation of multiple diffuse microemboli in the vascular system and haemorrhage resulting from the rapid depletion of clotting factors.

Common causes of DIC include:

- infection – septicaemia in particular
- shock associated with surgical trauma or burns
- malignancy – leukaemia and metastatic carcinoma
- obstetric emergencies such as septic abortion or eclampsia
- cardiac bypass surgery
- intravascular haemolysis associated with ABO-incompatible transfusion
- tissue rejection in transplantation
- liver disease such as cirrhosis.

DIC is the result of complex interactions involving an initial trigger such as damaged tissues, malignant cells or damaged endothelium. This trigger induces the activation of the coagulation cascade and platelet activation. Fibrin clots and strands form within the circulation and, in combination with activated platelets, cause partial blockage of the microcirculation, damaging red cells and inducing haemolysis. Localized clot formation in combination with this more generalized intravascular coagulation quickly leads to severe depletion of clotting factors. The liver is unable to compensate for this rapid depletion so that, as the circulating factors and platelets diminish and levels of fibrinogen degradation products (FDPs) increase, generalized bleeding ensues. There is then simultaneous bleeding and necrosis of the involved vessels and surrounding tissue.

Clinical characteristics

Diffuse bleeding may be evident as petechiae, haematuria, gastrointestinal bleeding, vaginal bleeding, epistaxis or persistent oozing from a surgical wound or needle puncture. The patient is often seriously ill and may be hypotensive and shocked. Pain may be experienced as a result of tissue ischaemia and bleeding. Organs such as the kidneys and lungs are particularly susceptible, and renal failure and acute respiratory distress are common features.

Management and nursing care

The diagnosis of DIC is made from the clinical picture and from a rapid laboratory evaluation of the patient's haemoglobin level and haematocrit (to establish possible haemolysis), platelet count, and the prothrombin and thrombin time as well as fibrinogen levels. Subsequent tests may include specific factor levels and FDP levels.

Prompt management of DIC is essential:

1 If at all possible, efforts should be made to eliminate the trigger factor.
2 Management of bleeding should be instituted to avoid hypotensive shock with red cell replacement. In the interim, plasma expanders or fluids may be required.
3 Coagulation replacement therapy in the form of fresh frozen plasma, cryoprecipitate and platelet infusion will be needed.

4 Intravenous antibiotics can be given if sepsis is suspected.

5 Central venous access should be considered to facilitate management.

6 Careful management of fluid replacement is important, particularly in the presence of renal insufficiency.

7 Respiratory management in the form of oxygen will be necessary; mechanical ventilation may be an option in some circumstances.

8 Cardiac function should be monitored and may also require support with inotropic agents.

9 Renal function should be closely monitored with careful measurement of output, and may also require support. In some instances, renal dialysis may be required.

10 Continuous monitoring of vital functions and regular assessment is an important nursing responsibility.

11 Pain management and comfort measures are also essential, as is the support of the critically ill patient and their family.

NURSING ASSESSMENT OF THE PERSON WITH A HAEMORRHAGIC DISORDER

Health history

It is important to ascertain at the outset the nature of the bleeding, the duration of bleeding, and any known or possible precipitating factors. The client may be asked to describe any abnormal bleeding such as rashes, bruising, swelling, tenderness or areas of discolouration on the skin or mucous membranes. Specific questions regarding changes that may have gone unnoticed for a period of time, such as nose bleeds, bleeding gums, increased menstrual bleeding, a bloodshot eye or a change in stool colour, may be helpful in establishing the possible history of the condition. A family history of bleeding may also help to elucidate the situation. For persons with known bleeding disorders, a history of recent episodes, expected severity of episodes, usual management strategies and commonly encountered problems may provide the healthcare team with valuable information for assessment and care strategies.

As bleeding is always a warning sign that something is wrong, the client may naturally feel anxious and concerned. Part of the health assessment may include assessment of the person's understanding and possible fears as well as support and relevant information giving to facilitate the client in coping with the situation.

Physical assessment

The person is examined for signs of bleeding. The clinical characteristics of bleeding that may be identified by inspection and palpation of the skin, mucous membranes and joints include:

● *Haemorrhage*. The bleeding may be external or internal. The amount of blood lost will depend on the size of the blood vessel(s), whether an artery or vein is ruptured, and the effectiveness of the body's clotting mechanism. External bleeding can be assessed by direct observation; the amount of blood that has soaked into the person's clothing or pooled on or under the affected part may be estimated. Arterial blood is bright red and spurts; venous blood is dark red and flows steadily. A gastrointestinal haemorrhage may lead to *haematemesis* (the vomiting of blood) or *malaena* (faeces that are black and tarry as a result of containing digested blood)

● *Petechiae*. These are small red spots about the size of a pinhead and may be seen in groups over various parts of the body. They are the result of an increased permeability of blood vessels that enables blood to extravasate (leak) into the surrounding tissue. They are a common feature of thrombocytopenia

● *Purpura*. Purpuric spots are caused by the same mechanism as petechiae, but are larger in size

● *Ecchymosis or bruise*. This is an area of extravasated blood beneath the surface of the skin that produces a patch of blue or purplish discoloration. It often occurs as a result of trauma or in platelet disorders

● *Haematoma*. This is a large bruise caused by infiltration of blood into the subcutaneous or muscle tissue as a result of a coagulation defect, trauma in thrombocytopenia or an overdose of anticoagulant. It is characterized by discoloration of the skin, swelling, pain and deformity of the tissue

● *Haemarthrosis*. This is haemorrhage into a joint, usually caused by a severe coagulation disorder such as haemophilia. It is characterized by pain, tenderness and swelling of the affected joint.

It is important to note the sites and extent of bleeding. If the person has a haemostatic defect, bleeding may occur at multiple sites. Bleeding at individual sites may also be indicative of local factors such as trauma. Baseline measurement of pulse, blood pressure and respiration rates are an important part of the initial assessment, as are blood samples for the full blood count (particularly the haemoglobin, haematocrit and platelets counts) and a clotting screen. Subsequent monitoring may then yield useful information on trends, indicating possible increased or continued bleeding as well as patient status.

Specific nursing needs of patients with haemorrhagic disorders vary with each individual and with the cause, associated symptoms and severity of the disease. Some nursing care issues are discussed under the relevant sections and further information can be obtained from the relevant texts in the reference list. Some common problems and considerations are presented in the care plan for patients with a haemorrhagic disorder shown in Box 14.5.

TRANSFUSION PRACTICE

TRANSFUSION OF BLOOD AND BLOOD PRODUCTS

The safe and effective supply of blood products depends on the availability of healthy volunteer donors and an

Box 14.5   Care plan: the person with a haemorrhagic disorder

Goal	Nursing intervention
Problem: Potential risk of bleeding due to a platelet disorder, deficiency of clotting factors, excess anticoagulant or a vascular defect	
• Bleeding will be limited due to prompt identification	1 Determine likely potential to bleed by checking current blood results (platelets, INR, etc.).
	2 Inspect the skin regularly for appearance of petechiae and purpura.
	3 Record any change in size or new areas of petechiae and purpura.
	4 Observe open lesions, incisions and intravenous and intramuscular injection sites for oozing or haematomas.
	5 Test urine and stools and examine vomit and sputum for blood.
	6 Examine joints for oedema, tenderness and limited movement.
	7 Assess symptoms of internal bleeding by recording changes in vital signs 4-hourly or as condition indicates.
	8 Observe for signs of cerebral dysfunction, confusion, disorientation or restlessness.
• Bleeding will stop with minimal blood loss and vital signs will be within normal range	9 Control overt bleeding with pressure and elevation of affected part if possible.
	10 Estimate and record blood loss in vomit, nasogastric drainage, stools, and on dressings and sanitary pads.
	11 Keep the person at rest in bed.
	12 Administer blood products and medications as prescribed, observing for potential reactions.
	13 Monitor and record vital signs regularly as indicated by person's condition.
	14 Maintain an accurate fluid balance record.
	15 Immobilize limbs or joints if bleeding is present in these areas.
• Patient will experience no further bleeding or long-term complications	16 Move the person gently to avoid causing tissue trauma.
	17 Remove objects that have the potential to cause injury from the immediate environment or ensure they are protected (e.g. cot sides may need to be padded).
	18 If there is bleeding into joints, immobilize in the optimal alignment.
	19 Provide a bed cradle to keep the weight of bedding off the affected part.
	20 Begin range of motion exercises 48 hours after bleeding stops.
	21 Use pressure-relieving aids on beds and chairs.
	22 Avoid invasive procedures, injections, etc. and minimize number of venepunctures.
	23 Apply direct pressure to venepuncture sites for 10 minutes.
	24 Take blood pressure only when essential, and rotate sites.
• Patient will express decreased fear and anxiety and actively participate in the treatment plan	25 Administer analgesia to relieve pain.
	26 Encourage questions and expression of anxieties.
	27 Encourage participation in decisions concerning treatment and care.

continued

Box 14.5 *Cont'd*	
Goal	**Nursing intervention**
• Patient will describe signs of bleeding, preventive measures and action to take if bleeding occurs	**28** Inform the person about causes, signs and symptoms of bleeding disorders (epistaxis, bleeding gums, petechiae, bruising, haematuria).
	29 Instruct patient and family to seek medical advice immediately if these occur.
	30 Discuss measures aimed at preventing tissue trauma, e.g. use of soft toothbrush, avoidance of constrictive clothing, use of electric razors for shaving, need to keep nails short and clean, need to prevent constipation and injury to rectal mucosa, need to avoid self-medication with any aspirin-containing drug.
	31 Review the safety of occupation and recreational interests and identify activities that are safe to continue and those to be avoided (e.g. contact sports).
	32 Provide information on community support available, self-help and support groups, etc.
	33 Instruct the person and family in first-aid procedures should bleeding occur.
	34 Advise the person to inform their dental practitioner of the bleeding problem before undergoing treatment.
	35 Inform patient of genetic counselling opportunities if appropriate.
	36 Suggest the need to wear a Medic Alert identification in case of emergencies if condition is prolonged.

established blood transfusion service. Both the World Health Organization and the International Society of Blood Transfusion support the principle of blood donation and collection that is not motivated by financial profit (Contreras and Hewitt 1999). It is possible that payment for blood may increase the risk of disease transmission and may also encourage concealment of relevant medical history or high-risk behaviours. However, others suggest that there is no conclusive evidence that payment increases the risk of contamination provided there is thorough screening of donors and adequate regulation to ensure safe and non-exploitative practice.

Most countries in western Europe, including the UK, as far as possible uphold the principle of non-profit provision of blood products, but in other parts of the world donors are paid for their blood donations. Worldwide, commercial companies are involved in the collection and supply of blood and, in particular, plasma products. One important factor is the relative scarcity of blood products combined with ever-increasing need. The social, political, scientific and practical issues involved in the provision of safe blood products are both a fascinating and complex subject, meriting careful consideration of the issues and debates.

The main indications for the transfusion of blood or blood products include:

• replacement of blood lost during surgery, trauma or haemorrhage
• the correction of anaemia, as in bone marrow failure, chronic diseases and haemoglobinopathies

• the correction of deficiencies in other blood and plasma components, such as platelets or clotting factors.

Donation

When blood is taken from the donor, it is collected into a sterile single-use collection pack containing a citrate-phosphate-dextrose-adenine (CPD-A) anticoagulant. Subsequent additions of plasma replacement solutions such as saline-adenine-glucose-mannitol (SAGM) permit the collection of large amounts of plasma from each donation and also increases the storage life of red cells to up to 35–42 days (Contreras and Hewitt 1999). It is important to remember the potential for interactions of these additives with drugs or other infusions. It is for this reason that safe practice guidelines dictate that no other solutions or additives be added to either the transfusion bag or giving set. Each unit of blood receives a unique identification number to enable it to be fully traced from donor to recipient. This is an important element of quality control in the event of a transfusion-related complication or an error in processing, storage or delivery. In the UK, as in many other countries, stringent quality standards are in place to ensure a safe blood transfusion service.

To minimize the risk of transfusion-related infections, donor blood is tested for HIV, hepatitis B and C and syphilis. Some donations are also screened for cytomegalovirus (CMV) to provide CMV-negative blood products for special recipient groups such as transplant recipients and neonates. All red cell and platelet products are currently also leucocyte depleted at source in view of the possibility of transmission of new variant Creutzfeldt–Jacob disease. Donors are also assessed at the time of donation for other potential problems such as a pre-existing illness or chronic conditions and for possible exposure to infections such as malaria. The donor's haemoglobin (Hb) is also tested to rule out anaemia. Each donation is typed for blood group and Rhesus factor and for the presence of alloantibodies for common blood group antigens. Other tests may be carried out according to need.

As another quality control measure, a standard label is used on each unit of blood. The ABO blood group and Rhesus factor, the date of collection and expiry, the additives used for collection and storage, and the unit's total volume as well as the unique identification number are clearly marked. Additional information specific to the unit such as CMV status, other blood groups such as Kell or Duffy, or leucodepletion will also be indicated, as required by the clinical situation. A label with the recipient details will be added at the time of cross-match to permit the correct identification of the unit and recipient in the clinical area.

To ensure compatibility between donor and recipient, a cross-match is performed. Initially the recipient's blood group and Rhesus status are determined and any antibodies to common blood group antigens identified. A number of units that appear suitable are then allocated. At this point, plasma from the recipient is mixed with red cells from the donation and observed for clumping, indicating incompatibility. If no agglutination occurs, the donation is considered to be suitable for transfusion to that particular individual. An ABO compatibility chart is shown in Figure 14.13 to serve as a general guide for red cell and platelet transfusions. Please note that this chart should *not* be used as a compatibility guide for the administration of plasma.

BLOOD AND BLOOD PRODUCT DERIVATIVES

Preparations used in transfusions (Table 14.6)
Whole blood
Whole blood is now seldom used but may be used to treat acute massive blood loss with hypovolaemia. The limiting factors in routinely using whole blood include the large volumes infused and the transfusion of potentially unnecessary blood products such as plasma, platelets and white cells with the risk they pose to the recipient, such as acute reactions or the development of alloantibodies. As donations of whole blood are routinely processed to provide a variety of other blood products, the frequent use of whole blood would also be an inefficient use of a scarce commodity.

Packed red cells
With the removal of a large volume of plasma from whole blood, a red cell concentrate can be obtained. This is

Donor blood group	Recipient blood group			
	A	B	O	AB
A	✓	✗	✗	✓
B	✗	✓	✗	✓
O	✓	✓	✓	✓
AB	✗	✗	✗	✓

Figure 14.13 ABO blood group compatibility. *Note*: plasma compatibility is the reverse.

Table 14.6 The administration of blood and blood products

Blood/blood product and composition	Administration	Common complications
RED CELLS **Whole blood** Red blood cells, leucocytes, plasma, platelets, clotting factors (500 mL/unit) **Packed red cells/concentrated red cells** Red blood cells, some leucocytes and platelets. Removal of some or most plasma gives a volume of 200–300 mL/unit **Other red cell preparations available** Red cells in optional additive solution (all the plasma removed)	Allow blood to warm at room temperature for 20–30 minutes but administer within 30 minutes of removal from the blood fridge. Check labels carefully according to hospital policy. Use a blood administration set with a blood filter inside the drip chamber. Use only normal saline (0.9% NaCl) solution for intravenous infusion before transfusion. Fill the drip chamber to cover the filter with the blood. Agitate the blood bag gently before and during administration.	Cold blood may induce venous spasm and slow or stop the infusion. Large volumes of cold blood may cause hypothermia. Transfusion reactions include: Fever Back pain Headache Restlessness Chills Dyspnoea Tachycardia Palpitations

continued

Table 14.6 *Cont'd*

Blood/blood product and composition	Administration	Common complications
Leucocyte-depleted red cells (most leucocytes and platelets removed) Red cells buffy coat depleted (leucocytes, platelets and plasma removed) Frozen red cells (washed red cells are frozen and stored for up to 10 years)	Begin the transfusion at a slow flow rate of approximately 1 mL/kg per hour and observe patient constantly for the first 15 minutes. Adjust rate if there are no adverse reactions. Record vital signs before each unit, every 15 minutes for 30 minutes, then every hour until complete. Discard any blood not transfused within 5 hours.	Thready pulse Hypotension Cold clammy skin Altered level of consciousness Risk of circulatory overload Haemoglobinuria
PLATELETS Platelets and some plasma, leucocytes and red cells (single unit packs 40–60 mL/unit) (pooled donation approximately 150 mL)	A platelet set is preferable but a blood administration set may be used. Administer as rapidly as tolerated (20–30 minutes/unit). Flush the line well with normal saline after infusion to ensure all the platelets are delivered.	Chills, fever. Alloimmunization producing rapid destruction of transfused platelets
PLASMA Fresh or fresh frozen – all plasma proteins and clotting factors (no RBC, WBC or platelets) (200 mL/unit)	Use a standard intravenous administration set. Administer as rapidly as necessary and tolerated for volume replacement. Administer fresh frozen plasma promptly after thawing to prevent deterioration of clotting factors. Requires ABO compatibility	Greater risk of allergic reactions than with whole blood. Risk of fluid overload with rapid infusions. Respiratory distress
GRANULOCYTES White blood cells and plasma with some red blood cells, platelets and other white blood cells (200–300 mL per suspension)	Use a standard blood administration infusion set. Administer first 50–75 mL slowly and observe for transfusion reaction. Administer over 1–2 hours. Use within 24 hours of collection.	Chills, fever, allergic reactions (urticaria, wheezing), hypotension, shock, respiratory distress
ALBUMIN (PLASMA PROTEIN FRACTION (PPF)) Albumin with plasma and normal saline (isotonic 4.5% or 5% in 50–1000 mL bottles; concentrated 20% or 25% in 20–100 mL bottles) PPF (plasma protein) – at least 85% albumin and saline (100, 250 and 500 mL bottles)	The rate of administration depends on the reason for administration. It is administered rapidly for volume expansion, but is usually given slowly. Use standard administration set with filtered air inlet.	Fluid volume overload, allergic reactions, hypotension, chills, fever
CLOTTING FACTORS Cryoprecipitated antihaemolytic factors	Administer by standard intravenous drip set. Administer promptly on thawing. Multiple units are usually administered.	Chills and fever
Factor VIII concentrate	Reconstitute freeze-dried powder with a small volume of sterile water for injection. Administer by syringe as an intravenous bolus through a butterfly needle. Use within 30 minutes of preparation.	Short half-life of factor VIII means several administrations of the concentrate may be required to control bleeding. Chills, fever, allergic reactions
Factor IX concentrate	As above	

commonly used to treat a variety of anaemias. One other advantage of packed red cells is that a greater number of cells can be transfused in a given volume as compared to whole blood, so that maximum benefit can be obtained from the transfusion with a lesser risk of circulatory overload.

Platelets

Platelets can be concentrated from individual units of whole blood or obtained directly from a donor using a cell separator. These are suspended in a small volume of plasma, and have a maximum shelf-life of 5 days. Platelets require storage at room temperature and a steady supply of oxygen for survival. They are generally stored in a platelet agitator and, once removed, should be administered promptly to ensure maximum platelet survival. Platelets are used to prevent or control bleeding in patients with thrombocytopenia. ABO and Rhesus compatibility is strongly recommended, particularly for patients requiring multiple or long-term transfusions, as there is a risk of alloimmunization with subsequent platelet destruction as well as febrile transfusion reactions. However, this is not always absolutely essential and may depend on availability of platelets. If Rhesus-positive platelets are transfused to an Rh-negative recipient, anti-D immunoglobulin may be considered to prevent alloimmunization.

Granulocyte concentrates

White blood cells from an ABO-compatible donor can be collected using an apheresis procedure. Alternatively, white cells can be obtained from whole blood collections. Blood is separated into its various components and white cells and platelets are found in a 'buffy coat' at the interface between the red cells and the blood plasma. White cells are very fragile and must be transfused within hours of collection. Transfusion of white cells may occasionally be considered in profoundly neutropenic patients with life-threatening infections, but are used infrequently because there is little evidence for their therapeutic effect (Mehta and Hoffbrand 2000).

Plasma

Fresh frozen plasma (FFP) is separated from whole blood shortly after collection and rapidly frozen to ensure the viability of certain clotting factors, namely factors V and VIII. FFP contains all of the coagulation factors and plasma proteins and, once defrosted, must be transfused promptly. Blood group-compatible FFP must be used. Single donor plasma is separated from whole blood up to 18 hours after collection and lacks the more fragile clotting factors.

Coagulation factors

Cryoprecipitate is prepared from plasma that has been frozen with subsequent controlled thawing, and contains fibrinogen and factor VIII. It can be used, for example, for patients with DIC or liver disease. Coagulation factor concentrates are available as high-purity freeze-dried powders. A variety of factors are available in this form, including factor VIII used in the treatment of haemophilia A and factor IX for haemophilia B. In many clinical situations, coagulation factor concentrates have superseded the use of cryoprecipitate.

Albumin

This is prepared from plasma and is available in different solutions. It is used to expand plasma volume rapidly in severe hypovolaemia, such as in burns or shock.

NURSING RESPONSIBILITIES

The safe administration of blood products is an important nursing responsibility. The nurse managing the transfusion should have sound knowledge of safe transfusion practice and the appropriate clinical skills to assist in the management of any adverse transfusion-associated reactions. The nurse should also have effective skills in the education and psychological support of the patient, who may naturally be anxious about the procedure and its possible side-effects. Patients are often particularly concerned about the risks of infection transmission and should have their concerns addressed to their satisfaction. Appropriate information and support can help clients make an informed decision about the procedure. During any transfusion, it is important to consider the client's comfort, particularly as mobility may be restricted for long periods. It may, for example, be feasible for the transfusion to be interrupted at an appropriate juncture to enable the patient to have uninterrupted sleep. It is in circumstances such as these that appropriate knowledge and effective teamwork and communication can improve the overall care of the client.

Collection and storage of red cells

It is important always to follow the local policy for the collection of blood, as this provides some important safety measures. Once collected, blood should be stored only in designated refrigerators and each unit of blood should remain in storage at 4°C until required for use. Individual blood bags should not be kept out of the refrigerator for more than 30 minutes before transfusion.

Checks prior to transfusion

It is important to remember that the systematic use of appropriate checking procedures and vigilance ultimately offers the final protection to the patient. Becoming familiar with and following local guidelines for the checking of blood products before transfusion are key safety elements. It is important that all the information on the transfusion request form, on the compatibility label, on the unit of blood and on the patient's identification bracelet correspond. If any discrepancies are noted – no matter how trivial they may seem – these should be challenged and the transfusion postponed until the discrepancy has been clarified. All queries should be referred promptly to the relevant staff and/or to the prescribing medical officer.

Administration

It is always important to use a standard blood administration set with an integral filter to prevent the transfusion of small clots or lysed cells into the patient's circulation. Giving sets should be changed every 12 hours or when a transfusion is complete and before the next one starts (BCSH 1999). The minimum infusion time is a clinical decision and depends on a variety of factors, including the client's general health and the reason for transfusion. The maximum infusion time for a unit of blood is 5 hours because of the risk of bacterial contamination and the deterioration of red cells (UK Blood Transfusion Services 2001). No medications or other infusion solutions should be added to the blood bag or the giving set during the transfusion, as there may be significant interactions or red cell lysis. Best practice dictates that other infusions should be given through a separate line. At the end of the transfusion it is important *not* to run normal saline through the giving set, as this can again introduce lysed red cells and small clots into the circulation.

Monitoring

Monitoring for signs of incompatibility or other adverse reactions is essential to good transfusion practice. Although reactions frequently occur during the first 20–30 minutes of the transfusion, it is imperative to keep vigilant throughout. Current guidelines (UK Blood Transfusion Services 2001) indicate the patient's baseline pulse, temperature, respiration rate and blood pressure are taken prior to the *start of each unit of blood*. At 15 and 30 minutes, the patient's pulse, respiration rate and temperature are again measured. Thereafter, frequent checks of the person's general condition should be made. It is likely, however, that individual Trusts will have local policies regarding monitoring, reflecting local risk assessments. It is also important to monitor fluid balance during the transfusion and to be alert for signs of circulatory overload. In the event of a transfusion reaction, it is important to store all of the used and/or partially used bags safely for return to the blood laboratory.

Documentation

Careful documentation of the checking process, the monitoring process, the patient's progress and the time element of the transfusion are all-important aspects of safe practice. This is particularly relevant as some complications of transfusion are delayed and careful record-keeping can then provide vital information.

Disposal

Empty blood bags are normally stored locally for at least 72 hours in case of a delayed transfusion reaction. Safe disposal of blood products is an important health and safety issue.

TRANSFUSION REACTIONS

The transfusion of a blood product carries with it some inherent risks. Any blood product could potentially generate an immune response in the recipient. This immune response may take the form of an allergic reaction, a new attack to what the body perceives as a foreign protein, or an antibody response to an unwelcome antigen. Other complex mechan-

isms underlie some of the potential complications of transfusion. Blood products can also transmit infections from donor to recipient and may create problems such as circulatory overload in the susceptible individual. The transfusion reactions discussed below include immediate and delayed haemolytic, febrile non-haemolytic, allergic, infection, circulatory and transfusion-related lung injury.

Haemolytic reactions

Intravascular agglutination of donor cells and their subsequent destruction (haemolysis) are key features of acute haemolytic reactions associated with transfusion. The destruction of donor red cells by recipient antibodies are, in almost all cases, an avoidable consequence of human error in the transfusion process. Rarely, antibodies fail to be detected in the compatibility tests (Contreras and Hewitt 1999). Usually, however, this is the result of a failure to follow strict protocol in the procurement or administration of blood products. Mistakes in sampling or failure to check the recipient and blood unit effectively are common reasons for this serious, and sometimes fatal, complication. A meticulous approach to procedure and systematic checks are imperative.

Occasionally, haemolysis may be a consequence of transfusing lysed cells from a unit of blood that has either been left to warm excessively for long periods or been incorrectly refrigerated and stored (Contreras and Hewitt 1999). The importance of following correct procedure cannot be overemphasized.

The severity of the ABO-incompatible haemolytic reaction will depend on a number of factors, such as the amount of blood transfused, the strength of the antibody response in the recipient and whether destruction is intravascular or occurs in the reticuloendothelial system. Such reactions typically occur within 20 minutes to 1 hour after the start of the transfusion. The timing is, in part, dependent on the speed of transfusion. The patient will typically complain of pain at the infusion site, headache, back pain, flushing, nausea and breathlessness, and may experience a sense of dread. There will also be a rapid rise in the heart rate and drop in blood pressure with possible rigors and pyrexia. The patient may collapse. Acute renal failure and abnormal clotting are possible serious consequences of the acute haemolysis. In very severe cases disseminated intravascular coagulation may exacerbate the problem.

Management of acute haemolysis includes immediate termination of the transfusion, careful monitoring of vital functions and renal function, maintenance of a satisfactory blood pressure and urine output and maintenance of vascular access. All urine should be saved for the first 24 hours and tested for the presence of haemoglobin. Blood samples should be sent and the unit of blood returned promptly to the laboratory for investigation and analysis. The event should be considered a medical emergency as it constitutes a major cause of serious transfusion-related morbidity and death. A list of actions to be taken in the event of an acute transfusion reaction can be found in Box 14.6.

Box 14.6   Management of a transfusion reaction

- STOP THE TRANSFUSION

- Maintain intravenous access with a slow infusion of normal saline

- Contact medical staff for urgent assessment and management

- Save remaining blood/blood product for prompt return to the blood bank for analysis

- Check patient identity, blood product and documentation for possible error

- Monitor patient continuously: pulse, blood pressure, temperature, oxygen saturations, urine output, evidence of bleeding

- Save all urine passed. Send sample for haemoglobin determination, as required.

Delayed transfusion reactions may occur as late as 7–10 days after transfusion. They are generally caused by a proliferation of a previously undetectable antibody to a red cell antigen in the transfused blood. Patients may often be at home by the time this develops, so appropriate information should be given to the client and family to alert them to the possible signs and symptoms. Fever, rapid anaemia, a degree of jaundice and general malaise are key features.

Febrile non-haemolytic reactions

These reactions are frequently a response to donor white cells; less frequently to donor platelets. They may occur at any point during the administration, but often at 30–90 minutes into the transfusion. Often, the patient will experience chills with a rise in temperature. Occasionally, a prolonged rigor will ensue and this can be very frightening for the patient. Management includes slowing down or temporarily stopping the transfusion, administering antipyretics and reassurance.

Once other causes for the reaction have been ruled out and the diagnosis confirmed, the transfusion can be restarted and administered slowly, with appropriate monitoring. Sometimes hydrocortisone and an antihistamine may be prescribed for a prolonged rigor. This is more commonly seen as a reaction to platelet transfusions. Leuco-depleted blood may also be prescribed for patients with a history of transfusion reactions. With the onset of a pyrexia or chill, it is important to rule out the possibility of a haemolytic reaction or bacterial infection.

Allergic reactions

A severe anaphylactic reaction with breathlessness, wheezing and possible shock is a rare but serious complication. In this circumstance, the transfusion is discontinued immediately and the patient should promptly receive medical treatment. Hydrocortisone, chlorpheniramine and adrenaline (epinephrine) should be available; bronchodilators may also be helpful. Careful monitoring of the patient's blood pressure, oxygen saturation and renal function is important. A severe reaction is a medical emergency. Mild urticarial reactions can be treated with an antihistamine.

Infection

The risk of transmission of infection has already been discussed. Bacterial infections, due to a contaminated blood product or to poor asepsis in the management of the intravenous infusion, can lead to a febrile reaction or to sepsis and shock. Current processing and storage techniques minimize the potential for contamination, and effective aseptic technique should always be maintained in the management of blood product administration. The patient may develop pyrexia and feel unwell; often the response to the pathogen or toxins may be dramatic and as potentially serious as that of severe haemolytic reactions leading to rapid collapse (UK Blood Transfusion Services 2001). In this instance, aside from the supportive care described previously, the patient will require prompt administration of appropriate antibiotics.

Circulatory overload

A rapid transfusion rate and/or the administration of large volumes of blood or plasma, except in patients whose intravascular volume is depleted (such as those with active bleeding), puts the patient at risk of circulatory overload. Individuals with cardiac or renal insufficiency, pregnant women and the elderly are at particular risk. Careful monitoring of the transfusion rate, the administration of diuretics and careful monitoring of pulse, blood pressure and respiration rates can minimize the risk. Signs and symptoms include breathlessness, coughing, cyanosis and anxiety. Patients may expectorate pink frothy sputum.

Transfusion-related lung injury

Occasionally, pulmonary oedema may develop even in the absence of compromised cardiac function. This transfusion-related acute lung injury (TRALI) is thought to be a consequence of sequestration of white cells in the lung microvasculature, leading to pulmonary oedema and respiratory distress. The underlying mechanisms are not fully understood but may in part be due to donor antibodies reacting to recipient white cells. Diagnosis is made from the clinical picture and the condition may initially be difficult to distinguish from circulatory overload. It can occur either during or after completion of the transfusion, and may even occur in the initial stages of the transfusion before any significant volume has been transfused. Treatment includes respiratory support and maintenance of haemodynamic status. This is an important but often difficult to diagnose complication of transfusion therapy with a high incidence of morbidity and death (SHOT Group 2000).

In 1996, the SHOT Group started a voluntary and confidential central reporting system for serious blood and blood-product transfusion-related complications. This has led to an increased awareness of the frequency of transfusion-related complications and to some of the factors involved in their occurrence. To date, the most common incident remains the transfusion of an incorrect blood component and between 1996 and 2000, there were 33 reported deaths in the UK directly attributable to blood transfusion (SHOT Group 2000). This highlights the need for systematic and careful procedures in the supply, issuing and checking of blood products before transfusion. A guideline from the British Committee for Standards in Haematology (BCSH 1999) aims to address some of the issues involved in the prevention of wrong blood incidents.

PATIENT REFUSAL OF TRANSFUSION

Although blood transfusion is a commonly used therapeutic procedure, it is important to bear in mind that blood is a potent symbol and that different cultures and religions may view the transfusion of blood or its derivatives very differently. Refusal of blood products on religious grounds is usually associated with the Jehovah's Witness community. The origins and functions of this doctrine are discussed by Singelenberg (1990), but it is based on certain biblical references. According to the Jehovah's Witness, the concern over blood products has been justified by what they perceive to be the lack of safety or clinical efficacy of blood transfusions and by the well documented transmission of infections such as HIV and hepatitis with the use of blood products. It is important to respect individual convictions, and most courts now recognize the right of adult Jehovah's Witnesses to make this choice for themselves. It has, however, usually been judged that parents and guardians do not have the right to refuse life-saving treatment for children, so that application for court order to protect a child whose parents refuse to consent to a transfusion may be considered appropriate in particular clinical circumstances.

When it becomes apparent that an individual may refuse a transfusion on religious or personal grounds, the use of blood and blood products should be discussed with the person at an early stage. The clinical team should offer a clear explanation of the consequences of refusing treatment, and any possible alternatives to treatment with blood products should also be considered. It is advisable to document the discussion process carefully and to obtain a signed and witnessed statement if treatment is ultimately refused. It is important to remember that other persons may have either general or specific concerns about the safety of blood product therapy and these must also be addressed. In all possible circumstances, appropriate informed consent must be sought prior to the use of blood products.

AUTOLOGOUS BLOOD TRANSFUSION

This technique involves collecting and transfusing the patient's own blood. In certain circumstances it may be an acceptable alternative for someone refusing transfusion. This technique has an important advantage in that it minimizes the risk of the complications of transfusion and, in particular, may reassure the individual who is particularly concerned about the transmission of infections such as hepatitis and HIV. It is also useful in elective surgery if there is a potential shortage of appropriate blood. Surgical procedures, such as major orthopaedic or vascular surgery, that have considerable requirements for blood are ones for which autologous blood transfusion (ABT) may most commonly be considered. In total, up to 2–4 units of blood may be collected over a period of time and stored for a maximum of 5 weeks. Alternatively, cryopreservation can offer long-term storage.

Although, in the right clinical circumstances, this technique can be useful, it is not without risk. First, the risks of bacterial contamination and errors in collection, storage and correct identification and administration are no less for this type of transfusion than for donor transfusions. Second, the patient needs to be fit for the removal of one or more units of blood in a finite time period. Third, there is no guarantee that the recipient will not require donor blood in addition to their own. Such procedures do require careful consideration of the risks versus benefits in the specific clinical context.

Two other techniques that allow the use of autologous blood are: (1) preoperative bleeding and isovolaemic haemodilution and (2) blood salvage. The first method involves the withdrawal of blood from the patient between anaesthesia and the start of surgery with fluid replacement. The venesected blood can then be re-infused after the operation. Blood salvage involves the collection and processing of blood lost during operation. This is then filtered and returned to the patient. This technique is not recommended for patients with bacterial infections, bacterial contamination or malignancy.

SUMMARY

The unique nature of blood – which is the body's only fluid tissue – and its functions, concerned with distribution, protection and maintenance of a constant internal environment, result in some aspect of the blood's composition and function being affected by almost any pathological process. As has been previously stated, blood tests are frequently the starting point for the investigation of a variety of health problems.

This chapter has focused on describing disorders that directly affect the haematological system, be it the blood cells themselves or constituents of the plasma. These disorders arise for a variety of reasons including deficiency in an essential nutrient, inherited genetic disorder, infection and malignant processes yet to be fully understood. They produce numerous acute and chronic symptoms resulting in disruption to the normal daily life of affected individuals. The problems commonly experienced by individuals include anaemia, a tendency to infection and a tendency to bleed.

Care and management of the individual with these problems is discussed in detail.

The nursing skills identified as essential to the nurse involved in caring for patients with haematological conditions specifically relate to management of:

- venous access
- the patient at risk of infection due to neutropenia
- the transfusion of blood and blood products.

Other non-specific skills of assessment, health promotion and patient education are as vital to the care of these patients as to all others. Symptom management and maintenance of independence are issues for many patients with blood disorders that are chronic in nature. In others, the course of the disease may be rapid and life-threatening, as in the acute leukaemias and lymphomas. For these patients there may be ethical issues about when it is appropriate to treat aggressively, for how long, and when to focus on palliative interventions. Many nurses find difficulty in caring for patients with haematological malignancies because patients may be actively treated or experiencing the sequelae of this treatment up to the time of their death. This requires the nurse to take account of ethical principles of autonomy, beneficience, non-maleficence and justice and to engage in analysis of the burdens and benefits of treatment with the individual, family members and other members of the multidisciplinary team.

Nurses are pivotal professionals in the patient's pathway from presentation, through treatment, during follow-up and on return to independent living. For families with children with blood disorders, nurses are an essential source of support and encouragement. Thus, the challenges of caring for individuals with blood disorders are many and varied and offer great opportunities for the development of specialist practice.

REFERENCES

Arif S, Mufti A (1998) Immune, blood, and lymphatic systems. London: Mosby.

Atkin K, Ahmad WIU, Anionwu EN (1998) Screening and counselling for sickle cell disorders and thalassaemia: the experience of parents and health professionals. Social Science and Medicine 47(11): 1639–1651.

Black J, Hawkes J (2005) Medical surgical nursing, 7th edn. Toronto: Elsevier Saunders.

Bouchier I (1998) Third report of the expert group on cryptosporidium in water supplies. Department of the Environment, Transport and Regions. Online. Available: http:www.detr.gov.uk/dwi/pubs/bouchier/index.htm

British Committee for Standards in Haematology (BCSH) (1997) BCSH guidelines on the insertion and management of central venous lines. British Journal of Haematology 98: 1041–1047.

British Committee for Standards in Haematology (BCSH) (1999) The administration of blood and blood components and the management of transfused patients. British Committee for Standards in Haematology, Blood Transfusion Task Force, Royal College of Nursing and the Royal College of Surgeons of England. Transfusion Medicine 9(3): 227–238.

British National Formulary (BNF) (2005) British National Formulary #49, 2005. London: British Medical Association/Royal Pharmaceutical Society of Great Britain.

Buchsel PC, Whedon MB (1995) Bone marrow transplantation – administrative and clinical strategies. Boston: Jones and Bartlett.

Cartwright RA (1998) Epidemiology. In: Whittaker JA, Holmes JA, eds. Leukaemia, 3rd edn. Oxford: Blackwell Science, p 1–21.

Contreras M, Hewitt P (1999) Clinical blood transfusion. In: Hoffbrand AV, Lewis SM, Tuddenham EGD, eds. Postgraduate haematology, 4th edn. Oxford: Butterworth-Heinemann, p 215–234.

Davies JM, Barnes R, Milligan D (2002) Update of guidelines for the prevention of infection in patients with an absent or dysfunctional spleen. Clinical Medicine: Journal of the Royal College of Physicians of London 2(5): 440–443.

CRITICAL INCIDENT

Mr and Mrs Ng are a Vietnamese couple who settled in this country after escaping from Vietnam. They have a take-away food business. Mrs Ng never learnt to read or write English and her spoken English is very limited. She always brings her husband to the hospital and he acts as her interpreter. They have one child who lives away from home and is studying at university. Mrs Ng was diagnosed as having a non-Hodgkin's lymphoma. She had been attending the oncology outpatient treatment suite for chemotherapy treatment and had her third course of CHOP chemotherapy was just over 2 weeks ago. It was very difficult to establish how she was tolerating this treatment as she apparently insists that all is well.

The last course of treatment had to be postponed for 1 week as her blood count was too low. Mrs Ng was admitted to hospital on Saturday in a collapsed state with septicaemia. You learn that she had been feeling unwell on Friday – cold and shivery, but thought she had caught a chill. Mr Ng had phoned his GP and made an appointment for Monday morning. He had not indicated, and had not been asked, what problem his wife was experiencing. Admission was instigated when Mrs Ng's daughter came home from university on Saturday morning.

Reflection

In reflecting on this incident it would be helpful to consider what factors contributed to the development of this life-threatening situation, what clues existed that all was not well prior to the incident described, and how the risks of this type of treatment might have been more effectively managed for this woman.

Department of Health (1992) Folic acid and the prevention of neural tube defects. London: DoH.

Erba H P (2003) Recent progress in the treatment of myelodysplastic syndrome in adult patients. Current Opinions in Oncology 15:1–9.

Gillespie G, Kevaney J, Mason J (1991) Controlling iron deficiency: nutrition policy discussion paper no. 9. Geneva: United Nations Administrative Committee on Coordination/Subcommittee on Nutrition.

Gluckman E (1998) Sources of haemopoietic stem cells for allogeneic transplantation. In: Apperley J, Gluckman E, Gratwohl A, eds. Blood and marrow transplantation – the EBMT handbook. Paris: European Blood and Marrow Transplantation and European School of Haematology, p 88–97.

Greer JP, Foerster J, Lukens JN, Rodgers GM, Paraskevas F, Glader BE Pine J eds (2004) Wintrobe's clinical hematology, Vol II. Philadelphia: Lippincott Williams and Wilkins.

Hamblin TJ, Oscier DG (1998) Chronic lymphocytic leukaemias. In: Whittaker JA, Holmes JA, eds. Leukaemia, 3rd edn. Oxford: Blackwell Science, p 105–135.

Haslett C, Chilvers W, Boon, Colledge N (2002) Davidson's Principles and Practice of Medicine, 19th edn. Edinburgh: Churchill Livingstone.

Hoffbrand AV, Pettit JE (1993) Essential haematology, 3rd edn. Oxford: Blackwell Scientific.

Hoffbrand AV, Pettit JE, Moss PAH (2001) Essential haematology, 4th edn. Oxford: Blackwell Scientific.

Howard MR, Hamilton PJ (1997) Haematology: an illustrated colour text. Edinburgh: Churchill Livingstone.

Luzzatto L, Gordon-Smith EC (1999) Inherited haemolytic anaemias. In: Hoffbrand AV, Lewis SM, Tuddenham EGD, eds. Postgraduate haematology, 4th edn. Oxford: Butterworth-Heinemann, p 120–143.

Marsh JCW, Ball SE, Darbyshire P et al (2003) Guidelines for the diagnosis and management of acquired aplastic anaemia. British Journal of Haematology 123(5): 782–801.

Medical Research Council Working Parties on Leukaemia in Adults and Children (2002) Acute Myeloid Leukaemia Trial 15. Protocol for patients aged under 60.

Mehta A, Hoffbrand V (2000) Haematology at a glance. Oxford: Blackwell Science.

Rees DC, Olujohungbe AD, Parker NE, Stephens AD, Telfer P, Wright J (2003) Guidelines for the management of the acute painful crisis in sickle cell disease. British Journal of Haematology 120(5): 744–749.

Roberts PJ, Linch DC, Webb DKH (1999) Phagocytes. In: Hoffbrand AV, Lewis SM, Tuddenham EGD, eds. Postgraduate haematology, 4th edn. Oxford: Butterworth-Heinemann, p 235–266.

SHOT (Serious Hazards Of Transfusion) Group (2000) Serious Hazards of Transfusion. Summary of Final Report 1998–99. Manchester: SHOT.

Simon B, Lee SJ, Partridge AH, Runowicz CD (2005) Preserving fertility after cancer. CA: A Cancer Journal for Clinicians 55(4): 211–28.

Singelenberg R (1990) The blood transfusion taboo of Jehovah's witnesses: origin, development and function of a controversial doctrine. Social Science and Medicine 31(4): 515–523.

Solzhenitsyn A (1968) Cancer ward. Harmondsworth, UK: Penguin.

Titmuss RM (1970) The gift relationship: from human blood to social policy. London: LSE.

Tuddenham EGD, Laffan MA (1999) Inherited bleeding disorders. In: Hoffbrand AV, Lewis SM, Tuddenham EGD, eds. Postgraduate haematology, 4th edn. Oxford: Butterworth-Heinemann, p 612–635.

UK Blood Transfusion Services (2001) Handbook of Transfusion Medicine, 3rd edn. Norwich: The Stationery Office. Online. Available: http://www.transfusionguidelines.org.uk/index

Weatherall DJ (1999) Genetic disorders of haemoglobin. In: Hoffbrand AV, Lewis SM, Tuddenham EGD, eds. Postgraduate haematology, 4th edn. Oxford: Butterworth-Heinemann, p 91–119.

While AE, Mullen J (2004) Living with sickle cell disease: the perspective of young people. British Journal of Nursing. 13(6): 320–5, 25 Mar–7 Apr.

FURTHER READING AND USEFUL WEBSITES

British Committee for Standards in Haematology, Blood Transfusion Task Force, Royal College of Nursing and the Royal College of Surgeons of England (1999) The administration of blood and blood components and the management of transfused patients. Transfusion Medicine 9(3): 227–238.
Important guidelines for anyone involved in blood transfusion.
British Committee for Standards in Haematology have a number of other guidelines. These are available online: http://www.bcshguidelines.com

Corner J, Bailey C (2001) Cancer nursing: care in context. Oxford: Blackwell Science.
This text provides a range of insights on cancer, its treatment and the management of cancer-related problems. Recommended for those interested in cancer care.

Dean Laura (2005) Blood groups and red cell antigens. Bethesda: NCBI. Online. Available: http://www.ncbi.nlm.nih.gov/books
Very readable and useful introduction to red cell antigens.

European Oncology Nurses Society Biological therapies and cancer: an educational resource for nurses. European Society of Oncology. Online. Available: http://www.cancerworld.org/CancerWorld/moduleStaticPage.aspx?id=2023&id_sito=2&id_stato=1
An online resource manual on biological therapies in downloadable modules.

Grundy M, ed. (2000) Nursing in haematological oncology. Edinburgh: Baillière Tindall.
This book provides a good overview of haemato-oncology and associated nursing issues. It is a useful text for nurses new to the field as well as being a source book for those already involved in the care of patients with haematological cancers. The first section relates to diseases, the second examines treatment issues, and there is a final section on nursing care issues. A second edition is due to be published soon.

Hoffbrand AV, Lewis SM, Tuddenham EGD eds. (2005) Postgraduate haematology, 5th edn. Oxford: Butterworth-Heinemann.
An excellent and comprehensive reference book.

National Institute for Health and Clinical Excellence (2003) Improving outcomes in haematological cancers – The Manual Online. Available: http://www.nice.org.uk/pdf/NICE_HAEMATOLOGICAL_CSG.pdf
National guidelines on the management and care of patients with haematological malignancies.

Ortin M (2005) Immunotherapy of hematological malignancies: what is new? Annals of Oncology 16(Suppl 2): ii53–ii62.

This article provides a detailed overview of the use of immunotherapy in the treatment of haematological malignancies.

Sickle cell disorders. Online. Available: www.scinfo.org\booksonline.htm

An excellent website on sickle cell disorders.

Thalassaemia. Online. Available: www.thalassemia.com

An excellent website on thalassaemia.

Thomas NT (ed.) (1997) Pain: its nature and management. London: Baillière Tindall.

This book provides a comprehensive holistic approach to pain and its management. Of particular interest are the chapters on sickle-cell disease pain and cancer pain; however, the reader will also find other chapters in the book relevant, interesting and useful.

UK Blood Transfusion Services (2001) Handbook of Transfusion Medicine, 3rd edn. Norwich: The Stationery Office. Online. Available: http://www.transfusionguidelines.org.uk/index

This handbook covers all aspects of blood and blood product transfusion, and is written in an accessible style. Recommended for all clinical areas involved in blood transfusion.

Whedon MB, Wujcik D (1997) Blood and marrow stem cell transplantation: principles, practice and nursing insights, 2nd edn. Boston, MA: Jones and Bartlett.

Although now a little out of date, there is still much content that nurses with an interest in transplantation would find valuable.

Weingard RJ, Bowden RA, eds (2003) Management of infection in oncology patients. London: Martin Dunniz.

This book has useful chapters on infection in patients with haematological malignancies.

15 Caring for the patient with a disorder of the gastrointestinal system

Alison Crumbie

INTRODUCTION

People who suffer with gastrointestinal disorders can experience the most profound discomfort and disruption to their daily lives. The problems can range form mild transitory symptoms to chronic difficulties that the patient has to learn to live with. Gastrointestinal problems can also present as acute life-threatening episodes and they can occur in patients of any age. Whatever area of practice you find yourself in, you will regularly be working with people who have gastrointestinal problems or those who have the potential to develop problems. Your work as a nurse will focus on relieving distressing symptoms and anticipating problems before they occur. This chapter aims to provide an introduction to many of the most common gastrointestinal problems you might encounter in clinical practice. Assessment, history taking, physical examination, goals of care and nursing interventions are considered and treatment options are explored. Skilled and empathetic nursing care can have an enormous impact upon the quality of life of patients who experience gastrointestinal disorders. This chapter aims to provide an introduction to the wide range of nursing interventions that are relevant to this area of practice.

OVERVIEW OF THE STRUCTURE AND FUNCTION OF THE GASTROINTESTINAL TRACT

THE GASTROINTESTINAL SYSTEM

The gastrointestinal system, frequently referred to as the alimentary tract, is divided into the mouth, pharynx, oesophagus, stomach and intestines. The primary function is to provide the body cells with a continual supply of nutrients, electrolytes and water in a form that is acceptable to the system. To do so, the gastrointestinal tract performs the functions of ingestion, digestion and absorption of food and fluid into the blood and elimination of residue and waste products.

Structural divisions of the gastrointestinal tract (Fig. 15.1)

Mouth

The mouth (sometimes called the oral or buccal cavity), is lined by a mucous membrane that secretes mucus to mix with the food, facilitating its movement through the pharynx and oesophagus. The entrance to the mouth is lined by the lips that are covered by squamous, keratinized epithelial

Figure 15.1 Structural divisions of the alimentary canal.

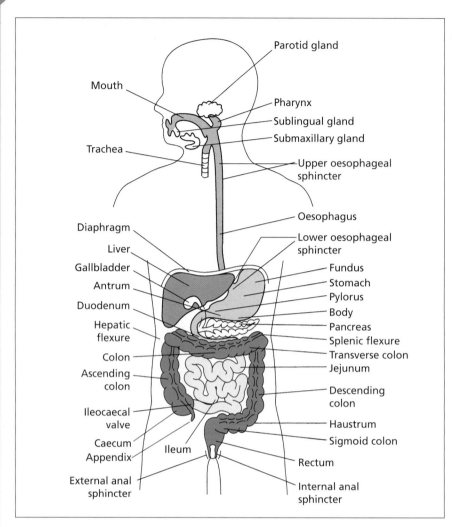

tissue which is very vascular, sensitive and has no sebaceous glands. The lips very quickly become dry and cracked in dehydrated patients. The inside of the lip is formed of mucous epithelial tissue and its superficial capillaries make this area useful in assessing for anaemia.

The tongue, teeth and salivary glands are contained within the mouth. The tongue is very vascular and is comprised of muscular tissue enclosed in mucous membrane. The superior surface is made up of papillae and over 10 000 taste buds, the undersurface of the tongue is anchored to the anterior floor of the mouth by a fold of skin called the frenulum. There are three pairs of salivary glands whose ducts open on to the surface of the mouth. The parotid glands produce a thin, watery secretion which includes an important digestive enzyme, salivary amylase. The sublingual glands secrete only mucus; the submaxillary glands produce both a watery and mucus secretion. The secretions of the salivary glands and the oral mucosa collectively form the saliva. The teeth tear, cut and grind food during mastication. Children have 20 deciduous teeth and adults have 32 permanent teeth.

Pharynx

The pharynx serves as a common pathway for food and air. Food and fluid are propelled from the mouth to the pharynx by the tongue and then are directed into the oesophagus, when the muscular tissue of the pharynx contracts. As the pharynx contracts, the band of striated muscle known as the cricopharyngeal or upper oesophageal sphincter relaxes, and the entrances to the larynx and the oral and nasal cavities are closed simultaneously.

Oesophagus

The oesophagus is a narrow muscular tube, approximately 20–25 cm long, that passes down behind the trachea, through the mediastinum and diaphragm to the stomach. Food is moved along the oesophagus by peristalsis, which is a series of ring-like contractions that occurs throughout the gastrointestinal tract. A thickened band of smooth muscle forms the lower oesophageal or cardiac sphincter, which opens when food is swallowed. Patients who have to eat when lying down or those who have increased abdominal pressure are likely to put additional strain on the cardiac

sphincter causing oesophageal reflux, which sometimes results in intense central chest pain.

Stomach

The stomach is located just below the diaphragm and is divided into three segments: the fundus, body and pylorus (or antrum) (Fig. 15.1). The mucous membrane lining is thick and lies in folds to allow for distension as the stomach fills. It contains numerous minute glands that sit in the highly folded surface epithelium. There are three types of secreting cells, zymogen cells that secrete gastric enzymes, parietal cells that secrete hydrochloric acid and intrinsic factor and mucous glands that secrete mucus. The glandular secretions are poured out into the stomach and collectively they form the gastric juice. In addition to its secretory function, the stomach acts as a reservoir for food, a site of absorption and works as a churn to mix the gastric contents into a semi-liquid substance called chyme. The opening into the small intestine is guarded by the pyloric sphincter.

Small intestine

The small intestine is the longest portion of the gastrointestinal system and is divided into the duodenum, jejunum and ileum. The duodenum is the proximal portion that originates with the gastric pylorus and measures approximately 20–25 cm in length. In addition to receiving chyme from the stomach via the pyloric sphincter, the duodenum receives bile and pancreatic enzymes from the common bile duct through the sphincter of Oddi.

The jejunum and ileum lie in loops and fill the greater part of the abdominal cavity.

The mucosal surface of the small intestine is highly folded and is covered with many finger-like processes called villi (Fig. 15.2), each of which contains a central lymph channel, and a network of capillaries. The villi have on their surface microvilli which serve to greatly increase the absorptive area of the gut. The small intestine contains many glands that secrete digestive enzymes and hormones and up to 3 L of digestive juice are secreted by the jejunum and the ileum each day. Nutrients pass from the lumen of the gut, across its wall and into the capillary network and in addition, approximately 8–9 L of water are transported from the gut into the blood supply daily. Most of the small intestine is attached to the posterior abdominal wall by a membrane called the peritoneum. The peritoneum supports the nerves, blood vessels and lymphatics that supply the small intestine.

Large intestine

The large intestine has a greater diameter than the small intestine and is divided into the caecum, colon, rectum and anal canal. The ileum opens into a pouch-like structure, the caecum, in the right lower abdominal quadrant. The appendix is a blind sac which protrudes from the end of the caecum. As the appendix is mainly made up of lymphoid tissue, it is often a site of inflammation and infection (appendicitis). At the junction of the ileum and caecum, an ileocaecal valve functions to allow contents to pass in one direction only: from the ileum to the caecum.

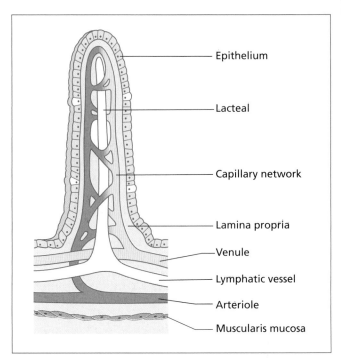

Figure 15.2 Schematic diagram of two sectioned villi and a crypt to illustrate the histological organization of the small intestinal mucosa.

The large intestine ascends the right side of the abdominal cavity from the caecum as the ascending colon, and flexes at the under surface of the liver to form the transverse colon. The descending colon passes down the left side of the abdomen and, because it takes an S-shaped course through the pelvis, becomes known as the sigmoid colon. The mucosa of the large intestine has no villi but has many goblet cells which secrete mucus.

The rectum is a continuation of the sigmoid along the anterior surface of the sacrum and coccyx. It is about 15–17 cm long.

The short terminal portion of the gastrointestinal tract, the anal canal, opens on to the body surface at the anus. The opening between the rectum and the anal canal is controlled by the internal anal sphincter, which is not under conscious control. The anus is controlled by the external anal sphincter which, after infancy, is under voluntary control.

The main function of the large intestine is to store unabsorbed foods. It is also responsible for the re-absorption of water, the active transport of sodium into the portal hepatic vein and the incubation of bacteria. The symbiotic bacteria that colonize the large intestine synthesize vitamin K, thiamine, riboflavin and folic acid although the amount produced is small and is probably not nutritionally significant.

DIGESTION

Digestion consists of both mechanical and chemical processes. The mechanical processes involve the movement of food through the tract, the mixing of it with digestive secretions, and the repeated breaking up of the food mass to

bring more of it in contact with the absorptive surface. These processes include mastication, swallowing, peristaltic movements of the stomach and intestines and defaecation. The chemical processes are chemical reactions catalyzed by enzymes to reduce the food to simpler compounds.

The digestive enzymes are substances secreted by the mucosal cells of the alimentary tract and by the associated digestive organs (pancreas and liver). They are classified according to the food they act upon. An enzyme that promotes the breakdown of protein is called a proteolytic enzyme or peptidase; one that acts upon starches is an amylase; and a fat-splitting enzyme is known as a lipase.

Digestion takes place within the lumen of the alimentary canal or the cells lining the tract. Most food undergoes several chemical reactions before it is reduced to a form that can be absorbed. The steps in the digestive breakdown of protein, carbohydrate and fat are as follows:

- *Protein*→Proteoses→peptones→polypeptides→amino acids
- *Carbohydrate*
  Polysaccharide: Starch→maltose→glucose
  Disaccharides:
      Maltose→glucose
      Sucrose→glucose and fructose
      Lactose→glucose and galactose
- *Fats*→Fat→glycerol and fatty acids.

The motility and secretions vary from one area of the digestive tract to another.

Digestion in the mouth, pharynx and oesophagus

Mechanical processes

The mouth performs mastication (chewing) and the initial part of swallowing. The pharynx and oesophagus are concerned only with swallowing. Swallowing involves certain reflexes occurring in rapid succession. When the larynx is raised, its opening is brought up against the epiglottis and the base of the tongue, thus preventing the food from entering the respiratory tract.

The reflex responses of the pharynx to the entrance of food or fluid may be depressed by local anaesthetic. To prevent aspiration following anaesthetization of the pharynx, food and fluid are withheld until the swallowing reflexes have returned. Depression of the swallowing centre in the medulla occurs with general anaesthesia, alcohol and drug intoxication, and following some cerebrovascular accidents, and can lead to aspiration of food and fluid.

Swallowed food is propelled through the oesophagus by the coordinated waves of muscular contraction known as peristalsis.

Secretory processes

The amount of saliva secreted from the salivary glands varies from approximately 1–1.5 L/day. The saliva is swallowed and much of the fluid is reclaimed by absorption. Saliva at rest has a pH of 6; with stimulation, this increases to 7.8. The alkalinity helps to retain the calcium in the teeth. Saliva consists of: water (97–99%), mucin, sodium, potassium, bicarbonate, calcium and chloride, an enzyme (salivary amylase), organisms, epithelial cells from the mucosa and antibacterial agents including lysozyme, which has an antiseptic action, and immunoglobulin A (IgA), which has a defensive action. The antibacterial agents help to prevent dental caries and halitosis.

Functions of saliva   One of the functions of saliva is to moisten the food and lubricate the oral cavity in order to facilitate swallowing. In addition, saliva has a cleansing effect, washing away food debris and maintaining oral hygiene. Saliva is necessary for the formation of a bolus, that is, a ball of partly broken up food that it is ready to be swallowed. It is also necessary for saliva to be mixed with food in order to stimulate the taste receptors in the pupillae of the tongue. Saliva contains a digestive enzyme, salivary amylase which converts polysaccharide starches into disaccharides (maltose and dextrins).

Regulation of salivary secretion   Control of the salivary glands is by the autonomic nervous system; each gland has both a parasympathetic and sympathetic nerve supply which deliver impulses from a salivary centre in the medulla of the brainstem. The presence of food in the mouth produces mechanical stimulation of the salivary glands and the impulse generated goes to the salivary centre in the medulla. Excitation of the parasympathetic nervous system results in an increased volume of a watery secretion containing the enzyme salivary amylase; sympathetic excitation causes a scanty flow of thick, viscous saliva. The generalized excitation of the sympathetic nervous system associated with fright or nervousness and stress will produce a dry mouth.

Digestion in the stomach

Gastric motility

The stomach retains the food and churns it about for a period of time until it undergoes certain chemical and physical changes. The fundus acts as a storage vessel, whereas the body of the stomach contracts rhythmically about three times per minute to mix the food with enzymes, producing a mixture referred to as chyme. The gastric contraction is continuous from the antrum to the pylorus and through to the duodenum. Continued contraction of the pylorus prevents reflux from the duodenum after chyme has been expelled into the duodenum.

Approximately 3–5 hours after the last meal, strong contractions, which originate in the lower oesophagus and stomach, sweep the entire length of the small intestine at about 90-minute intervals. They expel undigested residue and sweep debris along through the small intestines to the colon.

The presence of food in the stomach stimulates volume-sensitive nerve receptors as well as chemical receptors. Increasing volume stretches the stomach wall, which increases the force of contraction and secretion. The presence of proteins stimulates the release of gastrin and other

polypeptide hormones that increase motility and enhance antral contractions, forcing more chyme through the pylorus. At the same time, acid and enzyme secretion is stimulated. As chyme enters the duodenum, a negative feedback system operates to slow down gastric motility and secretion. To summarize, gastric emptying is controlled by the volume and consistency of the stomach content, the effects of the hormone gastrin in stimulating motor and secretory functions, and by neural and hormonal feedback from the duodenum.

Gastric secretion and digestion

The gastric glands secrete a clear, colourless fluid of high acidity (pH 0.9–1.5), which contributes to chemical digestion and changes the food to a more fluid consistency.

The constituents of gastric juice are:

- water (97–99%)
- hydrochloric acid (0.2–0.5%)
- enzymes:
  pepsinogen (inactive pepsin)
  renin
  gastric lipase
- inorganic salts of sodium, potassium and magnesium
- haematopoietic or intrinsic factor (promotes absorption of vitamin B_{12} from the terminal ileum)
- mucus.

The hydrochloric acid and enzyme content of gastric secretions are concerned with chemical digestion. Pepsinogen is converted into pepsin by the hydrochloric acid in the stomach. Once this conversion has occurred, pepsin acts on proteins to start their digestion. Proteins are broken down to polypeptides. The hydrochloric acid also destroys many bacteria which are ingested with food.

Regulation of gastric secretion The amount of gastric juice produced varies according to the types of food ingested, but with average meals, it is about 2 L/day. With fasting, the volume is reduced.

Secretion is influenced by mechanical, nervous and hormonal factors, and it is customary to describe gastric secretion as occurring in three phases: the cephalic, gastric and intestinal phases. The cephalic phase of gastric secretion occurs before the food reaches the stomach. When food is anticipated, tasted and chewed, sensory impulses from the mouth enter the central nervous system and result in parasympathetic excitation via the vagus nerve fibres, stimulating gastric secretion.

Food reaching the stomach further stimulates its secretion, producing what is known as the gastric phase. The food causes a direct mechanical stimulation of the gastric glands and initiates sensory nerve impulses that are delivered via vagus nerve fibres to the medulla, resulting in return impulses, via vagal motor fibres that increase the activity of the gastric glands. Chemical stimulation is by a hormone, gastrin, which is released by the gastric mucosa into the blood. A natural mucosal resistance prevents pepsinogen from digesting gastric tissue.

Histamine, which is produced, stored and released by enterochromaffin cells in the gastric mucosa, has been found to stimulate the parietal cells of the gastric glands, resulting in an increased output of hydrochloric acid. Two types of histamine receptors, H_1 and H_2 are present, and the H_2 receptors initiate the release of histamine which stimulates the secretion of hydrochloric acid. The administration of H_2 antagonists (e.g. cimetidine, ranitidine) aids in the treatment of ulcerative gastric disease by inhibiting histamine-stimulated acid secretion. More effective inhibition of hydrochloric acid secretion is achieved with a group of drugs that inhibit the proton pump in the parietal cells (e.g. lansoprazole, omeprazole).

The intestinal phase of gastric secretion involves an increase in the concentration of various hormones which have a number of effects including stimulation of the parietal cells to produce gastric acid; enhanced contraction of the lower oesophageal sphincter, preventing reflux; and the secretion of insulin and glucagon by the pancreas.

Digestion in the small intestine

Motility

Food moves slowly through the small intestine so that digestion may be completed and the simpler molecules absorbed. The small intestine terminates with the ileocaecal valve, which guards the opening into the caecum. The pressure in the small intestine forces open the valve and the fluid passes through into the large bowel. Muscular and villous activity of the small intestine is regulated by both an intrinsic and an extrinsic mechanism. The intrinsic control is by receptors that are associated with the plexuses, and are sensitive to stretch or irritation of the mucosa. The reflex response is contraction of the muscle tissues which initiates segmentation, peristalsis and movements of the villi. The extrinsic mechanism operates via parasympathetic impulses stimulating the muscle tissue and conversely sympathetic innervation which slows motility.

Secretion

The digestive juice in the small intestine includes external pancreatic secretions and bile as well as the secretions of the intestinal mucosal glands.

Pancreatic juice and bile Approximately 700–1200 mL of pancreatic secretions enter the duodenum daily and consist of:

- water (97–98%)
- enzymes:
  amylase (amylolytic)
  amylopsin
  proteinases (proteolytic)
  trypsinogen (inactive trypsin)
  chymotrypsinogen (inactive chymotrypsin)
  procarboxypeptidase (inactive carboxypeptidase)
  lipase (lipolytic)
  steapsin

- salts: principal ones are sodium and potassium bicarbonate and sodium alkaline phosphate.

Because of the salts, the pancreatic secretion is alkaline, with a pH of 7.5–8.4, and neutralizes the acid chyme. Bile does not contain a digestive enzyme, but the bile salts do facilitate the digestion of fat by the pancreatic lipase.

Regulation of pancreatic enzyme and bile secretion

Pancreatic secretion into the intestine is regulated mainly by hormones secreted by the intestinal mucosa. The entrance of the acid solution chyme into the duodenum causes the release of secretin (pro-secretin) into the blood. When secretin reaches the pancreas, it activates the cells to secrete a fluid high in sodium bicarbonate. Failure to produce this alkaline solution may result in damage to the duodenum by the chyme, which is strongly acid and contains pepsin. The duodenal mucosa is not as well protected by mucus as the gastric mucosa.

The liver cells secrete bile continuously, but the amount is increased when food is taken, especially fat and protein. It is thought that the hormone secretin, which excites the pancreas, may also cause an increased output of bile. The hormone cholecystokinin-pancreozymin, or CCK, causes the gallbladder to contract and bile flows into the common bile duct. It also causes relaxation of the sphincter of Oddi, and bile that has been stored in the gallbladder enters the intestine.

Intestinal juice (*succus entericus*) The mucosa of the small intestine produces 2–3 L of fluid per day. The solution, called *succus entericus*, is rich in bicarbonate, and the pH varies from 7.0 to 9.0, depending on the region of the intestine. *Succus entericus* contains:

- water
- salts
- mucin
- epithelial cells
- enzymes: enterokinase, which converts trypsinogen into the active form trypsin.

Most chemical digestion takes place in the small intestine. Any polysaccharides that have not been reduced by salivary amylase to maltose are acted upon by the pancreatic enzyme amylase (amylopsin). Disaccharidases reduce disaccharides to monosaccharides by hydrolysis, producing the simple absorbable sugars, glucose, galactose and fructose. The intestinal enzyme maltase hydrolyses maltose, lactase splits lactose, and sucrase breaks down sucrose. The final splitting of the disaccharides takes place at the microvillous level.

Protein digestion initiated in the stomach by pepsin is completed by several pancreatic and intestinal enzymes. The proteolytic enzymes reduce proteins to simpler forms, for example, trypsinogen is activated in the intestine by enterokinase and is then known as trypsin, which acts on polypeptides breaking them down to peptides. Aminopeptidases act on peptides to release free amino acids. Dipeptidases work on dipeptides and break them into single amino acids. Fat digestion is facilitated by bile, which emulsifies the fat.

Digestion in the large intestine
Motility
Contractions of the muscular tissue in the large intestine mix and knead the content as well as move it through the large intestine towards the terminal portion. Propulsion in the colon occurs as a mass movement three or four times a day, moving the content toward the rectum. When the content reaches the distal portion of the colon, it is then moved into the rectum. As the food proceeds through the mouth, stomach and small intestine, a large amount of water is added to it. Much of this water is reabsorbed in the colon, which changes the consistency of the remaining content. The latter becomes a soft, solid mass referred to as faeces.

Peristaltic movements in the large intestine are stimulated by the entrance of food into the stomach. This gastrocolic reflex results in the faeces being moved into the rectum, giving rise to the desire to defaecate. Material such as fibre holds water in the faeces and facilitates the mass movements. Lack of mixing contractions and diminished absorption combined with strong frequent propulsive contractile activity result in diarrhoea.

Faecal matter consists of unabsorbed food residue, mucus, digestive secretions (gastric, intestinal, pancreatic and liver), water and micro-organisms. The water content is progressively reduced by absorption as the faeces move through the large intestine so that, normally, on elimination, the stool is a formed mass. If the faeces are moved rapidly through the large intestine, less water is absorbed and the stool is unformed and liquid. If movement of the faeces and elimination are delayed, an excessive amount of water is absorbed and the stool becomes hard and dry.

Secretion and digestion
The large intestine is a major site of electrolyte and water absorption. It secretes a large amount of viscous alkaline mucus that lubricates the faeces, facilitating their movement through the large bowel. The mucus also protects the mucosa from mechanical and chemical injury, and its alkalinity neutralizes acids formed by bacterial action, which is considerable in the colon.

Irritation of an area of the large intestine results in an increased output of mucus as well as an outpouring by the mucosa of large amounts of water and electrolytes in an effort to dilute and wash away the irritant. This causes the condition known as diarrhoea (frequent liquid stools). The loss of fluid and electrolytes may cause dehydration and an electrolyte imbalance.

Intestinal micro-organisms Many micro-organisms inhabit the intestine, and colonic bacilli are present in large numbers. The tract is sterile at birth, but in a short time, organisms that have been ingested with food are present in the intestine. These organisms are useful in that they synthesize vitamin K, which is essential to the production of

prothrombin. A deficiency of vitamin K can result in uncontrollable haemorrhage. Intestinal bacteria also synthesize thiamine, riboflavin and folic acid. The organisms normally found in the intestine are non-pathogenic to the tract but may cause disease if they are carried into other tissues.

ABSORPTION

Absorption is the movement of food, water or drugs from the alimentary canal into the blood to make them available to the cells throughout the body. It is performed passively by the physicochemical processes of diffusion and osmosis, and by active transport by the cells. Like digestion, most absorption takes place in the small intestine. Its surface is especially adapted by the many circular folds in the mucous membrane to increase the surface area. The whole surface is also studded with millions of villi which contain epithelial mucosal cells that are specially adapted for both absorption and secretion. The network of capillaries and the central lymph channel of each villus take up much of the digested food.

Absorption in the stomach is negligible, although alcohol and some drugs are absorbed from the stomach. Minerals, vitamins, water, drugs, amino acids, simple sugars, fatty acids and glycerol are freely absorbed from the small intestine. Large amounts of water are absorbed in the colon. Approximately 500 mL of fluid passes from the small intestine into the colon daily. About 400 mL of water are absorbed from this, leaving 100 mL to be excreted in the faeces.

The water-soluble vitamins, B complex and C, are generally readily absorbed from the small intestine. The exception is vitamin B_{12}. For absorption of B_{12}, a substance called intrinsic factor is necessary and is secreted by the mucosa of the stomach. A deficiency of the intrinsic factor or of vitamin B_{12} causes a deficiency in the production of mature red blood cells. The fat-soluble vitamins, A, D, E and K, are absorbed from the small intestine if bile salts and pancreatic lipase are present.

SYMPTOMS ASSOCIATED WITH DISORDERS OF THE GASTROINTESTINAL SYSTEM

Disorders of the digestive system are many and varied; they may interfere with the ingestion, digestion, absorption of food and fluids, elimination of residue and/or with the immunological defence mechanisms of the body. The clinical characteristics depend largely on the location of the disorder in the system as well as the aetiology. Different diseases may cause similar disorders of function; making the symptoms non-specific and therefore challenging to diagnose. Health education places much emphasis on nutrition, and any interference with the ability to consume and retain food can create anxiety in the individual.

CLINICAL CHARACTERISTICS

The following section discusses some of the principal physical effects that gastrointestinal disorders have on the person. On reading this, you should consider how patient assessment may be influenced and guided by these pathological effects. Not only is it important to discover whether any of these signs or symptoms are present, but it is also important to consider how they may affect the person's life and what fears and anxieties may be generated by these physical signs of disorder. It is easy for the nurse to know that blood-stained stools are often associated with disorder of the rectum and anus, often without any malignant disease being involved; however, the patient may interpret this as a sign of cancer and understandably be very anxious and concerned. In addition, there are powerful taboos and beliefs associated with the act of defaecation that inhibit discussion of what is a very personal and embarrassing bodily function for many people. You must therefore display tact and sensitivity in assessing the patient for evidence of any of the clinical manifestations discussed below and remember that how the patient feels about any sign is just as important as the sign or symptom itself.

Pain

Pain caused by a digestive disorder may be due to strong contractions of muscle tissue, stretching of viscera, chemical or mechanical irritation of the mucosa, inflammation of the peritoneum, or direct irritation or pressure on associated nerves. It may occur in any part of the abdomen, and in some instances, the pain is referred to a site remote from its origin. For example, pain arising from a peptic ulcer or from the biliary tract may be referred to an upper area of the back.

Heartburn is a form of pain that is described as a burning sensation felt behind the sternum. It is usually attributed to irritation of the oesophageal mucosa by reflux of gastric acid fluid into the oesophagus and may be accompanied by regurgitation of some stomach content into the mouth.

A person may complain of a sense of fullness, especially after eating. Normally the stomach relaxes and distends to accommodate food without increasing the intragastric pressure. This accommodation may not occur if there is a disease, such as carcinoma, or if the patient is in an anxious state.

Significant characteristics of the pain must be noted and recorded. Meaningful clues include the duration, location and the nature and onset of the pain as described by the patient. Aggravating factors such as activity, the taking of food or medicine, or some specific experience or emotional stress may exist. Nausea, vomiting, flatulence and defaecation associated with the pain are pertinent observations. The effect of pain on each individual varies and also the pain experience varies with the cause and nature of the pain. For example, the patient experiencing gallstone or kidney stone colic writhes in agony, whereas the patient with peritonitis or paralytic ileus tends to remain immobile.

Anorexia

Anorexia is a loss of appetite for food and is a common complaint of patients with a digestive disorder, but is also associated with disorders in practically all parts of the body. It contributes to the general debilitation of patients. The individual may even express a revulsion to the odours of food. It may be functional in origin, resulting from an emotional upset.

Nausea and vomiting

Nausea is an unpleasant sensation producing a feeling of discomfort in the region of the stomach and the inclination to vomit. There may be nausea without vomiting, and vomiting may occasionally occur without being preceded by nausea. The involuntary muscular activity that precedes or accompanies vomiting is referred to as retching.

Nausea and vomiting are very common symptoms and are seen in a great variety of conditions. They may be manifestations of a digestive dysfunction, may represent hormonal changes such as occur in early pregnancy, or may accompany practically any acute illness or stressful situation.

The vomiting process is initiated by a vomiting or emetic centre in the medulla oblongata. This centre may be excited by sensory impulses originating in the stomach or intestines, by impulses of psychological origin when fright, unpleasant sights, odours or severe pain are experienced, or by impulses from a group of neurones referred to as the chemoreceptor trigger zone. The cells in the trigger zone are sensitive to certain chemicals in the blood and to impulses from the portion of the internal ear concerned with equilibrium. Vomiting in motion sickness, radiation therapy, toxaemia and as a side-effect of taking certain drugs (e.g. digoxin) results from impulses that arise from the chemoreceptor trigger zone. The sensitivity of the vomiting centre varies in different individuals; some vomit very readily and with little effort, whereas others are not affected even though the stimulus may be similar and of equal intensity. The nurse should be alert to the possible effects of vomiting, regardless of its cause. Considerable muscular energy can be expended in frequent vomiting and may result in exhaustion.

Obviously, nausea and vomiting interfere with normal nutrition and, if prolonged, malnutrition and loss of weight and strength occur. The reduced intake and loss of fluid may rapidly lead to dehydration. Loss of gastric secretion may deplete the body electrolytes and cause acid–base imbalance. Acidosis may develop as the patient becomes dependent on body fat as a source of energy. In conditions such as bulimia nervosa, tooth enamel may become eroded by persistent vomiting. The patient may complain of abdominal soreness from the retching and muscular effort, and may become increasingly anxious as a result of vomiting.

Regurgitation

Ejection of small amounts of chyme or gastric secretion through the oesophagus into the mouth without the vomiting mechanism being employed is referred to as regurgitation. It may occur as a result of incompetence of the lower oesophageal (cardiac) sphincter, as seen in infants or those with hiatus hernia, or it may be a symptom of organic disease.

Dysphagia

Dysphagia is defined as difficulty in swallowing. The patient may be able to swallow soft foods and liquids but may be unable to take firmer, more solid foods. Others may be able to swallow but complain of pain on doing so. Dysphagia may be due to mechanical obstruction, dysfunction in the neuro-muscular structures involved in swallowing such as motor neurone disease, or to diseases of the mouth, pharynx or larynx. Pain associated with swallowing can indicate an organic lesion such as an ulcer due to acid reflux from the stomach.

Interference with the transmission of food and fluid from the mouth to the stomach may be due to an abnormal condition within the oesophagus or to an extrinsic disorder. Swallowing may be impaired by a disturbance in innervation to the oesophageal muscle tissue, a decrease in or an obstruction of the lumen of the tube, or by mucosal irritation and inflammation. As the mouth, tongue and pharynx are involved in directing food and fluid into the oesophagus, it is obvious that disease in any one of these structures may interfere with the initial phase of swallowing. This may be seen in severe stomatitis, pharyngitis, tonsillitis, cleft palate and neoplastic disease of the mouth or tongue. The condition may actually interfere with the swallowing process or cause so much pain that the patient avoids swallowing.

Compression of the oesophagus by enlargement or neoplasms of neighbouring structures occurs rarely. Examples are goitre (enlargement of the thyroid), thoracic aortic aneurysm and enlargement of the mediastinal lymph glands. Dysphagia may result from a nervous system disorder that affects innervation to the central striated muscle tissue of the oesophagus. Damage to the swallowing centre in the medulla or to nerve fibres of the tenth cranial (vagus) nerve concerned with the swallowing mechanism may cause a partial or complete paralysis. Failure of the normal pharyngeal phase of swallowing may result in food passing into the trachea and the nasal cavities. The sphincter at the oesophageal opening may remain relaxed, allowing air to be drawn into the oesophagus during inspiration.

Conditions in which paralysis of swallowing is commonly seen include motor neurone disease (a progressive, degenerative disease of the central nervous system involving upper and lower motor neurones) and cerebrovascular accident (stroke). A congenital abnormality may occasionally be the cause of impaired swallowing in the newborn infant.

Loss of weight and strength

If food cannot be taken, digested or absorbed, body tissue cells are deprived of their requirements for normal functioning. Body stores and actual tissues are mobilized to meet the needs, but eventually these may be depleted. The person begins to lose weight and strength. If the problem is related to a specific food, symptoms characteristic of a lack of that particular food will appear. For example, the effects of a protein deficiency include muscle wasting, weakness, hypo-albuminaemia, oedema, anaemia and, in the child, delayed growth and development. If there is a disturbance in the absorption of vitamin K due to a lack of bile salts in the intestine, the deficiency may be manifested by bleeding, because prothrombin, which is necessary for blood coagu-lation, will not be produced by the liver.

Changes in the mouth

Changes in the mouth may be of local origin or may be associated with digestive or general disorders. General dis-orders can lead to disturbances such as a coated or furry tongue, dryness, soreness or halitosis. Changes due to local conditions may be caused by inflammation, infection, neo-plastic disease, ulcers or injury of the tongue, buccal mucosa or lips.

Hiccup (hiccough, singultus)

Persisting hiccups or frequent attacks of hiccups may be associated with organic disease of the digestive system. They are caused by intermittent spasms of the diaphragm due to digestive distension, irritation of the phrenic nerve, or a metabolic disorder such as uraemia or toxaemia, which affect the central nervous system. The frequency of the attacks and the effect of the hiccups on the patient should be noted. Dehydration, acid–base imbalance and malnutrition may develop, as hiccups may interfere with the taking of fluids and food. The hiccups may also lead to disturbed rest and the expenditure of muscular energy resulting in ex-haustion. A sedative may be prescribed if the hiccups persist.

Flatulence

Flatulence is an excessive amount of gas in the gastro-intestinal tract. The person may complain of a 'full, bloated feeling', pressure or actual pain. The abdomen may be dis-tended and the person may pass gas from the stomach through the mouth or pass (flatus) from the bowel. Exces-sive gas in the stomach or bowel is frequently due to swal-lowed air.

Excessive gas in the intestine may result from the inges-tion of excessive amounts of gas-forming foods (e.g. cabbage, turnips, onions) or from abnormal fermentation of the food due to bacterial action. Flatulence and distension occur with any obstruction in the gut and with paralysis of peristalsis.

Abdominal rigidity

Rigidity of any area of the abdominal wall due to excessively tense muscle tone may be evident in patients with disease of the gastrointestinal tract. The muscle contraction is usually a response to irritation of an underlying structure. Abdominal rigidity can be seen in advanced appendicitis where the inflammatory reaction has started to involve the peritoneum. The patient with abdominal rigidity will be in a great deal of pain and will often be unwilling to move.

Change in the normal pattern of bowel elimination

A disorder of the intestine may cause a retarded or acceler-ated movement of contents through the intestine. Delayed movement may cause constipation, whereas acceleration of the content causes diarrhoea. Whether the disorder is accelerated elimination or retarded elimination, a change in bowel habit is a significant symptom in a patient, which should always be taken seriously. This is particularly so in elderly patients who are more at risk of malignant disease and in whom changes in the pattern of bowel elimination may be the only sign that they have developed a malignancy.

Faecal incontinence

Involuntary defaecation is referred to as faecal incon-tinence. Involuntary defaecation may be caused by under-lying bowel disease, anal sphincter damage or neurogenic impairment. Faecal incontinence can also occur in patients who have a higher centre neurological disorder such as dementia, stroke or motor neurone disease. Soiling in chil-dren may not be related to a pathological process and instead may require behavioural training and psychological intervention.

Bleeding from the gastrointestinal tract

Bleeding in the alimentary canal may be manifested by the vomiting of blood (haematemesis), by melaena (the passage of a black, tarry stool containing blood pigments), or by the passage of frank blood from the bowel. Haematemesis and melaena occur as a result of bleeding in the upper digestive tract. Blood is a gastric irritant, and therefore swallowed blood, which might occur during an episode of epistaxis, may lead to vomiting. The characteristic black tarry appear-ance of melaena is due to the effect of the digestive enzymes on the blood as it passes along the gastrointestinal tract. Frank blood in the stool usually originates with bleeding in the colon, rectum or anal canal.

It may be necessary in some instances to examine the blood that has been ejected through the mouth to determine whether it has been coughed up (haemoptysis) or vomited. Blood from the respiratory tract is a brighter red and frothy because of the contained air; that from the stomach is usually darker and may contain small clots and food par-ticles. Melaena may be so slight that it goes unrecognized unless a stool specimen is examined for occult blood.

The most frequent cause of haematemesis and melaena is a peptic ulcer, but oesophageal varices, carcinoma, injuries or a blood dyscrasia may account for the bleeding. Any evidence of bleeding should be promptly reported. The patient who has haematemesis or a tarry stool maybe admitted to hospital or if they are already in hospital, they are likely to be put on bedrest. Monitoring of blood pressure, pulse, respirations, colour and general state (e.g. strength and consciousness) is important in the patient with haematemesis or malaena because the blood loss might be so great, it is important to assess for the signs of shock.

Frank bleeding from the lower part of the tract may be due to a number of conditions such as erosion of the mucosa, carcinoma, ulcerative colitis, an anorectal fissure or most commonly, haemorrhoids.

DISORDERS OF THE MOUTH

Disorders of the mouth and contained structures are numerous and may be of local origin or secondary to disease elsewhere in the digestive system or in some other system. Primary lesions may be due to bacterial, viral or fungal infection, chemical irritation, congenital malformation, injury or neoplastic disease. General diseases frequently accompanied by a mouth disorder include vitamin B complex or vitamin C deficiency, blood dyscrasias, metallic medication intoxication, infectious disease and any condition that interferes with the normal fluid and food intake or salivary secretion. Predisposing factors in mouth lesions are debilitation, poor dietary habits, excessive alcohol intake, smoking, poor oral and dental hygiene, dehydration, emotional stress and mouth breathing, or a side-effect of chemotherapy.

DENTAL CARIES

Tooth decay is a major health problem caused by the action of organisms on ingested refined carbohydrates; acids are produced which eventually destroy the enamel surface of the teeth. Tooth decay, cavity formation, inflammation and eventual loss of teeth result if measures are not instituted to prevent progression of the process. Toothache is the most common manifestation of a mouth disorder.

ACUTE TOOTH INFECTION

Infection of the dental pulp or development of an abscess at the 'root' of a tooth is very painful and may cause an increased temperature and general malaise. The person is advised to seek prompt treatment by a dentist.

PERIODONTAL DISEASE

This disorder affects the tissues that support the teeth. Development of periodontal disease is influenced by the build-up of plaque on the teeth, poor nutrition, poor oral hygiene, malocclusion of the teeth and by some metabolic disorders. Symptoms include inflammation, bleeding and tenderness of the gums and loosening of the teeth. Formation of plaque is prevented by regular brushing and use of dental floss and regular examination and care by a dentist. Bleeding of the gums or from a lesion may be present. An offensive breath may indicate sores or infection. Excessive salivation or dryness and/or disagreeable taste may be present. The individual may experience difficulty with clear speech or with swallowing.

STOMATITIS

This is a term applied to inflammation of the oral mucosa. In some instances, it may involve the gums and the lips. The mucosa is very red and tender, and ulcerative areas may develop.

THRUSH (MONILIASIS)

Thrush is caused by the fungus Candida albicans and may also be referred to as candidiasis. It may develop in the vagina as well as in the mouth. It occurs most frequently in infants and children and in the very old, but may also appear in debilitated persons. Areas of superficial ulceration occur in the oral mucosa or gums, and the membrane over the lesion becomes white and is easily detached. The condition is treated with nystatin, amphotericin or miconazole. Attention is directed to oral hygiene and also the person's diet in an effort to improve resistance and general condition.

GINGIVITIS

This is an inflammation of the gums (gingivae) followed by ulceration and necrosis. It is thought to be caused by proliferation of specific fusiform bacilli and spirochaetes which are present in only small numbers in healthy mouths. The gums are swollen and painful and bleed readily. Excessive salivary secretion and an offensive breath are usually present. There is a loss of marginal gum tissue and of the interdental papillae by the ulceration and necrosis. Lesions may develop on the buccal and pharyngeal mucosa. A smear may be made from the affected area to confirm the diagnosis. Predisposing factors are poor oral and dental hygiene, malnutrition and debilitation. It may be associated with dietary deficiencies, infections, alcoholism or a blood dyscrasia. Mouthwashes of warm saline are given frequently and normal oral hygiene measures are encouraged. The person is advised not to smoke, and a soft, nutritious diet of non-irritating foods is recommended. The patient will require treatment by a dentist as soon as the acute stage is over. The condition is infectious and can be transmitted to other persons unless precautions are taken.

LEUCOPLAKIA

This condition is characterized by patchy, yellowish-white, firm, thickened areas of the oral mucous membrane or of the tongue. The lesion results from hyperplasia of surface epithelial tissue and keratinization. The lesions are painless and are considered serious because they may be pre-cancerous. They occur most frequently in men after the fourth decade of life. The lesions usually develop in response to chronic irritation that may be mechanical, chemical, thermal or infective in origin. The lesions may disappear with elimination of the irritation. In many instances, the cause is unknown. Teeth are checked and defects corrected that may be causing irritation. Smoking should be discontinued. It is important to determine the histopathology of leucoplakia-type lesions by obtaining a biopsy to determine the exact histopathology. If malignant changes have taken place, surgical excision and radiation therapy are used.

CANCER OF THE MOUTH

Heavy smoking and alcohol consumption are the factors most associated with oral cancer. Poor oral hygiene and diet also contribute. The lesion usually appears as a small firm lump. Later the area breaks down, leaving a painful ulcer. If the condition goes untreated, swallowing and speech become difficult, hypersalivation develops, the mucosa becomes infected and the malignant growth metastasizes to the jaw and to the lymph nodes in the neck. As with all malignant disease, early recognition and treatment are extremely important.

Treatment involves surgical excision of the cancerous tissue, reconstruction using a skin flap and radiation therapy. Irradiation may be by interstitial implantation of needles or by external-beam radiation. When metastasis to lymph nodes is suspected, more radical surgery may be performed to include dissection of the cervical lymphatics, and chemotherapy may be employed. Extension of the malignant disease into the jaw may necessitate complete removal and reconstruction of the jaw. The specialized nature of the operation involved means that most patients are treated in regional units. Patients face major psychological problems in adjusting to the effects of the surgery and coming to terms with the life-threatening nature of the underlying disease. These may not become apparent until after discharge when multidisciplinary specialist skills are required to support patients. Adjustments in breathing, speech and nutritional intake may be needed as well as lifestyle changes in avoiding alcohol and tobacco use. The major oral surgical procedures that are performed most frequently for the treatment of carcinoma can be found in Box 15.1.

INFLAMMATION OF THE PAROTID GLAND

Inflammation of a parotid gland is the most common disturbance of the salivary glands and may be due to infection by the specific virus that causes mumps, or it may develop as a result of any non-specific bacterial invasion of the gland. Preventive measures include frequent mouth care and keeping the mouth moist by ample fluid intake. The disorder is treated by the parenteral administration of antibiotics. If secretion of pus develops, surgical drainage may be necessary.

OBSTRUCTION TO THE FLOW OF SALIVA

Obstruction of any one of the salivary glands may be due to intrinsic or extrinsic causes. Disease within the gland or duct may be infection, neoplasm or a calculus. Extrinsic causes such as a tumour or infection in neighbouring structures may

---

Box 15.1 Summary of the main oral surgical procedures

- Lip resection is the excision of a portion of a lip. It is usually done to remove a benign or malignant tumour

- Glossectomy is the removal of the tongue for the treatment of carcinoma

- Hemiglossectomy is the excision of part of the tongue in either the oral or the pharyngeal area

- Mandibulectomy is the removal of the lower jaw bone; it may be partial or complete

- Maxillectomy is removal of the upper jaw bone and may be partial or complete

- Buccal resection is the excision of a section of cheek (bucca)

- Radical neck dissection (*en bloc* dissection) involves the extensive excision of cervical lymph nodes and non-vital tissues on the side of a primary malignant neoplasm of the salivary gland, tongue, mouth or pharynx.

---

compress the duct, or scar tissue resulting from stomatitis may close off the duct orifice. The obstruction is manifested by swelling of the affected gland. The swelling is most pronounced during meals because of the salivary stimulation and may subside between meals. Pain and tenderness may be due to the pressure or to the condition causing the obstruction. Fever and general malaise may accompany infection.

A tumour in a salivary gland causes a more gradual swelling. It is treated by prompt surgical excision of the gland, as malignant neoplasms of the salivary glands are radiation resistant. Carcinoma involves radical surgery. In the case of cancer of a parotid gland, removal of the mandible and dissection of the cervical lymphatics may be necessary. Surgical excision of the submaxillary gland for malignancy includes dissection of the cervical lymphatics and possible resection of the mandible. Following such disfiguring surgery, a prosthesis may be constructed from a synthetic material or from the patient's own bone, grafted from the pelvis or forearm. This is implanted in the area to restore a normal appearance. The psychological trauma of such surgery is a major factor in patient recovery and extremely sensitive nursing care will be essential.

Following any operation on the parotid gland, the patient is observed for signs of facial paralysis because of the close proximity of the facial nerve to the operative site. In some instances, the facial nerve may be involved and is removed with the gland, leaving the patient with some permanent facial paralysis.

FRACTURE OF THE JAW

Fracture of the jaw is a relatively common injury in motor accidents, some sports and assault. In some cases, the patient does not need any intervention and simple analgesia and minimal conscious movement of the jaw is advised. If the fragments of bone are displaced, however, the patient's lower jaw is immobilized by wiring the lower jaw to the upper jaw or by attaching soft metal bars to the upper and lower teeth. These bars have hooks from which rubber bands extend between the upper and lower jaws, applying traction and fixation.

Following immobilization of the lower jaw, the patient is placed in a semiprone or lateral position to promote oral drainage and prevent aspiration of secretions during recovery from anaesthesia. A wire cutter is kept at the bedside; if the patient vomits, suction is applied and the wire or bands that immobilize the lower jaw must be released immediately so the mouth can be opened to prevent aspiration. A nasogastric tube may be passed and attached to low suction to remove gastric contents and reduce the risk of aspiration. Pharyngeal and oral suctioning with a small catheter may be necessary to remove secretions. Trauma and the resulting oedema of pharyngeal tissues may interfere with swallowing.

The patient will need a high-calorie fluid diet which may be given for a brief period via the nasogastric tube but as soon as possible, it should be taken orally through a straw. The patient's mouth will need cleansing thoroughly every 2 hours and after each feeding. Normal saline or a mild antiseptic mouthwash may be used, and the teeth brushed as normal using a soft paediatric toothbrush if necessary. The buccal mucosa and exposed area of the gums are examined twice daily for lesions and deposits of food, evidence of micro-organisms and epithelial elements.

Early ambulation is encouraged and the patient may be discharged from the hospital as soon as he or she can care for themselves. You should teach the patient and/or a family member the importance of good oral hygiene and how to carry out the necessary cleansing and inspection. The diet, with suggestions for variation, and its preparation and digestion are discussed in detail in consultation with a dietitian. When the wires are removed, the patient is urged to see a dentist.

History taking and physical examination of the mouth

History taking When taking a health history from a patient who has a problem with the mouth it is important to focus on specific questions associated with their oral hygiene and oral symptoms in addition to the more general questions associated with their general health and well-being. It is clear that general debility and poor nutrition will have an impact on the patient's oral health.

The following are key elements of the patient's health history relating to the mouth:

- current oral hygiene
- any pain and when it occurs
- changes in taste
- any excess salivation
- eating and drinking habits
- alcohol consumption
- smoking or use of chewing tobacco
- any previous dental or oral disorders.

General health status, current medications, occupation, medical history and family medical history are also important elements of the health history and these will be covered in the remainder of the general history-taking process.

Physical examination A tongue depressor and light are needed to inspect the oral cavity and tongue and it is important to wear gloves as you will be contacting the patient's body fluids. In a normal, healthy mouth:

- the lips are moist and intact
- breath is free from odour
- teeth are white, intact, firm and free from caries, jaggedness or plaque
- the gums are moist, pink, intact and adhere to the teeth
- the mucosa is moist, pink, soft and intact
- the tongue is pink and moist with minute papillae on the superior surface
- the uvula is central, moist and pink
- the tonsils are not enlarged.

On inspection of the mouth, it is important to look underneath the tongue and if necessary use your gloved hand to move the cheeks out of the way or to move the tongue to enable visualization of all areas of the oral mucous membranes. Observation of the mouth may elicit significant information as to the person's state of hydration and nutrition as well as manifestations of systemic disease and local disorders. The tongue and mouth are the first sites to reflect dehydration as they become dry and the tongue may be furred. Dryness in some instances may be a side-effect of a drug that is being administered. Bleeding of the gums may indicate a deficiency of vitamin C or an infection. Excessive salivation may be associated with a vitamin B deficiency, certain medications or a neoplasm in the mouth or neighbouring structure.

The lips are scrutinized for lesions (e.g. lumps, cracks, blisters, ulcers), dryness and abnormal colour, and palpated if necessary to determine the presence and extent of a mass.

Potential goals of nursing care

The individual will demonstrate:

1 Teeth that are white, intact and firm, or teeth that are in the best possible condition for the particular patient, e.g. properly fitting dentures and/or repair or reconstruction of teeth.
2 Pink, moist, intact gums, oral mucosa and tongue.
3 Understanding of the need for:
   a) daily oral hygiene
   b) dental check-ups every 6 months
   c) maintaining adequate intake of nutrition and fluid
   d) avoidance of excessive alcohol and smoking.

Nursing intervention

To maintain oral hygiene, use of a toothbrush and toothpaste is the method of choice. A soft paediatric toothbrush or foam sticks can be used by individuals who are unable to tolerate toothbrushing. These will not remove debris from the surface or between the teeth but will cleanse the oral mucosa. The stick, after immersion in appropriate mouthwash solution, should be rotated gently over the mucosa, teeth, gums and tongue, ensuring that the whole surface is used.

The choice of appropriate agent should be determined by assessing the person's needs and after assessment of the oral cavity. Turner (1996) points out that, although hydrogen peroxide is useful in dislodging debris, it has many disadvantages such as forming an excellent growth medium for candida, causing burns if not suitably diluted and causing tongue fissures. Saline solution has much to recommend it for safe effective mouth care. Petroleum jelly may be used sparingly on the lips to create an oil film, preventing loss of moisture.

You may need to provide artificial saliva and instruct the individual with a dry mouth or reduced saliva to use it to best effect. Lemon juice is particularly effective in helping to stimulate the production of the patient's own saliva.

Frequency of mouth care will be dependent on the needs of the individual and factors which increase mouth dryness, debris accumulation and plaque formation, such as continuous oxygen therapy, intermittent suction, no oral intake, or anaesthesia.

DISORDERS OF THE OESOPHAGUS

Symptoms associated with oesophageal disorders may gradually develop over time or may be present in the newborn as a result of malformation of the gastrointestinal tract. The most common malformations of the oesophagus include atresia, stenosis and tracheo-oesophageal fistula. Symptoms of oesophageal disorders that may develop over time include dysphagia (difficulty in swallowing), regurgitation, heartburn, substernal pain and bleeding.

REFLUX OESOPHAGITIS

The most common cause of oesophageal mucosal irritation is regurgitation of gastric content. Bacterial, viral or fungal infection may be imposed on the inflammation. Diagnosis is usually made on the basis of the patient's complaint of dysphagia, intolerance to hot, spicy foods, and substernal pain and heartburn. The pain may extend from the sternal area through to the patient's upper back. Endoscopy or barium studies may be performed to confirm the diagnosis. Biopsy and cytological examination of tissue of affected areas may be performed to exclude carcinoma.

If the lower oesophageal sphincter is incompetent, gastric contents reflux into the oesophagus, which leads to a burning sensation. The lower oesophageal sphincter is normally positioned within the abdomen (just below the diaphragm). In the patient with a hiatus hernia, the oesophageal sphincter is displaced into the thorax resulting in the pressure of the lower oesophageal sphincter being less than the intra-abdominal pressure, which ultimately causes reflux. Reflux can also occur in oesophageal sphincter incompetence which may be found in degenerative disorders of smooth muscle.

If a patient has chronic reflux oesophagitis, the discomfort might be relieved in part by elevating the head of the bed to reduce the reflux of acid gastric content during sleep. In addition, the administration of an antacid orally and inhibition of gastric secretion by a proton pump inhibitor such as lansoprazole or omeprazole might assist in relieving symptoms. A reflux suppressant such as Gaviscon can be used to protect the oesophageal mucosa and the patient can be advised to eat small amounts of food more frequently rather than infrequent large meals. Bending directly at the waste and any other manoeuvre that might increase the intra-abdominal pressure should be discouraged to help prevent the onset of symptoms. Smoking, alcohol, onions, tomatoes, spicy food and fatty meals should also be avoided.

The person is advised to remain upright for at least 2 hours after a meal and should avoid medication that could exacerbate the problem, such as salicylates, non-steroidal anti-inflammatories and anticholinergics. Drinking milk is contraindicated because the high calcium content stimulates gastric acid secretion. A weight reduction programme in the obese may help to reduce symptoms. If the cause of persistent oesophagitis is an incompetent lower oesophageal sphincter, surgical repair to prevent reflux may be necessary. The operative procedure frequently used is a fundoplication, in which the fundus of the stomach is wrapped around the lower end of the oesophagus and sutured to it, or a modified form of this may be performed.

Chronic oesophagitis may incur progressive formation of scar tissue leading to stricture. This may be treated by intraluminal dilatation or may necessitate surgical correction. Also, chronic reflux can lead to altered cell histology, known as Barrett's oesophagus, in the lower oesophagus. This is asymptomatic but highly increases the likelihood of developing oesophageal cancer.

OESOPHAGEAL ACHALASIA

This is the term used to describe the inability of the lower oesophageal sphincter to open in response to swallowing, accompanied by a lack of tone in the musculature above the sphincter and loss of peristalsis in that area. The cause of achalasia is unknown. The oesophagus gradually dilates above the denervated sphincter. The result is an accumulation and stagnation of food and fluids in the dilated segment.

The symptoms of the disorder are a full, uncomfortable feeling in the substernal region, heartburn, inability to belch, dysphagia, regurgitation and eventually weight loss. The person may also experience coughing and dyspnoea due to pressure on the trachea by the distended oesophagus or a disturbance in normal cardiac functioning. Pulmonary complications may also occur, due to inhalation of oesophageal contents (aspiration pneumonia).

Achalasia may be treated by repeated endoscopic dilation or by the surgical procedure oesophagomyotomy, which involves division of the muscle fibres at the lower end of the oesophagus. The food bolus then enters the stomach simply due to the effect of gravity. The patient then tends to develop reflux oesophagitis.

If dysphagia is accompanied by severe chest pain, the patient may undergo repeated cardiovascular examinations. A diagnosis of an oesophageal origin of the pain may reduce the anxiety and the dysphagia as emotional stress and anxiety tend to aggravate the disorder.

TRAUMA OF THE OESOPHAGUS

Dysphagia or aphagia may occur as a result of the ingestion of a caustic substance, foreign objects or too large a mass of food. When a caustic substance, such as a strong acid (e.g. sulfuric or nitric acid) or base (e.g. household bleach) is swallowed, serious corrosive burning occurs in the oesophagus. The larynx may also be affected, as well as the lips, mouth and pharynx. There will be evident corrosive burns on the lips and in the mouth; the voice may be hoarse and the patient experiences dysphagia and probably dyspnoea, and difficulty with speech due to laryngeal irritation and oedema. Shock may develop quickly. The mucosa becomes acutely inflamed and may manifest blisters, oedema and possible ulceration. If the chemical is not removed or neutralized promptly, burning and corrosion of deeper layers of tissue occurs. Later, with healing, scar tissue forms and the lumen of the oesophagus is constricted. Dysphagia progressively becomes more serious over several weeks as scar tissue is laid down.

Management of the person who has swallowed a caustic substance includes the following:

1 The chemical swallowed is immediately identified: the lips, mouth and clothing are examined if necessary for evidence. If a container of the chemical that was taken is available, the label is checked for suggestions as to an effective antidote. Milk may serve as a neutralizing agent.
2 Vital signs are assessed and treatment for respiratory insufficiency and shock commenced promptly.
3 An oesophagoscopy is done as soon as possible (within 12–24 hours) to determine the extent and depth of the burns.
4 An analgesic is prescribed for the relief of pain.
5 Oropharyngeal suctioning may be necessary to prevent aspiration of secretions.
6 Sips of water may be permitted. Gastric lavage and induced vomiting are contraindicated to prevent further damage to the oesophageal wall. An intravenous infusion is given to provide fluid and electrolytes.
7 A tracheostomy may be necessary if laryngeal oedema is indicated by respiratory distress and stridor. Blood gases are monitored.
8 A corticosteroid preparation is prescribed to reduce the inflammatory response and to lessen scar tissue formation and ensuing stricture. An antibiotic preparation is usually given to prevent serious infection.

9 A gastrostomy may be necessary in severe constriction in order to provide adequate food and fluids or the administration of parenteral feeding.
10 Stricture of the oesophagus is treated by bougienage; as soon as sufficient healing has taken place, bougies are placed into the oesophagus every day or two to dilate the lumen. The interval between treatments is gradually lengthened, but the dilatation may extend for over a period of 1 year or more.
11 If bougie therapy is not successful, surgical resection of the constricted area with an end-to-end anastomosis may be performed. When the area is extensive, surgical reconstruction of the oesophagus may be undertaken. A plastic tube or a section of intestine may be implanted to provide a patent passageway.

Trauma to the oesophagus may also occur as a result of injury caused by a rough or sharp foreign body. Such an injury may occur as the result of an accident when swallowing a fishbone for example or may result from an attempt at deliberate self harm by swallowing a razor blade or other harmful object. The person may experience choking and may become frightened and agitated, they may also experience dysphagia or aphagia. An oesophagoscopy is done and where possible the foreign body is located and removed. Depending upon the extent of the trauma the person may complain of soreness and dysphagia for some time.

NEOPLASMS OF THE OESOPHAGUS

Benign neoplasms

These occur rarely in the oesophagus. The most common of these are leiomyomas, which are tumours of non-striated muscle tissue. Those encountered less frequently are polyps, cysts, fibromas, adenomas and fibrolipomas. As the tumour imposes itself on the lumen of the oesophagus or interferes with normal muscle activity, dysphagia occurs. Usually the patient first experiences difficulty in swallowing the more solid foods, such as meat and bread.

Carcinoma

Cancer of the oesophagus tends to develop more often in the older age group. Its incidence is increasing and is more common in males aged 50–70 years. The lower-third of the oesophagus is the most common site. Oesophageal cancer is the ninth most common cancer in the UK and there are 7200 new cases of it each year (Cancer Research UK 2005a). The majority of malignant tumours of the oesophagus are squamous cell cancer. Adenocarcinoma may occur, but is most frequently secondary to gastric carcinoma.

The patient may complain first of dysphagia with solid foods which gradually progresses to difficulty with liquids. Substernal discomfort and pain, regurgitation and loss of weight and strength are experienced with steadily increasing severity. In advanced states, bleeding may occur. Structures adjacent to the primary lesion may become involved:

the disease may spread to the trachea, bronchi, stomach, diaphragm or associated lymph nodes, depending upon its location in the oesophagus. Diagnosis is made by oesophagoscopy and/or barium swallow. A biopsy and a smear from the lesion are taken for cytological study during the endoscopic examination.

Treatment may be by surgical resection and/or irradiation. Various surgical procedures may be employed, but many tumours are inoperable and only palliative treatment is possible. If surgical intervention is carried out, the affected part of the oesophagus is resected with a wide margin of normal tissue as well as the regional lymph nodes. If the lesion is in the lower part, the upper portion of the stomach is also removed (oesophagogastrectomy). The remaining proximal portion of the oesophagus is anastomosed to the stomach, which is drawn up into the thoracic cavity (oesophagogastrostomy). A nasogastric tube is passed and remains in place until the anastomosis is well healed and peristalsis is established.

If the tumour is located in the middle or upper portions of the oesophagus, surgical treatment involves excision and radical reconstruction of the oesophagus. This is a procedure which is associated with significant risk and therefore radiotherapy may be preferred. Relief from dysphagia in individuals with extensive disease may be achieved by the palliative surgical approach of inserting a stent or a feeding tube through the constricted area. As oesophageal cancer tends to be reasonably advanced at the time of diagnosis, prognosis can be poor. Survival depends upon the patient's general health and the stage of the tumour at diagnosis.

Nursing care of the person having surgery of the oesophagus

Preoperative care

Early involvement of other members of the healthcare team, such as dietitians, medical social workers, occupational therapists and physiotherapists, are of the utmost importance. The nurse has an important role in coordinating the multidisciplinary team, ensuring continuity and encouraging the individual to participate in therapy. Anticipatory grief and anxiety are real problems for both the person facing the operation and their family. The nurse must spend time assessing their understanding of the surgery and prognosis, provide information as indicated, identify their needs for emotional support, promote the development of coping strategies and help with the grieving process.

Preoperative preparation also includes emphasis on the promotion of respiratory function and teaching deep breathing and coughing techniques. Stopping smoking is essential for all patients who smoke. The establishment of good oral hygiene and the alleviation of infections and potential causes of oral infections are important aspects of care. The person is referred for necessary dental repairs before operation. Optimal fluid and nutritional status is an important goal, involving the administration of oral, nasogastric and/or parenteral nutrition as indicated. Fluid intake should be adequate and deficits corrected.

Postoperative care

The nurse can agree postoperative goals for nursing care with the patient and the patient's family. Principal patient goals in the postoperative period are that:

1 respiratory complications will be avoided
2 the wound will heal without complications
3 the patient will be free of pain
4 a fluid intake of 2.5 L/day will be achieved
5 weight loss will be avoided
6 the patient will be able to discuss plans for discharge and self-care.

OESOPHAGEAL VARICES

This serious condition is associated with cirrhosis of the liver and is discussed in detail in Chapter 16.

HIATUS HERNIA

The openings of the diaphragm that accommodate the oesophagus and aorta are potential sites for the herniation of abdominal viscera into the thoracic cavity. The hiatus through which the oesophagus passes is the most vulnerable area. When oesophageal content passes into the stomach it normally does not return to the oesophagus. If it does, it is referred to as reflux. The main causes of the defect in the diaphragm are considered to be a congenital weakness and the ageing process. The former probably results from a defect in the fusion of tissues around the opening. The incidence of hiatal hernia is much greater in middle-aged and elderly persons, and is probably due to weakening of the diaphragmatic muscle. The weakness or gap that occurs results in imperfect closure of the hiatus around the oesophagus. Rarely, the hernia may be caused by trauma such as a fractured rib or a perforating foreign object or the prolonged, extreme, intra-abdominal pressure that occurs in ascites or pregnancy.

The hernia may be classified as sliding (oesophagogastric) or rolling (paraoesophageal) (Fig. 15.3). A sliding hiatal hernia is one in which the oesophagogastric junction and a portion of the fundus of the stomach ride up into the thoracic cavity. In a sliding hernia, the lower oesophageal sphincter at the oesophagogastric opening (cardia) loses function, resulting in reflux of the gastric contents into the oesophagus. In a rolling or paraoesophageal hernia, a sac-like portion of the peritoneum and stomach herniates through into the thorax alongside the oesophagus. A section of omentum may also be extruded. The cardiac sphincter usually remains competent but the displaced portion of the stomach occupies space within the mediastinum and may cause respiratory distress or impaired cardiac function by direct pressure on the heart. Distension of the herniated segment or strangulation may develop, which demands emergency surgery.

The symptoms depend upon the size of the hernia and the amount of displaced viscera. Only intermittent mild

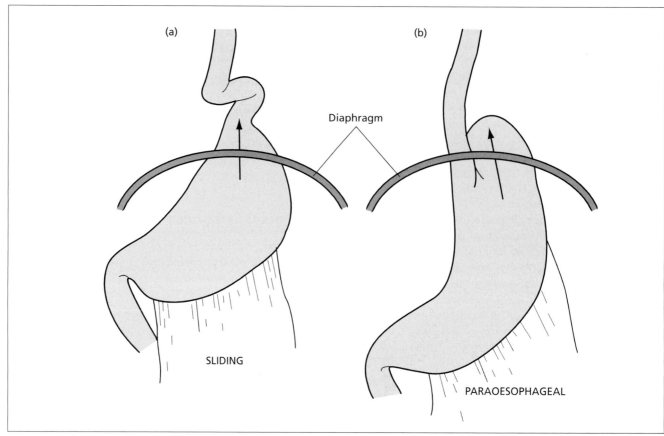

Figure 15.3   (a) Sliding hiatus hernia. (b) Paraoesophageal hernia.

digestive disturbances only may be experienced. The patient may complain of substernal burning pain or discomfort (heartburn), regurgitation of acid fluid, belching, a feeling of fullness and shortness of breath. The symptoms are frequently precipitated by the increased intra-abdominal pressure that occurs with stooping over, straining or a large meal. It may also be brought on when the patient is recumbent and may be relieved by sitting up. Frequent reflux may cause oesophagitis, ulceration and bleeding. Scarring may develop that causes some constriction and dysphagia.

Diagnosis is made by the person's history and by an oesophagogastroduodenoscopy (OGD) or barium swallow. The pain of reflux oesophagitis associated with hiatal hernia is often similar to that associated with angina pectoris and myocardial infarction.

Therapeutic management

Hiatal hernia can be managed medically and the principles of management are similar to those described for the treatment of reflux oesophagitis (see p. 439). In some situations, it is necessary to intervene surgically. If a loop of the intestine or a portion of the stomach becomes confined in the thoracic cavity, surgical treatment is necessary to return the viscera to the abdominal cavity. The surgical approach is usually made through the chest, but occasionally may be made via

the abdominal cavity. Following replacement of the viscera, the hiatus hernia is repaired. A nasogastric tube is likely to be introduced, and mild suction is applied to prevent vomiting and intestinal distension. Fluids are administered by intravenous infusion for the first day or two, and then gradually introduced by mouth when the gastric suction is discontinued.

Case Study 1 describes the management of a patient with hiatus hernia and gastro-oesophageal reflux.

CASE Hiatus hernia and gastro-oesophageal reflux

Mrs Vines, a 60-year-old widow was admitted as a day case to the endoscopy unit. On arrival, she explained that her husband died following a myocardial infarction a year ago. She has two adult children and three grandchildren, all of whom live some distance away. She has had symptoms of heartburn and 'indigestion' for over a year and attributed them to her being upset about her husband's illness and death. She was particularly disappointed to miss out on the retirement they had planned.

Mrs Vines was scheduled to have an oesophagogastro-duodenoscopy (OGD) to diagnose or exclude peptic ulcer, gastric carcinoma, gastro-oesophageal reflux disease and oesophagitis. She described the symptoms specifically as a central chest pain, which frightened her. This was associated with a burning sensation at the back of her throat before and after eating, and feeling full with only small amounts of food. She had lost weight (about 4 kg) over the previous 6 months. She was referred for OGD by her GP when ranitidine 300 mg daily at night had no effect, and a serum Helicobacter pylori test had proved negative.

Mrs Vines was accompanied by a neighbour who would take her home later. She had starved for 6 hours beforehand as advised, and had not taken ranitidine for 2 weeks prior to the OGD. Mrs Vines was naturally anxious about the procedure as the GP had briefly explained it to her. Having been assessed, she was seen by the person to perform the OGD and signed a consent form after a thorough explanation of the procedure. In the endoscopy room, she was seated on a trolley and the back of her throat sprayed with lidocaine (lignocaine) to numb it. She was then asked to lie down and a mouthguard was inserted to prevent biting of the endoscope. Sedation was given intravenously and oxygen administered via a face mask held by the nurse, who monitored her vital signs throughout the procedure. The OGD was completed without difficulty and revealed a sliding hiatus hernia of 3 cm, which could explain Mrs Vine's symptoms. Mild oesophagitis was noted from the reflux and biopsies were sent for histology. Her stomach and duodenum both appeared healthy.

Mrs Vines was then wheeled to the recovery area, where blood pressure, heart rate, respiratory rate, colour and percentage oxygen saturation were measured regularly until the sedation began to wear off. When she awoke, she was offered a cool drink. As Mrs Vines could drink this without pain or discomfort, she was given biscuits to eat. When able to move independently she was discharged home in the company of her friend. She was advised to rest for the day, and not to drive or sign any important documents for 48 hours. She was also asked to contact her GP in the event of sudden pain or fever within the next 24 hours, and to make an appointment after 2 weeks to discuss the findings of the procedure including the histology report. She was allowed to resume her medication that night.

The GP was advised of the diagnosis by the endoscopist and it was suggested that she be prescribed a proton pump inhibitor, such as lansoprazole 15–30 mg daily, and Gaviscon 15 mL as required up to four times daily after meals and last thing at night. Mrs Vines was to avoid heavy physical work or lifting. She should eat regularly three times a day, not within 3 hours of going to bed and have her main meal in the middle of the day. Tomatoes, onions, spicy foods, caffeine and excessive amounts (more than 2 units/day) of alcohol were to be avoided. If reflux continued to be a problem at night, she could consider raising the head of her bed 20–30 cm from the floor to facilitate stomach emptying and avoid reflux. Her symptoms needed to be monitored and a further OGD was indicated to check for changes in the oesophageal mucosa. Mrs Vines may require surgery in future if her lifestyle changes and the prescribed drug treatments are not effective.

History taking and physical examination of the patient with oesophageal disorder

History taking   The patient who has an oesophageal problem will tend to present with symptoms which could be related to disorders of the mouth or stomach. It is therefore important to make sure that your history taking is focused and accurate and that you listen carefully to the patient's story. In addition to the usual general history-taking process, specific questions should be focused on:

- dysphagia, when it occurs and what makes it better and what makes it worse
- pain, where does it occur, what makes it worse and what relieves it
- reflux, how long has it been present and what brings it on
- current medications (including over the counter medications)
- smoking and alcohol intake
- occupation
- medical history (particularly previous dyspepsia or oesophageal problems).

If the patient has been admitted to hospital they will probably have had a period of increasing difficulty in swallowing, leading to undernourishment. It is important to discover what foodstuffs can still be swallowed in order that the patient can be given an appropriate diet. Height and weight should be assessed and the patient asked whether they have lost weight recently. Serious undernourishment may be present and this can significantly reduce the patient's prospects of recovery; consequently, dietary supplements may be necessary and the involvement of a dietitian is important.

The person's mood and feelings about the illness should be explored. The inability to eat and subsequent loss of weight may lead to great anxiety and fear. The person may suspect cancer but not have been told the diagnosis; clearly, it is important to discover how the person feels about the illness and what questions he or she has. The patient may also see a significant change in his or her body, which constitutes a serious challenge to self-concept. The nurse needs to know how successfully the person is coping with this challenge and what methods are being used to adapt in order to approach the patient sensitively and give support.

Physical examination

Apart from assessing the patient's height, weight and body mass index, there is little physical examination that can be carried out to assess the patient's oesophagus and therefore more invasive investigations such as oesophagoscopy are necessary.

Oesophagoscopy

The oesophagus may be examined and a biopsy specimen obtained by oesophagoscopy if the patient has complained of dysphagia, gastric reflux, regurgitation, or haematemesis.

Oesophagoscopy is useful in localizing bleeding and is also used to remove a foreign body or a bolus that has lodged in the oesophagus.

DISORDERS OF THE STOMACH AND DUODENUM

GASTRITIS

The term gastritis implies inflammation of the stomach. The condition may be acute or chronic and the pathological process is usually limited to the mucosa.

Acute gastritis

The causes of acute inflammation may be the ingestion of large quantities of alcohol, contaminated foods or non-steroidal anti-inflammatory drugs (NSAIDs) (e.g. aspirin or ibuprofen). Infective gastritis is most frequently due to the ingestion of foods bearing staphylococci or salmonella organisms. The patient with acute gastritis becomes ill suddenly and suffers severe epigastric pain, nausea, vomiting and fever.

Depending upon the severity of the symptoms, the patient may be treated in the community setting where they are encouraged to drink clear fluids to maintain their hydration. As the symptoms subside, a bland diet of soft foods will be introduced and progressively increased until a normal diet is resumed. If the symptoms are more severe and if the patient has other co-morbidities and is therefore at risk of serious complications, the treatment may include giving the patient parenteral fluids and maintaining bedrest. Elderly patients or patients with chronic conditions such as diabetes could very rapidly become dehydrated if they develop gastritis and therefore intravenous fluid replacement and hospital care may be necessary.

Chronic gastritis

Chronic gastritis occurs with prolonged and repeated irritation of the mucosa and results in atrophic changes in the mucosa and glands. The symptoms of chronic gastritis are usually ill defined but may include anorexia, discomfort and a full feeling after meals, flatulence, heartburn, nausea and occasionally haematemesis. The patient may lose considerable weight as there is a tendency to restrict food intake to avoid the distress it may precipitate. Attention is directed toward improving the general nutritional status by encouraging a well balanced diet of non-irritating foods.

The causes of chronic gastritis may be unclear, as the condition may be associated with other diseases such as pernicious anaemia, and with the degenerative changes of ageing. The organism Helicobacter pylori (H. pylori) can be a significant factor in the development of chronic gastritis and peptic ulceration; indeed 90% of duodenal ulcers and 70% of gastric ulcers are thought to be associated with H. pylori infection (Livett 2004). H. pylori is a Gram-negative micro-aerophilic rod-shaped bacterium that resides in the gastric mucosa and can be acquired in childhood. Chronic gastritis may precede the development of gastric ulcer or gastric carcinoma and it is therefore a serious and important symptom.

Peptic ulcer

A peptic ulcer is the erosion of a circumscribed area of tissue in the wall of the gastrointestinal tract that is accessible to gastric secretions. The ulcer penetrates the mucosa and may invade the underlying submucosal and muscular tissues. The actual erosion is caused by the digestive action of hydrochloric acid and pepsin. The most frequent sites of an ulcer are the stomach (gastric ulcer) and the proximal portion of the duodenum (duodenal ulcer), but the oesophagus or jejunum or any other part of the gastrointestinal mucosa may be susceptible if the surface comes in contact with gastric secretions.

Normally, hydrochloric acid and pepsin are secreted but ulceration does not occur. This is attributed to a number of defensive factors. The mucosa secretes sufficient mucus to dilute the secretions and provides a protective coating that prevents mucosal digestion by the acid-pepsin action. The duodenum has the additional protection of the strong alkalinity of the bile and pancreatic and intestinal secretions which neutralize the acidic chyme. Still another defence is a healthy resistant mucosa which has a good blood supply and is capable of continuous rapid generation of the mucosal epithelial cells.

A peptic ulcer may develop when the secretory output of hydrochloric acid and pepsin is in excess of the normal or when the protective mechanisms are inadequate in relation to the amount of acid and pepsin produced. An ulcer is therefore caused by an imbalance between pepsin secretion and the body's natural defences. Stress is also involved as it causes capillary shutdown, decreasing the blood flow to the area, and a reduction in bicarbonate production, which results in an acid–base imbalance. H. pylori is thought to have a major role in the causation of peptic ulceration.

The following are potential contributing factors in the development of an imbalance between the secretion of hydrochloric acid and pepsin and the defensive mechanisms of the mucosa:

- *Stress*. Particularly associated with serious trauma and illness
- *Inflammation*. Gastritis and trauma of the mucosa reduce the resistance of the membrane to digestion. Cell destruction is accelerated and cell reproduction, which normally renews the superficial layers quickly, may be retarded
- *Heredity*. Genetic factors appear to have a role, as there is a tendency for peptic disease to occur in families
- *Medications*. Some drugs, e.g. NSAIDs (aspirin, ibuprofen) or corticosteroids (cortisone)
- *Bile reflux*. The reflux of bile and pancreatic enzymes into the stomach due to an incompetent pyloric sphincter may

lead to a gastric ulcer. The bile salts damage the gastric mucosa, predisposing it to ulceration
- *Endocrine secretions.* Rarely, severe peptic ulceration is caused by marked gastric hypersecretion that occurs in response to an excessive gastrin concentration in the blood. The gastrin is produced by a tumour of the islets of the pancreas or the submucosa of the duodenum and stomach or regional lymph nodes (Zollinger–Ellison syndrome). Peptic ulceration also develops in hyperparathyroidism. The disturbance is attributed to the altered serum calcium level
- *Histamine.* Histamine promotes stimulation of acid secretion; H_2-receptor antagonists, which inhibit histamine action, have been found in gastric parietal cells
- *Cigarette smoking and high alcohol intake* (Butler 1997).

The prominent symptom of peptic ulcer is epigastric pain with definite clinical characteristics. It may radiate to the back. The pain is usually described by the patient as gnawing or burning and of being rhythmic in its development and relief in relation to the ingestion of food. The onset of pain is variable, depending upon the location of the ulcer, and is relieved by taking food or an antacid. In the case of an oesophageal ulcer, the pain develops within a few minutes of the meal. It may be intermittent and the patient usually complains of heartburn and regurgitation. Pain associated with a gastric ulcer usually occurs 30 minutes to 1 hour after the ingestion of spicy or coarse food; that of a duodenal ulcer is delayed for approximately 2–4 hours.

The patient's rest is frequently disturbed by nocturnal pain, especially with a duodenal ulcer. Although the ingestion of food generally provides relief, in a few instances it may be the initiating factor of the ulcer pain, particularly if the food is coarse or highly seasoned. The association of eating with relief of pain ensures that the patient is not usually undernourished.

Vomiting is not a common symptom in peptic ulcer but may occur if the ulcer pain is very severe or if the ulcer is in the pyloric region. In the case of the latter, inflammation and oedema of the surrounding tissues, pyloric spasm or contracted scar tissue resulting from ulceration may narrow the lumen of the pylorus. This may delay the emptying of the stomach and may cause vomiting.

Clinical diagnostic measurements for patients with gastritis

Investigation of the patient for peptic ulcer may include OGD or barium meal, serum gastrin assays, exfoliative cytology, testing for H. pylori and stool examination for occult blood.

Endoscopy is now widely used for investigation of the upper gastrointestinal tract, for both chronic or acute disorders. The oesophagus is examined before passing the instrument through into the stomach where biopsy of any lesion and brushings for cytology may be carried out. It is possible in some instances to arrest haemorrhage by the direct application of electrocautery or a haemostatic preparation to the bleeding site. The endoscope is passed through the pylorus to examine the duodenum. The ampulla of Vater may be cannulated and viewed, and a radio-opaque dye injected to demonstrate the pancreatic and common bile ducts (cholangiopancreatography). Endoscopic examination may also be extended into the jejunum.

Nursing care in endoscopy Preparation for this diagnostic procedure should begin with an explanation to the patient of what to expect. The clinician who is responsible for carrying out the investigation may have described the examination but the patient will probably still have questions, which the nurse should be able to answer. Written consent for the procedure is required. The oesophagus and the stomach must be completely empty. No food or fluid is given for 4–6 hours before the procedure. In gastroscopy, the doctor may request a gastric lavage to be done several hours before the examination in patients in whom some pyloric obstruction is suspected. The dentures are removed and kept safe. Intravenous sedation may be given to minimize patient discomfort. The pharyngeal area may be sprayed with a local anaesthetic before the endoscopic instrument is introduced. The patient is unable to speak when the endoscope is in position and a mouthguard prevents them biting on the endoscope.

After the examination, the patient is allowed to rest. All food and fluids are withheld until the effect of the local anaesthetic has worn off and the gag reflex returns (usually 1–2 hours). Before giving any fluid, the reflex may be tested by gently touching the back of the throat with an applicator or spoon. The patient may complain of a sore throat or soreness in the mid-chest. Warm fluids may be soothing and may provide some relief. Any expectoration or vomiting of blood or severe pain should be reported promptly.

The nurse will generally encounter patients admitted with peptic ulcer in one of three situations:

1 The person is undergoing investigation and diagnosis.
2 The person is having an acute exacerbation with possible severe bleeding.
3 The person has been admitted for planned surgery as the ulcer is failing to respond to medical treatment.

Assessment will therefore tend to focus on different aspects of the patient in each of these situations.

The patient undergoing investigations may be very anxious and have fears of cancer being diagnosed. It is essential, therefore, that, in addition to the obvious physical parameters that are assessed, anxiety should be monitored and knowledge deficits explored. As health education about factors that predispose to ulceration will be a key part of the care plan, it is important to assess relevant areas of the person's lifestyle such as smoking and drinking habits, regularity and types of meals, and stress levels, all of which are amenable to health education. It is also important to discover the person's level of understanding and attitudes towards health education, as this will have a major influence upon the approach used.

In an acute emergency situation, physical parameters such as blood pressure and pulse are a high priority because of the risks of hypovolaemic shock and a major bleed which may be fatal. Close assessment of stools for melaena or occult blood, and of vomit for the presence of fresh or altered blood, is required. Pain must be assessed carefully so that appropriate relief can be given as required. The nurse should not lose sight of the patient's psychological condition, however, and should carefully assess levels of both fear and understanding in what can be a very frightening situation.

The patient being admitted for surgery should be assessed along the lines discussed in the first scenario above. He or she may be optimistic as surgery is seen as a cure for a long-term and distressing complaint. However, lingering fears of cancer may be present along with all the fears that can be conjured up by the prospect of any operation. Such topics need careful exploration during assessment as it is also important to discover whether the patient has a realistic view of the benefits surgery may bring and is aware of the various measures that will be needed to cope with the side-effects of surgery in the long term. Successful health education before discharge will depend on discovering such information.

Treatment of the patient is directed toward the relief of symptoms, healing of the ulcer and the prevention of complications and recurrence. A regimen of rest, non-irritating diet, avoiding alcohol, stopping smoking (and stopping the use of NSAIDs if applicable) is required. Medications are prescribed that are designed to promote healing by reducing gastric secretory and motor activity, diluting the gastric juice and neutralizing much of the hydrochloric acid in order to promote healing.

Diet Strict dietary control is not considered necessary. A regular, well balanced diet, free of foods that are upsetting to the individual, is recommended. Lengthy gaps between meals should be avoided. In the acute phase, small frequent meals will be more tolerable to the patient. These are gradually modified to the more customary three larger meals per day. In some instances, five or six smaller meals may have to be continued.

Medications Pain relief and healing of an ulcer are achieved by reducing the acidity at the ulcer site. However, it is important to diagnose infection with H. pylori in order to prevent a relapse when acid reduction is stopped. It is also important to avoid the use of NSAIDs. Current approaches to treatment for patients with peptic ulceration include antacids, antibiotics (if H. pylori-positive), proton pump inhibitors or H_2-receptor antagonists, and prostaglandin analogues.

Patients with H. pylori infection are usually given a one week course of 'triple therapy'. This consists of two of amoxicillin, clarithromycin or metronidazole, with a proton pump inhibitor (lansoprazole or omeprazole). Eradication rates are approximately 90% and the course of medication is usually well tolerated (Livett 2004). Maintenance therapy

with a proton pump inhibitor or H_2-receptor antagonist may be necessary for some weeks thereafter.

The use of NSAIDs (prescribed for chronic arthritic conditions) inhibits the production of prostaglandin E, which results in loss of the mucous layer protecting the gastric lining. Gastric protection can be achieved by prescribing a proton pump inhibitor at the same time as the NSAID but alternative forms of analgesia are preferable to prevent damaging the gastric mucosa.

Proton pump inhibitors are the most powerful gastric acid secretion inhibitors. They inhibit the adenosine triphosphate (ATP)-mediated pumping of potassium and hydrogen ions in parietal cells and have few side-effects. A single dose is usually given, before breakfast, on an empty stomach. Alternatively, they may be prescribed for both night and morning use. H_2-receptor antagonists block the histamine receptors in the parietal cells to prevent acid being secreted by parietal cells. They may be given either morning and night, or in a single dose at bedtime, to have effect when acid secretion is greatest, i.e. at night.

Antacids are used to neutralize the acid in the stomach. To be effective they must be taken frequently throughout the day. Examples include aluminium hydroxide and magnesium hydroxide. Magnesium and aluminium salts are absorbed minimally and should not cause any disturbances in electrolyte levels. Hypermagnesaemia and hyperalbuminaemia, can occur in patients with renal failure. Magnesium hydroxide can cause diarrhoea and aluminium hydroxide tends to cause constipation. Antacids may interfere with the absorption of certain drugs (e.g. ferrous sulfate, phenytoin, tetracycline) and it is usually recommended that the administration of antacids and other drugs be separated by at least 2 hours. Because of the inconvenience of taking antacids so frequently, these drugs should be used on an as needed basis rather than for long-term treatment.

Sucralfate is a sulfated polysaccharide that acts directly at the ulcer site. Sucralfate binds with the gastric mucosa and forms a barrier that inhibits the diffusion of hydrogen ions and the local action of pepsin. It is poorly absorbed and hence has few side-effects. Occasionally, constipation may occur. Sucralfate should be taken 30 minutes before meals and at bedtime. If prescribed with antacids, administration should be separated by at least 1 hour.

Surgical treatment

If the symptoms persist and the ulcer becomes intractable, or if there has been bleeding or the ulcer has resulted in some obstruction in the gastric outlet, surgical treatment may be considered necessary. Various operative procedures are used in the surgical treatment of an uncomplicated ulcer in order to reduce the potential gastric acid secretion. Current operative approaches include the following procedures.

Gastric resection (subtotal gastrectomy) This is the removal of a portion of the stomach, including the ulcer-bearing area and part of the parietal cell mass. Resection is performed because of the risk of the ulcer becoming malignant in the future. An anastomosis is then made between the gastric stump and the duodenum (gastro-duodenostomy; Billroth I) or jejunum (gastrojejunostomy; Billroth II) to restore gastrointestinal continuity.

Gastric resection plus vagotomy Vagotomy is a resection of the vagus nerve to reduce the stimulation of gastric secretion. It also reduces the motility of the stomach and may interfere with gastric emptying. For this reason, a highly selective vagotomy may be performed which leaves parts of the vagus nerve intact, particularly the sections that supply the antrum. Otherwise, vagotomy is combined with a gastric resection or with a gastroenterostomy to provide effective gastric emptying.

Vagotomy with pyloroplasty This involves a longitudinal incision made in the pylorus, which is then surgically closed transversely. This produces an enlarged outlet which compensates for the impaired gastric emptying resulting from vagotomy. In some instances, a gastroenterostomy may be done instead of the pyloroplasty.

For nursing management of the patient who requires gastric surgery, see p. 454.

Complications of peptic ulceration

The complications that commonly occur with peptic ulcer are serious and usually account for the deaths attributed to peptic ulcer. They are haemorrhage, perforation and pyloric obstruction.

Haemorrhage Peptic ulceration is the most common cause of haematemesis and melaena. The loss of blood is due to erosion of a blood vessel at the ulcer site. Most of the patients who have a haemorrhage are known to have or to have had an ulcer, but in a few, it may be the first symptom that prompts them to seek treatment. Vomiting of blood and the passing of black tarry stools are the prominent indications of serious ulcer bleeding together with the development of hypovolaemic shock. The patient experiences weakness, apprehension, dizziness and faintness, together with the classical signs of shock. If a large vessel is eroded, the signs and symptoms appear rapidly and collapse occurs quickly.

Management Management of the patient with haemorrhage may be conservative or include surgery. The complication of haemorrhage is serious and demands prompt resuscitation and treatment of the site of bleeding.

Nursing assessment Blood pressure, pulse and respirations are monitored frequently and the level of consciousness, colour and body temperature are noted. If a central venous catheter has been inserted, central venous pressure should be recorded from the same point, at regular intervals. Blood typing and cross-matching are done immediately. The haematocrit and haemoglobin levels are determined, initially to determine the extent of the blood loss then later, at intervals, to assess the patient's response to treatment.

Accurate recording of the volume and characteristics of the emesis and drainage via the nasogastric tube is impor-

tant. (Is the blood bright? Does the emesis contain clots?) An indwelling urethral catheter may be passed so that urinary output per hour can be monitored.

It is important to assess the person's reaction to the situation, because fear and anxiety aggravate the condition. The principal problem facing the patient is shock, and the main goals are that the patient's blood pressure and other vital signs will return to normal, indicating successful resuscitation.

Nursing intervention Nursing intervention for a patient with haemorrhage includes the following:

● A plasma expander such as Haemaccel is given intravenously until compatible whole blood is available. The rate of flow is usually slowed as the patient's blood pressure increases; too rapid an increase in the blood pressure has the risk of increasing the bleeding. The blood pressure may need to be measured every 15–30 minutes

● A central venous line may be inserted both to monitor central venous pressure and to provide wide, additional venous access for infusions

● Rest should be promoted by reducing disturbances, keeping nursing interventions to a safe minimum. A sedative may be prescribed to promote relaxation and an analgesic for pain relief

● The patient and significant others should be kept informed to allay anxiety. Information should be presented in short segments, without excessive use of medical terms, delivered in a calm manner, and regularly reinforced

● A nasogastric tube may be passed to remove blood and gastric secretions. Gentle aspiration of stomach contents will remove acid and pepsin which could further irritate tissues. Aspiration of blood may prevent vomiting (haematemesis), allow estimation of loss, and reduce trauma and discomfort

● OGD is usually performed to locate the bleeding site; injection of sclerosing agent (adrenaline/epinephrine), electrocautery or photocautery by laser, if available, may be used to control bleeding. If this is unsuccessful, emergency surgery may be necessary. If bleeding has ceased, close observation and fasting is usually continued until the person's overall condition is stable

● If treated conservatively, oral intake is permitted when bleeding ceases and the cardiovascular state is normalized. Once small volumes of water are tolerated by the person, intake is gradually increased to include clear fluids, liquid diet, soft food, and eventually an ordinary diet. Being able to take food and fluid again improves the patient's morale and lessens anxiety. Iron may be prescribed to promote replacement of haemoglobin

● Frequent mouth care is necessary because of the haematemesis, dehydration and the discomfort of extreme thirst.

Perforation A peptic ulcer may progressively erode the submucosal muscularis and serous layers of the gastrointestinal wall. When the serous membranous layer is penetrated, some of the stomach or duodenal content escapes into the peritoneal cavity and causes a generalized peritonitis by chemical irritation and infection.

When perforation takes place, the patient immediately experiences sudden, incapacitating abdominal pain that begins in the epigastric region but spreads through the abdomen as more of the peritoneum becomes irritated by the intragastrointestinal content. Pallor, a cold clammy skin, rapid pulse, shallow grunting respirations and probably nausea and vomiting may be evident. The abdomen becomes rigid and board-like.

Perforation demands immediate treatment; emergency surgery may be performed to close the perforation or resect the affected area. The surgical procedure may consist of gastric resection or simple closure of the perforation by suturing the serous layer and reinforcing the area with a patch of omentum. The peritoneal cavity is cleared of the intragastrointestinal fluid that seeped through the perforation. In addition to the usual preoperative procedures for emergency surgery, preparation will include the insertion of a nasogastric tube and an intravenous infusion of electrolytes and fluids. An explanation of the need for operation and what it entails will be made by the surgeon and reinforced by the nurse.

The patient's condition and history may be such that the perforation is treated by non-surgical conservative methods. Non-operative treatment usually includes parenteral administration of an analgesic such as morphine, aspiration of the stomach content using a large tube, followed by the insertion of a nasogastric tube and continuous gastric suctioning, intravenous electrolytes and fluids (fluids may include whole blood) and antibiotic therapy. If the patient's condition is satisfactory, continuous gastric suctioning is replaced by intermittent aspiration after 30–48 hours.

Pyloric obstruction   This may be caused by inflammation, oedema and spasm when the ulcer is in the acute stage, or by scar tissue that is formed as the ulcer heals. The ulcer may be gastric in the region of the pylorus, or it may be in the duodenum. The constriction causes gastric retention and dilatation.

The symptoms that the patient complains of include a 'full feeling' which causes greater discomfort toward the end of the day. Pain may be experienced after eating, as gastric contractions increase in intensity in an effort to overcome the obstruction. The contractions gradually decline and the stomach becomes atonic and dilates. Severe anorexia develops and the patient vomits large amounts irregularly. The loss of nutrients, water and electrolytes leads to loss of weight, weakness, dehydration and acid–base imbalance (alkalosis).

If the obstruction is due to the active ulceration process, it is treated conservatively by gastric aspiration and intravenous fluids.

Obstruction due to contraction of fibrous scar tissue is treated by operation. A gastric resection with a gastroenterostomy or pyloroplasty may be performed. For nursing care of the patient requiring gastric surgery, see p. 454.

CANCER OF THE STOMACH

In the UK, stomach cancer is the seventh most common cancer. It is the fifth most common cancer in men and the ninth most common in women, the incidence is slightly higher in men and rises rapidly from the age of 40 years. Each year in the UK, there are approximately 5800 new cases of stomach cancer in men and over 3300 cases in women (Cancer Research UK 2005b). Incidence has been falling; however, the fall has occurred more rapidly for males than females, revealing that the gender differential is narrowing (Cancer Research UK 2004).

Contributing factors

The cause of this cancer is unknown but certain conditions are considered predisposing. These include pernicious anaemia, achlorhydria, chronic gastritis, infection with H. pylori and benign gastric ulcer. It now seems likely that dietary carcinogens exist in some foods and contribute to the formation of gastric cancer.

Any region of the stomach may be involved, but the most frequent sites are the pylorus and antrum.

Clinical characteristics

The manifestations are vague and insidious. At first, the person may complain of some mild discomfort after eating but, as the disease advances, belching, regurgitation, nausea and vomiting may be experienced, and there is a progressive loss of appetite, weight and strength. Blood may appear in the vomitus and stool when there is ulceration at the tumour site. Pain is usually a late symptom. Unfortunately, because the early symptoms are mild and vague, the person tends to delay seeing a doctor, and the disease becomes well advanced before there is medical intervention. Nurses should be aware of this problem and, on learning that a person is experiencing even mild 'digestive' disturbances, should stress the importance of seeking medical advice.

Diagnosis

Investigation of the patient includes OGD and biopsy, barium meal radiography, cytological studies of gastric fluid, gastroscopy and biopsy, examination of the stool for blood, haemoglobin estimation and blood cell counts. Computed tomography of the chest and abdomen, and liver ultrasonography, may be performed to establish the extent of the tumour and infiltration or development of metastases in other organs.

Blood examinations will probably show some deficiency of haemoglobin and red blood cells, as anaemia is a characteristic of gastric cancer due to the chronic bleeding, reduced production of the intrinsic factor by the gastric mucosa, reduced absorption of iron because of the hypochlorhydria and nutritional deficits.

Metastases

Gastric carcinoma develops and metastasizes rapidly; all too often there has been a spread to some other structure(s) by the time of diagnosis. There may be direct extension to neighbouring organs (e.g. oesophagus, duodenum) or an indirect spread via the lymph and venous blood. The spleen, abdominal lymph nodes, peritoneum, liver, pancreas and lungs are frequent sites of metastases from gastric carcinoma. The left supraclavicular and axillary nodes may also be affected.

Treatment

Surgery is the treatment of choice but cure is possible only when the cancer is diagnosed in the early stages, i.e. before it has spread from the primary site or at least only to localized lymph glands. The surgical procedure used will depend on the site of the cancer and its extension or possible course of extension. A subtotal gastrectomy or, rarely, a total gastrectomy is performed and may include resection of the duodenum, excision of the areas of lymphatic spread (omentum, spleen), resection of the pancreas or resection of the lower oesophagus. In subtotal gastrectomy, the stomach is anastomosed to the duodenum (gastroduodenostomy) or to the jejunum (gastrojejunostomy) if the lower part of the stomach has been removed. With removal of the proximal portion of the stomach, the operation is completed by anastomosis of the oesophagus to the remaining stomach (oesophagoantrostomy). Total gastrectomy and resection of the oesophagus necessitate entrance into the thoracic cavity. Continuity of the alimentary tract is restored by an oesophagojejunostomy.

The preoperative and postoperative nursing care of the gastric surgical patient is presented on p. 454. Care of the patient following complete gastrectomy includes the care necessary for any patient who has had chest surgery (see Ch. 13). The patient who has had partial gastrectomy requires small frequent meals of easily digested foods because of the development of dumping syndrome (see below) and vitamin B_{12} injections.

DUMPING SYNDROME

Normally, the gastric content is delivered in small amounts into the intestine by the pylorus. Following a gastric resection, vagotomy or gastroenterostomy, the normal pyloric control of the volume moving from the stomach into the small intestine is absent and a small proportion of patients develop the **dumping syndrome**. This is caused by the precipitous passage into the small intestine of a relatively large amount of gastric content that has not undergone the usual dilution by gastric secretions and digestive changes. This leads to a rapid absorption of a large amount of carbohydrate and a consequent increase in insulin release, leading to hypoglycaemia-like symptoms 1–2 hours later. The following factors are also implicated:

- The sudden distension of the proximal portion of the small intestine initiates sympathetic reflexes
- The fluid that moved quickly out of the stomach is hypertonic, having a high concentration of sugar and/or electrolytes. The resulting hyperosmolarity on the intestine results in the movement of fluid from the intravascular spaces into the jejunum.

The effects on the patient are to produce faintness, sweating and palpitations immediately after meals, in addition to the symptoms referred to above, 1–2 hours later. The symptoms do tend to improve with time but in addition, the person is advised to drink less at mealtimes and to eat fewer foods with high sugar or carbohydrate content to minimize these distressing symptoms.

HISTORY TAKING AND PHYSICAL EXAMINATION OF THE PATIENT WITH A DISORDER OF THE STOMACH OR DUODENUM

History taking

The history should be focused on gastrointestinal functioning and factors that influence it:

- What is the usual diet of the individual?
- How has the diet changed in relation to symptoms?
- What strategies have been adopted to relieve symptoms?
- Does the person smoke or take alcohol or drugs such as aspirin or steroids?
- Has the individual experienced any particular stressful life events recently?
- What effects might the person's social circumstances have upon their diet?

Clinical symptoms
- Does the individual experience nausea, vomiting, epigastric fullness, discomfort or pain?
- If the patient has experienced vomiting, what does the vomit look like, is there any evidence of blood in the vomit?
- Where is the pain located? Does it move to the back or shoulders?
- What factors appear to increase discomfort?
- Is the pain or discomfort increased at night, when the stomach is empty or during any specific activities?
- How long have the symptoms been experienced? Have they changed?

General health status
- Has the person lost weight recently and how much?
- Have there been any other health problems such as breathlessness, reduced mobility or poor healing?

Physical examination of the abdomen

Physical examination of the abdomen is a relevant activity for patients who have symptoms associated with the stomach, intestines or any of the other structures within the abdomen. A general overview of the abdominal examination will be provided here to help guide the preliminary assessment of the patient. Nurses need to seek the advice of their experienced colleagues to make sense of the abdominal examination findings. Nonetheless, it is useful to be knowledgeable about the abdominal examination to enable prompt referral to others when abnormal findings are discovered.

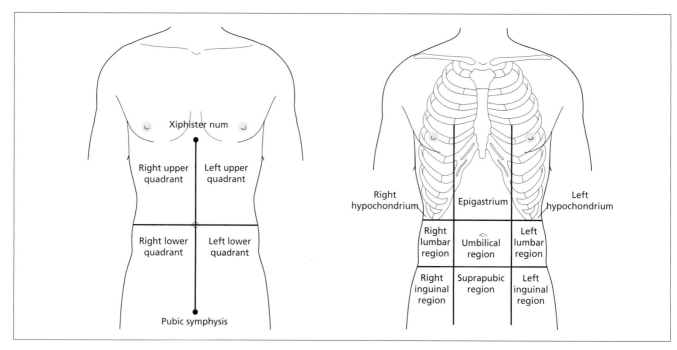

Figure 15.4   The four quadrants and nine segments of the abdomen.

The examination of the abdomen takes a structured step-wise approach. The abdomen can be split into nine or four anatomical areas (Fig. 15.4). It is important to have the patient in a relaxed position on the examination couch with a pillow behind the head whilst they lie supine with their arms down by their sides. The patient's dignity and privacy should be considered and the temperature of the room should be conducive to the exposure of the abdomen. The procedure should be explained to the patient carefully and in some cases, the patient may feel more relaxed if a partner or significant other is able to stay with them throughout the procedure.

Observation
Commence examination of the abdomen by deliberately observing the patient's hands for signs of nicotine staining, the nails for strength and structure and the dorsal surface of the hand for skin turgor and colour. Examine the patient's face for signs of pain, grimacing and particularly examine the sclera of the eyes for signs of jaundice. Ask the patient to stick their tongue out and examine it for signs of dehydration. Note the odour of the patient's breath and observe the colour and turgor of their skin for signs of malnutrition or anaemia.

Expose the abdomen from the xiphisternum to the groins. Initially just look at the abdomen noting signs of abdominal breathing, watching for the pulsation of an aortic aneurysm, noting any lack of symmetry in the contour of the abdomen and any superficial marks on the skin such as spider angioma (which can be a sign of liver disease, vitamin B_{12} deficiency or can be normal for a particular patient). It can be helpful to ask the patient to lift their head off the couch as this tenses the abdominal muscles and may

elicit pain in some patients and in others it may reveal a mass that had not been previously noticeable. After asking the patient to put their head back on the pillow and regain their comfort the remainder of the abdominal examination can take place.

Auscultation
There is debate over the value of abdominal auscultation with some suggesting that the abdominal sounds are so variable little information about the patient's health status can be obtained from listening to them. Others suggest that it can be helpful in determining the presence of bowel sounds after abdominal surgery and the high pitched sounds associated with early obstruction. It is worthwhile listening to the patient's abdomen so that you can become familiar with the different sounds and then make a judgement as to the significance of the sounds in relation to the remainder of your assessment. Place a warm stethoscope in the four quadrants of the abdomen, listening in each place for approximately 30 seconds. Clicks and gurgles should be heard at a frequency of about 5–35/minute.

Percussion
Percussion should be carried out in a systematic manner moving across the abdomen to cover all of the areas shown in Figure 15.4. Percussion elicits different sounds according to whether the area directly under the percussing fingers is fluid filled, air filled or solid. It is worthwhile practising percussion techniques on different surfaces to become familiar with the different sounds. In some patients, percussion may result in pain and it is therefore important to watch the patient's face throughout the examination so you can minimize the discomfort of the examination process.

Palpation

Palpation should once again cover the whole abdominal area. It is important to commence palpation in the area of the abdomen which is furthest away from the site of pain. Start with light, gentle palpation as you move across the abdomen using the palmar surface of your hand to a depth of about 1 cm. Then repeat the process with deeper palpation covering the whole area a second time but all the time being aware of areas of pain and watching the patient's face and reactions for signs of discomfort.

There is value in also palpating the lymph nodes in the groins and in the supraclavicular area as lymphatic drainage from the abdomen can be noted in these areas.

Explain your findings to the patient and then record them in the notes. Report significant findings to senior nurses or medical personnel to enable to patient's problems to be dealt with as efficiently as possible.

PATIENT PROBLEMS COMMON TO THOSE WITH DISORDERS OF THE STOMACH AND DUODENUM

- Dehydration due to nausea and vomiting
- Malnutrition due to increased gastric secretions, gastrointestinal discomfort, nausea, vomiting, and possibly surgical intervention
- Fear and anxiety that surgery may be necessary or that cancer may be present.

Potential goals of nursing interventions
The person will demonstrate or be able to report:

1 knowledge about the condition in terms of causes and treatment
2 absence or control of pain
3 absence or control of nausea and vomiting
4 awareness of dietary measures to relieve symptoms
5 an adequate nutritional intake, as shown by progressive increase in body weight towards normal
6 reduced anxiety levels and an ability to talk freely about the condition.

Nursing interventions
Alleviation of nausea and vomiting

Assessment   Assessment of the patient who is nauseous and is vomiting involves noting the following factors:

- Was the vomiting preceded by nausea?
- Was there retching or was the vomitus regurgitated without effort?
- Was pain associated with the vomiting?
- Was there any association with the ingestion of food or drugs?
- Do the nausea and vomiting occur at any time or are they more severe at a particular time of day?
- How frequent is the emesis?
- What is the quantity, consistency, colour and content of the vomitus?
- What are the effects (physical and emotional) on the patient?

Supportive measures   Sympathetic attention and understanding can mean a great deal to the patient. Stress and fear can perpetuate nausea and vomiting, and therefore the patient should be encouraged to express any concerns. The plan of care and any diagnostic and therapeutic measures should be explained to the patient; knowing that something is being done or going to be done can provide reassurance and help to relieve the anxiety. Support is also provided by remaining with the patient, supporting the head or painful site (e.g. incision), holding the basin, cleansing the mouth and lips, and making sincere efforts to relieve the discomfort.

Fluid and food   Oral intake is usually withheld for a period of time and is resumed gradually in small amounts. If vomiting is prolonged, an intravenous infusion of fluids may be necessary to prevent or correct dehydration and replace electrolytes. An accurate record is made of the fluid intake and output. The skin and oral mucous membrane are observed for dryness and skin turgor is assessed as an indication of dehydration.

Hygienic and comfort measures   The mouth is rinsed after each emesis and the basin emptied and disposed of promptly. Soiled bedding and clothing are changed and the room is ventilated. The odour or sight of vomitus may contribute to the patient's discomfort and may cause repetitive vomiting. The patient may be reassured by having tissues and a clean basin always within reach.

Rest, quiet and a minimum of disturbance may reduce the incidence of vomiting. Encouraging the patient to take several deep breaths may help to lessen nausea and offset vomiting. Nausea tends to increase with motion; any change of position should be made slowly. Positioning should facilitate drainage of the vomitus from the mouth to prevent possible aspiration. Subdued lighting may reduce external stimuli and be conducive to rest. Relaxation techniques including muscular relaxation, meditation, guided imagery and deep breathing exercises may help to decrease stress and relieve the nausea and vomiting. Some individuals find that food actually relieves nausea and prevents vomiting. Dry crackers or sips of soda water can be helpful.

Medication   An antiemetic or sedative may be prescribed. Diazepam may be administered orally or parenterally for sedation. Prochlorperazine or metoclopramide are examples of antiemetics that may be given, usually via the intramuscular or intravenous route depending on the drug. In the hyperemesis of pregnancy, the use of antiemetics or other drugs is restricted, to prevent any effects on fetal development. Some patients develop anticipatory nausea and vomiting and this may be controlled by preventive and regular doses of antiemetics. If the vomiting continues, gastric drainage by means of a nasogastric tube may be established.

Maintenance of adequate nutritional intake   Nutritional intake is maintained by decreasing stimulation of gastric secretions, adapting the person's diet to relieve the problem or using alternative routes to administer nutrients.

Dietary measures Measures to decrease stimulation of gastric secretions include withholding food for 24–28 hours to allow the stomach to rest. Fluids are given intravenously as even water taken by mouth will stimulate gastric acid secretion. Gastric intubation with aspiration may be used to remove gastric secretions to promote healing.

Recommended dietary modifications include the following:

- The patient should receive a nutritionally adequate diet
- Substances that stimulate gastric secretion (e.g. coffee, strong tea, highly seasoned foods, especially those with pepper, citrus fruit and alcohol) are avoided
- Meals are taken regularly at frequent intervals of about 3 hours to maintain the buffering action of food in the stomach
- Meals should be small to avoid gastric distension, which stimulates gastric acid secretion
- Foods that the person recognizes as actually precipitating symptoms are avoided
- The person should not smoke
- Drugs such as NSAIDs (aspirin, ibuprofen) that are known to damage the gastrointestinal mucosa are avoided.

Alternative routes for the administration of nutrients

Oral intake of food is preferred, but when this is not possible, nutrients can be administered intravenously or by nasogastric or percutaneous enteral routes.

Nasogastric tube feeding When a patient is unable to take fluid and foods by mouth, a fine-bore nasogastric tube may be passed, through which a specially prepared solution of essential nutrients is introduced directly into the stomach. This method of feeding a patient is known as enteral feeding and it can be used for up to 1 month (Holmes 2004).

Patients should always be nursed in an upright position whilst being tube fed to avoid the risks of reflux and aspiration.

Careful preparation of the patient before insertion will help in reducing discomfort and facilitate ease of insertion. The individual should have the procedure explained in full, including the sensations they will experience and how they can assist by swallowing when they feel the tube touching the back of the throat. The patient should be instructed to raise their hand if they want the procedure to stop (Best 2005). Measures that can reduce the unpleasant sensations include: application of sterile, water-soluble, lubricating jelly to the tube, deep breathing, relaxation techniques and swallowing.

Once the nasogastric tube has been inserted, it is essential to ascertain that it is in the correct anatomical location. A nasogastric tube can inadvertently be placed into the lung or remain part way down the oesophagus. The most accurate method of identifying the position of the nasogastric tip is to carry out an X-ray. However, it is essential that the findings should only be confirmed by a clinician with expertise in reading the X-ray results as these X-rays can be very difficult to interpret (Best 2005). Successful aspiration of gastric contents can also be used to confirm the correct placement of the tube. The aspirate should be tested with pH indicator tape and gastric placement is usually indicated with a pH <4. A further method of checking that the nasogastric tube is in the correct location is aspiration of visually recognizable contents. This test can only be carried out with a patient who is able to swallow and to take a drink orally. The patient is instructed to drink a fluid that can be visually recognized such as blackcurrant or milk and then the fluid is aspirated through the nasogastric tube.

Nasogastric tubes can easily be dislodged after placement and therefore it is important to secure the tube by applying hypoallergenic tape to the individual's nostril or by an adhesive patch to the cheek. The tube can be displaced by vomiting or coughing and it is therefore important to carry out regular checking of the tube position.

Enteral feeding involves close cooperation between medical, dietetic and nursing staff, who have an important role in supervising the diet. Commercially prepared feeds are commonly used because they have a known nutrient content, flow easily through the nasogastric tube, and are easy to prepare. They come sterilized and can be administered from a sterile reservoir through an administration tube attached to the nasogastric tube, reducing the potential for the introduction of contaminants.

The regimen is determined according to the individual's nutritional and fluid requirements, based upon their age, sex, body weight, medical condition and biochemistry. Continuous delivery of enteral feeding is the ideal as it minimizes side-effects, such as distension and nausea, and maximizes absorption, although intermittent feeding may be more convenient for some individuals.

When evaluating a feed, consideration is given to its osmolarity, caloric value and protein, carbohydrate, fat, vitamin and mineral composition. Nutrients are present in simple form, are easily digested and absorbed, and leave minimal residue in the bowel. Patients with some malabsorption disorders may not tolerate some of the prepared feeds. Functioning of the patient's digestive tract and hydration status are assessed before the preparation is selected.

For the initial feeding, an explanation of the procedure is given to the patient. The head of the bed is elevated to 35–40°. A continuous infusion of the feed is given via a giving-set attached to the nasogastric tube. The fluid feed is given slowly, and is allowed to flow into the stomach by gravity. To avoid air entering the stomach, a collapsible plastic feeding container is used. When the feed is completed, the tube is flushed with up to 50 mL of water and clamped. If regurgitation or vomiting occurs, it may be that the prescribed volume is too great. A smaller amount given more frequently may be tolerated.

The patient is encouraged to remain in a sitting position for at least 1 hour after each feed to decrease regurgitation and aspiration and to promote stomach emptying. Frequent mouth care is necessary, as is the care of the nostril through which the tube passes. Most medications are not licensed for administration through a nasogastric tube and so it is important that nursing staff communicate closely with medical staff and pharmacists to ensure that the appropriate preparations are selected for administration through the tube (Best 2005).

Gastrostomy This is the establishment of an opening into the stomach through the abdominal wall and the insertion of a tube through which fluids and liquefied food may be introduced directly into the stomach. Placement of a gastrostomy tube is indicated if enteral feeding is going to take place for longer than 30 days (Holmes 2004). Most commonly, this procedure is indicated for patients who have had a cerebrovascular accident (CVA). Insertion may be carried out under general or, most commonly in the UK, under local anaesthesia and intravenous sedation (Haboubi et al 2005). The stomach is visualized by an endoscope and the tube is inserted through the abdominal wall via a small stab wound. The tube is anchored with a flange in either side of the abdominal wall. This is often referred to as a percutaneous endoscopic gastrostomy (PEG).

A gastrostomy may be a temporary procedure during a period of corrective surgery or it may be permanent, for example in conditions such as multiple sclerosis, motor neurone disease or brain injury. The patient generally finds it difficult to accept a gastrostomy because the natural process of eating and its associated pleasures such as taste and sociability have been removed. Personnel caring for the patient, the family and friends should acknowledge to the patient that they understand any negative feelings.

Regular feeds are given according to the patient's needs. The food preparations used in gastrostomy are similar to those cited above for gastric tube feedings or are the person's normal diet, liquidized. The required amount of feed is given through an administration bag attached to the gastric tube. The patient's head and shoulders are elevated and he or she remains in this position for half an hour after the feeding to prevent regurgitation into the oesophagus and leakage around the tube.

Although a life-preserving intervention, PEG has complications and risks. Some of the main complications are:

- tube blockage
- infection at site of tube entry
- peritonitis
- dislodgement of the tube
- pulmonary aspiration
- diarrhoea
- gastrocolic fistula and
- haemorrhage.

One of the problems with gastrostomy tubes is the potential for them to block. If patients are on a continuous feeding regime, the tube should be flushed twice daily. If the patient is receiving bolus feeding, the tube should be flushed before and after each feed and after any medications (Holmes 2004).

Infection of the skin at the insertion site can lead to pyrexia, inflammation, drainage and swelling. The skin should be inspected regularly for signs of infection, necrosis or excoriation. A gauze or transparent dressing is applied to the wound, the escape of even a small amount of gastric juice from around the tube may irritate the skin because of its acid pepsin content. The gauze dressing is changed whenever there is drainage, and the skin is cleansed thoroughly with water and dried. Should excoriation occur, application of a hydrocolloid dressing or wafer following cleansing of the skin may both promote healing and protect the skin from further damage. Evidence of necrosis should be communicated to medical/specialist staff as soon as possible.

In a 2-year audit of patients who had insertion of a PEG tube Haboubi et al (2005) found that 47% of the patients had signs of aspiration. Migration of the tube upwards towards the oesophagus can cause vomiting and possible aspiration. If the patient develops aspiration pneumonia, treatment with antibiotics will be required.

Too much fat or carbohydrate may cause diarrhoea and therefore the feeds may have to be adjusted from time to time. Complaints of a full feeling or abdominal discomfort may necessitate a decrease in the amount of feeds given. A record of the patient's weight is made, which also serves as a guide in adjusting the caloric value of the feed's formula. This should be recorded twice weekly at the same time of day.

A further potential problem is bacterial contamination of enteral tube feeds. Poor hand hygiene, re-use of systems that should be disposable, poor cleaning of equipment and storage at incorrect temperatures are possible causes of enteral feeds being significantly contaminated.

If the patient is to be fed by gastrostomy over a long period while various stages of treatment are carried out, or if the gastrostomy is permanent, teaching in the correct techniques is essential for both the patient and family. Information should be provided regarding supplies of prescribed commercial feeding preparations and equipment. The nurse may direct the family to the appropriate community resources for the necessary assistance, or make the contact for them.

The patient's mouth will require special attention. Frequent cleansing and rinsing are essential. Close attention to the entry site, tube patency, patient positioning and any complaints of abdominal discomfort are essential, therefore, to minimize the potential complications of PEG.

Jejunostomy or duodenostomy A jejunostomy tube may be inserted and used for feedings when it is necessary to bypass the stomach as a result of surgery or reflux. A potential problem with a jejunostomy or duodenostomy is the occurrence of the dumping syndrome (see p. 449). The rapid entry of nutrients into the jejunum can cause the characteristic symptoms of tachycardia, sweating, weakness, syncope and abdominal pain. This can be managed by careful regulation of the flow of the feed (Holmes 2004).

Promotion of coping and control of stress
Emotional and physical stress affect gastric function, and ill-health of any type presents an additional stress to the individual. Whether stress is a contributing factor or a result of gastrointestinal disorder, the nurse can play a role in

identifying both the causes of the stress and the person's responses to it, and help that individual to explore, test and evaluate various coping strategies. Nurses can facilitate the expression and exploration of feelings, provide information and teach patients self-management skills to alleviate the stresses imposed by the illness. The exploration of coping strategies that work for the individual and the development of relaxation and other stress management programmes with the patient and family fall within the role of the nurse. They can inform the individual and significant others about resources available to them in their community and work setting. They can also help patients to identify stressors in their daily lives, to develop strategies to alter their lifestyles to avoid these precipitating factors or to implement coping strategies when these situations occur.

Evaluation

When evaluating the care delivered, it is important to remember that it is not just the individual's response to management of illness that is important but also their life situation and personal expectations. Each of the goals of nursing care should be considered and the patient's perspective should be sought. Nursing interventions for the patient who is receiving enteral feeding should be adjusted according to the patient's needs and will change as the patient and their family members become familiar with the technique of receiving nutrition through a feeding tube.

NURSING CARE FOR THE PERSON REQUIRING GASTRIC SURGERY

Special considerations applicable to the patient experiencing gastric surgery are outlined below. The amount of gastric drainage obtained after operation and the extent of the potential nutritional deficit resulting from the surgical intervention vary according to the type and extent of gastric tissue excised during the surgical procedure. In clinical practice, the care plan is modified to meet the specific needs of the individual.

Preoperative care

The goals for the patient during the preoperative period are to:

1 improve fluid and nutritional status
2 learn and practise deep breathing and coughing techniques
3 reduce anxiety experienced by the individual and significant others.

If the patient's nutritional and fluid status is poor, enteral or parenteral nutrition may be administered. Intravenous solutions may be given to increase the person's fluid volume and to correct electrolyte imbalances.

The incision will be in the upper abdomen below the chest; it is important therefore that the patient is competent at performing deep breathing and coughing techniques, and understands the importance of performing these after the operation. Introduction to the physiotherapist who will see the patient for chest physiotherapy after surgery is beneficial.

Explanations about the operation and hospital routines usually help to decrease anxiety in both the patient and family. The nurse should also take time to assess their learning needs and to determine their perceptions and expectations for the surgery and postsurgical outcomes.

Postoperative care

Health problems common to persons undergoing gastric surgery include:

● altered fluid and electrolyte balance due to gastric intubation and suction, and surgical fluid losses
● malnutrition due to preoperative nutritional deficits and decreased food intake after operation
● pain due to the surgical intervention
● altered breathing pattern due to incisional pain
● lack of knowledge concerning postoperative care and skills required to achieve self-care.

Goals

The patient will have:

1 a patent gastric drainage system
2 fluid volume intake of at least 2.5 L/day and output in balance
3 absence of pain
4 a clean, dry, intact incision
5 respirations, pulse and blood pressure within usual range
6 maintenance of nutritional status as shown by a weight loss of <2 kg
7 understanding of prescribed dietary regimen
8 understanding of plans for follow-up care.

Nursing intervention

Gastric drainage The patient will return from theatre with a nasogastric, nasointestinal or gastrostomy tube in place.

The characteristics of the drainage fluid are noted and the total volume is recorded at regular intervals. Intermittent aspiration or free drainage will be ordered. It is important that the patency of the tube be maintained to avoid a build-up of secretions in the stomach. The drainage will probably be coloured by blood at first, but this usually clears in a few hours. The doctor is notified if large amounts of blood appear or if the drainage continues to be blood coloured. The volume is an important factor in determining the fluid and electrolyte replacement needed. Loss of gastric secretions incurs a loss of hydrogen ions (H^+) and chloride ions (Cl^-) that may result in alkalosis. Loss of intestinal fluid may result in a severe loss of hydrogen carbonate and potassium, and cause acidosis. The number of days for which the nasogastric tube is left in and oral fluids are withheld varies and depends partly on the patient's progress. The nasogastric tube is usually removed when normal bowel sounds return and drainage volumes reduce. Antiemetic drugs (e.g. metoclopramide or cyclizine) may be given regularly to avoid postoperative nausea and vomiting. Not only is nausea unpleasant for the patient, but vomiting poses undue strain on the anastomoses of the surgical areas.

Removal of the tube   Before removal, the tube may be clamped and left in place while oral fluid is introduced. If the fluid is tolerated, the tube may then be removed. With a nasogastric tube, the patient is instructed to hold the breath to avoid possible aspiration of fluid or mucus that may escape from the tube into the oropharynx during removal whilst the tube is withdrawn gently and quickly.

An intestinal tube is removed slowly, a few centimetres at a time. The lumen into the air-inflated balloon is opened, and the air is allowed to escape. When slight resistance is encountered owing to the intestinal peristalsis, the tube is left for a few minutes and then withdrawal is resumed. The doctor should be notified if resistance to removal persists; force should not be used. If there is no resistance the tube may be pulled through the nostril and removed. As with the removal of the gastric tube, the patient is asked to hold the breath as the terminal portion of the tube is drawn from the oesophagus.

The mouth should be cleansed and rinsed immediately after removal of the tube. The patient may complain of soreness in the throat and nose, which usually subsides in a day or two.

Pain management   Considerable **pain** is experienced by the patient who has had gastric surgery. Analgesics such as pethidine are usually prescribed along with an antiemetic if necessary. Analgesia should be given regularly for the first few days and administered before activities that could increase discomfort, such as physiotherapy, turning and mobilization. Systems that allow self-administration of postoperative analgesia (patient-controlled analgesia; PCA) are increasingly used; these enhance patient control and increase participation in pain management (see Ch. 8). Continual assessment of pain levels is necessary in the postoperative period if the goal of a pain-free patient is to be achieved. Frequent regular change of position helps to relieve pain and discomfort.

Frequent cleansing and moistening of the mouth are necessary to lessen the patient's discomfort while the nasogastric tube is in place and oral fluids are restricted. The tube may cause irritation that results in mucus secretion which, if allowed to collect, might be aspirated. The nostril through which the tube is passed is cleansed and moistened, and given a very light application of mineral oil or water-soluble lubricant to prevent the accumulation and crusting of secretions; adhesive tape securing the tube should be changed regularly.

Promotion of respiratory function   If a total gastrectomy was performed, the incision may involve the thorax, and chest drainage tubes will have been inserted. Remind the patient hourly to take 5–10 deep breaths and to cough several times using the staged coughing technique to prevent undue tension on the suture line. Provide necessary encouragement and support by holding a small pillow lightly over the operative site and placing a hand on the patient's back during the coughing. Acknowledge the patient's distress but at the same time emphasize the importance of deep breathing and coughing in the prevention of other problems.

When vital signs are stable, the head of the bed may be gradually elevated to promote deeper breathing and gastric drainage. Change the patient's position at regular frequent intervals: side-to-side to back-to-side. Ambulation usually starts on the first postoperative day.

Fluid and nutritional intake   Parenteral fluids are used to sustain the patient over the first few days. Different procedures are used to introduce the first fluids into the gastrointestinal tract; the surgeon may have the nasogastric tube removed and small stated amounts of water given every half-hour or every hour. The amount is gradually increased if tolerated. The directive may be to introduce a specific amount of water at intervals through the nasogastric tube, which is then clamped.

If the patient tolerates the increased amounts of water without experiencing vomiting, pain or distension, liquids such as tea, fruit squash, soup and milk may be progressively introduced over 2–3 days, but only when normal bowel sounds are heard on auscultation.

With normal progress, the patient is usually receiving a soft diet by day 5–7. The volume given at any one time remains small because of the reduced capacity of the stomach. Foods high in calories and protein are selected and served frequently. The patient may benefit from fortified drinks between meals (Field and Bjarnason 2002). The patient's weight is recorded regularly, and the doctor is advised if there is a loss or a failure to gain weight. Inability of the patient to take the prescribed diet, any regurgitation, vomiting, abdominal distension, or fever or complaint of pain is reported.

By the time the patient is ready to leave the hospital, a light diet of high calorie/protein foods divided into five meals is usually tolerated. Fluids may be omitted from the meals and taken in between so that their volume does not prevent the patient from taking sufficient solid food. The patient is advised gradually to increase the amount taken at regular meals and, if no discomfort is experienced, eventually to resume three or four meals with fluids taken between them.

B complex vitamins and vitamin C and iron may be ordered, as the natural food sources of these will be restricted in the diet for a period of time.

Nutritional deficiency   Signs and symptoms of nutritional deficiencies include: the inability to maintain normal weight; insufficient food intake; and feelings of satiety or feeling full following a small amount of food.

The patient should be helped in developing a dietary plan that includes frequent high caloric intakes (small amounts at first and gradually increased as tolerated). Patients should be encouraged to take drinks between meals and to avoid drinks at meal times to avoid the sensation of fullness (Field and Bjarnason 2002). The patient's perception and responses to the necessary continuing dietary modifications after surgery should be assessed and discussed. The need for a period of time for the digestive system to adjust to the changes should be discussed.

Anaemia   Monitoring of the patient's red blood cell count and haemoglobin is done regularly after gastric resection, and information is elicited as to energy and food elements in the diet. The patient may develop an iron deficiency as a result of decreased iron absorption, which will be caused by measures that reduce acid secretion within the stomach. Normal absorption is facilitated by gastric hydrochloric acid which influences the change from ferric iron in the diet to ferrous iron, which is more easily dissolved and absorbed, mostly in the duodenum and jejunum. The bypassing of the duodenum by a gastrojejunostomy may therefore also reduce the amount of iron absorption. The deficiency may in some instances be due to a poor dietary intake of foods that provide iron (red meat, liver, leafy vegetables, whole milk, eggs and certain cereals). A supplemental preparation of iron can be prescribed and the diet corrected to contain the necessary sources.

Anaemia frequently develops as a result of a deficiency in the secretion of the intrinsic factor (due to the loss of gastric mucosa by the gastric resection) which promotes the absorption of vitamin B_{12}. It may develop within a few months or not for 2–3 years after the gastrectomy. The patient will be given weekly vitamin B_{12} (hydroxocobalamin) by intramuscular injection usually for 5 weeks initially and then a maintenance dose is given 3 monthly throughout the remainder of the patient's life.

Osteomalacia   This is characterized by decalcification of the bones and weakening of their structure, and is a rare complication following gastrectomy. It is attributed to decreased absorption of vitamin D and calcium. Associated symptoms include diarrhoea and steatorrhoea. Treatment involves the administration of vitamin D and calcium supplements.

Patient and family teaching   The patient and family are helped to develop a plan to modify the diet and activity to accommodate temporary and long-term limitations imposed by the surgery. The importance of frequent small meals of non-irritating foods high in calories and protein is explained. The size of the meals may be gradually increased when comfortably tolerated, as the remaining portion of the stomach progressively adapts to larger quantities. After several months, the person may find that three regular meals can again be managed. Written dietary instructions and outlines should be provided to reinforce verbal information. Involvement of the dietitian early on in the patient's care will help in the dietary education process.

The patient is advised to weigh him or herself regularly and to report to the clinic or doctor on scheduled dates. If pain, vomiting, progressive loss of weight or other distressing symptoms occur, the doctor is contacted promptly. Normal activities are resumed as tolerated and should not interfere with the regularity of meals.

Information should be given to the patient and significant others concerning support available in the community. Early referral to the community nursing service will promote continuity of care.

Evaluation

Evaluation is based on the goals determined for each patient. On discharge from the surgical unit, the patient and significant others should be familiar with the immediate dietary needs and what to expect as he or she adapts to the changes and gradually tolerates increases in the amounts and types of foods and liquids. The patient and significant others should be familiar with measures to take to alleviate the symptoms of dumping syndrome. They should be aware of community resources for dietary assistance and any required wound care. Follow-up medical supervision is planned, scheduled appointments are given to the patient and transport arrangements discussed.

DISORDERS OF THE INTESTINE

Disorders of the small intestine may cause disturbances in the movement of the content along the gut leading to problems of digestion or absorption that may threaten the patient's nutritional status.

Disturbance in the function of the large intestine interferes with the excretion of bowel waste and, if the right half of the colon is involved, the normal absorption of water and salts may be reduced and cause dehydration.

A disorder in motility, secretion or absorption rarely occurs independently; a disturbance in one is usually accompanied by dysfunction in one or both of the other intestinal functions. For example, increased secretion may accelerate motility, decreased absorption causes dysfunction in motility and elimination, and inflammation usually causes a disturbance in all three functions.

ALTERATION IN BOWEL ELIMINATION

The causes and clinical characteristics of problems relevant to altered bowel elimination are listed in Box 15.2.

Diarrhoea

The term diarrhoea implies an accelerated movement of content through the intestine with a decrease in mixing and absorptive processes resulting in frequent liquid or unformed stools. The faeces pass through the colon before the normal amount of water is absorbed while fluids and electrolytes may be secreted into the gut also.

Diarrhoea is a symptom of many different disorders which may be within the bowel or extrinsic to the intestine. Changes characteristic of organic disease may occur in the intestine and result in diarrhoea, or the bowel may be structurally normal with the hypermotility being functional. The most common causes of diarrhoea are presented here as

Box 15.2   Potential problems of patients with altered bowel elimination

Causes	Clinical characteristics
Diarrhoea	
Bacterial organisms and enterotoxins	Loose, watery stools
Intestinal neoplasms	Several bowel movements per day
Diet high in roughage, or spicy foods or alcohol	Dehydration: loss of skin turgor, weight loss, dry mouth
Allergy to ingested foods	Abdominal cramping and pain
Malabsorption syndrome	Weakness
Diverticulitis	Increased bowel sounds
Laxatives	Perianal excoriation
Antibiotics	
Inflammatory disorders of the intestinal tract	
Emotional stress	
Systemic diseases (e.g. hyperthyroidism, uraemia, endocrine tumours)	
Radiotherapy to the abdomen and pelvis	
Chemotherapy (5-fluorouracil, cisplatin)	
Constipation	
Disease of the bowel	Abdominal pain
Decreased intestinal motility	Abdominal distension
Altered innervation to bowel and anal sphincter	Sensation of fullness and pressure in rectum
Megacolon	Loss of appetite
Inadequate fluid intake	Headache
Lack of fibre or cellulose in diet	Dry, hard, formed stools
Physical inactivity	Infrequent bowel movements (less than three times per week)
Medication (e.g. opiates)	Straining on defaecation
Weakness of abdominal muscles and diaphragm	
Irregular habits of defaecation	
Loss of bowel tone from excessive use of laxatives	
Haemorrhoids	
Hypercalcaemia	
Pregnancy	
Tumour mass in abdomen or pelvis	
Alteration in mental state	
Impaction	
Altered tone, motility and sensation in bowel as a result of ageing process	Cramping pain
Immobility	Oozing liquid stools
Central nervous system disorders	Headache
	Loss of appetite
	Abdominal distension
	Dry, hard formed stools
	Palpable hard rectal mass
	Straining at defaecation
	No bowel movement for >3 days
Incontinence	
Constipation	Involuntary defaecation
Faecal impaction	Constant soiling of clothing
Excessive use of laxatives and enemas	Faeces soft and semiformed, or loose
Drugs (e.g. iron, methyldopa)	Absence of sensation or urge to defaecate
Diabetes	Diminished propulsive contractions on rectogram
Diverticulitis	

continued

Box 15.2   *Cont'd*

Proctitis
Carcinoma
Rectal prolapse
Regional enteritis (Crohn's disease)
Malabsorption syndrome
Ischaemic colitis
Neurogenic disorders
Sphincter damage

intrinsic or extrinsic, although there are many different aetiological classifications in medical literature.

Intrinsic causes

Normally, the stimulus for peristalsis arises within the intestine. It may cause direct stimulation of the muscle tissue, or may initiate sensory nerve impulses that are transmitted to the central nervous system, resulting in parasympathetic nerve impulses being carried out to the intestine which then stimulate its motility. Disease or irritation within the bowel that may increase either direct stimulation or reflex hypermotility include the following:

Malabsorption   Impaired absorption of foods may be due to incomplete digestion or to a defect in the absorptive process of the small intestine. Obviously, with reduced digestion and absorption, an increase in the bulk of the colonic content results and is a stimulus to intestinal motility. The stools are bulky, have an offensive odour and usually contain large amounts of fats, which are irritating to the bowel mucosa and initiate reflex peristalsis. The presence of unabsorbed osmotically active substances, such as glucose or a disaccharide, causes osmotic diarrhoea. The increased intraluminal osmotic pressure causes water to move into the intestine, producing diarrhoea.

Inflammation   Chronic inflammatory bowel diseases (Crohn's disease, ulcerative colitis and diverticulitis) all cause inflammatory processes in different parts of the gastrointestinal tract. Crohn's disease and ulcerative colitis, while progressive in nature, are characterized by periods of remission and exacerbation.

Laxatives   Many laxatives act by direct irritation of the intestinal mucosa, resulting in the content being hurried through the colon before the normal amount of water has been absorbed. Over use of laxatives is a reasonably common problem and should be considered as a possible differential diagnosis when the patient presents with diarrhoea.

Infection   Food or fluid contaminated by salmonella, shigella or staphylococcal organisms is the most common cause of intestinal infection and may be referred to as bacterial food poisoning. Meat or milk contaminated with *Escherichia coli 0157* has recently caused several serious community-based outbreaks of food poisoning. A vero cytotoxin produced by the bacterium causes haemorrhagic colitis and has profound systemic effects including renal failure. The shigella bacterium causes bacillary dysentery, and the primary source is usually the excreta of an infected person. This disease is rare, except under crowded and poor sanitary conditions.

Salmonella bacilli may inhabit the intestine of humans, fowl and animals, and may be the source of infection to others. They may be transmitted by the meat of infected animals and by food or water contaminated by the excreta of infected humans or animals. Sporadic outbreaks occur and may be due to a human carrier employed in the handling of food. Ingested salmonella or shigella organisms multiply, causing irritation and inflammation of the intestine, resulting in diarrhoea accompanied by crampy abdominal pain, fever, nausea and vomiting.

Neoplasms   Diarrhoea may be a symptom of a malignant neoplasm of the colon and may be alternated with periods of constipation. A change in bowel habit should always be taken seriously, particularly in the older population in whom the incidence of bowel cancer is most prevalent.

Dietary factors   An excessive amount of coarse foods or highly seasoned irritating food may produce hypermotility of the bowel. Occasionally, allergy to a certain foods may account for diarrhoea; if the intestinal mucosa is sensitive to the food, it becomes hyperaemic and oedematous and causes increased reflex hypermotility.

Antibiotics   Diarrhoea sometimes accompanies the administration of antibiotics. They may irritate the mucosa or alter the normal bacterial flora of the intestinal tract allowing infection by 'opportunistic' pathogens (e.g. *Clostridium difficile*). The most frequent offenders are the tetracycline and broad-spectrum antibiotics (e.g. co-amoxiclav).

Idiopathic inflammation   Patients with ulcerative colitis or regional enteritis experience severe diarrhoea. No specific cause has been recognized for either condition.

Extrinsic causes

Diarrhoea accompanies a variety of disorders in which the stimulus that results in increased parasympathetic innervation to the bowel originates outside the intestine.

Emotional stress   Anxiety or underlying tension may be associated with diarrhoea. Intestinal hypermobility and hypersecretion occur with both physical and mental stress. A study of the patient's total life situation may reveal a specific emotional conflict or ineffective coping that may account for the problem.

General or systemic disorders Frequently, diarrhoea is associated with general diseases, particularly if they cause toxaemia. Examples of such conditions are acute infectious disease, hyperthyroidism and uraemia.

History taking and physical examination of the patient with diarrhoea

History taking The health history should be specifically focused on the following information:

● the patient's previous bowel habits
● the number of bowel movements each day
● the volume and consistency of the stools
● whether the stools contain blood or excessive mucus
● whether the patient experiences abdominal pain
● whether there is exacerbation with certain foods or activities
● whether the diarrhoea is worse during the day or the night. Functional diarrhoea tends to occur during the day, while that associated with organic disease is generally as disturbing at night as during the day
● the systemic effects on the person:
   What is the hydrational status?
   Is the temperature increased?
   Is the person exhausted because of loss of sleep?
   Is the person losing weight?
   Are there any other associated symptoms such as nausea or vomiting?
● whether or not there are increased bowel sounds
● the individual's perception of, and reaction to, the diarrhoea
● the condition of the skin around the anus and over pressure areas.

Physical examination Physical examination for intestinal problems is the same as the abdominal examination outlined above (p. 450).

Goals

Potential goals for the patient with diarrhoea include:

1 formed stools
2 a return to the usual frequency of bowel elimination
3 fluid and electrolyte balance and absence of signs of dehydration
4 integrity of skin.

Nursing intervention

Measures to decrease peristalsis Peristalsis of the small and large intestines may be slowed by the following measures:

1 Removal of the cause of the diarrhoea. This may involve the administration of prescribed antibiotics for intestinal infection, avoidance of specific foods for the patient with a malabsorption disorder or an intestinal allergy, and avoidance of laxatives and treatment for systemic diseases such as hyperthyroidism or uraemia.

2 Changing the diet to eliminate spicy foods, fruit juices, raw fruits and vegetables and gas-forming foods.
3 Use of drugs. In particular conditions, various medications may be used in the treatment of diarrhoea:
   a) Drugs to reduce intestinal spasm and motility may be ordered. Examples are diphenoxylate hydrochloride (Lomotil) and loperamide hydrochloride (Imodium).
   b) Opiates such as codeine phosphate are believed to increase absorption by acting on the opiate receptors.
   c) Drugs to provide a protective coating on the intestinal mucosa or to provide an adsorbent, which condenses and holds irritating substances, can be used. Examples are kaolin, aluminium hydroxide gel and bismuth subcarbonate.
   d) An anti-infective drug may be ordered if the diarrhoea is persistent and of microbial origin.

Measures to promote rest The patient with diarrhoea feels weak and fatigued. Rest periods are provided and the person is encouraged to relax and pursue sedentary activities such as reading or watching television. If necessary, the patient is assisted to the bathroom, or a commode chair may be used at the bedside. The call-button should be answered promptly to avoid unnecessary effort or anxiety for the patient in attempting to reach the bathroom in time.

Some people are unable to relax and rest because of a constant fear of not getting to the bathroom in time; in such instances it may be helpful to make an exception and leave a covered commode at the bedside within the patient's reach.

Measures to maintain fluids and nutrition If oral intake is tolerated, the patient is encouraged to concentrate on drinking fluid. Small amounts of food can be taken if the patient feels hungry. Carbonated drinks and iced fluids may exacerbate the diarrhoea and if so, the patient should avoid these. If the patient is unable to tolerate oral intake, fluid and electrolytes are replaced by intravenous infusions.

The diet is expanded as soon as possible to reduce the possibility of nutritional deficiencies. A high-calorie, high-vitamin and high-protein diet is gradually introduced, and the patient is observed to determine the intestinal response. Roughage and gas-producing foods are restricted at first; whole-grain bread and cereals, raw fruits and vegetables and highly seasoned and fried foods should be avoided. Concentrated sweets and fats are likely to be poorly tolerated. Fibre-containing foods and roughage can be introduced gradually. If the diarrhoea is due to malabsorption, a gluten-free diet may be ordered in which foods are avoided that contain any wheat, rye, and barley grains or flour.

The first few mouthfuls of a meal may initiate a mass peristaltic wave, and the meal is interrupted by defaecation. The patient may require some persuasion to continue the meal because of fear of provoking another attack of diarrhoea.

Hygiene issues The patient who is mobile should be located as near to the toilet as possible on the ward and, if confined to bed, privacy should be provided so the patient is less embarrassed by frequent use of the commode.

The anal region should be left clean after each defaecation and, if the skin around the anus is irritated, it is washed and a protective cream applied. Soiled bedding or clothing is changed promptly. Provision is made for thorough washing of the patient's hands after each defaecation, and the nurse should also remember the importance of thorough handwashing. Commode or toilet facilities must be kept scrupulously clean. The patient may very well be embarrassed by the recurring episodes of diarrhoea. The nurse therefore should be sensitive and supportive, being aware of the demoralizing effects this problem may have on the patient. It may help to provide distractions for the patient, particularly if the patient has been confined to a side ward as a precaution against the spread of infection.

Control of infection Cases of acute diarrhoea are considered potentially infectious until indicated otherwise. Precautions should be used to prevent the possible spread of infection to others. It is important that all people who have been in contact with the patient should scrub the hands with soap and running water after each contact. Contaminated waste such as soiled dressings or swabs must be put into bags, which are sealed and labelled with a biohazard warning. When performing any nursing care procedures requiring contact with the patient's faeces, disposable gloves should be worn.

Acute infectious diarrhoea may readily spread throughout a family, school, hall of residence or neighbourhood because of a common source of infected food or water. The nurse may play an important role in the prevention of diarrhoea by alerting people to the hazards various foods, particularly meat and those with cream filling or topping. Opportunities may arise to emphasize the hygienic handling of food and the importance of thorough handwashing after going to the toilet and the handling of soiled clothing.

Carers should be informed of precautions to take to prevent spread to others. Should other individuals who live with that person develop acute diarrhoea, the likely source of the problem needs to be investigated.

If a large number of cases are found in a school or community, the local health authorities should be notified so that a systematic investigation as to the possible source may be instituted. Occasionally, acute diarrhoea may spread through the patients on one ward. The primary source of such an outbreak should be sought. Personnel are urged to practise strict precautions, for infection may be carried from one patient to another or from a member of staff to patients through failure to wash the hands thoroughly between patients.

Evaluation
Evaluation of the goals and outcome criteria is based on examination of the person's stools, documented evidence of a decrease in the frequency of defaecation, and absence of fluid and electrolyte imbalances, as well as on the patient's reported perceptions that the diarrhoea is decreased or absent. For individuals with chronic bowel disease that causes diarrhoea, success of the interventions may be determined when they resume active participation in social and recreational activities.

Constipation

The majority of persons normally defaecate once every 24 hours but there is considerable variance in the frequency among healthy persons. Some persons have more than one bowel movement daily, whereas others may have an evacuation of a normal moist stool once every 2–3 days. Such variances in frequency of bowel elimination are compatible with health. Constipation may be a delay in the passage of faeces through the colon, referred to as colonic constipation, or it may be due to prolonged retention of the faeces in the rectum. Constipation is a symptom not a disease (Thompson et al 2003) and can cause great discomfort to the patient.

A patient can be described as being constipated if they demonstrate two or more of the following within a 3-month period:

- straining for at least a quarter of the time
- lumpy or hard stool for at least a quarter of the time
- a sensation of incomplete evacuation for at least one-quarter of the time
- two or fewer bowel movements a week (Thompson et al 1992).

This is known as the 'Rome' diagnostic criteria.

Causes
The causes of constipation are many and varied. Constipation may be related to slow transit, obstruction or idiopathic causes (Rigby and Powell 2005) lifestyle factors, pharmacological factors, metabolic and endocrine disorders or neurological conditions (Thompson et al 2003). It may be associated with organic disease, or may be a functional disturbance.

Diseases associated with constipation Disease within the colon or rectum may narrow the lumen of the bowel and offer resistance to the forward movement of content. Common examples of diseases associated with constipation are:

- neoplasms of the intestine
- endocrine disorders such as diabetes or hypothyroidism
- neurological disorders such as multiple sclerosis, paraplegia, Parkinson's disease or cerebrovascular accident
- inflammation, which causes spasm, scarring and adhesions
- partial volvulus (twisting of the bowel).

Intra-abdominal pressure Severe ascites (accumulation of fluid in the peritoneal cavity) or a tumour, such as an ovarian cyst or uterine fibroid, may compress the colon and delay the movement of intestinal content.

Alteration in innervation of the intestine Failure of the normal propulsive movement may occur due to some disturbance or imbalance in the innervation of the intestine. The derangement may result in excessive tone and spasm in a segment of the bowel that retards the movement of the content. The spasm may be induced by a hypersensitivity of the colon or by anxiety. Constipation may be associated with injury or degeneration of the spinal cord or cauda equina, which affects the nerve supply to the colon and rectum.

Diminished food and fluid intake   Constipation may be associated with any illness in which there is diminished intake of food and fluid, or in cases where the diet is modified and lacks fibre, resulting in less residue in the stool. The lesser amount of food does not provide sufficient bulk to stimulate peristalsis. Dehydration causes a small, dry, hard stool that may irritate the colon, causing spasm, or may fail to stimulate normal colonic motility.

Medications causing constipation   Occasionally, drugs used in treatment may decrease intestinal motility and delay excretion. This increases exposure of the faeces to the absorptive surface of the intestines, resulting in dried out faeces and subsequent constipation. Common examples of such drugs are opiates, anticholinergic drugs, antiparkinson drugs, blood pressure medications (particularly calcium channel blockers), antacids, antidepressants, diuretics and iron supplements.

Muscular weakness   Expulsion of the faeces is aided by increasing the intra-abdominal pressure to compress the colon and rectum. This involves contraction of the muscles of the abdominal wall and diaphragm. Weakness of these muscles due to disease, ageing, malnutrition or inactivity may contribute to constipation. Similarly, lack of tone in the intestinal musculature or weakness of the levator ani muscles may impair peristalsis and expulsive power.

Habitual use of laxatives   Frequent causes of constipation in persons who are not ill are faulty defaecation habits, faulty diet and the habitual use of laxatives. The person may delay response to the defaecation urge because it is inconvenient or because toilet facilities are not available. If the urge to defaecate is ignored and evacuation delayed, the reflex becomes weak as the rectal mucosa adapts to the pressure of the content. Repeated failure to respond to the defaecation reflex may eventually result in the rectum becoming insensitive to the presence of a faecal mass and the reflex is not initiated.

Many persons have an inordinate concern about bowel elimination and think they must have a daily bowel movement or a frequent purge and resort to unnecessary, repeated use of a laxative. Loss of intestinal tone and reduced peristaltic response to normal food residue follow the use of a laxative, and then – too often – the laxative is repeated. The colon is not allowed to regain its natural rhythmic response to the normal faecal mass.

Dietary causes   A deficiency of foods with cellulose and fibrous content in the diet may be the cause of constipation. Refined foods and those that leave little residue after absorption, fail to produce sufficient bulk to stimulate colonic motility.

Constipation may cause considerable discomfort; the person may experience abdominal pain, a full feeling and abdominal distension. There is a loss of appetite accompanied by headache and eventually nausea and vomiting. The hard dry masses of faecal matter may damage the intestinal mucosa and lead to a fissure. Haemorrhoids are frequently the result of chronic constipation.

History taking and physical examination of the patient with constipation

History taking   Management of constipation can only be planned after a comprehensive assessment of the patient (Rigby and Powell 2005). The nursing history should focus on:

- the person's usual bowel elimination habits
- the person's perceptions of what is normal bowel elimination
- the person's eating habits – types of foods taken and the volume of fluid taken daily
- a description of the stool, its shape, colour, consistency and the presence or absence of signs of blood
- the duration, timing and severity of the problem recent changes in usual eating habits, fluid intake and physical activity
- pain, abdominal cramps, passing of gas associated with constipation
- history of disorders or medication therapy that may have altered food intake, digestion or absorption of foods, or bowel motility or sensation
- any unusual effort or stimulation used to promote defaecation including the use of laxatives or enemas
- the person's living arrangements and the availability of toilet facilities
- the family's knowledge of foods that contain fibre and the value of fibre in promoting bowel function; the need to maintain an adequate fluid intake; the benefits of exercise and activity; and the action and untoward effects of various types of laxatives.

The person may be asked to keep a record over 2–4 days to determine the frequency and time of bowel elimination, the volume and characteristics of the faeces. Any warning signs of constipation experienced by the patient such as abdominal cramps or flatulence should be noted, along with the patient's own feelings about the problem.

Physical examination   Physical examination for the person with constipation commences with the abdominal examination as outlined above (p. 450) and will include a rectal examination when appropriate. The patient needs to lie in the left lateral position for this examination with their knees bent up towards their abdomen. Some patients may find this position particularly uncomfortable and so thought should be given regarding the best possible position for a particular patient. The patient should be warned that this is not a painful examination but it may produce a feeling of 'fullness' in the rectum. This examination should only ever be carried out on a child by highly experienced clinicians for very specific and clearly documented reasons.

Commence the examination by observing the rectal area for signs of haemorrhoids and the health of the surrounding skin. Gently place the gloved, lubricated index finger of your dominant hand into the anal canal and rectum. Gently sweep the finger around assessing for the presence of hard stool or any palpable masses. The normal rectum should feel smooth and pliable. When you withdraw your gloved hand check the glove for the presence of stool or any other discharge including blood or mucus. Talk to the patient throughout the examination to allay anxiety and to ensure that they report any feelings of discomfort as the examination progresses. Findings should be documented accordingly and a plan of action developed accordingly.

Potential goals for the patient with constipation
The person will demonstrate:

1 understanding of the role of dietary fibre and fluid intake in stool formation and defaecation
2 awareness of the role of regular physical activity in the promotion of bowel elimination
3 a plan to increase dietary fibre and fluid intake and to obtain regular physical activity
4 awareness of the role of various medications in the cause of constipation
5 regular bowel elimination producing soft normal stools.

Nursing intervention
Box 15.3 lists the steps to be implemented in formulating a plan to develop regular bowel elimination habits for a patient.

Establishing a regular schedule   It is helpful to explain to the person in simple terms the physiological mechanism of defaecation so that the significance of responding to the initial urge for defaecation may be understood. The frequency of bowel elimination varies with the individual. It should be stressed to the patient that daily bowel elimination is not essential to health; defaecation every 2–3 days may be normal for some people.

Patients who are constipated due to a side-effect of their medication should be assessed for alternative treatments.

Dietary modifications   The nurse and dietitian work with the patient and family to evaluate current dietary habits and then help them to plan a diet that provides a liberal amount of fibre-containing foods, taking into consideration the person's food preferences, financial resources and daily routine. Emphasis is placed on whole-grain cereals and bread, fresh fruits and vegetables, and fruit juices. A daily fluid intake of 2000–2500 mL is recommended unless contraindicated by a cardiovascular or renal condition.

Peristalsis may be promoted by the drinking of a cup of hot water on rising in the morning (approximately 30 minutes before breakfast).

Techniques to promote defaecation   Box 15.4 lists various measures the person may use to promote regular bowel elimination; a scheduled time for defaecation is stressed as is the importance of prompt response to the urge to defaecate. Ensuring comfort and privacy during the defaecation attempt, contracting abdominal muscles, leaning forward and bearing down to increase abdominal pressure and, in some cases, application of manual pressure to the abdomen may be helpful.

The person is instructed to implement these techniques daily until defaecation occurs. If no bowel movement occurs in 2–3 days, glycerine suppositories may be used. If this is still not effective, a stool softener or bulk laxative may be administered. Once the person establishes a regular schedule, other laxatives or enemas should not be necessary.

Physical exercise   Some physical exercise is essential; walking is especially helpful and good tone in the abdominal muscles is important.

Box 15.3   Steps to establish regular bowel elimination habits

1 Identify factors contributing to constipation.

2 Gradually discontinue the use of laxatives and enemas.

3 Develop a diet plan to increase fibre and fluid intake.

4 Develop a plan to increase daily physical activity.

5 Establish a schedule for daily bowel elimination.

6 Implement diet, exercise plans and elimination schedule daily.

7 Evaluate the effectiveness of plan each day.

8 Modify plan as necessary.

Box 15.4   Techniques to promote bowel elimination

1 Increase the amount of fibre in the diet.

2 Increase daily fluid intake.

3 Increase daily physical activity.

4 Respond promptly to the urge for a bowel movement.

5 Drink a cup of warm liquid half an hour before the usual time of defaecation.

6 Go to the bathroom at the usual time for defaecation.

7 Sit comfortably on the toilet in an environment that provides privacy, quiet and warmth.

8 Use the following techniques to stimulate peristalsis:
   a) contract abdominal muscles, lean forward and bear down
   b) exert manual pressure downward on the abdomen.

9 If the above techniques are not successful in producing a bowel movement, consider use of the following:
   a) glycerine suppository
   b) emollient laxative or stool softener
   c) bulk-forming laxative, or
   d) enema.

Laxatives and enemas Laxatives, enemas and suppositories that the patient may be accustomed to using should be gradually discontinued. If increased dietary fibre, fluids and exercise are not sufficient at the beginning to establish normal bowel elimination, mild laxatives may be employed until the defaecation reflex is restored and bowel irritability and spasm are reduced. Glycerine suppositories placed in the rectum, and into stool if present, may be used 30 minutes before the usual time of defaecation to stimulate peristalsis and soften the stool. The suppository may be repeated daily for several days. If this is not effective, a stool softener may be prescribed to prevent severe straining at stool and injury to the rectal and anal tissues. The stool softeners in use are mineral oil and preparations of docusate sodium (which acts as both a softening agent and a stimulant). These latter preparations act as wetting agents, allowing water to penetrate and mix with the faecal mass. Mineral oil should not be used for prolonged periods because it may prevent normal intestinal absorption, especially of fat-soluble vitamins.

Bulk-forming laxatives may also be recommended. These preparations swell when combined with fluid in the gastrointestinal tract and have a stimulating effect. Examples of bulk-forming laxatives are bran and ispaghula husk. Use of these laxatives should be assessed carefully in the elderly if dehydration is present. Osmotic laxatives such as lactulose syrup are disaccharides that are not absorbed in the small intestine. They are broken down by bacteria in the colon and acidify the colonic contents, which then stimulates peristalsis and serves as an effective laxative for the elderly. Stimulant laxatives such as senna, bisacodyl, docusate and danthron cause rhythmic muscle contractions resulting in the expulsion of the faeces. All laxatives should be used with caution and prudence, as the aim of nursing interventions with patients who are constipated is ultimately to return them to normal bowel function without the assistance of laxatives.

Evaluation
A programme of increased dietary fibre, increased fluid intake, regular physical activity and a schedule for defaecation can promote effective regular bowel elimination for most adults as well as for the frail elderly. The use of laxatives is usually not necessary if a comprehensive bowel elimination programme is followed. In hospital and long-term care settings, the documentation of bowel patterns and laxative use on the same assessment tool facilitates regular review of the effectiveness of nursing intervention. Information from chart audits on a nursing unit as well as data provided by a quality assurance programme help nurses to analyse their clinical practice and to identify strengths and areas for change in relation to common health problems such as constipation.

Faecal impaction
Occasionally, faeces accumulate in the rectum, producing a hard dry mass that forms a partial or complete obstruction. It occurs most often in older persons and in those with central nervous system disorders. These patients frequently suffer a loss of intestinal musculature motility and sensation. It may be associated with dehydration, lack of dietary fibre and volume, immobilization or narcotics. Manifestations include cramping pain, the passage of liquid stools without expulsion of the hard palpable faecal mass. The patient may complain of headache, fatigue, loss of appetite, and pressure and discomfort in the rectal and anal regions. Faecal impaction is identified by the presence of a palpable hard mass in the rectum, the oozing of liquid stools without passing the faecal mass and the absence of a bowel movement for over 3 days.

Goals
The potential goals of nursing care for the patient with faecal impaction include:

1 regular bowel movements after relief of impaction
2 understanding of the role of dietary fibre and fluid intake in stool formation and defaecation
3 awareness of the role of physical activity in promoting bowel elimination
4 application of a programme to promote regular bowel elimination.

Nursing intervention
Relief of impaction The faecal impaction is treated by the administration of an oil retention enema to soften the impacted stool and by oral administration of an emollient laxative such as docusate sodium, which also softens the stools. The enema is followed in a few hours by digital breaking up and removal of the faecal mass. As described in examination of the rectum above (p. 461) the nurse lubricates a gloved finger and gently inserts it into the patient's rectum to loosen the impacted faeces. A cleansing enema of saline or tap water is then given. This process is usually both embarrassing and exhausting; following the enema, the patient is made comfortable and allowed to rest. Psychological support is very important.

Promotion of regular bowel elimination habits The patient experiencing faecal impaction should be assisted to develop a regular bowel elimination programme which includes dietary management, increased activity, a regular schedule and the use of techniques to stimulate peristalsis. Glycerine suppositories, stool softeners or bulk laxatives may be required initially. Impaction occurs most often in the elderly who do not eat adequate fibre and who have problems with mobility and experience difficulties in getting to the bathroom. The patient's living environment is assessed and the accessibility of the toilet taken into consideration. Assistance may be required from the district nurse, neighbours and friends to ensure the aged or incapacitated individual receives an adequate diet and necessary physical assistance. If the patient is in a hospital or nursing home, a plan for bowel elimination is an integral part of the patient care plan. Excessive bedrest is avoided and physical activity encouraged.

Evaluation

The nursing care of patients with faecal impaction can be assessed by the resumption of regular, spontaneous bowel movements and the absence of further episodes of impaction.

Faecal incontinence

Assessment

The nursing history is reviewed to determine the patient's usual bowel elimination habits. The problem of incontinence is assessed by observing and recording the frequency of defaecation, the consistency of the stools, and warning signs experienced or expressed by the patient related to defaecation. It is important to note whether the patient experiences an urge to defaecate, manifests abdominal discomfort, massages the abdomen, or provides verbal clues that defaecation is occurring. Mental alertness is evaluated to determine the patient's ability to respond to the urge to defaecate and to follow a bowel elimination schedule.

Goals

Potential goals for the patient with faecal incontinence are:

1 controlled and regular bowel evacuation
2 absence or decrease in episodes of faecal incontinence

and if these are not achievable:

3 the maintenance of personal hygiene and dignity.

Nursing intervention

Establishment of a regular bowel routine   Faecal continence can be established by developing regular bowel elimination habits, as discussed for the patient experiencing constipation, or by establishing a programme for regular bowel evacuation.

Programme to stimulate peristalsis   When the cause of the incontinence is constipation or faecal impaction, as commonly occurs in the older person, a programme to adjust the diet and activity, maintain regularity and stimulate peristaltic activity is usually effective.

Prevention of reflex bowel emptying   When neuromuscular control is impaired, management of incontinence is directed to preventing reflex emptying of the bowel in response to rectal distension by faeces. If the patient has a predictable pattern of defaecation such as after breakfast each morning, a schedule can be developed to ensure that the patient is assisted to the bathroom or to a commode each morning after breakfast. If the patient's pattern of defaecation is irregular, attempts are made to establish a regular time for bowel evacuation. A daily routine is established, similar to that described for the patient who is constipated. The techniques described in Box 15.4 to stimulate peristalsis are employed. If no bowel movement occurs, the routine is repeated the next day. A glycerine suppository may be used on the second or third day to further stimulate defaecation. If the patient usually defaecates every 2 days, this measure would be introduced on the second day before the expected involuntary defaecation. A stool softener may also be used.

Patients with spinal cord injury or neurological disease are usually able to establish a regular defaecation pattern and avoid episodes of incontinence. Routine enemas and laxatives are avoided. Patient participation in developing and implementing a bowel-retraining programme is important if long-term results are to be achieved.

Personal hygiene   Until regular bowel evacuation is established, the incontinent patient is kept clean and dry, and skin irritation is avoided. Following faecal incontinence, the skin is washed with soap, rinsed well and patted dry. Protective ointment may be applied to provide a coating over the skin. The clothing and bedding are changed as often as necessary to keep the patient clean. The nurse may reduce the patient's embarrassment and concern with reassurance that it is understood that the patient cannot control the bowel movements but that this can be achieved with a bowel-retraining programme. Episodes of incontinence may still occur if the patient develops diarrhoea or if the routine is changed, but most patients can achieve acceptable control if the programme is followed.

Irritable bowel syndrome

Irritable bowel syndrome (IBS) is a common but poorly understood syndrome characterized by multiple abdominal symptoms. It affects Western populations, and women are more likely to experience it than men. It is difficult to know how many people are affected but it is estimated that between 20 and 25% of the population have IBS symptoms and it accounts for 36–50% of all gastrointestinal consultations (Boyd-Carson 2004). IBS is a debilitating condition which has a significant impact upon people's lives. However, it is not associated with other gastrointestinal disorders such as cancer and it occurs in the absence of any organic cause.

Features of IBS include:

● cramping abdominal pain
● bloated abdomen
● altered and unpredictable bowel habit.

Abnormal colonic motility increases pressure in the large bowel. Spasmodic, non-propulsive contractions in the sensitive colonic muscularis result in cramp or spasm-like pain, but faeces may not be moved effectively through the colon. Consequently, they become hard, dry and pellet-like. Alternatively, very loose stool may be passed with urgency, but also with associated pain and bloating. The treatment of IBS depends upon the patient's particular symptoms. Antispasmodics (e.g. mebeverine) may help with severe cramping symptoms, osmotic laxatives may help patients with constipation and antidiarrhoeals may help those with diarrhoea as a predominant feature. Many people prefer to try to adapt their diet and lifestyle, or use complementary therapies to manage their symptoms.

People with IBS often fear they have cancer. IBS is often diagnosed only when all other differential diagnoses have been excluded by means of extensive investigation. Thus, the person can usually be reassured. Nursing support and encouragement to adapt lifestyle and manage symptoms is vital for people with IBS.

Malabsorption syndrome

Malabsorption involves failure to transport nutrients from the intestinal lumen to the vascular and lymphatic systems with loss of nutrients in the stool. It results from impairment of either the digestive or the absorptive process.

Nutrients are absorbed: (1) into the capillaries and from there are carried through the portal vein into the liver and then into the systemic circulation; or (2) through the lacteals into the thoracic lymphatic system and on into the systemic circulation. The absorptive cells of the intestinal villi are especially adapted for both absorption and secretion.

The causes of malabsorption may be:

- a lack of normal intraluminal digestion
- dysfunction of the absorptive cells of the intestinal mucosa
- impairment of the intestinal circulation or lymphatic system.

Clinical characteristics

The signs and symptoms of the malabsorption syndrome vary from severe to very mild; with the latter, the disorder may go undetected for years. The major manifestations are: weight loss; abnormal stools which are bulky, soft, light yellow to grey in colour and have a rancid odour; abdominal distension; anorexia; muscle wasting; peripheral oedema; weakness and skeletal disorders. Table 15.1 lists the signs and symptoms of malabsorption with their aetiological factors.

Digestive disturbances   Malabsorption due to digestive disturbances occurs with: liver and biliary tract disease, following a gastrectomy and with bacterial overgrowth in the small bowel. With liver and biliary tract disease, the primary symptom of inadequate digestion and absorption is the presence of steatorrhoea or undigested fat in the stool. Decreased synthesis or excretion of bile salts results in impaired digestion of fat and interferes with the absorption of vitamin D and calcium. Following a gastric resection, emptying of the stomach occurs more rapidly; the duodenum may be bypassed, decreasing the stimulation of pancreatic enzymes; mixing of bile salts may be inadequate; stasis of intestinal contents may occur; and protein intake may be decreased.

Bacterial growth in the small bowel is controlled by normal peristalsis. When intestinal motility is impaired, bacterial proliferation occurs, resulting in changes in the action of the bile salts. Fat absorption is impaired and steatorrhoea is present. Vitamin B_{12} absorption is also decreased due to its utilization by the micro-organisms.

Dysfunction of absorbing cells   Malabsorption due to dysfunction or destruction of the absorbing cells may be due to an inadequate absorptive surface resulting from extensive resection of the small bowel, intestinal bypass or extensive inflammatory disease. Patient management includes a high-calorie diet: high in carbohydrates and protein and low in fat. Vitamin and mineral supplements are administered. Drugs such as belladonna alkaloids and codeine may be given to decrease intestinal motility. Ranitidine may be given to decrease gastric acid secretion. Long-term parenteral nutrition may be required for some patients.

Enzyme deficiencies   The malabsorption syndrome may be due to enzyme deficiencies in the intestinal mucosal cells. Adult lactase deficiency is a common disorder which causes an intolerance to lactose – the sugar found in milk. Hydrolysis of disaccharides takes place on the glycocalyx of the microvilli of the intestinal cells. When lactase is deficient, lactose is not hydrolyzed to galactose, and glucose and is not absorbed; it remains in the intestinal lumen and draws water by osmosis into the lumen. Symptoms include abdominal cramps, distension, flatulence and diarrhoea following ingestion of dairy products. The diagnosis is made by taking a history and by a lactose tolerance test. The disorder is more common in African-Caribbean and Asian people than in Caucasians. Treatment consists of a milk-free diet; cheese contains a minimal amount of lactose and is tolerated by most patients.

Gluten-sensitive enteropathy   Gluten-sensitive enteropathy (coeliac disease) is an immunological disorder characterized by a reaction of the intestinal mucosa, particularly in the jejunum, to gliadin (a component of the gluten of wheat). The mucosa is damaged, the villi atrophy and absorptive cells are infiltrated by lymphocytes and plasma cells. Other enzyme alterations may occur. Mucosal damage results in decreased stimulation of pancreatic hormones, impaired absorption of water and electrolytes, and the excretion of unabsorbed fats.

Symptoms include weight loss, distension, diarrhoea and steatorrhoea. Patients often present with iron deficient anaemia and general lassitude. Coeliac disease can also be implicated in patients who have fertility problems, endocrine disorders, osteoporosis or dermatitis herpetiforms (Griffiths 2005). Serological testing for coeliac disease has almost 100% specificity and 98% sensitivity, although some patients may be diagnosed through biopsies during endoscopic investigations.

A gluten-free diet is recommended; wheat, rye, barley and oats are avoided. Rice, corn, soybean and potato flours are used as substitutes in the diet. Certain gluten free products are available on prescription in the UK. The advice and support of a dietitian is essential for patients with coeliac disease.

Drugs   Certain drugs may also interfere with intestinal absorption. Examples of drugs that affect the absorption in the intestine include antacids, anticonvulsants, biguanides and folic acid.

Table 15.1 Potential problems for the patient with systemic manifestations of malabsorption

Causes	Clinical characteristics
Nutrition less than body requirements	
Malabsorption of fat, carbohydrate or protein; calorie loss; and protein loss (albumin)	Muscle wasting, weight loss and oedema
Altered bowel elimination	
Impaired absorption or increased secretion of water and electrolytes	Diarrhoea, abdominal distension and flatulence, fatigue
Increased secretion of water and electrolytes with unabsorbed bile and fatty acids	Pale, bulky, odorous stools
Fluid and electrolyte load in excess of absorptive capacity of colon	Weight loss
Impaired carbohydrate absorption	
Impaired fat absorption and increased loss of fat	
Altered urinary elimination	
Delayed absorption of water; hypokalaemia	Nocturia and dehydration
Weakness and fatigue	
Impaired absorption of iron, vitamin B_{12}, folate; loss of electrolytes (potassium)	Anaemia and weakness
Increased potential for bleeding	
Impaired vitamin K absorption; increased prothrombin time	Bruising and haematuria
Altered muscle tone and sensation	
Impaired absorption of calcium and magnesium	Muscle cramps, tetany, and prickling and burning sensations
Impaired absorption of potassium	Muscle flaccidity, weakness, decreased tendon reflexes and cardiac arrhythmia
Increased potential for injury	
Impaired absorption of calcium and protein; demineralization of bone	Skeletal deformities and bone fractures
Altered sexuality patterns	
Impaired protein absorption; loss of calories	Amenorrhoea Decreased libido
Altered integrity of skin and oral mucosa	
Impaired absorption of iron, vitamin B_{12} and other vitamins	Dermatitis, glossitis and dry fissures of the lips
Altered visual acuity	
Impaired absorption of vitamin A	Night blindness

History taking and physical examination of the patient with a digestive disturbance

History taking Data collected from the patient during the health history focus on the diet, bowel habits and the symptoms being experienced.

Problems commonly encountered by patients are listed in Table 15.1; these should be borne in mind during the assessment and form the basis for a patient interview. The patient's perspective is very important in considering these problems and the effects they may have on everyday life.

Physical examination The nurse inspects the patient's skin for dryness, turgor and oedema. The specific characteristics of the patient's stools are observed and documented. The person's height and weight are recorded and their desirable body weight is determined. The perianal area should be examined discretely for soreness, excoriation, fissures and fistulae. Any episodes of faecal incontinence should be established, and how these were managed by the individual.

Goals

The person with malabsorption disorders will demonstrate:

1 achievement and maintenance of a desirable body weight
2 a decrease in diarrhoea
3 understanding of recommended dietary measures
4 integrity of skin and oral mucosa.

Nursing intervention

Health problems common to persons with malabsorption syndrome are listed in Table 15.1. As malabsorption syndromes are usually not curable, care for the patient is directed towards control of nutritional deficiencies and alleviation of symptoms.

Diet Dietary measures include elimination of the specific inabsorbable nutrient from the diet and administration of the unabsorbed nutrients by other routes if necessary.

The person with gluten-sensitive enteropathy should eliminate wheat, rye, barley and oats from the diet and substitute cornmeal and potato, rice and soyabean flour. The dietitian may provide recipes that substitute these products for the traditional wheat, rye and oat flours used in breads, pastries, cakes and pastas. The patient is also advised about health food stores and other outlets that carry gluten-free products.

The person with lactose intolerance should avoid dairy products, prepared foods and baked goods containing milk, butter and cheeses, instant coffee and chocolate. Some individuals with lactose intolerance are able to tolerate fermented dairy products such as yoghurt and cheese. Commercial products that are low in lactose or are lactose-free are available as substitutes for milk products in the diet or use as supplements.

Vitamins B_{12} and K are administered parenterally when deficiencies exist and persons with lactose intolerance may require calcium substitutes if dietary calcium is deficient.

Teaching The nurse and dietitian play a major role in patient and family teaching about the malabsorption disorder and dietary measures to manage the syndrome and associated symptoms. The person is taught to identify foods and food products containing the substances that cannot be tolerated and to avoid these in the diet. Skill and experience in reading product labels is emphasized. Individuals are also taught ways to alter the diet to incorporate substitute foods for the ones that are not tolerated. Patients also learn to identify their own symptoms and evaluate their diet to identify contributing factors and then to readjust their diet accordingly.

Evaluation

Symptoms associated with the malabsorption disorder should decrease as the person responds to the dietary changes that eliminate the responsible elements. Progress can be measured by changes in the stools and a decrease in diarrhoea, as well as by the establishment and maintenance of a desirable body weight.

INFLAMMATORY DISORDERS OF THE INTESTINES

Inflammation may develop in any area of the small and large intestines and alter motility, secretion and/or absorption. The most prevalent inflammatory intestinal diseases include the acute conditions of appendicitis and gastro-enteritis, and the chronic disorders of Crohn's disease and ulcerative colitis.

Appendicitis

The appendix, a narrow blind tube extending from the inferior part of the caecum, is a common site of inflammation, which may necessitate its surgical removal. The appendix has no essential function in the human and there is no change in body function when it has been removed.

Causes

The most common cause of appendicitis is obstruction of the lumen by a faecalith (a small, hard mass of accumulated faeces) or a solid foreign body, or by disease or scar tissue in the walls of the appendix. Secretion collects in the tube, causing distension that results in pressure on the intramural blood vessels. The mucosa becomes inflamed, ulcerates and readily becomes infected; the walls may become gangrenous because of the interference with the blood supply, and perforation is likely to occur. A ruptured appendix is serious; it allows the escape of organisms into the peritoneal cavity and may produce an abscess in the appendiceal region or a generalized peritonitis.

The disease may occur at any age but is more common in children over 4 years of age, adolescents and young adults. Early diagnosis and treatment of appendicitis is important to prevent serious complications.

Clinical characteristics

Manifestations of appendicitis are abdominal pain, nausea and vomiting, a moderate increase in temperature and a leucocytosis, with the increase being in the polymorphonuclear cells. At the onset, the pain may be diffuse or referred to the central portion of the abdomen or the lower epigastric region, and is described as crampy. As the inflammation involves the walls of the appendix, the pain becomes localized to the lower right quadrant or McBurney's point (the area about 5 cm from the anterior superior iliac spine on a line with the umbilicus, which corresponds to the normal position of the appendix). The area is tender on palpation, and rigidity gradually develops in the muscles (muscle guarding). Rebound tenderness may be present, and is determined by palpation of the left lower quadrant. With the sudden release of the pressure, the patient experiences pain or discomfort in the appendix region. The patient moves slowly and carefully to avoid jolting and movements that increase the pain, and tends to keep the right thigh flexed.

The omentum and adjacent bowel may become adherent to the inflamed appendix, walling off the area. If the appendix ruptures, an abscess will form in the walled-off cavity. If perforation occurs before the area is walled off, a generalized peritonitis develops; the patient complains of pain and tenderness over the whole abdomen, which becomes rigid and distended. The distension is due to inhibited bowel motility, and may be referred to as paralytic ileus.

Examination of the patient includes palpation of the abdomen and blood tests for full blood count to determine the white blood cell count. The doctor may also conduct a rectal examination, and a vaginal pelvic examination may be done on the female in order to rule out some of the important differential diagnoses.

The treatment of appendicitis is surgical excision of the appendix.

Nursing intervention

The person with abdominal pain should be urged to seek medical advice; self-treatment is discouraged, particularly the taking of a laxative or an enema which could be serious, because either could cause perforation of the appendix through stimulation of peristalsis. The patient is also advised not to take food or fluid until seen by the doctor. This is in case immediate surgery is necessary. In most instances, surgery is performed as soon as the diagnosis is established unless perforation is suspected. If the appendix was intact at the time of removal, the patient usually makes a rapid, uneventful recovery with a short period of hospitalization.

If an abscess is present, a drain is placed in the abscess cavity at the time of operation. The collecting bag attached to the drain allows observation of the discharge and accurate measurement of the volume of fluid draining. Antibiotics are prescribed and the patient should receive a minimum of 2.5 L of fluids daily. An accurate record of the intake should be kept and, if the patient cannot take sufficient quantities by mouth, the administration of intravenous fluids may be necessary. Close observations are made for possible extension of the infection and generalized peritonitis, such as abdominal distension, nausea and vomiting, lack of bowel sounds, a raised temperature and rapid pulse; these are brought promptly to the surgeon's attention.

Box 15.5 gives a care plan for a patient having an uncomplicated appendicectomy. Generally no follow-up is required for patients who have undergone straightforward appendicectomy.

Peritonitis

Peritonitis is a localized or generalized inflammation of the peritoneum and is most often a secondary condition. It is usually acute but may be chronic.

Causes

The inflammatory response may be due to bacterial invasion or chemical irritation caused by bile, pancreatic, gastric or intestinal secretions, urine or blood escaping into the peritoneal cavity. A common infectious agent is Escherichia coli that has escaped from the intestinal lumen.

Intestinal motility is depressed and the intestine becomes distended with gas and fluid. The peritoneal serous membrane becomes hyperaemic and oedematous, and there is an outpouring of fluid into the cavity that incurs serous fluid, electrolyte and protein imbalances.

Clinical characteristics

The patient experiences abdominal pain, nausea, vomiting and distension. The abdomen becomes rigid (muscle guarding) and progressively more distended. A leucocytosis and pyrexia may develop. The pulse becomes rapid and there is a decrease in blood volume due to loss of intravascular volume. The respirations may be shallow and rapid as a result of ventilatory interference by extreme abdominal distension. Unless quickly reversed, the patient shows signs of shock. Bowel sounds are absent as peristalsis ceases.

Treatment is directed toward the primary condition (e.g. an operation to close a perforated ulcer), relieving the distension and re-establishing peristalsis, combating infection and shock and replacing fluids and electrolytes.

Gastric and intestinal intubation with continuous drainage are established. Nothing is given orally. An intravenous infusion is administered and the solutions used may be based upon laboratory determinations of serum electrolyte levels. A blood transfusion may be given to counteract shock and replace protein lost in the inflammatory exudate. An antibiotic is administered if organisms are the causative factor of the peritonitis. The patient is very ill and requires constant supportive nursing care and monitoring.

Chronic inflammatory bowel disease

Crohn's disease and ulcerative colitis are examples of inflammatory bowel disease (IBD). Crohn's disease may affect any part of the gastrointestinal tract from mouth to anus but most commonly involves the terminal ileum and proximal colon. Patches of granulomatous inflammation and ulceration develop in segments of the intestine and involve all layers of the wall. The bowel may perforate and form fistulae into another loop of intestine. As the inflammation subsides, there is scarring and some stenosis, which may lead to a partial obstruction.

Ulcerative colitis is characterized by severe inflammation and ulceration of the mucosa of the rectum and of a part or all of the colon. The process begins in the rectosigmoid area and spreads up the descending colon. There is marked inflammation and oedema in the affected area, followed by ulceration. In affected areas, there may be infection and a loss of fluid, electrolytes and blood.

Incidence

Crohn's disease and ulcerative colitis mainly affect young adults and are much more common in the industrialized West than elsewhere in the world.

Contributing factors

The cause of IBD is unknown. It is believed that more than one mechanism contributes to the development of Crohn's disease and ulcerative colitis. Genetic and environmental factors seem to play a part (Nightingale 2004) and diet, infective agents, smoking and stress seem to play a role (Metcalf 2002). There are many misconceptions about possible causes of IBD such as dietary and personality factors, however, personality characteristics attributed to patients with the condition probably result from the disease and its pattern of exacerbations and remissions rather than contributing to its cause.

Box 15.5 Care plan for a patient undergoing appendicectomy

For a patient undergoing uncomplicated appendicectomy who does not live alone, the overall aim should be to be discharged home safely within 36 hours of operation. Such a patient's problems, the goals for care and the plan to achieve the goals are outlined below.

Problem	Goal	Action
Pain due to incision and resolving peritonitis	To be pain-free or at least to have a pain score of ≤1 (on a scale of 0 no pain, 10 worst pain imaginable). To be able to sleep, move and cough freely.	Administer prescribed analgesia regularly. Do not wait for the pain to develop first. Assess effectiveness of prescription and consult about a change if indicated. Administer oral analgesia as soon as possible, also on a regular basis to avoid the development of pain. As pain subsides, advise a reduction in dose before reducing frequency. Ensure the patient moves in bed every hour and gets out of bed, and undertakes activities of daily living independently.
Altered breathing due to discomfort and anaesthetic	Regular deep breathing; resting rate, <20/minute, >10/minute. No smoking	Deep breathing exercises hourly. Encourage coughing and expectoration. Show the patient how to support the abdomen with a soft pad while doing so. Advise continuing these exercises at home for at least 1 week. If a smoker, discuss the habit with a view to encouraging cessation.
Feeling weak after surgery	Blood pressure to be within the patient's normal limits as before operation. Heart rate <90 bpm or as before surgery. Homeostatic fluid and electrolyte balance to be restored as soon as possible.	Check vital signs regularly after operation for several hours until stable and goal attained. Check 6-hourly thereafter until discharge. Continue intravenous infusion (IVI) after operation until drinking and then discontinue. Check the patient has passed urine within 24 hours of operation and the volume is not more than 500 mL less than that taken in.
Altered gastrointestinal function following surgery	Resume oral intake of light diet and 1500 mL fluid as soon as possible	Clear fluids orally as able. If tolerated, may drink as likes. Remove IVI. Administer prescribed antiemetic if nauseous. When drinks tolerated, offer soup and pudding or light breakfast as appropriate, and light diet thereafter. Advise three light meals and 1500 mL fluid intake at home, introducing larger, high-fibre meals gradually. Counsel about healthy eating as required. Re-establishing bowel habit may take a few days but provided the patient follows advice about healthy eating and drinking and takes daily gentle exercise, this should resolve. Advise to consult GP if not.
Wound healing	Wound to heal by first intention within 2 weeks. Temperature to be <37.5°C.	Check the wound regularly after surgery for oozing and inflammation. Monitor the patient's temperature 6-hourly until discharge. Change the dressing as indicated and before the patient goes home. Advise the patient that it is safe to get the wound wet and demonstrate how to apply clean gauze if desired. If sutures are not absorbed, arrange appointment for practice nurse to remove them at surgeon's instructions (usually 5–7 days). Advise the patient to see their GP if there is any oozing or inflammation in the wound, or fever >37.5°C for more than 12 hours.

Clinical characteristics

Ulcerative colitis   The major symptom of ulcerative colitis is diarrhoea, the severity and frequency of which depend on the extent of colon involvement. Stools are usually liquid, occur with tenesmus (painful, ineffective straining), and may contain blood, mucus and pus. The number of stools per day may vary from as few as four to as many as 24. Accompanying the diarrhoea is a sense of urgency and cramping abdominal pain. The pain is usually located in the lower left quadrant and is colicky in nature. After defaecation, pain may subside.

Ulcerative colitis varies in intensity and severity of presentation, ranging from mild to severe. As the disease becomes more severe, malaise and fatigue occur. Weight loss is common and individuals may limit food intake in order to decrease bowel movements. In the more severe cases, tenderness in the left lower quadrant, guarding and abdominal distension may occur, as well as anaemia, leucocytosis, tachycardia, fever and dehydration.

Crohn's disease   The patient with Crohn's disease may have occasional acute episodes of illness; the clinical features are variable and determined by the site and severity of the disease (Nightingale 2004). Acute inflammatory symptoms include pain in the lower right quadrant, cramping, tenderness, spasm, flatulence, nausea, fever and diarrhoea. Unlike ulcerative colitis, there is often no visible blood in the stools. Borborygmi and increased peristalsis may also be present. The most severe pain may mimic acute appendicitis or bowel perforation. The more typical picture is the chronic type, which has more persistent but less severe symptoms.

Pain or discomfort accompanied by anorexia and malaise are the most common symptoms. The pain is usually peristaltic and intermittent, although a constant aching, soreness or tenderness usually indicates advanced disease. The patient may experience cramps and, unlike cramps associated with other colonic disease, relief does not occur after passing stool or flatus.

Diarrhoea is a consistent sign but is usually less severe than that associated with ulcerative colitis. The usual consistency of the stool is soft or semi-liquid. If steatorrhoea is also present, the stools will be quite foul smelling and fatty. A large amount of flatus is also likely to be a problem.

Abscess and fistula formation are common and may be characterized by a spiking fever and leucocytosis. Perianal disease, including fistulae and fissures, can occur. As Crohn's disease most often affects a portion of the small intestine, which then loses its ability to absorb nutritional matter, this can result in weight loss, malnutrition, cachexia, amenorrhoea in women and growth retardation in children. In addition, it is not uncommon for patients with Crohn's disease to experience mouth ulcers.

Extra intestinal manifestations of inflammatory bowel disease include:

- *Joints:* arthritis, ankylosing spondylitis, sacroiliitis
- *Liver:* sclerosing cholangitis
- *Skin:* erythema nodosum, pyoderma gangrenosum
- *Eyes:* uveitis, iritis, episcleritis, conjunctivitis

Comparison of the two disorders shows differences as well as similarities. Crohn's disease may affect any part of the gastrointestinal tract. The lesions are patchy in distribution and transmural in nature, resulting in thickening of the wall, fistula formation and perforation of the bowel. Ulcerative colitis affects the large intestine, the lesions are continuous and as they progress the bowel thickens, narrows and shortens. There is an increased incidence of gastrointestinal cancer with both disorders.

Patients may suffer from weight loss, anaemia, debility, fatigue, nausea, vomiting, and fluid, electrolyte and metabolic disturbances. Ulcerative colitis and Crohn's disease are both characterized by remissions and exacerbations. Both are very disruptive to the lives of the patients and their families. They affect the person's ability to eat and to participate in social situations and work activities.

Diagnostic investigations

The diagnostic process may be prolonged and cause considerable discomfort and inconvenience to the patient. The preparation for and the procedures themselves further aggravate the already troublesome bowel problems.

Stool examination   Stool cultures may be carried out to identify the presence of several microorganisms that can mimic IBD. In addition, the stool can be examined for presence of blood, mucus, for its consistency, odour and colour.

Endoscopy   Direct visualization of the bowel can take place with sigmoidoscopy or colonoscopy. The nursing care of patients undergoing endoscopy was explained earlier in this chapter (see p. 445). Endoscopy is particularly useful in the assessment of Crohn's disease; the pattern of the disease in the terminal ileum can be visualized (Metcalf 2002) and a tissue specimen (biopsy) may also be obtained at the same time. This procedure should never be carried out during an acute phase of the disease as this could lead to perforation of the bowel and hence a serious medical emergency.

Serological investigations   Active inflammation in the bowel is often associated with a raised C-reactive protein (CRP), raised erythrocyte sedimentation rate, an elevated platelet count and a low albumin concentration. In addition, patients with IBD are likely to have anaemia and therefore the full blood count will be abnormal and they may have deficiencies of iron, vitamin B_{12} or folate.

Radiological techniques and fluoroscopy   Introducing contrast medium (barium) into the lumen of the gastrointestinal tract allows it to be examined radiologically. The aim of the examination is to outline the lumen with the barium, utilizing its coating properties so that any mucosal destruction, distortion or deviation from the normal contour can be assessed. Lesions extending into the lumen are shown as filling defects or as an abnormal extension to the line of the mucosa. Failure of the barium to progress suggests obstruction.

The passage of barium may be followed in 'real time' by X-ray fluoroscopy. This yields useful information about function (e.g. the swallowing mechanism) and also facilitates the optimal position of the patient for a 'spot' radiography. The fluoroscopic image can be recorded on video for later analysis.

Barium may be used to examine the oesophagus (barium swallow), stomach and duodenum (barium meal), small bowel (small bowel meal or enema) and colon (barium enema).

Patient preparation for the barium study will vary, depending on the part of the gastrointestinal tract being examined. Instructions are issued by the radiology department directly to patients in the case of outpatient investigations, and to the ward in the case of inpatients. For barium swallows and meals, the patient has nothing by mouth from the evening before, as residual food or fluid interferes with the technical quality of the examination and hinders interpretation. Mild to moderate laxatives are given before small bowel studies to clear the bowel contents and help empty stool from the caecum, which facilitates the visualization of the ileocaecal region. More aggressive measures are needed for colonic cleansing prior to a barium enema, as even small amounts of faecal material can mimic polypoid lesions. These measures vary from place to place, but usually include food restriction for 24–48 hours before the examination, and a purgative. Some centres also use colonic lavage or enemas. Frail, elderly patients may tolerate the bowel preparation poorly (e.g. they may become dehydrated and/or hypotensive). In these cases, careful nursing supervision is required.

The majority of barium meals and barium enemas are performed using double contrast – a combination of barium and gas. This achieves distension and a thin mucosal coating of barium, facilitating the identification of small mucosal lesions. Gas is given in the form of effervescent granules for barium meals; for barium enemas, gas is delivered directly through the rectal tube.

After any barium study, the patient should be warned that the stools will be clay coloured until the barium has been eliminated. Fluids are encouraged as barium may become dry and thick, causing constipation. Should the patient suffer constipation or impaction of faeces following barium studies, an evacuation enema may be prescribed to relieve discomfort.

Treatment

Goals The goal of treatment for people with IBD is to maximize quality of life through the control of inflammation and through achieving an optimal nutritional state. Diet, pharmacological measures and surgery can be used to achieve this goal.

Diet The aim of dietary therapy is to rest the bowel by avoiding foods that have been found to provoke symptoms. An elemental diet can help to achieve remission in people with Crohn's disease and common food intolerances include, caffeine, dairy products, fats, fibre, wheat and yeast (Nightingale 2004). It is important to involve the dietetic team and to work collaboratively with the patient and their family.

Drug therapy Anti-diarrhoeal agents, anti-inflammatory agents, corticosteroids, immunosuppressants, antibiotics and biological therapies are options for the treatment of IBD. The choice of treatment depends upon the severity of the symptoms and the incidence of side-effects. There are differences in the approach to treatment for ulcerative colitis and Crohn's disease, however, many of the treatment options are the same.

Anti-diarrhoeals Drugs such as loperamide or codeine phosphate can be used to provide symptomatic relief of diarrhoea but they are not recommended for long-term use.

Aminosalicylates These drugs are anti-inflammatory and are thought to act through inhibition of prostaglandin synthesis (Grahame-Smith and Aronson 2002). Examples include: sulfasalazine, mesalazine and olsalazine. These drugs are used at the time of acute attacks and also to prevent remission. They also have a role in the prevention of recurrence after surgery (Nightingale 2004). Side-effects include headache, nausea, rashes and, in some men, reversible impairment of fertility.

Corticosteroids Examples of corticosteroids include hydrocortisone and prednisolone. These are prescribed for their anti-inflammatory and immunosuppressant actions. Corticosteroids can be taken either in oral form, intravenously or can be applied locally in the rectum. They have a role in the management of acute attacks when an initial dose of 40–60 mg of prednisolone is prescribed with a gradual reduction in the dose once the acute attack is over. A lower dose can be used in chronic active disease. One of the major problems with the use of corticosteroids is the potential for adverse side-effects. These include: increased appetite, weight gain and, in the long term, osteoporosis and diabetes. Some patients describe a feeling of euphoria whilst others report a sense of anxiety, irritability and difficulty with sleeping. Patients need to be monitored carefully for the potential side-effects of steroid use both in the acute phase and over the longer term.

Immunosuppressive therapy Azathioprine is used in chronic active disease either for those patients who cannot tolerate steroid therapy or in combination with steroids. This allows the patient to take a reduced dose of the corticosteroid. Azathioprine causes bone marrow suppression making the patient more susceptible to infections. Close monitoring of liver function and full blood count is essential throughout treatment as leucopenia and abnormal liver function can occur. Other side-effects include nausea, vomiting and, with long-term use, lymphoma, although the risk is small.

Antibiotics A fistula complicated by infection or a stagnant area or loop of intestine in which there is an overgrowth of bacteria may be treated with an antimicrobial agent. Options include metronidazole, ciprofloxacin and clarithromycin.

Biological therapies The monoclonal antibody infliximab has more recently been introduced for the treatment of severe active Crohn's disease when the disease has proved to be refractory to treatment with corticosteroids or immunosuppressants. It is administered in specialist centres and current guidelines suggest that it should be given in only the most severe cases (NICE 2002).

Surgical intervention Surgical intervention for persons with Crohn's disease or ulcerative colitis is reserved for patients who have not responded to medical therapy. Complications include the partial or complete obstruction of the intestine by the scar tissue, the formation of abscesses, perforation of the bowel and the formation of fistulae.

In patients with intractable ulcerative colitis, the diseased colon and rectum are removed and the ileum is brought through the abdominal wall to form an ileostomy. A portion of the ileum may be used to form an internal continent pouch (see p. 486) or the ileum may be anastomosed to the rectum. Strictureplasty to relieve obstruction (re-fashioning or release of narrowed areas) restores the lumen of the ileum without resection of small bowel. Surgery is usually effective but prognosis depends on the rate of development, severity and extent of the disease process. In patients with Crohn's, the disease process may recur after surgery, requiring further treatment and sometimes repeated surgical intervention.

Assessment

Assessment of a patient's quality of life provides insight into the problems that are most important for patients. Obtaining such information, while important to the understanding of the patient's adjustment to IBD, may be difficult because of the embarrassment about discussing such topics as bowel movements and incontinence, and because of fear of the disease. It is important for nurses to consider their own feelings about those issues in order to anticipate patients' anxieties sensitively.

Quality of life   Inflammatory bowel disease can have a major adverse impact on patients' lives. Numerous descriptions of the problems affecting patients with IBD have documented limitations in work and social activities, home and married life and emotional function. Patients tend to report symptoms that fall into five major categories: bowel symptoms, systemic symptoms, emotional function, social impairment and functional impairment.

Bowel symptoms   Problems most frequently cited by patients with IBD as having a significant impact on their lives include: frequent bowel movements, loose bowel movements, abdominal cramps, pain in the abdomen, abdominal bloating, passing large amounts of gas and rectal bleeding with bowel movements.

Systemic symptoms   Systemic symptoms include fatigue, feeling unwell overall, tiring very easily, waking up during the night and feeling weak.

Emotional function   Patients with IBD have sustained numerous losses, including loss of normal bowel habits, foods from the diet, body image, weight, relationships, work, leisure activities, familiar surroundings through hospitalization, income and self-esteem. They report feeling frustrated, depressed, discouraged, irritable, angry, anxious and impatient. They worry about not finding a toilet in time, about having to have surgery and about the next flare-up of symptoms.

Social impairment   Loss of normal bowel habits resulting in bowel frequency, incontinence and embarrassment about sudden calls to the toilet can lead to a change in activities. Patients with IBD tend to avoid social events where toilets are not close to hand; social engagements may be cancelled if a flare-up occurs, and sporting activity may be severely curtailed.

Functional impairment   Although some patients report an inability to attend work or school regularly, having to stop work or school, and difficulty doing housework, the majority of people with IBD lose little or no time from work over the long term. When symptoms are flaring, many patients have to get up earlier than usual in the morning because bowel actions can delay departure for work.

Serious disruption of personal relationships is a problem for only a few patients with IBD. The family may view the individual as a burden rather than as a capable, independent and functioning person who needs understanding and support during flare-ups. However, it is not uncommon for family members to be so attentive and wrapped up in the problems and needs of the individual with IBD that they tend to overlook their own personal needs. Such behaviour may result in increased family tension, fatigue, guilt feelings, resentment and a decreased ability to cope and offer support and reassurance over a long period of time.

In summary, symptoms of bowel disturbance such as frequent, loose bowel movements and abdominal cramps, as well as fatigue and malaise, have the most profound impact on the lives of patients with IBD. Disturbances of emotional function, including frustration and irritability, depression and discouragement, are common in patients with IBD. Impairment of social function is less frequent, with the majority of patients finding ways to cope with their job, social activities and family relationships.

Kelly (1992) describes the subjective experience of living with ulcerative colitis and, using autobiographical data, explains the personal strategies for coping with the disease. In his account, he describes adjusting to ill-health using the processes of denial, normalization and accommodation, and proposes that these strategies can be both 'healthy' and problematic. He argues that some well-meaning counselling approaches that break down an individual's denial of their illness could promote adoption of the invalid or sick role. His account also illustrates the miscommunication that can occur when the information given threatens the individual's personal construct of ill-health and the disease. This paper provides the healthcare professional, caring for the person with IBD, with insight into the experience of living with the condition and proposes approaches that can be adopted to encourage normal social development.

Nursing care

Potential patient problems:

- malnutrition due to the bowel inflammation, decreased absorption, diarrhoea, abdominal pain and lack of enjoyment of food
- dehydration due to diarrhoea and inadequate fluid intake
- diarrhoea due to the inflammatory process and disease complications
- stress and anxiety related to the disease process, and the impact on quality of life and resulting personality changes
- changes in body image and self-concept
- lack of knowledge concerning disease, treatment and long-term management.

Goals

The person will demonstrate:

1 understanding of parenteral nutrition
2 gradual, consistent increase in body weight
3 understanding of measures to promote adequate nutritional and fluid intake
4 acceptable management of diarrhoea
5 awareness of emotional responses
6 recognition of positive coping strategies
7 communication and sharing of significant others' concerns, and changes in sexuality patterns
8 understanding of the disease process and its recurrent nature
9 understanding of the treatment regimen and disease management.

Nursing intervention

Nutrition Nutritional deficits and weight loss are common to persons with IBD. When these are severe, all oral intake is withheld to decrease the mechanical, physical and chemical activities of the gastrointestinal tract.

Parenteral nutrition Parenteral nutrition (PN) is the infusion, into either a central vein or a large peripheral vein, of solutions of protein, glucose, electrolytes, trace amounts of essential minerals, vitamins and lipids (fat emulsions). This is carried out in sufficient concentrations to meet individual requirements for normal metabolism, tissue maintenance, repair and energy demands. Parenteral nutrition can be used with patients who have Crohn's disease or a bowel fistula that requires that the intestinal tract be rested. PN can be used as a form of treatment for some patients, although this is uncommon as medical regimens are used in the first instance.

The successful management of PN involves coordination of the efforts of all members of the multidisciplinary team. In some hospitals a special team – usually a specialist nurse, doctor, dietitian and pharmacist – coordinate activities. Their responsibilities may include teaching and preparing the patient to manage the feeding regimen at home.

Strict surgical asepsis is mandatory throughout the insertion of the catheter, when handling the solutions and tubes, and when caring for the site of insertion. Infection causes a serious problem; the line serves as an excellent culture medium and, because it leads directly into the blood, bacterial colonization will cause septicaemia.

It is important to prepare the patient, especially if PN is to be prolonged or permanent, with a detailed explanation of the procedure, its purpose and subsequent care. The patient and family are encouraged to ask questions and time is taken to answer them. They may require assurance that the patient will be able to eat normally after a period of being fed this way, if this is the case.

A large vein is used for administration of the highly concentrated (hyperosmolar) solutions, as they are irritating to the veins and can cause phlebitis in smaller peripheral veins. The rapid flow of blood in the large vessels dilutes the PN solutions and lessens the risk of phlebitis.

When the PN is to be used over an extended period of time, and particularly when the patient is to go home with the catheter in place, a long-term central venous catheter (e.g. Hickman) is inserted and tunnelled under the skin on the chest wall to decrease the incidence of infection. Usually a multi-lumen catheter is inserted to provide flexibility of use. A peripherally inserted central catheter (PICC) may be used to give PN to patients in hospital. This avoids the higher risk of inserting a CV line but cannot be used indefinitely. Certain simple PN regimens can be given via a peripheral vein for up to 1 week.

The frequency with which the intravenous tubing and/or filter(s) are changed is indicated by hospital policy. If contamination occurs or is even suspected, the following investigations are performed:

● blood cultures from the catheter and a peripheral vein
● full blood count
● midstream specimen of urine for microscopy, culture and sensitivity
● chest radiography
● other tests to eliminate potential sources of infection (e.g. wound swabs, throat swabs).

All tubing changes are made quickly while the catheter is clamped to prevent air entry and the risk of embolism. If the catheter cannot be clamped, the patient is instructed to bear down and hold the breath before tubing is disconnected and to breathe again once the connection has been made (Valsalva manoeuvre). The infusion line may contain one or two filters. Tubing connections are always luer locked to ensure maintenance of an intact line. PN solution consists of an amino-acid-dextrose solution, a fat emulsion solution and added vitamins, minerals and trace elements.

The rate of infusion is controlled by an automatic pump. This is essential because, if the infusion is too rapid, glucose will not be metabolized rapidly enough to maintain a normal blood glucose level. The glucose level will then exceed the renal threshold and glucose is excreted in the urine, taking with it essential water and electrolytes.

On dressing the site, strict aseptic technique is observed. Caution is necessary to avoid dislodging the catheter. The catheter site is inspected for redness, swelling or drainage; a swab is taken for culture if any irritation is observed. The skin is cleansed and re-dressed with an alcohol-based solution (chlorhexidine or iodine) and a sterile semi-occlusive dressing (e.g. OpSite) is then applied. The dressing of choice should be water- and bacteria-proof but permeable to air and water vapour. A transparent dressing permits frequent visualization of the area without disturbing the dressing, which can be left in place for 1 week as long as it provides a seal to a clean entry site.

Frequent mouth care is essential. Regular, frequent cleaning of the teeth followed by a mouthwash is very important. The lack of oral food and fluid intake causes discomfort and favours the growth of organisms present in the mouth, producing inflammation and tooth cavities. If the PN is prolonged or permanent, the patient may be permitted boiled sweets to suck, or a small amount of food which may be chewed and then expectorated. Some patients may be able to take small amounts of clear fluids or specified nutrients if their gastrointestinal tract is intact.

When assessing the patient the following observations are very important:

- The patient's blood pressure, pulse, respirations and colour are recorded frequently after the insertion of the catheter. Any complaint of pain or tightness in the chest or change in level of consciousness is reported promptly. Any such change may indicate air embolism, a pneumothorax or a haemothorax
- The temperature, pulse and respirations are recorded one to four times daily, always in the evening. An increase in temperature and pulse rate may indicate infection
- Blood specimens are usually taken daily for estimation of urea, electrolytes and glucose. Hyperglycaemia may develop, necessitating the administration of regular insulin
- The patient's weight is recorded daily. The intake and output are recorded and the fluid balance noted
- The site of insertion is examined carefully each time the dressing is changed and is inspected daily through the transparent dressing for inflammation, oedema, sloughing or purulent discharge
- Blood cultures are done and checked for fungi as well as bacteria
- 24-hour collections of urine may be made to check urine biochemistry.

Psychological support is necessary as the patient receiving PN for a prolonged period may report feeling 'very different'. Explanations of the purpose and value of the feedings are necessary. As the procedure becomes more familiar and better understood, it becomes more acceptable to the patient. Activity is encouraged as exercise promotes protein synthesis as well as improving the patient's psychological well-being. Any weight gain should be reported to the patient as this may help morale; however, a failure to gain weight may have the opposite effect.

Bowel elimination decreases and the patient should be advised that, as nothing enters the tract, this is not surprising. Appetite decreases during parenteral feedings. This is attributed to the calorie intake, decreased gastric motility and underlying disease.

Oral intake is gradually increased when PN is to be discontinued. When the patient can take sufficient calories and protein orally, the infusion rate is reduced gradually over 48 hours. The catheter tip is sent to the laboratory for culture on removal.

If this method of receiving nutrition is to be permanent or prolonged, the carers and patient need to be prepared for discharge from the hospital. They are taught how to put up the solutions, the maintenance of asepsis, indications of problems (e.g. symptoms of infection), care of the site of catheter insertion, how often the tube is changed and by whom, and that the solution should not be frozen. They are advised of the necessary supplies and how they are stored and obtained. They should also have contact telephone numbers and addresses in case of emergency.

Referral to the community nursing services is important on discharge. This will ensure early identification of difficulties or problems, monitoring progress, provision of support and assistance if necessary with aspects of care.

Most patients not only feel attached to the intravenous poles they have been pushing around for a period of time, whether as an inpatient, outpatient or on home care, they also feel protective of and dependent on their PN. They may require help in dealing with their ambivalent feelings of wanting to discontinue the feedings and anxieties over the loss. The patient needs positive reassurance to deal with the change in health status and what it will mean.

Oral intake   When oral intake is resumed, the patient may be given nutritionally balanced elemental feedings. These preparations are bulk and residue free and low in fat, making them easier to digest in the upper gastrointestinal tract. Palatability is enhanced by providing the feed chilled and in different flavours.

Nutrition of the patient requires a great deal of attention. The patient may develop serious nutritional deficiencies. Anorexia presents a problem, and there are serious losses of essential nutrients, fluid and electrolytes in the frequent stools. In many instances, the nurse must work at getting the patient to take sufficient nourishment; it may be necessary to provide frequent small meals. An effort is made to serve foods the patient likes, to provide variety, and to have the tray arranged attractively. A discouraging factor commonly encountered is that, as soon as the patient starts to eat, peristalsis is stimulated and he or she must get to the toilet.

Fluid and electrolyte replacement   An excessive loss of fluid in diarrhoea and a probable reduced intake by the patient because of abdominal pain and 'feeling sick' may lead to dehydration. The daily intake and output are recorded and the fluid balance is noted. The patient is encouraged and, if necessary, given assistance to take adequate amounts of fluid.

Serum electrolyte levels, especially potassium and sodium, are determined, as an abnormal amount may be lost in the stools or through fistula drainage. Replacement is made by intravenous fluids. A transfusion of packed red cells may be necessary to correct anaemia that has resulted from nutritional deficiencies. These develop due to insufficient food intake and/or impaired intestinal absorption. If the patient has PN in progress, additional intravenous fluids and blood products should be given by a separate peripheral line to avoid contamination.

Maintenance of skin integrity is an important role of the nurse when the patient is experiencing dehydration or malnutrition.

Bowel elimination: diarrhoea   The frequency, consistency, volume and colour of the patient's stools are recorded and the nurse and patient collaborate to identify foods, activities and emotional responses that increase or decrease the frequency and consistency of bowel movements.

Anti-diarrhoeal medications may be given after each loose bowel movement (see above, p. 459). The rectal and perineal area are inspected for irritation and redness. Should moist excoriation develop, the area should be kept dry. Soreness may be relieved by the application of a local anaesthetic gel. A barrier cream can be used to protect the skin.

Individual coping   The nurse must appreciate that dependence and insecurity may be encountered in persons with IBD and a great deal of tact and sensitivity is required in giving care.

Family coping   Family members, like professional caregivers, need help to understand the reasons for the person's changed behaviours and to appreciate the difficulties experienced in adjusting to a chronic illness that is probably progressive and definitely interferes with one's life. Awareness of the reasons for the behaviours and of the patient's needs provides a basis for understanding and the development of constructive coping strategies. The family may need assistance to identify and deal with their own needs as well as those of the patient.

Sexuality patterns   There is no evidence that IBD affects fertility, and pregnancy is possible. Sexual desire may be decreased by the disease and by the unpredictable bowel habits, odours and fatigue. The possibility of an ileostomy or colostomy raises additional worries about sex. The patient and partner may need support to discuss their concerns and to develop solutions to their particular situation.

Patient and family teaching   Assessment of patient and family learning needs is ongoing as needs change throughout the disease process. The possibility of a recurrence is reduced if the patient understands the illness. The patient is encouraged to return to work and to live as normal and useful a life as possible. A balance between rest, work and recreation is advisable.

Referral to the medical social work department may be useful in resolving domestic or socioeconomic problems. Some hospitals have a clinical psychologist or counsellor whose role is to assist the person with IBD and the family and significant others, to explore the ramifications and meaning of the disease and develop positive coping strategies. Self-help groups can also be a useful resource to assist in adaptation.

Emphasis is placed on the importance of a nourishing diet with the elimination of certain foods that are found to be irritating to the bowel.

Evaluation
Inflammatory bowel disease is characterized by remissions and exacerbation which, together with prolonged treatment,

interfere with the person's life and impact on the family and caregivers. Disease management and coping strategies vary according to the status of the disease and the person's responses and ability to cope with the chronic progressive illness. Evaluation is ultimately based on the patient's perceptions, how well they are feeling, and how they perceive they are coping with the latest treatment, symptom or complication.

Intestinal obstruction

Obstruction to the passage of intestinal content may occur in the small or large bowel and is a serious, life-threatening condition that demands prompt attention.

Causes
The cause of the obstruction may be within the wall or lumen of the intestine itself, or it may be extrinsic. It may be classified as mechanical, neurogenic, vascular or pseudo-obstruction and may be acquired or congenital (Box 15.6).

Strangulated hernia, is a condition in which a loop of the intestine escapes from the peritoneal cavity through a defect

---

Box 15.6   Causes of intestinal obstruction

Mechanical
- Inflammation and oedema of the intestinal wall
- Stenosis
- Constipation
- Strictures or scarring (narrowing the intestinal lumen)
- Adhesions (bands of fibrous scar tissue formed by the peritoneal tissue following inflammation and which may cause kinking and constriction of the intestine)
- Neoplasms (intramural and extramural)
- Foreign body
- Incarcerated hernia
- Volvulus
- Intussusception
- Congenital stenosis and atresia.

Non-mechanical
- Neurogenic disturbances:
  paralytic or adynamic ileus, dynamic ileus, chemotherapy
- Interrupted blood supply:
  mesenteric thrombosis, strangulation of blood vessels secondary to: incarcerated hernia, volvulus or intussusception
- Pseudo-obstruction:
  abdominal malignancy, renal failure, myocardial infarction, cerebrovascular accident and electrolyte disturbances.

in the abdominal wall. This results in constriction of the lumen of the bowel and a blockage, as well as compression of the blood vessels. The constriction may lead to necrosis of the protruding segment of the intestine.

Obstruction may result from intussusception, a condition in which a segment of the intestine is invaginated into the segment immediately below. This telescoping results in compression of the attached mesentery between the layers of intestine in the intussusception and interference with the blood supply to the bowel. Intussusception occurs mainly in infants and young children.

Volvulus, which is a twisting of a loop of bowel on itself, interrupts the passage of intestinal contents and the blood supply to the involved segment. Older persons are more often affected, and the twisted section of bowel is usually the sigmoid colon.

Congenital malformations may be responsible for intestinal obstruction in the newborn. The anomaly may be a stenosis or atresia in an area of the small or large intestine, or it may be an imperforate anus. The infant fails to pass meconium.

In neurogenic obstruction, peristalsis is inhibited by a disturbance in the normal nerve supply to the intestine. Often this is an imbalance in the autonomic innervation which results in a cessation of peristalsis. It may develop with peritonitis, pancreatitis, severe toxaemia as in pneumonia and uraemia, shock, or spinal cord lesions or after extensive abdominal surgery. An electrolyte imbalance in which the blood potassium level is below normal also predisposes to intestinal immobility. The inhibition of peristalsis due to impaired innervation causes the condition known as paralytic or adynamic ileus.

Obstruction of vascular origin is due to interference with the blood supply to a segment of the intestine and may be secondary to mechanical obstruction, or it may be primary and itself cause failure of bowel activity. Thrombosis and occlusion of a mesenteric artery may occur, blocking the blood supply to a large portion of the bowel and arresting peristalsis. The interruption in the blood supply may be secondary to an initial mechanical cause, as occurs in strangulated hernia, volvulus and intussusception.

Clinical characteristics

The symptoms and effects of obstruction depend on whether it is in the small or large bowel and whether or not the blood supply to the intestine is maintained.

The first symptom of mechanical obstruction is colicky abdominal pain due to the bowel spasms. The crampy pains are accompanied by high-pitched bowel sounds. In paralytic ileus, the pain is steady and is due mainly to the distension. There is an absence of bowel sounds in this type of obstruction. Once the faecal matter or gas which was below the obstruction has been evacuated, there will be no further evacuation from the bowel.

In small bowel obstruction, vomiting begins earlier and is frequent; the vomitus at first consists of stomach content and then of fluid containing bile. Eventually it becomes

dark brown and faecal in character as the intestine becomes distended with excessive fluids and gas that overflow into the stomach.

The abdomen becomes distended because of the accumulation of gas and fluids in the bowel. Intestinal secretions are increased and the loss of fluid and electrolytes in vomiting leads to severe dehydration and electrolyte imbalance. Extravasation of plasma from the capillaries adds to the accumulation of fluid in the intestine as the veins are compressed by distension. This depletes the circulating blood volume and causes shock.

The patient's general condition may deteriorate rapidly. Unless the bowel is decompressed and fluid and electrolytes are replaced, a serious state of shock develops, manifested by restlessness, anxiety, a rapid weak pulse, low blood pressure, subnormal temperature, greyish pallor and cold clammy skin.

If decompression of the intestine is not established, the pressure created within the intestinal lumen may increase until it exceeds venous and capillary pressure. This causes congestion, oedema and necrosis of the mural tissue and may lead to perforation of the intestine.

The colicky pain becomes continuous as peristalsis diminishes, and the intestine loses its tone because of the marked distension and strangulation. Bowel sounds diminish and the vomiting changes character; it is no longer preceded by nausea and retching; the vomitus comes up without effort and is simply regurgitated.

Peritonitis may develop as the weakened intestinal wall becomes permeable to organisms. Generalized abdominal pain and rigidity become evident.

Obstruction of the large intestine is less acute, and the symptoms develop over a longer period of time. Complete constipation (obstipation) and crampy abdominal pain are the patient's first complaints. Distension of the large bowel develops more slowly because fluid is absorbed, but eventually the distension may be very marked as the segment of the bowel is closed off by the obstruction at one end and the ileocaecal valve at the other. The ileocaecal valve will permit the entrance of content from the ileum, but not until the later stage does the content of the colon and caecum back up into the ileum. In the later stage, vomiting and the attendant dehydration and electrolyte imbalance occur.

Medical diagnosis

Blood samples are taken to determine the white blood cell count, urea and electrolyte balance and C-reactive protein. The results of these tests help to determine whether there are signs of infection, inflammation and help to assess renal function. There is much debate over the best radiological investigation to use in diagnosing intestinal obstruction (Hughes 2005). Plain X-ray of the abdomen can reveal the presence and levels of gas and can display a dilated bowel. Other options include, ultrasonography, computed tomography (CT scans), magnetic resonance imaging (MRI) and in some areas a contrast enema and X-ray might be used. Clearly accurate and timely diagnosis is essential for patients with intestinal obstruction and the relative merits of each investigation need to be balanced against the particular individual's needs. Availability of imaging equipment and cost implications should also be considered.

Treatment

In the absence of peritonitis and sepsis, patients with intestinal obstruction can be treated conservatively. This is considered to be acceptable when adhesions are thought to be the cause (Hughes 2005). Management includes nasogastric suction, pain relief, nil by mouth, fluid resuscitation and antiemetics. However, the majority of patients presenting with intestinal obstruction will require surgical intervention.

If there is evidence of interference with the blood supply to the obstructed intestine, emergency surgery is undertaken. In simple mechanical obstruction without strangulation, the operation may be delayed for a brief period during which medical treatment is used to improve the patient's general condition. Fluid and electrolytes are given intravenously to replace the losses; as much as 5–6 L may be administered daily. An accurate record of all fluid output and intake is necessary. The amount of intravenous fluid replacement is based on the volume of intestinal fluid lost in vomiting and aspiration. Once the patient is haemodynamically stable, surgery can take place.

The surgical procedure used in intestinal obstruction depends on the cause of obstruction and the patient's general condition. If the obstruction is due to adhesions, they are severed. The operation may involve resection of the affected area of intestine and anastomosis to restore continuity of the tract or a bypass of the lesion by anastomosing a part above the obstruction to a lower part (usually the colon). In the case of an incarcerated hernia, volvulus or intussusception, the obstruction is relieved and the intestine examined for viability. If the blood supply has been interrupted for some time or is not re-established, a segment of the bowel may be gangrenous, necessitating resection and anastomosis. The operation may entail an ileostomy, or colostomy. Ileostomy is an opening from the ileum on to the external surface of the abdomen. Intestinal content is eliminated through this opening. Colostomy is an opening through the abdominal wall from the colon. Faeces are diverted through this opening on to the external surface of the abdomen. Either of these procedures may be a temporary measure while an anastomosis heals or they may be carried out to establish drainage above the obstruction, making it possible to delay more extensive surgery until the patient's condition improves. In some instances, the stoma (colostomy or ileostomy) is permanent (see p. 485 for a more detailed overview of surgery for the formation of a colostomy or ileostomy).

Intestinal obstruction due to paralytic ileus is treated symptomatically. A nasogastric or intestinal tube is passed to drain gas and to fluid and to reduce distension. Fluid and electrolyte deficiencies are corrected; the serum potassium level receives special attention because hypokalaemia favours peristaltic dysfunction. Paralytic ileus is most frequently a secondary condition; as the primary disorder improves and decompression occurs, peristalsis is usually re-established gradually.

Cancer of the intestine

Bowel cancer is the second most common form of cancer in women in the UK and the third most common cancer in men (Cancer Research UK 2005c). There are about 35 000 new cases of bowel cancer each year in the UK and within the European Union it is the second most common cause of death (Borwell 2002). Most bowel cancers take between 5–8 years to develop. Cancer of the colon or rectum may occur at any age, although it is uncommon in people under the age of 40, and the incidence increases with increasing age. The incidence is high in Western countries and lower in less developed countries.

Contributing factors

The cause of colorectal cancer is believed to be multifactorial. Studies show an increased incidence in colorectal cancer in populations that have a high-fat, low-fibre diets and a lack of physical exercise. Low fibre diets result in a slow transit time of faeces through the intestines and this is thought to prolong the exposure of the intestinal mucosa to carcinogens (de Snoo 2002). Other risk factors such as obesity, tobacco smoking and high alcohol consumption have also been linked to the development of colorectal cancer. A prolonged history of inflammatory bowel diseases such as ulcerative colitis also carries an increased risk of developing large bowel and rectal cancer.

Approximately 20% of patients with colorectal cancer have a genetic or familial component to their condition (Coughlan 2005). Familial polyposis and hereditary nonpolyposis colorectal cancer are examples of syndromes that have a genetic element.

Types

The malignant growth may be papillary, soft and friable, or a firm nodular mass projecting into the lumen; it may be a ring-shaped (annular) mass of firm fibrous tissue, causing a constriction of the bowel, or it may be ulcerative and necrotic, leading to bleeding and perforation. The tumour is staged using the Dukes' staging system based on whether the disease is localized or has metastasized to other areas of the body.

Metastases

The malignant cells from bowel cancer spread by blood and lymph and by direct extension to neighbouring tissue and structures. Frequent sites of secondary growths are the liver, stomach, bones and peritoneal cavity. Direct extension may involve the bladder and reproductive organs.

Clinical characteristics

Manifestations vary with the location of the lesion in the intestine. If the neoplasm is in the small intestine, the symptoms develop insidiously and are vague and less noticeable.

They include anorexia, alteration in taste, nausea and vomiting, anaemia, loss of weight and strength and occult blood in the stool. The most common early signs are a change in bowel habit and blood in the stool. Any person presenting with either of these signs is urged to seek prompt medical attention.

There may be increasing constipation or perhaps alternating bouts of constipation and diarrhoea. The stool may gradually become smaller and ribbon-like in form and may be streaked with blood, mucus and pus. A continuous defaecation urge and the feeling that evacuation is incomplete after passing a stool may be experienced. The patient presents a general picture of ill-health with loss of weight and progressive anaemia. Laboratory examination of the stool will probably reveal occult blood and blood samples may reveal an unexplained anaemia. In cancer of the large bowel, abdominal pain is usually a late symptom; at first, the patient may have a vague discomfort and abdominal distension and later may experience a colicky pain which gradually becomes more severe. Unfortunately, if the cancer is in the caecum or ascending colon, the early symptoms are even more insidious and difficult to detect until the mass is large enough to be found by palpation. Occasionally, the first symptoms recognized are those associated with complications, such as obstruction or perforation of the bowel.

Screening and early detection

In the early stages of disease when the cancer is detected before lymph nodes become involved, the 5-year survival rate can be as high as 98%. However, if spread has occurred to the regional lymph nodes and beyond, the 5-year survival rate drops to <10% (Borwell 2002). This demonstrates the value of early detection of a malignant lesion before symptoms occur.

Screening for colorectal cancer at present is dependent upon occult blood estimation in stool samples. This test is estimated to produce a 25% false-positive result as foods that have been ingested such as raw vegetables, horseradish, rare meat and iron supplements can produce occult blood in the stool. Currently a screening programme using faecal occult blood testing for the UK population is being piloted.

Flexible sigmoidoscopy can be used to visualize the rectum and lower part of the colon. Colonoscopy can be used to visualize the entire colon. People with a positive faecal occult blood test result usually proceed to colonoscopy for diagnosis. Patients who are deemed to be at increased risk (IBD sufferers or those with a positive family history of familial polyposis) are screened, usually with colonoscopy, every 3–5 years.

There can be a strong history of colorectal cancer in certain families. Where this is the case, the patient is encouraged to attend a specialized family history and genetic screening clinic (Coughlan 2005). Some patients may progress to colonoscopy screening and all patients should be provided with lifestyle advice relating to smoking cessation, healthy diet with a high content of fruit, vegetables and fibre and increase in physical activity.

Diagnosis

A neoplasm in the small intestine may be recognized when barium sulfate is taken by mouth and the passage of the barium through the small intestine followed. Any delay at a given section may indicate narrowing of the lumen by a mass. The intraluminal contour of the small intestine is also recorded by radiography.

Investigation of the large intestine involves a colonoscopy, sigmoidoscopy or proctoscopy. A biopsy of the lesion, if it is located, is done at the time of the endoscopic examination. Radiography is done with a barium enema providing a contrast medium. The patient's haematocrit and haemoglobin level are checked for possible anaemia, and stool specimens are examined for blood, parasites and pus. Liver function tests may be done, to determine whether the malignancy has metastasized to the liver.

Treatment

Once the diagnosis of colorectal cancer has been made, the patient will be advised by the multidisciplinary specialist team regarding their options for treatment. In the early stages, surgery is the primary treatment and is potentially curative. The surgeon will remove the tumour, disease-free bowel on either side of it and the surrounding tissue including lymph nodes. The remaining ends of the bowel are usually anastomosed (joined) using a stapling device. If the tumour is within a few centimetres of the anus, a permanent colostomy will be formed and the rectum and anus excised. If the anastomosis is low in the rectum or the bowel is inflamed, a temporary stoma may be formed to facilitate healing at the anastomotic site.

Depending on the site and stage of the cancer diagnosed, patients may have radiotherapy and/or chemotherapy before or after operation. Various chemotherapy regimens are used, for example, Oxiplatin in combination with 5-fluorouracil and folinic acid can be used to shrink tumours prior to their removal. Chemotherapy can also be administered after surgery to destroy any remaining cancerous cells. Radiotherapy can also be used both before and after the operation.

Case Study 15.2 describes the management of a patient with colorectal adenocarcinoma.

CASE **Management of a patient with colorectal adenocarcinoma**

Mr England, at the time of his diagnosis, was 57 years old. He was divorced, had two grown daughters, and lived with his partner whom his daughters disliked. He worked as an insurance broker and described himself as a workaholic. He took little exercise, was slightly overweight and drank 42 units of alcohol a week. His parents were both dead, one from a stroke and the other from bowel cancer. In the preceding 6 months, Mr England had been experiencing bloating, constipation and then loose stools and more flatus than usual. The symptoms did not seem to be related to what he ate and after experiencing rectal bleeding on two occasions, he attended his surgery, partly at his partner's insistence. He was referred urgently to the gastrointestinal outpatient department.

After meeting with the consultant, Mr England proceeded to have a flexible sigmoidoscopy, which showed a mass at 8 cm from the anal margin, in the upper rectum. Having seen the GI clinic nurse and a consultant GI surgeon in the clinic, Mr England was referred for anorectal physiology measurement. Transrectal ultrasonography of the tumour showed invasion through the rectal wall, but Mr England's anal sphincter pressures were high and a low resection and anastomosis would be possible. This meant that he would avoid having the formation of a stoma which caused him great relief. Mr England was also seen by the colorectal cancer nurse specialist (colorectal CNS), who took time to explore the implications of his diagnosis with him. The specialist nurse also explained the treatment and possible outcomes and provided him with a contact number for ongoing support.

The plan for Mr England's treatment included radiotherapy to shrink the tumour before surgical resection. The surgery involved direct anastomosis. After recovery from the operation, a course of chemotherapy was planned in order to optimize his chance of remission from the cancer. Mr England was given external-beam radiation as an outpatient of the radiotherapy department, and the radiotherapy successfully reduced the size of the tumour.

Before admission for surgery, Mr England was seen in the surgical preadmission clinic by a nurse who took his history and blood samples, performed an ECG and ordered a chest X-ray. The nurse explained what to expect and that he would need a clean bowel for the operation. The bowel preparation prescription, dietary restrictions and high fluid intake were discussed.

Mr England was admitted for surgery and a low resection was undertaken as planned. The nurses on the surgical ward helped him to recover and encouraged him to take a healthy diet to help achieve a normal daily bowel habit.

Histological reports of the resected cancer showed an invasive rectal adenocarcinoma with local lymph node involvement.

Chemotherapy was commenced 2 months after the operation and was administered in the oncology day unit. During radiotherapy, surgery and chemotherapy events, the colorectal CNS saw Mr England and his partner in order to provide information and support, and to ensure that the treatment was progressing according to plan.

When the treatment was finally completed, Mr England made a full recovery and continued to be seen regularly by both the colorectal surgery and oncology teams, with the colorectal CNS maintaining contact.

Some 12 months later, after feeling unwell for a few weeks, Mr England was found to have liver metastases, which were not surgically resectable. A further course of chemotherapy was organized to delay the growth of the tumour. Mr England saw the same staff in the oncology day unit and was also seen by the colorectal CNS. After the chemotherapy, the colorectal CNS suggested a consultation with the palliative care nurse specialist, emphasizing that this was for symptom management and to anticipate this need in the future. This point proved difficult for Mr England and his family to accept as it implied 'the end' to them. With careful counselling and support, the acceptance of symptom management as opposed to 'terminal care' was made clear and accepted by the family so that they were familiar with the team members in advance of becoming reliant on them.

Mr England's symptoms were managed successfully for more than 1 year after diagnosis of the metastases. With the help of the colorectal CNS and the palliative care team, who coordinated with his GP and community nurses, Mr England and his partner and daughters learnt to work together to maximize the quality of his remaining life. Mr England died at home, 4 years after his initial symptoms became apparent.

This is a brief summary of Mr England's experiences during his illness. It could be valuable to reflect upon some of the important roles played by nurses throughout the course of this patient's illness and treatment. Consider how the initial presentation would have been managed in the general practice by a nurse practitioner; how the nurse in the outpatient clinic might have helped Mr England and his family during a period of uncertainty; how the clinical nurse specialist would have interacted with the family to inform them of the treatment plan and what to expect before and after surgery; and consider how the palliative care specialist nurses would have worked with the family to achieve the highest possible level of quality of life for Mr England in his last few weeks. Nursing care has a great deal to offer a patient who presents with colorectal cancer and it needs to be delivered in a skilled, sensitive and empathetic manner in an attempt to meet the needs, not only of the patient, but also his friends, family and wider acquaintances.

Critical pathway: colonic resection   Whilst it is important to individualize the care given to any patient, it is also useful to have a guideline for anticipated recovery from common illnesses and procedures (Table 15.2). This can inform patients and new staff and facilitates the collection of data relating to complications or delays in recovery that may be helpful in improving care.

Depending on their state of health (nutrition, hydration and other pathology), patients admitted for colonic resection, without stoma formation, will usually follow a predictable pathway of care and recovery. Admission before surgery will involve information-giving about the plan for the patient's stay in hospital and subsequent recovery. This period spent in hospital is relatively short and intensive, and it is important that the patients and their family are prepared for this. It is important that plans for discharge are based on information about the patient's home circumstances and commenced as soon as possible in order to maximize the opportunity for convalescence. Advice to be included in preparing patients to go home is summarized below.

Table 15.2 Critical pathway for a patient undergoing colonic resection

Aspect of care	Preoperative	Day of operation	Day 1	Day 2	Day 3	Day 4	Day 5	Day 6
Respiratory	Assessment of baseline rate, O₂% saturation. Teach deep breathing and coughing. Refer to physiotherapist if indicated (smoker or chronic obstructive pulmonary disease).	Administer prescribed O₂. Respiratory rate >12 per minute. Saturation at or above baseline level. Check colour and perfusion. Deep breathing every hour.	Wean O₂ to maintain O₂% saturation and respiratory rate. Deep breathing and coughing supporting the wound. Additional physiotherapy if required. Monitor regularly (2–4-hourly).	Deep breathing and coughing as previously. Monitor 4–6-hourly. Check any sputum produced. Report to doctors and culture if purulent.	As previously.	As previously. Monitor 8–12-hourly.	As previously. Monitor 12–24-hourly.	As previously. Should continue deep breathing and coughing at home until moving easily.
Circulatory	Baseline assessment of BP, HR, history of problems and medication. Bloods for FBC baseline, cross-matching for 6 units of blood. ID with appropriate labels.	Monitor BP and HR frequently and report deviation from preoperative baseline or parameters agreed with doctors. Check drainage from wound and wound drains frequently. If >300 mL in one drain in 30–60 minutes, inform doctors immediately.	Monitor BP and HR regularly. Check and record wound drainage for type and volume. FBC and check result.	Monitor BP and HR regularly. Check and record wound drainage for type and volume. If still fresh blood, report to doctors. FBC and check result if significant loss from drains.	As previously. If drains have drained <30 mL in 24 hours, remove. FBC and check result.	Check BP, HR 12-hourly. Remove remaining drain if <30 mL in 24 hours. FBC and check result.	Check BP, HR 12–24- hourly. Remove remaining drain if <30 mL in 24 hours. FBC and check result.	Check BP, HR 12–24 hourly. FBC only if previously <10 g/L or transfused.
Pain control	Explain measures for pain control and the importance of regular	Monitor use of PCA; adjust prescription as indicated. Ensure other prescribed	As previously.	As previously.	As previously.	As previously. Commence regular oral analgesia and wean PCA if able.	As previously. Stop PCA if not already.	As previously.

continued

Table 15.2 Cont'd

Aspect of care	Preoperative	Day of operation	Day 1	Day 2	Day 3	Day 4	Day 5	Day 6
	analgesia to enhance recovery. Assess ability to use PCA and teach technique.	analgesia regularly administered. Monitor effectiveness using pain scale						
Fluid balance	Assess current status (dehydration, use of diuretics, usual intake). Bloods for serum urea, creatinine and electrolyte (UCE) levels and check result. Ensure >3 L intake today (bowel preparation).	IVI to hydrate as prescribed (3 L/24 hours). Aim for urine output >30 mL/h. Consider other losses (gut, drains, perioperative fluid losses). Assess balance 6-hourly and consult if >500 mL positive or negative. Keep record of each 24-h balance and include in daily assessment	As previously. UCE and check result for appropriate IVI prescription.	As previously. Assess balance 24 hours. UCE as previously.	As previously. Decrease IVI rate as oral intake increases. Assess balance 24 hours. UCE as previously.	Remove IVI when drinking freely. Assess balance 24 hours. UCE as previously.	Stop monitoring fluid balance.	UCE if indicated.
Nutrition	Assess nutritional status. Clear fluid only; supplement protein and calories with fortified drinks if indicated (cancer, recent weight loss, sepsis).	Nil orally from 6 hours before surgery.	Sips of water or ice by mouth only. Increase volume if bowel sound present.	Increase volume of fluids by 30 mL increments hourly, as tolerated.	Free fluids by mouth including hot drinks as liked or tolerated when flatus passed. Use fortified drinks if indicated.	Free fluids, soup and soft pudding as tolerated.	Free fluids and a light diet.	As previously.
Excretion	Assess urinary function and screen urine with	Check urinary catheter patent and draining.	As previously. Check for bowel sounds.	As previously. Check for bowel sounds and	As previously. Check for bowel sounds and	Remove catheter; culture urine if indicated by	Check urinary function, volumes and frequency.	As previously.

continued

Table 15.2 *Cont'd*

Aspect of care	Preoperative	Day of operation	Day 1	Day 2	Day 3	Day 4	Day 5	Day 6
	dipstick test. Assess usual bowel habit (before and since symptomatic). Explain and administer bowel preparation having familiarized patient with bathroom facilities. Give barrier cream if perineal irritation present or develops.	Catheter care 12–24-hourly.		whether flatus passed.	whether flatus passed.	dipstick test or fever. Check for resumption of urinary function; measure volumes and frequency. Check flatus passed and whether bowels opened.	Check flatus passed and bowels opened. Consider lactulose prescription if difficult.	
Activity and rest	Assess usual exercise pattern and limits, sleep pattern. Assess skin integrity and use pressure-relieving appliances as indicated. Start bowel preparation early to minimize sleep disturbance prior to surgery. Teach leg and ankle exercises for postoperative use and the importance of early resumption	Fit antiembolism stockings before surgery. Commence prescribed anticoagulant therapy.	Help out of bed twice for as long as tolerated. Check calves for pain or inflammation. Hourly leg and ankle exercises. Prescribed anticoagulant therapy.	As previously. Also take short walk around the bed twice. Clean stockings.	As previously. Longer walk. Resume some independence in activities of daily living as able.	As previously. Clean stockings.	As previously.	As previously. Remove stockings before discharge.

continued

Table 15.2 *Cont'd*

Aspect of care	Preoperative	Day of operation	Day 1	Day 2	Day 3	Day 4	Day 5	Day 6
	of activity and independence. Describe activity targets for post-operative period.							
Regulation (endocrine, temperature, immunity, healing)	Check temperature for baseline. Inform anaesthetist if febrile and consider cause. Assess history of endocrine disease (diabetes mellitus) and establish usual management. Consider implications for wound healing.	Measure temperature 4-hourly after surgery. Consult with doctors if >38.5°C. Check wound for oozing and inflammation frequently. Administer antibiotics as prescribed (3 doses). Administer prescribed regimen and monitoring for diabetes if indicated.	Measure temperature 4–6-hourly. Consult if >38.5°C and culture wound, sputum and urine. Check wound for oozing and inflammation. Administer prescribed regimen and monitoring for diabetes if indicated.	As previously. Dress the wound if indicated. Dress drain-sites daily when removed (more frequently if dressings wet). Change i.v. cannulae	As previously.	As previously. Change i.v. cannulae if still required	As previously. Check temperature twice daily, always in the evening.	As previously. If wounds still require dressing either show patient how to care or arrange for community nurse/practice nurse.

continued

Table 15.2 *Cont'd*

Aspect of care	Preoperative	Day of operation	Day 1	Day 2	Day 3	Day 4	Day 5	Day 6
Self-image	Assess feelings associated with diagnosis and impending operation. Provide information, explanation, support and reassurance as indicated. Check informed consent given for operation.	Inform patient and family about outcome of operation as and when indicated depending on conscious level and need for further histology reports.	As previously. Encourage the patient to look at the wound when able.	As previously.	As previously.	As previously.	As previously. Establish all parties are satisfied with current available knowledge and situation.	As previously. Ensure appropriate referrals made and the patient and carer are fully aware of these.
Interdependence and discharge plan	Assess current situation at home; who is there and their level of ability to support the patient. Assess patient's current level of ability and what help is or may be required. Discuss and initiate appropriate referrals.	Provide information for the patient, family and friends as indicated and wanted. Pursue referrals for discharge plan and record progress.	As previously.	As previously.	As previously. Outline discharge plan.	As previously. Confirm discharge plan, arrange transport and appointments as required (GI surgical outpatients in 6 weeks).	As previously. Prescribe and order drugs to take home. Teach patient and family about convalescence using guidelines. Ensure clarity about drug regimens, appointments and when to seek help.	As previously. Confirm discharge plan in operation with all relevant parties.

BP, blood pressure; FBC, full blood count; GI, gastrointestinal; HR, heart rate; ID, identification; IVI, intravenous infusion; PCA, patient-controlled analgesia; UCE, urea, creatinine and electrolytes.

Discharge advice

- Take analgesia regularly and increase the dose as prescribed if you anticipate doing anything that may cause more pain. You should expect to exercise and cough regularly. Do not try to avoid taking analgesia. It will be more difficult to control the pain if you do. This could prevent you from sleeping or moving as easily as you should

- It is perfectly alright to wet the wound, although it should not be soaked. You should not require a dressing, but gauze could be taped over if the wound rubs or bothers you. If the wound still needs a special dressing when you go home, you will be shown what to do and/or the community nurse will be contacted to dress it for you. You should avoid direct sunlight to the scar and should not rub any creams into it. It is normal for it to feel itchy or numb for some weeks after the operation. If the wound becomes red or swollen, starts to drain fluid or you develop a fever (temperature 37.5°C or greater) for more than 12 hours, you should contact your GP

- Initially you should continue to eat a light diet at home. Regular meals of food you like eating will help to restore your appetite. You will benefit from eating little and often. Eating low-fat foods but a higher protein and calorie intake will help your body to recover from surgery. Include natural yoghurt in your diet to help your bowel restore its normal environment and gradually increase your fibre intake in the form of cereals and fresh fruit and vegetables by one helping at a time. Aim to establish a three-meals-a-day pattern of a high-fibre low-fat diet within 4–6 weeks of going home (if you can tolerate it)

- You will have opened your bowels before you go home but a regular habit may not yet be established. This is not unusual. You may find you go infrequently or your stool is hard and difficult to pass. Ensure you establish a routine for meals and going to the toilet and continue to take regular daily exercise. Drink at least eight glasses of decaffeinated and non-alcoholic fluids per day. If the problem persists, consult your local surgery who may prescribe you some laxatives to soften the stool and make it easier to pass

- You should not drive, lift, undertake heavy exercise or do sit-ups for 6 weeks. When you first resume these activities (particularly driving), ensure you have someone with you and stop if you develop pain or get tired. However, exercise and rest are both important. You should not take to your bed, but get up and dress every day. You should aim to walk daily, going a little further each day; take someone with you if at all possible until you feel confident about going out on your own. When you feel tired, take a rest and lie down for a nap in the afternoon if you need to. Slowly resume your usual activities and try to include some strenuous exercise at least three times a week when you are fully recovered. If you develop pain and swelling in your calf muscle, or sudden shortness of breath, contact your GP immediately.

In addition to the above it will be important to give advice about medications – when and how to take them and why, and to give advice about stopping smoking where applicable.

Nursing intervention

Prevention Evidence is accumulating in support of high dietary fibre as a protection against the development of colonic cancer. A low-fat diet is also recommended. The nurse's health education role can therefore make a substantial contribution to the long-term prevention of many cases of bowel cancer. By its very nature, such a contribution is not always apparent, and it requires long-term commitment by the individual for real benefits to accrue.

THE PERSON WITH FAECAL DIVERSION

ILEOSTOMY AND COLOSTOMY

The treatment of some intestinal disorders may necessitate surgery that establishes an opening into the bowel through which the intestinal content is discharged on to the surface of the abdomen. The opening may be temporary or permanent. A temporary diversion of the bowel content may be necessary for quick decompression and drainage in an emergency situation such as obstruction. A temporary diversion could also be created in order to allow an abnormal condition below the level of the stoma to be corrected. Later, the normal continuity of the tract will be restored and the stoma reversed. If the opening is permanent, the portion of the bowel below the opening is usually removed.

The operations performed to create an opening on to the abdominal wall are called ileostomy or colostomy.

Ileostomy

An ileostomy involves transection of the ileum, usually within the last 20 cm before the ileocaecal junction, and bringing the proximal end out to the abdominal surface to form a stoma. An ileal stoma usually protrudes 2–3 cm, which makes the management easier than with a stoma that is level with the abdominal surface. Because ileostomy effluent is liquid and corrosive to skin, if the stoma is flat, faecal fluid will leak under the appliance and cause excoriation. The removal of the distal severed portion of the bowel may be done at the same operation or may be postponed until the patient's condition is improved. If the lower part of the intestine is to be retained for a period of time, it is closed or, in some instances, the severed end may also be brought out to the abdominal surface. This second stoma is called a mucus fistula.

An ileostomy is most frequently performed for ulcerative colitis that does not respond to medical treatment. It may also be necessary for patients with Crohn's disease, multiple polyposis of the colon or an intestinal obstruction in the upper portion of the colon. Major advances in surgery now offer new procedures that overcome many of the obvious disadvantages of the traditional ileostomy. The first such procedure was the Kock continent ileostomy, which involved making a pouch or reservoir out of ileum (Fig. 15.5). This procedure is not performed on patients with regional enteritis (Crohn's disease) because the pouch may become affected.

The pouch serves as a reservoir for the intestinal content and is drained at regular intervals by the insertion of a catheter through the stoma. The capacity of the reservoir gradually increases, and may reach 400–600 mL over several months to 1 year. Continuous discharge and leakage of the fluid or semi-fluid between evacuations of the pouch is prevented by the formation of a valve-like structure at the internal end of the ileum which leads from the stoma to the ileal pouch.

More commonly, an ileal pouch is formed and connected to the anus (Fig. 15.6). This eliminates the need for a stoma and restores a normal means of passing faeces. The operation is performed in one or two stages. If the process is carried out over two stages, there may be a period when the patient has a temporary ileostomy. At the second stage, the ileostomy is closed and the pouch is activated to permit anal elimination. The sphincter muscles around the anus are conserved, permitting bowel evacuation in most patients via the anal route when the procedure is complete.

The postoperative period for patients with a pouch ileostomy is longer than that for patients who have had a conventional ileostomy. It involves gastrointestinal drainage via a nasogastric tube, intravenous fluids and continuous catheter drainage of the pouch for several days while the pouch heals. There may be a problem with anal incontinence for several weeks after operation as the pouch tissue continues to secrete mucus. Diarrhoea and anal soreness can be serious problems until reservoir adaptation has occurred, which may take 6–12 months. Eventually the patient will pass stool in a well controlled manner 4–8 times per day.

Colostomy

A colostomy is an opening of the colon on to the surface of the abdomen. It may be in the ascending, transverse, descending or sigmoid colon. The types of stoma include:

- permanent colostomy (usually called an end or terminal colostomy) carried out as a planned procedure with removal of all of the bowel beyond the stoma
- temporary colostomy to divert faecal matter away from the distal colon while healing occurs; they are often carried out in emergency situations.

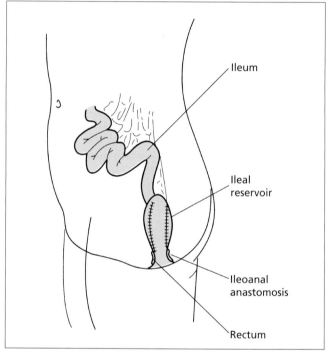

Figure 15.6   Ileoanal reservoir.

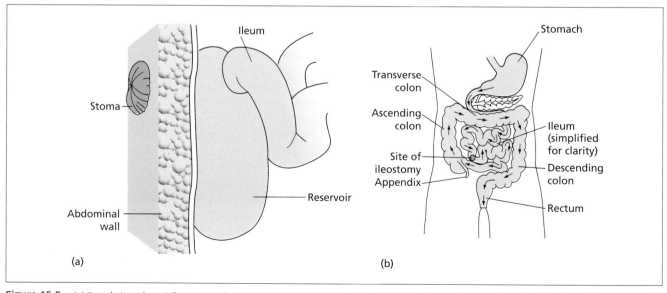

Figure 15.5   (a) Pouch (continent) ileostomy. (b) Diagram showing the location of the ileostomy. Arrows show the direction of movement of bowel contents.

Various techniques can be used to fashion these types of stoma such as:

- loop colostomy, where a section of the colon is brought out on to the abdomen, supported on the surface by a rod or bridge, opened longitudinally and the mucosal edges sutured to the skin
- double-barrelled colostomy, where the two ends of the colon are sutured together to make a spur and brought out on to the abdomen
- divided colostomy, where the proximal and distal ends of the stoma are brought out on to the abdomen to form two separate openings.

Nursing considerations in working with patients who have an ileostomy or colostomy

Differences between ileostomy and colostomy Certain differences exist between an ileostomy and colostomy that result in different problems and necessitate different types of care. For example, control of the discharge is determined by the location of the stoma; drainage from the ileum is of liquid consistency and is rich in enzymes that cause excoriation and erosion of the skin. Fluid from the ileum flows almost continuously, requiring the constant wearing of a receptive appliance unless an ileal pouch has been constructed. There may be quiescent periods but they are not predictable and cannot be controlled. Complications are a more common occurrence with an ileostomy than with a colostomy, and odour presents a greater problem if there is continuous drainage. Irrigations are not used with the conventional ileostomy; the introduction of anything into the ileal stoma is discouraged for fear of injury to the intestine.

Colostomy drainage is usually more manageable and less irritating to the skin unless the opening is into the ascending colon; the drainage then is similar to that from an ileostomy. The colostomy is more often in the transverse or descending colon, and much of the fluid and electrolytes has been absorbed from the faecal content, leaving it semisolid or solid by the time it reaches the stoma (Fig. 15.7). In some instances, the sigmoid colostomy may be so well controlled that it resembles normal bowel movement, and the patient does not have to wear an appliance continuously.

Intestinal activity in the individual with a colostomy or ileostomy may be influenced by diet, fluid intake and emotions – just as in any other person.

Psychological preoperative preparation When the doctor advises the patient before operation that a colostomy or ileostomy may or will be necessary, the patient may be quite distressed. If the colostomy is a temporary measure, it may be accepted more readily, but if it is likely to be permanent, the patient may be more concerned about this than about the operation or the primary condition. Assumptions about the patient's reactions can be misleading. The patient, for example, who is suffering much pain and disruption to their life from serious inflammatory bowel disease, may be relieved at the prospect of surgery. However, a patient with

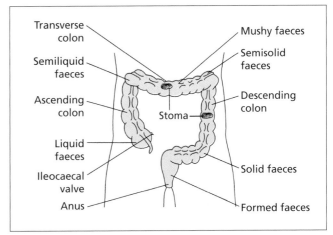

Figure 15.7 Colostomy sites and variation in faecal consistency within the colon.

only mild symptoms but a diagnosis of cancer may be devastated at the thought of surgery. The immediate response may be 'it would be better to die than have that'. The patient may become resentful or show marked depression, withdrawal and despair, perceiving this change to the body as making them unclean and unacceptable to society. There are fears because of odour and soiling. It is best to let the patient, family and partner express their feelings before attempting explanations. The nurse can help by being a willing listener, answering their questions and using every opportunity available to assure the patient that the 'ostomy' can be cared for without interfering with work and social life. When the patient recovers from the initial blow, discussions may then be held as to how to care for the ileostomy or colostomy. The patient should be actively involved in deciding the site of the stoma.

The stoma care nurse should be notified and meet with the patient and family before the operation. If no stoma care nurse is available, the nurse can encourage the patient and partner to handle the appliances, ask questions and look at literature or audiovisual resources on care and management of ostomies. It is important to reinforce that support and teaching will be available after surgery.

Some individuals, their families and significant others may welcome a visit from someone who has experienced a similar operation. Local branches of self-help groups such as the Ileostomy Association of Great Britain and Ireland (www.the-ia.org.uk) or the British Colostomy Association (www.bcass.org.uk) have a list of suitable visitors. Some centres develop their own group of ex-patients who can fulfil this function.

Physical preoperative preparation Physical preparation for the formation of a stoma is important. This will include siting of the stoma and bowel preparation. Correct siting of the stoma will ensure ease of mastery of the techniques of management and ultimately speedier adaptation to altered bowel elimination. Although the site may be chosen by the stoma care nurse or surgeon, the nurse may be involved in assessing the patient and identifying physical disabilities (e.g. poor eyesight or poor dexterity) that will influence where the stoma is sited. Box 15.7 outlines the sites that should be avoided. The nurse may also be involved in applying test patches of appliances, skin protective wafers and adhesives to avoid later problems with skin sensitivity.

Bowel preparation should be carried out according to local policy as methods vary. Whatever method is used, the nurse should prepare the person by explaining the procedure and the reason why it is necessary. Adequate privacy and hygiene needs should be provided, and monitoring of the patient for signs of dehydration, electrolyte disturbance, discomfort and exhaustion must be carried out. Bowel preparation can be psychologically traumatic, particularly if the individual experiences episodes of incontinence, as it may bring with it feelings of loss of control and realization of the impact of the planned surgery and future ramifications. The nurse should be supportive and encourage expression of anxieties about the future.

Nursing assessment

In addition to the usual surgical postoperative care, continuous assessment of the following is necessary:

- the patient's dexterity, eyesight and general ability to manage a stoma appliance
- the patient's perception of the ileostomy or colostomy
- the volume, colour, composition and consistency of the effluent (drainage)
- the patient's nutritional and hydrational status. The fluid intake and the quantity and composition of meals are noted. The patient's weight is recorded
- the condition of the stoma and surrounding skin surface
- the reaction to self-care
- the family's perception and reaction to the stoma
- the patient's ability to manage stoma care.

Box 15.7 Sites to be avoided when positioning a stoma

- Areas affected by skin conditions
- Bony prominences
- Fatty bulges or skin folds or creases (present on lying, standing or sitting)
- Groin creases
- Old scars
- Pubic area
- Site of surgical incision
- Site that cannot be seen by the patient
- Umbilicus
- Under large breasts
- Waistline.

Potential patient problems

Health problems common to the person with a stoma during the postoperative and early rehabilitation periods include:

- psychological distress at the stoma
- altered bowel elimination due to the faecal diversion
- potential for impairment of skin integrity related to leakage of intestinal or bowel contents on peristomal skin
- disturbances in body image due to the abdominal stoma, the surgical incision, changes in faecal elimination and control of odours
- altered sexuality pattern related to altered self-image, stoma, ostomy appliance, altered sexual responses
- lack of knowledge and lack of skill concerning self-management of the stoma.

Goals

The patient will demonstrate:

1 a healthy stoma with clean, intact peristomal skin
2 ability to look at and touch the stoma
3 active participation in care
4 ability to empty, clean, change, prepare and dispose of appliances
5 absence of diarrhoea, constipation, excessive gas and abdominal distension
6 awareness of how diet and fluid intake affect bowel function
7 recognition of the signs of complication and actions to take
8 ability to talk about feelings, concerns and to ask questions
9 awareness of community resources
10 understanding of how to obtain further supplies of appliances and accessories.

Nursing intervention
Physical management of the stoma

Postoperative assessment The patient usually returns from the theatre with a clear pouch in place to allow for observation of the stoma. Initially the stoma is swollen and oedematous, pink to bright red in colour, and shiny in appearance. A purple or dusky colour and coolness to touch indicate ischaemia. The volume of drainage is small. The baseline assessment data include the colour, temperature, size, type and location of the stoma. It is important to note whether the stoma is flush, retracted or prolapsed and to document the condition of the skin. The stoma is assessed at least every 8 hours for the first 24 hours after operation, and at least daily during the remainder of the hospitalization. The peristomal skin is inspected each time the appliance is changed. If a loop ostomy has been created, note the type of support system (e.g. rod, bridge, drain). It is important to label the pouch to alert others to remove the pouch gently if a rod is in place.

Selection of the drainage appliance Appliance selection is important for the person to be able to resume usual physical and social activities. The selected system should:

(1) be odour-proof, (2) protect the peristomal skin, (3) stay secure, (4) be readily available in the community, (5) be acceptable to the patient and (6) be invisible under ordinary clothing (Box 15.8). Drainage bags come as one- or two-piece systems. The one-piece appliances are used most commonly. The skin barrier is incorporated into the bag, eliminating the possibility of separation. Two-piece systems require that the drainage bag be snapped on over the solid skin barrier which is fitted around the stoma against the skin. The pressure of snapping the pouch in place can be uncomfortable against a newly operated area. There are two-piece systems available that avoid this pressure. After operation, all ostomy patients require a system with a drainable bag. An ostomy belt may be attached to the appliance to keep it secure during activities and to prevent undue pull on the seal, but is usually unnecessary.

The skin barriers often come in precut sizes and the bags are available in different shapes and sizes, clear or opaque, odour-proof and drainable. Some can be cut to fit, decreasing the need for hospitals to stock all options.

The size of the stoma is determined by a stoma-measuring card and bags of corresponding size are used. Too large an opening in the adhesive that attaches the bag exposes the skin to irritating drainage; too small an opening may traumatize or constrict the stoma.

The disposable bag is emptied when it is one-third to one-half full (whether of gas or faeces); if allowed to fill it becomes too heavy and the pull on the bag may break the seal of the stoma and cause leakage. The lower end of the bag is opened and the contents are allowed to drain into a receptacle. The volume and characteristics (colour, consistency and composition) of the drainage should be noted and recorded. The appliance is changed as regularly as necessary but at least twice weekly to permit inspection and cleansing of the peristomal skin.

The stoma care nurse will help the individual choose the system most suited to the individual's needs and to make any adjustments required because of variations in the size, characteristics or placement of the stoma. Persons with a colostomy may not require skin barriers because the stool is usually formed. A small stoma pouch or cap can be worn by persons who have achieved continency of a sigmoid colostomy. Persons with an internal continent pouch usually require only a stoma cap or gauze square with petroleum jelly over the stoma.

Colostomy irrigation A colostomy can in some circumstances be controlled entirely by diet, especially if the colostomy is in the descending colon or sigmoid. Irrigation may be used to achieve control when the colostomy exudes solid faecal material. The technique can be time consuming and requires motivation and dexterity to master. The purposes of irrigating the colostomy are to remove faeces, gas and mucus from the intestine and to establish a regular time of emptying the large bowel so that spontaneous, irregular drainage is less likely to occur and interfere with the person's activities and usual lifestyle. The technique usually

> **Box 15.8** Types of drainage appliance and indications for selection
>
> **One-piece closed pouch**
> - Suitable for solid effluent
> - Discarded after use once emptied
> - Changed once or twice daily
> - Patient may need to use a peristomal wafer if skin sensitivity occurs
> - Discrete appearance.
>
> **Two-piece system**
> - Skin sparing, because the baseplate or flange stays in place for several days
> - Interchangeable sizes of pouch:
>   activity pouch
>   closed pouch
>   drainable pouch
> - Can be used with a belt for extra security.
>
> **One-piece drainable pouch**
> - Suitable for liquid effluent
> - Wear times of 3–5 days can be achieved
> - Can be washed via emptying portal
> - Clip or clamp used to empty device
> - Can be used with a belt for extra security.
>
> **Colostomy plug**
> - Suitable for solid effluent, where stoma acts three or less times daily
> - Stoma should be less than 45 mm in diameter
> - Stoma should not protrude more than 6 mm from the skin
> - Manufacturer suggests that a 12-day training period is necessary
> - Patient may experience initial discomfort
> - Patient needs to be motivated and dextrous
> - Can be used with colostomy irrigation techniques
> - Discrete appearance.

takes approximately 30–40 minutes to perform and is usually done every 24–48 hours. It involves lavaging the terminal colon with 1 L of warm tap-water. The individual wears a long drainable pouch for the procedure but usually only wears a mini-pouch or cap to collect mucus or minimal faecal discharge at other times.

If the patient is constipated, it may be necessary to irrigate the colostomy. An irrigation set can be used or alternatively a funnel is attached to one end of a catheter;

the other end is lubricated and placed about 10 cm into the colon. Warm water is placed in the funnel, which is held above the level of the colostomy and the water is allowed to run into the patient. The catheter is then removed and the outflow runs into the toilet. All the water that was instilled into the colostomy must be returned before the process is complete. When evacuation is complete, the patient cleans the skin and applies a new drainage bag.

The irrigation is most effective early in the morning, as this approximates the normal time of defaecation. If bowel regularity is maintained, irrigation should be unnecessary unless the person decides to use irrigation as a means of stoma control.

Care of a Kock continent ileostomy Careful discussion preoperatively is essential to prepare the patient for surgery. The patient is returned from the operation with a catheter inserted through the stoma and valve into the pouch. The catheter is connected to a closed drainage system. It is important to maintain continuous drainage and prevent an accumulation of secretions, gas and faecal matter in the pouch in order to promote healing and prevent complications.

The colour of the drainage is checked frequently; it may be coloured by blood at first but the blood content progressively decreases over the first 2 days. The volume of the ileal discharge is also recorded. The faecal drainage eventually may become semi-liquid as the diet is increased and the capacity and retention of the pouch increase. Thicker pouch content may cause a drainage problem because 'solid' particles may obstruct the drainage tube, necessitating irrigation, increased fluid intake and adjustment in the diet.

A lightweight dressing with a slit for the catheter covers the stoma and surgical wound. This is changed daily and the stoma inspected for colour, swelling and oedema.

The nasogastric tube is attached to a drainage bag to prevent the possibility of gastric secretions and gas accumulating and distending the gastrointestinal tract. The catheter is left on open drainage for the first 10–12 days; thereafter it is clamped for progressively longer periods between drainage until it needs emptying only four times per day, utilizing the drainage catheter.

The capacity of the pouch gradually increases and in 6 months to 1 year, a capacity of 400–600 mL is achieved.

Food tolerance tends to be an individual matter; the introduction of 'new' foods one at a time makes it possible to identify those that are troublesome. Gas-forming foods, raw fruits and vegetables, foods with a high cellulose or fibre content, corn, celery, lettuce, beans, peas and cabbage are frequently among those not tolerated.

Care of an ileoanal pouch It is important that the patient understands this will not operate as a normal anal sphincter. Initial episodes of incontinence are common, with the mucus being discharged continuously from the pouch. The temporary stoma needs to be reversed in a second-stage operation; anal soreness can remain a problem and there is always the risk of the pouch becoming inflamed causing pain and frequent discharge.

Maintenance of skin integrity Each time the appliance is changed, the condition of the skin and stoma are noted. The latter should be bright red and moist; if it is bluish, or grey, or dry, the doctor is notified, as the change may indicate impaired circulation. The skin is examined carefully for possible excoriation or any break. Peristomal skin should be washed with warm water and gently patted dry. Skin irritation is treated promptly and a more effective protective barrier is provided. Fewer skin problems are encountered by the colostomy patient than the ileostomy patient.

Factors affecting the integrity of the peristomal skin include allergic responses, trauma, chemical irritants and infections. The individual may develop sensitivities to any of the products or appliances used to manage the ostomy. Known irritants are avoided and the method of use of each product is assessed and proper techniques taught. For example, skin barriers should be applied dry, not wet, to avoid moisture under the pouch and against the skin. The use of adhesive tape should be kept to a minimum.

Mechanical trauma most often occurs as a result of frequent, repeated changes of the pouching system. The pouch should be changed every 3–7 days and whenever leakage occurs. If the person is changing it more frequently, the nurse should assess the technique being used and consult with the stoma care nurse regarding other actions the person might use to overcome the identified problem. Perhaps a different system would be more appropriate for the person and their particular activity pattern, or there may be another type of adhesive that will hold better.

The location of the stoma affects the composition, consistency and quantity of the faecal discharge. The drainage from an ileostomy contains more proteolytic digestive enzymes, which quickly erode the skin. Skin barriers are sized or cut to fit snugly around the stoma to protect the skin from faecal drainage but should not cut into the stoma itself as this will cause local trauma. The bag should be changed regularly and the underlying skin cleansed and inspected to guard against hidden leakage. Soaps are avoided on the peristomal skin as they leave a residue. If solvents are used, care must be taken to ensure that the skin is well cleaned. Adhesive preparations should be applied sparingly.

Alterations in nutrition The ileostomy or colostomy patient usually starts out on a light, low-residue diet to which foods of a regular, normal diet are added gradually. Tolerance varies with patients but, by careful personal experimentation with foods, each person will recognize what can and cannot be taken. The foods that most often have to be excluded are those with a high-fibre or high-cellulose content. Nuts, prunes, celery, corn, pineapple, turnips, beans, cabbage and onions tend to be troublesome.

A well-balanced diet is encouraged and the person's weight followed. Patients are advised to eat slowly and to chew their foods well, which reduces the risk of a faecal bolus blocking the stoma.

Considerable water and salts are lost in ileostomy drainage, especially during the first 2–3 months. Gradually, the small intestine adapts to the lack of colonic function and absorbs more water and salts. Until then, extra water and food rich in sodium and potassium should be taken. The patient may erroneously think that limiting fluid intake will cause the intestinal drainage to be less fluid. Fluid intake should be more than 1.5 L/day.

Coping with the change in body function   As soon as practicable after the operation, the nurse concentrates on helping the patient to accept the 'ostomy' and on teaching the necessary care and management. Although there may have been considerable discussion of the modified method of elimination before operation, when the patient is actually faced with it, revulsion, discouragement and depression may occur. The patient with a temporary ostomy experiences the same feelings as the individual with a lifelong diversion. It is common for stoma patients to experience intense feelings of loss as they lose control of such a fundamental body function as elimination. The patient has a constant reminder that they are now different from other people; the stoma stigmatizes the patient. The individual may show evidence of passing through stages of the grieving process as he or she mourns these losses (see Ch. ***).

The patient will probably be concerned about future social acceptance. Acceptance comes first from the nurse, who willingly makes every effort to keep the patient clean and comfortable without any hesitation or aversion. Personal contact by touch, when bathing the patient and positioning and cleansing around the stoma for example, in a perfectly natural and matter-of-fact manner helps the patient to feel that the stoma is acceptable. The nurse should encourage the patient and gradually introduce self-care with an understanding of the patient's reactions to the adjustments that are required (see the Critical incident on p. 000). Competence in self-care of the ostomy promotes psychological adjustment. The patient may find it helpful to be visited by someone who has a stoma and is coping well. A visit by a stoma therapist should also be arranged well in advance of surgery.

Opportunities are created for the patient to interact and socialize with other patients on the ward. Return to normal activities and work are encouraged and may be achieved within 3 months.

Sexuality   The patient and partner are encouraged to ask questions about resuming normal sexual functioning, particularly as the partner may have more anxiety than the patient. Literature and pamphlets are available that may be given to the patient and partner regarding sex. Further opportunity for discussion should be arranged after they have read the information and formulated their personal questions and concerns.

Satisfactory sexual function improves the quality of life of the patient and promotes the closeness and sharing that the individual may perceive as lost or unattainable as a result of the alterations in body image and function. Identification of the patient's and partner's perceptions of the impact of the operation on their sexuality patterns and rela-

tionship should be assessed on an ongoing basis as they begin to cope with the realities of their situation. Box 15.9 lists the physical and psychological effects of ostomy surgery on sexual function. The patient and partner need help in understanding the meaning of these changes to their relationship. Misconceptions need to be identified, discussed and solutions explored.

The nurse plays an important role in helping the patient and partner adjust to the surgery and the effects of ongoing treatment and in the identification of problems related to altered sexuality patterns. If problems persist and interfere with the achievement of a satisfactory quality of life, the nurse should ensure that the patient and partner are referred appropriately and encouraged to utilize professional services.

Nurses can have a major role in encouraging discussion of issues related to sexuality and sexual functioning but it should be noted that it is an issue that is highly charged and requires sensitivity and understanding. Disclosure by the patient and the partner may threaten the attitudes and beliefs of the nurse, and, similarly, suggested strategies may frighten or disgust the individual's or partner's value system. If the nurse is unable to deal personally with this area, this should not be ignored. Encouragement to utilize other services (e.g. counselling) or to discuss problems with the stoma care nurse may be more advantageous in some circumstances in order to achieve a satisfactory outcome. In reviewing the literature, Allison and Stuchfield (1994) reported much evidence of positive adaptation between couples as well as acknowledgement of the major problems

---

Box 15.9   Sexual problems related to ostomy surgery

Direct effects
- Damage to sympathetic and parasympathetic nerves:
  erectile difficulty
  retrograde/no ejaculation
  change in ejaculatory amount or force
  orgasmic problems

- Penetration problems related to shortening or removal of vagina.

Indirect effects
- Altered expression related to:
  altered body image
  physical change
  lack of knowledge

- Fears:
  appearance of stoma or pouch
  noise and odour
  leakage
  rejection
  pain.

From Shipes (1987), with permission.

posed by stoma surgery. Some couples feel much closer as a result and others report such a dramatic improvement in the quality of life that sexuality has been enhanced.

Self-care A plan of education is developed to prepare the patient for assuming care of the ileostomy or colostomy and for living a healthy, active life. During the first few days after the operation, the patient's experience with pain and discomfort generally precludes concern about the stoma and future care and activity. Gradually, an awareness of the situation develops and the patient's reaction must be assessed. There may be a period of depression and withdrawal. Denial or suppression may be evident but this can all be a normal part of the adaptation process. The nurse should not challenge or confront the patient but rather work on building a supportive relationship so that eventually the patient can be helped to come to terms with their loss. In the meantime, the patient is unlikely to be receptive to any formal teaching. The nurse encourages expression of concern by being a good listener and accepting the patient's reactions and anxiety.

The preparation for the patient's discharge from the hospital should include a member of the family. Participation of a person with an ileostomy or colostomy who may have already visited the patient may be very helpful in reinforcing the information. Teaching includes explanations, discussions and demonstrations.

Management of the ileostomy and colostomy Active patient participation in stoma and appliance care is introduced gradually but as early as possible. On discharge, the patient should be engaged in self-care and be confident in the fact that support and assistance are available in the hospital and at home.

At first, as the nurse cares for the ileostomy or colostomy, each step of the procedure is clearly described. Then, gradually, the patient participates in the care until eventually, self-care is achieved. This progressive step-by-step approach takes time and patience but is less frustrating and discouraging for the patient. As self-care progresses, the community nurse should discuss any problems of self-care after discharge.

Necessary equipment and supplies A written list should be provided to inform the patients where the various parts of the appliance may be obtained from. Information regarding obtaining exemption from prescription charges should also be provided.

Care of the skin The need for thorough but gentle cleansing of the skin is stressed, as is the use of a protective skin barrier because of the irritating effect of the enzyme-containing discharge. Inspection for redness and excoriation is described and advice given as to what should be done if either is present.

Emptying the bag The role of regular emptying, changing and thorough cleansing of the appliance in controlling odour is discussed.

Problems or complications Problems such as excessive drainage, blockage of the stoma, excoriation, burning sensation or itching of the skin should be discussed with regard to possible causes, how they are recognized and the appropriate action.

Nutrition and fluids The patient is advised that foods high in cellulose and fibre and some raw vegetables and fruits may be troublesome. The importance of a well-balanced diet and the taking of additional amounts of sodium, potassium and water should be explained. It is suggested that one new food be added at a time so those that cannot be tolerated may be identified.

Bathing The patient may take a shower or bath with or without the appliance in place. Showering without the appliance is good for the skin and for cleansing the stoma. The patient must be sure that no soap is used on the peristomal skin. Bathing is usually done before applying a fresh appliance because the moisture is likely to loosen the adhesive disc. Some people with stomas may have sufficient confidence to go swimming – the appliance can be concealed by a bathing suit.

Activity Activity for the stoma patient is normal except for heavy lifting, which predisposes to prolapse of the stoma and hernia, and body contact sports, which could result in injury to the stoma. The patient can be encouraged to return to his or her occupation and recreational activities. Many people find that their general health is so much better than previously that they enjoy being able to participate in new activities.

The patient may be concerned about sexual relationships and is advised that the change in body image need not be a deterrent to satisfactory sex relations. If an abdomino-perineal resection has been done, injury to parasympathetic nerves may very occasionally result in impotence. A woman may experience some discomfort during intercourse for a period of time because of the perineal wound. This matter of sexual relationships is something the individual may wish to discuss freely with the stoma therapist. Further help may be available from SPOD (Association to Promote the Sexual and Personal Relationships of People with Disabilities).

Medications The patient should be informed that laxatives or other drugs should not be taken unless prescribed. If a medicine is prescribed by anyone other the gastroenterologist, the patient should remind the clinician about the stoma. Some preparations should be only in powder or liquid form to ensure absorption.

Sources of assistance The patient is likely to be very apprehensive about leaving the protective hospital environment. A list of persons or associations from whom advice or assistance may be sought can be provided, with telephone numbers. This list may include the stoma therapist, community nurse and the relevant associations and support groups.

Complications Potential complications of an ileostomy or colostomy include prolapse or retraction of the stoma, obstruction of the stoma, fluid and electrolyte imbalance, renal calculus and fistula.

In prolapse of the stoma, the mesentery of the remaining intestine is not secured sufficiently to the abdominal wall and/or the opening in the abdominal wall is too large. Increased intra-abdominal pressure results in a segment of the ileum or colon being forced out on to the abdomen. If several centimetres of the bowel are extruded, the patient should be placed in the dorsal recumbent position with the head and shoulders slightly raised and the knees flexed. A dressing moistened in sterile water or normal saline is placed over the area. The doctor may attempt manual replacement of the extruded segment or recommend surgical repair.

Retraction of the stoma occurs as the result of shrinking scar tissue in the supporting tissues of the abdominal wall. The opening becomes flush with the abdominal surface, making it difficult to protect the skin from the irritating effluent. Correction is by surgery.

Obstruction of the stoma may be caused by a faecal bolus formed as a result of insufficient mastication of food or the ingestion of fibrous or cellulose foods that are too bulky to pass through the stoma. The blockage may be relieved by an irrigation. An obstruction may also be caused by a volvulus of the ileum near the stoma. If there is no ileal or colostomy discharge, the doctor should be notified. Unless the obstruction is relieved, the patient will develop nausea, vomiting, crampy pain and abdominal distension.

Ileostomy dysfunction sometimes occurs and is characterized by sporadic free liquid drainage with a very offensive odour. It is associated with peristomal scarring and stenosis, which causes trapping of the intestinal contents until pressure and irritation result in the discharge. Dilatation of the stoma may be necessary.

Normally, much of the water and electrolytes contained in the small intestine content is reabsorbed in the colon. The person with an ileostomy loses considerable water, sodium and potassium in the ileal drainage and may develop fluid and electrolyte imbalance. The patient is encouraged to drink a minimum of 1500–2000 mL of fluid daily, to add salt to foods and to include potassium-containing foods (e.g. orange juice, bananas and meat) in the diet. If the ileal drainage becomes excessive, fluids containing potassium and sodium, such as fruit juice, are increased to compensate for the loss. If the excessive drainage cannot be controlled, the doctor should be notified. An anti-diarrhoeal drug may be prescribed, serum electrolyte levels determined and intravenous fluids administered to correct dehydration and electrolyte imbalance.

The ileostomy patient is predisposed to the formation of a renal calculus (kidney stone) because of the water and sodium loss in drainage. This further emphasizes the importance of a greater fluid and electrolyte intake for the person with an ileostomy or colostomy.

Rarely, an ileostomy or colostomy is complicated by a fistula. An opening develops in the ileum and the drainage forms a tract to the surface. This may be the result of a poorly fitting appliance or the recurrence of the primary disease. The drainage causes tissue irritation and erosion. Surgical intervention may be used to resect the tract and may include reconstruction of the stoma. Healing may necessitate complete rest of the intestine; the patient may receive parenteral nutrition until the area is healed.

Herniation of the intestine due to a weakness of the muscular tissue at the site of the stoma may occur. It is recognized as a bulging area. This should be assessed by the GI specialist team but a simple solution may be to provide support with the ileostomy or colostomy appliance.

Evaluation

Physical management of the stoma is an important step in the person's adjustment to the change in body image and altered control of an important body function. Ostomy surgery impacts on the person's total well-being and family and social relationships. Adjustment is slow and requires support from the nurse, other healthcare providers and the patient's spouse and family.

A variety of products and appliances is available for ostomy care. The stoma therapist and/or nurse should assist the patient in selecting a drainage system most suited to his or her individual needs. Achievement of self-management and an acceptable quality of life are realistic goals for most persons following bowel diversion surgery.

SUMMARY

The aim of this chapter was to give novice nurses, and nurses unfamiliar with the speciality, an insight into the effects of gastrointestinal disease and the syndromes that patients experience. With the imperative for evidence-based practice in mind, the text has sought to provide information about disorders and the current approaches to patients' care and treatment. Patients who have disorders of the gastrointestinal system are in need of skilled and empathetic nursing care. This chapter has provided some of the knowledge that is required to address the needs of patients in your clinical practice. More in-depth and specialist information for those wishing to explore the area further can be obtained by reading current papers in related nursing, medicine, surgery and pharmacology journals.

REFERENCES

Allison M, Stuchfield B (1994) Helping to adjust: an holistic approach to stoma care. RCN nursing update supplement. Nursing Standard 8(36): 3–13.

Best C (2005) Caring for the patient with a nasogastric tube. Nursing Standard 20(3): 59–65.

CRITICAL INCIDENT

Sarah is a 23-year-old student who has had Crohn's disease for 10 years. After numerous episodes of remission and exacerbation, she has undergone surgery to have a colectomy and formation of an end-ileostomy. It is 6 days since her operation and she has made a good recovery, even stating that it is a relief to have the ileostomy. She has just started to learn to deal with it and is emptying the bag without supervision. She helps to change the bag but is not doing it herself yet. She has a boyfriend of 1 year's standing who has been visiting her regularly but, as far as you are aware, she has not discussed the details of her operation with him yet.

You are on night duty and busy settling patients for the night. Sarah seems comfortable; you have given her analgesia and you have ensured that she has enough to drink during the night. You ask whether she has emptied the ileostomy and she says she has and there are no problems.

At 05:30 hours Sarah calls you. Her ileostomy bag has leaked; the odour and mess are obvious and Sarah is distressed to the point of not being able to move. You change the appliance for her and then help her to the bathroom. Whilst she is in the bath, you clean and re-make her bed and wash her nightclothes. You help her back to bed and quietly discuss what happened, when she is ready.

Points for reflection and discussion
Why did it happen?
- The bag became overfull (more than half full of either gas or faecal fluid) and movement caused it to leak by lifting the adhesive flange off the skin
- The bag was not well adhered and was beginning to lift off the skin anyway
- Movement in bed when asleep may cause the bag to lift off if it is becoming full, particularly with gas
- As Sarah is recovering, she will have begun to eat solid food and this will result in more flatus forming, which she will not yet be used to

How did it make Sarah feel?
- Disgusted by the mess?
- Appalled that this could happen to her?
- Reality shock – she had been doing well after the operation and this is the first pitfall she has encountered. She is not 'better' after all but has something else to deal with
- She has possibly been in denial about the change in her body image as indicated by her not discussing the details of the operation with her boyfriend or showing him her stoma. This event will confront her with that reality. It may well cause her to feel unattractive and depressed
- Angry – she did not realize this could happen.

How did it make you feel?
- Disgusted by the mess?
- Appalled that this could happen?
- Guilty?
- Disappointed that this episode has disrupted Sarah's recovery?
- Angry – you may be partly responsible for this happening.

What was bad about the situation?
- The mess?
- The distress it caused?

What was good about the situation?
- It gave Sarah the opportunity to overcome one of the practical and emotional aspects of her operation with your help and support
- It gave you an opportunity to consider your feelings and action in the situation which you will be able to act on productively in future.

What was learnt from the situation?
- Leaking stoma appliances cause significant distress for the patient and those around them
- Changes in dietary intake will affect the output of a stoma, particularly an ileostomy and need to be anticipated by the patient
- Ileostomy appliances need to be emptied regularly, of flatus or faecal fluid, and adhesion of the appliance should be checked whenever this is done
- New 'ostomists' need guidance and reassurance every step of the way despite seeming to be 'in control'
- Accidents happen to most ostomists sooner or later; learning to deal with them is an important part of the learning process and the adjustment to having a stoma.

What would you do differently in the future?
- Check new ostomists' appliances are empty and intact before their going to sleep – do so with them as a teaching opportunity
- Ensure new ostomists' learning and achievements are clearly documented so that all staff know what the patient is able to do independently, and where they need assistance, rather than making assumptions.

Discuss your practice and thoughts about such an incident with a stoma therapy nurse specialist.

Borwell B (2002) Bowel cancer in the older person. Cancer Nursing Practice 1(4): 32–38.

Boyd-Carson W (2004) Irritable bowel syndrome: assessment and management. Nursing Standard 18(5): 47–52.

Butler M (1997) Gastrointestinal bleeding In: Bruce L, Finlay TMD, eds. Nursing in gastroenterology. Edinburgh: Churchill Livingstone, p 119–139.

Cancer Research UK (2004) UK Stomach cancer incidence statistics. Online. Available: http://info.cancerresearchuk.org/cancerstats/types/stomach/incidence [Accessed 04.03.2006].

Cancer Research UK (2005a) Oesophageal cancer. Online. Available: http://www.cancerresearchuk.org/aboutcancer/specificcancers/oesophageal_cancer [Accessed 11.11.2005].

Cancer Research UK (2005b) Stomach (gastric) cancers. Online. Available: http://www.cancerresearchuk.org/aboutcancer/specificcancers/stomach_cancer [Accessed 04.03.2006].

Cancer Research UK (2005c) Bowel (colorectal) cancers. Online. Available: http://www.cancerresearchuk.org/aboutcancer/specificcancers/colorectal_cancer [Accessed 08.03.2006].

Coughlan C (2005) Screening for familial cases of colorectal cancer: a new practice environment. Gastrointestinal Nursing 3(4): 25–29.

de Snoo L (2002) Colorectal cancer. Cancer Nursing Practice 1(10): 32–38.

Field J, Bjarnason K (2002) Feeding patients after abdominal surgery. Nursing Standard 16(48): 41–44.

Grahame-Smith DG, Aronson JK (2002) Oxford textbook of clinical pharmacology and drug therapy. Oxford: Oxford University Press.

Griffiths H (2005) Coeliac disease: the nurse's role in investigative care. Gastrointestinal Nursing 4(5): 31–37.

Haboubi H, Hasan El-Hasan, Davies J, Lane S, Rowe P, Hurley M, Haboubi N (2005) Two-year audit of PEG patient follow up. Gastrointestinal Nursing 3(3): 25–30.

Holmes S (2004) Enteral feeding and percutaneous gastrostomy. Nursing Standard 18(20): 41–43.

Hughes E (2005) Caring for the patient with an intestinal obstruction. Nursing Standard 19(47): 56–64.

Kelly M (1992) Colitis. London: Routledge.

Livett H (2004) Test and treat Helicobacter pylori before endoscopy. Nursing Standard 19(8): 33–38.

Metcalf C (2002) Crohn's disease: an overview. Nursing Standard 16(31): 45–52.

National Institute for Clinical Excellence (NICE) (2002) Guidance on the use of infliximab for Crohn's disease. Technology Appraisal Guidance No. 40, April.

Nightingale A (2004) An overview of the diagnosis and management of Crohn's disease. Gastrointestinal Nursing 2(4): 31–39.

Rigby D, Powell M (2005) Causes of constipation and treatment options. Primary Health Care 15(2): 41–50.

Thompson MJ, Boyd-Carson W, Trainor B, Boyd K (2003) Management of constipation. Nursing Standard 18(14): 41–42.

Thompson WG, Creed F, Drossman DA et al (1992) Functional bowel disease and functional abdominal pain Gastroenterology International 5: 75–91.

Turner G (1996) Oral care. Nursing Standard 10(28): 51–56.

16 Caring for the patient with a liver, biliary tract or exocrine pancreas disorder

Sue Lee

INTRODUCTION

Disorders of the biliary system (liver and exocrine pancreas) account for many hospital admissions: the incidence of hepatitis C continues to grow worldwide (Grundy and Beeching 2004); non-alcoholic fatty liver disease has become a very common chronic liver condition (Adams et al 2005); and alcoholism and its concomitant pathophysiology and conditions continues to rise (Sargent 2005). There have been many improvements in the treatment of people with liver disease in recent years. Advances in surgical technique ('keyhole' or laparoscopic surgery) have reduced length of hospital stay for many patients with gallbladder disease, treatment with interferon is having an impact on patients with hepatitis (Centre for Reviews and Dissemination (CRD) 2001a, b). Improvements have also been made in the care of patients with acute pancreatitis (McArdle 2000, Abou-Assi and O'Keefe 2001). Organ transplantation, particularly of the liver and pancreas, is improving the morbidity and quality of life for many patients in developed countries (Grewal 2002). However, for those patients suffering from chronic or malignant conditions of the biliary system and pancreas, the outlook may still be bleak. This chapter aims to examine issues faced by patients with disorders of the liver, biliary tract or pancreas. The anatomy and physiology of the biliary tree will be reviewed briefly before entering into a discussion of the care and treatment required by such patients.

THE LIVER

The liver is situated in the right upper quadrant of the abdominal cavity immediately below the diaphragm. It is divided into four lobes and is highly vascular, receiving its blood supply from two sources. The *portal vein* carries blood from the stomach, intestines, spleen and pancreas into the liver. The *hepatic artery* delivers blood from the aorta. The blood from both sources leaves the liver by a common pathway, the hepatic vein, which joins the inferior vena cava.

The liver tissue is organized in functional units called lobules. The central veins from the lobules empty into sublobular collecting veins, which unite to form the hepatic vein. Minute ducts into which bile is discharged are also formed between the rows of hepatic cells within the lobules. The small lobular bile ducts unite to form larger ducts. Eventually, the bile from the lobules is transmitted in one main channel, the hepatic duct, which joins the bile duct from the gallbladder (cystic duct) to form the common bile duct (Fig. 16.1).

Functions of the liver

The liver performs a variety of very important complex functions which are vital in maintaining homeostasis and normal metabolism. The liver synthesizes, processes and/or stores many of the substances that are essential to normal body functioning. It also processes and excretes some substances that would be harmful if left in their original form or allowed to accumulate.

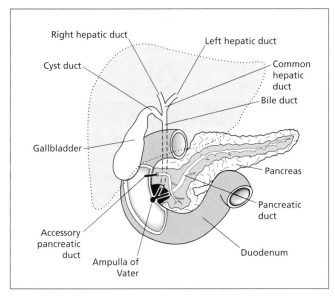

Figure 16.1   The pancreas and associated anatomy.

Bile production and excretion

The liver cells secrete 800–1000 mL of bile daily into the hepatic ducts. Bile is a yellow-green or brownish fluid that is strongly alkaline. The constituents of bile include water, cholesterol, various ions, bile pigments and bile salts:

- *Water (90–97%)*. The water content is reduced when the bile is stored in the gallbladder, where it is concentrated to ten times its original strength
- *Bile pigments*. The pigments resulting from the breakdown of red blood cells and from foods are excreted as the bile pigments of which *conjugated bilirubin* is the main component. Conjugated means it has been altered by adding glucuronic acid molecules. In the intestine, bile pigments are acted upon by bacteria and reduced to urobilinogen, a form of which is called stercobilin. This gives faeces their normal brown colour, consequently pale clay coloured stools indicate obstruction in the biliary tree leading to a lack of stercobilin in the colon. Some urobilinogen is absorbed through the intestinal mucosa into the blood where it is converted into urobilin and excreted in the urine
- *Bile salts*. These are sodium and potassium salts of certain amino acids that function in digestion and absorption. The bile salts emulsify fats, increase the digestive action of fat-splitting enzymes, and promote absorption of fats, fat-soluble vitamins and calcium salts. (Emulsification is the process whereby large fat droplets are dispersed into much smaller droplets.)
- *Other constituents*. Sodium and calcium salts, cholesterol, fatty acids and lecithin are other substances in bile.

Bile is discharged by the common bile duct into the duodenum through the sphincter of Oddi. The two main functions of bile are to promote the digestion and absorption of fats in the small intestine and, as it is alkaline, to neutralize the acidic chyme when it moves into the small intestine.

Metabolic functions

The liver has a role in the metabolism of carbohydrates, proteins and fats. Briefly, it converts glucose to glycogen (*glycogenesis*) and stores it, re-converting the glycogen to glucose, which is released into the blood when required to maintain an adequate blood sugar concentration. Glucose in excess of what can be converted to glycogen is converted to fat (*lipogenesis*) in the liver.

Lipids may be both synthesized and catabolized by the liver. Lipoproteins are a very important compound for transporting cholesterol around the body and they are made in the liver along with cholesterol. Conversely, fatty acids may be may be broken down to generate ATP.

Proteins are deaminated, a process in which the amine group (NH_2) is removed so the remaining amino acids can be used to make ATP or glycogen or fatty acids. This process forms ammonia (NH_3) which is converted to urea and released into the blood for elimination by the kidneys.

Storage

The liver stores glycogen, vitamins A, D, E, K and B_{12}, iron, phospholipids, cholesterol and a small amount of protein and fat.

Formation of certain blood components

Heparin and the blood proteins serum albumin, fibrinogen and α- and β-globulins are formed by the hepatic cells. The liver also synthesizes most of the blood-clotting factors; it is the primary source of prothrombin, fibrinogen and factors V, VII, VIII, IX, XI and XII.

Destruction of erythrocytes

Worn-out erythrocytes are broken down by Kupffer cells in the liver. The haemoglobin is released, the iron and globin are split off, and bilirubin is formed from the waste products and excreted in bile. The iron is reclaimed, combined with a protein to form ferritin and stored until it is needed for the formation of haemoglobin. White blood cells may also be removed in this way.

Detoxification of harmful substances

Certain drugs and chemicals that could be harmful (e.g. alcohol) are detoxified by the liver before being excreted by the kidneys. Normal liver function is therefore essential if drugs are not to accumulate in the body and cause problems. Abnormality of liver enzyme function can cause unwanted side-effects and complications during drug treatment.

The body itself produces certain chemicals (hormones) that, unless destroyed, would reach too high a concentration. Examples of physiological products that are destroyed in the liver are the antidiuretic hormone (ADH), progesterone and adrenocorticoid secretions. Some hormones, such as insulin and glucagon, undergo deamination in the liver, which renders them inactive.

The Kupffer cells also protect the body by destroying organisms that may have been absorbed from the intestine.

Heat production

The liver is second only to muscle tissue in the production of heat by its continuous cell activity. Under basal (resting) conditions, the liver is responsible for most of the body heat.

GALLBLADDER AND BILE DUCTS

The gallbladder is a sac on the undersurface of the liver with an average capacity of 40–50 mL. The cystic duct leading from the gallbladder merges with the hepatic duct to form the common bile duct. The latter unites with the pancreatic duct to form the ampulla of Vater, which opens into the duodenum. This opening is controlled by the sphincter of Oddi.

The functions of the gallbladder are to concentrate and store the bile. When the stomach and duodenum are empty of food, the sphincter of Oddi remains contracted. During this period, the bile that is continuously secreted accumulates in the gallbladder. Contraction of the sac to eject the bile is dependent upon hormonal stimulation. When food containing fat and partially digested protein enters the duodenum, a hormone called cholecystokinin-pancreozymin (CCK-PZ or CCK) is secreted by cells of the duodenal mucosa. It is carried in the blood and, on reaching the gallbladder, stimulates the smooth muscle tissue to contract and eject bile. CCK also produces relaxation of the sphincter of Oddi, which allows the flow of bile into the duodenum.

PANCREAS

The pancreas is an oblong gland; a thicker portion, referred to as the head, lies in the curve of the duodenum, and the remainder extends to the left directly behind the stomach. It has two distinct types of essential functional cells. Groups of one type (exocrine) secrete digestive enzymes and up to 1500 mL of pancreatic juice into small ducts that drain into a main channel running the length of the gland. This collecting channel is called the *pancreatic duct*; it passes out of the head of the pancreas to unite with the common bile duct to form the ampulla of Vater.

The other type of cell (endocrine) is scattered in groups, forming what are known as the *islets of Langerhans*. These cells produce hormones (e.g. insulin) and are classified as *endocrine* because their hormonal secretions are absorbed into the blood to be carried around the body where they have their effect.

Exocrine functions

The exocrine secretions pass through the ampulla of Vater and sphincter of Oddi into the duodenum. The pancreatic juice is strongly alkaline, owing to a high bicarbonate content. Several important digestive enzymes involved in the breakdown of proteins, carbohydrates and fats are contained in the exocrine secretion. Regulation of the secretion of these enzymes and their role in digestion is discussed on p. 431.

Endocrine functions

The endocrine portion of the pancreas produces insulin, glucagon and somatostatin. The effects of these hormones, particularly in relation to diabetes, are discussed on p. 555.

ASSESSMENT

Disorders of the liver, biliary tract and pancreas affect overall body functioning. The body's energy balance is affected when the supply and storage of nutrients is altered, fluid and electrolyte balance is disrupted, bowel and bladder elimination are altered, blood-clotting mechanisms are affected, and heat production diminishes. Patient assessment includes the collection of data on lifestyle, behaviour patterns, dietary habits and changes in physiological functioning of most body systems. Also, the nurse should have some understanding of the various examinations and tests carried out in order to explain them fully to the patient and discuss the implications of the results.

The signs and symptoms of biliary tract disorder may be very distressing to the patient. It is not sufficient therefore, to note that a patient appears jaundiced. The alteration in skin colour may make the patient embarrassed or ashamed and be a cause of great concern to the family. The person may have an inaccurate understanding of jaundice, or associate the condition with a fatal outcome; consequently patient education is required to relieve a great deal of possible anxiety and fear. Jaundice represents a significant alteration in body image which requires the patient to adapt to this change. The nurse therefore needs to assess how effectively the patient is coping, as maladaptive behaviour, if present, suggests the need for nursing intervention.

It is important, therefore, that the nurse considers the effects of the various clinical manifestations of biliary, hepatic or pancreatic disease on the whole patient, besides the obvious physical changes that are present. This consideration should be borne in mind while studying the rest of this chapter. The question 'What does the patient make of this?' should therefore be to the forefront throughout the assessment stage.

HISTORY

In taking a patient's history, the following areas should be looked at:

- *Jaundice* is a non-specific sign of disorder within the liver and biliary tree and therefore the patient should be asked if they have noticed any alteration of skin colour or yellowing of the sclera of the eyes if they have pigmented skin
- *Activity and lifestyle.* Data are collected on the type and extent of daily activities, how the person feels after activity, how leisure time is used, and the usual pattern and amount of sleep received

- *Nutritional history* includes identification of daily food intake, eating habits, and factors affecting eating. Daily food intake is analysed for adequacy of essential nutrients, vitamins, fluid volume and kilocalories. How the individual responds to food is elicited as well as symptoms that occur following ingestion of food. The presence of nausea, vomiting, anorexia, excessive thirst and changes in body weight are determined. Use of alcohol and drugs (prescription, over the counter and illegal recreational drugs must be included) is carefully recorded given the importance of the liver in metabolizing these substances
- *Elimination*. The person's usual bowel habits are determined and questions related to the nature, formation, colour and odour of stools are asked. The presence of steatorrhoea (fatty pale diarrhoea) or clay-coloured stools is noted as this indicates faulty lipid digestion and therefore problems within the biliary tree. Melaena or haematuria are significant points in the history as this indicates a bleeding tendency which could be caused by abnormal liver function failing to produce the necessary blood clotting factors. The volume and colour of urine and frequency of voiding are determined as well as the presence of nocturia
- *Environmental and occupational history* includes the identification of chemicals in the person's work and home environment that might be toxic to the liver
- *Pain and discomfort* are identified by questioning the patient about the location and duration of abdominal or epigastric pain or discomfort and factors which precipitate discomfort
- *The patient's psychological and social status* should also be assessed, including the patient's own perceptions of his or her health
- *Abnormal bleeding and bruising* should be explored as this indicates a failure to produce clotting factors in the liver.

PHYSICAL EXAMINATION

In a physical examination the following points should be noted:

1 *General appearance*. Changes in posture or weight distribution as seen with abdominal ascites are observed, as well as the general colour of the skin and the sclera of the eyes.
2 *Height and weight* are measured and recorded. Changes in body weight are noted.
3 *Temperature, pulse, respirations and blood pressure* are recorded. Body temperature reflects both liver function and cellular metabolism. Advanced liver disease may lead to intrathoracic complications; dyspnoea may result and should be observed and recorded (Oh et al 2000).
4 *The skin* is inspected for signs of petechiae or bruises, open lesions that have not healed, and jaundice as evidenced by a yellowish colour of the skin and sclera. There may be evidence of itching. Peripheral oedema is determined by pressing firmly for about 5 seconds with the thumb over a bony prominence such as the dorsum of the foot; on release of the pressure, the skin is observed and palpated for pitting or indentations and the rate at which it returns to normal. Oedema would be caused by a lack of plasma proteins due to liver failure.
5 *Abdominal ascites*. Inspection of the abdomen containing ascites will show distension, protrusion of the umbilicus and asymmetry when the patient shifts position.
6 Advanced nurse practitioners routinely carry out a full (medical) physical examination of the abdomen and are competent to palpate and auscultate. A diseased liver can be identified by palpation.

DIAGNOSTIC TESTS

Laboratory tests for liver, biliary and pancreatic function

Blood tests

Blood tests are designed to show up the biochemical markers of liver damage; liver function tests are often incorporated routinely into biochemistry panels rather than specifically ordered (Giannini et al 2005).

Serum bilirubin   This test gives an estimation of the concentration of bilirubin in the blood and indicates whether it is conjugated or unconjugated. Normally, the liver cells extract the pigment from the blood and conjugate it with glucuronic acid to make water-soluble conjugated bilirubin before excreting it in bile. In obstructive jaundice, the conjugated bilirubin level is increased as the liver cells are working normally and the problem stems from the bodies' inability to pass bile normally through the biliary tree. In jaundice caused by an abnormally rapid breakdown of red blood cells (haemolytic jaundice), unconjugated bilirubin is the predominant pigment in the blood as the bilirubin has not had chance to reach the liver where it can be conjugated. Malaria for example commonly causes a haemolytic jaundice as the infected red blood cells break down rapidly; damage to the liver makes the jaundice worse over time.

Serum alkaline phosphatase   Normally this enzyme is excreted in the bile by the hepatic cells. The blood concentration may be increased when there is liver disease or obstruction in the bile ducts (normal: 35–105 IU/L).

Serum enzymes (liver and pancreatic)

Liver enzyme tests   The liver cells contain the enzymes serum alanine aminotransferase (ALT; formerly referred to as serum glutamic-pyruvic transaminase (SGPT)) and serum aspartate aminotransferase (AST; previously called serum glutamic oxaloacetic transaminase (SGOT)). AST is also found in heart, skeletal muscle, kidneys, brain and red blood cells. ALT can be found in low concentrations in skeletal muscle and the kidney. As these enzymes are released into the blood when the cells are damaged, their concentration may be used to estimate liver damage (normal values: ALT 1–12 IU/L, AST 0–40 IU/L). Raised ALT levels are more specific for liver damage (than AST) given their low concentrations elsewhere (Giannini et al 2005). Opiates can cause a rise in ALT and AST levels. One of the problems with measurements of these enzymes is that the diagnosis of the severity of a condition based on the magnitude of the enzyme elevation may be misleading because a range of conditions overlap; the timing of tests is therefore crucial (Giannini et al 2005). For instance, ALT measurements may underestimate improvement that occurs following treatment (particularly with interferon), so patients may still need to undergo liver biopsy (CRD 2001c).

γ-Glutamyl transferase (GGT) is an enzyme found in greatest concentration in the liver and kidneys; it indicates liver cell dysfunction and alcohol-induced liver disease (normal: males 6–28 IU/L; females 4–18 IU/L). However, GGT activity can also be induced through the use of anticonvulsants and oral contraceptives. Furthermore, GGT levels may be elevated in such conditions as chronic obstructive pulmonary disease, renal failure and acute myocardial infarction (Giannini et al 2005). In alcoholic liver disease, GGT levels may be elevated whilst ALT levels may be normal or only slightly altered and is therefore useful for differential diagnoses of non-alcoholic fatty liver disease and hepatitis C (Giannini et al 2005).

Concentration of pancreatic enzymes   The pancreas has both endocrine and exocrine functions. Insulin and glucagon are produced as an endocrine function to regulate blood glucose. Pancreatic enzymes – amylase, trypsin and lipase – are produced as the exocrine function. Some of the enzymes secreted by the pancreas are normally absorbed into the blood and eventually are excreted in the urine. An increase in the serum levels of amylase and lipase occurs when there is an obstruction of pancreatic ducts and necrosis of cells, which is part of the process of autoingestion of body tissue, which results and causes pancreatitis (Hale et al 2000).

Serum globulin   This is produced in the liver and normally is of greater concentration than serum albumin. This situation is reversed in disease of the liver.

Prothrombin time   The liver is responsible for the synthesis of several clotting factors. The prothrombin time or activity reflects the effects of liver dysfunction on blood coagulation (normal: 11–15 seconds). The international normalized ratio (INR) is the ratio of the person's prothrombin time to a normal control and is commonly used to control warfarin anticoagulation therapy.

Blood lipids   The concentration of cholesterol and cholesterol esters in the blood falls in liver disease, when cell function is impaired, and rises in obstructive jaundice.

Blood ammonia   In severe impairment of liver function, the ammonia concentration in the blood is increased and may lead to hepatic coma.

Hepatitis tests   Viral hepatitis is caused by hepatitis viruses A, B, C, D or E. Serological tests on the plasma to identify known antigens and antibodies are available. The various tests for the hepatitis viruses are able to detect current infection and 'virus loading' (McCreaddie and Neilson 2001), long-term immunity or recent infection. However, they may have to be done in series, which can delay diagnosis (Shovein et al 2000).

Blood glucose concentration   Damage to the islets of Langerhans may cause a reduction in insulin secretion and resultant hyperglycaemia.

Leucocyte count   The white blood count is raised in pancreatitis, with a marked increase in the polymorphonuclear leucocytes in necrotizing and haemorrhagic pancreatitis.

Carbohydrate-deficient transferrin test   This test is a very specific indicator of high levels of alcohol abuse affecting the liver. Transferrin molecules are responsible for iron transport; they occur in high concentrations in the liver and become deficient in carbohydrate as a result of alcohol abuse (haemochromatosis) (Sargent 2005). Many employers now screen new staff for alcohol abuse and the carbohydrate-deficient test (CDT) test, which requires only a small blood sample, is proving attractive to occupational health departments.

Urine tests

Urinary bilirubin   A urinalysis may be requested for bilirubin. Normally, this bile pigment is not present in urine. Conjugated, or direct, bilirubin is water soluble and is present in the urine in obstructive jaundice and hepatocellular jaundice but absent in haemolytic jaundice.

Urinary urobilinogen   Conjugated bilirubin is changed to urobilinogen by bacterial action in the bowel. Most of the urobilinogen is then excreted in the faeces, and the remainder is absorbed. A small amount of the absorbed urobilinogen is excreted in the urine, but the larger portion is claimed by the liver to be excreted in the bile. If the liver cells are damaged they may not perform this latter function, and the amount of urobilinogen excreted by the kidneys is increased. The amount of the pigment in the urine may be decreased below the normal level in obstructive jaundice when bile is not reaching the intestine or when the bacterial content of the intestine is reduced, as it is in oral administration of antibiotics. If the individual is taking antibiotics this information should be noted on the laboratory form.

Stool test

Faecal fat test   Analysis of stool specimens made over a specified number of hours may be done to determine the fat content. Failure of pancreatic lipase to reach the intestine results in undigested and unabsorbed fat.

Ultrasonographic examination

Ultrasonography is a quick, safe and non-invasive method of assessing the patient for gallstones, hepatic cysts or tumours and other biliary problems. It is less reliable in obese individuals and in those with an excess of bowel gas.

Computed tomography

Computed tomography (CT) detects most liver lesions; information about their density and enhancement characteristics often allows a specific diagnosis to be made (e.g. in haemangioma). Watanabe et al (2000) have also used CT to study spleen size: splenic index can indicate both the severity of oesophageal varices and hepatic functional reserve in patients with liver cirrhosis. As with all radiological examinations, the patient must remain still during the procedure. CT is often used with ultrasonography to investigate the patient thoroughly.

Endoscopic retrograde cholangiopancreatography

A fibreoptic endoscope is passed into the duodenum. A catheter can then be passed via the ampulla of Vater into both the bile and pancreatic ducts, and a contrast medium injected to facilitate radiographic investigation. Retrograde cholangiography is performed to determine the cause of biliary problems, to diagnose cholestatic jaundice, and to remove gallstones that are obstructing the common bile duct. Radiographic films are taken during the procedure. A catheter (stent) or T tube may be inserted endoscopically to bypass the obstructive lesion and relieve the jaundice in some patients with malignant biliary obstruction.

When gallstones are removed by endoscopic retrograde cholangiopancreatography (ERCP) and sphincterotomy the patient will need blood coagulation levels measured, and blood typed and cross-matched. An antibiotic and intravenous fluid are usually administered before the procedure. The major problems that may occur are haemorrhage and infection, and the patient is assessed for any signs of these, following investigation.

Cholangiography may be used to aid diagnosis of the cause of jaundice, to determine the location of stones within the biliary tract, to diagnose cancer of the biliary system, and in the investigation of recurrent symptoms in individuals who have already had cholecystectomy.

Cholecystography

Radiography is also used in the diagnosis of gallbladder disease; the procedure may be referred to as cholecystography. A radio-opaque organic iodine compound that is eliminated in the bile is given orally or intravenously. The patient receives a fat-free evening meal which is followed by the administration of the contrast medium the night before the examination. Then the patient must not take anything by mouth until after the first radiograph has been taken. This procedure has increasingly been replaced by ERCP investigations.

Percutaneous liver biopsy

A small specimen of liver tissue may be examined microscopically to assist in the diagnosis of liver disease. The specimen is obtained by aspiration with a special liver biopsy needle. Using a lateral approach, the needle is passed through the right eighth, ninth or tenth intercostal space, or may be introduced below the costal margin if the liver is enlarged.

Before the procedure, the patient's blood coagulation is evaluated by determining the partial thromboplastin time (PTT) and platelet count. Blood is typed and cross-matched so that blood is available for transfusion if required. An explanation is made to the patient of the purpose of the biopsy and what will happen during and after the procedure. Pulse, respirations and blood pressure are noted by the nurse as a baseline for comparison following the biopsy.

The patient is placed in the supine position close to the right side of the bed. The area is cleansed, and an antiseptic and sterile drape are applied. A local anaesthetic agent is then injected at the puncture site. The patient is instructed to take two or three deep breaths, and then to stop breathing following exhalation. The doctor should quickly introduce the biopsy needle, aspirate and withdraw, taking only a few seconds.

Following the biopsy, absolute bedrest is necessary until the next morning. The patient is required to lie on the right side with a small pillow under the costal margin. This position places pressure against the biopsy site, preventing the escape of blood and bile. Close observation is made of the patient for haemorrhage for 24 hours. The pulse, respirations, blood pressure, colour, puncture site and general condition are noted and recorded every 15 minutes for 2 hours, then every 30 minutes for 2 hours. The interval is then gradually increased if there are no significant changes. Abdominal pain, tenderness and any rigidity are reported, because they may indicate irritation and inflammation of the peritoneum due to the leakage of bile from the liver. Severe pain and breathlessness are reported promptly as they may indicate that the lung or colon is perforated.

Transjugular liver biopsy

Transjugular liver biopsy may be carried out in patients at high risk of haemorrhage; it requires specialist facilities and expertise (Sargent 2005). A biopsy of liver tissue may also be obtained via the transjugular route. This is particularly appropriate for patients who have significant abdominal ascites or have developed coagulopathy, when complications from the percutaneous approach are more likely to arise. The procedure is undertaken within a radiology setting; the procedure is generally regarded as safe (Sargent 2005), although some complications may occur such as arrhythmias or bleeding.

Radioisotope liver scan

The Kupffer cells of the liver phagocytose small particles in the blood such as the isotope technetium-99m sulfur colloid. When injected intravenously, this accumulates in the liver (and spleen). Any lesion in the liver does not take up the radio-colloid and appears as a cold area in the γ-camera image.

CLINICAL CHARACTERISTICS OF DISORDERS OF THE LIVER AND BILIARY TRACT

Liver function is essential to life and, fortunately, this large organ has exceptional functional ability and regenerative capacity. If liver disease is limited and tissue damage is localized to one area of the organ, the body is not likely to suffer serious impairment of function. If there is diffuse disease and parenchymal damage, dysfunction is more marked. Liver disease may be acute or chronic, and disturbed function may be reversible or irreversible, depending on the amount of tissue involved and the nature of the cause.

Disorders of the gallbladder and bile ducts interfere with the flow of bile into the duodenum. They may be acute or chronic, and the intensity of the signs and symptoms parallels the severity of the condition. Like the liver, the pancreas has a large reserve capacity; a portion of the gland may be destroyed or become non-functional and the remainder will compensate sufficiently to maintain normal physiology.

Jaundice (icterus)

This is an indication of an excess of bilirubin in the blood, resulting in a yellowish staining of the tissues that may be seen in the sclerae, mucous membranes and skin. The cause may be intrahepatic or extrahepatic disease and, according to the cause, the jaundice may be classified as hepatocellular, obstructive or haemolytic (Table 16.1).

The *hepatocellular* type of jaundice is associated with intrinsic liver disease and is due to failure of the hepatic cells to take up the bilirubin resulting from the breakdown of red blood cells and excrete it as bile. Jaundice may not be present in chronic liver disease (e.g. cirrhosis), especially in the early stages, as regeneration of the hepatic cells may parallel the damage.

Obstructive jaundice is caused by an interference with the flow of bile in the extrahepatic ducts. It is most often due to the impaction of gallstones in the common bile duct, but may occur as the result of a stricture in the duct or neoplastic disease in neighbouring structures (e.g. pancreas) compressing the duct.

Haemolytic jaundice occurs when there is an inordinate destruction of red blood cells, resulting in excessive bilirubin formation.

The jaundiced patient's urine is likely to be dark because of the bilirubin or urobilinogen content. Urobilinogen is not present in obstructive jaundice, because it is formed in the intestine. The stools are pale grey in obstructive and severe hepatocellular jaundice.

Pruritus

The itching of the skin experienced by many patients with jaundice is attributed to irritation of the cutaneous sensory nerves by the retained bile salts.

General constitutional symptoms

The patient complains of a poor appetite, vague digestive discomfort and flatulence, and loses weight. McCollum (2000) reports a study in which appetite and nutritional intake in patients with chronic liver disease were assessed. No relationship was found between disease severity and nutritional intake. However, there was a strong association between liver disease and appetite suppression. Lassitude,

weakness and muscle wasting develop as a result of the impaired storage of carbohydrates and protein metabolism. A low-grade fever may be present.

Pain

Dull, aching pain in the right upper abdominal quadrant is a common symptom, especially in acute liver disease. Tenderness can be manifested on palpation.

The pain associated with gallbladder or biliary duct disease may be felt in the right upper abdomen or mid-epigastric region, or is referred to the right scapular area. It may be a persistent, dull ache, or very severe and disabling. The onset may follow a meal containing fatty foods. When it is very severe, causing the patient to writhe about, the pain is described as *biliary colic*. The pain of biliary colic or pancreatitis may be so severe as to interfere seriously with breathing (Hale 2000, Hughes 2004). Providing effective analgesia for patients with acute pancreatitis is notoriously difficult. Intravenous morphine may cause spasm in the sphincter of Oddi, increasing pain rather than relieving it initially. However, in some patients, the longer half-life of morphine means that it may provide a more consistent analgesia overall (Cole 2002).

Bleeding tendency

Inadequate production of prothrombin and other blood-clotting factors results in failure of the normal clotting process. Spontaneous bleeding may occur, manifested by purpura, epistaxis, bleeding of the oral mucous membrane and/or melaena.

Ascites and oedema

An accumulation of fluid in the peritoneal cavity develops with progressive liver disease, such as cirrhosis. The hepatic tissue damage, obliteration of blood vessels, and compression by the fibrous tissue (scar) replacement produce a resistance to the inflow and outflow of blood from the portal vein. The resulting increase in the blood pressure within the portal vein and its tributaries promotes the escape of fluid into the peritoneal cavity. The diseased liver produces less albumin and other plasma protein; therefore the person is unable to maintain the normal colloidal osmotic pressure of the blood which tend to pull interstitial fluid back into the circulation. This increases fluid loss to the tissues from the circulation and may lead to a more generalized oedema developing (Woodrow 2000). Some blood protein is also lost in the transudate in ascites. Reduced liver activity results in increased concentrations of antidiuretic hormone and aldosterone as these hormones are normally destroyed by the liver as it maintains homeostatic levels. Raised levels of these hormones promote sodium and fluid retention further contributing to oedema.

Dilated veins and varicosities

The portal hypertension associated with liver disease is reflected in changes within the veins that drain into the portal vein. They become dilated and **varicosities** develop.

Table 16.1 Characteristics of different types of jaundice

	Urine			Faeces		Plasma	
	Colour	Urobilinogen	Bilirubin	Colour	Stercobilinogen	Unconjugated bilirubin	Conjugated bilirubin
Haemolytic							
Increased bilirubin load (e.g. hereditary spherocytosis)	Normal	Increased	Absent	Dark	Increased	Increased	Normal
Hepatocellular							
Deficiency of transferase (e.g. Gilbert's disease)	Normal	Variable	Absent	Normal	Normal	Increased	Decreased
Cellular damage (e.g. infective hepatitis)	Dark	Variable	Increased	Paler than normal	Low	Decreased	Increased
Obstructive							
Intrahepatic fibrous obstruction (e.g. biliary cirrhosis)	Dark	Absent	Increased	Pale	Absent	Increased	Increased
Extrahepatic obstruction (e.g. carcinoma of head of pancreas)	Dark	Absent	Increased	Pale	Absent	Increased	Increased

From: Hinchcliff et al 1996.

The oesophageal and gastric veins are commonly affected and, because they are close to the surface, may rupture, resulting in massive haemorrhage manifested by haematemesis or melaena or both. Haemorrhoids develop because of the pressure and resistance to blood flow within the rectal veins.

Splenomegaly

The spleen enlarges because of the hyperplasia of the reticuloendothelial tissue and congestion, causing considerable discomfort for the patient.

Skin changes

In progressive chronic liver failure, several changes are likely to appear in the skin. 'Arterial spiders' (spider angiomas or naevi) may develop, in which a superficial arteriole gives rise to a series of fine, radiating branches readily visible on the surface of the skin. These lesions are seen predominantly on the face, neck, arms and chest, and are attributed to high oestrogen levels in the blood. Normally, oestrogen is destroyed in the liver.

Gynaecomastia and atrophy of the testicles may occur in males for the same reason. The palms of the hands are frequently mottled, bright red and warm because of capillary dilatation (palmar erythema). There is a loss of axillary and pubic hair in both sexes, and facial hair grows more slowly than usual in the male.

Neurological disturbances

Severe hepatic insufficiency leads to various mental changes. The patient may manifest irritability and behaviour not previously characteristic, such as becoming inactive, apathetic and forgetful. These symptoms may progress to confusion, lack of cooperation, stupor and eventually coma.

Twitching and a peculiar coarse tremor, referred to as *flapping tremor*, develop. Flapping tremor consists of a series of rapid, irregular alternating flexion and extension movements at the wrist and finger joints. The tremor may be referred to as *asterixis*. It occurs when the arms and hands are extended.

Ammonia toxicity is considered to be an important factor in producing the mental changes, coma and other abnormal central nervous system responses. The liver is unable to convert the ammonia that results from the breakdown of amino acids to urea.

Fetor hepaticus

In advanced liver disease, the breath has a faecal odour and the patient complains of a bad taste in the mouth. It is attributed to disturbed amino acid metabolism and abnormal bacterial action in the intestine.

Digestive disturbances

The patient with impaired bile transport may experience flatulence and an uncomfortable full feeling or nausea, especially after the ingestion of fatty or fried foods. Vomiting is usual if the patient has biliary colic or develops obstructive jaundice.

Fever

Chills and an increased temperature frequently accompany infection and inflammation within the gallbladder or bile ducts.

THE PERSON AT RISK OF A DISORDER OF THE LIVER AND EXOCRINE PANCREAS

ALCOHOL AND ALCOHOL ABUSE

Box 16.1 outlines statistics on the consumption of alcohol in England at the beginning of the twenty-first century.

The government has specified the recommended alcohol intake, and has provided guidelines in terms of daily units; this approach is believed to be more helpful and realistic for people, and aims to discourage binge-drinking (Box 16.2). Recent statistics indicate that alcohol intake has increased markedly in women and continues to fluctuate in the young. Alcohol misuse is discussed in Chapter 26, but the extent of the problem may be understood when it is considered that in the UK one-third of domestic violence incidents are linked to alcohol, it accounts for 22 000 premature deaths annually and up to 70% of all admissions to A&E at peak times are alcohol-related.

Nurses often hold negative attitudes towards individuals with drinking problems. This may be due to experiences of frequent A&E attendees, and inpatients with alcohol-related conditions who resume drinking despite advice to the

---

Box 16.1   Alcohol consumption in the UK

- In England, in 2002, around two-fifths of men (37%) had drunk more than 4 units of alcohol on at least 1 day in the previous week; just over one-fifth of women (22%) had drunk more than 3 units of alcohol on at least 1 day in the previous week

- In England, in 2002, 21% of men had drunk more than 8 units of alcohol on at least 1 day in the previous week; 9% of women had drunk more than 6 units

- In 2002, average weekly alcohol consumption in England was 17 units for men and 7.6 units for women

- In England, in 2002, 27% of men and 17% of women aged 16 drank on average more than 21 and 14 units a week, respectively. Drinking at these levels among men has remained stable at about 27% since 1992; for women it has risen from 12–17% in the same period

- In 2003, one-quarter (25%) of pupils in England aged 1–15 had drunk alcohol in the previous week; the proportion doing so has fluctuated around this level since the mid-1990s. In the UK, expenditure on alcohol as a proportion of total household expenditure has fallen from 7.5% in 1980 to 5.7% in 2003.

Source: Department of Health 2004.

contrary. However, we need a non-judgemental attitude; consider the case story of Pat with which we opened this book and you will realize blaming the patient for their alcohol problem is not going to help.

Nursing assessment of alcohol intake

Early identification and education may be effective with 'at risk' drinkers in reducing serious health problems and dependence. Nurses, as the largest group of healthcare professionals with the greatest patient contact, are ideally placed to promote healthy drinking behaviour. Given the harmful effects of excess alcohol intake, it should always be part of any patient health history.

Stewart and Richards (2000) and Compton (2002) suggest that the most direct approach is the best. They recommend that all patients should have their alcohol intake assessed by simply asking the patient: 'How much alcohol do you drink daily? Weekly? When was your last drink?' The units system should be explained in order to quantify the amount in a standardized way (see Ch. 26). A

glass of wine or a UK pub measure of spirits is 1 unit, a pint (540 ml) of beer counts as 2 units. In Chapter 26 we also explain the recommended safe weekly limits and the use of the CAGE and TWEAK screening tool to assess if the person has a drinking problem. Alcohol misuse, like misuse of other substances, is a complex problem which may involve behavioural and cognitive coping mechanisms (see Ch. 26). A non-judgmental approach that can help to educate and empower the person to seek help should be used (Box 16.3). The underlying mechanisms at work in alcoholism include denial, low self-esteem and poor self-care and are all well illustrated by Pat's story in Chapter 1. Chapter 26 contains another case study showing the problems of alcohol misuse (abstinence syndrome).

The issue of denial frequently interferes with the identification of alcohol-related problems and the acceptance of treatment. The first step towards dealing with an alcohol problem involves the person actually admitting they have one, rather than retreating behind statements such as 'I can handle this'. It is difficult for people to accept both their alcohol dependency and retain a positive self-concept if they have held a negative stereotype of 'alcoholics'. These issues are discussed in more depth in Chapter 26.

Nurses encounter persons with alcohol abuse problems in their daily practice, both in hospitals and the community. Unfortunately, the person may be seriously intoxicated and displaying antisocial behaviour. As their behaviour deteriorates and becomes abusive and threatening, so too the possibility of meaningful communication disappears. The person has lost control of themselves and the nurse has lost control of the nurse–patient interaction.

Box 16.2   Recommended daily alcohol intake limits

The Department of Health advises that men should not drink more than 3–4 units of alcohol per day, and women should drink no more than 2–3 units of alcohol per day. Alcohol should be avoided for 48 hours after an episode of drunkenness to give the body time to recover.

From: Department of Health 2006.

Box 16.3   The empowering approach

This approach centres around respectful attitudes, empathy and patient education.

State your concern about the consequences of the patient's behaviour on health and quality of life:

- Don't assume the patient understands the link between poor health and drinking

- Denial is common – you may have to point out the consequences several times in a respectful and open manner

- Don't show your anger or frustration with the patient – it rarely helps

- It is better to say: 'Coming into hospital must be scary and painful. Have you thought about getting help so this won't keep happening?' or 'Your GI bleeding is going to happen again unless you do something about your drinking. Would you be willing to talk to someone about it?'

- Don't threaten or isolate the patient.

Offer hope by assuring the patient that recovery is possible and they could feel better:

- For example, say: 'I realize that you might not know where to begin, given how seriously drinking has affected your life, but you can be sober and you can improve your health. It's not too late' Or:

- 'Maybe giving up alcohol is the last thing you want to do, but if you're fed up with coming into hospital, I know that there is help available to you. You don't have to go through this on your own'.

Be prepared to refer the patient to the appropriate resources for help:

- Your own hospital resources – check them out

- Community-based help and resources (e.g. Alcoholics Anonymous).

In such difficult circumstances the following key points are essential for nursing care of an intoxicated patient:

- There should be no ambiguity between what the nurse says and does
- There should be no difference between the nurse's verbal and non-verbal behaviour
- Reduce any environmental stimuli to a minimum
- Decide whether the planned therapeutic intervention warrants the risks involved
- Keep communication simple.

Meaningful discussions can occur only when the patient is sober.

DISORDERS OF THE LIVER

VIRAL HEPATITIS

This is an inflammation of the liver due to one of several viruses. Five viruses known as hepatitis A, B, C, D and E viruses are the most common causes, but other viruses such as the cytomegalovirus (CMV) or Epstein–Barr virus may also be implicated.

Hepatitis A

This type of hepatitis accounts for the greater number of cases. The disease may be epidemic and has a higher incidence in children and young adults. It has an incubation period of 3–5 weeks and is included in the list of *reportable diseases*. It is an acute, self-limiting disease which does not usually lead to chronic hepatitis or a carrier state.

Large amounts of the virus are eliminated in the faeces in the week preceding the onset of jaundice. The stools therefore constitute a low infection hazard once symptoms appear. Transmission is by the faecal–oral route and is therefore facilitated by poor hygiene. The virus, which is highly contagious, can also be spread by the ingestion of contaminated water or food (Shovein et al 2000). This disease may spread rapidly, especially in overcrowded and poor sanitary conditions.

Hepatitis B

Hepatitis B is caused by the type B virus (HBV), which consists of an inner DNA core enclosed in a protein coat. Both the inner core and the large surface mass contain distinctive antigens. The principal mode of transmission is by the injection of infected blood and blood products. Because of this, hepatitis B is a common problem among drug addicts who are sharing injection equipment. Needlestick injuries may result in transmission of the virus to healthcare workers. The same mechanism is also apparent in human immunodeficiency virus (HIV) infection. Hepatitis B can be transmitted like HIV, by intimate contact with carriers or those with acute disease. The virus can be found in saliva, semen and vaginal secretions, as well as blood. It may therefore occur as a sexually transmitted infection amongst homosexual males. The incubation period for hepatitis B ranges from 6 weeks to 6 months. It is more common in adults than children, whereas hepatitis A tends to have a higher frequency in children and young adults. Hepatitis B has an insidious onset; it may persist or become chronic, or produce a carrier state in which the individual may be asymptomatic but harbour the virus.

Hepatitis C

Hepatitis type C virus (HCV) is transmitted via the blood, but has a low risk of sexual transmission. The illness is usually relatively mild in the acute phase, although up to 70% of patients go on to develop chronic liver disease – chronic hepatitis, cirrhosis, end-stage liver disease or liver cancer (Parini 2001). HCV is still more common in southern Europe and Japan than in the UK. A report published in 2005 by the UK Health Protection Agency has highlighted growing concern about HCV as it estimated around 200 000 people in England alone may be infected with HCV of which 85% may be unaware they are infected. In around 4500 cases the person is suffering from severe liver disease. The HPA (2005) estimate approximately 80% of the infections are related to intravenous drug use at some stage. The report estimates 45% of current injecting drug users are infected. Some of these people were infected prior to 1991 from contaminated blood supplies, since when much more stringent screening procedures have eliminated this as a cause of HCV infection. Other countries with significant injecting drug user populations may be developing the same problem.

Hepatitis D and E

Hepatitis D requires the presence of hepatitis B for transmission. It is very rare in northern Europe, as is hepatitis E, which is found mostly in Asia and is transmitted by the enteric route.

Prevention and screening

Prevention of the transmission of viral hepatitis focuses on two areas: education of carriers to prevent transmission to others, and protection of at-risk groups against contamination of the virus. Nurses have an important contribution to make in giving advice to carriers and their significant others to allay fears, reduce anxiety, provide education regarding potential routes of contamination and abating misconceptions. However, this information should be relayed in such a way as to ensure reduction of risk to others but without promoting unnecessary restrictions or precautions that could cause distress. Nurses and other healthcare workers are also at risk of contracting hepatitis B and C – hence the importance of using universal precautions at all times when handling potentially infective material (De Palma 2000).

Education for drug users should focus on safe use and disposal of needles and syringes. Information regarding safe sexual practice, the use of condoms, etc., should be given and reinforced at every opportunity to homosexual males, sex workers and intravenous drug users as these people are most likely to engage in high-risk behaviours. Leaflets and other educational material can be useful for spreading sound information, and may be easily displayed in many health settings to which the public have access. The parallels with the prevention of the spread of HIV are obvious.

Screening for hepatitis is usually targeted on the following:

- all admissions to renal dialysis and transplant units
- individuals who have recently travelled to countries with high levels of hepatitis
- intravenous drug users
- individuals who have received blood or blood products
- the acutely or recently jaundiced
- staff who have sustained a needlestick injury
- pregnant women.

It is extremely important to remember that anyone who is screened for any of the hepatitis viruses must give their informed consent, irrespective of the circumstances of diagnosis (McCreaddie and Neilson 2001).

Clinical characteristics

Whatever the virus responsible, the subsequent illness is very similar. The virus attacks the hepatic cells, and inflammation and necrosis follow. The swelling and congestion interfere with normal bile formation and flow, resulting in intrahepatic obstructive jaundice and raised blood bilirubin levels. Serum enzyme levels of alanine aminotransferase (ALT) and aspartate aminotransferase (AST) rise sharply because of the necrosis, and the serum albumin:globulin ratio may indicate a reduced formation of albumin and an increase in the gamma globulin. The latter points to the acute infectious nature of the disorder. Urinalysis reveals an excess of urobilinogen, especially in the initial stage. The blood is examined for the presence of hepatitis virus antigens and antibodies that have been identified.

Fortunately, in most cases complete regeneration of the liver cells occurs on recovery, with a minimal fibrous tissue formation and scarring. However many patients go on to develop cirrhosis and there is a long-term increased risk of hepatic cancer following cirrhosis, especially with hepatitis C infection.

The signs and symptoms may vary in intensity from one individual to another. The onset is usually manifested by vague symptoms such as fatigue, loss of appetite, nausea, vomiting, headache, fleeting abdominal and joint pains and fever. After several days, abdominal tenderness and pain in the right upper quadrant are more predominant, the urine becomes dark, either constipation or diarrhoea may be troublesome, the stools may be abnormally light in colour and jaundice becomes evident. Hepatitis B is usually more prolonged and debilitating. Table 16.2 lists the clinical characteristics of viral hepatitis.

Diagnostic tests

- *ELISA* (enzyme-linked immunosorbent assay): detects anti-HCV (presence of HCV shows current or previous infection)
- *RIBA* (recombinant immunoblot assay): confirmatory test, done after ELISA but being replaced by PCR

Table 16.2 Assessment of the person with viral hepatitis

Pathophysiological alterations	Clinical characteristics
Liver structure and function	
Hepatomegaly	The liver is tender and enlarged on palpation Abdominal discomfort
Altered bile production, excretion and re-absorption	Pruritus Jaundice of skin and sclerae Urine, dark orange in colour Stools, clay-coloured Diarrhoea or constipation
Altered metabolism of carbohydrates, proteins and fats	Nausea and vomiting Anorexia Flatulence Malaise, weakness and fatigue Irritability Weight loss Muscle wasting Fever
Altered production and destruction of blood components	Spontaneous bleeding Purpura Melaena Haematuria
Extrahepatic	Skin rashes Arthralgia Headache Sore throat, cough, catarrh Depression

- *PCR* (polymerase chain reaction): this test has two components that confirm HCV infection and also the 'viral load' circulating in the bloodstream
- *Liver function tests* check for raised liver enzymes, e.g. alanine aminotransferase (ALT) and aspartate aminotransferase (AST)
- *Liver biopsy* to confirm liver damage – fibrosis and cirrhosis.

Treatment

There is currently no effective treatment for patients with hepatitis A, except for bedrest (the disease is debilitating), although children may be asymptomatic. There is some evidence to suggest that administration of interferon-α is helpful for some patients with chronic hepatitis B (CRD 2001b). However, less than 50% of patients respond to such treatment and relapse is common. Current NICE guidelines recommend the use of interferon alfa, ribavirin and lamivudine (NICE 2004). In the USA and, more increasingly in the UK, liver transplantation is being offered to patients with chronic hepatitis who then go on to develop liver failure (Grewal 2002).

Assessment

Health history   The person is questioned with tact and sensitivity regarding exposure to hepatitis viruses from blood transfusions, the use of contaminated needles, sexual activity and possible contact with infected individuals, and personal hygiene. Emphasis is placed on identification of the clinical symptoms the person is experiencing. As the course of the disease varies from asymptomatic and mild to acute, fulminating and life-threatening, symptoms vary considerably as to frequency and severity. The patient is asked specific questions related to gastrointestinal disturbance and changes in the colour of the skin and mucous membranes, sclera, stools and urine. Changes in the tendency to bleed are also noted.

Physical examination   This includes the measurement of the person's vital signs; observation of the skin, mucous membranes and sclera for changes in colour; observation of urine and faeces; observation of the skin and gums for signs of bruising and bleeding. Palpation of the abdomen to assess the size of the liver may be carried out by advanced nurse practitioners.

Nursing intervention

The *goals* of care are that the person will demonstrate:

1 alleviation of symptoms
2 fluid balance
3 maintenance of desired body weight
4 return of appetite
5 knowledge of self-management
6 resumption of usual daily activities.
7 understanding of the risk of transmission to others.

Rest   The person is encouraged and helped to get adequate rest and relaxation. Both at home and in the hospital, plans should be developed to provide uninterrupted periods of rest throughout the day as well as at night. Activity is resumed slowly, and the person observed for reactions. Liver function is monitored by repeated tests to detect any adverse effects of increased activity.

Medications   Many drugs (such as oral contraceptives and morphine) that are normally inactivated by the liver are not prescribed. The patient is advised against taking any drug that has not been prescribed during this illness. Alternative barrier methods of contraception and issues relating to safe sexual practices should be discussed.

Nutrition and fluids   In the acute stage it is difficult for the person to take sufficient fluids and food because of the nausea, vomiting and aversion to food. An increased daily fluid intake of at least 3000 mL is necessary because of the fever and to promote urinary elimination of the serum bilirubin. If the patient cannot tolerate fluids orally, intravenous fluids may be given. The patient is observed closely for signs of over-hydration manifested by sudden weight gain, oedema and respiratory distress. Fluid intake and output are recorded. Parenteral administration of vitamin K may be recommended if blood coagulation is impaired as a result of impaired absorption of vitamin K when bile salts are decreased.

A high-calorie diet of 3000 kcal is recommended daily; nutritional deficiency retards the liver's ability to overcome the infection and regenerate functional tissue. As soon as the nausea and vomiting are controlled, the patient is offered small amounts of high-calorie foods frequently. These are gradually increased until the ultimate goal of 3000 kcal is achieved. The diet consists principally of protein and carbohydrate. The fat content may be restricted while there is jaundice but is increased, as tolerated, by the addition of dairy products, which make the diet more palatable. Fried foods, fat meat and rich foods, such as pastries, are usually avoided for several weeks or months after recovery. The person is advised not to take alcohol for at least 6 months. The individual's weight is checked at regular intervals because there may have been a considerable loss in the early phase of the disease.

Skin care   Frequent bathing and changes of linen during the period of fever are necessary. The use of soap is avoided; emollients may be added to the bathwater to relieve the itching associated with jaundice. Calamine lotion may be used and fingernails are cut short and kept clean. Most people with cirrhosis of the liver have abused alcohol, although many alcoholics do not develop cirrhosis. It is not clear why this is the case.

Prevention of the spread of infection   All patients with viral hepatitis are treated as potentially infectious. Universal and body substance precautions are used with all patients, therefore no additional measures are required. Needlestick injuries pose the greatest threat to healthcare workers as HBV is transmitted through the blood. As with all patients, needles should never be recapped and only disposable needles and syringes should be used. Invasive procedures should be avoided whenever possible. Gowns and gloves should be worn whenever direct contact with blood or faeces is possible. Personnel caring for the patient are informed of the possible sources of the infective particles (faeces, vomitus, urine and blood) and of the fact that they are usually resistant to heat, antiseptics and prolonged exposure to cold and freezing.

The hands are scrubbed under running water with liquid soap after each contact. Bed linen contaminated with faeces or blood is placed in a clean bag at the bedside, which is identified as an isolation bag. No special precautions are necessary regarding dishes or glasses. The use of disposable equipment for procedures involving penetration of the skin (e.g. needles and syringes) is essential and gloves should be worn by those handling them. Used needles and syringes are placed in a puncture-resistant container used for all such supplies. Blood, urine, faeces and sputum specimens should be clearly labelled 'biohazard' to protect laboratory personnel.

The person is advised of the importance of thorough handwashing after going to the toilet. Gloves are worn when handling the patient's bedpan; excreta should be flushed promptly down the toilet. If the patient is being cared for at home, the patient and family are taught simple precautions and the importance of good handwashing.

Contacts Known contacts of infectious hepatitis A are advised to consult a doctor as soon as possible. An intramuscular injection of human immune serum globulin may be given to provide protection. It is effective against the virus A organism. Hepatitis B immune globulin is available for contacts of HBV. Its use is usually reserved for individuals exposed to HBV through needlepricks or other accidental injection. The γ-globulin may not always provide immunity, but is found to lessen the severity of the disease should the person develop it.

Vaccines for active immunization against hepatitis are recommended for high-risk groups, especially health professionals at risk of contamination with patient's blood. Hepatitis B vaccine is available to nurses in the high-risk groups and to all who wish it through most employee occupational health services. Immunization involves three intramuscular injections, with the second and third doses being given at 1 and 6 months, respectively. Antibodies persist for at least 3 years. Booster doses are given at regular intervals. HBV vaccine is also available in the community for individuals who are at risk for contacting the infection. High-risk groups include those with illness-related factors requiring repeated transfusions of blood or blood products, and those with lifestyle-related factors such as unprotected homosexual activity with multiple partners, intravenous drug use and prostitution.

Follow-up The person is encouraged to attend outpatient appointments; laboratory and physical examinations are carried out to detect possible progressive or residual impairment of liver function. Supervision is usually continued for 1 year. The intervals between visits to clinics or the doctor are gradually increased if the findings are favourable.

Evaluation

Achievement of the established goals for the individual with hepatitis is determined by ongoing assessment showing alleviation of the person's symptoms. The individual's body weight should be maintained at a desirable level. The patient and family should be able to describe plans for meeting nutritional needs and needs for increased rest, as well as precautionary measures to prevent transmission of the virus to others. They should be familiar with plans for follow-up care.

> **CASE** **Needlestick injury**
>
> Student nurse, Alice, was caring for 27-year-old Allan who had hepatitis B. Allan had been an intravenous drug user for some years but had only recently contracted the disease after sharing needles with his new girlfriend. Unfortunately, his condition was serious. Allan was tired, irritable and restless; he was experiencing extreme nausea and anorexia and had now developed coagulopathy. He was covered in bruises and had bleeding gums, and had been prescribed a vitamin K injection which Alice was giving under the supervision of staff nurse Joanne.
>
> Allan appeared to be half asleep as Alice and Joanne approached him. Alice explained what she was about to do and asked him to turn over. Allan turned over but as Alice gave him the injection, he shouted loudly in pain and brushed her hand out of the way. Although Alice was wearing gloves, she felt the needle scratch her finger, which she had used to position the skin around the injection site.
>
> The hospital policy was very clear. Although it was a barely perceptible scratch, Alice made the wound bleed and kept it under a running cold tap while Joanne completed the accident form. Alice then went down to the A&E department for a blood test.
>
> Both the initial ELISA and subsequent tests 3 months later showed that Alice had not developed anti-HBV. However, Alice found this a very distressing and protracted experience; during this time, she split up with her boyfriend and found it very difficult to concentrate on her academic work.
>
> 1 What could Alice and Joanne have done differently in relation to:
>   a) Preparing Allan?
>   b) Preparing Alice?
> 2 Is the hospital's policy for needlestick injury correct? Do you know what your placement's policy is?
> 3 What is the role of vaccination here?
> 4 What would the implications have been for Alice as a student nurse if she had developed HBV?
> 5 What would the implications be for Joanne had Alice developed HBV?

TOXIC HEPATITIS

Rarely, inflammation and degenerative changes in the liver occur as a result of a chemical. Carbon tetrachloride, phosphorus, sulfonamides, arsenical preparations and chloroform are examples of suggested offenders. The patient is treated by prompt withdrawal of the causative chemical, rest and supportive care.

CIRRHOSIS OF THE LIVER

The term cirrhosis denotes chronic diffuse degenerative tissue changes occurring in the liver. There is destruction of parenchymal cells and formation of excessive dense fibrous scar tissue. Blood, lymph and bile channels within the liver become distorted, compressed and effaced, with subsequent intrahepatic congestion, portal hypertension and impaired liver function. The fibrous tissue changes result in the liver becoming firmer. The surface is usually rough because of small projecting nodules of regenerated hepatic cells, and is frequently described as a 'hobnail surface'.

Incidence and causes

It is difficult to obtain an accurate figure for the incidence of cirrhosis but the scale of the problem may be gauged from the fact that it is the tenth leading cause of death in the USA and of those fatal cases, 45% were caused by alcohol. This is probably a reasonable estimate of the scale of the problem across the developed world. Elsewhere in the world, post-necrotic cirrhosis secondary to hepatitis is the most common type seen (Black and Hawks 2005). The incidence of cirrhosis is increasing in the developed world, mainly because of the lifestyle factors which lead to its development (Karsan et al 2004). Malnutrition increases the risk of alcoholic cirrhosis Black and Hawks (2005) Patients with cirrhosis of the liver are at high risk of developing hepatocellular (liver) cancer (Llovet et al 2003). The mechanisms responsible for cirrhosis of the liver are not clearly defined, although the following factors are known to be associated with the condition.

Alcohol abuse

Most people with cirrhosis of the liver have abused alcohol, although many alcoholics do not develop cirrhosis. It is not clear why this is the case. Ingestion of moderate to large quantities of alcohol over several years can produce fatty infiltration of the liver and liver dysfunction. The toxic effects on the liver develop more readily in the presence of malnutrition. Many persons show a marked improvement in the earlier stages of cirrhosis when alcohol ingestion is discontinued.

Hepatitis

Severe type B viral hepatitis (usually following injected drug use and/or unprotected sex) in which there has been extensive necrosis followed by considerable scarring may lead to cirrhosis.

Chronic cholestasis

Degenerative changes characteristic of cirrhosis may also occur with prolonged cholestasis (obstruction to the flow of bile). The cause is usually partial obstruction by a stone or stricture within the extrahepatic bile ducts, but may be intrahepatic as a result of infection or inflammation and subsequent stricture of the small ducts within the liver.

Autoimmune processes

Primary biliary cirrhosis is thought to be an autoimmune disease with progressive degenerative changes in the bile ducts within the liver, eventually resulting in liver failure. Mainly women are affected.

Hepatic infiltration

Fibrotic changes in the liver may be associated with the infiltration of certain substances. Examples include excessive glycogen which accumulates in the liver in the individual with von Gierke's disease; enlargement and fibrosis develop. Similarly, Gaucher's disease results from an abnormal reticuloendothelial cell content that incurs liver fibrosis and dysfunction.

Clinical characteristics

The liver has considerable reserve; early cirrhotic changes generally go unrecognized without apparent manifestations. With the characteristic insidious progress, signs and symptoms of impaired liver function appear gradually over a period of years. In the early stages the symptoms are vague digestive disturbances: the person experiences anorexia,

flatulence, nausea and loss of weight. Intense pruritus is often the presenting symptom. Later, jaundice, dependent oedema, spider angiomas, anaemia and increased abdominal girth due to ascites develop. Splenomegaly, neurological involvement (hepatic coma) and haemorrhage from oesophageal varices are characteristic of advanced cirrhosis and serious liver dysfunction.

The severity of liver dysfunction is determined by liver function tests as well as by history, symptoms and physical examination. Palpation of the liver and spleen provides significant information. The liver is enlarged and firm, and may have a rough surface; the spleen is enlarged owing to the resistance by the liver to flow of blood from the portal vein.

Treatment

The care required by the patient with cirrhosis depends upon the extent of the liver damage. There is no cure, as such, for cirrhosis. However, liver transplantation has been successful in patients with advanced disease (Karsan et al 2004).

Medications

There is no single recognized pharmacological agent for cirrhosis. However, some preparations have been used in an attempt to reduce mortality – propylthiouracil and colchicine do not now appear to offer any effective benefits. Pentoxifylline may offer some benefits if there is no renal involvement (Marsano et al 2003). Multivitamin preparations are prescribed. Parenteral vitamin K may be given if the prothrombin level is below normal and if a tendency to bleeding is manifested by petechiae, ecchymosis, epistaxis, melaena or haematemesis. Vitamin B_{12} injections may be necessary to correct anaemia.

Although the patient with cirrhosis usually develops oedema and ascites due to portal hypertension and decreased plasma oncotic pressure (because of reduced liver production of blood proteins), diuretics will be prescribed only with care. This is because of the risk of electrolyte imbalance, particularly excessive loss of potassium, as these patients often have low potassium levels initially. Fluid restriction is usual, depending on the level of serum sodium. Diuretics that are given initially are potassium-sparing diuretics (e.g. spironolactone), as hypokalaemia may precipitate hepatic encephalopathy. Cirrhotic ascites is often refractory and requires the use of a combination of diuretics and paracentesis (Gines et al 2004). Rapidly acting diuretics waste potassium and necessitate frequent determinations of electrolyte and fluid balance.

Potentially toxic drugs normally inactivated by the liver are avoided. Examples of these are paracetamol, diazepam, oral contraceptives and opiates.

Abdominal paracentesis

An abdominal paracentesis may be necessary if the fluid in the peritoneal cavity reaches a volume that is causing respiratory distress, compression of abdominal viscera and blood vessels, and considerable pain and discomfort. The nurse explains the aspiration procedure to the patient and makes sure the bladder is empty. The head of the bed is elevated and the patient is supported with pillows. The doctor may wish to have the patient sitting on the side of the bed with a support for the back and feet. A blood pressure cuff is made ready on one arm so that the blood pressure may be monitored during and after the paracentesis. The necessary sterile equipment and fluid receptacle are brought to the bedside. Following the application of an antiseptic and sterile towels, the doctor injects the site with a local anaesthetic before introducing the trocar and cannula. A tube is attached to the cannula to drain the fluid into the receptacle.

During the procedure, the nurse checks the patient's pulse, colour and blood pressure, and provides necessary psychological support. The doctor should be alerted promptly if the pulse becomes rapid and weak, pallor is noted, or there is a fall in blood pressure. No more than 1 or 2 L are withdrawn at one time. Removal of the fluid results in the loss of considerable plasma protein, especially serum albumin. Also, the sudden reduction of intra-abdominal pressure results in a dilatation of the abdominal blood vessels and a pooling of a large volume of blood, which may lead to circulatory collapse and shock.

A sterile dressing is applied to the site of the paracentesis when the cannula is withdrawn. The patient is returned to the dorsal recumbent position, and the head of the bed is lowered. The amount and character of the fluid are recorded and a specimen of the fluid is labelled and sent to the laboratory for examination. The abdominal site is kept clean and dry to prevent infection and discomfort. The pulse, colour and blood pressure are checked at frequent intervals for several hours. A plasma or whole blood infusion may follow the paracentesis to replace the lost protein. Increased diuresis may be observed with the decreased pressure on the renal blood vessels.

Peritoneovenous shunt
When ascites is persistent, a shunt may be placed between the peritoneal cavity and the superior vena cava. This draws ascitic fluid into the venous circulation and relieves the ascites.

Complications of cirrhosis and their management
Hepatic encephalopathy and coma, and oesophagogastric varices are common complications.

Hepatic coma
Before the patient with cirrhosis of the liver develops coma, neurological disturbances are manifested. These include mental dullness, slow responses, forgetfulness and disorientation. Muscle reflexes are exaggerated and muscular rigidity and asterixis (flapping tremor) are also present. The cause of the neurological involvement is failure of the liver to metabolize and detoxify nitrogenous substances; the toxic materials such as ammonia remain in the blood and are carried into the cerebral circulation. The failure may be due to hepatocellular necrosis or because portal blood bypasses the liver and reaches the central nervous system by being shunted directly into the systemic circulation.

Nursing measures used in the care of any unconscious person are applicable to the patient in hepatic coma. The condition is managed by reducing the level of nitrogenous substances. This is achieved by cleansing the gastrointestinal tract by administering lactulose orally and giving enemas (disposable magnesium sulfate). Sometimes a non-absorbable antibiotic (neomycin) is prescribed to suppress urea-splitting bacterial gut flora. Protein intake is restricted.

Portal hypertension
The flow of blood from the portal vein through the liver may meet with resistance due to disease and cirrhotic changes in the liver. Pressure rises within the portal venous system, causing portal hypertension. The increased pressure in the portal vein produces a back-up in the veins that normally empty into the portal system. Collateral circulatory channels develop between the portal vein and the systemic circulatory system to bypass the liver.

The veins most seriously affected by portal hypertension are those in the gastric cardia region and the lower part of the oesophagus. The veins become engorged and tortuous; the walls are weakened, predisposing them to rupture. These varicosed veins appear as large bulbous protrusions under the mucosa. The congestion in the mesenteric veins causes haemorrhoids and is also reflected in the apparent congested cutaneous veins around the umbilicus. In addition to varices, problems associated with portal hypertension include congestive splenomegaly and ascites.

The severity of portal hypertension may be assessed indirectly by evidence of oesophageal varices, which may be visualized using fibreoptic endoscopy or by liver scan.

Bleeding oesophagogastric varices
The oesophagogastric varices are frequently the site of rupture of the vascular wall and severe haemorrhage. The perforation and bleeding may be caused by mechanical trauma from 'rough' food passing over a varicosity, erosion and ulceration of the mucosa and venous wall by gastric acid secretion, or sudden increased intra-abdominal pressure associated with coughing, vomiting, straining at stool or physical exertion. Severe haematemesis occurs; some blood will enter the intestine and eventually the person passes tarry stools.

Prompt emergency treatment and care of bleeding oesophagogastric varices are necessary; the excessive loss of blood is life-threatening.

Control of bleeding   Various measures are used to control bleeding, including balloon tamponade, vasopressin infusion, sclerotherapy and surgical treatment.

Balloon tube tamponade   A balloon tube tamponade is achieved through the use of a special kind of nasogastric tube with three or four lumens. This is often referred to as a Sengstaken–Blakemore tube. This method is especially useful (life-saving) in active bleeding where visibility is obscured. One lumen ends in an elongated balloon that is inflated to exert pressure against the oesophageal wall;

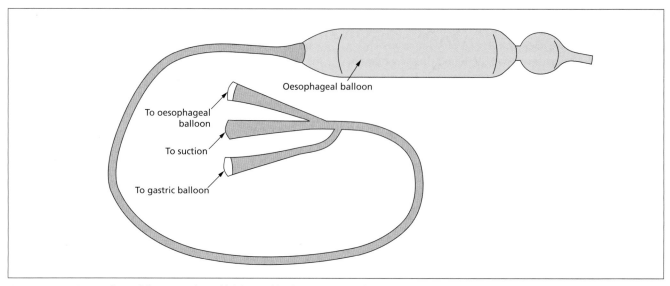

Figure 16.2 Sengstaken–Blakemore tube, which is used in the treatment of bleeding oesophageal varices. The tube has three lumens. One leads to the longer inflatable balloon that is positioned in the oesophagus to provide pressure. A second lumen ends in the smaller balloon that lies just within the stomach. The third lumen opens into the stomach to permit gastric aspiration.

another ends in a small balloon that is positioned just within the stomach and, when inflated, compresses varices in the cardia and anchors the tube in place (Fig. 16.2); and the third lumen opens into the stomach, extending well beyond the balloon in the cardia. The third lumen permits drainage or aspiration of the gastric content; its proximal end may be attached to suction. Removal of gastric contents reduces the amount of blood entering the intestine. Digestion of blood in the intestine produces nitrogenous wastes that, when absorbed, predispose the patient to hepatic coma. Some tubes have a fourth lumen which permits suction above the oesophageal balloon, for instance, the Minnesota balloon tube (Krige and Beckingham 2001).

Continuous suction is applied so as to aspirate any blood or secretions above the oesophageal balloon. Before the tube is inserted, the tube and balloons are tested for leaks. Before insertion, the tube is usually chilled, which makes it firmer and easier to manipulate, and is lubricated to ease insertion. The nurse makes sure that the proximal end of each lumen is identified and clearly labelled to prevent possible error in inflation or deflation of tubes after insertion. The pressures to be maintained within the balloons are indicated by the doctor and are usually 25–30 mmHg; excessive pressure can cause tissue ulceration (Fig. 16.3). Inadequate inflation is ineffective in checking bleeding and may also permit shifting of the tube. The gastric drainage is checked frequently for blood content, which should progressively decrease following the insertion of the tube.

The patient is observed closely for any indication of respiratory distress. Saliva or blood escaping around the tube into the oropharynx may be aspirated. The patient is unable to swallow saliva, so provision is made for suction or for expectoration into tissues or a basin.

The tube is positioned within the nostrils to exert a minimum of pull and pressure, and then secured. Frequent

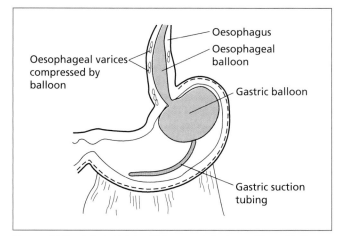

Figure 16.3 A Sengstaken–Blakemore tube in position with the oesophageal and gastric balloons inflated.

moistening and a very light application of a lubricant to the nasal mucosa may reduce the irritation. Some doctors position the tube via the mouth.

Compression by the inflated balloons is not usually continued for longer than 48 hours. Pressure for a longer period could cause oedema, ulceration and perforation of the oesophagus. The tube is left in position for continued gastric drainage and for the balloons to be re-inflated readily if bleeding should resume. In some instances, the doctor may order deflation of the balloons for 5 minutes at regular intervals to reduce the risk of tissue damage. Vomiting with the tube in place can lead to aspiration of the fluid – hence the extra fourth lumen which may be present.

Vasopressin infusion   Vasopressin (antidiuretic hormone; Pitressin) may be administered by an intravenous route. The vasopressin produces arterial vasoconstriction which reduces portal venous pressure by decreasing the volume of blood entering the portal system. The patient may experience cramping abdominal pain and be incontinent of faeces.

Sclerotherapy   This is the primary method of treatment. A coagulating substance is injected into the oesophageal varices. Visualization of the varices is achieved using fibreoptic endoscopy, and a coagulating substance is injected. The patient is closely monitored after the injection. The patient will be required to have this procedure repeated at regular intervals for 1–2 years.

Surgical treatment   If the measures cited above are not effective in checking the haemorrhage, emergency surgery may be performed. Different surgical procedures are used such as ligation of the submucosal veins that are involved in the haemorrhage by use of a stapling device. An incision is made for a gastrotomy and the target approached from below.

A transjugular intrahepatic portosystemic shunt (TIPS) may be more effective for patients with recurrent bleeding varices but should not be the first-choice treatment over endoscopic treatment (Krige and Beckingham 2001).

Assessment   The patient with bleeding varices is seriously ill and requires continuous attention and ongoing assessment.

The blood pressure and pulse are recorded every 15–30 minutes until the bleeding is controlled. The intervals are gradually increased as the patient's condition shows improvement and stabilization. The patient's respirations, colour and responses are noted at similar intervals to monitor for signs of hypovolaemic shock.

The pressures in the balloons are checked at frequent intervals and corrected if necessary to the prescribed pressure (30–40 mmHg). The gastric drainage is observed for amount and blood content. Persisting bright blood in the drainage is brought to the doctor's attention as this indicates continued bleeding. The fluid intake and output are recorded, and the balance determined daily. Stools are examined for blood content.

Supportive measures   The patient with bleeding oesophagogastric varices is critically ill and needs physical and psychological support.

Blood transfusion   Replacement of the blood lost is imperative. Fresh blood and fresh frozen plasma rather than stored blood alone is preferable in order to replace the thrombocytes and clotting factors lost.

Nutrition and fluids   A large-bore intravenous line is maintained until the patient is able to take fluids by mouth.

Fluids may be introduced via the tube in the stomach before it is removed. When the tube is removed, small amounts of nutritious fluids are given. The diet is progressively increased to a light diet as tolerated. Dietary fibre and raw fruits and vegetables are avoided. The patient is advised to chew food well, and in small amounts so that the bolus is small and less likely to cause trauma to a vulnerable area in the oesophagus or cardia of the stomach.

Rest and positioning   The patient is kept absolutely at rest to avoid displacing the balloons. Passive movements of the lower limbs and deep breathing are usually carried out to prevent circulatory stasis and to promote airway clearance. The head of the bed is elevated, unless contraindicated by shock. This position may reduce the flow of blood into the portal system.

Psychological support   The haematemesis, emergency measures and rapid loss of strength are very frightening to the patient. Fears and concerns should be acknowledged, and reassurance provided that everything possible is being done. Explanations are calmly made as to what is happening and what is going to be done. Sedation may be necessary to allay the patient's tension and anxiety and provide rest. The patient may be less apprehensive and more relaxed if a family member is present. The family should be kept informed about the patient's progress and what is being done.

Mouth care   The inability to swallow saliva and to receive anything by mouth necessitates special mouth care. Suction may be necessary to remove secretions. Tissues or a basin should be provided into which the patient may expectorate. The mouth is cleansed with moist applicators, and petroleum jelly or cold cream is applied to the lips to prevent irritation that may develop with the repeated use of tissues.

Nursing management (BOX 16.4)

Assessment

Health history   The patient who is admitted with bleeding varices will be acutely ill and initial assessment should focus on the vital signs and the ABC of resuscitation. When the situation has been stabilized and the patient's condition improved, the person's perceptions of symptoms and cause of the illness are obtained. Data are collected about changes in body weight and the appearance of ascites; nausea and vomiting and any loss of appetite; skin colour and itching; changes in mental status; changes in bowel habits; changes in energy level and feelings of tiredness.

Ongoing assessment includes recording of the person's fluid intake and output, and accurate assessment of nutritional intake. A mental status examination is performed frequently if there is indication of confusion, lethargy or altered level of consciousness.

The person is weighed daily as short-term changes will reflect changes in body fluid. The abdomen is examined daily for signs of ascites, and the presence of oedema should be monitored. The skin is inspected for changes in colour associated with jaundice and for petechiae and bruising, which indicate bleeding.

Nursing intervention

The *goals* of care are that the person will demonstrate:

1 adequate nutritional intake
2 absence of pain and discomfort
3 regular, rhythmic respirations
4 loss of weight associated with a decrease in the ascites
5 absence of signs of infection

Box 16.4   Care summary: Cirrhosis of the liver

Nurse
Admission assessment to include:

- Baseline observations of vital signs, neurological status, home and social circumstances, alcohol intake

- Weigh patient daily

- Daily measurement of abdominal girth

- Daily recording of blood pressure, pulse, temperature and respirations

- Daily neurological assessment

- Assess, observe and record nutritional intake

- Assess, observe and record bowel function

- Apply anti-pruritic lotions/moisturizers and medications as prescribed (change bedding at least once daily)

- Observe for bleeding tendencies, e.g. melaena, bruising and jaundice

- Assist with investigations, e.g. paracentesis

- Administer medications as prescribed: vitamin B_{12}, methotrexate

- Patient/family education

- Assist with nutritional intake

- Maintain fluid balance chart

- Encourage patient to maintain sitting position.

Doctor
Medical history:

- particularly alcohol intake, hepatitis, cholelithiasis

- blood tests: check full blood count and coagulation studies, urea and electrolytes, liver function tests

- prescribe medications: methotrexate, vitamin B_{12} injections, vitamin K

- tests: abdominal paracentesis

- patient/family education.

Dietitian

- nutritional assessment

- high carbohydrate, low sodium diet with vitamin supplements

- liaise with medical/nursing staff regarding patient's protein requirements

- potassium rich supplements

- patient/family education.

Social worker

- home social assessment

- initiate home support measures.

6 willingness to talk about feelings and concerns
7 understanding of and compliance with the treatment regimen.

Nutrition   As the progress of the disease is influenced by nutrition, a diet of 2500–3000 kcal/day, high in carbohydrates and vitamins is recommended. Protein content may be high (110–150 g), but can be restricted to 40 g, or eliminated according to the severity of the disease. Sufficient fat to make the diet palatable is added if the patient can tolerate it and is not jaundiced. Three small meals with in-between snacks will probably be more acceptable than three large meals. Sodium intake is restricted because of the tendency to develop oedema and ascites. Low-sodium protein concentrate and low-sodium milk are available and may be used to assist with the protein intake. Total abstinence from alcohol is very important.

If the liver insufficiency is serious and the patient is exhibiting neurological disturbances (e.g. depressed awareness, dulled mentation, confusion, asterixis/flapping tremor and hyperreflexia) and has increased blood levels of ammonia, protein is eliminated from the diet. The patient is sustained with carbohydrates. The disturbance of the nervous system is attributed to failure of the liver to metabolize the nitrogenous wastes; the ammonia level rises because it is not deaminized to form urea. If coma develops, intravenous infusions are used to support the patient.

Control of pain and discomfort   The person's skin should be kept clean and dry. Soaps and perfumed skin products are avoided. The skin is inspected for areas of redness or breakdown. Moisturizers are used to treat dryness and antipruritic lotions may be applied to alleviate itching. The person's nails are kept short and they are encouraged not to scratch. Diversional therapy may be useful. The person will be more comfortable in a cool environment and should be cautioned to avoid heat and heavy clothing that will increase itching.

The person will probably be more comfortable in a sitting position to alleviate discomfort from abdominal distension due to the ascites. The sitting position also alleviates respiratory distress. The person's respirations are monitored regularly as indicated and the patient is encouraged to carry out deep breathing and coughing exercises if respirations are impaired.

Prevention of infection   Resistance to infection is lowered in the patient with cirrhosis of the liver. Precautions should therefore be taken to prevent possible exposure to any source of infection.

Patient and family teaching   Significant changes in lifestyle are required after discharge and these should be carefully discussed with the patient and family. Strict adherence to diet, total abstinence from alcohol and the avoidance of infection and physical strain are stressed when interpreting the regimen to the patient and family. (If cirrhosis has been caused by alcohol misuse the nurse should encourage participation and commitment to therapy, and provide information and contact numbers and addresses of self-help groups such as Alcoholics Anonymous for the individual and significant others.)

The increased bleeding tendency associated with liver disorders makes it important to stress the need to avoid injuries and abrasions to the skin. A referral to the primary healthcare team will be necessary so that consistent support and supervision is ensured.

The prognosis for patients with cirrhosis depends on the degree of liver insufficiency. If treatment is instituted in the early stages and the patient is sufficiently motivated to adhere to the suggested care, a normal lifespan is still possible. If portal hypertension has developed with resultant ascites and oesophageal varices, the prognosis is grave.

Evaluation

The person with cirrhosis of the liver is assessed on an ongoing basis for relief from symptoms and absence of discomfort. The skin is inspected for signs of irritation, scratches, breaks and signs of bleeding. The client and family should understand dietary and comfort measures and recognize when to seek professional help. The patient and family should be comfortable talking about their concerns and anxieties, and be aware of the prognosis for the patient. They should be aware of support groups and palliative care in the hospital and the community.

TRAUMA TO THE LIVER

Any interruption of the capsule enclosing the hepatic tissue carries the risk of severe internal haemorrhage which may prove fatal before surgical intervention is possible. Urgent resuscitation is required together with surgical repair. Control of the bleeding is of prime importance. The area may be sutured or packed, or oxidized cellulose (Oxycel) gauze may be applied. The latter supplies fibres on which the clot may form more easily. In addition to the loss of blood incurred in injury, peritonitis may develop as a result of the chemical irritation caused by bile that may escape from the liver. Destruction of liver cells may also follow the injury, resulting in impaired liver function and serious clotting problems.

Non-alcoholic fatty liver disease

In this condition, a patient's liver shows evidence of fatty changes in the absence of excessive alcohol consumption. It is becoming an increasingly common disorder, is associated with insulin resistance and metabolic disorder. There are two causes of non-alcoholic fatty liver disease (NAFLD) – primary and secondary. Primary NAFLD is characterized by fatty changes in the liver cells – steatosis – and is more frequent in people with diabetes, being almost universally found in diabetic patients who are morbidly obese. Secondary NAFLD is associated with a variety of factors such as:

- nutrition (total parenteral nutrition, rapid weight loss, starvation)
- drug therapy (steroids, oestrogen, tamoxifen),

- poisons
- metabolic states and other disorders (inflammatory bowel disease and diverticulosis).

NAFLD is often asymptomatic. However, the disease may progress to liver fibrosis and cirrhosis leading to death, progression to fibrosis is usually slow and may take several decades to develop to its final stage. The aim of treatment is to slow the progression of the condition and to prevent liver-related illness and death. There is no specific pharmacotherapy at present. Interventions thus focus on weight loss and exercise, and controlling metabolic risk factors. Ultimately, liver transplantation may be the only option in end-stage NAFLD (Adams et al 2005).

NEOPLASTIC DISEASE

Benign and primary malignant neoplasms in the liver are less common than the more frequent metastatic growths. A primary tumour is usually associated with an already diseased liver (e.g. alcoholic cirrhosis). In the more frequent case where the growth is metastatic, the malignant cells will probably have been transported to the liver via the portal venous or hepatic arterial blood, or via the lymph. In many instances, secondaries in the liver are discovered before the primary source. The liver enlarges and signs of liver insufficiency develop. The patient experiences pain, food intolerance, anaemia, emaciation and ascites.

If a primary neoplasm is confined to one lobe of the liver, a hepatic lobectomy may be done. After the operation, the patient is observed closely for possible haemorrhage and biliary peritonitis. Chemotherapy may also be used.

LIVER ABSCESS

Infection with subsequent abscess formation occurs rarely and is most often associated with amoebic dysentery, especially in the tropics. Infection occurs through drinking water or eating uncooked food such as salads. The parasitic causative organisms (*Entamoeba histolytica*) infest the wall of the large bowel and produce chronic abdominal pains and bloody diarrhoea. They may be carried by the portal bloodstream from the bowel. Along with manifestations of impaired liver function, the patient has chills and a swinging temperature with frequent sweating episodes. The liver may enlarge and become tender while pain may be referred to the right shoulder. There may be one or multiple small abscesses which frequently coalesce, forming one large cavity. The pyogenic infection may also be caused by staphylococcus, streptococcus or *Escherichia coli*.

The patient is treated with metronidazole or tinidazole if acutely ill with diarrhoea but would be given the anti-amoebic drug diloxanide furoate if asymptomatic and a liver abscess has developed as a complication of amoebiasis (BNF 2005). The abscess is drained by aspiration followed by the injection of an antibiotic into the cavity. Open surgical drainage is avoided if possible because of the danger of dissemination of the infection within the peritoneal cavity and resultant peritonitis.

LIVER TRANSPLANTATION

The number of liver transplants being performed is increasing each year, although the procedure remains limited to a few centres. Donor organs are generally matched to the recipient according to body size and blood type, as the liver is not as immunologically active as other organs. The recipient's immune system is suppressed usually with ciclosporin in combination with low-dose corticosteroids. Patients and families require a great deal of emotional support and therapeutic intervention to help them deal with the transplant and the implications for the patient's life and the quality of life that can be anticipated.

As surgical techniques have become more sophisticated, with improved outcomes for transplantation patients, concerns have been raised in relation to the availability of transplant tissues. Demand far outstrips supply. As a means of improving supply, living donors have become more common and the evidence suggests that very nearly all the live donors achieve some psychological and spiritual benefit. However, there are some reports of donor death following liver transplantation (for example, of the right lobe). It is also clear that donors report more pain than anticipated and that postoperative recovery time is longer than expected. Clinicians must therefore make the risks of the process very clear to potential donors during the informed consent process (Surman and Hertl 2003). Liver transplantation for end-stage alcoholic cirrhosis remains controversial: is it

---

Box 16.5 Glossary of terms (extrahepatic biliary system)

Cholelithiasis – gallstones or calculi in the gallbladder

Cholecystitis – inflammation of the gallbladder

Cholecystectomy – surgical removal of the gallbladder

Cholestasis – stoppage or suppression of the flow of bile

Cholecystostomy – incision into the gallbladder and the insertion of a tube for drainage

Choledocholithiasis – gallstone(s) in the common bile duct

Choledochitis – inflammation of the common bile duct

Choledocholithotomy – surgical removal of stone from the common bile duct

Choledochotomy – incision and exploration of the common bile duct

Choledochoduodenostomy – anastomosis of the common bile duct to the duodenum

ethical for these patients to be offered an opportunity for transplantation, given the shortage of donor organs? Alcoholic liver disease is NOT medically contraindicated for transplantation and some studies report 'good' outcomes for former alcoholic patients.

DISORDERS OF THE GALLBLADDER AND BILE DUCT

CHOLELITHIASIS

Cholelithiasis is the term used for stones in the gallbladder (Box 16.5). The stones vary in shape and size and consist mainly of cholesterol and bile pigments. There may be one stone or many and, although they may develop in both sexes, they occur more often in middle-aged women.

Clinical characteristics

Cholelithiasis may not give rise to any disturbance in many persons; in others, the stones cause signs and symptoms ranging from mild digestive disturbances following fat ingestion to the severe, disabling pain of biliary colic. Gallstones may cause acute or chronic inflammation of the gallbladder (*cholecystitis*), or *cholestasis* (stasis of the bile) within the liver leading to impaired function of that organ. Small stones tend to cause more acute problems, as they may escape into the ducts. They may pass into the duodenum or may lodge in the cystic or common bile duct or the ampulla of Vater. Impaction of a stone in the common bile duct leads to obstructive jaundice and biliary colic – an intense, incapacitating pain.

Treatment and nursing intervention

Cholelithiasis is treated surgically by removal of the gallbladder (*cholecystectomy*) and exploration of the common bile duct for a stone or stricture. Stones may be removed from the common bile duct by means of the ERCP technique. Percutaneous removal of gallstones is indicated in patients who are at high risk in terms of anaesthesia, but recurrence of gallstones is common (although this may be asymptomatic).

Food and fluids by mouth are withheld, and the patient is given intravenous fluids. If vomiting and abdominal distension occur, a nasogastric tube is passed and regular aspiration is performed. After the acute episode and removal of the nasogastric tube, clear fluids are given and gradually increased to a light, low-fat diet as tolerated.

The patient is observed for signs of jaundice, and the colour of all stools is noted. The stools may be saved for examination for the presence of the stone, which may have passed from the biliary tract into the intestine. If the patient is jaundiced and the stools are a pale grey, indicating an absence of bile in the intestine, a daily dose of vitamin K is given parenterally to maintain prothrombin formation and prevent bleeding. Early surgical intervention has become much more common in recent years.

CHOLECYSTITIS

Inflammation of the gallbladder may be acute or chronic. Acute cholecystitis is most often associated with gallstones but may occur as a result of infection. The patient manifests pain and tenderness in the right upper abdominal quadrant or mid-epigastrium, fever, nausea and vomiting, and leucocytosis. The severity of the symptoms varies with the degree of inflammation. Jaundice may develop if the inflammation involves the biliary ducts.

Management

The treatment includes rest, intravenous fluids, analgesics and antibiotics. If the condition persists or worsens, it may indicate suppuration (empyema of the gallbladder), necessitating prompt surgery. A *cholecystostomy* (drainage of the gallbladder) or a laparoscopic *cholecystectomy* (removal of the gallbladder) may be done.

Chronic cholecystitis is characterized by a long history of vague digestive complaints. The person experiences abdominal discomfort and flatulence after a large rich meal or one high in fats. A dull, aching pain and nausea and vomiting may occur at times. The intensity and probably the frequency of the symptoms increase insidiously over months or years.

The chronic inflammation results in scarring and thickening of the wall of the gallbladder and cholestasis. If calculi are present, they progressively increase in size or number. The person may have subacute or acute exacerbations leading to nausea and vomiting, moderate fever and colic. The condition is usually treated surgically by removal of the gallbladder.

BILE DUCT DISORDERS

Obstruction of the common bile duct may occur as a result of a gallstone that has escaped from the gallbladder (*choledocholithiasis*), inflammation (*choledochitis* or *cholangitis*), neoplasm or a stricture formed by scar tissue following trauma and inflammation. The duct above the obstruction dilates and obstructive jaundice develops.

In the case of an impacted stone, ERCP may be done and the gallstone removed during the cannulation of the common bile duct. Surgery may be undertaken to open the duct and remove the calculus. When a stricture is present and the area is sufficiently small, it is resected and an end-to-end anastomosis performed. If the obstruction is due to primary carcinoma, excision may be undertaken and the duct stump anastomosed (joined) to the duodenum (*choledochoduodenostomy*) or the jejunum (*choledochojejunostomy*).

Extrinsic pressure on the bile ducts obstructing the flow of bile may occur with cancer of the pancreas or duodenum.

When surgery involves an extrahepatic bile duct, a T tube is inserted at the site of entry into the duct to maintain bile drainage during recovery of the tissues (*choledochostomy*). The stem portion of the tube is brought out on the abdominal surface through a stab wound or the incision and is attached to a drainage receptacle. Surgery on a bile duct is usually accompanied by a cholecystectomy, because the gallbladder is frequently the origin of the problem.

Nursing care of patients with extrahepatic disorders

The patient is kept at rest, and food is withheld as the patient is usually nauseous and vomiting. If there is vomiting, a nasogastric tube is passed and regular aspiration is performed. The temperature, pulse and respirations are recorded regularly. The patient should be checked for signs of obstructive jaundice and abdominal distension.

When the vomiting is controlled and the nasogastric tube removed, oral fluids are given and graduated, as tolerated, to a light, low-fat diet. Traditionally this conservative approach was followed by operation at a later date; however, early surgery is increasingly the favoured option.

Preoperative care

Preoperative preparation for surgery on the extrahepatic biliary system includes close observation for jaundice and the administration of vitamin K to raise the prothrombin level and improve clotting times. Special attention is given to having the patient understand the importance of the frequent coughing and deep breathing that will be required after the operation. Because of the site of the operation, the patient tends to take very shallow breaths to prevent pain and discomfort, predisposing to respiratory complications as insufficient lung expansion occurs, which may lead to an accumulation of secretions and atelectasis (consolidation of part of the lung). A nasogastric tube may be passed before the patient is taken to the operating theatre.

Postoperative care

The increasing use of laparoscopic techniques (so-called 'keyhole' surgery) reduces the need for lengthy postoperative recovery periods as the incision is much smaller and much less tissue is involved. Close observation of vital signs and pain is essential to detect any postoperative complications that may arise.

Exploration of the common bile duct for stones will still necessitate a special drainage tube (T tube) being used. This is inserted in the common bile duct and generally clamped during the transfer from the operating room. After the patient has been transferred, it is immediately attached to a drainage receptacle. The tubing leading to the receptacle is secured to the dressing, and should have sufficient slack to prevent traction and dislodgement. The patient is advised on how to turn to avoid a pull on the tube and of the need to be sure that the tube is not kinked or compressed. The drainage is observed frequently during the first 24 hours in case of haemorrhage. There may be a small amount of blood mixed with bile in the first few hours. Persistent bleeding is reported to the surgeon. The character and daily amount of bile drainage are recorded. If there is prolonged loss of bile, it may be given back to the patient through a nasogastric tube for the purpose of promoting more normal digestion and absorption in the intestine.

The dressing is checked frequently for possible bleeding or bile leakage. After a few days, the T tube is clamped for stated intervals and is removed when oedema of the common bile duct subsides. This is usually established by administration of a radio-opaque substance into the tube and the subsequent radiograph will show the outline of the biliary tract. Alternatively, the tube is clamped for 24 hours and, if the individual remains pain free, it is removed. After removal of the tube, the dressing is observed for bile seepage. If the dressing is soiled with bile, it is changed frequently; the skin and wound are cleansed. Should excoriation of the skin occur due to chemical irritation caused by strongly alkaline bile, a protective dressing such as a hydrocolloid wafer should be applied to the skin. If the drainage is heavy, application of a drainage bag may reduce soiling of clothing and reduce embarrassment or distress. The patient should be reassured that it will cease. The patient is also observed for signs of peritonitis, such as an increase in temperature, abdominal pain, distension and rigidity.

Until the procedures become less painful and the patient is less fearful, the nurse's assistance and support are required during the frequent, regular coughing, deep breathing and changes of position that are required. Early ambulation is encouraged, and provision is made for a small drainage receptacle that may be attached to the patient's dressing gown if there is a T tube in the common bile duct. The urine, stools, sclerae and skin are checked for any indication of obstructive jaundice.

The patient receives intravenous fluids until the nasogastric tube is removed and oral fluids and food are tolerated. The fat content of the diet is limited. In preparation for discharge, the patient's diet is discussed. The individual can usually gradually include fat as tolerated in the diet but the health advantages of a low-fat diet should be discussed.

An alternative technique introduced recently is to dissolve the stones with bile acids. This non-operative approach is suitable only for certain patients, such as those with stones that do not contain calcium.

CASE Jane was a 38-year-old woman who was brought to the A&E department at 17.00 hours by her partner, complaining of severe pain on the right side of her abdomen (right upper quadrant) and vomiting. She complained of feeling nauseated, hot and sweaty and was clearly in considerable distress with the pain.

The advanced nurse practitioner (ANP) took a brief history. Jane reported the pain as having come on after lunch (she had fish and chips). On questioning with a PQRST framework (see p. 128) she stated nothing seemed to bring the pain on and no matter how she sat, nothing seemed to alleviate it. She had taken two paracetamol and some ibuprofen with no effect. It was a sharp stabbing pain and while it started on the right side of her abdomen it now began shooting into her right shoulder (scapula). She rated the pain 10 on a 10-point scale. 'It's as bad as childbirth' she said 'and I thought nothing could be that bad, nothing seems to get rid of it, no matter how I sit or anything'. She had had the pain now for 5 hours; it started around 2 p.m. She stated she had been well with no significant medical problems and did not take any medication. She has had 3 children by a previous marriage and had been living with her current partner for 5 years. She does not smoke and only drinks 3–4 glasses of wine a week. There were no other symptoms such as headaches, visual disturbances, shortness of breath, chest pain or diarrhoea. The ANP took her vital signs and noted them as T 38.6C, BP 145/95, P 106, RR 20. Although unable to measure exact height and weight, the ANP noted she looked overweight.

The ANP continued to work up the patient by examining her abdomen. The appearance of the skin was normal. Auscultation revealed that bowel sounds were reduced. There was obvious tenderness in the right upper quadrant with guarding and rebound tenderness on deep palpation. She listened to the chest and noted normal breath and cardiac sounds.

At this stage, the ANP suspected an acute episode involving the right side of the abdomen or possibly the chest. She was considering a differential diagnosis of cholecystitis, hepatitis or liver abscess, pancreatitis, a peptic ulcer or appendicitis but was aware it could also be a right-sided pneumonia. Either way, the patient was an emergency who needed immediate medical intervention. After discussion with the A&E medical staff they referred her to the on-call surgical team. The referring doctor demonstrated a positive Murphy's sign as he obtained tenderness on deep palpation of the right upper quadrant as she took a deep breath in. He also did a rectal examination and noted a small amount of normal faeces on the glove which tested negative to occult blood.

Opioid analgesia was given with an antiemetic and she was transferred to the surgical admission unit where an ultrasound was organized. This showed stones within the gall bladder and cystic duct and thickening of the gall bladder walls. Blood revealed she had elevated levels of bilirubin, amylase, alkaline phosphatase and a leukocytosis (elevated white blood cell count) of 14 000. A full blood count, urea and electrolytes, a liver panel and blood clotting time were all ordered to give a full picture along with blood cultures.

She was initially kept nil by mouth and had an intravenous line established. Opioid analgesia was given together with a cephalosporin antimicrobial drug (i.v. cefotaxime) to deal with the likely pathological bacteria usually found in the bile in such cases. She had a laparoscopic cholecystectomy 2 days after admission from which she made an uneventful recovery.

Margenthaler et al (2004) support this approach to the management of gall stones, the degree of pain experienced by Jane before her treatment is typical of this condition and demonstrates the level of nursing support that patients in her situation need.

DISORDERS OF THE PANCREAS

Inflammation and neoplastic disease are the pathological conditions seen most frequently in the pancreas.

PANCREATITIS

Inflammation of the pancreas may be acute or chronic with recurrent acute episodes.

Acute pancreatitis

Acute pancreatitis is a potentially serious and life-threatening disorder; the severity of the inflammation varies. In the mild form the pancreas becomes swollen and oedematous and, with treatment, the patient is likely to recover within a few days. If the process is severe and persists, necrosis and haemorrhage ensue. Necrosis results from intrapancreatic activation of the proteinases and lipase, initiating auto-digestion of the pancreatic tissue and blood vessels. Enzymes and blood may escape into the surrounding tissue and peritoneal cavity; peritonitis, paralytic ileus or ascites may develop.

Cause

Pancreatitis is considered to be the result of some factor or change within the pancreas that effects activation of the pro-teinases and lipase of the exocrine secretion, with subsequent breakdown of the ducts, parenchymal tissue and blood vessels. The causative factor may be an obstruction to the flow of the pancreatic secretion within the ducts. The migration of a gallstone through the sphincter of Oddi is recognized as the most likely cause. It is suggested that such an obstruc-tion causes a reflux of bile into the pancreas, promoting activation of the enzymes and ensuing autodigestion.

There are many other possible causes, amongst which an acute relapse of chronic pancreatitis secondary to an episode of heavy alcohol intake is a strong possibility.

Clinical characteristics

Acute pancreatitis has a sudden onset, being preceded usually by only mild, vague digestive disturbances. The principal signs and symptoms are pain, gastrointestinal dis-turbances, obstructive jaundice, shock and hyperglycaemia.

Pain At first, constant severe incapacitating pain occurs in the upper abdomen, penetrating through to the back. It may be described as burning or boring. Later, with progression of the disease, the pain becomes more generalized in the abdomen.

Gastrointestinal disturbances Nausea and vomiting occur and persist. Constipation may be a problem. Abdom-inal distension and rigidity appear as a result of the dev-elopment of peritonitis. The latter is caused by chemical irritation of the viscera and peritoneum by the enzymes that escape from the pancreas. Peristalsis diminishes, and eventually paralytic ileus and intestinal obstruction may complicate the patient's condition further.

Shock Shock is attributed to the severity of the constant pain, the exudation of plasma into the peritoneal cavity that occurs with the peritonitis, and the loss of blood resulting from the erosion of vessels within the pancreas associated with necrotizing and haemorrhagic pancreatitis.

Vital signs The temperature may be raised in the early stage but may become subnormal if peritonitis and shock develop. The pulse is rapid and the blood pressure falls with the decrease in the intravascular volume. The patient is flushed at first, and then usually becomes pale. If peritonitis develops, a dusky or cyanotic colour is possible.

Obstructive jaundice If the head of the pancreas is involved, it may compress the common bile duct and cause obstructive jaundice.

Blood changes With the escape of enzymes into the pancreatic parenchyma and peritoneal cavity, fatty tissue is broken down into glycerol and fatty acids. The latter combine with calcium to form insoluble calcium compounds. The serum calcium level falls and may be severe enough to produce tetany (painful muscle spasm) and affect heart action (prolonged diastole). The serum bilirubin level may be increased after 2–3 days.

Haemoconcentration develops as a result of the loss of plasma. The prothrombin level falls because of the lack of absorption of vitamin K. Serum amylase and lipase levels are raised.

Disturbance in glucose metabolism A deficiency of insulin may develop when the islets of Langerhans are involved in the pathological process, and hyperglycaemia and glycosuria may be present.

Treatment

The patient with acute pancreatitis is critically ill. Care is directed toward the reduction of pancreatic secretion to a minimum, relief of pain, prevention of shock or correction if it has developed, prevention of electrolyte and fluid imbalances and prevention of infection.

Medications Analgesia should be given regularly to relieve pain and discomfort and promote rest. Pethidine is usually prescribed as it depresses the central nervous system and relaxes smooth muscle. Administration of morphine may cause contraction of the sphincter of Oddi in some patients (and therefore, more pain) but its longer half-life may help provide effective sustained analgesia for some patients. The patient may receive an anticholinergic drug such as propantheline bromide (Pro-Banthine) by intramuscular injection, which will inhibit vagal nerve stimulation of pancreatic enzymes and promote relaxation of the sphincter of Oddi. If an anticholinergic drug is prescribed, the patient will experience a very dry mouth, and close observations are made for the possible side-effects of urinary retention and paralytic ileus (Case Study 16.3).

Parenteral administration of vitamin K may be necessary to maintain normal prothrombin production and prevent bleeding.

CASE Pain management in pancreatitis

Paula, 55-years old, was admitted to the medical admissions ward with acute pancreatitis. This was her first admission with this condition. Her social history showed that she had some problems related to alcoholism. Paula was in severe pain and calling out constantly for analgesia, despite earlier administration of intramuscular pethidine. The nursing staff on duty were reluctant to administer any more analgesia because they suspected that Paula is 'crying wolf' because of her alcoholism. However, the nurse in charge made an immediate referral to the acute pain team, who visited Paula within 15 minutes, whilst the medical team was still present. The acute pain nurse explained that Paula's self-report of pain was valid and important; she initiated a pain assessment scoring system of 0–10; Paula said her pain was at 10.

The acute pain nurse was able to obtain a medical prescription for intravenous patient-controlled analgesia (PCA) with morphine. This was commenced immediately. With this regimen, and under her control, Paula's pain subsided into what she described as 'manageable' – a pain score of 3.

Often, pancreatic pain is resistant to opioid administration, however, but various combinations of analgesic drugs may be tried, along with anticholinergics. It is important to remember that this lack of response is about treatment failure, not drug-seeking behaviour.

Complications If *paralytic ileus* and intestinal obstruction develop, a nasogastric tube may be passed into the stomach and decompression suction established. *Obstruction of the duodenum* may develop because of the swollen oedematous pancreas. Escaping pancreatic enzymes may digest an area of the gastric or duodenal wall, causing *severe haemorrhage* as well as perforation of the eroded organ.

Renal failure may develop within 24 hours of the onset of acute pancreatitis, necessitating dialysis.

Another complication that may develop in pancreatitis is the formation of one or more *pseudocysts*. Accumulations of inflammatory exudate, liquefied necrotic tissue and secretions become walled off by a capsule of fibrous tissue. The cyst is atypical in that there is no epithelial lining characteristic of true cysts. This accounts for the term pseudocyst. The cyst may enlarge and impose on surrounding structures: the common bile duct may be blocked, the duodenum or stomach may be displaced, or the diaphragm may be elevated.

The symptoms depend on the size and location of the cyst(s). In some instances resolution takes place spontaneously, or the cysts may produce persisting pain, digestive disturbances, anorexia, loss of weight and mechanical interference with other organs. Percutaneous drainage of pseudocysts under ultrasonography or CT control is possible.

Surgical intervention Surgery is not usually undertaken during an acute episode unless the patient is critically ill with extensive pancreatic necrosis. Surgery on the pancreas may involve the removal of calculi in the pancreatic duct, drainage of a pseudocyst, or partial or complete pancreatectomy. Rarely, in severe chronic pancreatitis, the sensory nerves (splanchnic nerves) that transmit pain impulses from the pancreas may be interrupted to relieve intractable pain.

Where drainage may have contact with the skin, meticulous skin care and protection is essential to prevent excoriation. Use of skin-protective wafers or drainage bags with integral skin-saving adhesive plates may prevent problems. Early consultation with the stoma care nurse (if available) concerning skin care and appropriate appliances may prevent problems with skin integrity.

Nursing management

Assessment The person's condition may change rapidly with progressive necrosis and resulting haemorrhage. The *vital signs* and the *general response and appearance of the patient* are observed frequently. A rapid weak pulse, a fall in blood pressure, pallor and increasing weakness may indicate haemorrhage or shock and are immediately brought to the doctor's attention. An accurate record is kept of the *fluid intake* and *output*. A catheter is necessary for accurate hourly measurements of urine output. A urinary output of <0.5 mL/kg (35 mL for the average adult) per hour is indicative of impending circulatory collapse and must be reported to the medical staff immediately.

The *intensity and location of the pain* are noted, and the abdomen is examined for distension and rigidity. All *stools* are examined and, if they are bulky, greasy and foul-smelling or show other abnormalities, they may be saved for medical examination.

The *sclerae and skin* are observed for any yellow tinge that would indicate the development of jaundice.

Nursing intervention The *goals* of care are that the person with acute pancreatitis will demonstrate:

1 fluid and electrolyte balance
2 blood glucose levels within normal range
3 absence of pain and discomfort
4 absence of respiratory complications
5 gradual increase in self-care activities
6 knowledge of prescribed dietary and lifestyle measures
7 plans for follow-up care.

Gastric drainage A nasogastric tube is passed and regular aspiration is performed. This relieves vomiting and distension and prevents the acid gastric secretion from entering the duodenum, which would stimulate the release of the hormones secretin and cholecystokinin-pancreozymin. The colour, consistency and 24-hour volume of the drainage are recorded.

Fluids and nutrition The patient receives nothing by mouth to avoid stimulating the secretion of the pancreatic enzymes. The restoration and maintenance of normal blood volume is very important to prevent or correct shock. Plasma or whole blood may be given intravenously, in addition to electrolyte and glucose solutions. A close check is kept on the blood chemistry, volume of gastrointestinal drainage, urinary output and amount of perspiration to determine the specific electrolyte and fluid needs. Total parenteral nutrition may be prescribed during the acute and convalescent phases of the illness. Recent studies have indicated that enteral feeding via a nasojejunal tube is cheap, safe and effective (Abou-Assi and O'Keefe 2001). Frequent monitoring of

capillary blood glucose is necessary. McArdle (2000) argues that glucose levels should be tested as frequently as the patient's condition requires, which could be hourly, rather than according to a fixed schedule. Insulin may be administered in line with blood glucose levels.

When oral intake is permitted, fluids are introduced in small amounts. The principal nutrient given at first is carbohydrate; protein is added gradually, according to the patient's tolerance. Fats are avoided. The diet is progressively increased to a high-protein, high-carbohydrate, low-fat, light diet. Four or five small meals are recommended daily. A preparation of extract of pancreas (pancreatin) may be prescribed orally with meals to assist in digestion. Large meals are avoided, and total abstinence from alcohol is stressed.

Mouth and nasal care Frequent cleansing and rinsing of the mouth are necessary during the period in which oral intake is restricted because the antispasmodic, anticholinergic drug that the patient may be receiving suppresses salivary secretion. Oil, petroleum jelly or a cream is used on the lips to prevent cracking. The nostrils are cleansed with an applicator that has been slightly moistened with normal saline, and a light application of petroleum jelly or water-soluble lubricant is made to the nostril through which the tube passes to prevent irritation and excoriation.

Pulmonary care The person with acute pancreatitis may develop respiratory difficulties due to acid–base abnormalities, distended abdomen preventing full expansion of the lungs, or experience of pain on respiration causing reduced effort. Anticholinergic drugs may reduce normal secretions of the respiratory tract. The person should be nursed in a semi-upright position to reduce pressure on the diaphragm and promote full lung expansion. Deep-breathing exercises and coughing should be taught and the patient should be encouraged to perform them regularly. Should oxygen therapy be prescribed, humidification may prevent further drying of the respiratory tract, and the use of nasal cannulae rather than a face mask may improve tolerance.

Psychological support Support will be necessary throughout the illness as the experience is very stressful for the patient and family. This will only be compounded by worries and anxieties over social factors such as loss of earnings, or even job, while a history of alcohol misuse brings with it a whole sequence of psychological and social problems.

Follow-up care A long convalescence follows recovery from an acute episode of pancreatitis. The necessary care to avert an exacerbation is discussed with the patient and family. The importance of strict adherence to the prescribed diet, total abstinence from alcohol and the avoidance of large meals is explained. Verbal and written instructions are given about the content and preparation of the recommended low-fat, high-protein, high-carbohydrate diet.

Activities are gradually resumed and the individual may return to work in 1–3 months if the person's job has been kept available.

Evaluation

Evaluation of the outcomes of nursing intervention for the person with acute pancreatitis includes assessment of the person's symptoms and evidence that they have been alleviated; particularly important is the absence of pain. Vital signs and fluid and electrolyte balance should be returning to the person's usual levels. The patient should increasingly assume self-care activities. The patient and family should be able to describe the prescribed dietary measures, understand the need for rest, state plans to alter lifestyle factors such as alcohol consumption, and discuss plans for follow-up health care.

Chronic pancreatitis

Chronic pancreatitis may develop following an initial acute episode or may develop insidiously. It is frequently associated with alcohol misuse.

The chronic form of the disease is characterized by progressive fibrosing and calcification of areas in the pancreas following inflammation and necrosis. The degree of impaired function and the intensity of its signs and symptoms are proportionate to the amount of continuing inflammation or frequency of acute episodes and ensuing tissue damage.

Clinical characteristics

The person with chronic pancreatitis experiences recurrent attacks of pain in the epigastric region and right upper quadrant which progressively becomes persistent. Anorexia, nausea, flatulence and constipation are common problems. Episodes are frequently precipitated by the ingestion of alcohol or a large meal with considerable fatty content.

As more and more of the endocrine and exocrine cells become non-functional, the effects on the patient become more severe. A deficiency of enzyme secretion occurs in the intestine. Less fat and protein is digested; the person's stools become bulky, greasy and offensive (steatorrhoea) and there is a progressive weight loss. A deficiency of insulin secretion may result in diabetes mellitus.

Treatment and nursing intervention

The key intervention is to secure total abstinence from alcohol. A low-fat diet will help to reduce the diarrhoea associated with steatorrhoea.

Impaired digestion due to insufficient quantities of enzymes in the intestine may be corrected by the administration of pancreatic enzyme supplements (preparation of pancreatic extract). Vitamin supplements, including vitamins A, D, K, folic acid and B_{12} may be required.

Decreased insulin secretion may necessitate the giving of insulin to control glucose metabolism.

As the disease becomes more advanced, the pain experienced by the patient may indicate frequent doses of an analgesic. Not infrequently, this becomes complicated by the person's development of a tolerance for the drug, necessitating progressively larger doses or a change in the prescribed medication regimen.

NEOPLASMS OF THE PANCREAS

Carcinoma

Cancer of the pancreas usually arises from the ducts and, although it may occur in any part of the organ, it is most commonly seen in the head. It is usually fatal.

The patient experiences pain, progressive weakness and loss of weight. Obstructive jaundice develops if the neoplasm encroaches on the ampulla of Vater or common bile duct. The cancer may spread by direct invasion to adjacent structures or by metastasis to the liver.

Treatment

The condition is treated surgically if recognized sufficiently early and if it is the head of the pancreas that is involved. Neoplasms in the body and tail have usually metastasized by the time they are identified. Whipple's operation may be attempted in which the head of the pancreas is removed, along with the duodenum, with anastomosis between the common bile duct and jejunum, anastomosis between the pancreas and jejunum, and a gastrojejunostomy. Palliative operations may be carried out for inoperable tumours involving relief of jaundice by the placement of a stent to drain bile away to the small intestine, thereby relieving the obstruction caused by the tumour.

Preparation for surgery includes a high-calorie, low-fat diet if tolerated by the patient, intravenous rehydration, blood transfusions, and parenteral vitamin K if there is jaundice. Postoperative care includes gastrointestinal decompression to prevent distension of the jejunum and pressure on the sites of the anastomoses. The patient is supported by blood transfusions and intravenous fluids. Vitamin K administration may be continued.

Tumours of islet cells

A benign tumour may develop in non-β islet cells and may become malignant. The tumour cells secrete gastrin freely, causing the Zollinger–Ellison syndrome, which is characterized by gastric hypersecretion and persisting peptic ulceration. The treatment is surgical removal of the tumours or total gastrectomy.

Occasionally an adenoma develops from beta cells of the islets of Langerhans, causing an excessive secretion of insulin (hyperinsulinism) and hypoglycaemia. The adenoma is usually benign but, rarely, may be adenocarcinoma.

The symptoms presented by the patient are mainly due to the effect of the abnormally low blood sugar on the brain cells. Brain cells are more sensitive to glucose deficiency than other body cells. The initial symptoms are hunger, restlessness and apprehension. These progress to weakness, loss of coordination, tremors, diaphoresis, disorientation, convulsions and coma. The manifestations appear during a fasting period (early morning) or after extreme exertion. Prompt administration of some form of glucose is necessary to raise the blood sugar level. If the hypoglycaemia remains untreated, the glucose deficiency may result in permanent brain cell damage or death. When early signs are recognized, the patient is given sugar or orange juice with sugar. In the more advanced stage of hypoglycaemia, 50% glucose is given intravenously (via a central line – 50% glucose is hypertonic and would cause damage to a peripheral vein).

Surgical treatment may consist of excision of the adenoma or subtotal or total pancreatectomy. Preparation for the operation includes a high-carbohydrate, high-protein diet and intravenous infusions of glucose solution to restore glycogen reserves. The glucose infusion is continued during the operation. Following surgery, close observation is made for a recurrence of hypoglycaemia. If a total pancreatectomy is performed, the patient will receive supplemental insulin and pancreatic extract for the remainder of his or her life.

SUMMARY

This chapter has provided an overview of the structures and functions of the liver, biliary tract and exocrine pancreas. The clinical characteristics and the nursing assessment of alterations in function demonstrated by the person with disorders of the liver, biliary tract and exocrine pancreas have been discussed. Emphasis has been placed on the role of the nurse in the early detection and treatment of persons with alcohol abuse problems and the potential for preventing serious disorders of the liver and pancreas. The patient who has any of the disorders discussed in this chapter is usually seriously ill and in need of supportive care. The nurse needs to be sensitive to a whole range of patient needs, most particularly their pain management and the appropriate use of effective analgesia for their condition. Skilled and knowledgeable nursing care can have an enormous impact upon the person with the conditions discussed in this chapter and can relive the suffering and discomfort associated with disorders of the liver, biliary tract or exocrine pancreas.

REFERENCES

Abou-Assi S, O'Keefe S (2001) Nutrition in acute pancreatitis. Journal of Clinical Gastroenterology 32(3): 203–209.

Adams LA, Angulo P, Lindor KD (2005) Nonalcoholic fatty liver disease. Canadian Medical Association Journal 172(7): 899–905.

Black J, Hawks J (2005) Medical surgical nursing, 7th edn. St Louis: Elsevier Saunders.

BNF (2005) British National Formulary 49; London: BMA, RPSGB.

CRD (Centre for Reviews and Dissemination) (2001a) Interferon as treatment for acute hepatitis C: a meta-analysis. York: NHS Centre for Reviews and Dissemination, University of York.

CRD (Centre for Reviews and Dissemination) (2001b) The efficacy of interferon alfa in chronic hepatitis B – a review and meta-analysis, Vol. 1. York: NHS Centre for Reviews and Dissemination, University of York.

CRD (Centre for Reviews and Dissemination) (2001c) Correlation of biochemical response to interferon alpha with histological improvement in hepatitis C: a meta-analysis of diagnostic test characteristics. Database of Abstracts of Reviews of Effectiveness. York: NHS Centre for Reviews and Dissemination, University of York.

Cole L (2002) Unravelling the mystery of acute pancreatitis. Dimensions of Critical Care Nursing 21(3): 86–90.

Compton P (2002) Caring for an alcohol-dependent patient. Nursing 32(12): 58–64.

De Palma J (2000) HCV infection among nurses and surgeons: what are the odds? American Journal of Nursing 100(5): 28.

Department of Health (2004) Statistics on alcohol: England, 2004. Online. Available: www.dh.gov.uk/PublicationsAndStatistics/StatisticalWorkAreas

Department of Health (2006) Alcohol and Health. Online. Available: http://www.dh.gov.uk/PolicyAndGuidance/HealthAndSocialCareTopics/AlcoholMisuse [Accessed 08.04.2006]

Giannini EG, Testa R, Savarino V (2005) Liver enzyme alteration: a guide for clinicians. Canadian Medical Association Journal 172(3): 367–379.

Gines P, Cardenas A, Arroyo V, Rodes J (2004) Management of cirrhosis and ascites. New England Journal of Medicine 350(16): 1646–1655.

Grewal HP (2002) Impact of surgical innovation on liver transplantation. Lancet 359(9304): 368–370.

Grundy G, Beeching N (2004) Understanding social stigma in women with hepatitis C. Nursing Standard 19(4): 35–39.

Hale AS, Moseley MJ, Warner SC (2000) Treating pancreatitis in the acute care setting. Dimensions of Critical Care Nursing 19(4): 15–21.

Hinchcliff SM, Montague SE, Watson R (1996) Physiology for nursing practice. London: Baillière Tindall.

Hughes E (2004) Understanding the care of patients with acute pancreatitis. Nursing Standard 18(18): 45–52.

Karsan HA, Rojter SE, Saab S (2004) Primary prevention of cirrhosis; public health strategies that can make a difference. Postgraduate Medicine 115(1): 25.

Krige JEJ, Beckingham IJ (2001) ABC if diseases of liver, pancreas, and biliary system. Portal hypertension – 1:varices. British Medical Journal 322(7282): 348–351.

Llovet JM, Burroughs A, Bruix J (2003) Hepatocellular carcinoma. Lancet 363: 1907–1917.

Margenthaler J, Schuerer D, Whinney R (2004) Acute cholecystitis. Clinical Evidence 12: 571–580.

Marsano LS, Mendez C, Hill D, Barve S, McClain CJ (2003) Diagnosis and treatment of alcoholic liver disease and its complications. Alcohol Research and Health 27(3): 247–256.

McArdle J (2000) The biological and nursing implications of pancreatitis. Nursing Standard 14(48): 46–51.

McCollum J (2000) Appetite and nutritional intake in patients with chronic liver disease. Journal of Human Nutrition and Dietetics 13(5): 365–366.

McCreaddie M, Neilson M (2001) Hepatitis C: why all the fuss? Nursing Times 97(11): 34–41.

NICE (2004) Peginterferon alfa, interferon alfa and ribavirin for chronic hepatitis C. Online. Available: www.nice.org.uk/TA075

Oh Y-W, Kang E-Y, Lo NJ, Suh W, Godwin J (2000) Thoracic manifestations associated with advanced liver disease. Journal of Computer Assisted Tomography 24(5): 699–705.

Parini S (2001) Hepatitis C: speaking out about the silent epidemic. Nursing Management 32(6): 17–24.

Sargent S (2005) The aetiology, management and complications of alcoholic hepatitis. British Journal of Nursing 14(10): 536–562.

Shovein J, Damzo R, Hyams I (2000) Hepatitis A: how benign is it? American Journal of Nursing 100(3): 43–47.

Stewart KB, Richards AB (2000) Recognising and managing your patient's alcohol abuse. Nursing 30(2): 56–59.

Surman OS, Hertl M (2003) Liver donation: donor safety comes first. Lancet 362(9385): 674–675.

Watanabe S, Hosomi N, Kitade Y et al (2000) Assessment of the presence and severity of esophagogastric varices by splenic index in patients with liver cirrhosis. Journal of Computer Assisted Tomography 24(5): 788–794.

Woodrow P (2000) Intensive care nursing. London: Routledge.

FURTHER READING

McArdle J (2000) The biological and nursing implications of pancreatitis. Nursing Standard 14(48): 46–51.

This is a thorough and critically analytical review of the care of the patient with pancreatitis. Specific nursing issues are considered, especially capillary blood sampling, and protocols are suggested.

McCreaddie M, Neilson M (2001) Hepatitis C: why all the fuss? Nursing Times 97(11): 34–41.

A comprehensive, well presented account of hepatitis C and its implications for nurses and health care.

Sargent S (2005) The aetiology, management and complications of alcoholic hepatitis. British Journal of Nursing 14(10): 536–562.

This well-written and comprehensive article describes the pathophysiology and mechanisms of alcoholic hepatitis. The illustrations are clear. Management focuses on clinical interventions to control the physical symptoms.

Shovein J, Damzo R, Hyams I (2000) Hepatitis A: how benign is it? American Journal of Nursing 100(3): 43–47.

This article uses a clinical case study as a basis for an approachable but thorough discussion of the nurse's role in caring for a patient with hepatitis A.

17 Caring for the patient with a nutritional disorder

Sue Lee

INTRODUCTION

Nutrition is fundamental to growth, good health and well-being, and malnutrition is a potential cause of, or contributing factor in illness. Therefore, a sound knowledge of the principles of nutrition and the requirements of individuals in health and sickness is vital for nurses to give effective care. However, there are serious doubts about the standards of nutrition provided in care settings such as nursing and residential homes for the elderly and in NHS hospitals. This was highlighted by the Malnutrition Advisory Group (MAG) of the British Association for Parenteral and Enteral Nutrition (BAPEN) whose 2005 report claimed that 60% of hospital patients are malnourished; whilst in care homes the figure is 50%. Malnourished people are likely to stay in hospital longer and need more follow-up care after discharge due to their overall poor health. The BAPEN report estimated that the cost of hospital malnourishment was an extra £226m to the NHS (BAPEN 2005).

Amidst all the modern concern about the problem of obesity, it surprised many people when NICE (2006) issued guidelines stating that patients who are admitted to hospitals or care homes should be screened for malnutrition and urged the need for nutrition support. NICE argue this screening should be extended to include outpatients and also patients registering for the first time at their GP. This is aimed at rectifying the situation identified above by BAPEN

and others (Royal College of Physicians 2002, Savage and Scott 2005). This issue is as much about the key nursing activities of *helping* patients to eat and drink as much as it is the quality and quantity of the food with which they are provided. Nurses must be able to assess a person's nutritional status and feeding ability, relating data from a physical examination to that taken from a dietary history. They must have a knowledge of the requirements of a balanced diet, and the skills to be able to work with clients to devise and implement a plan to meet individual needs.

This chapter identifies the key components of any diet and describes how the body utilizes and metabolizes these nutrients. Means of assessing nutritional status are presented, together with the implications of the findings for nursing care. Recommendations for a balanced diet are identified, as well as a recognition of the needs of those who may be overweight or malnourished. There is a discussion of the ethical and legal difficulties associated with the nutrition of patients who are unable to take food or fluids orally, and who may be unconscious and therefore unable to verbalize their wishes. The cultural and religious influences on diet are also considered.

The provision of food and fluids has long been considered part of the nurturing role of nursing, although the evidence does suggest that nurses have neglected this aspect of caring for patients, particularly the elderly (Royal College of Physicians 2002, Holmes 2003). It has been suggested that this may be due to a growing emphasis on the increasingly expanded nurse's role, a lack of knowledge about assessment of nutritional status and a lack of clarity over responsibility and management (Savage and Scott 2005). Increasing pressure on the nurse's time may also contribute to this growing problem. Nurses need to be knowledgeable and skilful, and grasp the full implications of this aspect of care whether in hospital or the community. Liaison with dietitians and other healthcare professionals is vital, but ultimately it is nurses who are uniquely placed to identify needs and deliver appropriate care.

METABOLISM

PRODUCTION OF ENERGY

Food is essential to provide energy and to supply materials from which cells synthesize chemicals and bodily structures. Energy is required even at rest, when no voluntary physical activity is being undertaken. It is necessary for cellular activity, for the function of the organs of the body and for growth and maintenance of tissues. The amount of energy needed to maintain these involuntary functions at rest is known as the *basal metabolic rate* (BMR). The BMR varies with age, sex and body size, and is influenced by an individual's hormonal activity (especially the thyroid hormone). It is highest in children and adolescents because of their requirements for growth and declines with age. Women tend to have a lower BMR than men. Energy requirements for individuals vary greatly and are related to the BMR. When energy intake equals energy use, body weight is reasonably constant.

Food is taken into the gut and broken down by digestive processes into a form in which it can be absorbed into the bloodstream. From the blood, it is taken up into tissue cells. Some nutrients will be used by the cells to meet material requirements for the construction of tissue, for growth and repair, or for the production of hormones and enzymes. Much of the food, however, will be broken down to produce the energy the body requires.

Within cells, food undergoes the physical and chemical changes that comprise metabolism. When the cellular activity results in the synthesis of tissue substance, the process is referred to as *anabolism* or *anabolic metabolism*. The processes that break down the materials into simpler forms and release energy are called *catabolism* or *catabolic metabolism*.

Energy is stored inside the cells as adenosine triphosphate (ATP). ATP is generated by a mechanism called *phosphorylation* – the addition of a phosphate molecule to adenosine diphosphate (ADP), this reaction requires oxygen (aerobic metabolism).

Fuel + Oxygen + ADP + Phosphate →
Carbon dioxide + ATP + Water

ATP can react subsequently with water to revert back to ADP and a separate phosphate molecule, releasing the energy that was holding the ATP molecule together. It is this energy that drives the cell. The main nutrient that feeds this reaction is glucose and its role is described below.

GLUCOSE METABOLISM

Carbohydrates are absorbed as glucose, fructose and galactose and are the body's main energy source. Fructose and most galactose are converted to glucose by the liver. Some galactose remains as such, and is one of the components of the myelin sheath surrounding nerve fibres. Some glucose circulates in the blood to maintain a relatively constant blood glucose level.

Once glucose enters the cells it can be metabolized in three main ways:

1 It can be broken down completely to produce ATP.
2 It can be converted into glycogen and stored in liver and muscle cells.
3 It can be converted into fat and stored in adipose tissue.

The breakdown of glucose within the cells involves two main processes. *Glycolysis* involves the splitting of a glucose molecule into two pyruvic acid molecules and the release of some energy. The pyruvic acid is then broken down within the cell's mitochondria in a series of chemical reactions, controlled by enzymes, which is known as the *Krebs cycle* (or citric acid cycle). The end-result of the metabolism of one molecule of glucose is the production of water, carbon dioxide and energy (Fig. 17.1):

$$C_6H_{12}O_6 + 6O_2 \rightarrow 6H_2O + 6CO_{2+} + \text{ATP (32 molecules)} + \text{heat energy}$$

Some of the energy released is in the form of heat energy thereby maintaining body core temperature; the remainder is stored within the chemical bonding of the newly formed ATP. The glucose that is not needed to maintain the blood glucose level or as an immediate energy source is converted to glycogen and stored in the liver or skeletal muscle. The muscle cells store it for their own use during contraction. The liver stores glycogen and, as the blood glucose level falls, converts the glycogen back to glucose and releases it into the blood. If the absorbed glucose exceeds what the cells use, and what can be stored as glycogen, it may be converted to lipid (triglycerides) and stored in the fat depots of the body. Insulin plays an important role in both facilitating the transfer of glucose into the cell and in stimulating the deposition of lipid.

LIPID METABOLISM

Our body consists normally of 18–25% lipid or fat. Lipids in food are broken down in the gut into glycerol, fatty acids and monoglycerides. After entering the intestinal mucosa, these recombine into triglycerides, which in turn are coated by proteins to become *chylomicrons*. The chylomicrons enter the lymph system and eventually the blood, where they are

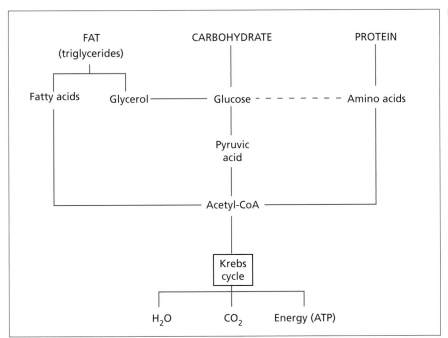

Figure 17.1   Metabolism of food to produce energy.

transported to the cells. Triglyceride molecules may be used by the body as an immediate or future source of energy, or for the synthesis of various compounds such as the eicosanoids (prostaglandins and leukotrienes). Phospholipids, lipoproteins, steroids, cholesterol and various vitamins such as E and K). When **fats** are used to provide energy, the triglycerides are first broken down by the liver into glycerol and fatty acids (lipolysis). Various hormones play a key role in lipolysis, especially epinephrine, norepinephrine, cortisol, thyroid hormones (T3 and T4) and insulin-like growth factors (IGFs). Conversely, insulin inhibits lipolysis.

If required as an immediate source of energy, glycerol is converted to glucose, broken down to pyruvic acid, and metabolized via the Krebs cycle (Fig. 17.1). The fatty acids are split by a series of reactions that occur mainly in the liver. In each reaction, two carbon atoms and energy are released. Two carbon atoms combine with co-enzyme A to form acetyl-CoA, which then enters the Krebs cycle to produce water, carbon dioxide and energy (ATP). Ketone acids are also produced and move out of the liver to be transported by the blood to cells in need of energy, where they are metabolized via the Krebs cycle. Under normal circumstances, the level of ketones in the blood is very low. However, if there is a shortage of glucose in the cells, there may be an increased use of fat as an energy source, resulting in an increase of ketone production. If ketone production exceeds ketone metabolism, *ketosis* will result. This condition may occur in starvation. It is also a feared complication of Type 1 diabetes mellitus where the absence of insulin inhibits the movement of glucose into cells and the state is then known as diabetic ketoacidosis (DKA, see p. 557).

Lipids that are not required for immediate use are stored in fat depots in the body. Most of the fat is deposited in the

subcutaneous tissue, in the abdomen, especially on the mesentery and omentum, around the kidney and between the muscle fibres. This is known as adipose tissue. A certain amount of stored fat is of value. The subcutaneous adipose tissue insulates the body against excessive heat loss and against the cold of the external environment. Adipose tissue also provides a protective cushion for the body against trauma.

Not all the absorbed lipids may enter the liver after a meal. Some of it moves directly into the fat depots so that the concentration of lipids in the blood is quickly lowered. These lipids which have been stored in the tissue can readily be mobilized when needed for energy. There is, therefore, a constant movement of lipid molecules in and out of adipose tissue.

PROTEIN METABOLISM

A normal lean body contains 12–18% by mass of protein. Proteins are extremely complex molecules built up from amino acids which in turn consist of NH_2 (the amino group), COOH (acidic carboxyl group) and a side chain. The side chain part of the molecule varies between amino acids and gives each one its individual chemistry. During digestion, protein in the diet is broken down into its constituent amino acids and in this form absorbed into the bloodstream. Amino acids are sometimes termed the body's building blocks. Tortora and Grabowski (2003) list the following types of protein with examples in brackets:

- structural (collagen in bone, keratin in skin, hair and fingernails)
- regulatory (hormones, neurotransmitters)

- contractile (myosin and actin fibers permit shortening of muscle cells)
- immunological (antibodies, interleukins)
- transporting molecules (haemoglobin)
- catalytic (enzymes).

Protein is not generally used as an energy source, as the essential amino acids are vital for growth and tissue repair. When inadequate supplies of carbohydrate or lipid are available however, for example in starvation, protein may be broken down to provide energy (ATP) (Fig. 17.1). Thus amino acids are used to:

- build and repair tissue and synthesize functional products
- produce ATP after deamination in liver
- convert into glucose or fat after deamination.

The liver is the main organ involved in the metabolism of amino acids. In a process called *deamination*, the amino radical is removed from the amino acid, forming ammonia. As ammonia could be toxic to tissue cells, it is combined with carbon dioxide to form urea, which is subsequently excreted via the kidneys. The residual elements of the amino acid are converted into glucose or fatty acids, which may be metabolized to meet energy requirements.

Some amino acids are described as '*essential*', that is they must be provided in the diet because the body cannot synthesize them in adequate amounts. Others, however, may be synthesized in the liver in a process called *transamination*; the amino group is removed from one amino acid and attached to a molecule of pyruvic acid or to another acid molecule formed during the Krebs cycle.

Protein metabolism is influenced by certain hormones. Growth hormone, thyroxine and testosterone stimulate the use of protein in the synthesis of tissue and cell products. The glucocorticoids promote mobilization of amino acids into the blood from cells and their conversion to glucose.

MEETING NUTRITIONAL REQUIREMENTS

A person requires food for energy and for materials to maintain the structure and functions of the body. These needs will be met by a number of different nutrients including carbohydrates and fats which are prime sources of energy. Protein and certain types of fats are essential for the body's structure and functions and a number of vitamins and minerals are also essential.

Different nutrients have different energy values (Box 17.1). Energy is expressed in joules (the SI unit; kj = kilojoules) or calories. The 'calorie' used in food science is, in fact, a kilocalorie, or 1000 calories. It is equivalent to 4.2 kJ.

CARBOHYDRATES

Sugars, starches and non-starch polysaccharides (NSPs) are known collectively as **carbohydrates**. They all contain

Box 17.1	Energy values of different nutrients
Carbohydrate provides	17 kJ (3.75 kcal)/g
Fat provides	37 kJ (9 kcal)/g
Protein provides	17 kJ (3.75 kcal)/g
Alcohol provides	29 kJ (7 kcal)/g

carbon, hydrogen and oxygen, in the basic unit of $C_6H_{12}O_6$. A monosaccharide (e.g. glucose) contains one such unit; disaccharides (e.g. sucrose) contain two units, and a carbohydrate with many units is described as a polysaccharide (e.g. starch). Sugars and starches may be broken down by the body to provide energy. NSPs are not used as an energy source, but help to maintain normal bowel function. Dietary fibre is more properly known as *non-starch polysaccharide*, and this is how it is labelled on many nutritional products.

Starch is found widely in grains, cereals, root vegetables and legumes. Due to the complex nature of starch molecules, it is digested at a slower rate than simple disaccharides, and therefore releases glucose into the bloodstream at a relatively slow rate. This is particularly in managing patients with diabetes. Dietary fibre is present in starchy foods in large quantities and includes a number of different substances, each with differing properties. As foods contain varying combinations of dietary fibre substances, it is important to eat a range of high-fibre foods.

Dietary fibre may contribute to good health in a number of ways. An increased consumption of it is directly correlated with an increase in stool weight, which in turn helps to prevent constipation. There is also some evidence that low stool weights are associated with increased risk of bowel disorders and gallstones, so that increasing the stool weight may afford some protection. Some types of dietary fibre, especially water-soluble components found in oats and beans, may help to lower blood cholesterol levels.

It is advisable to obtain dietary fibre from food rather than from unprocessed wheat bran, which may impair the absorption of some minerals (e.g. iron, calcium, zinc and copper).

Sugars

The food sugars most important in human nutrition are the monosaccharides, glucose and fructose, and the disaccharides, sucrose and lactose. The effect of sugar in the body is determined not only by the type, but also by the source. Sugars may be classified as *intrinsic* or *extrinsic* (Fig. 17.2).

No detrimental effects on dental health or health in general are attributed to lactose in milk and milk products or to intrinsic sugars. Non-milk extrinsic sugars (NMESs), however, play a significant role in the development of dental caries. It is not only the amount of sugar in sweets, drinks and snacks that is relevant, but also the length of time for which sugar is in contact with teeth. Sugar eaten as part of a meal may cause less decay because it is washed away by

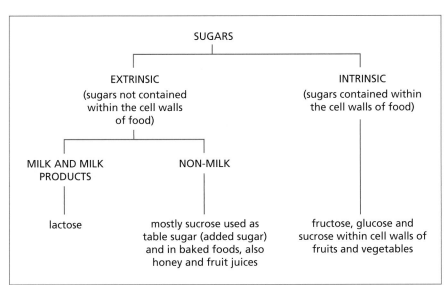

Figure 17.2 Classification of sugars. (From DoH 1991, with permission.)

other food and drink. It is particularly relevant to note that in people aged 65 years and over, the evidence suggests that the better a person's oral health is, including how many natural teeth they have, the better their diets and subsequent nutritional status (Department of Health 1998). Furthermore, the presence of natural teeth (in people not living in institutions) was significantly related to their intake of protein, intrinsic and milk sugars, fibre, calcium, non-haem iron, niacin and vitamin D. The amount of intake of intrinsic sugars and fibre has also been found to be related to the distribution of teeth.

FAT

Fat, as eaten in foods, is a mixture of triglycerides, each composed of a glycerol molecule and three fatty acid molecules. There are three main types of fatty acid:

- saturated fatty acid (saturates)
- monounsaturated fatty acids (monounsaturates)
- polyunsaturated fatty acids (polyunsaturates).

All fatty foods contain a mixture of these fatty acids, although some are more prevalent in particular foods.

Saturates
These are chemically very stable and are solid at room temperature. They are found mostly in foods of animal origin and in hard margarine. A high intake of saturates may contribute to an increase in blood cholesterol level, one of the main risk factors in the development of coronary heart disease.

Monounsaturates
These are found to some extent in meat and dairy products; olive oil and rape-seed oil are particularly rich sources. Substitution of saturates by monounsaturates reduces plasma levels of cholesterol but only to about the same extent as substitution by carbohydrates.

Polyunsaturates
These are chemically less stable. Some polyunsaturated fatty acids are known as *essential fatty acids* because they cannot be synthesized by the body and have to be provided in the diet. Different classes of polyunsaturates appear to have different functions in the body. The n-6 class, principally derived from seed oils and polyunsaturated margarines, reduces plasma cholesterol levels. It also contains essential fatty acids. The n-3 class of fatty acids has an important effect in reducing blood clotting, and therefore reducing a tendency for thrombosis development. These fatty acids are found mainly in oily fish (e.g. mackerel, sardines, herring, pilchard, trout and salmon). The n-3 class also contains essential fatty acids, found primarily in green leafy vegetables.

CHOLESTEROL

Cholesterol is a lipid essential for body function. Apart from being a key constituent of cell membranes, it is required for synthesis of steroid hormones (including sex hormones) bile salts and vitamin D. Most of the body's requirements are synthesized in the liver, although some cholesterol is present in the diet. A high intake of foods rich in saturates increases the synthesis of cholesterol in the liver and slows the breakdown rate, thus raising blood levels. Blood cholesterol levels are influenced more by the total fat content of food than by the amount of cholesterol present in food eaten.

PROTEIN

Protein in the diet is essential, as proteins form part of every cell in the body. Proteins are comprised of amino acids in various combinations. Twenty-two amino acids are used by the body to synthesize the proteins it needs. The liver can inter-convert amino acids, that is, it can synthesize some amino acids from others. There are eight amino acids, however, that are described as *essential* because the body cannot synthesize them and they must be provided in the diet.

Proteins that contain all eight essential amino acids have a high biological value. These proteins come mainly from animal sources such as milk, cheese, yoghurts, meat and fish. Proteins from vegetable sources tend to have a lower biological value. However, when proteins from different sources are eaten together, the relative surplus from one source can supplement the relative deficiency in another. The complementary effect is a mixture of proteins of high biological value. This combining of proteins is particularly important in vegetarian and vegan diets.

VITAMINS

These micronutrients are required for normal growth and maintenance and are involved in the normal metabolism of other nutrients. Nearly all **vitamins** must be obtained from the diet, as the body cannot synthesize them. They are derived from a variety of sources, and a varied diet is the most important factor in ensuring requirements are met. Some are fat soluble (A, D, E, K); others are water soluble.

MINERALS AND TRACE ELEMENTS

These are incorporated in many body tissues and fluids, and are essential components of many hormones, enzymes and transport molecules. Examples include iron, calcium and sodium.

RECOMMENDATIONS FOR HEALTHY EATING

DIETARY REFERENCE VALUES

The 1991 Committee on Medical Aspects of Food and Nutrition Policy (COMA) report on *Dietary Reference Values* (Department of Health 1991) presents advice on the intake of fat, carbohydrates, protein, salt, vitamins and nutrients; this COMA report was and remains significant as the dietary targets specified are still the benchmark.

The report also introduced a number of new terms, which replaced the previous recommended daily amounts (RDAs). These represented an estimate of the average requirements, together with upper and lower limits advocated for good health. These should make it easier to identify a person who is likely to be having insufficient (or possibly an excessive) intake of key dietary constituents.

The dietary reference values include the following terms:

- *Estimated average requirement (EAR)* – this is an estimate of the average requirement for energy or a nutrient. Some people need more and some less than average depending on factors such as pregnancy or recovery from illness
- *Reference nutrient intake (RNI)* – this represents the amount of a nutrient that will be sufficient for about 97% of the population. It is equivalent to the former RDA. This value will be higher than most people will need, and if

individuals are regularly consuming the RNI they are unlikely to be deficient in that nutrient
- *Lower reference nutrient intake (LRNI)* – this amount of a nutrient will be sufficient for only a few people with the lowest 2–3% of needs. Nearly all the population needs more than the LRNI. If an individual habitually eats less than the LRNI, they are at risk of becoming deficient in that nutrient
- *Safe intake* – this is the level of a nutrient that is judged to be adequate for almost everyone's needs, but not so large as to cause undesirable effects. The term is used when there is insufficient information to estimate requirements
- *Dietary reference value (DRV)* – this is a blanket term used to cover all the recommendations. All DRVs refer to the needs of healthy people.

Current advice on nutrition and health is much less prescriptive than before, focusing on achieving and maintaining health generally, and holistically, by following a *balanced* diet with plenty of fruit and vegetables and exercising regularly.

NUTRITIONAL REQUIREMENTS AND RECOMMENDATIONS

In the UK, the estimated nutritional requirements for the population have been described by COMA. The COMA group critically evaluates the evidence and makes recommendations which are then used to inform government policy, such as the Healthy Start initiative (Department of Health 2005a), the National School Fruit Scheme (Department of Health 2003), the Choosing a Better Diet guidance (Department of Health 2005b) and the national service framework for coronary heart disease (Department of Health 1998, 2000).

It is important to remember that nutritional requirements are described in technical terms, using the terminology and definitions provided earlier in this chapter. The *estimated average requirements* for calories, protein, carbohydrate and fat in different age groups and sexes are provided in Table 17.1. Nutritional requirements vary from person to person. Each nutrient has a particular function and all are needed in differing amounts. Our individual requirements are related to age, sex, level of physical activity and state of health. However, many people take in more energy than their bodies actually require, resulting in obesity and potential ill-health. The three main types of nutrient – fat, protein and carbohydrate – all provide energy, as can alcohol – although this should provide no more than 5% of total energy in a person's diet. A poor energy mix in a person's diet may be a factor in diseases such as coronary heart disease and some cancers (Davey-Smith 1998).

In 1994 the COMA report on nutritional aspects of cardiovascular disease was published (Department of Health 1994). This confirmed the government's targets for reduction of fat intake as appropriate. It also made a number of

Table 17.1 Dietary reference values

	Estimated average requirement (kcal/day)		Reference nutrient intake for protein (g/day)		Population average	
	Male	Female			Carbohydrate (as % energy)	Fat (as % energy)
0–3 months	545	515	12.5			
4–6 months	690	645	12.7			
7–9 months	825	765	13.7			
10–12 months	920	865	14.9			
1–3 years	1230	1165	14.5			
4–6 years	1715	1545	19.7			
7–10 years	1970	1740	28.3			
			Males	Females		
11–14 years	2220	1845	42.1	41.2		
15–18 years	2755	2110	55.2	45.0		
19–50 years	2550	1940	55.5	45.0	47	33
51–59 years	2550	1900	53.3	46.5	47	33
60–64 years	2380	1900	53.3	46.5	47	33
65–75 years	2330	1900	53.3	46.5	47	33
751 years	2100	1810	53.3	46.5	47	33
Pregnancy		1200		16		
Lactation						
1 month		1450		111		
2 months		1530		111		
3 months		1570		111		

From Department of Health 1991, with permission.

recommendations relating to dietary intake which are still appropriate today:

1 *Maintain a desirable weight* – a body mass index (BMI) of 20–25 is associated with an appropriate weight for most people (see p. 536 for calculation of BMI).
2 *Carbohydrates should contribute 50% of total daily energy intake*. Non-milk extrinsic sugars (Fig. 17.2) should form a maximum of 10% of total energy intake. Consumption of complex and fibre-rich carbohydrates should be increased (e.g. fruit and vegetables, bread and cereals) (Box 17.2).
3 *Dietary fibre intake should increase to 18 g/day*. This should follow from the increased consumption of fruit, vegetables and cereals and which should compensate for any reduction in dietary energy.
4 *Fat should form a maximum of 35% of total daily energy intake*. A maximum 10% of energy intake should come from saturated fats.

5 *Protein intake of 11% of total daily energy intake* should be ample to meet daily requirements (see Table 17.1 for reference nutrient intake).
6 *Salt intake should be on average no more than 6 g/day.*
7 *Antioxidant vitamin intake (E, C, β-carotene) should be maintained* as they may afford some protection against coronary heart disease (CHD).
8 *Energy levels should be maintained but daily exercise should increase* (for people of normal weight). Table 17.1 shows the estimated average requirements for total daily energy intake.

The recommendations given in the COMA report (Department of Health 1994) are designed to reduce risk factors associated with developing cardiovascular disease and stroke. For other potential disease, the risk factors may be reduced; for example, by increasing dietary fibre intake, problems associated with constipation and bowel disease may be decreased.

Box 17.2   Recommendations for 5 A DAY: portion sizes

Fresh fruit:
- Small-sized fruit: 2 or more, for example 2 plums, 2 satsumas, 3 apricots, 2 kiwi fruit, 7 strawberries, 14 cherries, 6 lychees

- Medium-sized fruit: 1 medium fruit, such as 1 apple, banana, pear, orange, nectarine or 1 sharon fruit

- Large fruits: half a grapefruit, 1 slice of papaya, 1 slice of melon (2-inch slice), 1 large slice of pineapple, 2 slices of mango (2-inch slices).

Dried fruit:
- 1 tablespoon of raisins, currants, sultanas, 1 tablespoon of mixed fruit, 2 figs, 3 prunes, 1 handful of banana chips.

Tinned fruit:
- Roughly the same quantity of fruit that you would eat as a fresh portion: 2 pear or peach halves, 6 apricot halves, 8 segments of tinned grapefruit.

Juices:
- A glass (150 ml) of 100% juice (fruit or vegetable juice or smoothie) counts as 1 portion, but you can only count juice as 1 portion per day, however much you drink. This is mainly because it contains very little fibre. Also, the juicing process 'squashes' all the natural sugars out of the cells that normally contain them, which can be harmful for teeth, especially if you drink a lot of it in between meals.

Green vegetables:
- 2 broccoli spears, 8 cauliflower florets, 4 heaped tablespoons of kale, spring greens or green beans.

Cooked vegetables:
- 3 heaped tablespoons of cooked vegetables such as carrots, peas or sweetcorn

Salad vegetables:
- 3 sticks of celery, 2 inch piece of cucumber, 1 medium tomato, 7 cherry tomatoes.

Tinned and frozen vegetables:
- Roughly the same quantity as you would eat as a fresh portion. For example, 3 heaped tablespoons of tinned or frozen carrots, peas or sweetcorn.

Pulses and beans:
- 3 heaped tablespoons of baked beans, haricot beans, kidney beans, cannelloni beans, butter beans or chick peas. Remember that beans and pulses do count, but only as 1 of the 5 portions, no matter how much you eat.

Potatoes and other related root vegetables:
- Because they are considered a 'starchy' food, potatoes do not count towards your 5 A DAY. (Starchy foods are foods like potatoes, rice, pasta and bread.) We are not suggesting you don't eat them, but they should form the 'starchy carbohydrate' part of your meal.

From Department of Health 2004.

However, the guidelines are not in a form that is readily accessible to the general public. It is very difficult to know exactly what to eat to enable 35% of the total energy intake to come from fats, or for 50% of the energy requirement to come from carbohydrates. In the past, this type of report has been criticized for not enabling people to make the practical changes in their diet that the report advocates.

FOOD GROUPS

If nurses are to be able to advise clients on a nutritionally appropriate diet, they must be aware of the nutritional value of foods that may be available to the client. For this reason, it is useful for nurses to become familiar with the four food groups devised by nutritionalists.

The Nutrition Task Force (NTF) guide emphasizes and clarifies the notion of a 'balanced diet'. However, rather than stating nutritional requirements in terms of DRVs, etc., it shows the different food groups and the different proportions a person should eat, including fats and sugary foods (Box 17.3). Although this has been perceived as a more user-friendly way of getting the healthy eating message across, it has also become obvious that people need more education to understand what constitutes a 'portion', so more specific guidelines have been developed (Box 17.2). In addition to this, the *Balance of Good Health* document recommends an 8-point plan for achieving a healthy diet (Box 17.4). These guidelines are useful and relatively easy to understand. However, proportion and types of foods also have to be considered. It is unnecessary to try to achieve a full balance

---

Box 17.3   Summary of food groups

Bread, other cereals and potatoes
- Recommendations: eat lots.

Milk and dairy foods
- Recommendations: eat and drink moderate amounts and choose lower-fat versions whenever you can.

Fruit and vegetables
- Recommendations: eat lots (at least 5 portions a day, excluding potatoes).

Meat, fish and alternatives
- Recommendations: eat moderate amounts and choose lower-fat versions whenever you can.

Foods containing fat, foods containing sugar
- Recommendations: eat foods containing fat sparingly and look out for the low-fat alternatives

- Foods containing sugar should not be eaten too often, as they can contribute to tooth decay.

From Department of Health 2004.

Box 17.4   Guidelines for a healthy diet

1 Enjoy your food.

2 Eat a variety of different foods.

3 Eat the right amount to be a healthy weight.

4 Eat plenty of foods rich in starch and fibre.

5 Don't eat too many foods that contain a lot of fat.

6 Don't have sugary foods and drinks too often.

7 Look after the vitamins and minerals in your food.

8 If you drink alcohol, drink within sensible limits.

From Department of Health 2004.

---

of all nutrients at one meal; instead, this should be considered over a full day or even a week (Department of Health 2005a). Foods are grouped according to their nutritional content, with foods in the same group having a similar range of nutrients, or similar role in the diet (Box 17.3). For example, foods in the milk group are a good source of protein, calcium and B group vitamins. For an adult, an adequate balanced diet would include a number of portions from each of the five groups.

The size of the portion would depend on the dietary requirements of the individual. Children, adolescents and nursing mothers require more portions (three or four) from the milk group, because of their need for calcium and protein. Within each of the groups there is scope for a wide variation of nutritional intake (Department of Health 2005a). Within the milk group, for example, a person could drink whole milk or skimmed milk, eat Cheddar cheese or cottage cheese; the difference in fat content of the alternatives would be substantial. The vitamin content of fruit and vegetables may vary considerably according to the storage and cooking. Nurses should advise on the importance of a balanced diet, including food from all five food groups. Whilst recommendations are to reduce fat intake, fats are essential to health and well-being and are an important source of vitamins. Severe diets, which exclude a range of nutrients, may cause health problems of their own.

It should be noted that; the *Dietary Reference Values* (Department of Health 1991), the *Health Start* (Department of Health 2005a) and *Choosing a Better Diet* (Department of Health 2005b) guidelines and suggested portions of the five food groups, refer to essentially healthy individuals. When illness or disease is present the ability or desire to eat may be absent or limited, and specific dietary regimens may be necessary to promote recovery. Often insufficient attention is paid to the dietary requirements of the ill (Best and Thomas 2001, Holmes 2003) and malnutrition in hospital is not uncommon.

It is therefore vital that nurses thoroughly assess their patients to determine their nutritional status and individual dietary requirements. If, as a result of this initial assessment, there appear to be problems associated with nutrition or metabolism, a further assessment by a dietitian and physician may be required.

FOOD ALLERGIES

It appears that the incidence of food allergies within the UK is on the increase and that these may involve life-threatening anaphylaxis (McKevith and Theobald 2005). Further evidence suggests that babies and children are more likely to develop a food allergy where there is a pre-existing history of eczema, asthma or hayfever and that exclusive breast-feeding for 6 months is recommended (Fewtrell 2004). Some foods are commonly involved in allergic reactions:

- milk
- eggs
- wheat
- peanuts
- nuts
- seeds (especially sesame)
- fish and shellfish.

Some people may be allergic to just one of these or to a range of foods. It is extremely important that anyone who has a suspected allergy seeks professional advice including referral to a specialist. There are a number of tests which can be performed; these should take place under close medical supervision. Once a diagnosis has been made, the particular food and anything containing it must be avoided; an auto-injector epinephrine (adrenaline) 'pen' should be carried in case of accidental ingestion. Obviously, avoiding such ingredients may be time-consuming and difficult and is dependent on the quality of food labeling. Optimal management must take into account the requirements of a nutritionally balanced diet and this may be extremely taxing when faced with multiple allergies.

FACTORS THAT INFLUENCE DIETARY PATTERNS

Dietary behaviour is influenced by physiological, psychological, sociocultural and environmental factors, as well as knowledge of food and food requirements. The consumption of food is usually a social activity; eating habits are very complex and are resistant to change as they become an integral part of the individual and family lifestyle.

Physiological factors influencing nutritional needs and eating behaviour include the individual's metabolic rate, growth phase, body excretions, reproductive functions and level of daily physical activity. Increased energy and nutrients are required by the individual during periods of rapid physical growth, pregnancy and lactation, increased metabolic rate (e.g. hyperthyroidism) and increased physical activity. Fewer kilocalories are needed by elderly individuals because of their lower basal metabolic rate and decreased activity, and by those with sedentary lifestyles.

The hypothalamus, the limbic system of the brain and gut hormones regulate food intake by influencing appetite, hunger and satiety. *Hunger* is a physiological phenomenon involving unpleasant sensations of abdominal discomfort and irritability, which prompt the individual to search for food. *Appetite* involves the conscious desire to eat. *Satiation* is the pleasant feeling of being fully satisfied after a meal. *Anorexia* is the abnormal loss of the desire to eat, and may be influenced by both physiological and psychological factors.

Emotions are important in determining eating behaviour. Food has different meanings for each individual, and responses to stress or happiness are often expressed as changes in eating habits. Some individuals respond to stress and decreased self-esteem by overeating, whereas others have loss of appetite and decrease their food consumption. It is possible that some people may experience both increases and decreases in consumption depending on the degree of stress perceived. Eating habits are believed to be formed early in life and become fixed responses.

Sociocultural factors influencing eating behaviour include religious and ethnic practices and the use of foods that have special meaning for the individual and family. The media also play an important role in influencing food consumption. Advertisements relating to specific foods have an impact on individuals and families; the portrayal of an 'ideal' body appearance greatly influences dietary intake and patterns of food consumption in girls and young adult females (Gilbert 1999). Sociocultural factors also influence the proportion of meals eaten in restaurants as opposed to the home, and the quality of restaurant chosen. 'Fast food' chains tend to have foods of higher saturated fat and salt than might be consumed in a meal prepared at home. Social class may affect diet, with knowledge about what constitutes a healthy diet being greater in higher social class families.

Environmental factors include the availability, cost and convenience of foods. The individual's income may be inadequate to meet the cost of the essential foodstuffs, or disability may limit a person's ability to prepare food or shop for food. The environment in which food is prepared and eaten also influences eating behaviour. Appetite is usually stimulated when eating takes place in a pleasant and relaxed social milieu.

Knowledge of dietary requirements and food values is an important factor in the individual's or family's eating patterns. In some instances, persons may not understand that in planning a balanced diet, expensive food elements can usually be substituted by less expensive items that will meet the essential dietary requirements.

These non-biological influences on the use of food may contribute to the development of nutritional disorders and are important restraining factors when attempting to change eating habits.

ASSESSMENT

HEALTH HISTORY

Any assessment of a person's nutritional status must obtain details about lifestyle and health status. A number of factors must be considered.

Age and sex
Both will influence a person's basal metabolic rate, and therefore their energy requirements, and may influence other dietary needs (e.g. for protein and calcium).

Typical diet
It is important to get the patient to describe their typical diet over 1 week, for example to gauge the extent to which they are eating a healthy diet or otherwise.

Alcohol consumption
This should be assessed as apart from its general health significance, alcohol is an important source of calories, especially beer.

Ethnicity, culture and religion
The types of food eaten may be influenced by family traditions and cultural identity, although people may not adhere strictly to the religious dictates on diet.

Activity and rest
The number of calories needed daily will be determined by energy expenditure. Occupation and daily activity should be noted, together with how the person feels following physical activity. Rest and sleep should also be assessed in relation to the normal pattern.

Elimination

Bowel habits should be determined, together with information relating to the nature, formation, colour, odour and frequency of stools. The use of laxatives or supplementary fibre should be assessed. The volume, frequency and colour of urine, as well as the presence of nocturia or urgency and frequency is important as is the use of diuretics, and the urine should be tested for abnormalities.

Medical history

Existing medical conditions or previous surgery or illnesses are important, together with the impact (if any) that these have had on the diet consumed and future dietary requirements. Check for any allergies and include medications (both prescription and over the counter).

Socioeconomic factors

Issues such as marital status and family grouping are important, as is the usual pattern of taking meals (e.g. in company or alone, eating out or eating at home). A key factor is who actually prepares the food, as any health education intervention aimed at improving a families' diet needs to start with the cook. Presence or lack of employment may be considered. Other social and economic factors may be relevant (e.g. whether the person has cooking facilities, and whether they are able to store and prepare food independently). The availability of shopping facilities and the ability to go shopping may be considered, together with economic factors relating to the ability to purchase sufficient food to meet the needs of the person and/or family.

PHYSICAL EXAMINATION

Table 17.2 gives an indication of clues you may pick up to suggest that a nutritional disorder or problem may be present.

- *General body appearance*, including the patient's general stature and posture, distribution of body fat and state of alertness. The skin is inspected for rashes, lesions, pet-

Table 17.2	Assessment of the patient's nutritional status		
	Characteristics of good nutritional status	**Characteristics of poor nutritional status**
Nutritional intake	Usual daily food intake contains basic food groups and all essential nutrients Fluid intake 1500–2000 mL/day Balanced calorie intake for size and activity	Some food groups and essential nutrients missing from diet Calorie intake less than or greater than that required for body size and activity Fluid intake <1200 mL/day Abuse of laxatives and diuretics
Physical examination		
General body appearance	Stands erect Alert Abdomen flat	Drooped shoulders Inattentive Abdomen protruded
Weight	Constant In proportion to height and body size	Variable >20% under or over suggested weight for height and body type
Body mass index	BMI 20–25	BMI <20 or >25
Skinfold thickness	Within 80% of standard value for age and sex	>20% above or below standard value for age and sex
Circumference measurement	Body muscle stores are within 90% of standard value for age and sex	Body muscle stores <80% of standard value for age and sex
Skin	Clean and intact	Dry, transparent, scaly with petechiae
Oral mucous membrane	Clean, moist and intact	Gums swollen and bleeding
Teeth	Clean, smooth, regular edges, straight and symmetrical and intact	Dental caries Discoloration Irregular edges Malpositioned and absent teeth
Lips	Smooth, intact	Red and swollen with fissures
Hair	Shiny and clean	Dull, listless and brittle
Nails	Smooth, shaped and intact	Brittle, ridged, irregular edges
Eyes	Clean, focused Conjunctiva pink and moist	Sunken Conjunctiva pale Discharge

echiae, bruises and change of colour. The oral mucous membranes, tongue, lips, teeth and gums are observed, as well as hair, nails and eyes

- *Height and weight* are measured and recorded, and changes in body weight over given periods are identified. The BMI can be calculated to give an indication of the appropriateness of the weight for height (Box 17.5). BMI is simply the weight in kilograms divided by the square of height (measured in metres)
- *Skin-fold thickness* is measured to determine the amount of subcutaneous fat. Callipers are used to measure the skin-fold thickness over the triceps. Results are compared with a table of normal values for age and sex
- *Mid-arm circumference (MAC)* measurements are taken. The circumference of the mid-arm muscle can be calculated by using this measurement and the triceps skin-fold thickness. This value can then be compared with a table of normal values. These calculations provide information on the body's muscle stores
- *A functional assessment* may be carried out to determine whether a patient is physically able to hold cutlery and feed him or herself. The patient's ability to chew food (noting whether their own teeth are adequate or dentures are well fitting) and ability to swallow food should also be considered.

DIETARY HISTORY

The history should include an account of the person's typical diet. Key aspects are:

- Times of meals and snacks, methods of preparing food and circumstances under which food is consumed
- An estimate of the quantity of foods eaten, using familiar measures (e.g. three egg-sized potatoes, two tablespoons of rice, a large glass of milk)
- Details about specific types of food consumed, for example type of milk (whole or skimmed), spread (butter, sunflower margarine, low fat spread), bread (white or wholemeal)
- Food preferences or dislikes; food allergies
- Average daily fluid intake and types of drink consumed, paying special attention to both alcoholic and fizzy soft

drinks both of which are prolific sources of calories. The latter also contain substantial amounts of caffeine which could be impacting upon behaviour, especially in teenagers, not to mention sugar which could have significant implications for dental health

- Appetite
- Whether there is a history of recurrent dieting
- Any consumption of dietary supplements
- Any consumption of snacks, type of snack and frequency.

The nurse or dietitian may wish to investigate further and the patient may be asked to keep a food record or diary for a few days (e.g. 3 days–1 week). The dietitian may estimate the amount of specific foods consumed daily and convert this into energy and nutrient intake in grams, milligrams or micrograms, using food tables. It is then possible to compare the client's nutritional intake with the dietary reference values, giving an indication of the adequacy of the diet.

As well as establishing what a person eats, the nurse must ascertain what a patient knows about the nutritional and energy values of food regularly consumed.

DIAGNOSTIC TESTS

Depending on the information obtained from the health and dietary histories and physical examination, it may be deemed useful to carry out blood and urine studies. These will reflect changes in the metabolism of carbohydrates, proteins and fats, and may be used to determine the level of vitamins and minerals.

OBESITY

Obesity may be clinically defined by a person's BMI (Box 17.5). The prevalence of obesity in the UK, as in the rest of the developing world, is increasing. It is now estimated that 75% of the UK population are overweight (BMI >25) or obese (BMI >30) while the number of clinically obese adults has increased by 400% since 1980. Not only that but one-quarter of British children have a weight problem that poses a risk to health (Gooding 2005).

HEALTH RISKS

There may be considerable risks to health from being obese. The incidence of CHD is high in obese men and women. The distribution of fat about the body appears to be relevant. Men and women with excessive abdominal fat (central obesity or apple shape) are at greater risk of CHD and diabetes mellitus than when the distribution is focused around the hips and thighs (peripheral obesity or pear shape) (Daniels 2002). It appears that abdominal fat is not just a passive layer of extra tissue but that it is metabolically active and in such a way as to predispose to a range of disorders that have given rise to the phrase 'metabolic

---

Box 17.5 Body mass index (BMI)	
The BMI is calculated by dividing a person's weight (in kilograms) by the square of their height (in metres):	
	Weight (kg) / Height^2 (m)
BMI <20	underweight
BMI 20–25	normal (desirable) range
BMI >25 but ≤30	overweight
BMI >30	obese
From Department of Health 1994, with permission.	

syndrome' (see Ch. 14). For this reason, the hip:waist ratio may sometimes be calculated (see Ch. 14).

Metabolic changes may be related to obesity. The linkage between obesity and type 2 diabetes is well known (see Ch. 14). Repeated unsuccessful attempts at weight loss may exacerbate these risk factors.

In addition to the metabolic changes and their associated increase in health risk factors, there is the psychologically stressful effect of being overweight. There are considerable social pressures to be thin, and those who are sensitive to the pressure to conform to the ideal may suffer from a poor body image and low self-esteem.

FACTORS RELATED TO OBESITY

Obesity results from an intake of energy that is in excess of the energy expended by the individual. The excess calories are stored, mainly as triglycerides, in the form of adipose tissue. There may be environmental, genetic, behavioural, physiological, psychological and socioeconomic factors influencing the development and/or maintenance of obesity. Of these factors, many are hard to control or influence. Those most readily amenable to change involve:

- the type of diet consumed (energy intake)
- voluntary physical activity (energy expenditure).

BMR is a major factor in determining energy expenditure, but is not amenable to change.

When the level of voluntary physical activity remains the same, it is ultimately the number of calories consumed that will determine the amount of fat stored. It is irrelevant as to which food source the calories come from, but it has been observed that diets high in fat may be more conducive to the development of obesity. Obesity contributes to several health problems including sleep apnoea, metabolic syndrome (including type 2 diabetes mellitus), joint and back problems such as osteoarthritis, varicose veins, stress incontinence and gall bladder problems (Pi-Sunyer 1999); even some moderate weight loss (3–8 kg) can reduce these debilitating and potentially serious problems (Drummond 2002). The cause of obesity for any individual will be a unique combination of factors. However, it is thought that lack of exercise, particularly in children, probably makes a bigger contribution to the problem than excess calorie intake. Before progress towards weight loss can be made, assessment of the person's health and dietary history is vital.

ASSESSMENT OF PEOPLE WHO ARE OBESE

Health history

In addition to the information gathered for a general nutritional assessment (Table 17.2), the individual should be questioned about their history of weight fluctuations, past attempts at weight control, and any pattern of restricted eating followed by binging. Any history of depression or drug and alcohol abuse or dependency should be noted. A family history of weight problems, hypertension, diabetes mellitus or heart disease should also be identified. The nurse should probe for dissatisfaction regarding body weight and shape. It is important to discern the daily pattern of eating, amount of food intake and crucially, the exercise pattern.

Physical assessment

Height and weight should be measured and the BMI calculated. Hips and waist may be measured for possible calculation of the hip:waist ratio. Blood pressure should be recorded.

Laboratory investigation

Medical assessment should include thyroid function, glucose tolerance, triglyceride, lipoprotein and cholesterol levels. Diagnosis and treatment of medical disorders is essential before actual treatment of obesity.

IDENTIFICATION OF PATIENT PROBLEMS

The exact nature of the problems will vary between individuals, but most are likely to have a mismatch between nutritional intake and body requirements. Self-concept and body image may also be disturbed.

POTENTIAL GOALS FOR THE OBESE PATIENT

The goals may be said to have been achieved if the patient is able to:

1 state the components of a nutritionally balanced diet
2 describe the potential effects of excessive weight and body fat on health
3 describe and implement a plan to increase physical activity
4 eat a diet containing essential food groups
5 space intake of food over the day
6 recognize feelings of hunger (as opposed to appetite) and satiety
7 state positive attributes of the body and self
8 resist weight preoccupation
9 state the dangers of severe food restriction.

NURSING INTERVENTION

Prevention of obesity is an important aim of nursing. However, given the many complex and multiple causes of obesity, the effectiveness of interventions will vary. The first treatment of choice for obesity is dietary management. However, if obesity is life-threatening, the treatment of choice may be hospitalization for gastric stapling surgery, calorie restriction and/or appetite-suppressant drug therapy. In this case, the role of the nurse involves emotional support and daily measurement of weight and food intake.

The majority of people with a weight problem are treated in the community. Nurses have a vital role in assessing clients and supporting them in their attempts to reduce or stabilize their weight. When assessment reveals that an individual's weight problem is related to overeating or lack of activity, the nurse can have an impact through education and support. This will be focused on three major areas: reducing energy intake, maintaining motivation and increasing exercise. Anti-obesity drugs may be necessary in the management of obesity for some patients. There is evidence to support improvements in weight loss with orlistat and sibutramine and sustained weight loss that continues after treatment albeit at a slower rate (NICE 2000, 2001).

Whichever approach to obesity management is taken, the patient is also going to need help with behaviour change and motivation (see Ch. 1 for an overview of Prochaska and DiClemente's (1986) cycle of change).

REDUCING ENERGY INTAKE

When working with a client on a weight reduction programme there are a number of dietary factors to consider (Drummond 2002):

1 The intake of energy must be reduced from the client's usual.
2 A balanced diet is essential.
3 Foods from each of the five groups should be eaten, but the following advice noted:
   a) *milk and milk products* – use low-fat varieties of products (e.g. semi-skimmed or skimmed milk, cottage cheese, low-fat yoghurts)
   b) *fruit and vegetables* – eat at least five portions daily
   c) *bread and cereals* – eat varieties high in dietary fibre; eat smaller portions
   d) *meat and meat alternatives* – trim all fat off meat, avoid products with high fat content.
4 Fat intake should be reduced (cooking methods may need to be changed).
5 Consumption of non-milk extrinsic sugars (Fig. 17.2) should be reduced.
6 Protein levels should be maintained.
7 A regular meal pattern should be established, usually involving three meals a day.
8 A list of foods to be eaten freely and foods to be avoided should be available.

MAINTAINING MOTIVATION

Nurses must consider a client's lifestyle, religious beliefs, financial restrictions and dietary preferences when advising about a diet. It is also important to stress the long-term nature of weight reduction and maintenance of a desirable weight. Weight loss need not be dramatic, but changes in dietary habits should be incorporated into a person's lifestyle and be sustainable over a period of time. Motivation is crucial to success. Targets for weight loss should be realistic and encourage the client to persevere with a steady weight loss. Clients should also be made aware that occasional lapses will not lead to excessive weight increases. The guilt feelings that accompany a lapse may cause the client to abandon the diet.

INCREASING EXERCISE

Increased exercise will hasten weight loss but, more importantly, will help a client to develop a positive attitude to their body and feel good about themselves. In those who are very obese, exercise should be introduced gradually and should not be strenuous because of the risks to the cardio-vascular system. It could include walking instead of using a car or public transport. For those who are only moderately overweight more vigorous exercise may be suggested, but this should be built up gradually and be within the limits of their health. Clients should be aware that vigorous exercise may increase their appetite, but maintaining a reduced energy intake is vital to weight loss.

For some clients who have a history of repeated dieting followed by weight gain, it may be preferable for them actually to stop weight reduction programmes, stabilize eating and increase activity levels.

EVALUATION

Prevention of obesity is of primary importance in preventing the numerous risk factors for ill-health. People with an established weight problem can be helped, but success becomes less likely as the degree of excess weight increases. Frequent evaluation of progress towards goals needs to be carried out by the patient and nurse in order to monitor progress, although measuring the patient's weight is only one method of evaluating success. The patient should be advised that maintaining weight (i.e. not gaining any more) is in itself an achievement. Changes to the plan should be made as necessary (see Case Study 17.1).

CASE **Obesity**

Mrs Shore is a 45-year-old woman with a long-standing history of obesity following the birth of her first child. She is 5 feet 6 inches tall and weighs 100 kg. She came to see the practice nurse for help and advice as she had recently been told she is a 'borderline hypertensive' (blood pressure 152/92 mmHg). Rather than start immediately on any antihypertensive treatment Mrs Shore had been advised to lose some weight. Mrs Shore was both angry and upset about this advice, stating that it was judgemental. Previously, she had attended various slimming clubs and lost varying amounts of weight. However, the weight always crept back on slowly over time. Mrs Shore stated quite categorically that she would not countenance 'counting calories' and that she did not want to do anything like going to a gym or health club as they were too expensive and time consuming and 'they're only for thin people, anyway'.

The practice nurse used her knowledge, skills and experience to assess Mrs Shore holistically. She knew that any goals and interventions must be decided upon with Mrs Shore's full participation and collaboration. She was also aware of the implications for Mrs Shore of developing hypertension, and of other potential health problems such as diabetes mellitus and coronary heart disease.

Between them, they decided that Mrs Shore's goal should be to eat healthily rather than 'go on a diet'. It was important for Mrs Shore not to become preoccupied with weight loss, so the practice nurse suggested that Mrs Shore weighed herself only once a week and should aim for a slow (1 kg per week) but steady loss over a long period of time. They discussed Mrs Shore's normal eating patterns and meal preparation and how these could be altered to make them healthier. Mrs Shore said she 'gets the munchies' quite late in the evening when watching TV, so ways of coping with this were addressed (treats were allowed as long as they were in small amounts; trying fruit and lower-fat alternatives). They also discussed shopping ideas. The practice nurse also provided some written healthy eating literature with recipes to support the discussion.

Mrs Shore has a dog and was amenable to taking brisk walks three times a week. The practice nurse encouraged her to take her family along, if possible, to make these more sociable and enjoyable.

Finally, Mrs Shore was encouraged to return to the surgery for weekly, then monthly, weigh-ins and blood pressure recordings. The practice nurse also suggested that, as time progressed, she would keep in telephone contact with Mrs Shore to see how her weight loss and motivation were being maintained.

It is important to remember what a demanding change this can be in a person's life and simultaneously what huge benefits they may gain by successfully making the appropriate changes in their life. It would be completely normal for Mrs Shore to have periods of relapse and this requires sensitive and empathetic nursing care in order to avoid any sense of blame or damaging effect on Mrs Shore's self esteem.

UNDERNUTRITION

Undernutrition occurs when the energy intake is less than the energy expenditure. Body fat is depleted for energy, and protein, mineral and vitamin deficiencies develop. The individual is likely to be underweight compared with ideal-weight charts.

RELATED FACTORS

Undernutrition may result from inadequate food intake or a pathophysiological condition. The cause of inadequate food intake may be:

- famine, unavailability of food
- poverty, which prevents the individual from obtaining sufficient food
- inability to shop for or prepare food, such as may occur in the elderly, disabled or housebound individual

- lack of knowledge of essential nutritional needs
- influence of the mass media in promoting nutritionally unbalanced 'junk foods'
- emotional disturbance (such as eating disorder, extreme fear of fat or desire to be thin)
- pathophysiological conditions. These include those that interfere with ingestion, digestion, absorption and/or metabolism of food; increase the body's requirements for energy; or result in loss of body fluids and their constituents.

IDENTIFICATION OF PATIENT PROBLEMS

The problem will be a nutritional intake of less than the body requirements. The exact cause of this will determine the precise goal and the nature of the nursing interventions.

POTENTIAL GOALS FOR THE UNDERNOURISHED PATIENT

The individual will be able to:

1 demonstrate understanding of basic nutritional needs of the body
2 gain weight progressively towards the normal range
3 where appropriate, express awareness of any underlying emotional disturbances
4 follow a prescribed dietary regimen where possible and, if indicated, with a counselling or psychotherapy programme.

NURSING INTERVENTION

When undernourishment is caused by pathological conditions, nursing care is directed towards alleviating the contributory symptoms such as nausea or diarrhoea. In palliative care, it may not be possible to meet the demands of the patient's nutritional needs (see Ch. 11) and in certain gastrointestinal disorders, the patient's ability to digest and absorb the necessary nutrients may be impeded (see Ch. 15) and they may even require parenteral nutrition (see p. 473). In some patients, malnutrition may arise from inadequate food intake which may in turn be caused by a variety of socioeconomic factors. This is a worldwide problem, existing in industrialized countries as well as in developing nations. Alleviation of this problem requires increasing the world's food supply and its distribution, as well as providing economic assistance to those in need. Individuals and families require knowledge of basic nutritional needs as well as assistance in the selection and preparation of foods to ensure an adequate diet within the limits imposed by their sociocultural and economic situations.

Assuming adequate food is available, the following interventions are needed for the underweight individual:

- providing information about basic nutritional needs of the body. This may be by discussion and the provision of pamphlets that outline a dietary plan containing the essential food groups (Box 17.3)

● identifying the causes of inadequate nutrition
● assisting the individual to develop a diet that will promote the development of body tissue.

Being thin may currently be fashionable, and peer pressure appears to reinforce the idea; girls go on diets more frequently than boys during the teenage years, the proportion increases to 16% of girls between 15 and 18 years of age (NDNS 2000). The appetite suppressing effect of nicotine may combine with the desire to be thin, to add the extra burden of smoking to poor diet in teenage girls. Simply increasing calorie intake may serve only to increase body fat; the diet should be balanced and contain extra protein as well as carbohydrates and fats. Calcium intake is important in order to build up bone mass as an insurance against the effects of post-menopausal osteoporosis in later life. However, it is very difficult to motivate teenage girls to make the link between what they eat today and their health in 40 years time. Meals should be regular and between-meal snacks of protein and complex carbohydrates encouraged. Moderate activity serves to build body tissue, but adequate and regular rest is essential to conserve energy and promote weight gain.

When emotional disturbances are the primary factor of malnutrition as, for example, in the patient with anorexia nervosa or bulimia nervosa, intervention is focused on identifying the underlying emotional cause. This is a long-term process that requires counselling and psychotherapy for the patient and usually the family as well. The person needs help to acquire a realistic appraisal of self and body, which may be distorted. Harmful and bizarre behaviours need to be identified and attitudes changed. The patient may have to be admitted to hospital at certain times during their illness.

EVALUATION

Evaluation of the undernourished patient should be based on a variety of factors including their psychological health, their self esteem and their physical well-being. Weight gain may be seen by the nurse as the ultimate goal of care, but an overemphasis on frequent weighing can cause disillusionment. Developing a knowledge of the nutritional needs of the body and the components of a balanced diet can be seen as progress. Sometimes the resolving of other physical or psychological problems, such as nausea or depression, will result in an improvement in nutritional status (see Case Study 17.2).

UNDERNUTRITION IN HOSPITALIZED PATIENTS

Undernutrition in hospital patients is a longstanding problem (Holmes 2000, Best and Thomas 2001, Holmes 2003, BAPEN 2005). It will require a multi-disciplinary approach which may involve re-organizing the way food is delivered to the bedside to rectify this situation. Inadequate food intake, especially when it is associated with illness, reduces the patient's nutritional status, slowing recovery and rehabilitation. Undernutrition in hospital patients may result in impaired wound healing (Shepherd 2003), an increased risk of infection (Ward 2002) and delayed rehabilitation (Gibbon 2002). Worse still, patients who are not provided with adequate nutrition are more likely to die (Royal College of Physicians 2002).

There may be many factors affecting patients' eating habits in hospital, in addition to those directly related to their medical condition. The quality of the food served, the presentation, quantity and temperature of the meal will effect food consumption. The presence or lack of company, and the position in which the patient eats the meal (leaning sideways out of bed, for example), can affect a person's ability to finish a meal. In many hospitals, the distribution of meals and collecting of plates afterwards is carried out by non-nursing staff. Nurses therefore have to be particularly vigilant to observe what patients eat and what they leave on their plates.

Savage and Scott (2005) have reported that given competing demands, nutritional assessment and subsequent interventions were not prioritized by nurses within a hospital setting. Their report highlights the fragmented nature of nutritional care and the implications of a clear lack of ownership which contribute to a patchy and probably under-funded aspect of care. Recognizing that there may be a constellation of problems contributing to patients' poor nutrition in hospitals the NHS has embarked on a series of initiatives to improve the services and the associated care under the banner of *Better Hospital Food*. For instance, *Protected Mealtimes* is designed to ensure that patients are provided with an undisturbed mealtime, to give them time to eat a meal without rushing or being disturbed; nurses should also have the time to be able to assist patients with eating.

This has now culminated in the NICE guideline referred to at the start of this chapter (NICE 2006). Apart from setting out a comprehensive list of the types of patients that should have their nutritional status assessed, the guidelines also require trusts to appoint a specialist nutrition support nurse and a nutrition steering committee. To be aware of patients' needs, a nutritional assessment should be made on admission and at regular intervals throughout the hospital stay. Frequent liaison with the dietitian is essential, so that action may be taken before patients become malnourished. Measures may be required to improve the nutritional status of many patients, particularly those in intensive care and during the postoperative period.

Savage and Scott (2005) identified a range of nursing responsibilities which must be fulfilled in order for nutrition to be improved. These included an initial nutritional assessment undertaken by nurses, with subsequent monitoring and referral to specialist staff where appropriate. The BAPEN

Malnutrition Universal Screening Tool (MUST) is available as a readily accessible screening tool (www.bapen.org.uk) that can be used for such a purpose. Nurses have an obvious role in helping patients to complete menu cards and should also ensure that patients receive their chosen meal, including special diets. Nursing staff should help to serve meals with the help of domestic staff, such as housekeepers. Ward staff should also be able to provide snacks (such as toast and tea) for patients. Nurses should be available to help patients who may need help with eating, and nursing work should be organized around protected patient mealtimes in order to gain maximum benefit from this.

CASE **Undernourishment in hospital**

Mr Booth, aged 72, was admitted to hospital following a severe stroke. He had a right hemiparesis, including difficulty swallowing and speaking. He also had diet-controlled diabetes (diagnosed last year). Mr Booth's clothes hung loosely; his daughter said he looked as if he had lost a lot of weight recently; his wife died 6 months ago and he had been depressed ever since.

The staff nurse who admitted Mr Booth fully understood his nutritional needs and the potential difficulties involved. She knew that it was important to obtain Mr Booth's body mass index (BMI) so that his progress could be monitored. As Mr Booth was unable to stand, she ascertained his height by measuring his arm span (Ward and Rollins 1999) and then weighed him using the ward sit-down scales. A BMI of <20 meant that Mr Booth was, in fact, underweight and his score was 18.5.

Because of Mr Booth's dysphagia and dysphasia, he was referred to the dietitian so that his swallowing reflex could be assessed. Initially, he was commenced on nasogastric feeding but, as his swallowing reflex improved over the following 3 days, the nasogastric feeding was withdrawn and Mr Booth was given thickened supplements to help him swallow. Daily weighing showed an initial weight loss, and Mr Booth developed two small (2 cm) grade 2 pressure sores: one on his right buttock and the other on his right heel.

The occupational therapist was involved at an early stage and Mr Booth was provided with specially adapted cutlery and crockery to help him feed himself. At first, a student nurse stayed with and helped Mr Booth cut up his food and eat. It was a time-consuming process: Mr Booth did not like to feel rushed and it took him time to chew his food properly. However, the student nurse was very patient and gave Mr Booth time and support. She also encouraged him to choose from the hospital menu. Mr Booth began to put weight back on slowly – he gained 2 kg while in hospital. The pressure sores also showed signs of improvement.

Before discharge, the dietitian discussed Mr Booth's dietary requirements with him and his daughter. Mr Booth's daughter was very pleased to discover that her father would not need 'sloppy food' and understood how to use the modified cutlery provided.

This case study demonstrates the complex interplay between social situations, psychological status and physical conditions that can lead to undernourishment. Mr Booth would require further support in the community from the district nursing team, community occupational therapist and the extended primary healthcare team to continue with his steady progress. He may also need assessment by the social worker and may benefit from involvement in community groups and activities. Skilled nursing care can have an enormous impact on patients like Mr Booth making your role in his rehabilitation process extremely important. Box 17.6 provides a summary of care for the undernourished patient, and highlights the need for liaison with all members of the multidisciplinary team.

UNDERNUTRITION DUE TO WITHHOLDING OF NUTRITIONAL SUPPORT

ETHICAL ISSUES

The withholding of nutritional support from a patient is one of the more controversial dilemmas faced by patients, families and healthcare professionals. The provision of food and water holds moral and emotional significance, and the symbolic value of providing nourishment may be far greater than any resulting therapeutic benefit. Advances in medical technology make it possible to offer nutritional support via a nasogastric tube, a gastrostomy tube or central venous catheter to patients who would otherwise die as a result of their inability to swallow fluids and diet. This poses the dilemma as to when nutritional support should be given, and whether it is ever ethically justifiable to withhold food and fluids.

LEGAL IMPLICATIONS

There are no clear guidelines for doctors or nurses in the UK. The position in law is unclear, and decisions regarding whether nutritional support is given or withheld are generally made by doctors in consultation with the family. The case of Anthony Bland has clarified the situation a little, but left it unclear in other respects.

Anthony Bland was crushed at a football match (the 'Hillsborough Disaster') and suffered brain damage. His brainstem functions were intact, he could breathe unaided, cough, blink and respond to loud noises, but he had no higher brain activity. He remained unconscious and was diagnosed as being in a persistent vegetative state (PVS). He was fed and hydrated via a nasogastric tube. He was not brainstem dead, but there was no possibility of his condition improving. His parents fought to have the artificial nutrition and hydration withdrawn, and the case of *Airedale NHS Trust v. Bland* was taken to the House of Lords in 1993. The Law Lords upheld both the Court of Appeal and High Court decisions, stating that 'it was not unlawful for doctors to

---

Box 17.6   Critical summary: the undernourished patient

Nurse

1   Record patient's height and weight; calculate BMI (weight in kg/height in metres^2).

2   Weigh patient daily.

3   Pressure sore risk calculation; re-assess according to level of identified risk.

4   Liaise with multidisciplinary team members.

5   Ensure patient has access to food, appropriate cutlery and crockery.

6   Monitor and record all food and supplements intake, including snacks.

7   Ensure that patient is given time and appropriate assistance to eat; involve relatives (as per patient's wishes).

8   Monitor and record bowel movements, particularly diarrhoea.

9   Monitor and record nausea and/or appetite.

10   Discuss discharge dietary needs with patient and carers.

Occupational therapist

1   Swallowing assessment within 48 hours (for patients with stroke or motor neurone disease).

2   Assessment and monitoring of consistency of food required.

3   Assessment and monitoring of progress of motor coordination and activities of daily living (e.g. muscle strength).

4   Provision of modified cutlery and other aids to assist food intake.

Dietitian

1   Calculate and record calorific and metabolic requirements.

2   Order dietary supplements and discuss food preferences with patient.

3   Liaise with pharmacy re: dietary supplements and feeds required.

4   Calculate actual calorific intake.

5   Discuss discharge dietary needs with patient and carers.

Doctor

1   Initiate referrals to multidisciplinary team members.

2   Assess and discuss causes for poor nutritional status.

3   Prescribe parenteral feeds if necessary.

4   Review patient's progress.

Pharmacist

1   Liaise with dietitian re type and amount of feeds and dietary supplements required.

2   Provide feeds and dietary supplements.

---

withdraw life-supporting medical treatment, including artificial feeding from a patient in a PVS who had no prospect of any recovery or improvement, when it was known that the discontinuance of treatment would cause the patient's death within a matter of weeks'. The ruling stressed that it was applicable only to the case in question, and that in any future cases an application should be made to the courts. However, shortly afterwards, in the case of *Frenchay Health Trust v. S*, the courts allowed an emergency declaration that the health authority refrain from providing life-saving treat-

ment for a patient in a PVS, on the basis that it was in the patient's best interests.

The United Kingdom Central Council for Nursing, Midwifery and Health Visiting (UKCC) was asked to give evidence to the Select Committee on Medical Ethics (House of Lords 1993) following the Bland case. The terms of reference stated that the Committee was appointed 'to consider the ethical, legal and clinical implications of a person's right to withhold consent to life prolonging treatment, and the position of persons who are no longer able to give or withhold consent' (House of Lords 1993, p. 140). The UKCC highlighted the dilemma facing many nurses in caring for patients requiring life-supporting measures, and the difficulty in making a distinction between 'killing or letting die', when the action taken in withholding support results in the patient's death. The judgement in the Bland case was made on the basis of the patient's 'best interests', but the UKCC noted that this raises the question of who is to be regarded as the arbiter of the best interests of the patient. The views of relatives may at times be in conflict with those of healthcare professionals. The UKCC recommended that all relevant professionals should discuss the way forward, seeking to take account of those closest to the patient (who may or may not be relatives). If no consensus emerges, then the case may need to be taken to court, but this should not normally be necessary.

One other situation that is occasionally encountered by nurses working within the prison service concerns the patient who goes on hunger strike and refuses any food. This is a grey area but the general approach taken in the UK is that if the person is lucid (i.e. not psychotic) it would be assault to attempt to force feed such a person. Consequently, they should be allowed to starve themselves to death if necessary, as happened for example in the case of IRA hunger striker, Bobby Sands. Other countries may take a different position on the legality of force feeding a hunger striker.

CLINICAL FACTORS

The issue of withdrawal or withholding of nutritional support is related to many more patients than those in a PVS. Patients who have suffered a cerebrovascular accident may have lost their ability to swallow, and patients with cancer of the larynx or oesophagus may be unable to swallow food or fluids. In terminal illness, particularly in the end stages, patients may lose the desire and ability to eat. Patients with acquired immune deficiency syndrome (AIDS) often have severe weight loss in the terminal stages of their illness, and gastrointestinal dysfunction prevents adequate intake of nutrients. Patients who are unconscious for whatever reason will require artificial hydration and nutrition. In every situation where patients are unable to meet their own hydration and nutritional requirements, a decision will need to be taken as to how these requirements will be met.

For each patient there will be a balance between the benefits and burdens of nutritional support. It is important that the patient is consulted; fluids and food should be given, or not given, according to the patient's wishes, provided that he or she is mentally competent to make the decision. Tube-feeding causes discomfort and may not be in the best interests of terminally ill elderly patients as it carries the risk of aspiration pneumonia, and diarrhoea is a common side-effect (Eberhardie 2002).

For terminally ill patients, the provision of good nutrition in the end stages is unlikely to prolong life, and the aim is the maintenance of comfort and dignity. There is an ongoing debate as to the merits of continuing to hydrate patients who cannot drink or eat in the last few days of life. Some contend that a reduced fluid intake may result in a potentially painful and distressing state of dehydration, which requires artificial hydration therapies (i.e. administration of intravenous, nasogastric or subcutaneous fluids). Other workers suggest that dehydration may actually benefit patients by relieving distressing symptoms; incontinence may be reduced, and a reduction in pulmonary secretions will lessen coughing and reduce the need for tracheal suction. Eberhardie (2002) discusses the evidence both for and against hydration in the terminally ill patient as this remains a controversial topic, and makes the point that the relative's perception that the withholding of nutrition and fluids from their family member may cause distress and they may feel it has directly contributed to an earlier death. Decisions regarding the provision or withdrawal of food and fluids must be made with the patient and their relatives. The more aggressive forms of hydration and nutrition support, such as intravenous feeding, can be distressing to relatives, and they may be afraid of going near the equipment or disturbing it. This may prevent them from getting close to the dying patient. For these patients, it may be that local measures to relieve thirst and a dry mouth, such as sucking ice-chips, may be more appropriate.

ETHICAL DECISION-MAKING PROCESS

In 1999, the British Medical Association produced some guidelines for ethical and legal decision-making when considering treatment withdrawal. First, clinical staff have a duty of care towards any patient who is able to swallow, and in such cases food and drink should be offered. Any mentally competent adult also has a right to information about his/her condition or illness, so that they can make their own decision about their treatment, refusing it if they so desire. Patients should be consulted with regard to their treatment plans, and carers may be involved in this wherever appropriate. It is clear that tube feeding is now understood in the law to be a medical treatment. Finally, where a patient is not mentally competent, then the consultant in charge of that patient's care is responsible for all therapeutic decisions, including any to withdraw nutrition and hydration.

When it is identified that an individual's nutritional state is inadequate or deteriorating, the nurse should discuss this with the dietitian and doctor. If an ethical conflict arises regarding the provision of nutritional support, all responsible individuals should participate in determining its resolution. Patients and their families may be unaware of the options for nutritional support and nursing staff should initiate discussion appropriately and facilitate enquiries. If the patient is conscious, every effort should be made to fulfil the patient's wishes, involving them in discussion as appropriate. The intent of a patient's behaviour (e.g. when turning their head away, or not opening their mouth, or pulling out tubes) is often difficult to assess, but the team must work alongside the patient and relatives to try to find the most acceptable way forward. If the patient is unconscious the clinical team, together with the relatives, need to make a decision. However, relatives cannot make a decision *on behalf of* a patient (Lennard-Jones 2000). The patient may have made a 'living will', expressing a desire to avoid being dependent on life support systems. These statements, however, rarely refer to nutrition and hydration support. Accurate records summarizing discussions (as fully and clearly as possible) and identified wishes must be kept in the patient's notes.

Intravenous feeding is expensive, and the nursing hours involved in caring for an unresponsive patient for weeks, months or even years are considerable. The cost implications are very significant. The UKCC, in its evidence to the select committee, emphasized its opposition 'to decisions being led on the grounds of cost and economics'. It stressed that 'it must always be the patient's best interests and not the financial position of a purchasing authority or agent that is the determining factor' (House of Lords 1993, p. 141). Eberhardie (2002) suggests that when the patient's condition falls into the early palliative care stage, then providing good nutritional care should be prioritized as this contributes to overall sense of well-being and may enhance recovery enough to facilitate the patient finalizing legal and personal matters.

IMPLICATIONS FOR NURSES

The provision of nourishment to patients may be viewed as symbolic of the caring and nurturing nature of nursing. The withholding or termination of nutritional support to patients may provoke strong feelings in the nurse and may be morally offensive. In certain clinical situations, nurses may feel that, by providing food and fluids by technical means, they are prolonging a person's dying rather than supporting life. In other situations, they may feel that the lack of adequate nourishment is contributing to the patient's death.

Ethical decisions about a patient's care should be made by the healthcare team in collaboration with the patient or family. Whilst the decision may be, in the words of the Bland case, 'to withdraw life-supporting *medical* treatment', in practice it is *nursing* care that is being withheld. Nurses must therefore ensure that they are active in continuing to give the patient all the care they require in support of this decision. Moistening the patient's lips and frequent cleansing of the mouth are necessary to prevent and alleviate any feelings of thirst or discomfort. Continual psychological support to the patient and relatives is essential.

NUTRITIONAL NEEDS OF THE OLDER PERSON

There is evidence that a lifelong good diet is an important determinant of good health in older people (Holmes 2000). The nutritional requirements of older people vary only a little from those of younger adults, but older people may be more susceptible to malnutrition. There are a number of factors that may influence their desire and ability to eat and absorb food:

- *Teeth* may be in poor condition or dentures ill-fitting
- *Appetite* may be reduced as the senses of taste and smell deteriorate with age
- *Social circumstances* influence the desire to eat: cooking for one and eating alone may seem a waste of effort. Cooking facilities may be limited. Income may be low and ability to purchase a balanced diet may be limited
- *Functional ability* may be impaired, and the ability to buy food, cook and eat may be restricted
- *Knowledge* of nutritious foods and requirements of a balanced diet may be poor; individuals may never have needed to cook before their spouse died
- *Health* – ill-health may impinge on the appetite or ability to eat
- *Digestive processes* – the ability to absorb foods may decrease with age (see Ch. 15).

The consequences of poor nutrition in elderly people are well documented in terms of susceptibility to infection, increased risk of developing pressure ulcers, delayed wound healing and a variety of deficiency disorders that significantly reduce quality of life.

Nurses need to be aware of the nutritional needs of their older clients and to be able to advise on ways in which they can maintain a good nutritional status, bearing in mind any limitations of the circumstances or abilities. The dietary requirements are similar to those of any adult. Patients should be advised about the benefits of fruit, vegetables and fish and added salt in the diet should be reduced. However, such advice needs to deal with the reality of the low incomes which many pensioners have to survive on. The need to maintain moderate levels of physical exercise such as walking should also be stressed.

The Department of Health (2005b) recommendations on reducing fat and sugar intake are relevant, but balance is very important. In the context of elderly patients with poor appetites, this means that advice which suppresses food or nutrient intake (even where theoretically too much saturated fat or inadequate amounts of fibre are consumed) is potentially harmful. In elderly patients, maintaining a good appetite is extremely important. Although elderly people do sometimes have more difficulty in maintaining a regular bowel habit, increasing their non-starch polysaccharide intake too markedly may reduce their energy intake.

For hospitalized patients, nurses have a vital role in assessing nutritional status, liaising with the dietitian if appropriate and ensuring that patients receive an appropriate diet. Nurses are responsible for making sure that patients have appropriate food and for recording the amounts of food eaten. If insufficient amounts of food are consumed, dietary supplements may be recommended. However, supplements should be used by nurses according to local guidelines or on the specific advice and prescription of a dietitian, as recommended by Savage and Scott (2005). This paper makes a number of other suggestions to help maximize food intake, including paying attention to the mealtime environment in hospitals. With a little consideration to decor, freedom from interruptions and seating arrangements, patients may be tempted to eat a little more. In 2001, Best and Thomas reported on their experience of improving practice with a nurse nutrition team. They found that team activities could be used effectively as a basis for making 'significant changes' in the way that staff provided nutrition for their elderly patients.

CULTURAL AND RELIGIOUS INFLUENCES ON DIETARY HABITS

Food is one of the most obvious aspects of an individual's cultural identity, and is closely related to religious, social and economic circumstances. Within the UK today, there is a wide diversity of ethnic, religious and cultural backgrounds and a corresponding variety of preferred dietary behaviour. All over the world, societies have developed traditional eating patterns, based on locally available foods and influenced by cultural and religious beliefs (Chappiti et al 2000).

HEALTHY ASPECTS OF TRADITIONAL DIETS

Many of the traditional diets of people from minority ethnic groups now living in the UK could be considered healthy in the light of the 2005 Department of Health guidance *Choosing a Healthy Diet* action plan. People from Bangladesh, African-Caribbean and Mediterranean countries, for example, have a tradition of eating a large variety of fish and seafood products. The Department of Health exhorts us to eat more oily fish. Regular consumption of a great variety of fresh fruits and vegetables is a healthy aspect in the diet of many people from black and minority ethnic groups, again recommended by the Department of Health. Many millions of people in the Far East and Asia eat vegetarian diets. These are healthy when nutritionally balanced, and involve complementary foods such as beans or pulses with cereals, and are eaten with adequate fresh fruit and vegetables.

The amount of fat in the average British diet is considered by the government to be too high. Yet the diets of many people from minority ethnic groups have much lower fat contents and a higher ratio of polyunsaturated to saturated fats. Many people from African and African-Caribbean communities eat soup and stews regularly. These are prepared with cereals, beans and root vegetables, and therefore are high in fibre and low in fat. These cooking methods also help to reduce the loss of some vitamins and minerals.

POSSIBLE CAUSES FOR CONCERN IN TRADITIONAL DIETS

The diet of many societies evolved over generations is often very healthy. However, the effects of coming to a colder climate, and many traditional foods being unavailable (or expensive), together with the influences of a British diet can have adverse effects on the health of individuals. In some diets, for example in Chinese cuisine and African-Caribbean diets, a lot of salty foods or added salt is used. This may be appropriate in a hot climate to compensate for loss of sodium through perspiration, but can be a contributor to hypertension when sodium loss is minimized. Rickets (caused by vitamin D deficiency) is now relatively uncommon in the white population of the UK, partly due to the fortification of margarine with vitamin D. However, for Asians who use ghee (clarified butter) instead of margarine, and who may be vegetarian, there may be an increased incidence.

The variety of fruit and vegetables may have become severely restricted for many people compared with what they may have been used to. There is often a very good range of traditional fruit and vegetables in shops and markets serving communities where there is a large minority ethnic population, and supermarkets do stock a wide variety. However, because of the need to import the fresh produce, it is generally more expensive. This may lead to vitamin deficiencies.

Although a vegetarian or vegan diet can be nutritionally balanced, there is some risk that there may be deficiencies, particularly of protein, vitamin B_{12}, riboflavin, vitamin D and calcium (Chappiti et al 2000). Deficiencies are more likely in a group that has moved away from its country of origin, as subtle changes may occur, and even if one or two commonly consumed foods are missing this may cause deficiencies. Changes in the source of foods can also have an effect. For example, rice in south-east Asia is a good source of calcium and iron, containing 600% more calcium and 380% more iron than rice quoted in British food tables (*Effective Health Care* 1997).

There is evidence that people, particularly young people from black and other minority ethnic communities, have an increased consumption of snacks and other processed foods, such as crisps, biscuits and high-fat take-aways. The consumption of refined sugar has also increased, especially of fizzy and sugary drinks, sweets and the consumption of tinned fruit in syrup (*Effective Health Care* 1997). This is in marked contrast to the traditional diets in many countries, where fresh fruit would be eaten as snacks rather than commercial products. There is a high incidence of diabetes, coronary heart disease and hypertension in African-Caribbean and Asian communities in the UK. No clear contributory factors have emerged, and their diets do not appear to be, on average, higher in fats than that of Europeans, although there may be a relatively high consumption of refined sugar in some diets. However, it is clear that for many communities in the UK the 'Westernization' of their diet may bring increased health risks (Chappiti et al 2000).

THE INFLUENCE OF RELIGION ON DIET

Food is not only a way of obtaining nutrients. For nearly all people, meals are important, having social and possibly religious significance. Food is central to celebrations and commemorations, but the preparation and presentation of everyday meals are related to social and cultural norms. In many countries, cooking is a time-consuming activity and (often) the women in the household may spend a large proportion of their day in food preparation. With changing economic trends and more women in employment, there have been inevitable changes in the pattern of meals consumed and the relative value placed upon them.

For some minority ethnic groups there are special concepts surrounding the nature of food, and for others there are clear religious codes that dictate the preparation and serving of a meal. However, it is important to remember that there is wide diversity in these communities and many members may be quite relaxed about their observation of food-related rules. The individual's preferences must be assessed at all times and no automatic or stereotypical assumptions made.

In general, Hindus will not eat beef, and are often vegetarian. Some may eat mutton, poultry, fish and eggs, whereas others follow a vegan diet. Sikhs will tend not to eat beef or pork, but usually eat mutton, poultry, fish, eggs and diary products. Islam provides directives relating to food preparation and eating. Food laws are derived from the Koran, which forbids the consumption of alcohol, pork, carnivorous animals and some birds (see Case Study 17.3). All meat consumed by Muslims must be from animals killed by ritual slaughter (Halal), and utensils that have come into contact with pork or pork products cannot be used for cooking. Buddhists are vegetarian or vegan, eating no food of animal origin.

'Observant' Jews also have regulations governing the consumption and preparation of food. They will not eat pig products or shellfish, and only kosher meat from a kosher butcher should be eaten. Milk and meat foods must be kept apart in cooking and eating. All utensils used in the preparation and serving of either food must be washed and kept separately (e.g. crockery, cupboards, ovens and tea-towels). Meat and milk dishes may not be served at the same meal, and a period of 3 hours must elapse after a meat meal before foods containing milk can be consumed. However, many Jews do not follow the strict dietary dictates of Orthodox Judaism outlined above, just as in other religions there will be a wide range of diversity in religious observance.

CASE

'Hot bread!'

Mrs Kay, a 68-year-old Muslim, was admitted to the female orthopaedic ward at 10 p.m., with a fractured neck of femur having been in the A&E for 4 hours waiting for a bed. She spoke very little English; her 18-year-old granddaughter acted as an interpreter and informant but was sent home when Mrs Kay was settled into the ward.

That night Mrs Kay slept well but became very agitated at breakfast time when she was given porridge and orange juice on a tray. She spat the porridge out, failed to open the orange juice carton and pushed the tray away, which was then removed. 'Bring me "hot bread!"' she demanded, 'hot bread!' The nursing staff gave her a bread roll with some butter and jam; this was also refused.

The dietitian visited Mrs Kay later that day as she had already refused her entire lunch of ham salad, demanding 'hot bread' again. Although the dietitian understood the requirements of a Muslim diet, she was unable to ascertain Mrs Kay's preferences, nor did she understand the request for 'hot bread'.

By this time, Mrs Kay was very upset and shouting at everyone. She was transferred, still protesting loudly, into a single side-ward. Her family visited early in the evening, just as Mrs Kay was being served curry and rice (as ordered by the dietitian). Mrs Kay took one bite and refused the rest. She had eaten nothing for 36 hours and had drunk very little. Her urine output was poor and her vital signs were at the lower end of the normal range.

Mrs Kay's granddaughter spoke to the nurse in charge and explained that her grandmother did not like very spicy food. She was appalled and very annoyed that her grandmother had been offered a ham salad. She also explained that 'hot bread' meant 'toast'. A letter of complaint was received by the hospital 2 days later: it alleged neglect, lack of knowledge and racism.

Reflection
- What are the issues here and who for?
- How and when could these needs and problems have been identified?
- What nursing actions could have prevented these problems arising?
- What potential physiological complications could ensue here?

THE IMPORTANCE OF BALANCE IN TRADITIONAL DIETS

The observance of these directives will vary between individuals and communities. There are, however, other concepts that may significantly affect an individual's eating habits, but are unfamiliar in Western diets. These concepts often involve balance. Many people from Bangladesh, India and Pakistan hold to the concept of 'hot' and 'cold' foods. The actual temperature of the food is unimportant. 'Hot' foods are meat, ginger, dates and spices – they have pungent, acidic and salty tastes. 'Cold' foods are milk products, cereals, potatoes, fruits and leafy vegetables. The latter are foods that are sweet, bitter, sour or astringent. Groups of people who use this Unani system believe that sickness is produced by an imbalance of humours. Healing can be achieved by eating foods containing the opposite qualities to those of the humour that is out of balance.

In traditional Chinese medicine, good health similarly depends on maintaining a balance of two opposite elements, 'yin' (cold) and 'yang' (hot). When this balance is altered, a person may become ill. To help a person's recovery, an appropriate diet is very important. Some foods have 'heating' (yang) and others 'cooling' (yin) properties. Other foods are neutral. The property of a food is not related to its temperature when eaten, although boiling and stir-frying tends to make foods 'colder' (more yin), and stewing, roasting and deep frying all increase the food's 'heat' (its yang properties). Yang foods include meat, herbs, alcoholic drinks, ginger, pepper, spices, oils and fats. Fish, rice and some vegetables are regarded as neutral (yin yang), and yin food includes some fruits and vegetables.

These concepts may be unfamiliar to Western thinking, where associations with foods do not appear to have any such spiritual or symbolic significance. Yet a knowledge of the Unani (hot/cold) system, and yin and yang concepts is particularly important for people involved in the provision of food to those who are ill. These food beliefs and preferences may strongly affect what people will eat. What may seem a nutritionally appropriate meal to a nurse, may be quite unacceptable to an ill patient. Even in health, it is very important. A pregnant Bangladeshi woman is considered to be in a 'hot condition', and would therefore eat fewer 'hot' foods, such as chicken, meat and eggs, but aim to restore balance in the body by eating more 'cold' foods such as milk, cereals, fruit and vegetables.

IGNORANCE AND APATHY?

There is a relative lack of understanding and provision for the needs of black and other minority ethnic groups within the UK. Progress is being made and the provision of traditional foods in nurseries, schools, hospitals, day centres and workplace canteens is slowly increasing. In hospitals, the provision of adequate food of a type that can be consumed by ill patients is vital. In the community and in hospital, the detection of health problems that may be related to diet is essential and cultural and religious influences should be considered when a patient is assessed. There has been only a brief consideration here of some of the cultural and religious influences on diet. Nurses, whatever their cultural background, must explore the specific dietary needs of the people with whom they are in contact, and recognize the centrality of food in the maintenance and restoration of health.

SUMMARY

In every contact with clients, in hospital or in the community, nurses have a unique opportunity to assess needs, liaise with other health professionals, plan and implement care in order to ensure that individuals' nutritional needs are met. To do this, nurses must have a knowledge of the metabolic processes whereby food can be transformed and used by the body. Nurses must know how to undertake an assessment of nutritional status and how to use the information gathered to plan care. They must be familiar with recommendations for a healthy diet and know how these can be related to the diets of clients with whom they are working. There are increasing numbers of obese people in our communities, and nurses should be aware of their needs and how to help individuals gain and maintain a desirable weight. Conversely, there are many who are vulnerable to becoming malnourished and underweight, and nurses have a duty to help this client group. Nurses also have a particular responsibility towards those who are unable to maintain their own nutrition. The provision of nutrients by either enteral or parenteral routes may, however, be surrounded by ethical dilemmas. Nurses should not shy away from these issues, but must be involved in the resolution of these difficult decisions in each individual case. Nurses should have an awareness of the needs of people whose diet may be influenced by their religious beliefs or their cultural heritage. A detailed knowledge of their eating patterns, beliefs, and possible causes for concern in the diet will help nurses to ensure the individual's needs are met in a positive and supportive manner.

Nutrition is vital to the maintenance of health and wellbeing, and to the restoration of good health. Nurses have a fundamental responsibility to promote good nutrition and to address the complexity of factors that are known to have an impact on the nutritional status of the patients with whom they work.

REFERENCES

BAPEN (2005) The cost of disease related malnutrition in the UK and economic considerations for the use of oral nutritional supplements in adults. British Association of Parenteral and Enteral Nutrition. Online. Available: www.bapen.org.uk

Best C, Thomas S (2001) Improving practice with a nurse nutrition team. Nursing Standard 15(19): 41–44.

Chappiti U, Jean-Marie S, Chan J (2000) Cultural and religious influences on adult nutrition in the UK. Nursing Standard 14(29): 47–51.

Daniels L (2002) Diet and coronary heart disease. Nursing Standard 16(43): 47–52.

Davey-Smith G (1998) Influences throughout the life course: from early life to adulthood. Social inequalities in coronary heart disease: opportunities for action. London: National Heart Forum and The Stationery Office.

Department of Health (1991) Dietary reference values for food energy and nutrients for the United Kingdom. Committee on Medical Aspects of Food and Nutrition Policy. Report on Health and Social Subjects 41. London: HMSO.

Department of Health (1994) Nutritional aspects of cardiovascular disease. Committee on Medical Aspects of Food and Nutrition Policy. Report on Health and Social Subjects 46. London: HMSO.

Department of Health (1998) Health service circular HSC 1998/074: national service frameworks. Leeds: NHS Executive. Online. Available: www.open.gov.uk/doh/coinh

Department of Health (2000) The national service framework for coronary heart disease. London: Department of Health.

Department of Health (2003) The national school fruit scheme. London: Department of Health.

Department of Health (2004) What counts. Portion sizes. London: Department of Health. Online. Available: www.5aday.nhs.uk/WhatCounts/PortionSizes.aspx

Department of Health (2005a) Healthy start. Information for health professionals. London: Department of Health.

Department of Health (2005b) Choosing a better diet: a food and health action plan. London: Department of Health.

Drummond S (2002) The management of obesity. Nursing Standard 16(48): 47–52.

Eberhardie, C (2002) Nutrition support in palliative care. Nursing Standard 17(2): 47–52.

Effective Health Care (1997) The prevention and treatment of obesity, Vol. 3, No. 2. York: NHS Centre for Reviews and Dissemination, University of York.

Fewtrell MS (2004) Breastfeeding as a prophylaxis against atopic disease prospective follow-up study until 17 years old. Lancet 346: 1065–1069.

Gibbon B (2002) Rehabilitation following stroke. Nursing Standard 16(29): 47–52.

Gilbert H (1999) Weight watching. Nursing Standard 14(6): 12.

Gooding L (2005) The Big Question. Nursing Standard 19(46): 25–26.

Holmes S (2000) Nutritional screening and older adults. Nursing Standard 15(2): 42–44.

Holmes S (2003) Undernutrition in hospital patients. Nursing Standard 17(19): 45–52.

House of Lords (1993) Minutes of evidence taken before the select committee on medical ethics, 15 June. United Kingdom Central Council for Nursing, Midwifery and Health Visiting. London: HMSO.

Lennard-Jones J (2000) Legal and ethical aspects of feeding. NT Plus 96(17): 7.

McKevith B, Theobald H (2005) Common food allergies. Nursing Standard 19(29): 39–42.

National Diet and Nutrition Survey (NDNS) (2000) National diet and nutrition survey: young people aged 4–18 years – Vol. 1: report of the diet and nutrition survey. Norwich: The Stationery Office.

NICE (2000) Orlistat for treatment of obesity in adults – full guidance. Online. Available: http://www.nice.org.uk/page.aspx?o=15724 [Accessed 31.03.2006].

NICE (2001) Guidance on the use of sibutramine for the treatment of obesity in adults. Online. Available: http://www.nice.org.uk/page.aspx?o=23017 [Accessed 31.03.2006].

NICE (2006) Nutrition Guideline, National Institute for Health and Clinical Excellence. Online. Available: www.nice.org.uk

Pi-Sunyer F (1999) Comorbidities of overweight and obesity: current evidence and research issues. Medicine and Science in Sports and Exercise 31(11): 602–608.

Prochaska JO, DiClemente CO (1986) Towards a comprehensive model of change. In: Miller WR, Heather N, eds. Treating addictive behaviours: processes of change. New York: Plenum.

Royal College of Physicians (2002) Nutrition and patients: a doctor's responsibility. London: Royal College of Physicians.

Savage J, Scott C (2005) Patients' nutritional care in hospital: an ethnographic study of nurses' role and patients' experience. London: RCN Institute.

Shepherd AA (2003) Nutrition for optimum wound healing. Nursing Standard 18(6): 55–58.

Tortora G, Grabowski S (2003) Principles of anatomy and physiology, 10th edn. New York: Wiley.

Ward J, Rollins H (1999) Screening for malnutrition. Nursing Standard 14(8): 49–53.

Ward D (2002) The role of nutrition in the prevention of infection. Nursing Standard 16(18): 47–52.

FURTHER READING AND USEFUL WEBSITES

British Association for Parenteral and Enteral Nutrition website: www.bapen.org.uk

Contains much important information about hospital nutrition and also their Malnutrition Universal Screening Tool (MUST)

Chappiti U, Jean-Marie S, Chan J (2000) Cultural and religious influences on adult nutrition in the UK. Nursing Standard 14(29): 47–51.

This article could prove to be especially useful to nurses who would like to be able to offer appropriate dietary advice to patients/clients from other minority ethnic groups and provides some basic level information which links dietary needs to religious belief. Some very useful resources for different ethnic groups are indicated.

Ellis J, Cooper A, Davies D et al (2000) Making a difference to practice: clinical benchmarking, Part 2. Nursing Standard 14(33): 32–35.

This is the second of two articles that explore the use of clinical benchmarking in nursing practice. Nutrition benchmarking factors and benchmark statements of best practice are identified. The article is relevant to nurses who are thinking of benchmarking as a way of addressing continuous quality improvement, and ensuring the effectiveness of nursing practice.

Lennard-Jones J (2000) Ethical and legal aspects of fluid and nutrients in clinical practice. Nursing Times Clinical Monograph no. 37. London: NT Books.

This monograph is excellent value at £4.95; it summarizes the legal and ethical positions succinctly and in jargon-free language. The author links the underpinning pathophysiology with the professional concerns.

McKevith B, Theobald H (2005) Common food allergies. Nursing Standard 19(29): 39–42.

This is a really interesting and welcome article which describes common food allergies, the testing and diagnostic process and the management of food allergy. Given the increasing incidence of food allergies in the population and the lack of specialist services, it is extremely likely that nurses will find themselves dealing with a patient (or colleague or relative) with this condition. The article provides a useful overview as well as links to appropriate organizations.

National Obesity Forum website: www.nationalobesityforum.org.uk

Gives a review of the obesity problem. Alternatively, visit the Association for the study of Obesity at www.aso.org.uk

NICE guideline on malnutrition screening (2006) Online. Available: www.nice.org.uk

Savage J, Scott C (2005) Patients' nutritional care in hospital: an ethnographic study of nurses' role and patients' experience. London: RCN Institute.

This is a well-written and focused piece of primary research investigating nurses' and patients' experiences of nutritional care. In terms of UK nurses, this is extremely comprehensive and written in jargon-free language. The underpinning clinical problems are accounted for and the

findings are clear and well-related to real-life practice. It is available via the public section of the RCN website.

The Better Hospital website: http://195.92.246.148/nhsestates/ better_hospital_food/bhf_content/introduction/home.asp
This website contains much useful information both for patients and professionals interested in nutrition. It is an easy site to navigate with good external and internal links and some excellent resources, including recipes and information on initiatives such as protected mealtimes.

5 a day: http://www.5aday.nhs.uk/
This NHS website is very clear and user-friendly with lots of advice and helpful tips for professionals (and the public). Portion sizes are explained, recipes are presented, there are downloads and resources, as well as some games for use with reluctant fruit and vegetable eaters. The health professionals area has sections for data and evidence and discusses the barriers to the 5 a day recommendation.

18 Caring for the patient with a disorder of the endocrine system

Wendy Fairhurst-Winstanley

INTRODUCTION

A gland is an organ that extracts substances from the blood and produces one or more new chemical substances, referred to as secretions. Glands may be classified as exocrine or endocrine. The secretion of an *exocrine gland* is carried along a duct into a body cavity or to the external surface of the body. Examples of such glands are the salivary, gastric, mammary and sweat glands. *Endocrine glands* do not have ducts; their secretions, which are called *hormones*, pass directly into the blood and act on remote tissues.

The glands usually cited as composing the **endocrine system** are shown in Figure 18.1. Unlike other body systems in which the component organs are located close together and are connected, the glands are situated in various parts of the body.

Coordination and integration of the development and functions of the body that maintain homeostasis are dependent upon the nervous system and the endocrine system. The endocrine system is concerned mainly with growth, maturation, metabolic process and reproduction. The action of each hormone is specific. One hormone may modify the activity of all body cells (e.g. thyroxine); others affect the activity of only one particular organ (e.g. adrenocortico-trophin). The site of action of any hormone is referred to as the *target organ* or *tissue*.

Target cells contain *receptors* for which specific hormones have an affinity. Some hormones are necessary for survival (e.g. adrenocorticoid hormone); others are not essential to life (e.g. gonadal secretions).

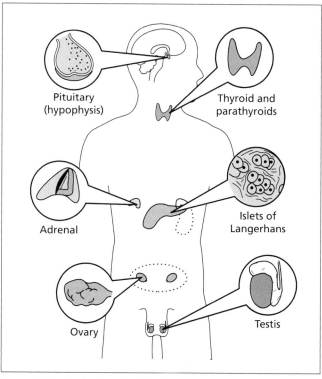

Figure 18.1 Endocrine glands in the body.

MECHANISM OF HORMONE ACTION

Hormones are transported in the blood either freely in solution or in combination with a carrier protein. The water-soluble hormones bind with the receptors on the surface of the target cells. The steroids and thyroid hormones require a carrier for transportation to the target cells and bind with intracellular receptors.

Hormones that bind with surface receptors on the target cells act by altering a membrane-bound enzyme which stimulates the production of a 'second' messenger in the cell; the second messenger then activates enzymes within the cell to produce the specific cellular functions. The second messenger is believed in most instances to be cyclic adenosine monophosphate (cAMP).

Steroid hormones cross the membrane of cells containing their specific receptors and bind with the intracellular receptors. The receptor is altered by the hormone, allowing it to enter the cell nucleus and combine with the chromatin of certain genes. The messenger ribonucleic acid (RNA) is formed and migrates to the cell cytoplasm, where it influences the synthesis of specific peptides and proteins. These peptides and proteins carry out the metabolic functions of the cells that were in the past attributed to the steroid hormones.

REGULATION OF SECRETION

The production of endocrine secretions is generally controlled according to the need for their action; that is, production and release into the bloodstream are stimulated when their action is needed and are inhibited when the effect is achieved. Secretions by the pituitary gland are regulated by either hormonal or nervous signals originating in the hypothalamus. The control mechanism may be influenced by the blood concentration of secretions from the target organ, or by physicochemical processes. For example, regulation of secretion by the thyroid, adrenal cortices and the gonads is maintained by hormones that are produced by the anterior pituitary gland and liberated in response to the blood concentration of the hormones of those glands. A hormone that stimulates the secretion of another hormone is referred to as a *trophic hormone*.

DYSFUNCTION

Disorders of an endocrine gland may incur an excess or deficiency of its hormone(s). Signs and symptoms of the disorder are predominantly manifestations of dysfunction in the target organ or tissues. Enlargement or out-growths of a gland may also impose on neighbouring structures, interfering with their function(s).

PITUITARY GLAND (HYPOPHYSIS)

The **pituitary** gland is a very small gland located at the base of the brain in the sella turcica, a depression in the sphenoid bone. It is attached to the hypothalamus by a stalk, the *infundibulum*, which contains nerve fibres and blood vessels. The gland has two distinct parts: the anterior lobe (or anterior pituitary) and the posterior or neural lobe (posterior pituitary).

The cells of the anterior pituitary are truly glandular in that they extract substances from the blood and secrete new chemicals (hormones). The posterior pituitary consists mainly of many terminal nerve fibres which originate with nerve cells (neurones) in the hypothalamus. The hormones released by the posterior pituitary are secreted by the neurones of the hypothalamus and are released at the nerve endings in the posterior pituitary.

Anterior pituitary lobe (adenohypophysis)

The anterior pituitary secretes the following **hormones**:

- *thyroid-stimulating hormone* (TSH)
- *growth hormone* (GH)
- *prolactin* (PRL), which affects lactation
- *adrenocorticotrophic hormone* (ACTH), which stimulates the adrenal cortex
- *related peptides* – β-lipotropin (β-LPH), α-melanocyte-stimulating hormone (MSH), which increases pigmentation of the skin and mucous membranes
- β-*endorphin* (a substance with morphine-like actions)
- *follicle-stimulating hormone* (FSH), which stimulates the development of mature Graafian follicles in women and stimulates spermatogenesis in men
- *luteinizing hormone* (LH), which stimulates the development and maintenance of the corpus luteum in women; in men, where it is called *interstitial cell-stimulating hormone* (ICSH), it affects secretion of testosterone.

The hormones TSH, ACTH, FSH and LH stimulate other glands; GH, PRL and MSH act directly on tissues of the body.

Regulation by hypothalamic hormones

Hypothalamic hormones control, by stimulation or inhibition, the release of hormones from the pituitary gland. The hypothalamic hormones comprise:

- growth hormone-releasing hormone (or factor) (GHRF)
- growth hormone release-inhibiting hormone (somatostatin; GHRIH)
- thyrotrophin-releasing hormone (or factor) (TRH)
- corticotrophin-releasing hormone (CRF)
- gonadotrophin-releasing hormone (GnRH)
- prolactin release-inhibiting hormone (PIH).

Functions of the anterior pituitary hormones

Figure 18.2 summarizes the metabolic functions of anterior pituitary hormones.

Growth hormone Growth hormone is concerned with the growth of the body and plays an important role in determining a person's size. The most striking effect of the hormone is evidenced in the skeleton. Bones increase in length and thickness until late adolescence, the muscles

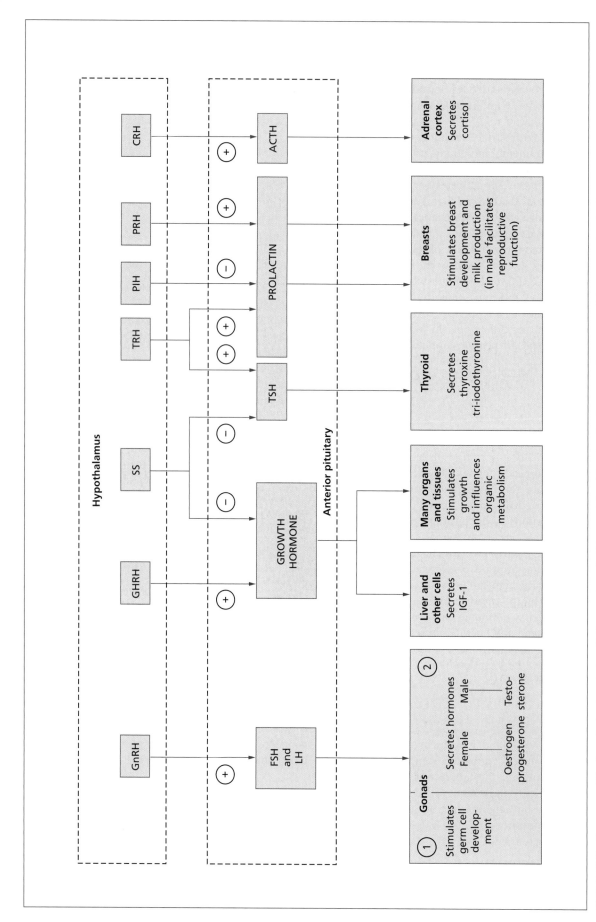

Figure 18.2 Summary of the hypothalamic-anterior pituitary system. GnRH, gonadotrophin-releasing hormone; GHRH, growth hormone-releasing hormone; SS, somatostatin; TRH, thyrotrophin-releasing hormone; PIH, prolactin release-inhibiting hormone; PRH, prolactin-releasing hormone; CRH, corticotrophin-releasing hormone; FSH, follicle-stimulating hormone; LH, luteinizing hormone; TSH, thyroid-stimulating hormone; ACTH, adrenocorticotrophic hormone; IGF-1, insulin-like growth factor 1. (Modified from Vander et al 1990. Reprinted by permission of the McGraw-Hill Companies, Inc.©)

enlarge and there is a corresponding growth of the viscera. Growth is also dependent upon the secretion of normal amounts of other hormones. The thyroid hormones are necessary to maintain an adequate metabolic rate, and insulin must be available to promote glucose metabolism for the provision of energy. Growth hormone is diabetogenic; it increases the breakdown of glycogen in the liver, promotes the release of glucose into the blood and also produces an anti-insulin effect in muscles. This promotes the synthesis and conservation of protein, conservation of glucose and utilization of fat.

The secretion of GH is controlled by the hypothalamus, which produces two regulating hormones: one stimulates the release of GH and the other, somatostatin, inhibits the release of GH by the anterior pituitary. The secretion of GH is influenced by the state of nutrition; hypoglycaemia, fasting, exercise, stress and trauma increase its production. Hyperglycaemia and high concentrations of cortisol decrease the secretion.

Thyroid-stimulating hormone Thyroid-stimulating hormone promotes the growth and secretory activity of the thyroid gland, the function of which is the production of hormones that regulate the metabolic rate of all tissues. The production of TSH is regulated by a negative-feedback mechanism. A decrease in the blood concentration of thyroid hormones increases the secretory output of thyrotrophin; conversely, when the thyroid hormones reach a normal or above normal level, there is a reciprocal decrease in the release of thyrotrophin.

Adrenocorticotrophic hormone Adrenocorticotrophic hormone has as its target organ the adrenal cortices, influencing their secretory output of several cortical secretions. ACTH secretion is regulated by an ACTH-releasing factor produced in the hypothalamus in response to a decreased blood level of cortisone, or to nerve impulses initiated by biological stress (e.g. trauma, pain).

Follicle-stimulating hormone Follicle-stimulating hormone causes the development of the ovarian follicle and the secretion of oestrogen. The secretion of FSH is inversely related to the blood level of oestrogen (see Ch. 23).

Luteinizing hormone Luteinizing hormone promotes ovulation and is necessary for the formation of the corpus luteum in the ruptured follicle. When the corpus luteum develops and secretes progesterone, the production of LH is suppressed. In the male, this hormone may be called the interstitial cell-stimulating hormone (ICSH) because it stimulates the production of the male hormone testosterone by the interstitial cells of the testes.

Prolactin Prolactin stimulates the corpus luteum to secrete progesterone and initiates and stimulates the secretion of the mammary glands which have undergone preparatory changes in response to the oestrogen and progesterone blood levels.

Posterior pituitary lobe
Functions of the posterior pituitary hormones
Two hormones, antidiuretic hormone (ADH) and oxytocin, are released by the posterior pituitary gland.

Antidiuretic hormone Release of ADH by the posterior pituitary lobe is regulated by osmoreceptors in the hypothalamus. When the osmotic pressure of the blood is increased, for example because of dehydration, the neurones sensitive to changes in the osmotic pressure of the blood transmit impulses to the posterior pituitary to release ADH into the circulating blood. This reduces urine output as a result of increasing water reabsorption in the kidneys. ADH has this effect by increasing the permeability of the distal and collecting tubules. This hormone therefore plays an important role in maintaining normal fluid balance.

Oxytocin Oxytocin excites contractions of the pregnant uterus, especially during the latter part of gestation. This hormone also plays an important role in lactation; suckling initiates afferent nerve impulses which, on reaching the hypothalamus, bring about the liberation of oxytocin from the posterior pituitary gland. The hormone is carried by the blood to the mammary glands, stimulating the release and flow of milk.

THYROID GLAND

The **thyroid** is situated in the neck and consists of two lateral lobes, one on each side of the trachea immediately below the larynx. These lobes are connected by a band of tissue, the thyroid isthmus, lying across the anterior surface of the trachea (Fig. 18.3). The lobes contain numerous vesicles or follicles, and the walls of the follicles are composed of a layer of secreting cells. The follicles contain a clear, colloidal protein-iodine compound called *thyroglobulin*. The gland has an abundant blood supply; paired superior and inferior thyroid arteries arise from the external carotid and subclavian arteries.

Three hormones are produced and released into the blood:

- tri-iodothyronine (T_3)
- thyroxine (T_4)
- calcitonin (thyrocalcitonin; TCT).

Tri-iodothyronine and thyroxine are produced by the follicular cells, and calcitonin is secreted by the parafollicular cells. Thyroxine (T_4) occurs in greater amounts than T_3.

The thyroid hormones (T_3 and T_4) increase the metabolic rate in most of the cells by stimulating oxidative processes. There is a notable increase in cellular activity, oxygen consumption and heat production. The hormones are essential for normal physical growth, maturation and mental development. The production and release of the thyroid hormones are controlled by TSH secreted by the anterior pituitary. A negative-feedback relationship exists between TSH and the thyroid hormones. When the blood concentration of the thyroid hormones decreases, the hypothalamus produces a

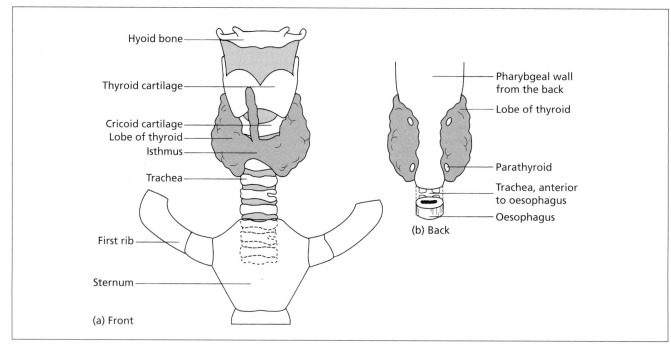

Figure 18.3   (a) Front and (b) back views showing the position of the thyroid.

releasing factor (TRH) which alerts the anterior pituitary to release TSH.

Calcitonin is secreted in response to an above-normal increase in the blood level of calcium or an excess of glucagon in the blood. It lowers the serum calcium and phosphate levels by promoting their excretion in urine and movement into the bones.

PARATHYROID GLANDS

The parathyroid glands are small oval bodies attached to the posterior surface of the lateral lobes of the thyroid. The number may vary but is usually four. The principal secretion of the parathyroid glands is **parathyroid hormone** (PTH), which regulates the concentration of calcium and inorganic phosphorus in the blood through its action on the intestine, bone tissue and kidneys. It promotes absorption of calcium in the intestine, and the demineralization of bone and movement of the calcium into the extracellular fluid. In the kidneys, the hormone increases the excretion of phosphorus by decreasing its reabsorption from the glomerular filtrate and, conversely, the reabsorption of calcium is increased, decreasing its excretion in urine.

A normal concentration of calcium is essential for the normal structure of bones and teeth, coagulation of blood, maintenance of normal cardiac rhythmicity, normal neuromuscular excitability and cellular membrane permeability. The greater part of the absorbed calcium is deposited in bones.

The rate of secretion of the PTH is controlled by the concentration of calcium in the blood. When the calcium level rises above normal, the glands are inhibited and less hormone is produced. A fall in the blood calcium level stimulates the glands, resulting in an increased output of PTH.

ADRENAL GLANDS

The two adrenal, or suprarenal, glands are situated immediately above the kidneys. Each is enclosed within a capsule and consists of two distinct parts: the cortex and the medulla. The adrenal glands have an abundant blood supply through branches of the aorta and the inferior phrenic and renal arteries.

Adrenal cortex

The **cortex** forms the outer part as well as the greater portion of the gland and produces hormones essential to life. These are steroids and collectively are called the *adrenocorticoids*, corticosteroids or corticoids. Those secreted in physiologically significant amounts fall into three classes: mineralocorticoids, glucocorticoids and sex hormones. The steroids in each of these classes have some predominant characteristics or actions, but may overlap into another class.

Mineralocorticoids
Mineralocorticoids are essential to life. The most significant is *aldosterone*, which influences electrolyte concentrations and fluid volume.

The secretion of aldosterone is regulated in the interest of maintaining a normal sodium concentration and normal fluid volume. Factors that influence the amount of aldosterone released are the blood sodium and potassium levels and the blood volume. A decrease in the sodium concentration stimulates an increased output of aldosterone, and vice versa. Aldosterone acts by stimulating the renal tubules to reabsorb sodium and excrete potassium; consequently, the effect of changes in serum potassium levels is the reverse of that of sodium. Decreases in renal arterial blood pressure such as occur in shock, physical trauma and haemorrhage increase renin secretion by the kidneys. The production of angiotensin II that results from the release of renin stimulates the adrenal cortex to secrete aldosterone.

Glucocorticoids

Several glucocorticoids have been recognized, but *cortisol* (hydrocortisone) is considered to be the most important, because it is more potent and is produced in much greater amounts than the other cortical hormones. Cortisol influences the metabolism of glucose, protein and fat, and is involved in the body's responses to physical and mental stress. Its actions are complex and not clearly understood; for example, it enables a person to deal more effectively with stress, but how this is achieved is not known. Cortisol increases the blood sugar level and the liver glycogen stores are increased. Tissue protein is broken down and the amino acids are converted to glycogen or glucose in the liver (gluconeogenesis). Fat is also mobilized, some of which is also converted to glucose.

Glucocorticoids are secreted in response to circulating ACTH. In turn, the production and release of ACTH by the anterior pituitary depends upon the release of corticotrophin-releasing hormone (CRH) which is secreted by the hypothalamus. The production of CRH is influenced by a negative-feedback mechanism; that is, a low concentration of adrenocorticoid secretions in the blood initiates the hypothalamic responses. With an increase in the blood level of glucocorticoids, the output of ACTH is depressed. Physical and psychological stress and hypoglycaemia also stimulate the release of CRH through impulses delivered from the cerebral cortex or midbrain to the hypothalamus.

A concentration of cortisol in excess of the normal is of clinical significance because it suppresses local inflammatory responses to irritating substances (anti-inflammatory effect), delays healing through depressed fibroplasia and reduces tissue sensitivity reactions to antigens (antiallergic reaction). Other effects also associated with an excess of cortisol include a decreased production of antibodies and an increased secretion of gastric hydrochloric acid and pepsinogen which predisposes to the development of ulcers.

Adrenal sex hormones

The adrenal cortices of both sexes secrete both male and female hormones: *androgens, oestrogen* and *progesterone*. Oestrogen and progesterone are produced in lesser amounts than the androgens but, normally, the quantity of any of these hormones is considered to be physiologically insignificant compared with the amounts produced by the gonads.

Adrenal medulla

The **medulla** forms the central portion of each adrenal gland and is composed of specialized neurones which secrete two hormones, *adrenaline* and *noradrenaline*. Because of their chemical composition, they are frequently referred to as *catecholamines*. During any stress or threat to the organism, the hormones are released and serve with the autonomic nervous system to produce defensive reactions throughout the body. Their production is controlled by nerve impulses transmitted to the medullae by sympathetic nerve fibres, and their effects are similar to those produced by sympathetic innervation.

Adrenaline causes constriction of the peripheral and renal blood vessels and dilatation of the coronary and skeletal muscle blood vessels. The rate and force of contraction of the heart and skeletal muscle is increased. The smooth muscle of the bronchioles, gastrointestinal tract and urinary bladder relaxes. The dilator muscle fibres of the irises contract, resulting in dilatation of the pupils. The blood sugar level is raised by increased glycogenolysis (conversion of glycogen to glucose) in both the liver and skeletal muscles. The metabolic rate is accelerated and there is an increased alertness and awareness due to stimulation of the brain. Adrenaline also promotes the release of ACTH, which in turn increases the secretion of glucocorticoids.

Noradrenaline causes a more generalized vasoconstriction and does not produce dilatation of any vessels. Because of this action, it is more effective in raising the blood pressure; both systolic and diastolic blood pressures rise.

PANCREAS (ISLETS OF LANGERHANS)

The **pancreas** is both an exocrine and an endocrine gland. Its exocrine secretions are carried by a system of ducts to the duodenum and contain enzymes that play an important role in digestion. The islets of Langerhans form the endocrine component of the pancreas and consist of irregularly scattered groups of cells that are totally independent of the pancreatic system of ducts. The islets are highly vascularized and consist of four types of cell:

1 α *cells*, which secrete the hormone **glucagon**
2 β *cells*, which produce **insulin**
3 δ *cells*, which may secrete small amounts of gastrin and **somatostatin** (growth hormone release-inhibiting hormone (GHRIH))
4 F *cells*, which secrete pancreatic polypeptide.

Insulin and glucagon are proteins and are rendered inactive in the gastrointestinal tract by the proteolytic enzymes; when prescribed, they must be administered parenterally.

Secretions and functions
Insulin
This hormone plays a dominant role in carbohydrate, fat and protein metabolism, especially in the liver and muscular and

adipose tissues. Knowledge of the ways in which insulin promotes specific metabolic cellular activities is incomplete, but it has been established that it binds to receptors in cell membranes and stimulates the following actions:

1 The transfer of glucose into most cells and its metabolism by those cells.
2 The formation of glycogen by the liver and muscle cells.
3 The synthesis of fatty acids and storage of fat in adipose tissue.
4 The uptake and incorporation of amino acids into cell proteins.
5 An increased uptake of potassium by cells.

These activities result in a lower concentration of glucose in the blood.

The concentration of blood glucose is the major controlling factor in the secretion of insulin. An increase raises the production of insulin and, conversely, a decrease below the normal blood level of glucose suppresses its secretion. Thus, a negative-feedback mechanism is established which controls the output of insulin in order to maintain the blood sugar level within a normal range. The synthesis of insulin is also stimulated by an excess of growth hormone and glucocorticoids, but somatostatin is an inhibitor of both insulin and glucagon secretion. The amount of insulin circulating in the blood increases when carbohydrate foods are ingested; this is attributed to the effect of the gastrointestinal hormones on the β cells. Glucose given intravenously does not produce the same effect as when it is taken orally.

Other factors that result in an increased insulin level include vagal nerve stimulation and oral antidiabetic agents.

Glucagon

This hormone may also be referred to as the hyperglycaemic factor, because its primary effect is stimulation of glycogenolysis (the conversion of glycogen to glucose) and the release of glucose into the blood by the liver to increase the blood glucose concentration. Its secretion by the α cells is stimulated by a low blood sugar level. An oral intake of proteins initiates an increased secretion of glucagon, greater than that seen in response to the intravenous administration of amino acids. This suggests a gastrointestinal hormone that stimulates the secretion of glucagon. Sympathetic nervous stimulation of the pancreas also increases the glucagon output.

Somatostatin (growth hormone release-inhibiting hormone (GHRIH))

This hormone is found in cells of the hypothalamus, where it passes down the portal vessels to the anterior pituitary, gastrointestinal tract and islets of Langerhans. It inhibits the secretion of insulin, glucagon, pancreatic polypeptide, GH and various gastrointestinal hormones. It interferes with carbohydrate absorption and possibly with the absorption of protein and fat.

Pancreatic polypeptide

This hormone is known to decrease glycogen concentration in the liver and to slow the absorption of food. Release of the hormone is stimulated by protein ingestion, fasting, exercise and hypoglycaemia.

Blood glucose level

The normal blood glucose level 3–4 hours after a meal varies from approximately 4 to 6 mmol/L depending upon the type of meal consumed and the amount of energy expended. The types of food taken also influence the degree of change; a meal high in carbohydrate produces a greater concentration of glucose when compared with a meal with a low carbohydrate content. An increase in the blood sugar level above the normal is known as *hyperglycaemia*. A level below normal is referred to as *hypoglycaemia*. Blood sugar level is therefore determined principally by the hormones secreted in the islets of Langerhans, although some other endocrine secretions also have an effect, such as the glucocorticoids.

DISORDERS OF THE ENDOCRINE SYSTEM

GENERAL

Signs and symptoms of endocrine dysfunction may be non-specific, resulting from changes in the widespread target tissues and are common to many disorders. They include the following:

Alterations in growth. *Delayed growth* can occur from endocrine and metabolic disorders as well as genetic factors. Delayed growth from endocrine disorders usually occurs during a specific period of development. *Excessive growth* may result from endocrine disorders in which an excess of adrenal, ovarian or testicular, or pituitary hormones is produced. Excessive pituitary secretion of growth hormone causes gigantism.

Obesity. Obesity can be associated with hormonal disorders and may be a causative factor (as in diabetes) as well as a result of a disorder.

Appetite changes. These include anorexia and polyphagia. Excessive eating (polyphagia) is most often seen with hyperthyroidism and occasionally with uncontrolled diabetes or hypothalamic disorders.

Polyuria and polydipsia. Excessive urinary output and abnormal thirst are frequently the result of uncontrolled diabetes mellitus.

Weakness and exhaustion. Excessive weight loss, muscle wasting, weakness and exhaustion may be seen in patients with uncontrolled disorders of the pancreas, thyroid or adrenal glands.

Skin pigmentation. Changes in skin pigmentation may develop in patients with disorders of the pituitary, parathyroid and adrenal glands.

Hirsutism. Changes in the distribution and texture of body hair occur with several endocrine disorders. Facial hair in the female may occur with adrenal or ovarian disorders.

Sexual disturbances. Impotence, menstrual disorders and infertility may be associated with endocrine disturbances. Impotence may occur in men who have had diabetes mellitus for several years. The onset of puberty and delay in the development of secondary sex characteristics may occur with deficiency of growth hormone and gonadal dysfunction.

Bone and joint disorders. These may accompany changes in the secretion of growth hormone, thyroid hormones and adrenocorticoids.

Renal colic and stones. These may be associated with excess secretion of parathyroid hormone leading to hypercalcaemia.

Hypertension. There are numerous contributing factors to the development of hypertension; hyperactivity of the adrenal cortex can be one of the causes.

Personality changes. Behavioural changes, including lethargy, confusion, nervousness, restlessness, convulsions and coma, may result from acute metabolic disorders associated with uncontrolled diabetes mellitus as well as with disorders of secretions of the pituitary gland, adrenal gland and thyroid.

THE PERSON WITH DIABETES

DIABETES MELLITUS

Diabetes mellitus is a heterogeneous group of disorders of carbohydrate, fat and protein metabolism characterized by chronic hyperglycaemia, degenerative vascular changes and neuropathy. It tends to accelerate degenerative changes throughout the body by widespread vascular changes in the large blood vessels and the microvessels.

Characteristics and epidemiology

Diabetes is diagnosed when the patient has the symptoms of diabetes (such as polyuria, unexplained weight loss and excess thirst) and a random plasma glucose level ≥11.1 mmol/L. Random refers to the fact that the blood sample has been taken at any time of the day regardless of the last meal. A fasting plasma glucose ≥7.0 mmol/L (no food in the previous 8 hours) in the presence of the classical symptoms is also diagnostic of diabetes (Watkins 1998). In the absence of symptoms, a glucose tolerance test (GTT) should be carried out to determine the patient's response to the ingestion of a precisely measured quantity of glucose.

There are two principal types of diabetes which have different aetiologies. *Type 1 diabetes (previously referred to as insulin-dependent diabetes mellitus)* is caused by the destruction of β cells in the islets of Langerhans. The destruction is an autoimmune response associated with environmental and genetic factors. The onset of type 1 diabetes can be very rapid.

Type 2 (previously referred to as non-insulin-dependent diabetes mellitus) covers a multitude of different disorders. The basic problem is that either the islets of Langerhans gradually diminish their insulin output or there is increased peripheral resistance to the action of insulin or there is a combination of decreased insulin secretion and increased insulin resistance. The onset tends to be slow and patients frequently live with the disease for a number of years before diagnosis. Obesity and lack of exercise are the commonest causes of insulin resistance and hence of type 2 diabetes (Springhouse Corporation 2000), although a small portion of people with type 2 diabetes are of normal weight and are reasonably active. The most common age of onset is 50–70 years. There is a strong genetic influence, and as a result, certain families and ethnic groups are much more likely to have type 2 diabetes. For example in the UK, Pakistanis and Bangladeshis are more than five times as likely as the general population to have diabetes, while Indians are three times more likely (Erens et al 2001).

There are approximately 2.5 million people in the UK with diagnosed diabetes and approximately 600 000 people who remain undiagnosed (British Heart Foundation 2006). The complications of diabetes are a greater public health problem than any infectious disease, particularly as many of the patients who develop complications do so before their diabetes is even diagnosed.

In addition to primary diabetes (types 1 and 2), there is also secondary diabetes. This is due to a range of conditions such as pancreatic disease or hormonal disorders such as Cushing's syndrome (see p. 594), it may occur as a side-effect of medication such as steroid therapy or it may occur during pregnancy when it becomes known as *gestational diabetes*.

Whatever the cause, the result is a deficiency of insulin or inadequate insulin function. This leads to an inadequate transfer of glucose into the cells; the utilization of glucose for energy and cellular products and its conversion to glycogen or fat and storage as such are depressed. Glucose accumulates in the blood, causing hyperglycaemia.

Fat may be mobilized from adipose tissue and broken down to provide a source of energy. The mobilized fat is withdrawn from the blood by the liver and broken down to glycerol and fatty acids. The fatty acids are oxidized by the hepatic cells to ketone bodies, which are then circulated and may be metabolized by cells to produce energy, carbon dioxide and water. Only a limited amount of ketone acids can be utilized by the cells. If ketogenesis proceeds rapidly, exceeding the rate at which they can be metabolized, the ketone acids accumulate in the blood, causing ketosis or ketone acidosis.

Tissue protein may also be broken down to amino acids which are used in gluconeogenesis, contributing to the hyperglycaemia. Both the uptake of amino acids by the cells and body protein synthesis are decreased.

The patient excretes an excessive volume of urine (*polyuria*) as a result of the increased concentration of glucose in the glomerular filtrate. The glucose increases the osmotic pressure of the filtrate, preventing the reabsorption of water. As a result of the excessive water loss, the patient experiences a persisting thirst (*polydipsia*), and dehydration and electrolyte imbalance may develop. The blood glucose concentration exceeds the capacity of the renal tubules to reabsorb it from the glomerular filtrate, and glucose is excreted in the urine (*glycosuria*). The maximum capacity of the renal tubules to reabsorb glucose represents what is referred to as the glucose renal threshold. The normal value is 10–12 mmol/L.

Weakness and fatigue are common complaints because the glucose cannot be utilized to produce energy. There is a loss of weight which is attributed to the mobilization of fat from adipose tissue and the breakdown of protein. Some patients also experience an increased appetite (*polyphagia*).

Female patients may develop pruritus of the vulva, usually due to infection by fungi (candida) that thrive on the glucose deposit from the urine. The vulva becomes swollen and inflamed. Balanitis is a similar problem affecting the glans penis in men.

Table 18.1 lists the clinical characteristics of persons with the two major types of diabetes mellitus.

Chronic complications of diabetes

The blood vessels of practically all people with diabetes undergo degenerative changes to some extent. These changes may be both microvascular and macrovascular. Hyperinsulinaemia and/or increased insulin resistance is considered to be fundamental to vascular complications in diabetes (Winters and Jernigan 2000). Microalbuminuria is a significant marker for many vascular problems being a precipitating factor in insulin resistance, along with raised low-density lipoprotein (LDL) cholesterol levels and hypothyroidism (see p. 577). These three factors are important indicators or markers for microvascular and macrovascular complications according to Winters and Jernigan (2000).

Microvascular degenerative changes

Microvascular degenerative changes are specific to diabetes; the basement membrane in the capillaries and arterioles thickens. The retinae, kidneys and skin are the areas most affected by microvascular changes. The long-term quality of diabetic control plays a major part in determining the rapidity of onset of such complications.

Diabetic retinopathy occurs in the form of minute aneurysms in the retinal vessels. These dilatations are prone to rupture and cause a haemorrhage into the eye. The resultant visual loss varies with the location and proliferation of the lesions. Poor diabetic control, increased diastolic blood pressure, impaired renal function, deterioration in motor nerve conduction and raised triglyceride levels increase the risk for diabetic retinopathy. It is estimated that comprehensive screening and treatment for diabetic retinopathy could prevent 260 new cases of blindness per year in the UK (York 1999).

Renal function may be slowly impaired by changes in the glomerular capillaries (intercapillary glomerulosclerosis, or Kimmelstiel–Wilson syndrome) and by sclerotic changes in the larger renal vessels. There may be no clear symptoms reported by the patient until renal disease is far advanced and the kidneys are close to failure. Approximately 25% of patients with type 2 diabetes develop microalbuminuria and a further 15% have proteinuria (Melville et al 2000). Microalbuminuria is the earliest indicator of diabetic renal disease. Microalbuminuria relates to values of albumin in the urine which, although small are above normal ranges. Microalbuminuria is reversible if blood pressure is strictly controlled. In addition to being a marker for the development of renal disease, the presence of microalbuminuria also predicts total mortality, cardiovascular mortality and cardiovascular morbidity. In short, if microalbuminuria is present the patient is at risk of developing other complications of diabetes.

In order to test for microalbuminuria, an early morning urine sample is necessary. This can either be sent to the laboratory or near patient testing strips are available. If microalbuminuria or proteinuria is present, urine should be repeated twice more within 1 month (NICE 2002). Serum creatinine should be measured concurrently. Results will indicate the albumin/creatinine ratio. (Abnormal =

Table 18.1 Classification of diabetes mellitus

	Type 1	Type 2
Synonyms	Juvenile onset	Maturity onset
Age of onset	Usually before 30 years	Usually after 40 years
Type of onset	Frequently sudden	Usually gradual
Presentation	Polydipsia, polyuria	Often asymptomatic
Body weight	Thin	Usually (85%) obese
Ketoacidosis	Ketosis-prone	Ketosis-resistant
Control by diet alone	Not possible	Possible
Control by oral agents	Not possible	Frequently possible
Long-term complications	Frequent	Frequent

>2.5 mg/mmol for men and >3.5 mg/mmol for women.) A positive finding indicates damaged kidneys associated with microvascular pathology and raised blood pressure, which should be treated with ACE inhibitors whether the blood pressure is within a normal range (140/90 mmHg) or not (Melville et al 2000, York 2000). Diabetic renal disease is also associated with hypertension, which exacerbates further renal damage, setting up a vicious circle.

Macrovascular degenerative changes

Macrovascular degeneration involves the development of *atherosclerosis* (deposits of the fatty substance cholesterol) in the arteries, narrowing their lumen. Atherosclerosis of the coronary arteries frequently leads to angina pectoris and myocardial infarction, especially in older persons.

Defective circulation due to vascular changes in the lower limbs may lead to abnormal coldness of the extremities, numbness, discolouration, muscular cramps, weakness, burning pain or a small ulcer that does not heal. Proteinuria indicates a high risk of such large vessel disease (Watkins 1998). Something as trivial as a wrinkled sock or a poorly trimmed toe nail, a superficial injury or a pressure sore on the heel may precipitate an infected lesion and ultimately gangrene, leading to the amputation of a foot or leg. A combination of poor peripheral blood supply and/or nerve damage (diabetic neuropathy; see below) leads to some 15% of people with diabetes developing foot ulcers. Infected diabetic foot ulcer is the second most common reason for amputation after trauma (York 1999). It is estimated that some 40–50% of lower-limb amputations in diabetic patients are, however, avoidable (Umeh et al 1999). Screening for the two main predictors of gangrene and amputation – peripheral vascular disease and peripheral neuropathy – should therefore form part of the long-term management of all diabetic patients.

Diabetic neuropathy

Neuropathy may be defined as a non-inflammatory, non-specific pathological or functional disorder of the peripheral nervous system. This complication affects all parts of the nervous system except the brain. Peripheral neuropathy is usually bilateral and worsens at night. The patient may experience muscular cramps, tingling and burning sensation as well as pain.

Deep tendon reflexes are absent and the patient's vibratory and positional senses may be impaired. Foot problems are most common due to accidental injury as the person gradually loses sensation in the lower limbs. Injuries are compounded by poor circulation, which delays healing (see above). A Diabetic Foot Screen tool is available for screening peripheral sensation and involves the use of a calibrated nylon filament mounted on a handle that buckles at 10 g of pressure when applied perpendicular to the skin (a monofilament). This monofilament is applied systematically to each foot at the required pressure while the patient has their eyes closed. The foot is 'at risk' if the patient cannot consistently and accurately report the touch of the monofilament as it is applied (Umeh et al 1999). Autonomic

neuropathy can also occur and leads to diarrhoea, vomiting and postural hypotension. Impotence and retrograde ejaculation may occur in the male.

Box 18.1 shows the main risk markers for vascular complications in diabetic patients. The prevention of complications depends upon identifying which of these are present and working with the patient to reduce or eliminate them (Winters and Jernigan 2000).

Metabolic syndrome

Diabetes or impaired glucose tolerance is part of the metabolic syndrome which is a cluster of factors that have been shown to increase the risk of cardiovascular disease. There are various definitions of metabolic syndrome in the literature, which tend to feature the following factors:

1 Fasting plasma glucose >6.1
plus two of the following:
2 Central obesity (excessive fat distribution around the abdomen which is measured by calculating the hip:waist ratio – people with a low hip:waist ratio are sometimes referred to as being apple shaped). Central obesity is strongly associated with the presence of metabolic syndrome and the presence of coronary heart disease (Marchesini et al 2004)
3 Raised triglycerides
4 Low HDL cholesterol
5 Raised blood pressure
6 Microalbuminuria.

Additionally, blood markers of inflammation (C reactive protein (CRP)) have been implicated in the syndrome. Minimum criteria for the metabolic syndrome are met in most patients with type 2 diabetes (Marchesini et al 2004). A knowledge of metabolic syndrome enables us to target screening to people with one or more of the indicators for each of the others, for example, someone with hypertension

---

Box 18.1   Risk markers for diabetic vascular complications

- Sedentary lifestyle
- Obesity
- Increased blood viscosity
- Raised blood glucose and haemoglobin A_{1c} levels
- Hypothyroidism
- Tobacco use
- Hyperlipidaemia
- Raised blood pressure
- Microalbuminuria and proteinuria
- Vision changes
- Skin lesions on feet and diabetic neuropathies.

or low HDL cholesterol should be screened annually for diabetes by having a measurement of their blood glucose.

Prevention of diabetes mellitus

Primary prevention

Diabetes mellitus is not a single entity but a group of heterogeneous disorders caused by a combination of genetic, environmental and viral factors. Additionally, measures can be taken to prevent and/or correct obesity and stop smoking. This is especially important for those with a family history of diabetes. Haslett et al (1999) point out that the only cost-effective way to deal with diabetes is to prevent it. Health promotion aimed at reducing obesity and increasing fitness could therefore be of immense benefit to the whole population in the prevention of diabetes (Connor et al 2003).

Secondary prevention

Once diabetes has been diagnosed in a patient, health education aimed at preventing or at least delaying the development of complications is essential. Such secondary prevention can greatly improve the quality of life of the patient and bring about enormous savings in cost to the National Health Service. Once again, nurses are in the forefront of such work, especially practice nurses and diabetes nurse specialists who have developed considerable expertise in the field of diabetic care.

Management and education of the diabetic patient and family

Although inroads are being made in the prevention of diabetes, to date no cure exists. Individuals must therefore live with this chronic disorder and the potential complications. The diabetic patient may be dependent on health professionals for restoration of health when the disease is first diagnosed and during episodes of acute illness. As the individual acquires knowledge and skill to make alterations in lifestyle to regulate the hyperglycaemia, greater independence may be achieved. Individuals with diabetes mellitus must alter their lifestyles and health behaviours if they are to minimize the impact of the disease.

Management of diabetes mellitus

The principal aims of management are to establish and maintain metabolic control and to control hypertension (UK Prospective Diabetes Study 1998) in order that treatment may:

● save life
● alleviate symptoms
● prevent long-term complications.

This also involves reducing risk factors such as obesity and smoking.

The main therapeutic interventions aimed at achieving these goals consist of diet, insulin, other medication aimed at reducing blood glucose levels, medication for the reduction of hypertension, medication for the reduction of cholesterol and lifestyle modification such as weight reduction, smoking cessation and exercise. Ideally, this should all be carried out within a framework of patient self-care, allowing individuals to take the maximum responsibility for managing their condition.

Blood glucose levels, hypertension and raised cholesterol levels are controlled by balancing the person's energy intake with energy utilization or out-put; dietary measures, medication and physical activity are adjusted to achieve the best possible control for the individual.

Diet The goals of dietary advice are:

1 to maintain or improve health through the use of appropriate health choices
2 to achieve and maintain optimal metabolic and physiological outcomes, including:
   – reduction of risk for microvascular disease by achieving near normal glycaemia without undue risk of hypoglycaemia
   – reduction of risk of macrovascular disease, including management of body weight, dyslipidaemia and hypertension
3 to optimize outcomes in diabetic nephropathy and in any concomitant disorder (Connor et al 2003).

Diet is a major factor in the control of diabetes and is the first line of management in type 2 diabetes. The prescribed 'diabetic diet' has been replaced by an individualized diet regimen with the patient assuming responsibility for planning, implementing and adjusting the diet to needs and lifestyle. Basic dietary principles are the same as any healthy eating plan for people without diabetes and focus on being low in fat and low glycaemic index. The glycaemic index is a ranking of foods based on the speed of absorption. Slowly absorbed foods have a low glycaemic index and foods that are absorbed more quickly have a high glycaemic index (Diabetes UK 2006a). Foods that are absorbed slowly avoid the sharp rise in blood glucose which is associated with foods that are absorbed quickly.

Initially, if the type 2 patient is overweight, the objective will be to bring about a gradual and steady loss of weight until a realistic weight is achieved. A weight loss of 10% is realistic for many people and confers major health benefits (Connor et al 2003). Although the patient may find it difficult to make any sense of the recommendations on daily intake of calories it is useful for the nurse to know that the proportion of prescribed calories allocated to each food type is approximately 45–60% carbohydrate, not greater than 1 g/kg of body weight of protein, <10% of energy intake of saturated and transaturated fat, <10% of energy intake of polyunsaturated fat, 10–20% of energy intake from mono-unsaturated fat. Interestingly, recent guidelines suggest that up to 10% of daily energy intake may come from simple sugars (sucrose) as long as this is included as part of a general healthy diet, although it should be avoided by those trying to lose weight (Connor et al 2003). Refined carbohydrates should be substituted for unrefined carbohydrates with fibre, such as whole-grain breads and cereals, fruit and vegetables and carbohydrates with a low glycaemic index should be promoted. Foods high in soluble fibre are thought to improve glucose tolerance, lower insulin secretion, reduce glycaemia and glycosuria and reduce LDL levels. These include oat, rice, corn, bran, legumes and lentils. Carbohydrate intake is distributed over the day to avoid abnormal fluctuations in blood glucose concentrations and in the selection of fat, the substitution of monounsaturated fat for saturated fats and polyunsaturated fat, because these are less implicated in the development of atherosclerosis. It is recommended that oily fish is eaten once or twice weekly because it is high in omega 3 which is thought to protect against heart disease (Connor et al 2003).

Food intake is usually best divided into at least three main meals. The carbohydrate intake is usually divided across meals and snacks distributed throughout the day and evening. Careful education and the availability of good eating guides permit the diet to be varied and take into account the availability of foods as well as the person's preferences. Cookery books, extensive information about food values, and general dietary guidelines are available from the charitable organization 'Diabetes UK'.

It must be impressed upon the person that all of the daily food allowance should be eaten, especially if insulin or a hypoglycaemic drug is being taken. If the insulin-taking patient is unable to take his or her usual diet, the carbohydrate requirement is made up in some way (e.g. orange juice, milk) in order to avoid hypoglycaemia. Meals should be taken regularly: the delay or missing of a meal may upset the blood glucose level and promote the breakdown of fat.

Non-caloric sweeteners such as aspartame and saccharin may be used safely by diabetics. These sweeteners are found in many low-calorie beverages and prepared foods.

Sorbitol (a sugar alcohol) has been used as a sweetening agent, as has fructose (crystalline fruit sugar). Both are virtually all absorbed and metabolized, but the rate of absorption from the gut is slow and so sorbitol and fructose have less effect on blood glucose levels than glucose. Both are often used in the manufacture of 'diabetic' jams, boiled sweets, biscuits and chocolate. Because they do not offer any energy savings, they should not be used for slimming purposes or by people with diabetes whose main therapeutic aim is to reduce weight. They also have the disadvantage of possibly lulling the patient into a false sense of security with regard to diet. The use of artificial non-nutritive sweeteners and the bulk nutritive sugar substitutes are not necessary in the management of diabetes, but many people find their use improves the quality of their life and helps make dietary restrictions more acceptable.

The diabetic person's diet is very much an individual affair. Adjustments in the total calorie intake and distribution of food throughout the day are often necessary. Adjusting to lifestyle change involving changes to diet and weight reduction can be very difficult. Common problems experienced by patients include the need for continual self-discipline, the influence of other people especially when eating out, time constraints and dealing with their own emotions and self-image. Negotiation and shared decision-making between nurse and client are important to achieve concordance and a management plan which is acceptable to the patient. Patients may need assistance with behavioural management techniques and require psychosocial support during the adjustment period. Above all, a non-judgemental, non-confrontational approach is needed to build a rapport with the patient.

Naquib (2002) found that self-management programmes which are individualized, realistic and which assist patients in coping with everyday life, produce better long-term outcomes than more traditional didactic approaches. The most effective self-management programmes were found to:

- include behaviour change strategies
- recognize and understand the importance of the patient's personal and unique experience of living with diabetes
- be patient-centred
- take social, emotional, cultural and psychological aspects into account
- include personalized goal setting
- include social learning variables such as problem-solving skills and self-efficacy
- involve health professional and patients working as partners.

The key dietary points important for individuals with diabetes mellitus to note are listed in Box 18.2.

Medication The *goal* of drug therapy is that the patient will maintain therapeutic glucose levels by increasing endogenous insulin production and utilization; or by maintaining serum insulin levels through the administration of exogenous insulin.

Box 18.2 Key points regarding diet for the person with diabetes mellitus

- The diet provides approximately 45–60% of calories as carbohydrate, not >1 g/kg of body weight as protein and <35% as fat (emphasis on monounsaturated fat)

- Total calorie intake will be adjusted as necessary for the individual to achieve and maintain a desirable weight

- Calorie intake is adequate to provide for optimal growth and development (childhood, pregnancy and lactation)

- Carbohydrate intake is evenly distributed throughout the day and consistent from day to day

- The diet should consist of normal foods, with a preference for foods that contain unrefined carbohydrates and are high in soluble fibre

- Food intake is adjusted to accommodate changes in lifestyle (e.g. illness, physical activity, emotional stress, eating out and travel)

- Meal plans are individualized and consider social, cultural and ethnic values of the patient and family.

Insulin This is prescribed for all people with type 1 diabetes. Type 2 diabetes is a progressive disease and people with this condition may require insulin as the disease progresses. Additionally insulin may be required during periods of stress (e.g. infection, surgery, pregnancy, a cardiac event or if the patient requires steroid treatment). Insulin is prescribed for the individual whose plasma glucose level cannot be controlled at acceptable levels despite weight control and adherence to dietary regulation, and for the treatment of ketoacidosis and non-ketotic hyperglycaemia. The main actions of insulin are summarized in Box 18.3.

Because it is a protein, insulin is destroyed in the gastrointestinal tract by proteinases; therefore, it must be given parenterally. Several types are available and may be classified as rapid acting with a shorter duration of action, as intermediate acting with a longer duration of action, as long acting with a prolonged duration of action or biphasic with a mixed length of duration of action.

Over the past decade, insulin analogues have been developed in order to try to overcome problems with hypoglycaemia which may result when tight control of blood sugar is strived for. The molecular make-up of more traditional insulins results in a delayed onset and wide variability of absorption. This means that they are not immediately responsive to changes in blood glucose. Insulin analogues (such as insulin lispro) are insulin molecules with slightly altered composition which are more quickly absorbed. Thus, administration of short-acting insulin analogues mimics more closely the normal physiological action of insulin (Barnett 2001a).

Biphasic insulins are available which are a mixture of rapid-acting and intermediate insulins. The use of two different insulins has the advantage of combining an immediate effect with a more long-lasting sustained effect. The National Institute of Clinical Excellence (NICE) suggest that biphasic insulins should be used for those who want them, people who find adherence to lunch-time injections difficult and people with learning difficulties who may require assistance (NICE 2004). It is important for the nurse caring

for or counselling people with diabetes to be familiar with the action characteristics of the various types of insulin so that appropriate instruction can be given and the patients assisted in monitoring their medication. The average action profile of some of the different types of insulins can be found in Figure 18.4.

Administration of insulin Insulin is measured in units. Each patient's regimen is determined individually in relation to a particular schedule and diet plan in an attempt to achieve a normal physiological level of glucose throughout a 24-hour period. The regimen is organized so that insulin action coincides with major meals and also provides action overnight. Diet and activity may have to be readjusted with the insulin routine to facilitate physiological control. Blood glucose levels are normally lowest during the night and begin to rise in the early morning hours. Most insulin regimens consist of combinations of rapid-acting and intermediate-acting insulin. Patients may use a multi-injection regimen with an intermediate-acting insulin and a rapid-acting insulin administered with meals. Typically, people with type 1 diabetes will have a regime involving a long-acting analogue with rapid acting analogues given with meals. Most patients can be taught to adjust or supplement their insulin regimen in response to changes in their blood glucose levels, changes in activity, portion and carbohydrate content, stress or illness.

Insulin is given by subcutaneous injection below the subcutaneous fat. The arms, thighs and abdomen are the areas used (Fig. 18.5). Injections should be at least 2.5 cm apart and rotation of sites is important. Too frequent use of one site can cause fibrosing, scarring, lipodystrophy or lipohypertrophy which can delay absorption as well as make the injection more difficult.

The use of an injection 'pen' makes the process of injecting more convenient and discreet. The device, similar to an ordinary cartridge pen, is loaded with a prefilled cartridge of insulin. The 'nib' of the pen is a disposable needle. Alternatively, the pen is pre-filled and completely disposable. The dose of insulin required is selected on the dial on the body of the pen, or clicks are counted, and the insulin is injected. Individual regimens are planned with the patient according to needs and abilities. Occasionally, disposable syringes with non-detachable needles of fine gauge are used with a capacity of either 0.5 mL (50 units insulin) or 1 mL (100 units). The injection site should be clean, but there is no need to swab it with an alcohol wipe as this has no effect on the normal bacterial population living on the skin and may lead to hardening of the skin. The injection should be given at 90° to the skin. An alternative is subcutaneous administration via a small electrically driven pump attached to a belt. The patient 'tops up' the insulin level with a subcutaneous injection just before meal times. Although this is by no means a usual method of insulin administration, it is suitable for some patients and is becoming more common.

> **Box 18.3** Main actions of insulin (adapted from Walton and Brand 1994)
>
> 1 Stimulates glucose uptake by cells, thereby making it available for energy production.
>
> 2 Increases the storage of glucose as glycogen in liver and muscle.
>
> 3 Inhibits release of glucose from glycogen stores.
>
> 4 Stimulates conversion of glucose into glycerol, which then combines with fatty acids to form triglycerides which are stored in adipose (fatty) tissue.
>
> 5 Increases uptake of amino acids by cells and hence facilitates protein synthesis.

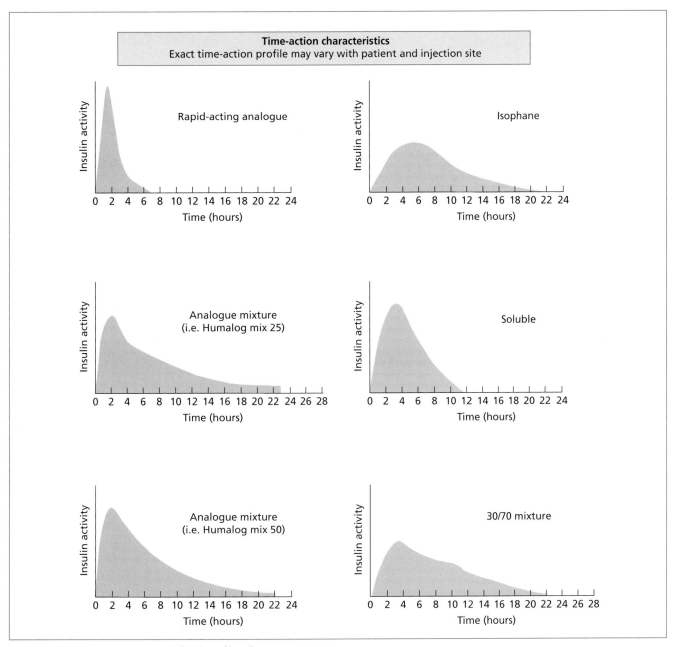

Figure 18.4 Action and duration of action of insulins.

All insulins other than clear insulin must be thoroughly mixed before use to ensure uniform suspension and concentration throughout. This is done by rotating the pen or bottle and inverting it slowly from end to end; vigorous shaking is avoided to prevent the formation of froth. Each vial, cartridge or pre-filled pen of insulin should be kept in the refrigerator and bears an expiry date beyond which the content should not be used. Insulin in use should be kept at room temperature and out of direct sunlight and has a life expectancy of 28 days. Insulin pen devices should be stored without a needle as this prevents leakage. Each needle is recommended for single use only.

Complications of insulin therapy Various local and general reactions to insulin may occur. The *local reactions* are minor in nature and include local sensitivity, lipodystrophy, lipohypertrophy and fibrosis. Frequently, when insulin therapy is first started, sensitivity may be manifested at the site of injection because the insulin is a foreign protein and antigenic. The area becomes red, swollen and itchy, but the response is generally temporary and disappears as the patient becomes desensitized by the repeated doses of insulin. The local action of insulin on the adipose tissue cells may incur a swelling of the fatty tissue followed by atrophy, which leaves a hollow space in the area. These atrophic areas need

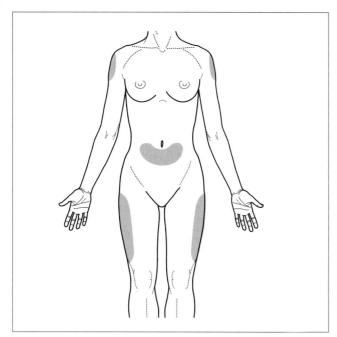

Figure 18.5   Sites for insulin injection.

to be avoided as injection sites until healed which may take months. Fibrous tissue has poor vascularization which decreases the rate of absorption of insulin. This complication may be prevented by systematic rotation of the injection sites and avoiding the use of any one spot more often than once every 4 weeks.

Antidiabetic drugs   Several groups of drugs are used in conjunction with dietary control in the treatment of type 2 diabetes. The term 'non-insulin-dependent diabetes' is misleading as up to 50% of patients with type 2 diabetes ultimately require insulin therapy (Barnett 2001b). The main drugs used are described briefly below.

Biguanides   The biguanides act by reducing the production of glucose in the liver and increasing glucose uptake in muscle. The person has to be manufacturing at least some insulin for these drugs to work. The only member of this group licensed in the UK is metformin, which has the disadvantage of causing gastrointestinal side-effects such as nausea, diarrhoea and flatus. These side-effects usually disappear after 2 weeks of treatment and are minimized if metformin is introduced slowly.

Sulphonylureas   They stimulate the β cells in the islets of Langerhans to secrete more insulin and as a result can be very effective in reducing blood glucose levels in the early part of the disease. Commonly used examples are gliclazide and glipizide. An important side-effect with these drugs is the potential for hypoglycaemia.

Thiazolidinediones (glitazones)   These drugs increase the sensitivity of the body to insulin, thereby having an insulin-sparing effect. The two licensed UK products are rosiglitazone and pioglitazone, and they should be used in conjunction with either a sulfonylurea or metformin (British National Formulary 2005).

Meglitinides   The first drug in this group to be used in the UK is repaglinide, which is a derivative of glibenclamide. It is taken just before a meal, has a short duration of action and can be used with metformin (British National Formulary 2005).

Non-sulfonylurea insulin secretagogues (nateglinide) This drug should be taken immediately before each meal and in the presence of food; it appears markedly to enhance insulin secretion, thereby reducing sharp rises in glucose level immediately after a meal. It is licensed for use only with metformin (British National Formulary 2005).

α-Glucosidase inhibitors   Intestinal enzymes known as α-glucosidases are important in breaking down carbohydrate molecules into short sugar chains. Competitive inhibition of these enzymes has a mild effect in reducing blood glucose levels. The only UK-licensed drug in this group is acarbose, which, due to the problem of causing severe flatulence, is used rarely.

Activity   The *goals* of activity and exercise for the person with diabetes mellitus are to:

1   establish a daily activity and exercise pattern to promote metabolic control
2   reduce the risk for cardiovascular and peripheral vascular complications
3   assist in weight control.

Physical activity promotes health and its importance is shown by the fact that 25% of diabetes is attributable to lack of exercise (Lehmann 1998). Apart from reducing obesity, activity promotes the uptake of glucose to muscle for a period several times longer than the period of exercise and hence reduces blood glucose levels (Pullen 2000). It also stimulates and improves the circulation, helps to maintain muscle tone, and promotes a sense of well-being. Some people with diabetes have sufficient exercise in their occupation, but those in sedentary jobs or who are retired should have a planned programme which is introduced gradually. As the prescription for diet and a hypoglycaemic agent is based on the patient's physical activity, the regimen should be approximately the same each day to minimize fluctuations in the blood glucose concentration. When variations in daily energy expenditure are necessary, adjustments in the diet may be needed. Extra carbohydrate in the form of fruit or bread may be added if activity is increased, or even more concentrated carbohydrate forms may be required if activity is strenuous or prolonged. When the usual amount of activity is decreased for some reason (other than illness or infection), some decrease in the calorific and carbohydrate intake is usually indicated.

Active exercise at regular intervals is encouraged during hospitalization if at least a moderate degree of glycaemic control has been achieved. With an anticipated increase of activity on discharge from the hospital, the insulin dosage may be decreased and the food plan amended accordingly. For the older person with diabetes a daily routine of walking and light home chores (house and garden) is recommended.

The aim is to maintain a balance between energy expenditure and the prescribed treatment (diet with or without medication). More than the usual amount of exercise lowers the blood glucose level; less than the usual amount will raise it.

The person with diabetes participating in strenuous activity, particularly if on insulin therapy, is likely to face several problems. The impaired physiology of diabetes may mean that they tire very quickly. If the person is insulin dependent, injected insulin is not inhibited by adrenaline and noradrenaline as happens with the non-diabetic person, lowering insulin levels, during exercise. Abnormally high levels of insulin therefore inhibit three normal mechanisms of energy release: growth hormone and cortisol release, the conversion of fatty acid glycerol to glucose and glucagon production (Pullen 2000). Hypoglycaemia may ensue as the uptake of glucose by muscles is unimpaired but the ability to mobilize glucose is poor. Careful, controlled experimentation under medical supervision with diet and insulin and frequent blood glucose monitoring are essential if the diabetic person is to achieve optimum performance in sporting events. However, the remarkable Olympic achievements of the oarsman Steve Redgrave, are a testimony to what can be achieved.

Patient and family education

The overall *goals* of diabetic education are to:

1 impart the knowledge and skills necessary to maintain optimal glycaemic control
2 develop and foster the attitudes, beliefs and behaviours that are conducive to metabolic control
3 promote a quality of life whereby the individual's disease and lifestyle are harmoniously balanced.

The person with diabetes mellitus has a chronic lifelong disease and is ultimately responsible for the self-management of health care. To achieve a state of health and an acceptable level of functioning, the person must learn to coordinate the treatment regimen of diet, activity and medication into a daily routine of work or school and recreation to achieve and maintain normal physiological blood glucose levels. To do this, adequate knowledge and skill to be able to make informed decisions about health problems are required.

Nursing intervention   The nurse, with the doctor, dietitian and pharmacist, is responsible for assessing learning needs, helping the patient to set realistic goals, providing knowledge, teaching necessary skills, identifying relevant learning resources and evaluating the outcomes of teaching. Diabetic education programmes benefit from a team approach.

All nurses should possess a sound working knowledge of diabetes as, whatever area of care you practice in, a significant proportion of your patients will be diabetic. Some nurses have however, built up considerable levels of expertise in the specialist field of diabetic care and manage patients in primary care with a high degree of autonomy.

Assessment of learning needs   Assessment of what the patient already knows, learning capability and lifestyle factors that will influence learning and cooperation with the therapeutic plan is important before a learning plan can be developed. For a previously diagnosed person with diabetes, information is required about the usual diabetic routine at home, work or school, how usual activities have changed, community resources used, and what further information and skills are needed.

Assessment should include the patient's perceptions (which may be very different from the nurse's), their interpersonal relations, the social systems they live within (family, work, etc.) and finally the health state and usual capabilities of the person. This is a holistic approach to health that, while maintaining the importance of key physiological parameters such as blood glucose levels, brings in a host of other psychosocial factors that influence the health of persons with diabetes and their ability to cooperate with treatment. The patient's own goals for diabetes management can be made visible in this way. Coping strategies therefore need to be explored carefully with the patient as part of the assessment process. How the person lives with diabetes should be a major concern of the nurse.

Educating a patient does not, however, guarantee that there will be any observable change in behaviour. McIntyre and McDowell (1994) described an illuminating case study involving a 55-year-old Asian Muslim woman, Mrs R, who had had diabetes for 17 years. She was considered to be at risk of developing foot problems, so a teaching programme was instituted concerning foot care. The authors concluded that after 9 weeks, her knowledge of diabetic foot care had increased significantly; however, her practice of it remained minimal. Similar findings were made for other aspects of self-care resulting in consistently high blood glucose levels and continued smoking. McIntyre and McDowell considered that Mrs R had not accepted that diabetic care was within her own control and consequently did not take responsibility for her own self-care. They speculated whether her Muslim religion encouraged a fatalistic view of life and health care, perhaps explaining her lack of self-care. This case study underlines two important points:

1 Diabetes care and health education in general must encompass the whole individual and their psychosocial framework.
2 Outcomes must be demonstrated that show changes in behaviour and health status before any health education programme can be claimed a success. Simply increasing patient knowledge is not sufficient on its own.

The patient's responses to diagnosis and treatment influence readiness to learn. Initial responses to the diagnosis may include fear, withdrawal or anger. Assessment of learning needs continues as patients work through their immediate reactions to reach a phase in which they may talk about their feelings and are prepared to listen and accept the reassurance that their disease can be controlled and that the necessary treatment and care can soon become a routine part of their life without seriously altering it.

Development of a teaching plan   Once learning needs have been identified, the nurse, with the patient and family, sets priorities. These may be dictated by the fact that the patient will be discharged in a few days and will be responsible for preparing meals and/or administering insulin. The knowledge and skill necessary for safe functioning assumes priority and must be adjusted according to the readiness of the patient to learn. Information available from 'Diabetes UK' may provide further support after discharge home.

In planning the instruction, it is necessary to know the patient's background so that care can be adapted as much as possible to normal living patterns. The amount of information given at one time depends on the patient's ability and willingness to receive it. Generally, brief periods of discussion are more effective than the presentation of a large amount of information at one time. Group instruction may be used in the hospital or clinic for some topics, but it must be remembered that each person's treatment and lifestyle are unique. A large part of the discussion must be on an individual basis. Patient negotiation and learning contracts are useful strategies to assist individuals with the development of self-management skills.

Teaching is begun as soon as possible to avoid giving too much at one time, leading to confusion and discouragement, and to allow time for the patient to practise self-care, read and ask questions.

Explanations are made in simple lay terms, and demonstrations are broken into steps, made slowly, repeated as often as necessary, and sufficient opportunity is provided for the patient to practise. Follow-up discussion of signs and symptoms experienced during episodes of hypoglycaemia and hyperglycaemia, and responses to interventions, helps the patient to develop the problem-solving skills needed for self-management. Illustrations, videos and written material should be used for clarification and reinforcement of teaching. The 'Diabetes UK' website (www.diabetes.org.uk) is a source of excellent teaching material.

An educational programme should cover the areas listed in Box 18.4.

Implementation of the teaching plan   How the teaching plan is implemented depends upon the immediate patient situation and the agreed goals and plan. Rarely does one nurse have the opportunity to work with a patient and family throughout the learning process. Teaching carried out in hospital, whether with the newly diagnosed patient or with an established diabetic patient and family, requires evaluation and supplementation in the community as the

---

> **Box 18.4**   Areas to be covered in an education programme for the patient with diabetes
>
> - An explanation of diabetes – types and effects on everyday living
>
> - Diet – meal plans, foods to avoid, a plan to achieve correct body weight
>
> - Insulin therapy or oral medications, if appropriate – demonstrate correct technique for insulin injection, explain storage, time and dosage of insulin, or explain name, dosage and timing of oral medication
>
> - Skin integrity – advice about foot and skin care
>
> - Activity – balance of insulin and exercise
>
> - Assessment of glycaemic control – if appropriate, explain and demonstrate technique for blood glucose monitoring, explain significance of variation in blood glucose levels
>
> - Metabolic emergencies – discuss causes of hypoglycaemia and hyperglycaemia and strategies to prevent or cope with problems
>
> - Diabetic identification card
>
> - Regular health supervision – discuss long-term complications, signs to look out for and how to prevent them and explain the importance of regular blood pressure monitoring, eye examination, urine testing for microalbuminuria and cholesterol checks
>
> - Sources of information, assistance and advice such as prescription exemption certificates, guidance on implications for driving and advice relating to occupation.

---

person has the opportunity to apply knowledge and skill and learning needs continue to evolve.

The following is presented as an example from which the nurse can select the content relevant to an individual patient in a given situation.

What is diabetes mellitus? A simple basic explanation is made of the nature of diabetes, relating it to the symptoms experienced by the patient. To illustrate, the patient may be told that sugar and starches (such as bread and cereal) are converted by digestion to a simple form of sugar called glucose, which is the body's chief source of energy. In order for the cells to extract glucose from the blood and use it, the chemical insulin is necessary. There are two types of diabetes. In type 1 diabetes, there is not sufficient insulin being produced to use the amount of sugar and starches being taken, so glucose accumulates in the blood in excess of the normal. The kidneys remove some of the excess, which is why the person with diabetes voids a lot of urine that contains sugar. The loss of large amounts of urine results in thirst. Weakness, fatigue and hunger occur because the sugar is not being 'burned' to produce energy. The body, in an effort to provide energy, may breakdown body tissue, causing a loss of weight. Daily insulin injections and dietary measures are necessary to control this disorder.

With type 2 diabetes, enough insulin to handle the amount of sugar may be produced but the cells cannot effectively utilize the glucose. This type of diabetes can be controlled by diet and activity to achieve a desirable body weight. Some patients may require oral medication, although some may eventually require insulin.

Diet The patient and health professional discuss and agree on a target or ideal body weight for the person. A plan to achieve and/or maintain the desirable weight is mutually developed and should include plans for regular weight checks. The diet must be clearly and carefully interpreted to the patient and family. The initial instruction is sometimes given by a dietitian, but considerable clarification and reinforcement by both ward and community nurses is necessary. The dietitian explains the diet and reviews the principles of healthy eating. It is helpful for the patient to plan meals with the dietitian, gaining assistance and support in making healthy choices. The purchase and preparation of food and how it may be worked in with the family meals should be discussed.

Adjustment of diet and medications in relation to increased stress and changes in lifestyle is important. Diabetic patients can be taught to adjust their diet and medication in relation to change in demand for glucose and insulin. Blood glucose monitoring by patients makes it possible for them to achieve good glycaemic control during illness and to be more flexible in their eating patterns, activity and travel.

Eating out and delayed meals may also necessitate changes in food intake. Whenever possible, people with diabetes should maintain their usual eating pattern, including the time of meals and the content of each meal. They quickly learn to select appropriate meals from menus or from the selection offered by friends and relatives. When eating out, they should be prepared for delays and the possibility of hypoglycaemia by carrying dextrose tablets or other sources of quickly absorbable carbohydrate. When aware that meals will be delayed, the patient is instructed to have a small snack before leaving home. People using insulin and with a good understanding of their disease and its management may be provided with guidelines from their doctor on the use of compensatory insulin supplements before large meals. Patients using insulin pumps and blood glucose monitoring quickly learn to take an extra bolus of insulin with an unusually large meal.

The patient is encouraged to read and obtain for personal use, books and pamphlets that contain considerable detail on diabetic dietary plans.

Drug therapy If the patient is on *insulin* therapy, advice is required on equipment and where it may be obtained. An explanation is made of what insulin is, types available, the name and nature of the insulin prescribed and how it is identified. Unit dosage is explained and measurement by units is demonstrated. The injection technique (see p. 562) is described and demonstrated to the patient who is then encouraged to practise under supervision until competent. Storage and maintenance of an adequate supply of insulin are discussed. The need to plan and breakdown all this information into small logical teaching units or blocks is again emphasized. If discouragement and frustration are evident, further instruction is delayed and another approach considered.

If *oral medication* is prescribed, the importance of taking the drug in the exact dosage at the times prescribed is stressed. Written directions are given, and the patient is advised that if headache, nausea, vomiting or other disturbances are experienced, the general practitioner should be contacted. The patient is reminded not to experiment with the dosage of the drug and that adherence to the prescribed diet is most important even though medication is also being received.

Illness will affect medication. People with diabetes are instructed on how to manage their disease during illness. If nausea and vomiting are present, the diet plan may be converted to liquids. A balanced diet may still be obtained. Vegetables and fruit may be ingested in the form of juices or soups. If oral intake is not possible, parenteral fluids are administered. All people with diabetes should continue to take their medication during an illness (this is called the 'sick day rules'). Larger doses of insulin with more frequent supplementary doses may be required. Insulin dosage should be adjusted according to prescribed guidelines in relation to blood glucose determinations. Insulin may be switched to short-acting insulin for the duration of illness.

Travel may also necessitate changes in drug therapy. The person with type 1 diabetes needs to take precautions to avoid hypoglycaemia while travelling. If travelling by car, snacks or juices are kept available. On planes and trains, while meals may be obtained if delays occur, it is still important to carry some food in the hand-baggage in case there are problems. Additionally, luggage in the baggage hold of an aircraft can experience very low temperatures which may damage insulin. Travelling through several time zones should not pose any difficulties, provided a plan is developed ahead of time. People using insulin must remember to carry insulin and syringes and be prepared to inject insulin wherever required. It is important for the patient to take a sufficient quantity of insulin and supplies for insulin administration and blood glucose monitoring or urine testing for the duration of any stay, as products may vary or be difficult to obtain in different countries. Insulin should be refrigerated whenever possible but will be quite safe if kept in a small insulated container to prevent exposure to high temperatures and bright light.

Activity Regular activity is beneficial and an integral component of the person's diabetic control. The nurse and patient should review usual activity patterns and develop plans for the person to receive consistent exercise. The person who participated in extended exercise activities before diagnosis is helped to develop a modified routine until glycaemic control is achieved and the skill of balancing diet and insulin in relation to activity has been learnt.

Precautions to avoid exercise-induced hypoglycaemia or hyperglycaemia and hyperketonaemia include:

- regulation of food and insulin intakes in conjunction with exercise
- regular monitoring of blood glucose levels
- a readily available source of carbohydrate
- a decrease in insulin dosage before extended exercise
- use of an injection site that is not active during exercise (e.g. the abdomen)
- regular monitoring of blood glucose levels
- avoiding exercise when glycaemic control is poor.

These points are general guidelines and may be altered for people who are embarking upon intense sporting activities. Patients who have diabetes and enjoy sport should be advised to seek specialized support and advice for their particular personal needs.

Skin integrity People with diabetes have an increased risk for infection and skin breakdown, particularly in their feet. The person is taught to keep the skin clean, warm and free of irritation and pressure as far as possible. Precautions are taken to prevent cracks and breaks in the skin. Cuts and abrasions of the skin are cleaned and protected with a dressing. The use of strong antiseptic (such as iodine) and adhesive is avoided. Prolonged exposure to sunlight and the use of local heat applications (hot water bottle) are discouraged.

The patient's feet require regular special attention because of the increased susceptibility to circulatory disorders and loss of sensation. The patient is directed to bathe the feet daily with warm (not hot) water, using a mild soap and a small amount of bath oil, and to dry them thoroughly, especially the areas between the toes, using gentle pressure rather than vigorous rubbing. If the feet are dry and scaly, a light application of lanolin or prescribed lotion can be applied. The toenails are cut straight across with scissors and, where appropriate, regular foot care should be carried out by a registered chiropodist. Calluses and corns should be treated by a state-registered chiropodist who is advised of the person's diabetes. The patient is cautioned against attempting to remove them by cutting or applying commercial preparations. Stockings or socks should fit well to avoid any constriction or wrinkles that might cause irritation or pressure, and are changed daily. To prevent possible interference with the circulation, garters are not worn. Shoes should be well fitting so there is no irritation or pressure on any part of the foot, and new shoes are worn only for brief periods until 'broken in'. Walking barefoot and the application of heating appliances are discouraged. The feet should be examined daily for breaks in the skin, discolouration and dryness. Numbness, persisting coldness, dis-

colouration, a burning feeling, pain or any unusual condition of the lower limbs should be reported immediately.

Assessment of glycaemic control *Urine glucose monitoring* is not adequate to enable good control of glycaemia. It does not identify hypoglycaemia and may not reveal hyperglycaemia; the latter is detected only when the blood glucose levels exceed the renal threshold, which is variable and may change in older people and those with renal complications. Testing the urine for ketones is, however, useful when the blood glucose test result is raised, during periods of illness or stress, in pregnancy, or when oral hypoglycaemic therapy is being commenced.

Blood glucose monitoring is easily perfected by most patients once they have adjusted to the invasive aspect of pricking their finger to obtain a drop of blood. Self-monitoring of blood glucose levels may facilitate understanding of diabetes and give the patient an active role in the management of the disorder. Satisfaction is generally high; infections and other complications due to self-monitoring are negligible. However, once well-controlled, patients with type 2 diabetes may be advised that they need to monitor blood glucose less frequently. For them blood glucose control can be monitored successfully by 3–6 monthly HbA$_{1c}$ blood tests. For people with type 1 diabetes, self-monitoring remains an important part of the management plan enabling them to adjust insulin dosages throughout the day according to activity.

Most monitors are intended to be used only with capillary blood and therefore should not be used with either venous or arterial blood as they will give false readings due to the differing partial pressure of oxygen that the sample will contain. Results can also be affected by abnormal haematocrit readings, and equipment will have a stated range within which the machine should be used. This is particularly important in areas such as intensive care and maternity units (Batki 1999).

Monitoring of blood glucose levels may be done continually to build up the blood glucose profile of a 'typical day' to assess glycaemic control. This allows adjustment of diet, exercise and medication to achieve better control of blood glucose levels. It may also be done as a spot check for hypoglycaemia or during episodes of illness or when other problems occur. Self-monitoring of blood glucose is carried out using a reagent strip and a machine that gives a digital display of the result. It is important to follow the manufacturer's instructions precisely, particularly with regard to calibration, accuracy and timing. It is a common mistake to use the test strips after the recommended expiry date or to fail to store the strips in the airtight container.

The hand is washed in warm water to improve circulation and remove any contamination from the skin which, if transmitted to the blood drop, can affect the reading. A single-prong lancet pricks the skin either manually or as part of an automated device. A drop of blood large enough to cover the reagent pad is placed on a reagent strip, which is inserted into the machine and left for the period of time recommended by the manufacturer. The machine provides a digital readout of the result.

The person should be given information and teaching on the various types of equipment and their use. Pamphlets, audiovisual presentations and individualized instruction are usually available from the supplier. The newly diagnosed person with diabetes may not grasp the significance of the results initially; however, involvement in the decision-making process about disease management will help to promote responsibility for self-care. The person should begin to keep a record of the results of the blood glucose tests while in hospital. The nurse and doctor discuss these with the patient each day, comparing results with the previous day and exploring factors that influenced any changes. This process is continued after discharge.

A very important method of assessing diabetic control is to measure glycated haemoglobin (HbA_{1c}) concentrations. Measurement of this fraction of haemoglobin gives a good indication of overall blood glucose levels over the previous 12 weeks and offers a validation check on the results the patient produces in their own diary. The results are expressed either as the percentage of HbA_{1c} alone (normal value 4–6%) or as the percentage of total glycated haemoglobin (HbA_1) including all other subfractions (a+b+c), which gives a normal range of 5–7% (Watkins 1998). HbA_{1c} is most commonly used in UK laboratories.

Knowledge of metabolic emergencies (hypoglycaemia and hyperglycaemia)   The diabetic person who is receiving insulin or an oral hypoglycaemic agent should know that under certain circumstances the blood glucose level may fall below normal, resulting in what is called an insulin or *hypoglycaemic* reaction. The patient and family should be familiar with the symptoms, which usually begin to appear when the blood glucose level falls below 3.3 mmol/L. A hypoglycaemic reaction in a person receiving soluble insulin usually occurs approximately 2–6 hours after the injection. In a person receiving intermediate-acting insulin, the reaction happens more commonly in the afternoon or evening. Hypoglycaemic reactions to the newer isophane insulins are less common than the more frequent reactions with the old-style long-acting insulins. It is possible for persons receiving sulphonylureas to develop hypoglycaemia.

Symptoms vary from one person to another, but each individual usually has similar symptoms with each reaction. The early signs and symptoms include sweating, tremor, apprehension, hunger, weakness, rapid pulse and palpitations. More advanced symptoms are faintness or dizziness, blurring of vision or diplopia, headache, slow reactions, uncoordinated movements, twitching, disorientation and confusion. The possible causes of hypoglycaemia are the delay or omission of a meal following administration of insulin or oral medication, excessive energy expenditure with prolonged and/or strenuous exercise, an overdose of insulin, anorexia, vomiting or diarrhoea, increased utilization of glucose and weight loss without readjustment of insulin dosage.

The person is instructed that on experiencing early symptoms carbohydrate should be taken immediately. With more pronounced symptoms, a quick-acting form of carbohydrate will be required, for example 2–3 dextrose tablets, tea or coffee with 2–3 teaspoonsful of sugar, 2–3 small sweets, orange juice or grape juice (120 mL) or 2 teaspoonsful of honey or syrup may be used. If the symptoms do not disappear in 10 minutes, the administration is repeated. The patient on insulin is advised always to carry dextrose tablets, boiled sweets, glucose tablets or GlucoGel (formerly known as Hypostop). GlucoGel, HypoStop or any of the treatments for hypoglycaemia should only be used on people who are conscious and able to swallow, as placing anything in the mouth of someone unable to swallow or unconscious could cause them to choke (Diabetes UK 2006b).

The family should know that if the person cannot swallow or retain sugar, glucagon should be administered or a 999 call made. Friends and associates as well as the family should know that the person takes insulin and may experience a reaction. Hypoglycaemic attacks should be reported to the doctor as the insulin dosage or diet may require adjustment.

In addition to the immediate treatments for hypoglycaemia, patients should be instructed to take a longer acting snack such as a sandwich. This prevents a relapse into a second incident of hypoglycaemia once the fast acting carbohydrate has been used up by the body.

The patient should also be able to recognize early symptoms of uncontrolled diabetes, which cause *hyperglycaemia*. If not corrected in the early stage, hyperglycaemia may lead to the serious complications of diabetic ketoacidosis or hyperosmolar non-ketotic coma. Hyperglycaemia and dehydration with or without ketosis develop more slowly than hypoglycaemia, usually over several days. The disturbance is usually manifested by loss of appetite, nausea, vomiting, thirst, weakness, abdominal pains, drowsiness and general malaise. Glucose will be present in the urine and blood glucose levels are greatly increased. They are frequently associated with infection or stress, or may be due to prolonged dietary indiscretion or omission of insulin or oral hypoglycaemic agent. The patient is advised that they should seek help as soon as symptoms are experienced. Until medical attention is obtained, the patient should remain in bed, keep warm, and try to drink clear fluids *without sugar*, to avoid dehydration and electrolyte imbalance, even if this causes vomiting. If possible, someone should remain with the patient. In this instance, it is useful if the patient has been instructed to test their urine for ketones as this provides extremely useful information regarding the severity of their problem.

Health maintenance   The newly diagnosed patient will be required to make more frequent visits to their general practice. These will become fewer as the disease and treatment are stabilized. The nurse in either situation checks how the patient is managing and gives the patient the opportunity to ask questions. Some aspects of care may require repetition and reinforcement. In the case of older persons, assistance may be necessary in making arrangements for regular follow-up.

It is advisable for the diabetic person to have an annual *eye examination* because of the risk of diabetic retinopathy, which is the most common cause of blindness in advanced industrial countries. Up to 40% of people with diabetes have some retinopathy when type 2 diabetes is first diagnosed (York 1999). The fundus is frequently examined by the use of a retinal camera which takes a photograph of the retina. The photograph is then examined by a specialist and provides a record for future comparison.

Diabetic identification card Every diabetic person should carry a diabetic identification card at all times so that their condition can be made known quickly in the event of a reaction, illness or accident. Cards that carry appropriate information are available from the hospital, doctors, the diabetic clinic and 'Diabetes UK' or its local branches.

Sources of help and information The patient should be informed about available sources of help and information. These include the national and local diabetic associations, which patients are encouraged to join. This entitles them to the regular periodical and additional literature published by 'Diabetes UK'.

Evaluation of patient and family teaching Studies of diabetic education use a variety of outcome measures to evaluate the effectiveness of education programmes and individual teaching. *Knowledge* of the disease and its management can be evaluated using tested tools. However, this knowledge has to be translated into positive behaviour. Auditing the frequency of hospital admissions, A&E attendances or clinic visits related to diabetes control and complications also gives a useful indication of how well the person is managing their diabetes.

Glycaemic control can be evaluated using blood glucose levels. These are useful for daily monitoring by the patient as well as by health professionals. The determination of glycosylated haemoglobin levels (see above) gives an accurate picture of long-term glucose control over the preceding 3 months. It is possible that the patient may have deliberately recorded false values, showing much lower levels, in their diary. Such a situation needs great tact and good communication skills if it is to be resolved satisfactorily.

Attention must be given to the *patient's attitudes to diabetes* and what it means to them. Patient education should help the person with diabetes achieve the highest standards of glycaemic control, but this should be accompanied by satisfactory emotional adjustment and social fulfilment. Diabetes educators need to address the affective or attitudinal aspects of coping with this lifelong condition.

The nurse in any clinical setting should always use the best source available to evaluate the effectiveness of *teaching the patient and family*. Only the patient and those close to him

or her can determine whether the knowledge and skills taught meet their needs and whether the teaching contributed to their psychological and social adjustment to diabetes.

Two clinical situations are described in Case Studies 18.1 and 18.2.

CASE Grace Cook is a relatively inactive 60-year-old woman who enjoys baking and gardening. She is 10 kg overweight. She was having a problem with a cut on her right middle finger that 'just won't heal'. She had also been experiencing blurring of her vision, had less energy than usual and, when questioned, thought that she had been urinating more frequently. Her fasting blood glucose level was 13 mmol/L and her urine was negative for ketones when tested by her practice nurse.

Mrs Cook's doctor referred her to a dietitian for dietary assessment and a diet for type 2 diabetes. The dietitian found that Mrs Cook drank a lot of fruit juices. She skipped breakfast but ate a very large evening meal with her husband and continued to eat snacks throughout the evening while watching television.

Discussion

Mrs Cook is typical of many persons with type 2 diabetes. Her symptoms developed slowly, she had the major risk factor of obesity and she was within the age group of 50–70 years, when over 50% of type 2 diabetics are diagnosed. Symptoms of hyperglycaemia experienced by Mrs Cook included decreased energy, urinary frequency, blurred vision and impaired healing. Her fasting blood glucose level was raised.

The patient's overall goals were to return to a normal body weight for her age and height, and to have blood glucose levels within normal limits.

Goals

Mrs Cook should:

1 decrease her body weight by 10 kg over the next 6–8 months
2 establish a regular pattern of exercise
3 alter her eating habits to decrease calorie intake, increase dietary carbohydrate and fibre and eat three meals a day
4 have a HBA1c level below 7
5 have a blood pressure below 130/80 mmHg.

Intervention and evaluation

The dietitian prescribed a weight-reducing diet which included three meals a day. She helped Mrs Cook to select foods that were high in complex carbohydrate and fibre. She told her to drink water or diet fizzy drinks rather than fruit juices for thirst. Mrs Cook was able to lose 1 kg in the first month of her diet and her fasting blood glucose level dropped to 10 mmol/L.

Exercise recommendations for people with type 2 diabetes include low-intensity exercise over 40–60 minutes on at least

5 days each week. Mrs Cook began taking a walk after breakfast. She did this for 30 minutes almost every day and was able to lose a further 0.5 kg in the second month. Her fasting blood glucose dropped to 8.7 mmol/L.

CASE   Tom Tolly is a recently married 22-year-old construction worker. He experienced a weight loss of 9 kg in the previous 2 weeks, had been very thirsty and had been urinating large amounts. He had been getting up at night to urinate and to drink fluids. He stated that his vision was blurred and that he was tired and lacked energy. His appetite had been very poor for a few days and he had experienced nausea and stomach pain.

Tom went to his general practitioner whose practice nurse carried out a random capillary blood glucose measurement, which was over 30 mmol/L. His urine tested positive for glucose and ketones. Tom was sent to hospital for blood glucose tests. The results were: blood glucose, 36 mmol/L; positive ketones, pH 7.0; bicarbonate level, 17 mmol/L.

Tom was admitted to hospital with a medical diagnosis of severe diabetic ketoacidosis. The medical goals of care were to rehydrate him and to treat his diabetes with insulin.

The priorities for nursing care related to the patient's hyperglycaemic state. Although diabetic ketoacidosis can be resolved in 24 hours, it may be life-threatening. Nursing actions included immediate and continuous assessment of Tom's metabolic state and the identification of associated health problems, as well as collaborative activities related to the implementation and evaluation of medically directed care. The long-term goal for Tom and his wife was to control and achieve self-regulation of his diabetes.

Tom's hyperglycaemia was related to diabetic ketoacidosis and was due to inadequate production of insulin associated with his undiagnosed type 1 diabetes mellitus. He demonstrates the characteristic clinical picture of a person with diabetic ketoacidosis. His symptoms, which developed over a 2-week period, included thirst, polyuria, blurring of vision, weakness, loss of appetite, nausea and gastrointestinal discomfort. The results of diagnostic tests showed that Tom had glycosuria, as evidenced by the presence of glucose and ketones in his urine, and that he was hyperglycaemic; his blood glucose level was raised and ketones were present. His bicarbonate level was decreased (normal range 24–32 mmol/L) and his pH below normal (normal: 7.35–7.45). As the nurse, you expect to observe changes in respirations. *Kussmaul breathing* (rapid, deep respirations) is usually present in diabetic ketoacidosis when the pH is below 7.2. When the bicarbonate level decreases, hyperventilation occurs in order to drive off excess carbon dioxide in an attempt to maintain the pH at a physiological level. When the pH is less than 7.0, the compensatory mechanisms change and slower respirations result. Tom was in a very vulnerable state with a pH of 7.0.

The nurse must also be alert for the development of drowsiness and confusion as Tom's metabolic state was no longer compensated and increases in the partial pressure of carbon dioxide (PCO_2) would have a depressing effect on his central nervous system.

The *goals* for Tom on admission to hospital were that:

1 he would achieve fluid, electrolyte, acid–base and metabolic balance
2 he and his wife would develop a basic understanding of his diabetes and resulting ketoacidosis.

The actual and potential *patient problems* on admission to hospital and the care plan developed for a patient with ketoacidosis are listed in Table 18.2.

Evaluation   On admission to hospital, Tom was acutely ill and required skilled care from knowledgeable, experienced nurses. The nurses worked in collaboration with the doctors to manage the acute medical problems. Many of the patient problems discussed in Table 18.2 fall primarily into the realm of nursing. The patient usually makes a good recovery with prompt care and is normally awake, self-caring and mobile within 48 hours of admission.

Teaching plan

A teaching plan was developed with Tom and his wife. Teaching was carried out in short intervals throughout the day to accommodate Tom's limited physical tolerance and shortened attention span. Teaching sessions with the dietitian, pharmacist and nurse were arranged for late afternoons when Mrs Tolly could be present. Because of the overwhelming quantity of new knowledge and skills faced by Tom and his wife, care was taken to limit teaching to that which they needed to know to function safely on discharge. The following expectations were agreed:

Goals

The reader is referred to the list on p. 566. Additional goals which might be incorporated in a teaching package include the ability for Mr and Mrs Tolly to:

1 experience a gradual increase in weight for Tom from his present 65.5 kg to his ideal body weight of 72 kg
2 understand how insulin works
3 describe the role of exercise in diabetes management
4 discuss with health professionals the adjustments to insulin dose as a result of changes in blood glucose levels
5 verbalize awareness of complications of diabetes
6 describe the relationship between diabetes control and the development of complications
7 talk about the meaning of the diabetes to themselves, their new relationship and their future lifestyles
8 confirm that their major concerns have been addressed
9 describe an agreed plan for continuing education and medical supervision on discharge.

Tom's major expressed difficulties were: (1) how can he continue his current job, which often does not have regular coffee and lunch breaks and is very physically demanding and (2) acceptance of the fact that he has diabetes when he is a young, healthy man, recently married and enjoys sports and drinking alcohol with friends.

Table 18.2 Care plan for a patient with ketoacidosis

Goals	Nursing intervention	Rationale
Patient problem 1: Fluid volume deficit due to polyuria and glycosuria		
1 Fluid intake and urine output will be in physiological balance. 2 Mucous membranes will be moist. 3 Blood glucose levels will decrease towards normal.	Administer 0.9% saline at 650 mL/hour for the first 2 hours as ordered. Adjust rate as indicated Accurately record fluid intake and output hourly Assess for signs of fluid overload: dyspnoea, pulmonary crackles and wheezes, increased central venous pressure	The severe dehydration is life-threatening. Isotonic fluids are administered rapidly to restore the intravascular volume and increase cardiac output
	Assess blood pressure, pulse and respirations hourly	Hypotension and tachycardia occur in response to hypovolaemia and decreased tissue perfusion
	Record patient's temperature 2–3-hourly	Dehydration produces a rise in body temperature
	Provide mouth care regularly	
Patient problem 2: Metabolic imbalance: ketoacidosis related to decreased production of insulin		
1 Serum glucose level will be 5.6–7.8 mmol/L. 2 Serum ketone level will be in the normal range. 3 Urine will be negative for glucose and ketones.	Administer regular insulin by continuous i.v. infusion (8 units/hour) and adjust rate as ordered Monitor blood glucose and ketone levels, urine glucose and ketones and urinary output hourly	Low-dose infusions of insulin are effective in decreasing the catabolic process and promoting glucose uptake by the cells. The rate of flow (dosage) is determined by blood glucose levels and decreased ketosis
	Assess hourly for signs of hypoglycaemia	Sudden reduction in blood glucose levels can cause tachycardia and symptoms of hypoglycaemia
Patient problem 3: Ineffective breathing pattern related to hyperventilation in response to metabolic acidosis		
1 Respirations will be 20–24/minute and regular. 2 Blood gases, pH and bicarbonate levels will return to normal range.	Assess respiratory rate, depth and rhythm hourly Change position 2-hourly and assess response to position change	Hyperventilation occurs with acidosis. Respirations decrease with pH<7.0
	Administer oxygen by nasal cannulae as ordered Evaluate blood gas level	To increase tissue perfusion
Patient problem 4: Sensory/perceptual deficits due to ketoacidosis, central nervous system depression, and blurring of vision		
1 pH will be within normal limits. 2 Serum glucose levels will be within normal limits. 3 Patient will respond appropriately to the environment and to verbal commands.	Assess level of consciousness and pupillary responses, reflexes and behavioural responses 2-hourly and record Call by name Explain all procedures and activities and describe what is happening	Cognitive and perceptual changes are multifactorial in origin and can develop in response to aggressive rehydration and treatment of acidosis
	Explain that vision will clear when diabetes is controlled Keep cot sides in place on bed	Awareness that blurring of vision is transient helps to decrease fear

continued

Table 18.2 *Cont'd*

Goals	Nursing intervention	Rationale
Patient problem 5: Alteration in nutrition: intake less than body requirement due to inability to utilize glucose as a result of insulin deficit, loss of appetite, nausea and gastrointestinal discomfort		
1 Abdominal distension and discomfort will be absent. 2 Gastrointestinal sounds will be present on auscultation. 3 Patient will take oral fluids with no discomfort.	Assess for abdominal distension and signs of increased abdominal discomfort Pass nasogastric tube Document amount and colour of aspirated gastric content Following removal of nasogastric tube, administer small amounts of clear fluid and assess for distension and discomfort Answer questions regarding diabetic diet and explain that the dietician will see the patient before discharge	Gastric mobility is impaired with ketoacidosis To decompress gastrointestinal tract and reduce discomfort
Patient problem 6: Impaired physical mobility related to weakness, fatigue and restrictions of treatment		
1 Peripheral pulses will remain palpable. 2 Peripheral skin will be normal and warm to touch. 3 Patient will move to bedside chair within 24 hours. 4 Rehydration will be evident by urine output of >1.5 L/day and normal vital signs.	Assess peripheral skin colour and peripheral pulses 2-hourly Provide antiembolic stockings if prescribed Perform passive leg exercises 2-hourly while awake until fully mobile Mobilize patient as soon as possible	Patient is at risk for developing vascular thrombi due to decreased intravascular volume with dehydration and acidosis, increased blood viscosity, decreased tissue perfusion, decreased cardiac output and increased adhesiveness of platelets
Patient problem 7: Lack of knowledge about diabetes mellitus, ketoacidosis and their management		
1 Patient and family will be able to describe the causes of ketoacidosis and signs of hyperglycaemia. 2 Patient and family will verbalize plans to begin learning about diabetes and its management.	Assess level of understanding of diabetes and ketoacidosis Provide explanations of all procedures and activities Answer questions from patient and family Develop an initial learning plan with the patient and family as soon as they are able to participate	If the patient and family are knowledgeable about the signs and symptoms of hyperglycaemia and appropriate interventions, future episodes of ketoacidosis are largely preventable

In this case, the nurse should discuss Tom's concerns with him and arrange for the dietitian to talk with him about possible solutions to the irregular meals and snacks he will experience at work. It will be possible for him to learn to adjust his insulin administration when he knows that meals will be delayed. He can also carry snacks with him to take when meals are delayed. Although his present insulin dosage is being regulated according to his restricted activity in hospital, this will be increased and regulated according to the demands of his usual work activity. He should be referred to the occupational health department in his place of work. He should be told that he will still be able to participate in active sports. It is important that Tom has regular, consistent exercise. When exercise is extended or excessive, he will have to take glucose supplements such as fruit and sweets and adjust his insulin. He is assured that he will have the opportunity to learn these skills once metabolic control is re-established and after he has learnt the basics of diet, insulin and exercise management. The doctor and diabetes specialist nurse will help him with regulation of the insulin and work will continue with Tom and his wife when he returns home.

Another area to explore with Tom concerns intercourse, as he may have experienced difficulty in maintaining an erection due to his diabetes. It should be explained that the severely high blood glucose levels he experienced with the uncontrolled diabetes may cause impotence and that this will resolve when metabolic control is re-established. The diabetes will not affect his sexual desire but when the diabetes is uncontrolled, he may be unable to achieve or maintain an erection. As this problem may impede progress, alter self-concept and affect his new role as a husband, the nurse should encourage him to discuss this with his wife. The initial and later changes in sexual function associated with diabetes can represent the most difficult adjustments faced by persons with diabetes. The reality of impotence, concerns about infertility and the stress these place on the relationship, are major concerns for any patient and family. The nurse may give Tom a pamphlet on sexual health and diabetes, and plan to reassess his concerns and discuss them further before his discharge.

ACUTE METABOLIC EMERGENCIES

Diabetic ketoacidosis

Diabetic ketoacidosis is a serious metabolic complication that develops when there is too little insulin and an excess of glucose.

The cause of insulin deficiency may be inadequate production of insulin in the undiagnosed diabetic patient, inadequate administration of insulin or an increased need for insulin resulting from emotional or physical stresses such as infection. Excess glucose may result from increased hepatic production of glucose, decreased utilization of glucose by peripheral tissue and increased ingestion of glucose in the diet.

The production of **ketone bodies** involves processes occurring in adipose tissue, liver and muscle. The glucose in the blood cannot be utilized by the cells, and fat is broken down to provide energy. Fat is mobilized and broken down rapidly, producing ketone bodies (acetoacetic acid, β-hydroxybutyric acid and acetone) in excess of the ability of tissue cells to metabolize them. Alterations in liver metabolism lead to further ketone production. This process is accelerated when glucagon levels rise. An associated decrease in the ability of muscle tissue to utilize these organic acids further contributes to ketoacidosis. The acids and acetone accumulate in the blood. At first, the normal pH is maintained by the buffer systems, but eventually the alkali reserve becomes depleted and the pH of the body fluids falls, resulting in acidosis. At the same time, the increased concentration of glucose causes an increased output of urine (osmotic diuresis) and dehydration develops. The increased osmotic pressures of the extracellular fluid result in the movement of fluid out of the cells accompanied by electrolytes. Serious sodium, potassium and phosphate deficiencies develop.

Symptoms

Ketoacidosis has an insidious onset over several days, being preceded by symptoms characteristic of uncontrolled diabetes (polyuria, thirst, glycosuria, weakness). The symptoms related to the accumulation of ketones and reduced alkalinity of body fluids include anorexia, nausea, vomiting, deep and rapid respirations, drowsiness, weakness which progresses to prostration, and abdominal pain or muscular cramps. The skin and mouth are dry, and the eyeballs are soft because of dehydration. The patient may appear flushed in the early stages but later becomes pale owing to hypotension. The pulse is rapid and may be weak because of severe dehydration and the reduced intravascular volume. Unless the condition is recognized and treated promptly, the blood pressure falls, the patient becomes comatose, and brain damage will occur unless the situation is reversed quickly. Even though the patient may be fully conscious and walking when presenting in the health centre or medical admissions unit, he or she is seriously ill with the risk of a rapid deterioration in their condition leading to coma, brain damage and possible death.

The patient's urine shows a high concentration of glucose, while blood glucose levels are well above normal. Ketones will be found in the urine related to increased levels of ketones in the blood. Reduced serum bicarbonate levels (12 mmol/L) indicate severe acidosis associated with the raised ketone levels in plasma. The patient's reserves of sodium, potassium and chloride are greatly reduced as a result of the loss of fluid and dehydration. The leucocyte count is generally raised as part of the stress response. There may be no correlation between the blood glucose levels and the severity of the ketoacidosis; only moderately increased blood glucose levels may be associated with a life-threatening ketoacidosis.

Treatment and nursing intervention

The treatment and nursing intervention for the patient with diabetic ketoacidosis requires emergency care that is directed toward stimulating the utilization of glucose by the cells and decreasing the production of ketone bodies by the administration of insulin, and correction of dehydration and the electrolyte imbalance. Any causative disorder is also treated.

An indwelling catheter may be inserted if the patient is comatose, to enable monitoring of urinary output. If the patient is comatose, a nasogastric tube is passed to avoid risk of aspiration of vomit. The patient receives an intravenous infusion of soluble (rapid acting) insulin. Continuous cardiac monitoring is necessary to detect cardiac arrhythmias due to abnormal blood potassium levels. Intravenous fluids are given to correct electrolyte deficits as well as dehydration. The initial solution used is usually normal saline, 1 L in 30 minutes, followed by 0.5 L in 30 minutes and then 0.5 L in 1 hour. As potassium moves out of the cells in this situation, first the serum concentration may be misleadingly normal or even raised. With the administration of the intravenous infusions and insulin, plasma potassium moves into the cells and hypokalaemia develops, which may necessitate the administration of potassium chloride supplements to the intravenous infusion. Repeated blood electrolyte, glucose and ketone determinations are necessary. When the blood glucose level approaches normal, the frequency of administration and the dosage of insulin are decreased, and an intravenous glucose solution (5% in water or saline) may be ordered. If the patient's blood pressure is low and shock is present, plasma or plasma expanders may be given. Unless the cause of the ketoacidosis was evident at the onset, efforts are made to determine why it occurred.

A clinical situation of diabetic ketoacidosis is described in Case Study 18.2.

Hyperglycaemic, hyperosmolar, non-ketotic diabetic coma

This serious metabolic complication is characterized by severe hyperglycaemia with no significant ketosis or acidosis. Serum osmolarity is increased; insulin is deficient but not absent; and severe dehydration and hypovolaemia exist.

Hyperglycaemic, hyperosmolar non-ketotic coma is most likely to occur in elderly people and carries a mortality rate of 40% or more (Haslett et al 1999). The patient may not even have been diagnosed as a diabetic when they present in a collapsed condition, usually to A&E or a medical emergency admissions unit. The onset of hyperglycaemic, hyperosmolar non-ketotic coma is insidious, occurring over several days. The patient demonstrates weakness, polyuria and polydipsia. As intracellular dehydration progresses and fluid shifts to the extracellular spaces, symptoms of neurological involvement, lethargy, confusion, convulsions and eventually coma develop.

Treatment

Treatment is directed toward reversing the hyperosmolar state with fluid replacement and correcting underlying causes. The prognosis for patients with this condition is generally poor but is improved with prompt treatment. Treatment differs in three ways from that of ketoacidosis:

1 Hypotonic saline solutions (0.45%) are given intravenously instead of the isotonic solutions (0.9%) used to treat ketoacidosis. Central venous pressure monitoring serves as a guide to the rate of infusion.
2 Insulin is administered intravenously, but lower doses are required than for ketoacidosis.
3 Thromboembolic problems are common; therefore, heparin should be given.

Nursing intervention

Nursing intervention is similar to that outlined in Table 18.2 for the patient with diabetic ketoacidosis. Careful monitoring and recording of the large volumes of hypotonic parenteral solutions that are administered is important. The patient is assessed for signs of fluid overload, which include dyspnoea, pulmonary crackles and wheezes, and increased central venous pressure. The low doses of insulin prescribed are administered using an infusion controller to regulate the dosage carefully. Observations should be made for signs of hypoglycaemia as a precaution.

Care of the patient with altered levels of consciousness is discussed in Appendix 1. Nursing intervention includes measures to maintain a patent airway, personal safety and pressure area care.

The patient and family's level of understanding of diabetes, the causes of metabolic complications, general disease management and actions to take when complications occur are assessed. An individualized teaching plan is developed, implemented and evaluated; referrals are made to the community nurse where appropriate. Attempts are made to determine the factors precipitating the episode and to institute measures to prevent future episodes of hyperosmolar, non-ketotic coma.

Hypoglycaemia

Hypoglycaemia implies an abnormally low blood glucose concentration. The onset of symptoms varies with individuals and consequently different people develop symptoms at different blood glucose. People with either type 1 or type 2 diabetes can have hypoglycaemic episodes; the most frequent cause of the problem is inadequate patient education. The patient may take their normal medication but miss or delay a meal or eat a meal that is inadequate in carbohydrate content. Unexpected exercise or excess alcohol intake can also provoke an episode. Errors in self-medication or deliberate self-harm caused by manipulation of the dietary or hypoglycaemic medication regimen may also lead to hypoglycaemia. Nocturnal hypoglycaemia may occur if the patient has a poorly designed insulin regimen. Patients tend to have a certain pattern of symptoms but sometimes the pattern changes and the patient is taken unawares. This can happen with ageing or in patients who have had diabetes for more than 15 years. Some patients experience hypoglycaemic symptoms with blood glucose levels which would usually be considered to be in the normal range, these patients have adapted to high levels of glucose and over time their receptors respond to a fall at a higher level than would normally be expected.

A hypoglycaemic reaction occurs in a patient who is on insulin at a time that relates to the duration of action of the insulin. It is therefore important to familiarize yourself with the range of different insulins and their duration of action. It is also important to check that the patient has been educated about the onset of action and the peak time of action for the insulin they are using. It is also possible for the patient receiving an oral hypoglycaemic agent such as a sulphonylurea to develop hypoglycaemia.

The signs and symptoms manifested by an abnormally low blood glucose level are a reflection of its effect on the central nervous system. The brain is very dependent on a constant, adequate supply of glucose. Any deprivation, even for a relatively brief period, may seriously impair cerebral activity and result in permanent damage. It has been suggested that repeated occurrences of hypoglycaemia, especially in children, may incur some permanent cerebral impairment. The manifestations of hypoglycaemia vary from one patient to another but tend to be the same with each reaction for the same person, which makes it more easily recognizable by the individual. The earlier signs and symptoms include sweating, tremor, apprehension, hunger, weakness, tachycardia and palpitation. Symptoms usually do not appear until the blood glucose level is 2.8–3.3 mmol/L. More advanced symptoms are faintness or dizziness, blurring of vision or diplopia, headache, slow reactions, uncoordinated movement which occasionally leads to mistaking the patient's condition for alcohol intoxication, muscular twitching that may progress to convulsions especially in children, disorientation and confusion, stupor and eventual loss of consciousness. The urine is usually negative for glucose, although, occasionally, a trace may be found if the bladder has not been emptied for a few hours. All diabetic people, their immediate family and close associates should be familiar with the early signs and symptoms of hypoglycaemia and should know what to do.

If the patient can still swallow, some form of rapidly absorbable concentrated sugar should be given; 10–20 g of carbohydrate are usually sufficient to restore the blood glucose level. Two or three glucose tablets, a cup of tea with 2 teaspoons of sugar, a sweet drink such as 50 ml Lucozade, 100 ml Coca Cola or a mini bar of chocolate (25 g). This represents 20 g of carbohydrate and should be sufficient to treat an attack. GlucoGel ampoules can also be used. After eating, the person should measure the blood glucose level 15–20 minutes later. If there is no improvement, the administration is repeated. If the patient is unconscious or uncooperative, 30–50 mL of 50% glucose are given intravenously. Glucagon (1 unit) subcutaneously may be ordered to promote hepatic breakdown of glycogen (glycogenolysis) and subsequent increase in blood glucose. Family members may be taught to administer the glucagon. A venous or capillary blood specimen is collected as soon as possible and is repeated at frequent intervals for blood glucose determinations until the patient is stabilized.

Following a reaction, the patient is encouraged to rest for several hours in order to decrease the utilization of blood glucose. Carbohydrate administration may be repeated with some form of protein (a cheese sandwich for example) to provide additional glucose that is absorbed more slowly as a result of protein metabolism. The nurse should check with the doctor before giving the next scheduled dose of insulin. If the patient is at home, instructions should be given not to take more insulin or hypoglycaemic agents at that time. Adjustments are usually made in the carbohydrate content of the diet and in the insulin dosage.

Most diabetic patients and their families are taught which symptoms signal hypoglycaemia or hyperglycaemia. Evidence suggests that people miss hypoglycaemia or hyperglycaemia symptoms and erroneously believe that their blood glucose levels are within normal range, or feel they are hypoglycaemic or hyperglycaemic when they are not. Self-monitoring of blood glucose, while readily available and used by many diabetic patients, is not necessarily used appropriately to confirm subjective symptoms. The individual's ability to distinguish good predictors of blood glucose levels can be improved through systematic education. The person may be helped to review documented daily blood glucose levels and associated symptoms and to identify which cues are predictive of the actual blood glucose levels. This problem-solving approach requires that the patient and a family member or close associate be knowledgeable of the symptoms, the measurement of blood glucose levels, the associated risk factors and the treatment of hypoglycaemia. The patient and family member will learn from the experience if

encouraged to examine the reaction in retrospect. A discussion of the possible cause and the early symptoms may be helpful in preventing further reactions and in having the patient recognize hypoglycaemia at the onset.

The *Somogyi effect* occurs in people with type 1 diabetes who are treated too aggressively in an attempt to normalize blood glucose levels. The hypoglycaemia resulting from administration releases counter-regulatory hormones, producing a rebound hyperglycaemia. The insulin produces a decrease in blood glucose concentration, which triggers the sympathetic nervous system to release ACTH. The liver releases glycogen and the blood glucose level rises. Further administration of insulin causes a repeat of the cycle. Sudden falls in blood glucose levels followed by rebound hyperglycaemia are characteristic of the Somogyi effect. Treatment consists of gradually decreasing the insulin dosage. The phenomenon is less common in patients whose diabetes is controlled by insulin infusion pumps.

THE PERSON WITH A DISORDER OF THE THYROID GLAND

Disease of the thyroid may cause a hyposecretion or hypersecretion of the thyroid hormones and a change in the size of the gland. A deficiency in the secretion is called *hypothyroidism*; an excessive secretion is referred to as *hyperthyroidism*. The normally functioning gland is referred to as *euthyroid*.

ASSESSMENT

Assessment of the person with a disorder of the thyroid gland begins with a comprehensive health history. The health problems experienced by the individual usually develop gradually and are vague and general in nature. Knowledge of the clinical characteristics of altered thyroid function assists the nurse to organize data collection, to formulate specific questions for the health history and to identify patterns of responses demonstrated by the patient. Table 18.3 lists the common health problems experienced by persons with thyroid disorders and the clinical characteristics of hypothyroidism and hyperthyroidism.

Health history
The patient is asked about changes in physical appearance, activity tolerance and energy level, skin moisture, muscle tone, body weight, diet, menstrual cycle and thought processes. Specific questions related to usual and current daily routine and activity patterns and how the individual organizes the day may provide clues to subtle changes and how the person is compensating. With questioning, the person may recognize that they have become more forgetful and have compensated for the changes by instituting reminders for themselves to keep appointments and fulfil commitments. They may also recognize insidious changes in physical activity and usual exercise patterns. Other specific information includes any difficulty in swallowing, episodes

Table 18.3 Assessment of the person with altered thyroid function

	Clinical characteristics	
	Hypothyroidism	**Hyperthyroidism**
Nutrition and metabolism	Pulse rate decreased Blood pressure low Respirations decreased Appetite poor Weight gain Serum cholesterol raised	Pulse rapid and bounding Palpitations Increased blood pressure Respiratory rate increased Appetite increased Weight loss Serum cholesterol decreased
Activity tolerance	Weakness and fatigue Slow movements Dyspnoea Decreased muscle tone and reflexes	Weakness and fatigue Weakness of eyelid muscles Shortness of breath on exertion Tremor of hands Increased muscle tone and reflexes
Skin integrity	Skin dry, thick and pale Eyelids oedematous Lips and tongue enlarged Hair coarse and sparse Interstitial oedema	Increased sweating Skin warm and moist Eyelids retracted Hair loss
Thought processes and emotional responses	Slow mental processes Increased sleep and lethargy Speech hoarse, slow and monotonous Depression Mental disturbance	Anxiety, apprehension Restlessness Irritability Emotional instability Insomnia
Bowel elimination	Decreased gastrointestinal motility Constipation	Increased gastrointestinal motility Diarrhoea
Thermoregulation	Sensitivity to cold Decreased body temperature	Sensitivity to heat Increased body temperature
Sexuality patterns	Metrorrhagia Amenorrhoea Low sex drive Infertility	Oligomenorrhoea or amenorrhoea Low sex drive Impotence

of palpitations, prescription and non-prescription medications taken and any family history of thyroid disease. It is important to identify the onset and duration of the symptoms.

Physical examination

Physical examination begins with observation of the person's *general appearance*. Changes that may indicate decreased thyroid function are paleness, facial puffiness and a non-expressive appearance. The person with increased thyroid function may appear anxious and agitated and their eyeballs may protrude. The *skin* and *hair* are inspected for dryness, brittleness and texture. The density and pattern of hair distribution are noted. *Vital signs* are measured because changes in respiratory rate and depth, blood pressure and cardiac rate and rhythm may be present.

HYPOTHYROIDISM

Hypothyroidism is a common disorder characterized by a hypometabolic state. It is more common in females and can occur at any age but the incidence is higher in the elderly.

Causes and contributing factors

The deficiency of thyroid hormones may be primary, due to a disorder in the thyroid itself, or may be secondary as a result of a pituitary or hypothalamic disturbance. If the dysfunction is congenital or develops in infancy or early childhood, it gives rise to cretinism which is characterized by a failure to achieve normal physical growth and mental development. In the adult it produces myxoedema.

Primary hypothyroidism accounts for about 95% of the cases of hypothyroidism in adults. It is due to destruction of thyroid tissue by disease, surgery or radioactive iodine treatment of hyperthyroidism. Autoimmune thyroid disease (Hashimoto's thyroiditis) is the most common cause of hypothyroidism. A less common cause is iodine deficiency, which produces an enlargement of the thyroid gland known as a goitre. The enlargement of the thyroid in iodine deficiency occurs because of stimulation by an increased release of thyroid-stimulating hormone (TSH) by the anterior pituitary in response to the low thyroxine concentration of the blood. The follicles increase in number and size and the thyroid becomes more vascular.

A deficiency in the natural supply of iodine in the water and soil occurs in inland areas distant from the sea. The addition of iodine to the salt used in food has largely eliminated this once common cause of hypothyroidism in the UK.

Clinical characteristics

A decreased production of tri-iodothyronine (T_3) and thyroxine (T_4) influences most metabolic processes of the body, resulting in many and varied manifestations.

The symptoms and the rate at which they develop correspond to the degree of thyroid inactivity. An abnormal decrease in thyroid hormone causes a general reduction in cellular metabolism, producing mental and physical sluggishness. The person gradually exhibits apathy and slowness in responses. An abnormal deposition of a mucopolysaccharide, which tends to hold water, occurs in the subcutaneous tissues, giving the person an oedematous appearance. The skin becomes dry and thick, the face (particularly the eyelids) appears puffy and the lips and tongue enlarge. The person experiences weakness, fatigue and an increased sensitivity to cold, and appetite is poor, although there may be a gain in weight. The temperature, pulse and blood pressure may be abnormally low. Mental processes are slow and the patient sleeps a great deal. Impaired function of the reproductive system is manifested by menstrual disorders, such as menorrhagia, amenorrhoea, and loss of sexual drive. Hoarseness and slow, monotonous speech may be noted (Elliot 2000). Because of complacency and dull mental processes, the condition may appear to be of much less concern to the patient than to the family or friends witnessing the changes. Allowed to progress, the disorder may lead to cardiac insufficiency, depression or the patient may pass into a comatose state.

Older persons with hypothyroidism are more predisposed to develop coma, particularly in response to cold weather when body temperature may fall to hypothermic levels and respiratory insufficiency may develop.

With a goitre, the enlarged gland may cause disfigurement which creates embarrassment for the person. More serious symptoms are pressure on the larynx and trachea, manifested by a chronic cough and respiratory difficulty, interference with swallowing, and compression of nerves in the area.

Treatment

Hypothyroidism is treated with thyroid hormone replacement therapy, usually thyroxine in uncomplicated cases. In cases where there are complications, such as ischaemic heart disease, tri-iodothyronine (T_3) may be given. T_3 acts very rapidly, but the effect is sustained for a shorter period than that of thyroxine (T_4), which is not fully effective before 7–10 days. The dosage is usually small to start with and is increased gradually to guard against too sudden and excessive a demand on the heart by rapid acceleration of metabolism. The pulse is checked and recorded frequently until the maintenance dose is established. Symptomatic relief for the patient will usually be reported within 2–4 weeks of beginning replacement therapy, but it takes up to 6–8 weeks for steady-state levels of thyroid hormones to be achieved (Elliot 2000). Patient and family should therefore be advised that there will be only a gradual improvement in symptoms. Adverse effects are almost entirely related to under-replacement, with the symptoms of hypothyroidism remaining, or to over-replacement, producing symptoms of hyperthyroidism. Allergic reactions are rare.

The maintenance dose is individualized on the basis of the person's responses and on levels of TSH and T_4 and T_3. Elderly persons usually require smaller doses. Drug replacement is lifelong.

Nursing intervention

It may be necessary for the nurse to explain the condition to the patient and family and emphasize that replacement therapy must be continued indefinitely. The patient may neglect to take the medication if feeling better. During the myxoedematous state, it is important that the family appreciate that the patient's lethargy and dullness are a part of the disease. The nurse, the patient and the family must be tolerant of this slowness, and encouragement and time should be given to complete responses and activities. Early indications of improvement and response to the drug therapy may be pointed out as reassurance that the physical condition is reversible, although depression does not always resolve.

Much of the nursing care is symptomatic. For example, extra warmth is provided because of the patient's lower heat production and consequent decreased tolerance to cold. Without extra clothing and bedding, the person may be uncomfortable in an environmental temperature that is comfortable to others. A minimum of soap is used on the patient's skin, and oily lotions or creams are applied to relieve the dryness. The diet should be low in calories to decrease and/or maintain body weight; low in fat and cholesterol because of the accompanying increase in serum cholesterol concentration; and high in fibre with increased fluid intake to promote bowel function. Laxatives or enemas may be necessary to maintain adequate bowel elimination. The hypothyroid patient is seen at the outpatient clinic or in their general practice at regular intervals; adjustment of the drug dosage is necessary from time to time.

The patient with hypothyroidism must learn self-management in relation to the drug therapy and symptom control. Teaching is individualized and planned according to the identified needs of the individual. This takes into account the severity of symptoms, the impact the disorder is having on the person's life and daily functioning, and the ability of the family to adjust to the changes in the patient before control is achieved and during episodes when readjustment of the treatment plan is necessary.

Despite treatment, survey evidence from O'Malley et al (2000) suggests that 75% of patients remained overweight, whereas 80% reported still feeling depressed even though their thyroid hormones had been returned to normal levels. The areas of weight and mood therefore remain problematical even though other symptoms will probably be largely relieved by hormone therapy. A clinical situation of hypothyroidism is described in Case Study 18.3.

CASE Jane Green is a 34-year-old wife, mother and office manager. She and her husband Robert, an engineer, usually share household tasks and childcare activities and like to participate in outings which include their 4-year-old and 8-month-old sons.

Jane made an appointment to see you as practice nurse. She told you that she was having difficulty balancing her job and her family life since returning to full-time work after the birth of her last child. She was constantly tired and fell asleep each evening while reading bedtime stories to the children. She felt pressured by the demands of her job and was concerned that she was becoming forgetful and disorganized.

You question Jane about any physical and emotional changes she experienced since the birth of the baby and discover that Jane had not been able to lose the extra weight she had gained; her menstrual periods were still not regular; her hair and skin had become very dry; she felt cold and wore an extra sweater, socks or other clothing to keep warm; she was frequently constipated; and felt she was pushing herself to get through the day. She stated that her husband complained about her disinterest and felt that she was not fulfilling her share of household tasks. Following discussion with the GP you take blood, and arrange for Jane to see her GP.

On Jane's next visit to the surgery, her GP, on reviewing the health history and the results of laboratory tests, concluded that Jane has primary hypothyroidism. T4 was reduced and thyroid stimulating hormone (TSH) was raised. Jane was to begin thyroid replacement treatment with thyroxine 0.025 mg daily. The dose was to be adjusted in 3–4 weeks according to her serum TSH level and response to drug therapy.

You meet with Jane and mutually set the following learning objectives. Jane should be able to:

- understand the reasons for the physical and behavioural changes she has been experiencing
- take her prescribed hormone replacement regularly, safely and knowledgeably
- recognize the clinical signs and symptoms of hypothyroidism
- discuss actions to take to alleviate the health problems she is experiencing related to changes in activity tolerance, temperature regulation, nutrition, constipation, skin integrity, sexual pattern and thought processes.

Jane's lethargy, decreased attention span and distress at her diagnosis are impeding her ability to comprehend instructions at this time. It was agreed that you should review her medication plan and answer immediate concerns.

Thyroid hormone replacement

The medication was taken daily on an empty stomach. Jane decided that she would take her tablet as soon as she woke up each morning. You told her not to exceed the prescribed dose and explained the importance of continuing with drug therapy. You reviewed the signs of under-replacement, which were the same symptoms that Jane was experiencing. The half-life of thyroxine is 6–7 days, so Jane should not expect immediate relief from her symptoms. You explained to Jane that her blood pressure and pulse rate are be monitored on each visit. She was currently hypotensive and her pulse was slow at 60/minute. As her hormone levels rise, her pulse and blood pressure should return to her usual levels. As Jane was not taking any other prescription or non-prescription medications she did not need to be cautioned about the fact that thyroxine potentiates the effects of anticoagulants, insulin and oral hypoglycaemic agents.

It was agreed that at a later visit you would discuss the symptoms of over-replacement and any concerns Jane had after starting her hormone replacement.

Evaluation

Jane returned to the surgery in 3 weeks with her husband. At this time, her symptoms were beginning to abate. She was still extremely tired and sensitive to cold but was taking more interest in family and work activities. You discussed the function of the thyroid gland and its hormones, and helped Jane and her husband to understand the cause of her symptoms. You emphasized that, although she would require hormone replacement for life, her symptoms could be controlled and she should return to her previous level of functioning. She would require regular medical supervision to monitor her control and to make periodic adjustments in hormone replacement.

Jane's husband was encouraged to learn about her responses to decreased thyroid hormone levels and the symptoms of hyperthyroidism so he could help Jane to recognize changes and seek further medical evaluation. An appointment was made for Jane to meet the dietitian to discuss her dietary needs. She was taking her medication regularly. The increase in the dose prescribed by her GP was explained to her. Her blood pressure was 115/80 mmHg and her pulse rate 72/minute. Arrangements were made to review Jane's learning needs on her next visit.

HYPERTHYROIDISM

Hyperthyroidism implies an excessive secretion of the thyroid hormones and may be called *thyrotoxicosis*, *toxic goitre*, *exophthalmic goitre* or *Graves' disease*. The terms exophthalmic goitre or Graves' disease are reserved for hyperthyroidism that is accompanied by exophthalmos (see p. 580) and extreme nervousness.

Causes

The exact cause of hyperactivity of the thyroid in most patients is not clear. In many cases, it is thought to be due to autoimmunity. Thyroid-stimulating immunoglobulins (TSIs) are found in almost all people with Graves' disease. There may also be a genetic factor in Graves' disease (Springhouse Corporation 1998). Excessive secretion of TSH by the pituitary gland may also cause enlargement of the thyroid gland and thyroiditis. Over-replacement of thyroid hormones is the most common iatrogenic cause of hyperthyroidism. Hyperthyroidism affects females more often than males and is rare in childhood.

Clinical characteristics

Some enlargement of the gland may be evident owing to a diffuse hyperplasia of the gland or the development of one or more adenomas. It may be readily seen to move upward with the larynx in swallowing.

The increased blood level of thyroid hormones accelerates the metabolic rate. Thyroid stimulating hormone (TSH) is reduced. The patient's appetite increases and, unless the food intake keeps pace with the rapid metabolic rate, there is a loss of weight. Lowered heat tolerance and excessive sweating are manifested. The hyperthyroid patient is uncomfortably warm in an environmental temperature acceptable to others.

Nervousness, apprehension, emotional instability and restlessness are evident, and the hands are *warm* and moist in contrast to the *cold*, moist extremities associated with anxiety. Despite eating more, the patient may complain of weakness and fatigue. The pulse is rapid and exhibits a sharp rise on exertion. The increased pulse rate is due to the increased metabolic demands and the effect of thyroxine on the sympathetic nervous system. Shortness of breath on exertion and palpitations are experienced as a result of the increased metabolic rate. The diastolic blood pressure is usually lower than normal because of widespread vasodilatation. A fine, rapid tremor develops in the hands and is accentuated when they are outstretched. Diarrhoea, resulting from increased gastrointestinal activity, may be troublesome. Menstrual disorders, such as oligomenorrhoea (scant flow) or amenorrhoea, are common.

Eye changes may appear in hyperthyroidism. *Exophthalmos* may be evident when the upper eyelids are retracted, showing the upper sclerae, and the eyes appear to be protruding. This is due to the accumulation of mucopolysaccharides and fluid in the retro-orbital tissues, which forces the eyeball outwards. The lids fail to follow the movement of the eyes when the person looks down (lid lag).

Treatment

Hyperthyroidism may be treated by antithyroid drugs, radioactive iodine (I^{131}) or surgery.

Drug therapy

The drugs most commonly used suppress the formation of the thyroid hormones. They may be used alone or as an interim treatment before surgery; they include carbimazole and propylthiouracil, although much larger doses of the latter drug are required. The drug is generally taken over a prolonged period of 1–2 years if the patient remains free of side-effects. These antithyroid drugs are potentially toxic. Side-effects that may develop are dermatitis, agranulocytosis and fever. The patient is advised to report promptly a sore throat, swollen tender 'neck glands', fever or a rash. The patient must be taught the importance of taking the drugs regularly and at the hours suggested in order to obtain the desired effect and prevent a remission. Some compensatory enlargement of the gland may occur and the patient is reassured that this is not serious.

The patient is followed closely; weekly visits to the general practitioner or clinic are usually required for 4–6 weeks and the interval is gradually lengthened. A blood specimen is taken for determination of serum levels of T_4, T_3 and TSH, and a leucocyte count is made on each visit. The reports may indicate a need for an adjustment in the dosage of the antithyroid drug.

Short-term drug therapy may be given to reduce the cardiac effects of excess T_3 and T_4 levels and other symptoms; for example, a β-adrenergic blocking agent may be prescribed to decrease the heart rate.

Radiation treatment

Iodine-131 therapy of hyperthyroidism is widely used. The radioiodine is given orally and is trapped in the thyroid, where its radiation destroys tissue, reducing the functioning mass. Improvement is usually evident in 3 weeks and the metabolic rate is expected to reach a normal level in 2–3 months. Antithyroid drugs are usually prescribed during this period. Radioiodine is never given during pregnancy. The therapeutic dose is not considered large enough to constitute a radiation hazard to those in the person's environment.

The patient is observed closely for signs of aggravation of the disease and thyroiditis, manifested by tenderness and soreness in the area of the gland. Rarely, a thyroid crisis may develop (see p. 584). After receiving the I^{131}, regular visits to the clinic or the doctor are necessary. The patient is examined for remission of the disease and for hypothyroidism, which can frequently occur as a side-effect. The serum T_3, T_4 and TSH levels are determined. If hypothyroidism is indicated, a replacement preparation (e.g. a thyroxine preparation) is prescribed.

Surgical therapy

A partial thyroidectomy may be done if radioactive iodine is contraindicated, for example if the patient is young, if antithyroid drug therapy has failed, if there is the possibility of carcinoma, if sensitivity precludes its prolonged administration, or if the gland is very large, causing disfigurement or pressure on the respiratory tract or oesophagus. In hyperthyroidism, approximately three-quarters of the gland is removed; in the case of cancer of the thyroid, a complete thyroidectomy may need to be done, which necessitates continuous replacement drug therapy during the remainder of the patient's life. The patient must be euthyroid before surgery can be undertaken.

Nursing assessment

An accurate record of the person's temperature, pulse and respirations is made at least every 4 hours, and the responses and degree of restlessness and agitation are noted frequently. This is necessary so that an early indication of increasing thyrotoxicosis and cardiac insufficiency may be recognized and receive prompt attention. The patient is told that the vital signs will be checked at regular intervals, to avoid undue apprehension associated with such frequent checking. The patient is weighed daily or every second day to determine whether calorie intake is keeping pace with metabolic rate.

Patient problems

The patient with hyperthyroidism is expending energy in excess of the body's ability to produce energy. Metabolic processes are increased, requiring more calories to prevent excessive weight loss. Environmental stimuli increase energy demands further. Health problems that are experienced by the person with hyperthyroidism are listed in Table 18.3 (p. 577).

Goals

The patient and family will be able to:

1 understand the reasons for the physical and behavioural changes
2 recognize the clinical signs and symptoms of hyperthyroidism
3 describe the prescribed medication and/or treatment plan
4 describe the expected and possible adverse responses to therapy
5 discuss actions to take to alleviate the health problems experienced in relation to changes in thought processes and emotional responses, nutrition, activity tolerance, thermoregulation, skin and eye integrity, sexual pattern and body image
6 describe plans for ongoing therapy and health supervision.

Nursing intervention

Altered thought processes and emotional responses

The *goal* is that the patient will appear less anxious:

● *Environment* – Because of the patient's nervousness and hyperexcitability, quietness is very important. An established routine may prevent unnecessary disturbance, which only aggravates the condition. If the patient is being cared for at home, the family is made fully aware of these needs. They are advised that irritability, restlessness and emotional lability are characteristic of the illness and are helped to develop coping strategies to avoid upsetting the individual. In the hospital, careful consideration should be given to placement on the ward. Exposure to very ill, talkative or otherwise disturbing patients should be avoided

● *Information* – You should explain all procedures and medical treatment to the patient and family and answer questions regarding care, and work in a calm, quiet, competent manner

● *Identification of additional stresses* – You should work with the patient and family to identify additional stresses that may have resulted from the patient's illness or may have existed previously. Referrals to community resources are made if relevant

● *Visitors* – Visitors and family members require information on the need for limiting visitors and suggestions as to how they can best contribute to the patient's well-being and avoid aggravating the condition.

Altered nutrition

The *goal* is that the patient will maintain or increase body weight:

● *Diet* – The patient requires a high-protein, high-carbohydrate, high-calorie diet (4000–5000 kcal) to prevent tissue breakdown caused by the high metabolic demand and to satisfy the patient's increased appetite. A snack between meals and at bedtime is provided. Tea and coffee are usually restricted to eliminate caffeine stimulation. Decaffeinated coffee may be used as a substitute.

● *Fluids* – The patient's excessive heat production and resultant perspiration increases fluid loss, necessitating extra fluids. Also, there is an increased production of metabolic wastes, requiring dilution for elimination by the kidneys. A minimum fluid intake of 3000–4000 mL daily is recommended, unless contraindicated by cardiac or renal dysfunction. An explanation of the importance of this amount of fluid is made to the patient to gain cooperation, and a variety of fluids is provided.

Hyperactivity and fatigue

The *goal* is that the patient will decrease energy expenditure:

● *Rest and activity* – Activity is restricted because it increases the metabolic rate, but the patient's nervous excitability makes it difficult to rest. Efforts are made to engage the patient's interest in activities which expend little energy. The occupational therapy department may be very helpful in this goal. The patient is helped to plan activities and daily routines to obtain sufficient rest. Activities requiring fine motor movements are kept to a minimum. When necessary, assistance is provided by the family or nurse.

Altered thermoregulation

The *goal* is that the patient will state that he or she feels comfortably cool:

● As the patient is producing more than the normal amount of body heat, comfort will be achieved only in an environment of lower temperature than normal. Lightweight clothing is used and the room is kept well ventilated and cool

Altered skin and eye integrity

The *goals* are that the patient will maintain skin integrity and avoid injury to the eyes:

● *Skin care* – A daily bath is necessary because of the profuse perspiration. If the patient is extremely restless, has lost weight and has decreased mobility, special attention is given to the pressure areas

● *Eye care* – If the patient has exophthalmos, the eyes should be protected from irritation by sunglasses. Methylcellulose (a conjunctival lubricant) drops (0.5–1%) may be recommended to prevent drying of the conjunctiva and cornea. The patient's vision is tested frequently, especially if the exophthalmos is progressive; compression of the optic nerve and artery may occur, with ensuing visual impairment.

Altered sexual patterns and self-image
The *goal* is that the patient will be able to express concerns regarding alterations in body image and changes in sexual patterns:

● The patient and partner are helped to understand that the changes in menstrual cycle, low sex drive and/or impotence are a result of the hyperthyroidism and that they will abate or disappear once thyroid hormonal balance is achieved
● Repeated explanations of the causes of the physical changes and assurance should be given. There is a prolonged phase of gradual improvement of the eyes once the hormone imbalance has been corrected. It should be said, however, that the eyes may not return to the normal state. Good grooming and attractive dress promote self-confidence and the feeling of wellness.

Lack of knowledge about the disease process, therapeutic plan and self-management
The *goal* is that the patient will achieve self-management of the therapeutic regimen and self-care:

● The patient and family are given information about hyperthyroidism, causes, manifestations and treatment. Learning needs are assessed and they are assisted in developing a plan for home care of the patient. The dietician may be consulted about diet and meal planning.

Evaluation

The physical and behavioural changes that the person is experiencing should begin to diminish with treatment. With drug therapy, clinical improvement should be apparent after several weeks. The dose of the medication will then be decreased by the doctor according to symptomatic changes and decreases in the T_4 level. The person should begin to regain weight. As weight approaches the person's desirable level, and energy expenditure is consistent and within usual parameters, the diet is adjusted and calorie intake decreased.

The patient and family should demonstrate understanding of the hyperthyroidism, the treatment plan and medication regimen. They should be able to describe and implement measures to alleviate symptoms by: (1) the provision of a quiet, cool environment; (2) the avoidance of undue stress; (3) provision for sufficient rest and sleep and decreased physical activity; (4) adequate calorie and fluid intake; (5) maintenance of dry clean skin; and (6) protec-

tion of the eyes. The person should verbalize a decrease in anxiety and begin to take responsibility for self-care.

THE PERSON HAVING THYROID SURGERY

In caring for the patient who has had a thyroidectomy, pertinent factors to be kept in mind are:

● the location of the gland in relation to the trachea and larynx
● its proximity to the recurrent laryngeal nerve, which controls the vocal cords
● its abundant blood supply
● that the parathyroid glands, which influence neuromuscular irritability through their control of the blood calcium level, lie on the posterior surface of the thyroid. The nurse must be constantly alert for manifestations of disturbances due to these factors.

Preoperative preparation

The hyperthyroid patient who is to have surgery is given an antithyroid drug for several weeks before operation to reduce the metabolic rate and return the gland to as near the euthyroid state as possible. During this period, whether at home or in the hospital, the care cited in the preceding section is applicable. The antithyroid drugs produce some compensatory enlargement of the gland and an increased blood supply. When the metabolic rate has been reduced to a satisfactory level, the drug is discontinued. Then, in a few days, a course of potassium iodide is commenced and continued for approximately 10 days. This reduces the size and vascularity of the gland, facilitating surgery and lessening the problem of bleeding. As potassium iodide has a disagreeable taste and may also irritate the mucous membrane, it is well diluted in fruit juice or milk.

Preparation includes electrocardiography to obtain further information about the patient's cardiac status, and blood typing and cross-matching for transfusion. The patient may have some concern regarding the cosmetic effect of the operation but they can be assured that consideration is given to this and that the scar becomes barely perceptible in a few months. During the interval, it may be concealed by a scarf or necklace. Remembering that the hyperthyroid patient may be hyperexcitable and apprehensive, judicious explanations are made of what may be expected after the operation. Demonstration and practice in supporting the head with the hands while turning in bed is carried out to decrease stress on the neck.

Preparation to receive the patient after operation

Special equipment to be assembled and ready for use when preparing to receive a patient following a thyroidectomy includes:

1 sandbags or small firm pillows to immobilize the head
2 suction equipment and catheters for clearing mucus from the throat

3 sterile clip removers or stitch cutters in case of a haematoma at the site of surgery obstructing the trachea by compression

4 a humidifier to relieve tracheal and laryngeal irritation and facilitate the removal of mucus

5 intravenous infusion equipment

6 a sterile emergency intubation and tracheostomy tray in the event of respiratory obstruction

7 equipment for obtaining a blood specimen quickly for blood calcium determination

8 ampoules of calcium chloride or calcium gluconate, with the necessary equipment for intravenous administration in the event of the complication of tetany (hypocalcaemia) due to inadvertent parathyroid damage.

Postoperative care

Patients are usually very apprehensive, and serious complications may *develop rapidly*. They should therefore be placed on the ward in a position where they are readily visible at all times.

Assessment

Vital signs are recorded every 15 minutes; the frequency is gradually reduced if the patient remains stable. The body temperature is recorded every 4 hours. The degree of restlessness and apprehension is noted and, if not relieved by the prescribed sedation, is brought to the surgeon's attention. Particular attention is paid to the patient's respirations; any complaint or sign of respiratory distress and cyanosis is reported promptly, because it may indicate laryngeal paralysis or compression of the trachea by accumulating blood. Some hoarseness is common and is due to irritation of the larynx by the operation and the endotracheal tube used in maintaining the airway during surgery. The doctor is advised if the hoarseness and weakness

---

Box 18.5 Potential patient problems following thyroid surgery

- Obstructed airway, because of:
  - oedema, decreased head and neck mobility and tracheal-bronchial secretions from the anaesthetic, which all contribute to difficulty in expectorating secretions
  - haematoma formation behind the wound site pressing on the trachea

- Pain related to surgical intervention

- Impaired mobility of head, neck and shoulders related to surgical intervention, pain and discomfort

- Inadequate nutrition because of difficulty in swallowing

- Complications as a result of the surgical intervention (e.g. haemorrhage, respiratory distress, loss of voice or tetany)

- Inadequate knowledge about follow-up care

---

of the voice persist beyond 3 or 4 days. Potential patient problems are listed in Box 18.5.

Goals

Following thyroid surgery, the patient will be able to:

1 maintain a patent airway

2 state that pain is absent

3 show vital signs within normal limits

4 assume self-care activities

5 achieve and maintain desirable body weight

6 demonstrate ability to perform neck exercises safely

7 describe a plan for follow-up care.

Nursing intervention

Potential obstruction of the airway   The *goal* is that the patient will maintain a patent airway:

- The patient is assisted to a sitting position with support given to the head and neck in order to help the patient to cough and expectorate. Suction of the oropharynx is carried out if the accumulation of secretions is severe. Deep breathing and coughing should be encouraged several times each hour. Pulse oximetry may be used to monitor oxygen saturation

- You should observe the wound and ensure free drainage from the wound drains is maintained to prevent the formation of a haematoma.

Pain   The *goal* is that the patient will state that pain is absent. Opioid analgesia and an antiemetic may be required to keep the patient comfortable and less apprehensive during the first 48 hours. Analgesia should be administered regularly and consistently to control pain. Respirations are assessed for evidence of a decrease in rate or depth.

Wound healing   The *goal* is that the wound will heal and the patient will maintain the range of movement of the neck:

- After recovery from the anaesthetic, the patient is placed on his or her back and the head of the bed is moderately elevated to facilitate breathing. The head and neck are supported by a pillow and are positioned in good alignment, preventing flexion and hyperextension. When the patient's position is changed, the nurse lifts and supports the head, preserving good alignment. The patient is taught to lift and support the head by placing the hands at the back of the head when wishing to move

- The patient often returns from the operating theatre with surgical drains inserted. These should be checked at intervals to ensure that they are functioning. While a large accumulation of blood behind the wound site can cause respiratory obstruction, smaller haematomas may increase vulnerability to infection and delayed wound healing

- If the vital signs are stabilized and normal, the patient is assisted out of bed on the first postoperative day. After removal of the drains, sutures or skin clips and firm healing of the incision, head exercises, which include flexion (forward and lateral), hyperextension and turning, are gradually introduced with the surgeon's approval. To prevent contraction of the scar, the patient may be taught to massage the neck gently twice daily, using lanolin, cold cream or an oily lotion.

Inadequate nutrition The *goal* is that the patient will maintain adequate nutritional intake:

● Some difficulty in swallowing is usually experienced for a day or two, but fluids by mouth are encouraged as soon as tolerated. Intravenous fluids are given until an adequate amount can be taken orally. The patient progresses through a soft diet to a full diet in 2–3 days.

Potential complications The *goal* is that complications will be promptly identified and corrected:

● The nurse must be aware that haemorrhage, respiratory difficulty, loss of voice and tetany are serious complications that may occur following thyroid surgery. The first three may develop with startling rapidity and are usually seen within 48 hours of operation.

Haemorrhage may be manifested by a rapid pulse, fall in blood pressure and evident bleeding. The bleeding may be discovered only by frequent checking of the dressing and by sliding the hands under the shoulders and behind the neck. Blood may collect quickly within the tissues and cause pressure on the trachea. The patient may complain of a choking sensation and shortness of breath; cyanosis and dyspnoea develop and, unless the pressure is relieved quickly, asphyxia may occur. The surgeon is notified immediately at the earliest sign of change. The dressing is loosened to promote freer, outward drainage. Instruments for removing the sutures or skin clips should already be at the bedside and the emergency tracheostomy tray is made ready, because the surgeon may consider an immediate tracheostomy necessary. On reporting the situation, the nurse may be instructed to remove the skin clips to allow the escape of blood. A thick sterile dressing is then applied until the surgeon arrives. The patient will probably be returned to the operating theatre to bring the bleeding under control.

Occasionally, *injury to one or both recurrent laryngeal nerves* may occur during thyroid surgery. These nerves control laryngeal muscles, the opening of the glottis and voice production. Injury to one nerve produces hoarseness and weakness of the voice but no serious respiratory disturbance. Bilateral nerve injury causes paralysis of muscles on both sides of the larynx, resulting in closure of the glottis and respiratory obstruction. The patient is unable to speak and stridor occurs (i.e. respirations become shrill and crowing), cyanosis develops and loss of consciousness ensues unless respirations are quickly re-established. Prompt endotracheal intubation or emergency tracheostomy is done, and oxygen is administered via either tube. The injury and paralysis are rarely permanent; function is usually gradually restored and the tracheostomy tube is removed.

During surgery, interference with the blood supply to the parathyroid glands or injury or removal of parathyroid tissue may occur which depresses secretion by the glands. Decreased parathyroid hormone concentration leads to *hypocalcaemia*, resulting in increased neuromuscular irritability and the condition known as *tetany*. Early signs of this complication include complaints of numbness and tingling in the hands or feet, muscle twitching and spasms, and gastrointestinal cramps. A change may be evident in the voice; it may become high pitched and shrill, because of spasm of the vocal cords. A blood specimen is obtained for serum calcium determination with the appearance of early symptoms. Calcium gluconate 10% may be slowly administered intravenously by the doctor; then, an oral preparation is given until normal parathyroid function resumes. The patient is encouraged to take milk and calcium-containing foods.

Thyrotoxicosis or thyroid crisis rarely complicates the postoperative period following a thyroidectom; however, as an important manifestation of thyroid disease it is worthwhile mentioning here. This emergency situation is attributed to: (1) the release of a large amount of thyroid hormone into the circulation to produce a hypermetabolic state and (2) adrenergic hyperactivity which may potentiate the hypersecretion of thyroid hormone. The patient's symptoms develop abruptly and include irritability, tremor, tachycardia, vomiting, visual disturbance, vascular collapse, hypotension, pyrexia, coma and death. Rapid notification of medical staff, electrocardiography (ECG), temperature and vital sign monitoring are essential as this is a rare but life-threatening crisis (Springhouse Corporation 1998).

Inadequate knowledge concerning follow-up care The *goal* is that the patient will verbalize understanding of a plan for post-hospital care and follow-up:

● The patient's hospitalization is usually brief if no complications develop. Information regarding the amount of activity that may be resumed is discussed with the patient. Extra rest will still be necessary, and the patient is advised to continue neck exercises until there is freedom of movement without any feeling of pulling. Follow-up is usually at the outpatient clinic for about 1 year, checking for any residual laryngeal damage, hypoparathyroidism, recurring hyperthyroidism or developing hypothyroidism. If no problems develop during that year, an annual check-up is then recommended. Information is provided on the administration and effects of prescribed thyroid hormone replacement. Following a total thyroidectomy, hormone replacement will be lifelong.

Evaluation

The patient should show absence of complications; the serum calcium level will be within the normal range. There will be no muscle twitching, hoarseness or breathing difficulties. The patient and family will describe plans for follow-up care and demonstrate understanding of the prescribed neck exercises, medication schedule and other self-care activities.

THE PERSON WITH A DISORDER OF THE PARATHYROID GLANDS

Primary hyperparathyroidism has a prevalence of about 1 in 800 and is found predominantly in people aged over 50 years of age, in women more often than men, and is usually caused by a single parathyroid adenoma (Haslett et al 1999). Serum calcium levels increase in response to the excess parathyroid hormone (PTH) secretion. Secondary hyperparathyroidism occurs when the gland secretes excessive amounts of PTH to try to compensate for hypocalcaemia caused by any abnormality that inhibits the effect of PTH, such as chronic renal failure, thiazide diuretic use or vitamin D deficiency. Hypoparathyroidism occurs due to a rare autoimmune genetic disorder or more frequently due to damage to the glands during thyroid surgery.

ASSESSMENT OF PARATHYROID FUNCTION

The *health history* begins with the collection of information related to the health problems experienced by the individual. Table 18.4 lists health problems common to individuals with increased and decreased parathyroid function. The nurse asks specific questions to determine the presence, duration and severity of the associated signs and symptoms; vitamin D and calcium intake; the use of drugs such as thiazide diuretics; and any history of renal calculi.

HYPOPARATHYROIDISM

Clinical characteristics

The deficiency of parathyroid hormone (PTH) causes hypocalcaemia. Symptoms of increased neuromuscular excitability and tetany are usually the first manifestations (muscle cramps, carpopedal spasms, laryngeal spasm affecting the voice, dysphagia, convulsions). Wheezy respirations may be heard due to bronchospasm. Less calcium than normal is excreted in the urine because of the low blood calcium level, and the bones tend to become more dense. Renal excretion of phosphorus is reduced and the serum phosphate level is raised, which predisposes the patient to acidosis. If the hormone deficiency is prolonged, calcium deposition may develop in the lens and conjunctiva of the eyes, the brain, lungs or gastric mucosa. The hair becomes thin and grey, areas of alopecia and loss of eyebrows are common. The skin becomes coarse and scaly and the nails are brittle and have horizontal ridges. Mental changes include depression, fatigue, psychosis and intellectual impairment.

Treatment

The hypocalcaemia is corrected initially by the intravenous administration of 20 mL calcium gluconate 10%. The patient is then given regular oral doses of a calcium salt, along with a preparation of vitamin D to promote the absorption of the calcium. The patient is followed closely; frequent determinations of blood phosphorus and calcium levels are made in

---

Table 18.4   Assessment of the person with altered parathyroid function

| | Clinical characteristics | |
	Hypoparathyroidism	Hyperparathyroidism
Activity tolerance	Muscular cramps and spasms Numbness and tingling of extremities Tetany	Muscle weakness and fatigue Decreased muscle tone Bone tenderness and pain on weight-bearing Pathological fractures
Thought process and emotional response	Irritability, agitation Depression Psychosis Slow mental processes Anxiety	Lethargy Drowsiness Impaired memory Disorientation
Nutrition	Nausea and vomiting Abdominal cramping	Loss of appetite Nausea and vomiting Abdominal discomfort Weight loss
Elimination	Constipation or diarrhoea	Constipation Increased urinary output
Skin integrity	Skin coarse, scaly and dry Alopecia Loss of eyebrows Nails brittle with horizontal ridges	
Breathing pattern	Laryngeal spasm Wheezing	

order to adjust vitamin D dosage. Overdosage may cause renal damage. Phosphorus-containing foods may have to be limited to avoid complications: these are principally dairy products. An alternative may be the prescription of aluminium hydroxide gel which binds the phosphorus in the intestine, preventing its absorption. The patient is encouraged to take extra fluids to promote renal excretion of phosphorus.

HYPERPARATHYROIDISM

Clinical characteristics

The high PTH concentration in the blood causes decalcification of the bones, and hypercalcaemia occurs. The blood level of inorganic phosphorus falls as its renal excretion increases, and the concentration of calcium in the glomerular filtrate is higher than normal, predisposing to the formation of renal calculi. Neuromuscular excitability is depressed and loss of muscle tone is evident. Demineralization of the bones may be so marked that fibrous cystic areas develop which frequently lead to deformities and pathological fractures. In some instances bone tumours consisting of an overgrowth of osteoclasts develop. When bone changes occur, the disorder may be referred to as *von Recklinghausen's disease* or *osteitis fibrosa cystica*, and the patient may experience tenderness and pain in the bones, especially with weight-bearing. Muscular weakness, loss of appetite, nausea, vomiting and constipation may develop. The urinary volume is usually increased because of the excessive amounts of calcium and phosphorus to be excreted. Renal function may become impaired; the tubular epithelium may be damaged by the excessive excretion of calcium or the formation of renal calculi. Frequently, the disease is recognized only when some deformity develops or a pathological fracture occurs.

Treatment

If the patient is very ill as a result of increased serum calcium levels (malignant hypercalcaemia), rehydration with up to 6 L of normal saline is needed. Bisphosphonates (e.g. intravenous pamidronate) are given to reduce serum calcium levels, together with further intravenous saline and furosemide (frusemide) to achieve a forced diuresis aimed at further reduction of serum calcium concentration. Fluid intake and output are monitored carefully. Foods containing calcium are restricted in the diet.

Hyperparathyroidism is treated by surgical excision of all four glands. Normal residual parathyroid tissue may be allografted into a muscle to preserve as much of the patient's parathyroid function as possible. After the operation, the patient is observed closely for the early signs of possible hypocalcaemia (tetany). Frequent serum calcium and phosphorus determinations are made. A diet high in calcium and phosphorus may be necessary to restore normal bone structure.

THE PERSON WITH A DISORDER OF THE PITUITARY GLAND (HYPOPHYSIS)

ASSESSMENT

The signs and symptoms of pituitary dysfunction are varied and reflect not only the increase or decrease in the production of one or more of the pituitary hormones, but also the resultant changes in the target tissues. Pituitary hormones, their functions and associated disorders are listed in Table 18.5.

Health history

The health history should include questions related to the following:

- *Growth and development* – Questions relate to changes in growth pattern and perceived changes in appearance or clothing size. The development of secondary sex characteristics and abnormalities of secondary sex characteristics may be explored. A great deal of sensitivity is required as these are all very personal areas. For the female, questions are asked about changes in the menstrual cycle. For the male, questions relate to sexual dysfunctions, in particular difficulties in attaining and maintaining an erection and any changes in body hair growth and distribution
- *Appetite and body weight* – Recent changes in appetite and the pattern of weight gain or loss are determined. It is important to ask questions about the volume of fluid intake and whether thirst is relieved. Alteration in heat tolerance may also be present with metabolic changes
- *Elimination patterns* – Changes in the volume, frequency and pattern of urinary elimination are determined. The person is asked specifically about getting up at night to void. Changes in bowel habits, constipation and/or diarrhoea are identified
- *Skin and hair* – Alteration in skin colour, texture, dryness, bruising and ability to heal may be caused by pituitary dysfunction. The patient can validate the nurse's observations as he or she is in the best position to recognize changes
- *Activity tolerance* – Questions are asked about feelings of tiredness or exhaustion related to usual daily activities and on exertion. Knowledge of the person's usual pattern of daily activity provides a basis for comparison
- *Cognitive/perceptual function* – Changes in memory, ability to concentrate, decreased attention span and visual losses may result from pituitary disorders or altered function of the target tissues. How the person usually responds to stressful physical and emotional events is elicited in detail and recent changes in these responses are also recorded.

Physical examination

The following areas are assessed:

- *General appearance* – The patient's general appearance, body build and fat distribution provide valuable infor-

Table 18.5 Pituitary gland hormones

Hormone	Functions	Disorders
Anterior pituitary		
Growth hormone (GH)	Growth; aids in determining size; accelerates metabolism; diabetogenic	Pan-hypopituitarism Gigantism – increase in GH level in childhood Acromegaly – increase in GH level in adulthood Short stature – decrease of GH level in childhood
Thyroid-stimulating hormone (TSH)	Promotes secretory activity of thyroid	Hyperthyroidism secondary to increase of TSH Hypothyroidism secondary to decrease of TSH
Adrenocorticotrophic hormone (ACTH)	Stimulates secretion of adrenal cortices	Cushing's syndrome and excess TSH Addison's disease secondary to pituitary disorder
Gonadotrophins: a. Follicle-stimulating hormone (FSH)	In women: development of ovarian follicle and secretion of oestrogen In men: promotes production of spermatozoa	Tumours Amenorrhoea Infertility
b. Luteinizing hormone (LH)	In women: induces ovulation, stimulates secretion of progesterone In men: stimulates production of androgens	
c. Prolactin	Initiates and sustains lactation	Galactorrhoea Infertility
Melanocyte-stimulating hormone (MSH)	Pigmentation of skin cells	Increase in pigmented areas
Posterior pituitary		
Antidiuretic hormone (ADH)	Increases permeability of distal and collecting tubules of kidneys (i.e. increases re-absorption of water)	Tumour
Oxytocin	Contracts pregnant uterus; stimulates release and flow of milk	

mation about pituitary abnormalities and overall growth and development of the individual

- *Body weight and vital signs* – The patient's weight, height and vital signs are recorded
- *Skin, hair and nails* – The skin is observed and palpated for pigmentation, dryness, oiliness, elasticity, hydration, temperature and breaks in the integrity and any resulting discharge. The pattern of distribution and amount of body hair are observed and the texture and dryness noted. Nails are observed for thickness and changes in growth
- *Genitalia and breasts* – The genitalia of the male and female are observed for size and shape, and the breasts are examined to assess development and maturation
- *Neurological examination* – Changes in sensation, pain, discomfort and muscle tone are noted. The patient's speech is carefully listened to for huskiness, slurring, hoarseness, volume and pitch, and rationality.

Diagnostic measurements

Apart from taking bloods to measure hormone levels, medical staff may carry out other tests such as those involving the osmolarity of urine and serum which are influenced by ADH levels. A key investigation is the adrenocorticotrophic hormone (ACTH) stimulation test, which is used if there is suspicion of a pituitary tumour. It will also help to diagnose primary or secondary adrenal insufficiency. The patient receives an intramuscular injection of 250 mg tetracosactin and blood samples are taken immediately and 30 minutes later to assess plasma cortisol levels. In people with no disorder of the pituitary or adrenal glands, the response should be a plasma cortisol level greater than 550 nmol/L, 30 minutes after the injection. Such a result indicates normal adrenal function (Haslett et al 1999).

Radiological studies

These include magnetic resonance imaging (MRI) and computed tomography (CT). Larger tumours may be identified with CT, but MRI is needed for smaller microadenomas.

PATIENT PROBLEMS

Problems associated with disorders of the pituitary vary greatly, depending on which lobe is involved, the nature of the disease (hyperplasia, neoplasm or destruction of tissue) and the particular type of cell of the anterior pituitary that is involved. Dysfunction may be manifested in one or more of the gland's target organs, reflecting either an excessive or deficient output of one or more pituitary hormones. Secondary neurological disturbances may also occur as a result of pressure on neighbouring brain tissue by a pituitary neoplasm. For example, early manifestations may include altered perceptual/visual function. The visual disturbances frequently occur because of the proximity of the visual tract. Conversely, primary pathological lesions in the brain, especially in the hypothalamic region, may cause secondary involvement of the pituitary.

The more commonly recognized disease entities associated with the anterior pituitary include:

- gigantism, the result of an excessive secretion of growth hormone (GH) in childhood
- acromegaly, due to an excessive secretion of GH commencing in adulthood
- dwarfism, resulting from a deficiency of GH in childhood
- Cushing's disease, the result of a hypersecretion of steroid hormones
- Simmonds' disease (pan-hypopituitarism), which occurs when there is a deficiency of all the anterior pituitary hormones.

Hyperthyroidism (Graves' disease) may also be secondary to an excessive production of TSH or an abnormal form of the hormone, and is discussed in the section on disorders of the thyroid.

The most common disorder associated with the posterior pituitary is *diabetes insipidus*, which is a result of a deficiency of ADH.

HYPERSECRETION OF GROWTH HORMONE: ACROMEGALY

An overproduction of GH before closure of the epiphyses and skeletal maturity causes a rapid overgrowth of the bones, producing the condition known as *gigantism*. **Acromegaly** results from an excess of growth hormone after puberty, usually due to a GH-secreting pituitary adenoma. It is a rare condition affecting four people per million of the population. The person has usually had the disease for several years before diagnosis, typically around the age of 40 years (Carr 2001).

Clinical characteristics

A person with gigantism may attain a height of 2.1–2.4 metres. Most cases are attributed to an adenoma. When the person passes adolescence, acromegaly is superimposed on the gigantism.

If the adenoma develops after the epiphyses have closed, longitudinal growth cannot occur, but marked thickening of the bones occurs and acromegaly develops. Enlargement of the head, jaws, hands and feet becomes apparent. Increased growth of cartilage produces an increase in the size of the

nose, ears, costal cartilages and larynx. Hypertrophy of the larynx may be accompanied by a deepening of the voice, and the change in the costal cartilages results in an increase in the thoracic circumference. The skin, subcutaneous tissues and lips thicken, the chin lengthens and the lower teeth separate because of the overgrowth of the mandible. Viscera enlarge and may become overactive, leading to disturbances.

As well as the evident skeletal changes and alteration in appearance, the patient experiences lethargy, weakness, increased metabolic rate and excessive sweating due to hypertrophy of the thyroid. Common complaints are joint pains, stiffness in the limbs, and tingling or numbness in the hands. Impaired carbohydrate metabolism and hyperglycaemia develop owing to the diabetogenic effect of GH. Pressure from the causative expanding neoplasm may cause headache, insomnia and loss of visual acuity and fields. Increased gonadal function may be associated with the early stage of acromegaly but, later, loss of libido and amenorrhoea are common. Osteoporosis (rarefaction of bones due to loss of calcium) may develop, especially in the vertebrae, and kyphosis (forward curvature of the spine) may be seen in the advanced stage. Hypertension is a common complication. The course of the disease varies considerably from one patient to another; it may develop slowly over many years in some, but in others, it may prove fatal in 3–4 years. Destruction of pituitary tissue by progressive growth and spread of the tumour may cause a general hypopituitarism.

Diagnostic investigation involves radiography of the skull in which the sella turcica is checked for widening.

Treatment

Acromegaly may be treated surgically by a hypophysectomy or transsphenoidal microsurgery to remove the hyperfunctioning tissue. A nasal, transsphenoidal approach is used by the surgeon. Radiotherapy is a second line of treatment. Internal radiation may be achieved by the implantation of radioactive yttrium (^{90}Y) seeds in the pituitary; a proton beam may be used for external irradiation. Patients may require long-term injections of somatostatin (hypothalamic release-inhibiting hormone) analogues, which lower GH levels. Octreotide or lanreotide are licensed for use but they have significant adverse gastrointestinal side-effects. During treatment, GH-producing pituitary tumours can still expand and the patient should be monitored carefully for reports of visual disturbance which would indicate such a problem is developing (British National Formulary 2005). Substitution hormonal preparations are prescribed if a hypophysectomy is done or if the patient manifests insulin, thyroid, adrenal or gonadal insufficiency in the advanced stage of the disease. Treatment arrests further changes but the changes in bony structures are irreversible.

Nursing intervention

Health problems experienced by the person with acromegaly vary with the stage and type of therapy and the impact of the disorder and treatment on the individual's lifestyle. Common problems include the following:

- *anxiety* related to the operation and treatment
- *altered self-esteem* related to changes in physical appearance
- *sexual dysfunction* related to possible amenorrhoea, decreased libido or impotence
- *altered nutrition* related to increased physical growth and metabolic rate
- *perceptual deficits* related to visual impairment
- *knowledge deficit* related to surgery or radiation therapy and possible long-term hormone replacement therapy
- *social and career disruption* caused by frequent visits to hospital and time off work due to symptoms such as joint pains.

Long-term support and counselling are needed. The reasons for the physiological changes are explained and the patient is taught about both short- and long-term therapy. The nurse helps the patient and family to develop a self-care plan that includes a diet that is well balanced but high in calories and plans for long-term hormone replacement therapy.

PANHYPOPITUITARISM (SIMMONDS' DISEASE)

This disease denotes a deficiency of all the anterior pituitary hormones. The condition may be the result of a primary lesion, such as a tumour or cyst, within the anterior lobe itself, or it may be secondary to a space-occupying lesion in neighbouring structures or to interference with the blood supply to the gland. The latter may occur with thrombosis of the hypophyseal vessels associated with postpartum shock. This remains the most likely cause of Simmonds' disease (Rees and Williams 1995). A tumour will compress and destroy the secreting cells as it enlarges. Surgical excision or irradiation of the gland for the purpose of suppressing the secretion of certain hormones in the treatment of carcinoma of the breast or acromegaly may incur hyposecretion of all the adenohypophyseal hormones.

Clinical characteristics

The multiple hormone deficiency results in a lack of stimulation to the thyroid, adrenal cortices and gonads. Secondary atrophy and hyposecretion of their hormones ensue. If the condition occurs in childhood, failure of the secretion of GH along with the other hormones produces dwarfism. Growth and development are arrested, the skin becomes wrinkled and the child develops an appearance characteristic of a 'wizened old person'.

In the adult, there is also a general wasting of all body tissues and the person exhibits emaciation and severe weight loss. The skin is dry and wrinkled and may assume a yellowish cast. The body hair becomes sparse. Decreased thyroid activity causes a reduction in the metabolic rate, leading to a subnormal temperature and extreme weakness. Arrested function of the gonads results in failure of ovulation and amenorrhoea in the female, and an absence of spermatogenesis and impotence in the male. Concomitant

hypoglycaemia and hypotension are seen and may lead to shock and coma. The low blood sugar level is attributed to the decreased GH and adrenocorticoid secretions. If the panhypopituitarism is due to an expanding neoplasm, the posterior pituitary and the infundibulum may become involved, manifested by polyuria and extreme thirst, which is characteristic of a deficiency of antidiuretic hormone (ADH). An expanding lesion may impose itself on the optic tract, impairing vision. The hypothalamus may also be affected, and varied neurological disturbances become evident; for example, the patient may experience severe anorexia.

Treatment

Treatment includes the administration of substitution hormones of the target glands. The patient receives corticosteroids and thyroid hormone in dosages adjusted to individual needs. Thyroid hormone is prescribed only when the patient is receiving corticosteroids. Gonadal hormones may be prescribed, depending on the patient's age. Testosterone (male hormone) may be administered to both sexes for its anabolic effect. Oestrogen may be used in the female to preserve female secondary sex characteristics.

If the cause is a tumour, it is removed by trans-sphenoidal microsurgery and/or treated by irradiation.

Nursing intervention

The nurse assists the patient and family in setting realistic long-term goals to promote adjustment to the chronic endocrine dysfunction. Patient and family concerns are identified and explored in depth, because the disorder has profound effects on both the individual and family, particularly if it is after a post-partum haemorrhage.

The nurse plays an important role in encouraging patients at home to take a high-calorie, high-vitamin diet. As anorexia is a common problem, resourcefulness is necessary to ensure adequate nourishment. Various methods and approaches must be tried. It is usually helpful to provide small servings of high-calorie foods at frequent intervals. Varying the foods, adding concentrates to fluids, determining the patient's preferences, having favourite 'dishes' prepared at home, eating with others and a change of environment are just a few suggestions that may prove beneficial.

The lethargy and apathy generally associated with Simmonds' disease predisposes to the patient's immobility. Prompting the patient to change position and exercise is necessary to stimulate circulation and prevent complications.

ANTIDIURETIC HORMONE HYPOSECRETION: DIABETES INSIPIDUS

Causative factors

The causative factor in this disorder may be a deficiency of ADH (vasopressin) or failure of the renal tubules to respond to ADH. A deficiency of ADH is most commonly due to hypoactivity or destruction of a part of the hypothalamic-posterior pituitary system resulting from primary or metastatic neoplasms or infection, such as encephalitis, meningitis or brain injury. In some instances, no apparent cause can be identified.

Clinical characteristics

Diabetes insipidus is characterized by a very large urinary output (polyuria) and extreme thirst (polydipsia). The daily output may range from 5 L to 20 L and the patient may experience anorexia, headache, muscular pains, loss of weight and strength, and electrolyte imbalance. The urine has an abnormally low specific gravity and does not contain any abnormal constituents. If fluid is withheld or does not keep pace with the output, an excessive loss of urine continues, leading to severe dehydration and shock. The persisting symptoms of polyuria and polydipsia day and night interfere with rest and normal activities.

Diagnosis

Investigation of the disorder usually involves water deprivation tests. A period of 8 hours without any fluids to drink will produce a significant rise in urine concentration in the normal person, but not in a person with diabetes insipidus.

Investigative procedures may also include neurological examination, radiography of the skull, visual field tests and CT.

Treatment

The patient is treated by replacement therapy with hypotonic parenteral fluids and unlimited oral fluids; a preparation of posterior pituitary extract or vasopressin is prescribed. The preparation used is normally desmopressin, an analogue of vasopressin. It is given as either an intranasal spray (10–40 mg daily in one or two doses) or by injection.

The patient is usually hospitalized during diagnostic investigation and regulation of medication.

Nursing intervention

Nursing care focuses on the two major health problems demonstrated by individuals with diabetes insipidus: (1) dehydration due to polyuria and (2) a lack of knowledge concerning hormone replacement therapy.

Dehydration

The nurse is responsible for the ongoing assessment of the person's fluid balance and for teaching the patient and family to recognize signs of dehydration and hypovolaemia. Vital signs, mental status, intake and output, urine specific gravity and skin integrity are assessed and recorded regularly. Daily weights are determined.

Provision of adequate fluid intake is achieved by the intravenous administration of hypotonic fluids, which serve to reduce the existing hypertonic state, and unlimited oral fluids. When the thirst mechanism is intact, the person will seek fluids, which should be readily available. If the person lacks the desire to drink, the nurse must be creative to ensure that the oral intake is maintained and/or supplemented with parenteral fluids.

Patient and family teaching

Lifelong dependence upon medication is not an easy fact for the patient to accept. The nurse can help the patient to plan for necessary readjustments, while giving reassurance that a normal pattern of life can be resumed.

The patient and a family member are taught the details of how to administer the drug. The instructions are also given in writing. Further explanation of the disorder may be required for appreciation of the importance of regular administration of the drug, and it should be advised that vasopressin is ineffective when taken orally because of inactivation by digestive enzymes. The patient is advised to record their weight every 2 or 3 days, and to note the urinary volume. Water retention indicated by weight increase and scanty urine may necessitate a decrease in vasopressin dosage.

ANTIDIURETIC HORMONE HYPERSECRETION: SYNDROME OF INAPPROPRIATE ANTIDIURETIC HORMONE

Causes

Inappropriate production of ADH may be caused by malignant tumours, respiratory and central nervous system infections, head trauma or positive-pressure ventilation. The exact mechanisms producing the excessive ADH secretion are not fully understood.

Clinical characteristics

The clinical characteristics of syndrome of inappropriate antidiuretic hormone (SIADH) are those of water intoxication. The blood volume increases, haemodilution results, and serum sodium level and osmolarity are decreased. Oedema is absent as a result of the hyponatraemia. The person's urine is concentrated and the volume is diminished. Weight gain, nausea and vomiting, and a decreased level of consciousness and seizures may be present.

Treatment

Treatment depends on the severity and duration of the water intoxication. In an emergency situation, intravenous hypertonic saline solutions are administered along with diuretic drugs such as furosemide (frusemide). In less acute situations, the restriction of fluids to 500 mL daily may be sufficient. Demeclocycline may be prescribed because it inhibits the renal response to ADH. The underlying cause of the increased ADH secretion must be treated.

Nursing intervention

Nursing care is directed toward: (1) management of the fluid volume excess; (2) assessment and control of the altered thought processes that occur as water moves into the cerebral cells; (3) patient teaching for the person with chronic SIADH.

Fluid volume excess

Assessment of the person's fluid balance includes monitoring vital signs, serum electrolytes, urine osmolarity, fluid intake and output, body weight and mental status. Oral fluids are restricted to 500 mL/day. Intravenous infusions are monitored closely and administered slowly to prevent further fluid overload and aggravation of the neurological manifestations.

Mental status

The patient's level of consciousness is assessed regularly. If it declines or if seizures are likely, safety precautions are implemented. The side-rails should be up on the bed and the patient should be visible at all times.

Patient and family teaching

The patient and family are helped to understand the disease and to recognize signs and symptoms of water toxicity. Information is provided about Medic Alert identification. The patient is instructed to monitor body weight and changes in the amount of urine output.

PITUITARY ABLATION

The anterior and posterior pituitary gland may be removed or destroyed because of hyperfunction or a neoplasm of the gland. Hypophysectomy is also employed in the treatment of cancer of the breast and prostate, and is often supported by the sex hormones oestrogens and androgens respectively. Removal of the source of gonadotrophic hormones reduces support for the primary neoplasm and its metastasis. Withdrawal of the hormones does not cure the disease, but usually produces a remission for a period of several months.

Pituitary ablation may be carried out by radiation therapy, surgical excision or destruction by cryosurgery (freezing). Irradiation may be from an external source or radioactive yttrium-90 may be implanted. Access to the gland is usually by a nasal-trans-sphenoidal approach, but a transfrontal approach may be used if the tumour is large and has spread.

Hypophysectomy results in the withdrawal of ACTH, TSH and probably ADH, as well as the gonadotrophins. In some instances, the neural stalk, which transmits the nerve fibres from the hypothalamus to the posterior pituitary gland, may be preserved at operation, thus preventing diabetes insipidus. The patient requires cortisone, thyroxine and possibly ADH replacement for the remainder of his or her life. Gonadal function ceases and the patient becomes infertile. If the operation was done because of disease of the pituitary gland, the male patient may be given testosterone to prevent impotence.

Preoperative preparation

The patient and family are likely to be very apprehensive. The nurse should therefore encourage them to talk about their fears and ask questions, and provide necessary emotional support. The permanent results of the operation will have been explained by the doctor, but the nurse, knowing what the patient has been told, should be prepared to answer questions and explain the hormonal replacement.

The patient is advised that nasal packing will be inserted if a transsphenoidal approach is used. The patient is taught deep-breathing techniques, encouraged to practise mouth breathing before operation and is cautioned against nose-blowing, sneezing and coughing after surgery. A corticosteroid preparation is usually given the day before operation and again before going to the operating theatre.

Postoperative care

The care following a hypophysectomy is similar to that of any patient who has had intracranial surgery. Close observation is made for early signs of acute adrenal insufficiency (see below) or fluid imbalance. An adrenocorticoid steroid is given intravenously until the patient can tolerate it orally. The dose is gradually decreased until the maintenance dose is established. Vasopressin may be necessary to control the fluid loss; the dosage is adjusted to the urinary volume. Thyroid replacement may be started orally on the second or third postoperative day.

The intravenous infusion is usually discontinued the morning after operation. Oral fluids may be started the evening of surgery or the next morning. If a transsphenoidal approach was used, the incision will be above the front teeth. The patient is instructed not to brush the teeth until the incision is healed and the sutures are removed. Mouthwashes are used to maintain dental and oral hygiene. The patient is taught to carry out meticulous oral hygiene regularly until healing has taken place in about 4–6 weeks. The period of hospitalization is relatively short; instruction about the taking of the necessary hormones (cortisone, vasopressin and thyroxine) is carried out throughout the postoperative period and, if necessary, a referral is made for follow-up instruction and supervision by a community nurse.

THE PERSON WITH A DISORDER OF THE ADRENAL CORTICES

As with other endocrine glands, dysfunction of the adrenal cortices may involve hyposecretion or hypersecretion of their hormones. Adrenocortical hypofunction produces Addison's disease. Hyperfunction may cause Cushing's syndrome or primary aldosteronism.

ASSESSMENT OF ADRENOCORTICAL FUNCTION

Assessment of the person with altered adrenocortical function includes the identification of health problems common to persons with increased or decreased production of the adrenocortical hormones (Table 18.6).

Common characteristics identified during the *health history* include progressive fatigue and weakness, and changes in appetite and weight. The patient and family are questioned regarding changes in emotional responses including irritability, lability or depression. Questions are posed to identify changes in sexuality patterns in both males and females.

The *physical examination* focuses on observation of the skin and secondary sex characteristics.

The *skin* is inspected for signs of oedema or dehydration; increased bruising and pigmentation may be present on the palms and exposed body surfaces, joints, genitalia and oral

Table 18.6 Assessment of the person with altered adrenocortical function

	Clinical characteristics	
	Adrenocortical insufficiency (Addison's disease)	**Adrenocortical hyperfunction (Cushing's disease)**
Nutrition and metabolism	Hypoglycaemia Anorexia, nausea Abdominal pain Weight loss	Hyperglycaemia Abdominal discomfort Weight gain
Fluid and electrolyte balance	Dehydration Increased serum potassium level Decreased serum sodium level Hypotension	Oedema Decreased serum potassium level Increased serum sodium level Hypertension
Skin and hair	Skin dusky, bronze Increased pigmentation	Purple striae Bruising Thinning of skin and hair Hirsutism
Activity tolerance	Weakness Constant fatigue	Weakness, fatigue Muscle atrophy
Potential for infection		Delayed wound healing Suppression of usual signs of infection
Sexuality patterns	Decreased pubic and axillary hair in females	Secondary male sex characteristics in females Amenorrhoea Development of breasts in males
Individual coping	Depression Irritability Restlessness	Depression Apathy Mood changes

mucosa. The abdomen is observed for the presence of purple striae. The development of a 'moon face' and the existence of fat deposits, particularly a 'Buffalo hump' (cervicodorsal fat), are characteristic signs that may be observed in hypersecretion.

Changes and deviations in the structure of the breasts and in the distribution and amount of body hair, particularly scant pubic and axillary hair and excessive facial hair in the female are noted.

Body height and weight are measured and alterations in normal growth and development assessed.

ADRENOCORTICAL INSUFFICIENCY (ADDISON'S DISEASE)

Causes

Primary failure of the adrenal cortices to produce corticosteroids is rare; it is most often the result of atrophy of the glands but may be caused by congenital adrenal hyperplasia, tubercular infection, adrenal haemorrhage or a neoplasm. Atrophy of the glands is attributed to an autoimmune reaction and affects females twice as often as males. Secondary hypofunction of the adrenal cortices occurs with hypopituitarism and the concomitant deficiency of ACTH,

and with excessive administration of steroids. Adrenal insufficiency may also occur in patients with acquired immune deficiency syndrome (AIDS) as a result of fungal or cytomegalovirus infections.

Clinical characteristics

In Addison's disease, there is a deficiency of cortisol which interferes with the maintenance of a normal blood sugar level; the body cannot compensate by gluconeogenesis, liver glycogen is depleted and hypoglycaemia develops, especially between meals. There is a general depression of metabolic activity and energy production. The ability to cope with even mild stress is greatly diminished and minor infections, slight injuries, exposure to extremes of temperature or emotional problems that are relatively insignificant to the normal person may prove very serious to these individuals.

The patient complains of weakness and constant fatigue, which becomes progressively more severe and incapacitating. Listlessness, irritability and impaired mental ability may be manifested. Anorexia, nausea, abdominal pain and constipation alternating with diarrhoea are common complaints. Increased sensitivity to cold develops. The patient loses weight. The skin takes on a dusky, bronze hue and brown pigmented areas appear, especially in sites normally exposed to light, pressure or friction. Patchy areas of pigmentation may also be observed in the oral mucosa and conjunctivae.

The adrenocortical insufficiency causes an outpouring of the hormone ACTH, which results in overproduction of melanocyte-stimulating hormone (MSH). As a result, pigmented areas of the skin are common in the patient with Addison's disease.

The aldosterone deficiency leads to decreased reabsorption of sodium by the renal tubules with a consequent excessive loss of water as well as sodium in the urine. Severe dehydration may develop, leading to a depletion of the intravascular volume and ensuing reduced cardiac output, hypotension and shock. Hypotension is inevitable and it would be unlikely that someone with a systolic blood pressure above 110 mmHg would have the disease. The patient is often diagnosed only after presenting in a collapsed and critically ill condition known as an *Addisonian crisis* (see below).

Treatment and nursing intervention

Addison's disease is treated by maintenance doses of corticosteroid preparations. The glucocorticoids are replaced by the oral administration of a cortisol preparation (hydrocortisone) two or three times daily. The deficiency of mineralocorticoid (aldosterone) associated with primary adrenocortical insufficiency is met by giving fludrocortisone (synthetic aldosterone) orally once daily. The patient with secondary adrenocortical insufficiency does not require the aldosterone replacement.

The nurse caring for a patient receiving corticoid preparations must be familiar with the potential adverse effects of these drugs. If the patient receives corticoids in doses even slightly in excess of the amounts normally secreted, certain changes are likely to occur, especially with prolonged administration. Constant observation is necessary for early signs of side-effects. Restlessness, insomnia, euphoria and swings in mood may be manifested. The patient's susceptibility to infection may be markedly increased by the drug's suppression of lymphocyte and antibody production and local inflammatory responses. Muscle wasting and weakness may occur as a result of an excessive protein breakdown and increased loss of potassium in the urine. Sodium and water retention may be evidenced by oedema. Increased fat deposition on the trunk and face may develop, changing the patient's general appearance. Increased fullness and rounding of the face produces the characteristic change referred to as the 'moon face'. Females may develop secondary male characteristics accompanied by growth of hair on the face, and growth of the breasts in males is occasionally seen. Prolonged administration of corticoids in excess of normal secretion may produce hyperglycaemia and glycosuria. The patient also becomes predisposed to the development of gastrointestinal lesions, such as peptic ulcers.

The patient with Addison's disease is encouraged to take a high-carbohydrate, high-protein diet. The danger of hypoglycaemia which may occur with glucocorticoid deficiency may be offset by the patient taking nourishment between meals and at bedtime. In primary adrenal insufficiency, the patient may require additional sodium chloride. A directive as to the amount of salt to be included in the diet should be received from the doctor; the average amount served with meals may be sufficient. The patient with secondary adrenocortical insufficiency will not require additional salt.

Acute corticoid insufficiency, which is also referred to as *Addisonian crisis*, may develop when corticoid replacement is inadequate or omitted, or it may be what brings the patient for medical attention before the disease is diagnosed. Frequently, a crisis is precipitated by some physical or psychological stress such as infection, exposure to extremes of temperature, gastrointestinal upset (e.g. vomiting and diarrhoea), fever, profuse perspiration, strenuous activity, anxiety or grief. Acute insufficiency is serious and, unless treated promptly, can rapidly lead to death. Early symptoms are nausea, vomiting, diarrhoea, abdominal pain, fever and extreme weakness. Severe hypoglycaemia and dehydration develop rapidly; the blood pressure falls, and shock and coma may follow. Blood glucose, sodium and cortisol levels are low and the potassium and urea concentrations are markedly increased.

Addisonian crisis is treated by continuous intravenous infusion of normal saline to which hydrocortisone (cortisol) is added for at least the first 24 hours. Intravenous dextrose is required if hypoglycaemia is present. Hydrocortisone is also given orally as replacement medication. The large doses of hydrocortisone that the patient receives usually exert a sufficient sodium-retaining effect, eliminating the need for supplementary administration of a mineralocorticoid preparation such as fludrocortisone in the short term.

Frequent recordings of the blood pressure, temperature, pulse respirations and level of response are made. The patient is kept at absolute rest to avoid expenditure of energy and is turned, bathed and fed by the nurse. He or she is kept flat and any change of position is made slowly because of the hypotension. Frequent high-carbohydrate feedings are given as soon as they can be tolerated. When the patient's blood pressure and other vital signs have returned to normal and are sustained, and the condition that precipitated the crisis has been controlled, the corticoid dosage is gradually reduced to maintenance level.

Patient and family teaching

The overall goals are to learn self-regulation of the disease and to maintain a satisfactory level of functioning.

Goals The patient and family will be able to:

1 state the purpose of lifelong steroid replacement therapy
2 describe a plan for taking medications daily and state the names, dosage, frequency, actions and side-effects of each prescribed medication
3 describe the effects of stress on the disease and plans to minimize stress

4 discuss plans to minimize exposure to infection

5 describe symptoms that indicate Addisonian crisis and actions to take if symptoms develop.

Nursing intervention

As primary adrenal insufficiency requires lifelong replacement therapy, an important nursing function is teaching the patient and family about the disease and necessary care. A simple explanation is given of the nature of the condition with reassurance that, although hormone replacement will be necessary for life, if the prescribed therapeutic regimen is followed, a relatively normal life can be expected.

Activity tolerance The importance of regular and adequate hours of rest, stopping activities short of fatigue and avoiding exposure to cold are stressed, indicating the effect of exposure and overexertion on cellular activity and the blood sugar level.

Medication therapy No medications, including laxatives, except those ordered by the doctor should be taken. Detailed teaching is carried out regarding the taking of prescribed corticoid preparations, including the importance of taking the exact amounts at the correct times. The patient is warned of the dangers of being without medication. Increased doses of medication may be recommended during periods of stress.

Nutrition The high-carbohydrate, high-protein diet with the amount of sodium recommended by the doctor is discussed in detail, explaining the need for nourishment between meals and at bedtime to maintain a normal blood sugar level.

Prevention of infection The patient and family are advised of the need to avoid contact with those with an infection as much as possible, and suggestions are made as to how this may be achieved.

Individual coping Patients should understand that a stressful situation or illness demands more corticoids. To prevent a serious crisis or acute corticoid insufficiency, prompt medical attention is necessary with any disorder such as a respiratory infection, vomiting, diarrhoea, fainting or sudden weakness. The role of worry and emotional situations in precipitating a crisis is emphasized.

Safety measures The patient with Addison's disease should always carry a steroid card or wear a Medic Alert bracelet or pendant that clearly indicates the presence of corticoid insufficiency and what should be done in the event of injury or sudden collapse.

In teaching, the nurse does not attempt to provide all the necessary information at one time. The instruction is planned to cover several sessions; salient points are clarified and reinforced by repetition, and opportunities are provided for the patient and family members to ask questions and to participate actively in the learning process.

Evaluation The patient and family should be able to administer the prescribed corticosteroid replacement therapy safely and to recognize side-effects of over- or under-replacement. The patient should be able to describe plans to receive adequate rest, to decrease exposure to infection, to minimize the effects of added physical and emotional stress and for ongoing health care and supervision. The patient should maintain a desirable body weight and quickly identify fluctuations in weight pattern.

ADRENOCORTICAL HYPERFUNCTION (CUSHING'S SYNDROME)

Causes

This is a rare disorder which is more common in females and results from an excessive secretion of adrenal corticoids. It may be due to primary hyperfunction of one or both of the adrenal cortices or may be secondary to a pathological hypersecretion of ACTH by the anterior pituitary gland which ultimately causes an over secretion of the steroid hormones from the adrenal glands. Primary hyperactivity of the adrenal cortex is usually caused by a neoplasm, most frequently an adenoma, but may also occur as a result of unexplained hyperplasia. The most common cause, however, is iatrogenic: the excessive administration of glucocorticoid hormone.

Clinical characteristics

These will vary in individuals according to age and the amount of corticoid being produced in excess of the normal. The increased output of cortisol causes excessive protein catabolism, gluconeogenesis, an abnormal distribution of fat and atrophy of lymphoid tissue. The person manifests a decreased glucose tolerance, hyperglycaemia, and muscle wasting and weakness. The appearance changes because of the increased deposition of fat on the trunk, thin wasted limbs, and a round, bloated-looking face ('moon' face). Purple striae may appear, notably on the abdomen, buttocks and thighs, and are due to increased fragility of the blood vessels and atrophy of the skin. Ecchymoses are common. The production of lymphocytes is suppressed, increasing the patient's susceptibility to infection. Osteoporosis may occur, usually in the vertebrae, because of calcium mobilization; the patient frequently complains of backache.

The excessive secretion of mineralocorticoids results in electrolyte, fluid and acid–base imbalances. Hypernatraemia, water retention and hypokalaemia develop. The increased reabsorption by the renal tubules of sodium ions in exchange for hydrogen ions depletes the acid ions, producing alkalosis. The low blood level of potassium may cause extreme weakness and cardiac dysfunction. Hypertension due to the sodium and water retention is common.

As a consequence of the increased production of androgens, women develop secondary male characteristics. There is a marked growth of hair on the face, the voice deepens, breasts atrophy, amenorrhoea occurs and the clitoris may enlarge.

Treatment and nursing intervention

The treatment of Cushing's syndrome is urgent as the disease carries a 5-year mortality rate of 50% (Haslett et al

1999). This depends upon whether the hypersecretion of corticoids is due to primary dysfunction of the adrenal cortices or is the result of a hypersecretion of ACTH. In the case of an adrenocortical neoplasm, the affected gland is removed. The patient is prepared medically with drug therapy before operation to reduce cortisol levels, and then receives hormonal replacement therapy after surgery as outlined for Addison's disease. If the condition is secondary to a pituitary tumour, the tumour is usually treated by irradiation or removed surgically via the trans-sphenoidal route.

Nursing care of the patient with Cushing's syndrome is mainly symptomatic (Table 18.6). Precautions are necessary to prevent accidental falls, which may occur because of weakness. The fluid intake and output are recorded to determine the amount of water retention, and sodium intake is restricted. The blood pressure and pulse are taken at regular intervals so that early changes may be detected. Changes in mood and behaviour are common and should be recorded. Exposure to persons with infection is avoided because of the patient's lowered resistance.

HYPERALDOSTERONISM

An excessive production of aldosterone is usually caused by an adenoma or hyperplasia of the particular adrenocortical cells that secrete the hormone. The most striking features of the disease are the excessive renal loss of potassium, retention of sodium and hypertension. The person experiences severe generalized muscular weakness due to the hypokalaemia. Depletion of the body potassium reduces the kidneys' ability to concentrate the urine, and polyuria occurs. Despite an increased retention of salt, there is no corresponding retention of water or oedema. This is attributed to an increased glomerular filtration rate and the polyuria. As a result of the hypernatraemia and polyuria, the person usually experiences severe thirst. An increase in arterial blood pressure is characteristic. In addition to hypernatraemia and hypokalaemia, laboratory investigation reveals raised urinary and plasma aldosterone levels and normal renin concentration. Treatment consists of surgical removal of the adenoma or affected gland preceded by administration of potassium salts.

Secondary hyperaldosteronism due to an excessive secretion of renin by the kidneys may occur. It may be treated with spironolactone, an aldosterone antagonist, or renal surgery.

THE PERSON WITH A DISORDER OF THE ADRENAL MEDULLAE

ASSESSMENT OF ADRENAL MEDULLARY FUNCTION

The *health history* focuses on identification of the person's usual responses to stress and documentation of episodes of excessive stress reactions (flight or fight reaction).

Physical examination involves the documentation of fluctuations in and excessively high blood pressure readings.

Excess of adrenaline and noradrenaline (phaeochromocytoma)

Disease of the adrenal medullae is rare and most commonly occurs in the form of a neoplasm known as a phaeochromocytoma, which produces an excessive amount of adrenaline and noradrenaline. The tumour is usually unilateral and benign, and causes hypertension, hyperglycaemia and hypermetabolism. The increased liberation of large amounts of the hormones is usually paroxysmal at first, lasting from a few minutes to hours, but is likely eventually to become persistent. The patient frequently complains of a pounding headache, nausea, vomiting, palpitation, air hunger, nervousness, tremor and weakness. Sweating, pallor, dilatation of the pupils, tachycardia and a sharp rise in the blood pressure are also manifested. The increased glycogenolysis and subsequent raised blood sugar level may result in glycosuria.

Tests used to establish the diagnosis of phaeochromocytoma include the estimation of the blood and urinary content of the hormones or their major metabolite, vanillylmandelic acid (VMA). CT is carried out to localize the tumour.

The patient with phaeochromocytoma is treated by surgical removal of the tumour of the affected gland. Sympathetic blocking agents are administered before operation to decrease blood pressure and reduce other symptoms.

Nursing in adrenal surgery

Surgery of the adrenal glands may be performed on patients with hypersecretions of hormones due to hyperplasia or tumours of one or both glands. The procedure may involve the removal of both adrenal glands (bilateral or total adrenalectomy), the removal of one gland (unilateral adrenalectomy) or resection of part of a gland (subtotal adrenalectomy). Bilateral adrenalectomy is occasionally undertaken in patients with cancer of the breast and occasionally in those with cancer of the prostate. Malignant disease of these organs is dependent to some extent on sex hormones, and because the adrenal cortices produce both oestrogens and androgens, removal of the cortices eliminates a source of the supporting hormones. In the case of cancer of the breast, adrenalectomy is preceded by oophorectomy (removal of the ovaries). Occasionally the patient with cancer of the prostate undergoes orchidectomy (removal of the testicles) before adrenalectomy is considered.

Preoperative preparation
Preparation of the patient for adrenal surgery includes the general preparation for surgery. Blood studies are done to determine electrolyte concentrations, and corrections are made as indicated. Because of an excessive potassium excretion, a solution of potassium chloride may be ordered to restore the normal level of potassium in the blood. The blood sugar level and glucose tolerance are investigated. The patient is given a high-protein diet because of the protein

depletion due to excessive glucocorticoid secretion. The fluid intake and output are measured, and the balance is noted. The blood pressure is recorded at least once daily to serve as a postoperative comparative baseline. The patient with hyperfunction of the adrenal cortices frequently has experienced hypertension for some time. Phenoxybenzamine hydrochloride (an α-blocker) may be prescribed before surgery for 6 weeks to reduce vasomotor tone and restore normal plasma volume.

If both adrenal glands are to be removed, the patient and the family must understand that constant hormone replacement will be necessary for the remainder of the patient's life.

After operation, the patient's respirations tend to be shallow because the incision is close to the diaphragm. Careful teaching about postoperative breathing and coughing exercises are therefore essential.

The surgeon's approach to the adrenal gland is usually through a high flank incision or occasionally through the abdomen. When a bilateral adrenalectomy is carried out, two incisions are made, unless the transabdominal approach is used.

Hydrocortisone may be administered before and during as well as after the operation to prevent adrenal insufficiency in the immediate postoperative period. An intravenous solution is run slowly and continuously. This is in preparation for prompt administration of corticosteroids or a vasopressor, as indicated.

Postoperative care

Assessment and management of medication and fluid therapy   During the first few postoperative days, and until the maintenance dosages of hydrocortisone and fludrocortisone are established in the case of adrenalectomy, special attention is paid to the patient's blood pressure, fluid balance and blood chemistry. Constant nursing care is necessary until the vital signs and the corticoid, sodium and potassium concentrations are stabilized. The blood pressure, respirations and pulse are recorded every 15 minutes for several hours and the interval is gradually lengthened if they remain satisfactory. Any rapid or significant fall in blood pressure, dyspnoea or tachycardia is reported promptly. The fluid intake and output are accurately measured, and any imbalance is brought to the doctor's attention. Frequent checks are made of the blood sodium, potassium and glucose levels, which influence the amount of corticoids given. Vomiting, increased weakness, dehydration, hypotension and an increased temperature may indicate acute corticoid insufficiency.

Intravenous corticoids are given continuously for a day or two with the dosage and rate of flow adjusted to the patient's clinical condition and electrolyte and fluid balances. Oral doses of hydrocortisone and fludrocortisone are started as soon as tolerated by the patient. The dosage of both corticoid preparations is gradually tapered off until maintenance amounts are established. When the intravenous corticoids are withdrawn, an intravenous infusion of glucose in water or normal saline is continued slowly even though the patient may be tolerating fluids by mouth. The purpose of this is to keep the route available for quick administration of corticoids or a vasopressor (e.g. metaraminol or noradrenaline (norepinephrine) acid tartrate) if needed. The patient's condition tends to be labile and may change quickly. The nurse must be constantly alert for signs of corticoid insufficiency or indications of excessive corticoid administration.

When surgery is performed to remove a phaeochromocytoma, monitoring of the blood pressure is necessary every 30 minutes–1 hour for at least 36–48 hours; severe fluctuations may occur. A marked rise may occur during or immediately after operation because of excessive liberation of catecholamines from the tumour during removal. An adrenergic blocking agent such as phentolamine is kept available for quick intravenous administration to neutralize the medullary hormones.

More often, the problem following surgery is severe hypotension and concomitant shock. The blood pressure is maintained by giving a vasopressor such as noradrenaline (norepinephrine) acid tartrate or metaraminol in an intravenous solution. The rate of flow must be carefully controlled and adjusted according to frequent blood pressure recordings and the doctor's directives. The patient is kept flat and any change in position achieved slowly.

When unilateral adrenalectomy or a subtotal resection of one or both glands is done, the patient may receive some hydrocortisone following operation. Less will be required than in total adrenalectomy, and it is gradually withdrawn.

After adrenal surgery, the patient usually stays in bed until the blood pressure remains at a satisfactory level. Before commencing ambulation, the head of the bed is elevated and the blood pressure checked. The patient should not be left unattended during mobilization and frequent blood pressure checks should be carried out. If a significant decrease in blood pressure occurs, the patient is returned to bed and kept flat.

Patient teaching   In preparation for discharge, the patient who has had a bilateral adrenalectomy receives the same instruction as the patient with Addison's disease. If one gland has been removed or a subtotal resection done, the patient is cautioned to avoid over-fatigue, exposure to extremes of temperature (especially cold), infections and emotional disturbances as much as possible. It is possible that stress may precipitate an acute adrenal insufficiency or crisis because the remaining adrenal tissue cannot meet the increased hormonal demand. If the patient experiences weakness, fainting, fever, or nausea and vomiting, the general practitioner should be contacted immediately; a corticoid supplement will be required.

After any adrenal operation, the patient should resume activity very gradually, and should be followed closely as an outpatient. Usually several months are required to adjust the hormonal replacement satisfactorily. The patient who has had hypertension due to phaeochromocytoma may not regain a stable blood pressure level for 3–4 months.

SUMMARY

The endocrine system contributes to the homeostatic control of many body functions. Disorders of the endocrine system and its interrelated components are of three major types:

1 Increased production of one or more hormone(s)
2 Decreased production of one or more hormone(s)
3 Failure of the target organ or tissue to respond to the hormone.

Clinical characteristics of endocrine disorders are varied, subtle and slowly progressive. The patient and family are the best source of assessment information as they are usually aware that something is wrong before a pattern of characteristic signs and symptoms can be recognized. The health problems common to most persons with endocrine disorders include: altered nutrition and metabolism, changes in activity tolerance, altered thought processes and emotional responses, altered sexuality patterns, altered fluid balance, impaired skin integrity and impaired thermoregulation.

The person with a hormone imbalance is at risk for the development of life-threatening as well as chronic complications. The nurse provides intensive care during acute episodes and assists the patient and family to recognize the early warnings of endocrine imbalances and actions to take to prevent complications.

The discussions in this chapter focus on the more common endocrine disorders of type 1 and type 2 diabetes mellitus, and hypothyroidism and hyperthyroidism. Individuals with disorders of the pituitary gland, parathyroid and adrenal glands experience similar and equally devastating problems. Many persons with endocrine disorders require lifelong hormone replacement therapy as a result of decreased production of hormones with disease and/or therapeutic destruction of the involved gland. All are faced with the need to make major adjustments in their lives. The patient ultimately becomes responsible for self-management of the endocrine disorder.

The growing body of nursing knowledge available to resolve patient health problems is useless if it is not transmitted to patients and their families to enable them to assume control of their own care. Throughout this chapter, the importance of patient and family teaching has been stressed. Emphasis is placed on the provision of information about the survival skills or the basic knowledge and skill required by the person to function safely. Nurses are also responsible for evaluating the effectiveness of health teaching and for determining whether the patient and family understand the need for continuing therapy.

Advanced teaching and counselling skills are needed to help people change their habits and lifestyles. Although not all nurses have the opportunity to follow individuals for an extended period of time to enable them to provide this level of teaching, they can ensure that all persons with long-term endocrine disorders are aware of the many resources available in the community.

REFERENCES

Barnett A (2001a) Insulin made easy. London: Medical Education Partnership.

Barnett A (2001b) New therapies for the management of type 2 diabetes. Nursing Times 97(6): 34–36.

Batki A (1999) Selecting blood glucose monitoring systems. Professional Nurse 14(10): 715–723.

British Heart Foundation (2006) Overall prevalence of diabetes. Online. Available: http://www.heartstats.org/datapage.asp?id=1106 [Accessed 06.01.2006].

British National Formulary (2005) British National Formulary. London: British Medical Association/Royal Pharmaceutical Society of Great Britain.

Carr S (2001) Acromegaly management in the community. Nursing Times 97(2): 32–33.

Connor H, Annan F, Bunn E, Frost G, McGough N, Sarwar T, Thomas B (2003) The implementation of nutritional advice for people with diabetes. Diabetic Medicine 20(10): 786–807.

Diabetes UK (2006a) Glycaemic index. Online. Available: http://www.diabetes.org.uk/faq/GI.htm [Accessed 06.01.2006].

Diabetes UK (2006b) HypoStop – name change to GlucoGel. Online. Available: http://www.diabetes.org.uk/infocentre/guidance/HypoStop.doc [Accessed 07.01.2006].

Elliot B (2000) Diagnosing and treating hypothyroidism. Nurse Practitioner 25(2): 92–105.

Erens R, Primatesta P, Prior G (2001) Health survey for England; the health of minority ethnic groups. London: DoH.

Haslett C, Chilvers E, Hunter J, Boon N (1999) Davidson's principles and practice of medicine, 18th edn. Edinburgh: Churchill Livingstone.

Lehmann R (1998) The effects of exercise on cardiovascular risk factors in type 2 diabetes mellitus. Practical Diabetes International 15(5): 151–156.

McIntyre M, McDowell J (1994) Educating a patient with diabetes about foot care. British Journal of Nursing 3(2): 75–78.

Marchesini G, Forlani G, Cerrelli F, et al (2004) WHO and ATPIII proposals for the definition of the metabolic syndrome in patients with Type 2 diabetes. Diabetic Medicine 21: 383–387.

Melville A, Richardson R, Lister-Sharp D (2000) Complications of type 2 diabetes: renal disease and the promotion of patient self management. Nursing Times 96(17): 37–38.

Naquib (2002) A question of choice – compliance in medicine taking, a preliminary review. In: Carter S, Taylor D, Levenson R, eds. Medicines Partnership. Online. Available: www.medicines-partnership.org [Accessed 12.08.2005].

NICE (2002) Clinical guidance F Management of type 2 diabetes, renal disease-prevention and early management. NICE.

NICE (2004) Clinical Guideline 15. Type 1 diabetes: diagnosis and management of type 1 diabetes in adults. NICE.

O'Malley B, Hickey J, Nevens E (2000) Thyroid dysfunction: weight problems and the psyche, the patients' perspective. Journal of Human Nutrition and Dietetics 13(4): 243–248.

Pullen M (2000) Exercise for the person with diabetes. Professional Nurse 16(2): 888–891.

Rees P, Williams D (1995) Principles of clinical medicine. London: Edward Arnold.

Springhouse Corporation (1998) Handbook of medical-surgical nursing. Springhouse, PA: Springhouse Publishing Corporation.

Springhouse Corporation (2000) Handbook of pathophysiology. Springhouse, PA: Springhouse Publishing Corporation.

UK Prospective Diabetes Study 38 (1998) Tight Blood Pressure Control and risk of macrovascular and microvascular complications in type 2 diabetes. British Medical Journal 317: 703–713.

Umeh L, Wallhagen M, Nicoloff N (1999) Identifying patients at high risk for amputation. Nurse Practitioner 24(6): 5670.

Vander AJ, Sherman JH, Luciano DS (1990) Human physiology: the mechanism of body function, 5th edn. New York: McGraw-Hill.

Walton J, Brand S (1994) Diabetes mellitus: implications for nursing care. British Journal of Nursing 3(9): 442–445.

Watkins P (1998) ABC of diabetes, 4th edn. London: BMJ Books.

Winters S, Jernigan V (2000) Vascular disease risk markers in diabetes: monitoring and evaluation. Nurse Practitioner 25(6): 40–65.

York CRD (1999) Complications of diabetes: screening for retinopathy, management of foot ulcers. York: York NHS Centre for Review and Dissemination.

York CRD (2000) Complications of diabetes: renal disease and the promotion of self-management. York: York NHS Centre for Review and Dissemination.

Caring for the patient with a disorder of the renal and urinary systems

Mike Walsh and Alison Crumbie

INTRODUCTION

In England, national standards for the care of people with chronic renal disease have been developed by the Department of Health (2004, 2005). The aim of these documents is to help the NHS and its partners manage demand, increase fairness of access and improve choice and quality in dialysis and kidney transplant services and to limit the development and progression of chronic kidney disease; minimize the impact of acute renal failure, and extend palliative care to people dying with kidney failure. The nurse has an important role to play in working with patients and their families to achieve these aims. This chapter will help to provide an introduction to the renal and urinary systems. Understanding these systems can be complex and challenging. Delivery of expert, comprehensive care to the person with a disorder in either system is essential in order to gain a full understanding of the impact of that disorder on the individual's quality of life. The purpose of this chapter is to give an overview of the normal kidney and urinary tract and common disorders. The effect of these disorders on the rest of the body will also be considered. This will assist the nurse to understand the impact of disease and how to deliver care and will help to achieve the standards set out in the National Service Framework for Renal Services (Department of Health 2004, 2005).

THE RENAL SYSTEM AND URINARY TRACT

STRUCTURE OF THE KIDNEYS

The kidneys are paired organs that lie retroperitoneally against the dorsal abdominal wall. Each kidney is enclosed in a fibrous capsule and is embedded in fatty tissue. It consists of approximately 1 million *nephrons, collecting tubules*, and a *pelvis*. The kidney is anatomically divided into an outer portion called the *cortex* and an inner section lying between the cortex and the pelvis called the *medulla* (Fig. 19.1). The blood vessels, nerves and ureter enter or leave the kidney at the *hilum*, the indentation on the medial surface.

Nephron

The nephron is the functional unit of the kidney. It consists of a narrow, convoluted tubule and a tuft of capillaries referred to as a *glomerulus*. The upper end of the tubule is dilated and invaginated to envelop the glomerulus and is called *Bowman's capsule*.

The tubule is divided into three segments: the *proximal convoluted tubule*, the hairpin-like *loop of Henle* and the *distal convoluted tubule* (Fig. 19.2). A major function of the tubules is to convey water and solutes in either direction across the tubular cells between the interstitial fluid and the tubular content. The thickness and structure of the walls differ from one segment to another; this arrangement accounts for

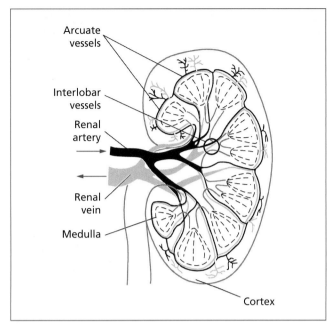

Figure 19.1   Cross-section of the kidney.

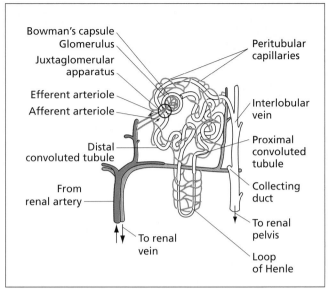

Figure 19.2   A renal unit, or nephron, of the cortex of the kidney.

different substances being re-absorbed and secreted in different sections of the tubule.

The proximal convoluted tubule is the longest portion of the nephron and has thin walls consisting of a single layer of cells. The loop of Henle varies in length and lies mainly in the medulla. Its terminal portion approximates the glomerulus of the nephron, of which it is a part, and its afferent arteriole. The distal convoluted tubule is shorter than the other portions of the tubule. The cells in most of the tubule are sensitive to the concentration of antidiuretic hormone (ADH) and adrenocortical steroids, which influence re-absorption of substances by the distal tubule.

Collecting tubules

The distal tubules coalesce to form straight collecting tubules, which unite to form progressively larger collecting tubules. Groups of the larger tubules come together to form a pyramid-like structure in the medulla. The apex of each pyramid is known as the *papilla* and contains the terminations of collecting tubules through which the urine passes into a cup-like pouch (calyx) of the renal pelvis. The ureter drains the kidney via the renal pelvis.

Blood supply

The renal artery to each kidney arises from the abdominal aorta. When the artery enters the kidney, it progressively subdivides to become afferent arterioles. Each *afferent arteriole* enters a nephron to form a glomerulus. The glomerular capillaries unite to form the *efferent arteriole*, which terminates in a second capillary network in which the tubule is invested. The blood pressure in this second set of capillaries is much lower than that in the glomerulus. The blood is then collected into venules and eventually into a renal vein which carries it to the inferior vena cava.

A large volume of blood is circulated continuously through the kidneys. It is estimated that the renal blood flow averages about 1000–1200 mL/minute in an adult. Receiving an adequate blood supply under the appropriate driving pressure is critical to maintaining kidney function.

A group of special cells is located just before the afferent arteriole becomes the glomerulus. These are known as *juxtaglomerular cells*. They are responsible for the production of the chemical *renin*.

RENAL FUNCTION

Normal functioning of the body cells is greatly dependent upon a relative constancy of the internal environment. The kidneys play a major role in maintaining this constancy by regulating the water and electrolyte content and the acid-base balance of the body; they *conserve* appropriate amounts of essential substances vital to normal cellular function (e.g. glucose) and *excrete* excesses, the waste products of metabolism, toxic substances and drugs in the urine.

The kidneys also have an important *endocrine role*: the production of renin and erythropoietin, and their release into the blood when needed. In addition, the kidney is the major organ responsible for the production of the most active vitamin D metabolite (calcitriol). Its major effect is to stimulate calcium absorption from the gut, thereby assisting in the maintenance of healthy bone. The processes involved in these functions performed by the kidneys are filtration, selective re-absorption, the transport of substances from the interstitial fluid to the tubule and endocrine secretion (Box 19.1).

FILTRATION

The permeability of the glomerular capillaries is greater than that of capillaries elsewhere in the body. The same

---

Box 19.1 Renal functions

Overall function
Homeostasis – the maintenance of a suitable environment for optimum cellular function

Principal function
To regulate the volume and composition of the extracellular fluid
The kidney maintains homeostasis by performing the following roles:

1 Production:
vitamin D metabolite (calcitriol)
erythropoietin
renin.

2 Regulation:
volume of water in extracellular fluid
concentration of electrolytes in extracellular fluid
osmolality of extracellular fluid
concentration of hydrogen ions in the extracellular fluid.

3 Excretion:
endogenous – end-products of protein catabolism
exogenous – medications.

---

principles that govern the movement of fluid out of the arteriolar ends of the capillaries throughout the body are applicable to the filtration process in the glomeruli. The hydrostatic pressure of the blood in the glomerular capillaries is approximately 60 mmHg, which is considerably higher than that in the other capillaries of the body. This hydrostatic pressure is opposed by the osmotic pressure of the blood proteins (approximately 28 mmHg) plus the hydrostatic pressure in Bowman's capsule (about 18 mmHg). The net filtration force is 14 mmHg:

> hydrostatic blood pressure (60) subtract (colloidal osmotic pressure (28) plus capsular hydrostatic pressure (18) equals 14 mmHg

The average volume of filtrate in both kidneys is estimated to be about 180 litres each day. The glomerular filtration rate (GFR) is directly proportional to the filtration force; the normal rate is approximately 125 mL/minute. Factors that may alter the GFR include:

- change in glomerular capillary hydrostatic pressure, which may be incurred by an increase or decrease in systemic blood pressure or by constriction or dilatation of the afferent and efferent arterioles
- increase or decrease in renal artery blood volume
- increase or decrease in the hydrostatic pressure within Bowman's capsule due to compression by ureteral obstruction or disease within the kidney, causing swelling confined within the renal capsule
- decrease or increase in the oncotic pressure (concentration of plasma proteins)

- increased glomerular permeability due to disease, such as nephrotic syndrome
- decrease in glomeruli due to pathological destruction.

Many solutes escape from the blood in the glomerular filtrate, but small amounts of only a few of them appear in urine. The formed elements and plasma proteins of the blood do not normally pass out of the glomeruli; the composition of the filtrate is the same as that of plasma minus the plasma proteins.

Tubular re-absorption

Re-absorption and secretion are complex renal activities. The composition and volume of the filtrate that enters the Bowman's capsule differ markedly from those of urine. Of the 180 L of filtrate produced in 24 hours, only about 1.5 L are excreted as urine. Most of the water and many of the solid constituents of the filtrate are needed by the body to maintain homeostasis and normal cell metabolism. Other substances, such as urea, creatinine, uric acid, sulfates and phosphates, are waste products of metabolism and are excreted in the urine. The tubule cells selectively reabsorb according to the body's needs. Certain substances, such as glucose and amino acids, are completely re-absorbed when their plasma concentrations are within normal range but appear in the urine when the normal is exceeded. About 99% of the water in the filtrate is reclaimed. Re-absorption of the inorganic salts (e.g. sodium, chloride, calcium, potassium, bicarbonate) is variable, depending mainly on their plasma levels.

The *proximal convoluted tubule* is responsible for the greatest amount of re-absorption. All of the glucose and amino acids and a large proportion of the water and other essential substances are re-absorbed here. Only about 35% of the total volume of filtrate enters the loop of Henle.

The *loop of Henle* seems to be concerned principally with the transport of sodium chloride ions and water. The ascending limb is impermeable to water. It actively transports sodium and chloride ions out into the interstitial fluid, and the tubular fluid becomes hypotonic. The descending limb of the loop of Henle is permeable to water; water moves out to the interstitial fluid which has become hypertonic. At the same time, sodium and chloride ions diffuse into the descending limb.

The maintenance of the volume and concentration of body fluids within a narrow range is largely controlled by the ability of the kidney tubules to concentrate or dilute the urine. When body fluids are diluted by an excess of water or diminished solute intake (especially sodium), the urine becomes dilute and the volume is increased. Conversely, if the concentration of body fluids is raised to above the normal level by an excessive intake of solutes or an extrarenal loss of water, water re-absorption from the filtrate is increased, concentrating the urine and decreasing the output volume.

The dilution and concentration of urine depend principally on two factors: (1) the osmotic pressure of the peritubular fluid, which in turn is mainly dependent on the normal functioning of the loop of Henle and the distal convoluted tubules and (2) the concentration of ADH in the blood.

The fluid entering the distal tubule is hypotonic, but the volume and osmolality are modified selectively as the fluid proceeds through the distal and collecting tubules.

Re-absorption of water from the hypotonic filtrate in the distal convoluted and collecting tubules is regulated by ADH. This hormone is produced by the hypothalamus in the brain, and is stored and released into the blood by the posterior pituitary gland (see p. 658).

The re-absorption of sodium by active cellular transport in the distal and collecting tubules is influenced by the adrenocortical hormone *aldosterone*. A high concentration of aldosterone stimulates the distal tubular cells to reabsorb increasing amounts of sodium. Aldosterone also affects the amount of potassium reclaimed and excreted. Increased concentrations of the hormone promote excretion of potassium, and a deficient amount of aldosterone produces excessive retention of potassium.

Tubular secretion and excretion

Tubular cells are capable of actively transporting some substances from the blood into the filtrate – a reverse process to that of re-absorption. The potassium concentration of plasma is regulated by this process. Practically all of the potassium that escapes from the plasma into the filtrate is re-absorbed in the proximal tubule. Any excess in the blood is then actively secreted by the distal tubules and is excreted in exchange for sodium ions.

Cells of the distal tubules play an important role in maintaining a normal *acid–base balance* in the blood and extracellular fluid. In association with the respiratory system, the kidneys regulate the body's systemic arterial pH within a narrow range of 7.35–7.45.

The first lines of defence against alteration in body pH are the extracellular and intracellular buffers. The major extracellular buffer is bicarbonate and the buffering capacity of the $HCO_3–CO_2$ system is greatly extended by the regulation of carbon dioxide gas tension by the respiratory system.

The kidney's role in acid–base homeostasis is to stabilize the balance between H^+ and HCO_3^- in the blood. This is accomplished by four processes:

1 secretion of hydrogen ions
2 re-absorption of sodium and bicarbonate ions
3 acidification of phosphate salts
4 synthesis and secretion of ammonia.

All these mechanisms serve to restore the hydrogen ion concentration so that the pH of the blood is maintained within normal limits.

Endocrine renal secretions

The kidney produces two endocrine secretions: renin and erythropoietin.

Renin reacts with an inactive precursor fraction of the plasma globulin (angiotensinogen), producing a substance called angiotensin I which is converted to angiotensin II by another enzyme in the lungs. As angiotensin II circulates, it causes vasoconstriction of the systemic arterioles and stimulates the secretion of aldosterone and, to a lesser extent, glucocorticoids.

The principal mechanism responsible for the release of renin is a drop in blood pressure and circulating blood volume, although falling sodium and chloride levels in the distal tubule can have the same effect.

A second hormone produced by the kidneys is the *renal erythropoietic factor* (REF; erythrogenin). It is produced and secreted into the blood mainly in response to hypoxia and functions in the maintenance of normal erythrocyte production by the bone marrow. REF reacts with a plasma globulin to produce *erythropoietin*, which stimulates the bone marrow to produce and release blood cells.

CHARACTERISTICS AND COMPOSITION OF URINE

When the filtrate flows into the main collecting tubules and renal pelvis, it becomes **urine**. The average volume excreted in 24 hours is approximately 1.5 L, but varies with fluid losses through other channels (e.g. sweat) and fluid intake. The reaction of urine is usually acid, with a pH of about 6.0, but may range from 4.5 to 8.5 with a varied dietary intake. The acidity increases with high protein ingestion and tissue catabolism, whereas a vegetable diet produces an alkaline urine.

The specific gravity, which gives a rough estimate of the concentration of solids, ranges from 1.003 to 1.040. The composition of urine varies with dietary intake and metabolic wastes produced. Normally, about 90–95% of urine is water. The chief solutes are urea, creatinine, uric acid and the chlorides, phosphates and sulfates of sodium, potassium, calcium, magnesium and ammonia.

URETERS, BLADDER AND URETHRA

Ureters

Each of the two **ureters** is a tube, made up mainly of muscle tissue, 25–30 cm in length, extending from a kidney to the bladder. They are situated behind the parietal peritoneum and enter the posterior wall of the lower half of the bladder obliquely. The slanted entrance forms a flap in the bladder wall which serves as a valve to prevent a reflux of urine as the bladder fills or contracts.

The function of these tubes is simply to convey urine from the kidneys to the bladder. Contraction of the ureteral muscular tissue produces peristaltic waves which move the urine along the tube and into the bladder in spurts.

Bladder

The urinary bladder serves as a temporary reservoir for the urine, which it expels at intervals from the body. It is a collapsible muscular sac that lies behind the symphysis pubis. Three layers of plain muscle tissue form the bladder walls. The fibres are arranged in longitudinal, circular and spiral layers. Collectively, these layers are referred to as the *detrusor muscle*. The ureteral orifices in the posterior wall and the urethral opening outline a triangular area called the *trigone*. When the bladder is empty, the mucous membrane lining falls into folds (rugae) except in the area of the trigone (Fig. 19.3).

Urethra

The urethra is a slender tube that conveys urine from the bladder to the exterior. It has a thin layer of smooth muscle tissue and is lined with a mucous membrane which is continuous with that of the bladder. The opening from the bladder is controlled by two sphincters: an internal one which is under autonomic (involuntary) nervous system control, and an external one which is voluntarily controlled by the cerebral cortex. The external urethral orifice is known as the *urinary meatus*.

In the female, the urethra is about 4 cm long and lies anterior to the vagina. The male urethra is approximately 20 cm in length and, on leaving the bladder, passes through the prostate gland. As well as conveying the urine, the male urethra receives the semen from the ejaculatory ducts of the reproductive system, transmitting it through the meatus (Fig. 19.3).

Micturition

This is a term used for the elimination of urine from the bladder. The process involves both autonomic (involuntary) and voluntary nervous impulses. When 300–400 mL of urine collect in the bladder, receptors that are sensitive to stretching initiate impulses that are transmitted by afferent nerve fibres into the lower part of the spinal cord. A reflex response via parasympathetic nerves to the bladder results in contractions of the detrusor muscle and relaxation of the internal sphincter.

The initial impulses from the stretch receptors are also relayed via a spinocortical tract to the cerebral cortex, producing an awareness of the need to void. When a person is prepared to empty the bladder, voluntary impulses are initiated that descend the cord and are carried out to the external sphincter, causing it to relax. With both sphincters relaxed, the detrusor muscle contracts and urine flows from the bladder through the urethra. Voluntary micturition may also be accompanied by relaxation of the perineal muscles and contraction of abdominal muscles. Infants and very young children empty their bladder whenever the micturition reflex is initiated, as they have not yet developed voluntary control over the external sphincter. Obviously, any interruption of the spinocortical impulse pathway interferes with control of the external sphincter, resulting in involuntary voiding or retention.

ASSESSMENT OF RENAL FUNCTION

The investigation of renal dysfunction may include examination of urine specimens (which may be voided or obtained by bladder or urethral catheterization), blood chemistry determinations, renal function tests, radiography and ultrasonographic procedures.

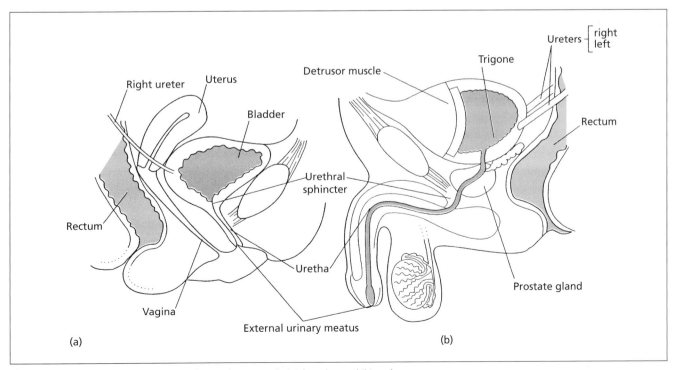

Figure 19.3 The bladder, ureters, urethra and prostate in (a) females and (b) males.

URINE OUTPUT

Perhaps one of the most crucial nursing functions in the care of the person with renal dysfunction is the accurate measurement of urine output and fluid balance.

URINE COLOUR

It is important that the nurse be aware of the colour of the urine being eliminated. Changes from the normal amber, clear urine can be an indication of many things, such as urinary tract infection (cloudy urine), bleeding into the urinary tract (blood-stained urine) or dehydration (darker, more concentrated urine).

ROUTINE URINALYSIS

Routine urinalysis is usually a nursing responsibility; it is relatively fast, simple and accurate because of the wide availability of reagent strip tests that allow the nurse to test for protein, glucose, ketones, acetone, blood and bilirubin, as well as to measure pH. It is important to use the reagent strips according to the instructions and to be aware of the potential factors that could affect the results (Wilson 2005). Table 19.1 is a summary of some of the factors that can affect the quality of a urine specimen.

URINE FOR BACTERIOLOGICAL EXAMINATION

This is achieved by culturing the urine; the organism is identified by means of a microscope. Sensitivity to antibiotics is determined by placing impregnated discs of specific agents upon the culture plate and observing the colonization pattern. Areas where colonies of microorganisms fail to grow indicate sensitivity to the specific antibiotic.

Urine specimens for bacteriological examination should be fresh, or refrigerated after collection. The first morning specimen is the most concentrated and therefore most likely to reveal abnormalities. A clean-catch mid-stream specimen (MSU) is the most effective method of obtaining urine for bacteriological examination. The patient should be given clear instructions on which part of the urine stream should be collected. The individual should start passing urine and, once the urine is being voided, a sterile container should be used to collect it. The first part of the stream should be avoided.

In the catheterized patient, the specimen should be obtained using a syringe and needle from the rubber portal on the collecting tube, not from the reservoir or collecting bag.

24-HOUR URINE COLLECTION

A 24-hour urine specimen means collection of all the urine that a person produces in a 24-hour period. Collection is begun first thing in the morning, with the urine of the first void being discarded. For the next 24 hours, all the urine must be saved and collected in a container, including the first void of the next day. Serious errors in the results may occur if strict attention is not paid to timing the 24-hour period or if the patient voids urine that is not collected. The urine can be examined to determine the amounts of specific substances that the person's kidney is capable of excreting, based on calculations that include height, weight and total volume excreted during the 24-hour period. By making a quantitative determination of the 24-hour creatinine clearance, a statement can be made about the glomerular filtration capacity of the kidney. The container should be refrigerated during the period of collection. Some 24-hour collections may be needed for specific tests, and a stabilizer or preservative may be added to the receptacle before collection.

BLOOD CHEMISTRY DETERMINATIONS

Impaired glomerular filtration and loss of the tubular ability to reabsorb and excrete discriminately lead to alterations in plasma composition. Blood specimens may be requested to determine the concentration of a number of substances. The nurse is often the first healthcare provider to be informed of results, and should therefore have an understanding of normal serum concentrations so that abnormal levels can be promptly passed on to medical staff. The following normal values are of particular importance for patients with renal disorder:

- urea nitrogen – normal: 2.5–6.6 mmol/L
- creatinine – normal: 55–120 mmol/L
- urate – normal: 0.42–0.48 mmol/L
- sodium – normal 135–145 mmol/L
- potassium – normal 3.5–5 mmol/L.

Table 19.1	Issues affecting the quality of a urine specimen (Wilson 2005)
Time of urine collection	Early morning specimen is preferable as the urine will be more concentrated
Contamination	The urine should be passed directly into a clean container
Sample collection	A sterile container should be used to transport the specimen
Labeling errors	The specimen should be labeled accurately
Time lapse	Test the sample immediately but at least within 4 hours of collection
Concurrent use of medications	Certain drugs will mask results ((high doses of ascorbic acid mask the presence of glucose) others will change the colour of urine (nitrofurantoin colours the urine brown)

HAEMATOLOGICAL TESTS

The haemoglobin concentration and haematocrit are determined, as anaemia is a common problem. If infection is suspected a leucocyte count is done, and a platelet count and prothrombin time may be needed in advanced chronic renal failure.

RENAL FUNCTION TESTS

In renal function, the removal or clearance of substances from the blood is achieved by glomerular filtration and tubular cell activity. If a substance passes freely through the glomeruli, and is neither re-absorbed or secreted by the tubules, the quantity appearing in the urine is the same as that filtered by the glomeruli. The 24-hour urine collection test referred to earlier is used for renal function tests, usually to estimate creatinine clearance. By measuring the amount excreted in the urine in a specified period of time, information is obtained about the efficiency of glomerular filtration.

The nurse needs to understand what is involved in these tests for two reasons: first, to ensure the patient is properly prepared and cared for before and after any procedure; second, to reduce anxiety and fear by answering questions and giving explanations to the patient.

Glomerular filtration rate

To determine the glomerular filtration rate (GFR), an estimation of the GFR (eGFR) can be calculated from the serum creatinine level or a creatinine clearance tests can be used.

Estimated glomerular filtration rate

The eGFR is calculated using the patient's serum creatinine level, age, sex and race. Most local laboratories in the UK are now providing a report on the eGFR which is a more accurate reflection of kidney function than serum creatinine alone (Renal Association 2006). The eGFR can be used to determine the stage of kidney failure and these results are summarized in Table 19.2. The eGFR is only an estimation and it is important to be aware of other evidence of chronic kidney damage when interpreting the results. Other evidence includes the presence of microalbuminuria, proteinuria, haematuria, structural abnormalities of the kidneys (e.g. polycystic kidney disease) or the presence of glomerulonephritis.

CASE Mr Moore is an 83-year-old gentleman who lives alone in a large house in a rural setting. He was diagnosed with

hypertension 20 years ago. He had a heart attack 15 years ago and subsequently suffered with periods of angina. He continued to live alone but found that his increasing physical disability caused him problems when he was trying to look after his dog and his large garden.

Mr Moore was regularly reviewed at the surgery in the cardiovascular clinic. He had regular checks of his blood pressure which on occasion was found to be as high as 190/100 mmHg and at other times it was 130/85 mmHg. His blood pressure gradually settled over a number of years and is currently 131/76 mmHg. As part of the routine review in the clinic at the Health Centre Mr Moore's creatinine was checked and was first found to be raised 5 years ago at 178 μmol/L. It was noted that this gradually increased and the most recent reading was 237 μmol/L (normal range 62–115). His eGFR was calculated at 18–34 indicating stage 4 chronic kidney disease. He showed no signs of renal failure, although he regularly described tiredness and difficulty with managing his home and garden. The nurse practitioner was concerned about Mr Moore's deteriorating renal function and so referred him to the nephrologists.

The nephrologist assessed Mr Moore's renal function and concluded that it was deteriorating steadily and slowly. He reassured Mr Moore that this was probably not going to be a problem to him and that his ischaemic heart disease was perhaps of more concern. The cardiologist and nephrologist both agreed that a focus on blood pressure management was perhaps the most important intervention for Mr Moore. As Mr Moore's blood pressure was reduced with increasing medication, he became dizzy and had even more difficulty managing around his home and garden. The nurse practitioner worked with him to strike a balance between well controlled blood pressure and the best possible quality of life.

Mr Moore's blood pressure is currently under control with a combination of, felodipine, doxazosin and bendroflumethiazide and he takes atorvastatin, isosorbide mononitrate and clopidogrel for his heart problems and omeprazole for indigestion and ferrous gluconate for chronic anaemia.

This case study illustrates the way kidney failure can gradually and slowly develop in a patient who has other evidence of vascular disease (i.e. heart disease and hypertension). Mr Moore has to take numerous medications. What issues do you think this might raise for this patient? Mr Moore and the nurse practitioner had to agree a compromise between perfectly controlled blood pressure and quality of life. What implications do you think this might have for this patient and his family?

Table 19.2 Estimated glomerular filtration rate (Renal Association 2006)	
GFR >90 mL/minute/1.73 m²	Normal or stage 1 Chronic kidney disease
GFR 60–89 mL/minute/1.73 m²	Normal or stage 2 Chronic kidney disease
GFR 30–59 mL/minute/1.73 m²	Stage 3 Chronic kidney disease
GFR <30 mL/minute/1.73 m²	Stages 4 and 5 Chronic kidney disease

Creatinine clearance test

Another way of assessing creatinine clearance is with a 24-hour urine collection, this may take place in hospital settings but is rarely used in primary care. The patient maintains normal but not excessive activity, because endogenous creatinine is produced in muscular activity. No special diet is necessary but excessive intake of tea, coffee and meat is avoided for a 24-hour period before the test. A 24-hour specimen of urine and a venous blood specimen are collected for determination of creatinine concentration. The rate of urinary excretion per minute is calculated. The normal amount of creatinine excreted in 24 hours varies with age: in an adult the normal range is about 1.2–1.7g, and in a child it is approximately 0.36g. Calculations are made to determine the volume of plasma cleared of creatinine per minute, which is the GFR.

Tubular function

To maintain homeostasis, normal kidneys are able to vary the concentration of solid wastes and the volume of urine according to the volume of body fluids. When there is an excessive loss of body fluid by other channels or a restricted intake, more water is re-absorbed by the renal tubules; the solid wastes are excreted in a smaller volume of urine and the specific gravity is high. Conversely, with a large fluid intake, less water is re-absorbed by the tubules, the volume of urine is greater and the specific gravity and osmolality are lower than usual. This ability to vary the volume and concentration of the urine appropriately is impaired when there is tubular damage.

The standard test involves collecting an early morning sample for estimation of osmolality (normal value 550 mmol/kg or above; younger people usually have values of 750 mmol/kg or above). Below-normal values indicate the need for concentration tests to estimate specific gravity. Protocols vary between hospitals, so you are advised to consult your own pathology laboratory directions.

RENAL SCANNING (DMSA SCAN)

The use of radioisotope scanning techniques may demonstrate areas of renal dysfunction and is becoming increasingly widespread as an investigative procedure. DMSA stands for di mercapto succinic acid, the substance that is used with the technetium tracer to view the kidneys. There are no special preparations for this test. It involves the injection of the tracer into a vein in the arm and then a gamma camera is placed over the abdomen to detect the radiation as it passes through the kidneys. It takes about 2–3 hours for the tracer to reach the kidneys and the radiographer usually takes about 4–6 different views over about a 30-minute period (Royal College of Radiologists 2003).

ULTRASONOGRAPHY

There is no preparation for ultrasonography, and no X-rays or injections are needed, although if the person is not anuric a full bladder may be requested as it provides a good 'landmark' for the radiographer. The examination is used to look at the size and structure of the kidneys and other organs. Renal lesions seen in polycystic kidney disease and hydronephrosis can be distinguished. Ultrasonography is also widely used in determining the position of a kidney for renal biopsy.

INTRAVENOUS PYELOGRAPHY (IVP) OR INTRAVENOUS UROGRAPHY (IVU)

This procedure involves the intravenous administration of a radio-opaque contrast medium. This fluid concentrates in urine and, as it is excreted through the kidney (pyelography) and the ureters and bladder (urography), radiographs are taken. Patient preparation varies, but fluids are usually restricted 4 hours before the procedure; sometimes a laxative is administered the night before the examination. This avoids bowel content or gas obscuring the outline of the urinary tract. It is important to ascertain whether the individual has a history of allergies, particularly to iodine preparations, as severe reactions to the contrast medium can occur.

CYSTOSCOPY AND RETROGRADE PYELOGRAPHY

Cystoscopy involves the passage of a cystoscope through the urethra into the bladder. The instrument is equipped with a light which permits direct visualization of the internal surface of the bladder. A long, fine catheter may also be introduced into each renal pelvis through the cystoscope (ureteric catheterization), and a urine specimen collected from each kidney. Ureteric catheterization may be used to obtain specimens from one or both kidneys for microscopic examination and culture, or in renal function tests when the function of each kidney is to be determined.

A radio-opaque iodide preparation may then be introduced into the catheters, and radiographs which outline the renal pelvis and ureters are taken. This procedure is referred to as *retrograde pyelography*. The examination is used to exclude or delineate a ureteral obstruction when excretion of contrast by the kidney during an IVP is poor.

Preparation of the patient for a cystoscopy includes an explanation of the procedure. The patient's signature indicating consent for the examination is required. The procedure may be performed under local, epidural or general anaesthetic; food and fluid therefore are restricted for 6–8 hours preceding the examination and intravenous fluid is administered to ensure hydration and hence urinary flow.

If a general anaesthetic is contraindicated, the procedure may be performed under sedation.

Upon completion of the examination, the person rests in bed for a few hours. Additional fluids are encouraged. It is important that the nurse examine the urinary output for haematuria, and any severe pain or persisting bright blood in the urine is reported to the doctor. Should the individual report inability to pass urine it may be necessary for an indwelling catheter to be inserted. Severe haematuria may

necessitate catheterization and irrigation of the bladder with fluid to control bleeding and flush debris and blood clots.

COMPUTED TOMOGRAPHY

Computed tomography (CT) is used in the detection of renal tumours and cysts. The patient is given an oral contrast medium before the scan to opacify the bowel; food is not allowed for 4 hours before the procedure.

RENAL ANGIOGRAPHY

Renal blood vessels may be outlined on an X-ray film following the administration of a radio-opaque substance into the vascular system. The procedure is performed under local anaesthesia by a radiologist; it is used to explore the blood supply to the kidneys. The main indication for renal angiography is for a diagnosis of renal artery stenosis or to differentiate renal masses (e.g. tumours or cysts). As the person may be sensitive to the radio-opaque iodide preparation, the same precautions as cited for intravenous urography should be followed. Preparation of the patient is similar to that for intravenous urography.

After the procedure, the radiologist will place firm pressure over the site of catheter introduction into the femoral artery and will apply a firm dressing. Frequent inspections are made for bleeding. The person may be on bedrest for several hours after the procedure to reduce the risk of bleeding. The site is also observed for local swelling, redness and tenderness. The temperature of the lower limbs is noted and the popliteal and pedal pulses are checked so that any indication of impaired circulation may be reported promptly.

MAGNETIC RESONANCE IMAGING

This technique is also being developed to permit investigation of the kidneys and has been shown to have an important role in the detection of abnormalities of renal tissue.

PERCUTANEOUS RENAL BIOPSY

A biopsy is a valuable test in diagnosis and assessment of the effects of treatment but carries with it the risk of haemorrhage. It is frequently used to determine the underlying pathology of renal dysfunction so that appropriate treatments may be selected. Renal biopsy is also performed in selected cases in renal transplant patients in order to diagnose rejection. It is contraindicated if the person has hypertension, a bleeding tendency, only one kidney, or suspected perirenal abscess. Before a person is booked for renal biopsy, coagulation, bleeding and prothrombin times are determined. If these are satisfactory, the person's blood is grouped and cross-matched, and compatible blood is kept available in the event of haemorrhage. An explanation is given to the person of what to expect and that he or she will be put in the prone position over a firm pillow (kidney elevator) for a brief period.

The exact location of the kidney is identified by radiography, which may include intravenous urography or ultrasonography, and the position is indicated on the skin surface. The skin is cleansed and local anaesthesia is infiltrated. The person is instructed to hold the breath during insertion of the needle and the actual taking of the specimen. Following removal of the biopsy needle, pressure is applied to the site for a few minutes.

The blood pressure and pulse are recorded every 15 minutes for 1 hour, then every 30 minutes for a period of 1–2 hours, and then every 4 hours for 24 hours. The risk of heavy bleeding after the procedure is very real, so the nurse must observe the person carefully for signs of shock, and assess the urine for prolonged haematuria. Any undue pain, haematuria or change in vital signs should be reported immediately. The person is kept on bedrest in the dorsal recumbent position for 18–24 hours or until the urine is cleared of blood.

CLINICAL CHARACTERISTICS OF RENAL DYSFUNCTION

In impaired kidney function, the constancy of the internal environment (homeostasis), which is essential for the normal functioning of all body cells, is disrupted. The normal volume, composition and reaction of the body fluids may be altered by the inability of the kidneys to conserve essential substances and excrete excesses, metabolic wastes and toxic substances; disturbances in the functioning of other organs readily develop. Consequently, the signs and symptoms of renal insufficiency are varied, and many are not directly referable to the urinary system. Whether the disease is acute or chronic, and whether it affects the glomeruli or the tubules, will also affect the manifestations.

As the nurse assesses the patient the physical signs listed in Box 19.2 must be borne in mind as evidence of significant renal dysfunction. The nurse should be alert to the possible psychological sequelae of these clinical signs as such effects may be a cause of great distress requiring urgent nursing intervention, for example a change in the colour of a person's urine.

ABNORMAL URINARY VOLUME

Oliguria or anuria may develop, especially in acute and advanced renal failure:

- *Oliguria* means that <500 mL of urine is formed in 24 hours
- *Anuria* implies a urinary output of <250 mL in 24 hours and is sometimes referred to as a renal shutdown.

The diminished urine formation may be associated with decreased glomerular filtration due to renal disease (e.g. glomerulonephritis), hypotension as in shock and dehydration, decreased renal blood flow or an obstruction within the tubules.

Box 19.2   Physical signs of renal dysfunction

- Abnormal urinary volume
- Abnormal constituents in the urine (e.g. protein, blood, casts, pus, organisms)
- Abnormal urine colour
- Uraemia
- Fluid, electrolyte and pH imbalances
- Changes in vital signs
- Gastrointestinal disturbances
- Headache and pain
- Visual disturbances
- Neurological manifestations
- Skin changes
- Haematological changes.

Polyuria, a volume of urine in excess of the normal (over 2000 mL in 24 hours), may also indicate renal disturbance in which the ability of the tubules to reabsorb water and concentrate the solid wastes is limited. It is seen most often in patients with chronic kidney disease, or may be secondary to diabetes insipidus as a result of a deficiency in the secretion of vasopressin (antidiuretic hormone). Polyuria may not be a manifestation of renal disease but may indicate a disorder elsewhere. Frequently, polyuria is the symptom that may cause an individual to go to a doctor where, on investigation, diabetes mellitus is diagnosed.

Nocturia (voiding during the night) usually accompanies polyuria and the person becomes desperate for undisturbed sleep.

Hyposthenuria is the inability of the kidneys to reabsorb the normal amount of water and to concentrate the wastes. As well as the excessive volume, a low specific gravity of the urine persists because the impaired tubules cannot concentrate or vary the amount of solids.

ABNORMAL CONSTITUENTS IN THE URINE

Abnormal constituents revealed in urinalysis vary with the underlying renal disease. They include protein (usually albumin), blood, casts, pus and organisms.

The large molecular structure of serum albumin inhibits its filtration through normal glomeruli. *Albuminuria* usually indicates inflammation and almost always indicates damage to the glomeruli. If significant amounts of protein are lost in urine, this leads to the development of nephrotic syndrome. Protein loss leads to a range of symptoms of which oedema, increased risk of blood clotting, raised cholesterol levels and increased infection risk are the most common (Haslett et al 1999).

Haematuria denotes blood in the urine and may be macroscopic or recognized only by microscopic examination after a positive dipstick test. Wilson (2005) comments that false-positive dipstick test results may occur in the presence of contaminants such as peroxidase released by bacteria or if a woman is menstruating at the time the test is carried out. False-negatives can occur if the patient is taking ascorbic acid tablets or certain medications such as captopril. Haematuria indicates a systemic problem (such as a clotting disorder or excess dosage of warfarin) or some pathological process within the kidneys or the urinary collecting system. A clear history from the patient may give important clues about the possible cause of such a finding. For example, the most common cause of macroscopic haematuria in men aged over 60 years is benign prostatic hyperplasia (BPH). A history of difficulty in passing urine coupled with haematuria in a man of that age suggests BPH as a probable cause. In a young woman, haematuria is most likely to be due to a bacterial infection of the urinary tract.

Urinary casts are microscopic cylindrical structures formed in the distal and collecting tubes by the agglutination of cells and cellular debris in a protein matrix. They are moulded or cast in the shape of the tubule. Depending on their composition, casts are usually classified as red blood cell, epithelial, hyaline, granular or fatty. They point to the presence of some inflammatory or degenerative process within the tubules. Obviously, *pus* and *bacteria* in the urine indicate infection in the kidneys or urinary tract.

The presence of protein, blood and casts together in the urine is strongly suggestive of disease of the renal parenchyma, especially in the presence of peripheral oedema and/or hypertension.

ABNORMAL URINE COLOUR

Abnormal discolouration of urine may be associated with infection within the urinary tract, but more often occurs with a disorder extrinsic to the kidneys and urinary tract. Examples of disorders in which the urine is discoloured are: obstructive jaundice, where the urine appears a dark colour due to the presence of bilirubin; haemoglobinuria, which may develop following a blood transfusion reaction in which there is a breakdown of erythrocytes and the release of haemoglobin; and treatment with certain medications such as nitrofurantoin will change the colour of the urine (Table 19.1).

It should be remembered that urine can sometimes be discoloured by the contrast media used in intravenous X-ray examination, or by the eating of foods such as beetroot.

URAEMIA

Metabolic wastes accumulate in the blood when renal function is impaired. Urea, creatinine and uric acid levels are usually raised. In acute failure and anuria, the levels rise rapidly. In chronic kidney disease, even though there may be polyuria, the blood urea progressively rises as the kidneys are failing to excrete the waste products of metabolism.

FLUID, ELECTROLYTE AND PH IMBALANCES

Generalized *oedema* may be one of the early symptoms of renal insufficiency and usually becomes apparent first around the eyes. It may be due to decreased glomerular filtration and the retention of water and sodium, or to an abnormal permeability of the glomeruli to plasma proteins, especially serum albumin. The loss of plasma protein causes a decrease in the colloidal osmotic pressure of the blood, and an excess of water remains in the interstitial spaces. The urine is high in albumin, and the plasma protein concentration is abnormally low.

In some instances of chronic renal failure due to impaired tubular function, the excessive volume of urine excreted (polyuria) may lead to *dehydration* unless there is a corresponding increase in the water intake. Fluid balance is an important sign which must be monitored carefully in any acutely ill patient, whatever the cause. Daily fluid loss of up to 800 mL can occur in evaporation from the skin and in exhaled air, together with a further 100 mL in faeces. Urine output alone therefore does not convey an accurate picture of the patient's true fluid balance (Sheppard 2000).

Deficiencies or excesses of electrolytes may occur, depending on the nature of the renal disturbance and the degree of tissue damage. Failure of impaired tubules to secrete potassium ions is a serious development in renal insufficiency. Abnormal concentrations of sodium and calcium as well as hyperkalaemia may develop, and may seriously affect cardiac function and threaten the patient's life.

Failure of the kidneys' capacity to excrete hydrogen ions by the formation and excretion of acid sodium phosphate and ammonia results in their accumulation in the blood, causing *acidosis*.

VITAL SIGNS

An increase in blood pressure occurs in most patients with renal insufficiency associated with parenchymal disease of the kidneys. It is attributed to an increase in the blood volume as a result of the retention of sodium and water, or to a decrease in the renal blood flow and consequent secretion of renin by the juxtaglomerular cells. The renin results in the formation of angiotensin I and II, which cause vasoconstriction of the arterioles and increased aldosterone release.

Central venous pressure (CVP) monitoring is an invasive technique for monitoring fluid load and how well the heart is coping with the work it has to do. The CVP is obtained by measuring blood pressure in the venous circulation and it is used in critical care areas (see p. 264). Jugular venous pressure (JVP) may be measured without any specialist equipment and gives an estimate of fluid overload or dehydration. It is therefore a useful guide, in the same way as the CVP reading. A raised JVP indicates fluid overload, whilst dehydration is associated with a lowered JVP.

The *pulse* may become weak because of heart failure, which may result from hypertension, excessive fluid load or electrolyte imbalance.

The patient may experience *dyspnoea* due to pulmonary oedema. *Kussmaul's breathing* (deep rapid respirations), characteristic of acidosis, may be manifested. In advanced renal failure, the breath has an ammoniacal or 'uraemic' odour.

Pyrexia is associated with infection in the kidneys or secondary infection, such as pneumonia, that may develop readily if pulmonary oedema is present.

GASTROINTESTINAL DISTURBANCES

The patient experiences anorexia and, in the later stages of renal dysfunction, nausea and vomiting. Diarrhoea may also be troublesome in the acute stage. Hiccups may develop in advanced failure, and the oral mucosa may become sore and ulcerated.

HEADACHE AND PAIN

Headache is an early complaint as a result of the hypertension and cerebral oedema. Pain and tenderness in the back between the lower ribs and iliac crest occur in acute kidney disease because of the stretching of the renal capsule.

VISUAL DISTURBANCES

The patient may complain of 'spots before the eyes' or blurred vision, which are attributed to oedema of the optic papillae (papilloedema).

NEUROLOGICAL MANIFESTATIONS

Signs of both irritation and depression of the nervous system appear in renal failure. The patient becomes irritable, lethargic and drowsy. Family members may be distressed at perceived personality changes in the person. Short-term memory may also be affected, hence clear explanations and repetition will be necessary. It is important to assess the level of consciousness as the person may become disoriented and progress to a comatose state. Muscular twitching may be noticeable and, in advanced kidney disease, may be an indication of ensuing convulsions.

SKIN CHANGES

Dehydration alone leads to turgid, dry skin, a dry tongue and oral membranes (Sheppard 2000). However, in progressive renal insufficiency, the skin may take on a yellowish-brown appearance. Dryness and scaliness, known as *xerosis*, are common with chronic disease and polyuria. The patient may complain of pruritus, and excoriated lesions may appear from scratching. Pruritus is often persistent and there is no treatment that appears to have a lasting effect. Consequently, pruritus can be a debilitating and depressing experience.

In advanced failure, urea frost may be manifested, although this will be seen only in those persons for whom dialysis intervention is not possible. As the individual becomes progressively uraemic, deposits of small white crystals of urea are excreted by the sweat glands. The frost is usually first seen around the mouth.

HAEMATOLOGICAL CHANGES

Most patients with prolonged renal disease show a reduction in the production of red blood cells, a shortened red cell survival time with a resultant anaemia. Normal kidneys, as well as the liver, contribute erythropoietin which stimulates erythropoiesis. In renal dysfunction, this activity may be decreased.

With uraemia, the patient develops a bleeding tendency; the platelets are defective and the bleeding time increases. Petechiae, purpura or bleeding from mucous membranes, particularly the gums, may be present. The person with renal dysfunction is most likely to notice an increased propensity to bruising.

THE PERSON WITH IMPAIRED RENAL FUNCTION

Renal dysfunction may be due to a primary disease within the kidneys or may be secondary to a disorder elsewhere in the body. When kidney function is impaired, dysfunction of extrarenal systems ultimately develops. Similarly, primary dysfunction in other systems may readily affect renal function.

RENAL FAILURE

When the kidneys are unable to excrete metabolic wastes and perform their role in fluid, electrolyte and acid–base balance, renal failure exists. Homeostasis of the internal environment is no longer maintained. The retention of the waste and excess products normally excreted in the urine may be referred to as *uraemia*. The latter is not a disease but rather a syndrome or complex of symptoms reflecting failure of the kidneys to carry out their role. Renal production of renin, erythropoietin and vitamin D_3 is also disturbed. With failure of fluid volume regulation, the patient becomes either oedematous or dehydrated and the acid–base imbalance leads to metabolic acidosis. Electrolyte imbalances occur and an accumulation of nitrogenous wastes produces increased blood levels of non-protein nitrogenous substances such as urea, creatinine and uric acid. The disturbance in the secretion of hormones leads to alterations in blood pressure, erythrocyte production and calcium absorption by bone tissue. As renal efficiency diminishes, symptoms develop reflecting impairment of function in other body systems. Renal failure may be acute or chronic.

The population of patients in renal failure is ageing, in line with the general population. Bevan (2000) estimates that 60% of patients in Europe receiving kidney transplants are over 65 years old. The nursing care of the person with renal failure, whether acute or chronic, is complex. The working relationship between patient and nurse must begin with an assessment and baseline physical examination to establish an appropriate, individualized healthcare plan.

Health assessment

In assessing the patient, the nurse needs to explore the physical, psychological and social effects of the illness on the person's normal functioning. Not only should the patient's self-caring or adaptive abilities and family resources be examined, but it is also important to discover the patient's own perceptions and understanding of the illness and health status.

Physical assessment

The physical assessment of the patient with acute or chronic renal failure will focus upon collecting information on the effects of renal impairment on extracellular fluid volume and the body systems. The nurse should begin by making careful observation of the person's overall appearance, noting the skin's colour, turgor, intactness and texture. General activity and comfort level should be assessed by noting posture, movement, gait, strength and restlessness. Mental status is assessed by noting the level of consciousness, orientation, anxiety and any signs of agitation.

As fluid volume assessment is critical in acute and chronic renal failure, the nurse looks for distinctive changes that might suggest circulatory overload or dehydration. Records of fluid intake, urine output and daily weights might show trends that indicate gains or losses. The nurse then assesses the pulse and blood pressure for hypertension. Circulatory overload may manifest as breathing difficulties, such as dyspnoea and orthopnoea. Pulmonary congestion and oedema can result from renal disease. The nurse should observe the individual for breathlessness, alteration in respiratory effort, restlessness, sounds accompanying breathing, and engorgement of jugular veins.

The skin at the base of the spine should be inspected for oedema, particularly in the patient who is critically ill and is in a dependent position in bed: extracellular fluid expansion may manifest itself in oedema at the base of the spine rather than at the periphery. It is crucial for the nurse working with the hospitalized renal patient to perform a fluid volume assessment on at least a daily basis.

The increasing number of older people who reach end-stage renal failure means that, when assessing patients, changes that occur naturally with ageing must be taken into account, such as loss of skin turgor. Older people have a raised thirst threshold; therefore they have a reduced thirst response when dehydration develops. Although the GFR declines with age, so does muscle and body mass, and as a result lower levels of creatinine can be expected when compared with a younger person. Sodium excretion slows down with age, whereas potassium is more readily lost – factors that are important in considering the effects of diuretics (Bevan 2000).

Acute renal failure

Acute renal failure (ARF) is a sudden, severe interruption of kidney function that, in most instances, is a complication of another disorder and is reversible. A biochemical definition of ARF is an increase in plasma creatinine concentration to above 200 mmol/L (Haslett et al 1999). As ARF is often associated with serious other pathology, mortality rates are high although, if the patient survives, renal function frequently returns to normal.

Causes

The primary or initiating causes of ARF are many but the basic mechanisms causing the failure, in most instances, are tubular necrosis due to inadequate tissue perfusion and hypoxia, or acute inflammation of glomeruli. Causes may be classified as prerenal, intrarenal or postrenal.

Prerenal   Prerenal refers to extrarenal disorders that cause inadequate renal perfusion as a result of a decrease in vascular volume or cardiac output or obstruction of a renal artery. The renal insufficiency is secondary to a condition that reduces the blood supply to the kidneys. The condition may be haemorrhage, dehydration, shock (due to major trauma, cardiac failure or burns) or renal artery occlusion by thrombosis. The frequent association of ARF with major trauma leads to many situations where the patient suffers major tissue destruction and hence is in a hypercatabolic state. The patient's energy requirement may be much greater than the normal supply, leading to breakdown of fats and proteins to make good the shortfall in energy supply (Garrett 1995). This process is known as *catabolism* and, when it exists alongside ARF, it poses major problems.

Intrarenal   Intrarenal refers to disorders in which there is actual renal tissue irritation and destruction which impairs renal function; examples are acute inflammation of the glomeruli (glomerulonephritis), acute tubular necrosis, and acute inflammation of the kidney tissue and renal pelvis (pyelonephritis). The primary renal tissue damage may be induced by a chemical or biological product or an infectious agent.

Renal failure may be the result of glomerulonephritis which is secondary to an extrarenal *Streptococcus haemolyticus* infection. The antigen complexes formed in response to the infection are trapped in the glomeruli and initiate the inflammatory process.

Nephrotoxic agents that are possible causes of a renal shutdown may be endogenous or exogenous in origin. Epithelial cells are destroyed; the tubular lumens are obliterated by swelling and oedema of the tissues as well as by casts formed from the sloughed cells. Examples of endogenous nephrotoxins are haemoglobin, released in haemolysis of erythrocytes following incompatible blood transfusion, and myoglobin, released from muscle cells in crushing injuries. The molecules of haemoglobin pass through the glomeruli and become concentrated in the tubules, obstructing the flow of filtrate. Similarly, the tubular necrosis that follows a crushing injury is attributed to the myoglobin accumulating in the tubules and causing an obstruction, as well as to shock. The individual who has been 'pinned down under a weight' for a period of time or who has been subjected to limb ischaemia may appear to be in a satisfactory condition

when released, but should be put to bed under close observation. Severe shock, acute renal failure and gross oedema of the injured part may develop hours later.

Exogenous nephrotoxins may be poisonous chemicals or drugs. Poisons, which may be taken accidentally or with suicidal intent, include carbon tetrachloride, ethylene glycol (a constituent of antifreeze), bichloride of mercury, chloroform and lead. Common pharmaceuticals that may prove toxic and damaging to the tubules include sulfonamide preparations (e.g. sulfadiazine), analgesics such as aspirin, non-steroidal anti-inflammatory agents, a cephalosporin and furosemide (frusemide) combination, and aminoglycoside antibiotics (e.g. kanamycin, gentamicin, tobramycin). Interstitial nephritis may be produced by methicillin and some analgesics. Obstructive disorders may result from cytotoxic drugs.

Post-renal   Post-renal causes of acute renal failure are conditions that result in an obstruction to the outflow of urine. Calculi, a neoplasm or prostatic hypertrophy may obstruct collecting tubules, the pelvis, a ureter or the bladder; the accumulation of fluid within the kidney compresses blood vessels and nephrons, seriously reducing kidney function.

Clinical characteristics

Patients with acute renal failure fall into two distinct categories:

1 Those who are oliguric, passing <500 mL of urine per day.
2 Those who are never oliguric but who continue to pass 1000–1500 mL of dilute urine per day.

The effects of a decreased urinary output are retention of an excess of certain biochemical substances in the blood and a decrease in the pH of body fluids, indicating increasing acidosis. Additionally blood urea and serum creatinine, potassium and sodium chloride concentrations are raised.

The first sign of acute renal failure may be oliguria, which may progress rapidly to anuria. The oliguric phase may last for 7–10 days and the urine contains blood and protein. An output of <30 mL per hour is an indication for concern and should be reported immediately. If oliguria and anuria persist for a few days, manifestations of water retention and disturbances of blood chemistry are likely to develop. Sodium and water retention cause oedema and, unless the fluid intake is controlled, overhydration may lead to cardiac failure and pulmonary oedema.

The increase in serum potassium concentration becomes a serious threat to cardiac muscle. In addition to the fact that potassium is not being eliminated by the kidneys, haemolysis and the breakdown of tissue cells by the primary condition (trauma, burns, sepsis, etc.) increase the concentration of potassium ions in the blood. Metabolic acidosis, which also develops in acute renal failure, promotes the movement of potassium out of the cells. Cardiac arrhythmias are common, and cardiac arrest may occur.

The rate of the accumulation of nitrogenous wastes (urea and creatinine) in the blood varies with the cause of the renal insufficiency. If there is rapid catabolism, as in infection, fever and pathological destruction of tissue, the blood concentration of nitrogenous wastes may rise more quickly. The onset of the uraemic state is usually marked by mental changes, nausea and vomiting, and probably hiccups. The patient may complain of pruritus.

Metabolic acidosis develops because the hydrogen ions produced in metabolism are not being eliminated by the renal tubules. Respirations are increased in rate and depth, and an acidotic odour of the breath becomes noticeable.

Leucocytosis may be present and anaemia is likely to develop fairly quickly. If the renal failure persists, the patient may develop a bleeding tendency. Ulcerated areas in the mouth are common and may bleed. Vomit and stools may contain blood, and petechiae and ecchymoses may appear. As the condition worsens, disseminated intravascular co-agulation (DIC) may develop (see p. 414).

The patient becomes drowsy and may progress to a comatose state. Muscle twitching and convulsions may also develop.

The outcome in acute renal failure is unpredictable. Many patients do recover; tubular healing and repair occur within 2–6 weeks and there is no serious functional impairment. Those who do not recover do not necessarily die from renal failure alone; frequently, the cause of death is the severity of the underlying cause or the combination of several associated disorders and complications. The patient with renal insufficiency is very susceptible to infection, especially pulmonary. Fluid in the alveoli (pulmonary oedema) and the retention of secretions due to inability to cough because of weakness predispose to pneumonia. Early recognition of renal insufficiency and prompt treatment are important. The nurse may play an important role in early recognition by being familiar with the possible causes of renal failure and by being alert to any significant decrease in a patient's urinary output.

Diuretic phase   If the renal failure is reversible, the patient experiences a period of diuresis following the oliguric period; large volumes of urine are excreted. The tubules are unable to concentrate urine and serum creatinine and blood urea levels remain raised. A diuretic phase may not be observed if the patient has been treated by dialysis.

Recovery phase   Improvement in renal function continues over 3–12 months. As function returns, the urine becomes more concentrated but some residual impairment often remains.

Complications

Complications that commonly develop in renal failure include hyperkalaemia, cardiac insufficiency, convulsions and coma.

Hyperkalaemia   Normal serum potassium levels of 3.5–5.0 mmol/L can be maintained until the 24-hour urine output falls below 500 mL with a decreased GFR. There are few visible signs of hyperkalaemia that the nurse may observe until the serum concentration reaches 7–8 mmol/L. At this increased level, severe electrocardiographic changes may rapidly occur. Cardiac function becomes impaired, and failure or sudden cardiac arrest may occur.

The nurse should be aware of the possible clinical symptoms of potassium intoxication which include:

- generalized muscular weakness
- shallow respirations
- complaints of a tingling sensation or numbness in the limbs and around the mouth
- a slow irregular pulse
- a fall in blood pressure.

Electrocardiographic (ECG) changes are an important indication of potassium intoxication. The critical aberrations include tall, tented T waves, ST segment depression, prolonged P-R interval and broadening of the QRS complex, with eventual ventricular fibrillation and cardiac standstill.

As the outcome of hyperkalaemia can be life-threatening, its management focuses on prevention, early detection and treatment of emergencies.

As well as ensuring that no potassium is ingested in fluid or food, preventive measures may include the oral or rectal administration of a cation-exchange resin, such as calcium resonium. The resin preparation combines with the potassium in the gastrointestinal secretions, preventing its absorption. Care must be taken to give a stool softener with it, as constipation and occasionally bowel obstructions are complications. Potassium loss via the gastrointestinal tract is effective only if a regular and effective bowel habit is established.

If hyperkalaemia develops, an intravenous infusion of 50 mL glucose (50%) cation-exchange resin, such as calcium resonium with a dose of human soluble insulin may be given if hyperglycaemia occurs. Alternatively, a 10–20% glucose solution may be given 4–6 hourly. This is to promote the deposition of the glucose as glycogen, a process that utilizes potassium. A solution of 1.26% sodium bicarbonate (500 mL 6–8 hourly) may be given to correct acidosis, and 10–20 mL calcium gluconate (10%) given intravenously to reduce the risk of cardiac arrest (Haslett et al 1999). An antiarrhythmic drug may also be prescribed. The only permanent and effective way for potassium to be removed from the body is by dialysis.

Cardiac insufficiency   Heart failure may occur as a result of the retention of sodium and water (see Ch. 12). If hypertension is associated with the renal failure, it may also be a factor in heart failure. Urgent fluid removal by ultra-filtration is required to ensure the safety of the patient.

Convulsions   Convulsions may occur and are usually preceded by muscular twitching, persisting severe headache, severe hypertension, increasing oedema and rising blood urea level. Benzodiazepines (e.g. diazepam) may be prescribed to control the seizures.

Coma   Increasing drowsiness may indicate increasing uraemia and may progress to disorientation and coma. The delirious patient requires constant attendance, and a sedative such as diazepam may be prescribed. If the patient becomes comatose, the care appropriate for any unconscious patient is applicable. At this stage, an urgent decision needs to be made either to refer the patient for dialysis or to institute palliative care.

Management

Medical management of acute renal failure is aimed at regulating fluid and electrolyte balance, controlling nitrogen imbalance, maintenance of nutrition and treatment of the underlying cause. Dialysis is initiated before the uraemic state develops to re-establish a normal homeostatic environment for tissue repair and restoration of renal function. Haemodialysis is considered necessary to deal with the hypercatabolic state encountered in severe renal failure (see p. 610). (Also, see the discussion of haemodialysis and peritoneal dialysis, on pp. 618, 619.)

Daily dialysis is usually required but the frequency will vary according to the rate of catabolism and the fluid imbalance. Excess fluid may be removed by haemofiltration using continuous, slow ultrafiltration. The use of ultra-filtration filters permits continuous fluid removal from the patient's intravascular content without the side-effects of sudden fluid loss, and without altering serum osmolality as occurs with diffusion dialysis. *Ultrafiltration* can be monitored by the nursing staff in an intensive care unit and has the advantage of allowing intravenous fluids and medications to be given to treat the cause of the patient's acute renal failure while controlling the fluid balance.

Fluid intake is restricted to 500 mL plus the previous day's output. The dietary protein should not be severely limited to decrease the production of nitrogenous wastes but maintained to provide adequate resources for tissue repair, and the patient should be dialyzed as often as necessary to keep nitrogenous wastes at an acceptable level. In other words, dialysis is performed as often as needed to 'make room' for a healthy protein intake. This will often mean daily dialysis. The calorie intake is maintained by the administration of glucose. The electrolyte balance is closely monitored, sodium and potassium are restricted and dialysis is used to lower the potassium level.

Patient problems

The nursing management of persons with acute renal failure is challenging and complex. Virtually every body system will be affected and the nurse must be able to assess how the disease process is affecting the patient as a whole. Table 19.3 lists actual and potential health problems and outcome criteria for care relevant to most persons with acute renal failure.

Nursing intervention

Assessment   The patient with acute renal failure is seriously ill and requires constant nursing care and *close observation* for changes, which may occur suddenly.

Fluid intake and output   Accurate measurements are essential. The daily fluid intake is limited to 500 mL plus an amount equal to the urinary output of the preceding 24 hours. The 500 mL replaces the obligatory loss through the skin and lungs. The fluid that may be given will depend on the laboratory findings. An explanation of the fluid restriction is essential if the patient is to understand the reasons for such severe limits on fluid intake.

Vital signs and blood tests   The *pulse, respirations* and *blood pressure* are checked frequently. Cardiac function may be impaired by the retention of potassium and fluid or by hypertension, which may accompany renal parenchymal disease. Blood tests are carried out at least every 4 hours to detect changes in the serum potassium level (hyper-kalaemia). Continuous ECG monitoring may be established if the plasma potassium level remains raised.

Any oedema is noted, and the patient's weight recorded daily as a gain usually indicates fluid retention. Breathing is observed for signs of developing pulmonary oedema, which may result from overhydration and cardiac failure. A noticeable increase in the volume and depth of respirations may point to acidosis.

The blood pressure is recorded at frequent regular intervals to provide information on the patient's progress. A progressive rise in excess of normal levels is reported immediately; it may point to increasing fluid volume. The temperature is taken every 4 hours, even if normal, as a sudden increase may occur and indicate complicating infection.

Frequent laboratory determinations of blood urea and serum creatinine levels and electrolytes are followed closely. The sodium and potassium levels are especially important in decisions relating to the types of solutions to be administered, and the patient's fluid balance and weight are used to determine the daily volume of fluid to be given.

Responses to drugs   Patient responses to medications are carefully assessed. Administering a drug to a patient in renal failure requires knowledge of the metabolic and excretory course of the drug, that is, what happens to it within the body. Drugs with which renal cells normally react or which are excreted by the kidneys are not given or, if used, are administered in a lower dosage than usually prescribed, and levels are monitored. Drugs containing potassium or sodium are avoided.

Neurological signs   Muscular twitching, increasing drowsiness and disorientation are recorded, as they may be manifestations of uraemia, cerebral oedema and approaching convulsions and coma.

Nutrition   A minimum of 100–200 g of potassium-free carbohydrate is given daily to reduce the amount of tissue protein and fat broken down for energy. The patient may lose 250–300 g of protein/day from muscle breakdown (catabolism), yet even when dialyzed, patients can cope with only 70–100 g of protein daily. Intakes in excess of these amounts will therefore only exacerbate uraemic symptoms (Haslett et al 1999). Often patients initially do not tolerate large amounts of food and so are fed naso-gastrically or intravenously until they have a desire to eat.

Essential amino acids as well as hypertonic glucose may be provided by the administration of total parenteral nutrition (TPN). Adequate protein is necessary for the synthesis of body tissues, enzymes and antibody production.

Table 19.3 Actual and potential health problems of persons with acute renal failure

Patient problem	Goals	Outcome criteria
1. Excess circulating fluid volume due to inability of kidneys to excrete water.	The patient will achieve a state of fluid balance with intake and output within normal limits	The patient's weight will be stable and within 2 kg of usual weight Fluid intake and output are balanced and within normal volumes
2. Alteration in electrolyte levels, particularly life-threatening hyperkalaemia, due to inability of kidneys to maintain normal serum electrolyte levels.	Electrolyte levels will be within normal limits	Serum electrolyte concentrations, pH and osmolality will be within normal range
3. Loss of lean body mass due to malnourishment.	No loss of lean body mass will occur	The patient experiences no true weight loss Serum creatinine and blood urea nitrogen levels are within an acceptable range for the patient
4. Potential impairment of oral mucosa and skin integrity due to oedema and increased excretion of waste through the skin.	Patient's skin and oral mucosa will be clean and intact	The oral mucosa will have a normal healthy appearance
5. Potential for infection and bleeding due to effects of uraemia on patient's resistance to infection and clotting mechanism.	Infection and bleeding will not occur	Temperature <37°C; respiration <20/minute No evidence of petechiae, haematuria or melaena
6. Anxiety due to lack of knowledge and loss of control over events.	Patient will be able to talk about anxieties and ask questions	The patient states that he or she is less anxious and shows some understanding of the disease process and its implications
7. Potential for injury due to confusion.	No injury will occur	The patient does not injure self despite altered cognition or level of consciousness
8. Dehydration due to excessive fluid loss associated with diuresis or diuretic therapy.	The patient will not become dehydrated	The patient will be in fluid balance Signs of dehydration (e.g. dry mouth, loss of skin elasticity) will be absent
9. Lack of knowledge about plans for future management.	Patient will be aware of long-term implications of the illness for future life	The patient and family understand how to manage convalescence The patient is aware of support services within the community and how to use them to promote recovery

The delivery of these nutrients requires the administration of a considerable volume of fluid, so parenteral administration of nutrients is used if the patient is treated by ultrafiltration to remove the excess fluid and prevent overloading the heart.

Activity Activity is not restricted but most patients are initially very ill and therefore need help with all activities. Early involvement of the physiotherapist and occupational therapist is important, so a coordinated exercise regimen, including active and passive exercises and use of appropriate devices and aids, is used to support and assist activities and so enhance independence. The family should be consulted to determine the usual level of pre-illness function. Preparations for rehabilitation and discharge should be initiated early, involving other appropriate healthcare professionals and referral to community services so that recovery is supported both in hospital and at home.

Skin and oral mucosa In renal failure, the mouth requires special care. The tongue becomes coated, salivary excretion is reduced, and the mucosa and lips are dry and frequently encrusted. Ulcerative lesions may develop, and the patient may be distressed by the disagreeable taste frequently associated with uraemia. Mouth lesions predispose to respiratory infection, local mouth infections and parotitis.

Frequent cleansing of the mouth is necessary. Petroleum jelly or cold cream is applied to the lips. The limited fluid intake and dry mouth are frequently a source of great distress to the patient. Resourcefulness on the part of the nurse may reduce the discomfort. Rinsing the mouth with ice-cold mouthwash or water is more acceptable than using lukewarm solutions. Occasional rinsing of the mouth with ice-cold fruit juice or ginger ale provides a change.

The patient is bathed daily to remove the increased wastes that may be excreted in sweat and to provide comfort. Regular assessment of pressure risk should be carried out, with inspection of at risk areas at frequent intervals. Meticulous pressure area care is essential.

Anxiety   Acute renal failure that is secondary to some serious disorder heightens the patient's fear and anxiety. Giving information to the patient and creating time in which the patient can ask questions or just talk about feelings are essential aspects of care. Relatives are kept informed of the patient's progress and encouraged to visit. They require support in understanding changes observed in the patient's behaviour and level of awareness.

Potential for injury   Cot sides may be kept in position because the uraemic patient may become drowsy and disoriented. Uraemia frequently leads to convulsions and coma, but regular dialysis will prevent this.

Fluid volume deficit (diuretic phase)   Improvement in renal function is manifested by a steady increase in the volume of urine. The latter may rise rapidly to as much as 6000–8000 mL in 24 hours. The diuresis is accompanied by marked losses of potassium, sodium and water because the tubules have not yet regained their ability to regulate the volume and composition of urine. Frequent serum electrolyte determinations continue, and necessary replacements are made either orally or intravenously. The fluid intake is increased to cover the volume lost. The nitrogenous waste concentration (urea) decreases more slowly. The patient is offered a soft diet and then a light diet. The nurse continues to record the intake and output.

Patient education   Preparation for discharge requires a multidisciplinary approach in order for the anticipated needs of the individual, family and significant others to be met. The patient and family should be actively involved in discharge preparation to promote a sense of personal control and to ensure cooperation with ongoing management. The nurse may be a key member of the team, ensuring coordination and reinforcing information so that it is fully understood. Early involvement of the dietician is important so that dietary restrictions can be discussed against a background of the individual's food preferences, usual eating patterns and food preparation practices at home.

Education should include information concerning recognition of the signs and symptoms of volume overload and hyperkalaemia, and monitoring of dialysis access sites for bleeding and infection. Written and verbal information and contact addresses and telephone numbers should be provided. Community services such as district nursing should be discussed and organized. Again, written and verbal communication with the community services will assist in ensuring continued and appropriate support. Discharge planning should also include outpatient follow-up plans so that the person clearly understands when progress will need to be reviewed.

The prolonged convalescence frequently causes socioeconomic problems for the person and family. The nurse may be able to assist by a referral to a medical social worker. It is important to understand the uncertainty of this period because many patients may be discharged before renal function is fully recovered. Consequently, the nurse who is working with the individual, planning the discharge, must be sensitive to the need for continued emotional support of the patient within the community.

Chronic renal failure

Chronic renal insufficiency is due to progressive disease of both kidneys. Irreversible damage to nephrons occurs which eventually leads to the retention of many waste and toxic products of metabolism, fluid and electrolyte imbalances, metabolic acidosis, anaemia, hypertension and decalcification of bone tissue (renal osteodystrophy).

Causes

The most frequent causes of chronic renal failure (CRF) are given below with approximate percentages (Haslett et al 1999):

- *Glomerulonephritis* (19%) – This involves a variety of immunologically induced diseases that cause inflammation, fibrosis and destruction of glomeruli, with tubular degeneration
- *Diabetes mellitus* (17%) – Diabetic nephropathy involves extensive glomerular and arteriolar impairment. The glomeruli lose their structure and no longer act as filters
- *Interstitial disease* (14%) – Includes chronic pyelonephritis and reflux nephropathy
- *Polycystic kidney disease* (7%) – Progressive enlargement of the cysts compresses functional renal parenchyma, increasing renal insufficiency in this inherited disease
- *Vascular disease* (6%) – Renal artery stenosis
- *Hypertension* (4%) – This involves a nephrosclerosis secondary to hypertension
- Other causes (15%)
- Cause uncertain (18%).

It should be noted that the incidence of *diabetes* varies substantially in different ethnic groups. Diabetes is five times more common amongst Asians living in the UK than amongst Caucasians. It is not surprising, therefore, that end-stage renal failure is six times more common and death from renal failure three times more common amongst Asians than amongst Caucasians in the UK (Whyte 2000).

Clinical characteristics

Regardless of the cause of the chronic renal failure, the disease progresses through three stages:

1 *Diminished renal reserve*, characterized by an asymptomatic decrease in renal function.
2 *Renal insufficiency*, demonstrating slightly raised serum creatinine and blood urea levels, and a GFR of about 25% of normal.
3 *End-stage renal failure or uraemia*, which occurs when the GFR is less than 10% of normal, and functional disturbances are apparent.

The patient may pass through the early stage of chronic kidney impairment without the renal disease being recognized. It may first be discovered in a routine physical examination, revealed by an increase in blood pressure and by albuminuria. The rate of destruction of functional tissue varies among individuals and with the primary causative factor. Some persons live a normal active life for many years because the functioning nephrons compensate for those destroyed. Others, whose disease progresses rapidly, may enter the advanced uraemic phase in a matter of a few months. In compensation, the GFR per nephron is increased, as are the re-absorption and secretory functions of the tubules. However, a deficit still exists which progressively increases.

Gradually, with increasing nephron destruction, the patient enters the phase in which renal compensation can no longer maintain homeostasis. The normal total GFR for an adult is 80–120 mL/minute; when this rate has dropped to 20 mL/minute or less, symptoms become apparent. Filtration is impaired and there is a loss of tubular ability to vary the composition and volume of urine according to the need to conserve or eliminate urinary solutes and water.

The signs and symptoms vary considerably in individuals in the early stages of uncompensated insufficiency, but tend to become similar in the more advanced stage when all the body systems become affected (Box 19.3). An increase in blood pressure, lassitude, headache and loss of weight may be the earliest manifestations. Urinalysis reveals albumin due to increased permeability of glomeruli. The loss of plasma protein as the disease progresses may be severe enough to produce the nephrotic syndrome (see p. 630). As more and

---

Box 19.3   Physiological alterations related to chronic renal failure

Fluid and electrolyte alterations
- Volume overload or depletion
- Hyperkalaemia or hypokalaemia
- Metabolic acidosis
- Hypercalcaemia and hypocalcaemia
- Raised serum phosphorus concentration.

Cardiovascular and pulmonary alterations
- Arterial hypertension
- Heart failure
- Pericarditis
- Pulmonary oedema.

Neurological alterations
- Fatigue, lassitude
- Headache, irritability
- Impaired cognition
- Seizures
- Peripheral neuropathy.

Gastrointestinal alterations
- Anorexia, nausea and vomiting
- Weight loss
- Peptic ulcer
- Gastrointestinal bleeding.

Haematological alterations
- Anaemia
- Bleeding tendency
- Increased potential for infection.

Musculoskeletal alterations
- Muscular twitching and weakness
- Renal osteodystrophy
- Calcium deposition in muscle tissue.

Skin alterations
- Pruritus associated with xerosis
- Thinning, loss of elasticity
- Increased potential for bruising
- Increased potential for skin breakdown and infection
- Calcium deposition in the skin.

Metabolic and endocrine alterations
- Hyperlipidaemia
- Sex hormone disturbances
- Secondary hyperparathyroidism
- Hyperglycaemia.

more nephrons are destroyed, decreased filtration results in the retention of metabolic wastes. The blood urea and serum creatinine levels rise and a formal medical diagnosis will be made depending upon the GFR.

With a progressive decrease in GFR and the development of hypertension, the patient experiences increasing fatigue and lassitude, more severe headaches and loss of weight. Nausea, especially in the mornings, and anorexia become troublesome. Fat and glucose metabolism are impaired, as well as protein metabolism. Serum triglyceride levels increase and a moderate hyperglycaemia occurs.

Initially, in chronic renal failure the 24-hour urinary volume is increased and the patient experiences nocturia as a result of tubular inability to concentrate the glomerular filtrate. The concentration of solutes in the urine is invariable, producing a fixed specific gravity. If the fluid intake does not cover the increased fluid loss, the patient develops a negative fluid balance and the retention of solid wastes is increased.

Tubular destruction causes electrolyte imbalances. There is usually an excessive loss of sodium, which may produce hyponatraemia unless there is adequate replacement. Potassium retention is not usually a problem until the terminal oliguric phase. In moderately severe failure, metabolic acidosis develops and hypocalcaemia may also be a problem, contributing to muscular twitching and general weakness.

Eventually, the urinary output is reduced, hypertension becomes severe, and the nitrogenous waste and potassium blood concentrations rise sharply. The patient is pale, and the haematocrit and haemoglobin determinations indicate anaemia, which accounts in part for the fatigue and reduced activity. In chronic renal failure a bleeding tendency is also manifested; the thrombocyte count is low and the prothrombin time is abnormal. Petechiae, ecchymoses and bleeding of mucous membranes may be observed.

The central nervous system is affected by the retained wastes: the person is irritable; memory, reasoning and judgement are impaired and the attention span is shortened. In the advanced uraemic stage, the patient manifests confusion, disorientation, drowsiness and stupor. Restlessness and twitching may be observed and frequently precede convulsive seizures. Retention of phosphate and decreased synthesis of the active metabolite of vitamin D by the kidney alter bone metabolism, producing renal osteodystrophy (osteomalacia, osteitis fibrosa, soft tissue calcification and osteosclerosis).

Pruritus may be a severe problem for the person with renal failure; it is attributed to the precipitation of retained phosphates into the skin.

Alterations in ovulatory and menstrual patterns occur in women experiencing renal failure. Although pregnancy has been reported, few women can successfully continue a pregnancy to term because of the overwhelming physiological changes in the body. Both women and men often experience changes in sexual desire and expression. This is for a variety of reasons but fatigue, lowered self-esteem and changed perceptions of attractiveness to their partners appear to play a great part.

Late symptoms are anuria, generalized oedema, persistent headache of increasing severity, nausea and vomiting, hiccups, diarrhoea, muscular twitching, convulsions, ulceration of the mouth, fetid breath, rapid deep respirations indicating acidosis, drowsiness, disorientation and coma. As a result of the severe hypertension and water retention, a cerebrovascular accident or cardiac failure and pulmonary oedema may supervene.

Management

It is necessary to create a positive relationship so that the nurse and patient can work together to meet patient-centred goals effectively. The more involved the patient is, the more successful therapy is likely to be.

The primary cause of renal failure is treated to retard progression of the disease (e.g. hypertension, pyelonephritis). The therapeutic plan includes measures to correct the body biochemistry and modify symptoms.

Conservative treatment Conservative treatment is reserved for patients who can be maintained without dialysis or kidney transplantation. The dietary and fluid intake are adjusted to maintain water and electrolyte balance and to reduce the retention of nitrogenous waste. Dietary protein may be decreased to around 60 g/day and limited to proteins high in essential amino acids (eggs, meat, fish and poultry) and to proteins from vegetables and grains. Carbohydrate intake is increased to provide adequate calories and to prevent the catabolism of body protein. Polyunsaturated fats are recommended and cooking with fats is avoided. A normal sodium intake is maintained if the patient has no signs of oedema or hypertension, but is restricted if these symptoms develop. Dietary potassium is usually restricted and potassium-exchange resins are prescribed if hyperkalaemia persists. Serum phosphate levels are controlled by the use of phosphate binders such as *aluminium hydroxide gel* and restricting the intake of high-phosphate foods such as cheese and milk. Multivitamin tablets are prescribed daily to prevent deficiencies of water-soluble vitamins which may develop when the diet is low in protein and potassium. Serum calcium concentration is monitored closely and, if generalized bone pain, muscle weakness or radiological evidence of bone changes are present, vitamin D in the form of 1α-hydroxycholecalciferol is given and calcium supplements may be prescribed if the phosphate level has been lowered. Balancing the sometimes contradictory requirements outlined above in a diet that prevents malnutrition, and which the patient can adhere to, is often very difficult.

The patient is monitored closely for symptoms of complications, and treatment is initiated promptly to control hypertension, fluid and electrolyte imbalances, metabolic acidosis, anaemia and altered bone metabolism.

Dialysis When conservative treatment will no longer adequately control the blood concentration of wastes and the fluid and electrolyte balance within limits compatible with life, regular *dialysis* may be employed to maintain the patient, and a kidney transplant is considered.

The person undergoing dialysis

When the person with renal failure is being cared for on a conservative therapeutic regimen, he or she will be monitored closely for manifestations that suggest that dialysis needs to be initiated. When the serum creatinine level reaches 800–1200 µmol/L, dialysis will probably need to be instituted. However, blood concentrations alone do not indicate clinical need for dialysis. The signs and symptoms that the nurse must be aware of and that should be reported are progressive hypertension, fluid retention, anorexia, nausea, vomiting, twitching and/or pruritus. These symptoms are often experienced to a degree of debilitation that indicates that dialysis needs to be initiated. In the UK, there are presently over 37 000 patients who are receiving treatment for established renal failure (UK Renal Registry 2003).

Standard four of the National Service Framework for Renal Services Part One recommends that all types of dialysis treatments should be available to all patients based on their individual needs and choices (Department of Health 2004). Dialysis is a therapeutic procedure used in acute and chronic renal failure to lower the blood level of metabolic waste products (urea, creatinine, uric acid) and toxic substances, and to correct abnormal electrolyte and fluid balances. Two methods currently in use are *continuous ambulatory peritoneal dialysis* (CAPD) and *haemodialysis*. The latter dialysis takes place outside of the body using a dialysis machine to which an artificial kidney is attached. Although the procedures in the two types of dialysis differ, the purposes and principles are basically the same. In haemodialysis, a semipermeable membrane separates the patient's circulating blood from a specially prepared solution known as the *dialysate*. In CAPD, the peritoneum is the membrane that separates the dialysate from the person's interstitial fluid, the dialysate being introduced into the peritoneal cavity. By using the principles of osmosis and diffusion, the dialysis procedure can partially replace some of the excretory and regulatory functions of the nephrons of the kidney. It is important to understand that the endocrine function of the normal kidney cannot be replaced by either haemodialysis or peritoneal dialysis.

Continuous ambulatory peritoneal dialysis Approximately 26% of the patients with established renal failure in the UK receive continuous ambulatory peritoneal dialysis (CAPD) (UK Renal Registry 2003). This technique may be used for most people with symptomatic renal failure and a healthy peritoneal surface area. The dialysate is introduced into the peritoneal cavity, which is lined by a membrane, the peritoneum. This acts as a dialysis membrane. Osmosis removes fluids whilst other metabolites are also gradually removed. CAPD is effective in removing small and middle-sized molecules, sodium, potassium and water, and in controlling hypertension and anaemia. The dialysate is replaced four times a day. Scheduling of exchanges is flexible and the equipment is portable to permit travel, work and schooling. This method is used particularly in children and the elderly, and patients may be maintained for up to 10 years with CAPD. A recent innovation involves automated peritoneal dialysis, which consists of a machine able to perform the exchanges during the night while the patient is asleep. As a result, the patient does not have to dialyze during the day.

CAPD involves the following steps:

1 Connection of the catheter to tubing from a plastic bag containing the dialysate solution
2 Instillation of the dialysate
3 Folding of the plastic bag into a waist, leg or pocket pouch worn under the clothing
4 Drainage of the peritoneal cavity by gravity into the plastic bag about 6 hours later
5 Disposal of the filled bag
6 Connection and instillation of a fresh bag of dialysate (Fig. 19.4).

Bags containing 2 L of dialysate are exchanged 3–5 times a day, 7 days a week. The exchange schedule may be adjusted allowing 6 hours between two exchanges, 4 hours between the next exchange and an 8-hour interval at night to permit uninterrupted sleep.

Peritoneal catheters A permanent peritoneal catheter is required for CAPD. A catheter with several openings in the tip, such as the Tenckhoff catheter is inserted into the peritoneal cavity. Tissue cells (fibroblasts) grow into the two Dacron cuffs on the subcutaneous section of the catheter in 2–3 weeks, stabilizing the catheter position and decreasing the incidence of infection and escape of fluid. The procedure is usually carried out in the operating theatre under either a local or a general anaesthetic.

Dialysis cycles Each exchange of dialysate is divided into three stages:

1 instillation time
2 dwell time
3 drainage time.

The solution is warmed to body temperature and infuses fairly rapidly into the peritoneal cavity by the force of gravity.

The *instillation time* for the 2 L of solution usually used for an adult requires approximately 10 minutes. *Dwell time* is the period of time the dialysate remains in the peritoneal cavity. For CAPD this varies from 4 to 6 hours, and exchanges are carried out continuously, 7 days a week. Smaller molecules such as blood urea nitrogen equalize in 2–3 hours; larger molecules take longer to equalize. The osmolarity of the solution influences the dwell time required to remove water. Dextrose concentrations above 1.5% increase the osmolarity of the dialysate above that of the plasma and promote water removal. Higher concentrations of dextrose (3.86%) remove larger volumes of water in less time than solutions of 1.5% dextrose. *Drainage time* is the period in which the solution drains from the cavity. It takes up to 20 minutes.

Complications of peritoneal dialysis

Peritonitis This is the major complication of peritoneal dialysis. Symptoms include abdominal pain and tenderness,

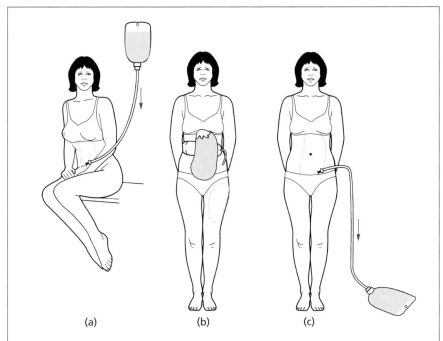

Figure 19.4 Continuous ambulatory peritoneal dialysis. (a) Fluid flows from bag into peritoneal cavity through permanent access tube. (b) Patient wears bag around waist or leg and resumes normal activity. (c) Bag is lowered and fluid drains out. Bag is then discarded and the procedure is repeated with fresh fluid.

(a) (b) (c)

cloudy effluent, fever, diarrhea and occasionally vomiting and paralytic ileus. The peritoneal effluent is cultured for identification of organisms and white blood cell count. Antibiotic therapy is required and if this is not successful the catheter may require re-siting.

Catheter complications. Leakage around the catheter, obstruction of the catheter, retention of fluid and infection of the exit site are the most common complications associated with the catheter. Maintenance of regular bowel elimination helps to prevent problems with the flow of solution into the peritoneal cavity.

Dehydration. This may result from use of large volumes of 4.25% dextrose dialysate. The patient will be hypotensive, manifesting pallor, weakness, fainting and a rapid, weak pulse, and will experience muscle cramps and may also be hyperglycaemic.

Pain. This may be due to the tip of the catheter pressing on viscera or overheating of the dialysate.

Social factors. Social isolation can be a problem with peritoneal dialysis as the patient's life becomes governed by the ongoing procedure to manage their condition. They may become depressed and may have difficulty adhering to the regimen. A reduction in appetite and restrictions on dietary intake can disrupt family meal times and lead to further feelings of isolation and rejection. The patient needs sensitive nursing care and support at these times and need to be helped towards acceptance and understanding of their condition.

Others. There are many other potential complications associated with CAPD, these include; fluid overload, malnutrition, obesity, hernias, lumbar back pain, cardiovascular

and lipid problems and constipation (Redmond and Doherty 2005).

Nursing care of the person undergoing long-term peritoneal dialysis Because of its relative simplicity, nurses often make the assumption that the person undergoing long-term peritoneal dialysis should adjust quickly and easily. However, it is wrong to imply that peritoneal dialysis is 'easy', as it involves skill, problem-solving ability and fine motor coordination. Learning the technique takes time and the patient needs a gradual, well supported, approach. By careful assessment, the nurse can begin to work with the patient to promote self-care as independently and safely as possible. The nurse can assist patients to develop new methods of self-care which are unique to their particular needs and situation. At all times the nurse must be aware of the patient's perspective of the illness.

Before dialysis is started, an explanation of the procedure and its purpose is given to the patient and family. Assessment of their continued education needs is crucial, because the effects of uraemia, by interfering with cerebral function, may prevent the patient from understanding what is being taught.

While the patient is learning CAPD, frequent assessment is very important and should include recording of blood pressure, pulse, respirations, temperature and weight in order to establish a baseline for physical signs. Signs of oedema, respiratory distress and dehydration should also be noted. The area around the exit of the catheter is observed for redness, drainage and infection. It is important to assess how the patient is feeling and how the forthcoming dialysis is viewed. When outflow is completed, the volume of fluid drained should be measured and recorded in order to ensure all dialysate is drained. Long-term complications reported by Bevan (2000) in older patients include hernia formation, constipation and the potential for malnutrition due to excess protein loss in the dialysate draining from the peritoneum

Haemodialysis Haemodialysis can remove water and catabolic wastes at a faster rate than CAPD. Because of this efficiency, it may not always be used for patients who are haemodynamically unstable, as can be the case in certain cardiac diseases. It is a complex procedure that requires expensive and sophisticated equipment.

In haemodialysis an extracorporeal dialyzing system is used to remove toxic wastes. During haemodialysis the person's uraemic blood is purified by drawing it from an artery, passing it through a sterile extracorporeal circulation, through a dialyzer in which dialysis takes place, and returning it to the venous system in its purified state. It is within the dialyzer that the actual exchange of material across the dialysis membrane takes place. Figure 19.5 illustrates the relationship of the patient to the equipment. During routine haemodialysis, clearance of body toxins and filtration of water occur simultaneously.

In haemodialysis, both solute and solvent transfer across the membrane under the force generated by hydrostatic pressure, in addition to that created by osmotic pressure.

The dialysate is an aqueous solution that contains varying concentrations of the body's normal extracellular and intracellular cations and anions. The cations commonly found in dialysate are sodium, potassium, calcium and magnesium. The anions found in dialysate may be acetate and bicarbonate.

The concentrations within the dialysate solution promote the removal of toxic substances, such as excess urea, creatinine and uric acid, from the body, as well as excess potassium, sodium, phosphate and water. Because of the semipermeable nature of the dialysis membrane, it readily allows the passage of small molecules such as urea, potassium and sodium, while retaining such large entities as proteins, glucose and red blood cells. The small molecules that can pass through the pores of the membrane will always travel from the area of greater to lesser concentration so that there is equal composition and concentration on both sides of the membrane. Because of the hydrostatic pressure across the membrane, excess water can be removed as the water flows toward the dialysate solution, which is of greater osmolality.

Vascular access Maintenance haemodialysis requires direct access to the circulating blood by the extracorporeal dialyzing system. The requirement for vascular access in persons with renal failure can be either permanent or temporary. Patients using long-term haemodialysis will need a permanent access because the duration of the treatment will be months or many years. Access is usually via an

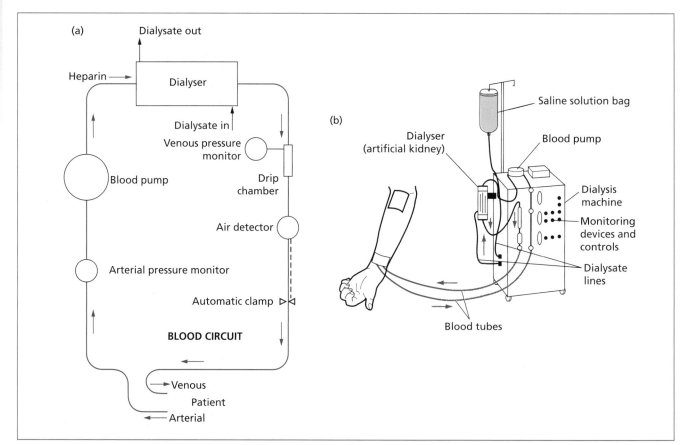

Figure 19.5 (a) Diagrammatic representation of haemodialysis. (b) Relationship of the patient to the equipment.

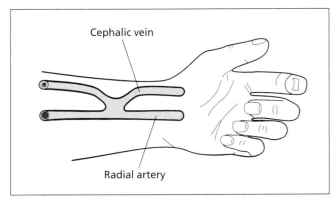

Figure 19.6 An arteriovenous fistula.

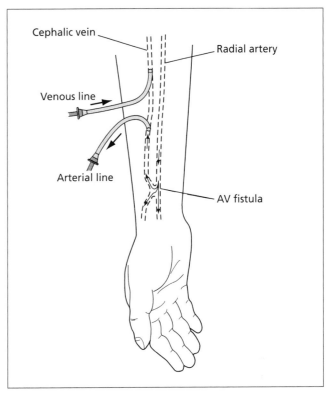

Figure 19.7 The position of needles when an arteriovenous fistula is established for haemodialysis.

arteriovenous fistula. Each access requires specialized nursing care, the focus of which should include assessing the access for patency, pain, signs of infection, tissue trauma or oedema, and bleeding. The nurse will also work with the patient to ensure that he or she can monitor the vascular access thoroughly and independently. The need for long-term vascular access is often problematic in older patients because of the adverse effects of ageing on their blood vessels.

Arteriovenous fistula. This is surgically constructed by a side-to-side or end-to-end anastomosis between an artery and a vein in the forearm. The anastomosis may be between the cephalic vein and the radial artery, or between the cephalic vein and brachial artery (Fig. 19.6). This redirects arterial blood through the vein, thereby causing enlargement of the vein in response to the increased rate of blood flow and the higher pressure of arterial blood now passing through it. This engorgement of the arterialized vein requires 6–12 weeks to 'mature' before it is able to withstand the changing pressures against its vessel wall and the repeated insertion of dialysis needles.

Haemodialysis with an arteriovenous (AV) fistula involves the insertion of two large bore needles. One needle is connected to the arterial line of the dialyzer and the second is connected to the tube that returns the blood from the dialyzer. Blood flows out from the distal needle through the dialyzer and back via the proximal needle (Fig. 19.7). The limb in which an AV fistula is developed should not normally be used for taking blood pressure or blood samples, as either may jeopardize the patency of the fistula.

The AV fistula is the preferred access for long-term haemodialysis because it has several distinct advantages. It is completely subcutaneous, thus lessening the possibility of infection and reducing the risk of haemorrhage and thrombosis during everyday activity. Temporary vascular access can be gained via alternative methods in some clinical situations. For example, the normal access may have failed and the patient may need urgent dialysis before a permanent access can be re-established. In these cases, the patient may undergo haemodialysis with a *subclavian catheter* or prefer-

ably a *femoral catheter*. In either case, access is gained to the circulation by percutaneous insertion of a cannula.

Box 19.4 outlines issues for the immediate postoperative care of the patient with a newly created AV fistula or temporary access.

Nursing intervention in haemodialysis Nurses responsible for the care of patients receiving dialysis require specialized preparation. Dialysis is a complex therapeutic procedure used to correct a life-threatening body dysfunction. Staff on general medical and surgical units and in the community should also have an appreciation of the implications for and the concerns of the renal patient and family. Personnel working in dialysis units usually assume responsibility for the specialized needs of dialysis patients being cared for in other areas of the hospital.

Emotional and socioeconomic concerns. When the person's chronic renal failure necessitates haemodialysis, it is natural that the patient and family will be concerned. The need for dialysis is likely to have many implications; knowing that the disease has progressed to this stage and that life has become dependent upon the procedure is extremely threatening. Severe anxiety may be manifested due to concern for the future and life expectancy. Acceptance may be very difficult for some patients and they may show resentment and anger at first, followed by a period of depression. A regular schedule of dialysis two or three times weekly imposes modifications on the patient's and family's

> **Box 19.4** Guidelines for nursing care of the patient with a permanent or temporary vascular access for haemodialysis
>
> 1 Elevate affected arm or leg on pillow to minimize tissue swelling.
>
> 2 Check dressing for any bleeding; document and report to the doctor.
>
> 3 Check warmth, colour and mobility of fingers or toes for circulation.
>
> 4 Oedema is expected after operation but excessive oedema should be reported to the doctor.
>
> 5 Access insertion is a painful procedure, so analgesia should be given as required during the postoperative period.
>
> 6 Teach the patient to monitor own access for bleeding and swelling, and to report pain.
>
> 7 No blood specimens, intravenous infusions, blood pressure monitoring etc. to be performed on access arm.
>
> 8 Psychological support should be given to the patient at all times.

life pattern. Treatment may mean changing occupation or giving up employment or, at best, working only part-time unless home dialysis can be provided. The adjustments that have to be made may cause both social and economic changes for family members. Special diet requirements and transport to and from the dialysis unit or the need to accommodate dialysis equipment in the home may incur worrisome additional expense. A referral to a social worker may be helpful.

It is important for the nurse to be a willing listener and encourage the patient and family to reveal their concerns and problems; these vary from person to person and from family to family. An understanding of their situation and recognition of their reactions are essential to providing the appropriate support and care, and in assisting them to accept necessary modifications in lifestyle. A positive attitude on the part of the healthcare team promotes realistic patient and family acceptance and adaptation. Many people obtain support and pleasure through socialization and the establishment of close relationships with other dialysis patients.

Gradually, as the uraemic toxicity is reduced, the person experiences physical and emotional improvement and, by degrees, becomes more active and interested in living and may lead a relatively normal productive life.

Predialysis responsibilities. The patient and family should receive a simple explanation of the purpose of dialysis and what to expect during the procedure. Many units have prepared brochures and audiovisual programmes to provide information and reinforce verbal explanations

and instruction. If the patient is to be dialyzed at home, an extensive home-training programme is planned. Prior to the initial treatment, if the patient's condition permits, he or she should visit the dialysis unit, meet the dialysis staff and may have the opportunity to chat with a patient on a regular dialysis programme. Such preparation is helpful in reducing the person's fear.

For dialysis, the patient is positioned comfortably in a bed or a reclining chair with the limb with the AV fistula exposed and supported. Temperature, pulse, respirations, lying and standing blood pressure and weight are recorded before the dialysis is commenced to provide a baseline. Blood specimens are obtained when the needles are introduced (or cannulae are opened) for laboratory determination of the haematocrit, electrolyte (K^+, Na^+), blood urea and creatinine levels, and clotting time. Anxiety is often greatly reduced if the patient and a relative are actively involved, even for the first dialysis. This might mean helping to set up the machine or preparation of the patient's dialysis access. A working knowledge of the equipment often greatly reduces fear.

The vascular access site is examined for signs of a haematoma or infection. Observations are made of the person's colour and the condition of the skin (dryness, turgor, abrasions) and for oedema. Weight is compared with that recorded following the last dialysis to check fluid accumulation. Weight changes, as well as blood chemistry and physical findings, determine the desired fluid loss and the appropriate dialyzer, dialysate and flow rate.

Responsibilities during dialysis. During dialysis, the patient is monitored continuously for indications of the effectiveness of treatment and signs of complications. Each unit or home programme will have a schedule for observing and recording vital signs, equipment used, rate of flow, composition and temperature of dialysate, heparinization and blood-clotting times, as well as ongoing monitoring of the functioning of the equipment. The person is observed closely for signs of dehydration or overhydration. Changes in blood pressure and respirations are recorded and the flow rate through the dialyzer is regulated accordingly. If there is a rapid, excessive loss of water into the dialysate, the ensuing reduction in the intravascular volume causes a sharp fall in the blood pressure. Overhydration may be indicated by respiratory distress, moist sounds and an increase in the blood pressure.

Headache, vomiting and twitching may develop if the patient becomes dehydrated and should be brought to the doctor's attention. The first dialysis should be short (i.e. 2–3 hours) to allow a gentle clearance of nitrogenous waste. This prevents the complication of cerebral oedema associated with disequilibrium syndrome, which may present as disorientation or a convulsion.

The length of time the patient is kept on the dialyzer varies with the patient's condition and type of machine used. The average range is 4–6 hours. The frequency also varies with patients. In acute renal failure, daily dialysis may be necessary until renal function is re-established.

Persons with chronic renal insufficiency are dialyzed two or three times weekly and may lead a relatively normal, productive life for the remainder of the week. The dialysis programme may be long term, extending over years, or may be a temporary measure for the individual who is awaiting a kidney transplant.

Post-dialysis care. Upon completion of the dialysis, the arterial line is clamped and as much blood as possible in the dialyzing circuit lines is returned to the patient. Dressings are applied to the needle sites and the area observed until there is no evidence of bleeding; it may be necessary to apply some pressure for a brief period. The patient's weight, blood pressure (lying and standing), pulse and temperature are recorded for comparison with the original baseline observations.

Patient education. When a regular dialysis programme is recommended, the person and a relative receive detailed instruction concerning diet and fluid intake, care of the fistula site or cannulae, activity, and recognition of disturbances that should prompt immediate notification of the dialysis unit. The brochure given out by the dialysis unit that explains dialysis also discusses these factors.

The diet prescribed varies from person to person and with doctors. The food intake must be balanced with the renal capacity to eliminate protein waste and prevent excesses of electrolytes (K^+, Na^+) and water. The protein content may be 60–80 g/day, allowing 0.75–1 g/kg body weight if dialysis facilities are limited; otherwise a normal diet is encouraged and dialysis hours are adjusted to control nitrogenous waste.

Nursing the person with chronic renal failure
Patient problems Patients are particularly vulnerable to reactive depression, feelings of powerlessness and loss of control, social isolation and a whole host of physiological complications. This is illustrated by the work of McCann and Boore (2000). They found fatigue and lack of vitality associated with sleep problems, poor physical health, anxiety and depression were closely interrelated in a study of 39 adult patients undergoing haemodialysis. Box 19.5 lists actual and potential health problems common to most patients with chronic renal failure. The needs of patients and their families will also vary as the disease progresses.

Nursing intervention
Altered fluid and electrolyte balance Assessment of fluid and electrolyte balance is continuous. The patient and family should be taught to identify signs and symptoms of fluid excess or dehydration and to adjust fluid intake accordingly. The patient is also taught to recognize the signs of hyperkalaemia and other electrolyte imbalances and to adjust diet as necessary.

In the early stages of chronic renal failure, tubular re-absorption of water is decreased so the intake must be increased to approximately 2000 mL per day to avoid dehydration. When oliguria is present the fluid intake is limited to 400–500 mL plus the measurable loss (e.g. urine and vomit). Fluid restriction may be minimal for the person

---

Box 19.5 Actual and potential health problems of the person with chronic renal failure

1 Altered fluid and electrolyte balance.

2 Nutritional intake lower than body requirements.

3 Potential for infection and bleeding.

4 Activity intolerance.

5 Impaired skin integrity and altered oral mucosa.

6 Clouding of consciousness.

7 Ineffective individual and family coping patterns.

8 Lack of knowledge about:
   a) kidney function
   b) methods of treatment (dialysis or transplant)
   c) self-care measures
   d) necessary alterations to lifestyle.

---

on CAPD because fluid is removed continuously; however, fluid restrictions may be introduced if the individual on CAPD exhibits signs of fluid volume expansion that could jeopardize cardiovascular integrity.

Nutrition The prescribed diet varies with the severity of disease and the type of maintenance treatment used. In the early stages, protein restrictions may be based on the glomerular filtration rate (GFR), but when the GFR decreases to 4–5 mL/minute, protein restrictions are no longer effective in reducing the retention of nitrogenous wastes and dialysis is required. Protein is lost during CAPD and the loss is greater if peritonitis develops. Less protein is lost during haemodialysis, but some free amino acids escape with this treatment. The protein intake must be adjusted to compensate for the loss and prevent catabolism of body protein. Calorie intake must be sufficient to permit activity without breakdown of tissue protein.

Electrolyte balance is maintained by adjusting the dietary intake according to serum electrolyte levels. As impaired tubular re-absorption results in an excessive loss of sodium, salt is not restricted in the diet unless there is oedema or hypertension. Dietary sodium is restricted following a transplant as corticosteroid therapy leads to sodium and water retention. Foods high in potassium are restricted for most renal patients because potassium is not effectively removed by impaired kidneys. The serum phosphate level is usually controlled by the use of phosphate binders, such as an aluminium hydroxide antacid, and avoidance of foods high in phosphorus.

Nutritional management in chronic renal failure is complex. As diet is such an important part of disease management, the individual and family require considerable teaching and prolonged support from the nurse as well as the dietician. It is essential that a person's previous meal patterns and food preferences be incorporated into any management plan.

Dietary management becomes more complex for the person with chronic renal failure who experiences sudden stress such as infection, surgery or trauma. Food and fluid intake must be closely monitored and adjusted to body needs.

Preventing infection and bleeding Immunosuppressive drugs or uraemia affect white cell activity, making the person prone to infection. Preventive measures and prompt treatment of infection are essential. Uraemic blood also has altered clotting ability and the patient therefore needs to be monitored for signs of bleeding from the dialysis access, mucous membranes or surgical sites.

Activity intolerance The individual with chronic renal failure experiences considerable fatigue and lethargy; anaemia may contribute to the decreased energy. The anaemia may be due to decreased erythropoietin production, depression of the bone marrow associated with uraemia, or to blood loss due to increased tendency to bleed and through dialysis. It develops gradually and may not be symptomatic at first.

The nurse working with haemodialysis patients should therefore take precautions to minimize blood loss during dialysis. Promising research results suggest that the monitored administration of a manufactured form of erythropoietin, *recombinant human erythropoietin (EPO)* or *novel erythropoiesis stimulating protein (NESP)*, may be instrumental in increasing haemoglobin concentrations (National Kidney Federation 2002). This will improve the person's energy level and quality of life dramatically.

Enquiry should be made concerning joint and muscle pain and any changes in range of motion or mobility. Signs of hypocalcaemia, tetany, carpopedal spasm, seizures, numbness and tingling of extremities, or confusion should be noted and reported to medical staff.

Skin and oral mucosa Assessment of the skin of the patient with chronic renal failure may show pallor, a yellow-grey colour, dryness, bruising and decreased sweating. The patient complains of itching. The hair is dry, becomes brittle and the nails are rigid and dry. The mouth should be inspected regularly for signs of inflammation and bleeding.

The patient is taught to care for skin, mouth, hair and nails; this includes following the dietary regimen to control serum calcium and phosphorus levels and avoiding tissue trauma.

Clouding of consciousness Changes in the patient's level of awareness usually develop gradually as uraemia increases. Rapid progression of the disease produces severe disturbances in behaviour and cognition. Dialysis should be started before the progression of these neurological complications.

Early symptoms may include headache, lethargy, dizziness, euphoria, depression, apathy, sleeplessness or drowsiness. Recent and remote memory and attention span are decreased and decision-making is impaired. In the late stages of renal failure, confusion, slurred speech, stupor, coma and convulsions may develop.

The patient is assessed for orientation to time, place and person. Changes in behaviour as perceived by the patient and family are noted and relatives are helped to understand that the patient cannot always control behaviour.

Cognitive abilities should be evaluated before patient teaching is started. Explanations of procedures should be simple, broken down into steps and repeated frequently. It is possible that the patient's home environment may need modification to promote safety.

Coping patterns Adaptation to chronic renal failure is a complex process and varies with each patient, the degree of loss of renal function, the type of treatment selected and support available.

Assessment of the patient's coping includes learning about pre-illness personality and the degree of independence in daily life. The patient will have to cope with many losses such as loss of job and financial security; position in the family; stamina; and sense of well-being. The patient will experience a loss of freedom due to dependence on a machine coupled with loss of self-esteem, and will have to cope with a reduced life expectancy. Further changes in family roles and relationships are increased by decreased sexual function. The previously independent person has the most difficulty in adjusting initially, but measures to prevent feelings of helplessness and dependence can be effective.

Information about how the patient coped with stress in the past helps in assessing present coping responses and in developing new coping strategies. Some coping mechanisms used every day are dangerous when employed by the person with chronic renal failure. For example, a period of denial or non-adherence to the management plan is often seen in persons with chronic illness as they strive to deal with the staggering life changes necessary. The nurse should accept this as the patient works through the denial period, and should work with the person in exploring thoughts and feelings about the impact of chronic illness on lifestyle.

Changes in cognitive ability and behaviour affect the patient's perceptions of the illness, ability to comprehend what is happening, to understand and adhere with treatment and make informed, rational judgements about care. Chronic fatigue and lethargy together with increased dependency on others further impair the patient's ability to cope. The presence of family and other support groups enhances positive coping; consequently, family members are very important in supporting the patient. The family requires knowledge of the disease, understanding of the patient's responses and understanding of the treatment plan so that they can be informed participants in care and support.

The patient starting dialysis must acknowledge dependence on machines to sustain life. Transplantation usually results in an initial state of euphoria, which is followed by reactions to living with a foreign body, before eventual acceptance of the graft occurs. These patients live with a lifelong need for medication and constant fear of graft rejection. Even with a successful transplantation, the patient needs help adjusting to the changes imposed by this lifelong process.

Lack of knowledge As the patient and family must assume the responsibility for following the prescribed regimen, formal and informal instruction is planned. Patient education is started at the time of diagnosis and the teaching is adjusted as the patient's needs change with progression of the disease and revision of the treatment plan. The decision about home or hospital dialysis influences the degree of responsibility the patient and family assume for self-care and the resources needed to help them.

When a patient with chronic renal failure is admitted to hospital, it is important that the nursing staff assess the patient's understanding of care and support the individual's achievements by encouraging active patient participation in care. Taking away the patient's control on each hospital admission retards progress already made and contributes to feelings of dependency.

Goals for education should be established for each patient and teaching should draw upon a range of different methods such as pamphlets, detailed instructions for technical tasks, videos, group sessions and practical demonstrations. Content includes the function of the kidneys, types of treatment (dialysis or transplant), self-care measures and lifestyle adaptations.

Necessary alterations to lifestyle. Helping the person adjust his or her lifestyle is an individual process. The teaching programme includes consideration of the following:

● *Work*. The person's treatment plan, chronic fatigue and lethargy may limit the ability to retain gainful employment. Liaison with the individual's employer and occupational health service, if available, or employment counselling may assist the person to continue working
● *Sexuality*. Counselling of the patient and partner helps them to understand the reasons for changes in sexual desire and expression. Many persons do not ask about the effects of renal disease on this aspect of their lifestyle. The nurse therefore needs to be sensitive to the couple's need to discuss this issue. Contraceptive information is necessary because pregnancy is possible, although there is a high likelihood of spontaneous abortion in the second trimester. Many couples affected by renal disease are able to have a satisfying sexual relationship by exploring alternative ways of expressing affection. The nurse should encourage the couple to participate in decision-making and care, and assist them in establishing and maintaining open communication, thereby fostering the solidarity of the emotional and sexual relationships
● *Holidays*. The person and family are helped to plan holidays and are informed of resources available. These include portable machines that may be borrowed, a directory of renal units in other cities nationally and internationally, and trips and camping facilities available through the local or National Kidney Federation (www.kidney.org.uk)

● *Exercise*. The patient is helped to plan an activity schedule that includes moderate exercise and is taught that regular exercise improves circulation and appetite and promotes rest and a sense of well-being
● *Social activities*. Alterations in social activities, such as eating and drinking, that are required by the treatment regimen need to be discussed fully. Encouragement from staff and family is needed for the person to initiate and increase social interaction.

Kidney transplantation

The development of donor selection by tissue typing and the steady progress that has been made in managing the rejection process have resulted in an increase in the number of kidney transplants.

An advantage of a kidney transplant for the person who has severe renal failure is the discontinuance of the demanding dialysis schedule; considerable time is saved, and the individual's employment is uninterrupted and more productive. Dietary restrictions are lifted and constraint of activity is slight. The patient must be aware of the possible adverse effects as well as the benefits of transplantation before deciding on this mode of treatment. Some experience few complications and their quality of life is greatly improved. Others experience side-effects from the drugs used to control the rejection process and graft rejection. Transplantation requires major surgery and a lifelong dependency on immunosuppressive drugs. Rejection of the transplant necessitates return to dialysis and consideration for retransplantation.

Transplant recipients The patient and family should be informed of the available types of treatment for chronic renal failure and the risks and benefits of each, as well as the implications for their well-being and quality of life. Given such understanding, the person makes the final decision whether to have the transplant or not.

The number of people waiting for an organ transplant in the UK far exceeds the number of donors (TalkTransplant 2006). In 2006, NHS Direct states that there are over 7000 people in the UK waiting for organ transplantation most of whom are waiting for a kidney (NHS Direct 2006). On 31 March 2005 there were 5423 people waiting for a kidney transplant (UK Transplant 2005a). The criteria for the selection of transplant candidates have become more liberal in the past few years. A set of evidence-based rules has therefore been introduced to decide priorities when kidneys become available for transplant. All patients with end stage renal failure should be considered for transplantation (UK Transplant 2006), although certain patient groups are prioritized immediately, such as children and people with high levels of sensitization to human leucocyte antigens (HLA, see below). There are some absolute contraindications to transplant including patients who have a predicted survival of <7 years, for example those with malignant disease, cardiac failure, HIV that has progressed to AIDS or is not being treated and people with cardiovascular disease with a poor prognosis. Patients who are unable to comply with immunosuppressant therapy or where immunosuppressant therapy is predicted to cause life-threatening side-effects will also be considered to have a contraindication to transplant. Each person is considered individually and their particular circumstances are reviewed. Additional issues such as a BMI >30 further reduce the chance of successful transplantation (UK Transplant 2006). Factors such as length of time on waiting list, similarity in age with donor organ, ease of matching and the distance between donor and recipient centre are also issues that are considered.

Immunological factors The greatest hazard associated with any organ or tissue transplant from another person is the incompatibility of the recipient's tissue with that of the donor, and the ensuing rejection process. Secondary to this are the effects of the immunosuppressive drugs used to depress the rejection process; the most formidable is the recipient's increased susceptibility to infection.

The rejection process is an antigen–antibody reaction or immune response; the recipient's immune system recognizes the graft as a foreign substance, and specific antibodies and sensitized lymphocytes attack the foreign tissue.

The antigenicity and compatibility of the donor and recipient in tissue and organ transplants are determined by heredity. The antigens of concern, being determined by genes, are specific for each individual and are located on the surfaces of nucleated cells and red blood cells. Erythrocyte antigens compose the ABO antigen system used in blood typing and matching in blood transfusions, and may be present in vascular endothelium of the graft. Blood groups must be identical in the UK for organ transplant.

The donor–recipient relationship is an important factor in influencing acceptance or rejection of a graft. In the 12 months preceding 31 March 2005, a total of 1783 people received a kidney transplant in the UK, of which 475 (27%) were given their kidney by a friend or relative (UK Transplant 2005b). The closer the relationship, the greater the possibility of compatibility. Because cellular proteins and antigens are specific for each individual, donor tissue is rejected by the recipient's body unless it is taken from an identical twin. In this case, the transplant is compatible because the antigens of both the host and donor are identical, having been determined by the same genetic blueprint of a single fertilized ovum. Such a graft (with identical cellular proteins and antigens) is referred to as an *isograft*. A graft between two genetically dissimilar persons is known as an *allograft* or *homograft*.

The antigens located on the nucleated cells belong to the system designated HLA (human leucocyte antigen). These antigens, present on cell membranes of most tissues, are easily detected on leucocytes, which are readily accessible for tissue typing and clinical tests for histocompatibility of potential donor tissue. Histocompatibility may be understood as the ability of cells to be accepted and to function in a new situation. Normally, the HLA antigens would be recognized as foreign by the T lymphocytes of the recipient's immune system. This would lead to the production of killer T cells and subsequently antibody-secreting B lymphocytes.

Tissue typing is the typing of antigens of the recipient and each potential donor. Antigens are identified by mixing lymphocytes with a series of standard sera that contain HLA antibodies. The reaction of the donor's and patient's cells to each serum is observed; lysis of the cells indicates that the antigen is specific to the known antibody. The patient's HLA typing is then compared with that of the donor. The closer the match, the less the T-cell response and the better the chance of a successful outcome. It is estimated that this technique improves the success rate by at least 10% or, put another way, permits some 200 extra transplants each year in the UK alone (Dyer 2000).

The importance of HLA tissue typing becomes apparent when the high incidence of renal failure amongst the Asian population of the UK is recalled (see p. 615). Because of the presence of certain very low frequency HLA antigens in the Asian population, tissue typing is difficult. The situation is exacerbated by the low frequency of donors amongst the Asian population owing to the mistaken belief that their religion forbids it. The opposite is true as Hinduism, Islam and Sikhism all approve of the practice (Whyte 2000). As Dyer (2000) has pointed out, this means that if transplant centres are to carry out transplants on Asian patients they have to accept an HLA mismatch and possibly lower success rates.

ABO blood typing identifies the red blood cell antigens present in the recipient and donor. Antigens are identified when agglutination occurs on exposure of red blood cells to serum containing identified antibodies.

Donor In early transplants, the kidney was always obtained from a live blood relative. Now, cadavers serve as the principal donor source. The cadaver is frequently an accident victim or someone who has had a sudden death and who is known to have been in good health.

If a living donor is used, he or she is usually related to the patient. The donation is more likely to be successful if the relative is close (e.g. sibling, parent) than if the donor is a genetically non-related person (e.g. cousin).

The demand for kidneys is much greater than the supply, and locally available kidneys may not be immunologically compatible. An established central service or register is maintained; persons with end-stage renal failure are registered with their tissue and blood types. When a locally available kidney is not compatible, one that matches may become available in another part of the country and is obtained through the UK transplant centre based in Bristol. Because of the demand for kidney transplants, various educational programmes have been organized to alert the public to the need for donors.

Legal and ethical considerations include the need for donation consent and the determination of death. Organ donation cards making a gift of any organ for the purpose of transplantation in the event of death can be completed and carried at all times. These cards are available from surgeries, most healthcare settings and public buildings, and are sometimes displayed in shops and public houses. In addition, people in the UK can now let their wishes be known when they register with at a new GP surgery or when they renew their driving license. In January 2005, 12 million people in the UK were registered with the organ donor scheme (UK Transplant 2005c). Nurses can play a significant role in encouraging the general public to participate in this programme, particularly by working with Asian communities where the problem is most acute (see above). The next of kin may also provide written authorization for the donation of organs if death is imminent. Laws in most countries define brain death, and policies are established to ensure independence of the doctors treating the donor patient from the transplant team. Most regions now have a transplant coordinator who is responsible for coordination of organ transfer. This person will often meet the potential donor, next of kin and ward staff, and is responsible for feedback of information to them after the transplant. The coordinator also has a very important role in the education, not only of the medical and nursing staff, but also of the general public to encourage greater referral of potential donors.

When death occurs, the kidneys are removed with their arteries, veins and ureters. The blood vessels are flushed out with an 'extracellular' electrolyte solution such as Ringer's lactate.

The organs are kept cool during transport and storage, until implantation. Transplantation should be done within 72 hours of obtaining the kidney from the donor. Storage for up to 2–3 days requires pump oxygenator perfusion. When a cadaver kidney is used in transplant, the source remains anonymous to the recipient and the family.

Transplant procedure   The donor kidney is placed in the recipient's iliac fossa, usually on the side opposite to that from which it was taken: that is, a left donor kidney is placed in the recipient's right iliac fossa (Fig. 19.8).

The patient's own kidneys are removed if there is recurrent infection or uncontrolled hypertension. Polycystic kidneys may need to be removed to provide room for the graft. Usually this will have been performed while the patient awaits transplantation.

When a person is selected as a candidate for a renal transplant, a full and detailed discussion with the surgeon is necessary. The patient and family are informed of what is entailed in the operation: that the kidney graft may be rejected, necessitating the resumption of a maintenance dialysis programme; that continuous drug therapy and close supervision will be needed; and that precautions against infections will be necessary. The patient is encouraged to be as fit as possible whilst awaiting a transplant. This may involve taking calorie supplements to improve nutritional status.

If the patient's anaemia is severe, blood transfusions may be given. Controversy exists as to whether blood should be

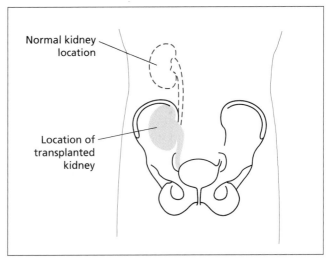

Figure 19.8   Location of a transplanted kidney.

given; transfusions are believed to increase graft survival but may also cause pre-sensitization.

The patient's family's level of anxiety is assessed. The patient receiving a cadaver graft will have little notice before the actual operation. Preparations must be made quickly but opportunity is provided for the person to review the decision and to ask questions and share feelings. A consent form will be completed.

Deep breathing and coughing are taught and practised and the patient is informed about what to expect after the operation. If the person is known to have respiratory problems, baseline blood gases will be measured before surgery. Immunosuppressive drug therapy is commenced before operation and maintained afterwards. The regimen consists of a number of medications including, azathioprine, prednisolone and ciclosporin. A central venous pressure line will be established under anaesthetic so that the intravascular fluid volume can be monitored during and after operation. A retention (Foley) catheter is introduced into the bladder in the theatre under strict aseptic conditions for accurate monitoring of urine output.

Nursing intervention   The nursing care of the patient who has received a kidney transplant includes measures to maintain fluid balance, kidney function, prevention of infection and assessment for possible graft rejection and other complications. The immediate care is the same as that for any patient recovering from anaesthesia.

Assessment   Vital signs, urinary output, fluid intake and electrolyte concentrations are monitored, and frequent observations are made for bleeding from the wound and early signs of infection and rejection. A renal scan is performed the day after operation to provide a baseline for graft function.

Maintenance of fluid balance and kidney function
The retention catheter is connected to a sterile closed-drainage system; the urinary output is recorded hourly.

Frequent urinalyses and cultures are made and 24-hour urine specimens may be obtained for measurement of creatinine clearance.

The transplanted kidney usually begins to excrete urine soon after the operation. The volume may increase rapidly, resulting in profuse diuresis. The patient may experience bladder spasm and pain with the large urine volume, because the bladder has not been used to receiving urine for some time before surgery. If the transplant fails to excrete sufficient urine for several days, haemodialysis or peritoneal dialysis may be used until kidney function improves. Fluid and electrolyte restrictions are required until adequate urine volume has been achieved. Once kidney function appears to be stabilized, the hourly measurement can be discontinued. The catheter is removed, normally at about 4–5 days. The person is encouraged to void frequently to avoid overdistension of the bladder and pressure on the ureteral implantation area. If the patient's own kidneys have been retained, consideration must be given to their usual output when assessing the function of the graft kidney. The patient's weight is recorded daily and changes noted.

Prevention of infection   The person is receiving immunosuppressive medications and is at greater risk of infection. The application of good asepsis is stressed; thorough handwashing is important before each contact with the patient. Infection risk remains high in the long term and problems such as pneumonia, food poisoning, chickenpox, urinary tract infections and late infection with cytomegalovirus (CMV) some 6 months after transplant are cause for particular concern. Late CMV infection is an opportunistic infection that can lead to loss of the transplanted organ (Hasselder 1999).

Because the patient's immune system is suppressed, normal inflammatory responses to infection may not occur. The patient's skin and oral mucosa are examined frequently for redness, swelling, drainage, warmth and tenderness. The temperature is taken every 4 hours and the patient is asked to report any pain or discomfort. The white blood cell count is monitored frequently and, if severely depressed, protective measures may be instituted and immunosuppressive therapy decreased for a brief period.

The patient is required to carry out regular frequent periods of deep breathing and coughing, and ambulation is encouraged. Early removal of central venous lines and the urethral catheter eliminates potential sources of infection and facilitates ambulation. Mouth care should be carried out regularly, particularly after meals.

Rejection   Early manifestations of the rejection process may occur on the second or third day. There may be swelling and increasing tenderness over the kidney, fever, general malaise, headache, an increase in the leucocyte count, anorexia, decreased urinary output, hypertension, oedema and raised levels of serum creatinine, sodium and potassium, and of blood urea concentration.

The intensity of the rejection process and the rapidity with which it develops correspond to the degree of difference between the recipient's and donor's cellular antigens; the greater the difference, the more severe and rapid is the rejection:

Hyperacute rejection occurs within minutes or hours of the transplant, due to preformed antibodies attacking the homograft. This severe type of reaction may be attributed to presensitization to donor antigens as a result of previous transfusions or several pregnancies.

Acute or early rejection may develop up to months after the transplantation. Oliguria and increasing blood urea and creatinine levels are manifested. Rejection can usually be reversed by increased dosage of immunosuppressive drugs.

Late rejection develops insidiously after 3 or 4 months, or it may occur several years after the homograft was received. This type of rejection is characterized by arterial impairment due to intimal hyperplasia. It is attributed to chronic reaction between circulating antibodies and the antigens of the vascular endothelial cells. This process cannot be reversed with medication.

Prevention of rejection   The dosage of azathioprine and prednisolone is adjusted according to the leucocyte count and the patient's reactions to these drugs. It is necessary for the nurse to be familiar with their side-effects. Azathioprine may depress the bone marrow production of leucocytes and produce leucopenia. Ciclosporin A is severely nephrotoxic and so blood levels are monitored closely. It may also produce hepatic impairment and lymphomas.

Immunosuppression can lead to the development of glucose intolerance in 20% of patients and even diabetes in some; consequently, blood glucose levels should be monitored closely (Hasselder 1999).

When rejection is suspected, the patient is given higher doses of prednisolone, which may be given intravenously as well as orally. Plasma exchange may be carried out to remove antibodies and immune complexes and thus reduce the rejection response. This will depend on the patient's original disease. If the reaction is severe and there is marked fluid retention and an increase in serum potassium and creatinine and blood urea levels, dialysis may have to be resumed. Fluid intake and dietary restrictions may also be necessary.

If the rejection process is irreversible, the immunosuppressive drugs are discontinued and the graft may be removed. The patient may well become discouraged and the nurse should be prepared to offer support and reassure the patient that a second graft may be considered.

Other medications   Most medications are eliminated through the kidneys, so as few drugs as possible are given following renal transplantation. Small doses of an analgesic may be prescribed, if necessary, for the relief of pain and discomfort when nursing measures do not provide adequate palliation.

Patient education for health management   The patient may become apprehensive about leaving the hospital and becoming independent. The need to follow a prescribed pattern of living indefinitely, and the need to be constantly alert for early signs of rejection and complications, may provoke considerable anxiety. Consequently, a good teaching programme for both patient and family is essential. The patient should fully understand the drug regimen that will be required after discharge. Careful self-monitoring of weight and fluid output is essential, and the patient should be advised about simple measures to reduce the risk of infections (e.g. regular handwashing).

The early signs of rejection are reviewed with the patient and family. By this time, the patient is usually quite familiar with them and realizes that prompt action is necessary. The patient and family are cautioned to report immediately a cold, sore throat, fever, dysuria, frequency or other disturbance that may indicate infection. The patient is also urged to contact the unit promptly if there is a sudden gain in weight (e.g. 1 kg in 1 day), swelling of the ankles or puffiness of the face, pain, tenderness and/or swelling in the area of the graft, decrease in urinary output, headache, unaccounted for fatigue, or increased temperature.

After discharge, the patient is followed closely by visits to the outpatient department at least once a week, because constant surveillance plays an important role in progress and the development of acceptance of the situation with less fear. If progress is satisfactory, and understanding and efficient management of care are demonstrated, the intervals between visits are gradually lengthened. The patient and family may appreciate information regarding self-help organizations such as the British Kidney Patient Association.

Complications   Complications include all those associated with steroid therapy and the risk of rejection.

The National Kidney Federation (2001) estimate that over 90% of live donor kidney transplants are still working well after 12 months; 10 years after transplantation 84% of grafts from a living sibling with an identical HLA match are still working, as are 80% of those with a half match. If the kidney has been retrieved from a cadaver, only 47% will have survived after 10 years. Grafts from unrelated donors have a 6-year graft survival of 78%.

OTHER DISORDERS OF RENAL FUNCTION

Glomerulonephritis

This disease is usually characterized by a diffuse, non-infectious inflammation of the glomeruli of both kidneys. As the blood supply that supports the tubules normally passes through glomerular capillaries before reaching them, fibrous scarring and obliteration of some glomeruli lead to secondary degenerative changes in the associated tubules, blood vessels and interstitial tissues.

Causes

The glomerular injury is usually caused by immunological processes. Three major immunological mechanisms are recognized:

1 Antigen-antibody complexes formed extrarenally are trapped in glomeruli and initiate the inflammatory process; this is a common reaction responsible for glomerulonephritis.
2 Antibodies are formed against an antigen in or produced by the glomerular basement membrane, initiating glomerular inflammation.
3 Activation of the alternative complement pathway.

A common cause of glomerulonephritis is the β-haemolytic streptococcus, although a wide range of other infectious organisms have been implicated as possible causes. The patient's history usually reveals that the renal disturbance follows an infection, such as a sore throat or respiratory infection of some form, by a latent period of 2–4 weeks. In some instances, the infection may have been so mild that little or no attention was given to it at the time.

Clinical characteristics

The onset of glomerulonephritis is generally abrupt but in some instances may be insidious. The affected glomeruli are partially or completely obstructed, resulting in reduced filtration. Some glomeruli rupture, permitting the escape of blood into the tubules. The permeability of the glomeruli that remain patent is increased. The scant output of urine is cloudy and contains albumin, blood cells and casts.

Oedema develops and is usually seen first in the periorbital areas and ankles. The patient complains of pain and tenderness in the back, headache and weakness. Visual disturbances may also be manifested. The blood pressure is raised, and decreased filtration results in a gradual accumulation of nitrogenous wastes in the blood; the blood urea and serum creatinine levels may be increased.

Neurological signs and symptoms corresponding to the degree of hypertension may be present. Unless the renal insufficiency is reversed, uraemia, pulmonary oedema and cardiac failure may ensue.

Management

The treatment of patients with acute glomerulonephritis consists mainly of rest, fluid and diet regulation, and chemotherapy to eliminate possible residual streptococcal infection. The daily fluid intake is restricted to 400–500 mL in excess of the urinary output of the previous 24 hours. The blood chemistry is followed closely and the sodium, potassium and chloride intake regulated according to the findings. The patient receives a high carbohydrate diet to reduce the breakdown of tissue protein. Protein may be provided in the form of essential amino acid or keto analogues to achieve nitrogen balance. Similarly, salt restriction in the diet is regulated according to the degree of oedema and hypertension.

If the low output of urine is prolonged and the blood potassium and nitrogenous waste levels are progressively increasing, diuretic therapy is initiated or peritoneal dialysis or haemodialysis may be instituted.

Plasma exchange may be carried out to remove antibodies and immune complexes because the disorder is usually caused by immunological processes. Precautions are necessary to protect the patient from exposure to infection. A superimposed infection could aggravate the disease or cause pneumonia that could prove fatal.

The frequent association of glomerulonephritis with respiratory infections emphasizes their potential danger and the importance of prevention and prompt, adequate treatment of such infections. Too often they are ignored, considered as unavoidably seasonal and treated very lightly. Women who have a history of acute glomerulonephritis are advised to consult a doctor before planning a pregnancy, as they are more likely to develop toxaemia and eclampsia.

The majority of patients with acute glomerulonephritis associated with infection (e.g. streptococcal) recover with no residual kidney disease. These patients generally show an increase in the volume of urine and a decrease in the blood pressure and serum urea levels within 1 week. The albuminuria and microscopic haematuria may persist for much longer. A few patients progress through a subacute phase to chronic glomerulonephritis. Others may be asymptomatic for a period of months or years and then experience an insidious development of the chronic disease which may progress to chronic renal failure.

Pyelonephritis

This is an inflammation of the pelvis and parenchymal tissue of the kidney due to infection. The predominant causative organism is *Escherichia coli*. Other causative agents are the *Proteus* species, *Klebsiella*, staphylococci or streptococci. The infective organisms have usually invaded the lower urinary tract and ascended to the kidney via the ureters. In rare instances, the pathogen, such as the staphylococci or streptococci, may be blood-borne.

Significant predisposing factors are defective urinary drainage and reflux of urine from the bladder into the ureters. Obstructions to the flow of urine from the kidney may be the result of a renal calculus, neoplasm, stricture of a ureter due to pressure, scarring or congenital anomaly. Stasis of urine in the lower urinary tract due to bladder or urethral dysfunction may increase the intravesical pressure sufficiently to produce a reflux into the ureters.

Pyelonephritis is more common in females than males. The incidence is relatively high in female infants and children, due perhaps to faecal soiling and *E. coli* contamination of the urethral meatus. Its frequent occurrence in pregnant women is attributed to stasis of urine incurred by pressure from the enlarging uterus and atonia of the ureters due to the effect of progesterone. It may also occur following urethral catheterization; infection introduced into the bladder may ascend through the ureters to the kidney. Pyelonephritis in males in the later years of life is generally associated with defective urinary drainage as a result of an enlarged prostate.

Clinical characteristics

The onset is usually sudden. In children, it may be accompanied by a convulsion. Manifestations include chills, fever, headache, nausea and vomiting, pain and tenderness in the loins, leucocytosis, and frequent and painful micturition (dysuria). The urine is cloudy and contains bacteria, pus, blood and epithelial cells.

Treatment

The patient is encouraged to take liberal amounts of fluid unless there is complete obstruction of urinary drainage. An accurate record of the fluid intake and output is necessary. A culture will be made of the urine and the causative organism antibiotic sensitivity determined. Antibiotic therapy is prescribed.

Unless there is complete eradication of the infection, pyelonephritis may become chronic with insidious destruction of nephrons, leading to chronic renal failure and uraemia. After the initial episode of acute pyelonephritis, the patient generally undergoes a thorough investigation for a predisposing obstructive lesion. Antimicrobial therapy and a high fluid intake are needed beyond the disappearance of acute signs and symptoms in order to ensure complete eradication of the infective organism. Specimens of urine are examined and cultured at regular intervals after the antimicrobial drug is discontinued.

Tuberculosis of the kidney

Tubercular infection in the kidney is usually secondary to tuberculosis elsewhere in the body; most often the primary site is a lung or lymph node. It is, however, very rare in the UK. The tubercle bacilli are carried by the blood to the kidneys. Scattered characteristic granulomatous lesions (tubercles) develop, eroding renal tissue and leaving cavitations. The infection may spread to involve the bladder and multiple strictures may develop in the urinary tract.

The patient receives a prolonged, intensive course of anti-tuberculous drugs and should be observed for possible reactions to the drugs, which may take the form of dermatitis, fever, dizziness and impaired hearing. A nutritious full diet is encouraged without restrictions if there is adequate renal function to prevent oedema, hypertension and the accumulation of wastes in the blood. Frequent urine smears and cultures are made to determine the progress of the patient's disease. Treatment is continued for a period of 12–18 months even if the cultures become negative for tubercle bacilli.

The nephrotic syndrome (nephrosis)

The characteristic symptoms of the nephrotic syndrome are proteinuria (more than 3.5 g protein in 24 hours), hypoproteinaemia and oedema. It may develop in a patient with primary renal disease, or may be associated with other conditions in which kidney involvement is secondary. Systemic disorders (e.g. diabetes mellitus, systemic lupus erythematosus and amyloidosis), circulatory disturbances and infections are some of the causes.

The proteinuria, which is chiefly albumin, is the result of some change in the glomeruli that causes an increase in their permeability to the plasma proteins. Obviously, the loss of the proteins reduces the colloidal osmotic pressure of the blood, contributing to increased movement of fluid into the interstitial spaces as well as to its decreased re-absorption into the capillaries. The resulting decrease in intravascular volume leads to retention of sodium and water by the kidneys.

The urine is reduced in volume and usually contains casts as well as large amounts of albumin. In contrast to other forms of impaired renal function, the blood pressure and nitrogenous waste levels of patients usually remain within a normal range in the absence of advanced damage to glomeruli.

The severity of the nephrotic syndrome is variable. In some, the oedema may cause only slight puffiness in the periorbital areas and ankles, yet in others, it may be so extreme that ascites (accumulation of fluid in the peritoneal cavity) and pleural effusion develop. The oedematous areas are generally soft and readily pit on pressure. The patient is usually pale, may be breathless, complains of fatigue and may experience anorexia, which further complicates the problem of hypoproteinaemia. Susceptibility to infection increases and the incidence of venous thrombosis is greater as anticoagulant substances are lost in the urine. The onset may be insidious or abrupt.

Treatment

When the nephrotic syndrome is secondary, the treatment is directed towards the likely prime cause and inducing diuresis, reducing oedema, producing and maintaining a normal serum albumin level. Diuretics will help reduce oedema and the patient's diet should contain a full quota of protein.

The patient is particularly susceptible to infection because of the lowered resistance of oedematous tissues and reduced plasma g-globulin which is essential in the formation of antibodies. Precautions are necessary to avoid exposure to infection.

The patient is not usually hospitalized once a satisfactory therapeutic regimen has been established, nor confined to bed; activity is encouraged. Treatment is generally required over a long period, and frequent medical check-ups are necessary.

Nephrolithiasis (renal calculi)

Stones or small concretions may develop in the collecting tubules, calyces or the pelvis of a kidney. They are formed by the precipitation of various substances in the urine; if retained, the initial precipitation forms a nucleus or matrix which promotes further precipitation and calculus enlargement. The substances commonly involved in calculus formation are calcium, oxalate, phosphate, uric acid, cystine, xanthine and ammonia, but most often the stones are of mixed composition (e.g. mixed phosphates and oxalates). They vary in size from tiny particles to large smooth or irregular masses. The irregular stone that forms in the pelvis and has projections into the calyces is referred to as a *staghorn calculus*. The usual composition of the latter type of calculus is phosphate.

Causes

The constituents of renal calculi are present in normal urine; any condition that increases their concentration, reduces their solubility or promotes retention of the urinary salts favours their precipitation, calculus formation and possible obstruction to urinary flow. Conditions favourable to their formation include hypercalcaemia, as occurs with hyperparathyroidism, excessive vitamin D, an excessive ingestion of milk or an alkali, and prolonged immobilization. Other causes include dehydration, a highly acid urine and infection by *Proteus* (Gram-negative bacteria usually associated with faeces). *Proteus* infection makes the urine alkaline; this results in the precipitation of phosphates, forming what may be referred to as a *struvite calculus*.

Symptoms

The manifestations of renal calculus depend upon the size of the stone and whether it remains stationary. It may remain latent over a long period, producing no symptoms. Small gravel-like stones may be passed without any disturbance.

The majority cause some pain, haematuria, infection and, if large, kidney damage and renal insufficiency. Renal calculi may obstruct renal drainage by impaction of the tubules, by completely filling calyces and the pelvis, or by lodging in a ureter. The urine accumulates in the pelvis and tubules, dilating them and creating a back pressure; this condition is known as *hydronephrosis*. Compression of the blood vessels and nephrons by the mass of fluid leads to their destruction and obliteration, and to renal insufficiency.

The patient may complain of pain in the back, which may be caused by irritation of tissues by movement of the stone or by the back pressure and accumulation of fluid if the stone is obstructing renal or ureteral outflow. A small stone may enter the ureter and initiate *ureteric colic*. The patient complains of excruciating pain radiating from the back to the front along the groin into the genitalia; this may be associated with pallor, sweating, restlessness and vomiting.

Haematuria results from injury to the membranous lining of the pelvis or ureter. Infection is frequently associated with a calculus and, if present, chills, fever, leucocytosis and pyuria are likely to be manifested.

Complete obstruction of the kidney outflow is eventually reflected in renal insufficiency and a palpable mass in the renal area as a result of the hydronephrosis. The total volume of urine is less than normal, and blood investigations indicate reduced elimination of waste products.

Investigation of the patient for nephrolithiasis includes: midstream specimen of urine for culture and sensitivity, ultrasonography, abdominal radiography, intravenous urography or pyelography, and sometimes cystoscopy with retrograde pyelography. Serum calcium and uric acid levels are determined and renal function tests may be done. Investigation includes 24-hour urine studies for calcium, phosphorus, uric acid, creatinine and sodium oxalate.

Treatment and nursing intervention

If the urogram indicates that the calculus is small and may be passed by the patient, activity and large amounts of fluids are encouraged. All urine is strained through several layers of gauze or a filter paper and is observed. All sediment or solid particles passed are saved and submitted for identification of their composition.

During an attack of ureteric colic, the patient usually receives an analgesic, such as pethidine, to relieve the pain, and an antiemetic. When the pain subsides, fluids should be encouraged once nausea is no longer a problem.

Modern techniques have made direct surgical removal of stones rare events. Percutaneous stone removal involves the introduction of a needle and other instrumentation under radiographic control, through the loin and into the kidney. Laser or ultrasound probes can be used to disintegrate the stone, permitting its piecemeal removal. This technique can be employed with access being gained via the urethra and bladder (retrograde removal). An alternative approach is known as *extracorporeal shockwave lithotripsy* (ESWL). Ultrasound shockwaves are focused on the stone to shatter it, the fragments then being passed naturally.

Calculi are prone to recur in patients with a history of previous episodes. In an effort to prevent the formation of new stones or the enlargement of existing stones a high fluid intake of at least 3000 mL daily is essential to maintain a dilute urine. A portion of this should be taken at bedtime and during the night to prevent the concentration of urine that normally occurs at night. High levels of uric acid are associated with calcium oxalate stones in some patients, and the administration of potassium citrate may help. This makes the urine alkaline and increases the solubility of uric acid, reducing the risk of uric acid crystals acting as the nuclei of new stones.

If the patient should become ill, prolonged immobility should be avoided as the effects of immobility on calcium metabolism increase the probability of stone formation.

Neoplasms in the kidneys

Neoplasms in the adult kidney are of lower incidence than those in many other areas of the body. When they occur, they are usually malignant and are seen more often in males than in females. Cancer Research UK (2006a) states that cancer of the kidney is a relatively rare cancer. Nonetheless, they estimate that the incidence is on the increase and that 6600 people are diagnosed annually and 3600 people die each year from the condition. Tumours may arise in parenchyma or the collecting system of the kidney. The most common form of parenchymal tumours in adults is adenocarcinoma. It readily invades the blood vessels, causing early metastases to bones, lungs or liver, which may be the lesion that brings the person to the doctor. Tumours that arise in the renal pelvis and ureter are the same histologically as bladder cancer; 85% are transitional cell in origin, the remainder being squamous cell or adenocarcinoma-type cancers. Tumours of the renal pelvis and ureter are ten times less common than those developing in the bladder.

Clinical characteristics

In the adult, the first symptom is usually haematuria. As the neoplasm enlarges, the kidney becomes a palpable mass and the patient experiences pain, abdominal discomfort from pressure, anorexia and loss of weight. Ureteric colic may occur as a result of a blood clot entering the ureter. Polycythaemia develops in some patients because of an overproduction of erythropoietin by the affected kidney. Others may have marked anaemia.

A cystoscopy with ureteric catheterization is done to determine whether the source of the bleeding is unilateral or bilateral. Radiological studies are undertaken, using intravenous or retrograde pyelography to determine filling defects and the location of the neoplasm. Renal angiography may also be done to assess the extent of blood vessel involvement. Renal ultrasonography may be performed to assess the nature of the lesion and allow visualization of the lesion to facilitate aspiration.

Treatment

Nephrectomy is the usual treatment for parenchymal tumours; treatment may also involve local lymph node dissection. When nephrectomy is not performed arterial embolization of the kidney may be used to cut off the main blood supply to the tumour. This is not a cure and is reserved for advanced disease (Cancer Research UK 2004). Radiotherapy may be used but its effectiveness with these tumours is debatable, except for prophylaxis of metastatic symptoms. Chemotherapy is only used in clinical trials as currently there is no evidence that it has a place in the treatment of cancer of the kidney. Immunotherapy with treatments such as interferon or interleukin 2 is currently being investigated to determine their value in treating these cancers but at this time, it use is restricted to patients with advanced disease (Cancer Research UK 2004).

Polycystic disease of the kidneys

This disorder is characterized by the widespread distribution of cysts of varying sizes throughout both kidneys. The disease is congenital and familial, and affects both sexes. It is predominant in infants and adults over 40 years of age. In infants and young children, other abnormalities may be present. The disease is often found in more than one member of the family and in successive generations. Because of the distinct difference in the age of the groups in which the disease is manifested, it is suggested that there are two different genetic types. When it occurs in infants and young children, it is considered to be autosomal recessive, but the polycystic disease that becomes manifest in adults is autosomal dominant.

THE PERSON WITH A DISORDER OF THE URINARY SYSTEM

CLINICAL CHARACTERISTICS

Clinical characteristics of impaired bladder function and urinary elimination include abnormal constituents in the urine and altered patterns of urinary elimination (functional, reflex, stress, total and urge incontinence, and urinary retention). Alterations in voiding may be related to infection in the urinary tract, emotional stress, a neurological disorder, bladder calculi, obstructive disease of the bladder or urethra and, rarely, chemicals excreted in the urine.

Abnormal constituents in urine

Blood, pus, microorganisms and mucus may be present in the urine as a result of inflammation, tissue necrosis or a malignancy in the lower urinary tract. The urine may be cloudy or blood coloured and have an ammoniacal odour.

Alteration in patterns of urinary elimination

Symptomatic changes in voiding include:

- frequency
- urgency
- nocturia
- dysuria
- residual urine
- alterations in urinary stream
- hesitancy
- retention
- incontinence.

Frequency, urgency, nocturia and dysuria

Irritation of the bladder or urethral mucosa may give rise to an abnormally frequent desire to void, urgency and painful micturition. Frequency due to a urological disturbance is generally accompanied by an *urgency*, which implies that there is an intense desire to void immediately. The normal voluntary control to retain the urine cannot be maintained, and some urine may escape before the person can reach the toilet or use a bedpan. *Dysuria* refers to the abnormal discomfort, pain, burning or smarting sensation that may accompany voiding. *Strangury* is a term used occasionally when the dysuria is unusually severe and there is increasing frequency of decreasing amounts of urine.

Residual urine

Micturition may not completely empty the bladder, leaving a residue of urine. This problem is diagnosed, and the amount determined, by catheterizing the patient immediately after voiding. Residual urine is usually the result of an obstruction to the bladder outlet and causes a stagnation that predisposes to bladder and kidney infection and calculus formation.

Alterations in the urinary stream and hesitancy

The person may have difficulty in initiating the urinary flow. This symptom of hesitancy is usually due to some obstruction in the bladder-urethral orifice or the urethra. Pressure within the bladder must be increased beyond the normal to force the urine past the obstructing lesion. Because of resistance to the urinary outflow, the muscle tires before the bladder is empty; after a few moments, it contracts again and voiding is resumed.

Retention of urine

The inability of a person to void is a relatively common problem. The distension of the bladder and stasis of urine predispose to the development of ureteric back pressure, reflux of urine into the ureters, and infection of the bladder and kidneys. The reaction of the bladder to progressive obstruction of the outflow is hypertrophy of the detrusor muscle. Diverticulae may develop; these are saccular protrusions of the mucosa between the muscle fibres. The sacs fill with urine, which becomes stagnant and readily infected. Calculi may also form within the diverticula.

Retention of urine is suspected if the person has had a normal fluid intake and has not voided within a period of 8–10 hours or if there is distension of the lower part of the abdomen. A distended bladder may also be present with frequent voiding of small amounts (30–50 mL), which is termed *retention with overflow*. The person may experience a constant desire to void but efforts to do so are ineffective.

URINARY INCONTINENCE

Incontinence is a symptom not a disease (Colley and Pomfret 2001). Estimates of the prevalence of urinary incontinence give a wide range of values. This is due to the difficulty in defining exactly what is meant by the term and reliance upon self-reporting with little external validation. Notwithstanding this difficulty, Dorey (2000) cites evidence showing a range of estimates of between 3.6% for men aged over 45 years up to 28% in men aged 90 years or more. The figures seem to be higher in women, and Brittain et al (2001) present data from various studies showing a range from 9% in women aged 20–59 years to 47% in a sample of women aged 30 years or more, the average being around 25–30%. It is difficult to extrapolate from these studies to the whole population with any precision, but we can estimate that several million people are affected by problems of urinary continence in the UK.

Incontinence probably goes untreated or unassessed because of embarrassment associated with social interaction and can exert severe stress both on the individual, partner and carers. Williams (2004) points out that, on average, it can take a woman up to 5 years to present with symptoms of stress incontinence. Urinary incontinence presents a real challenge to nurses to assist in improving the quality of life of a significant proportion of the population.

The classification of types of urinary incontinence can be confusing. It is better, therefore, to focus on the causes, which may be grouped under three headings (Cheater 1995):

- physiological causes
- extrinsic factors affecting bladder function
- intrinsic factors affecting bladder function.

Causes

Physiological

Instability of the detrusor muscle leading to spontaneous contraction, or contraction in response to a stimulus such as coughing, leads to micturition occurring with little or no warning. Urgency, frequency and substantial volumes of residual urine (i.e. urine left in the bladder after micturition) occur commonly.

Genuine *stress incontinence* is the other main physiological cause. It occurs when pressure in the bladder exceeds that in the urethra and is usually associated with a sudden rise in intra-abdominal pressure (e.g. sneezing or laughing). It is more common in females.

Other causes include damage to the spinal cord (neurogenic bladder) and obstruction of urinary outflow which leads to large volumes of residual urine and overflow.

Extrinsic

Limited mobility and dexterity, difficulty of access to toilet facilities, low expectations of carers and confusion can all contribute to incontinence.

Intrinsic

Faecal impaction can lead to compression of the bladder, exacerbating continence problems. A urinary tract infection or an endocrine disorder such as diabetes which causes polyuria can cause incontinence.

Urinary incontinence is a major health problem. It brings with it many hardships; not only is there the cost, but also the effort involved in maintaining hygiene and containing the problem, together with the emotional hardships in relation to the isolating and demeaning aspects of the problem.

It is generally acknowledged that most people with urinary incontinence can benefit from treatment, yet many receive only palliative remedies of protective pads and urinary appliances while the basic problem remains unidentified and untreated.

Nursing assessment

Urinary elimination is a personal and private activity; social norms and personal habits influence how individuals respond when problems develop with urinary emission. Patients may be uncomfortable and embarrassed discussing their problems and delay seeking assistance until some event finally triggers action. The main triggering events found by Brittain et al (2001) amongst a sample of 112 patients were:

- raised awareness of the issue and a service that could help as a result of publicity
- deterioration of their symptoms
- personal factors such as emotional difficulties, embarrassing events, anxiety over hygiene and awareness of age
- worries about their health
- the impact of incontinence on their social life.

The key findings here are that publicity campaigns which raise awareness of the problem can lead to many people seeking help. In assessing the patient, the nurse has to be sensitive to the personal significance of the problem to the patient and the impact it has on significant others in their life. Assessment should therefore include the individual's level of anxiety, feelings of discomfort or embarrassment; the nurse should acknowledge awareness of these feelings and reassure the patient that everything possible will be done to ease any embarrassment and provide privacy. It is also important to establish the terms and expressions used by the patient to describe the act of voiding and to ensure that the terminology used by the nurse is understood.

Patient history and subjective data

The person should be asked about their perception of the problem and how it affects their life. Tactfully, they should be asked to describe the symptoms they experience and to estimate how often and how much leakage occurs. Bowel habit should be discussed together with any previous surgical or medical history. Particularly relevant are any *family or personal history* of urinary system disorders or infections, diseases affecting the urinary system such as diabetes mellitus or hypertension, and the past use of drugs (either prescribed or bought over the counter). Women should be asked about their obstetric history because of the effects of pregnancy on the pelvic floor muscles. Functional factors such as whether a male patient is able to stand to void, ease of access to toilet facilities, and manual dexterity with buttons and zips should be explored (Dorey 2000).

Specific information about the person's usual and present *pattern of urinary elimination* is obtained. Information includes frequency of voiding, volume of urine excreted at each voiding and in a 24-hour period, and usual times of voiding. Any changes in the usual pattern of elimination such as nocturia or frequency are identified. The person is asked about the colour, odour and clarity of urine and whether there is any discomfort or pain associated with voiding. It is important to determine for how long the incontinence has been present.

Factors influencing urinary elimination

- *Past experiences and attitudes.* Urinary habits vary with each individual. The nurse should discuss the person's usual habits and attitudes to urinary elimination. The person may associate urinary incontinence with loss of control of body function, and see the problem as regression towards infancy; sensitivity on the nurse's part is therefore of paramount importance
- *Diet and fluid intake.* The volume of fluid intake has a direct effect on the urinary output. The person who suffers from incontinence may well restrict fluid intake in order to try to reduce the problem. Unfortunately, this may lead to dehydration and an increased risk of urinary tract infection (UTI). For patients with renal disorders it is important to identify usual eating habits and the relative amounts of protein and sodium in the daily diet
- *Lifestyle factors* that influence elimination include accessibility of toilet facilities, privacy and any unusual stresses associated with voiding
- *Activity, mobility and dexterity.* Physical activity is necessary to maintain muscle tone and normal amounts of calcium in the bones. Bedrest and immobility predispose to the formation of calculi. Impaired mobility and dexterity may interfere with the individual's ability to get to the toilet quickly enough to use it effectively

- *Level of awareness and orientation.* Confusion, disorientation and difficulty following directions may interfere with the individual's ability to respond appropriately to the urge to void as well as to meet fluid and nutritional needs
- *Medications.* The name, dosage, frequency and duration of use of any medications being taken are recorded. Diuretics have a direct effect on urine production, whereas sedatives may alter cognition.

Physical assessment

General appearance The patient is observed for general state of health, lethargy, fatigue and degree of alertness.

Urinary meatus and perineum The urethral orifice is observed for signs of drainage, oedema, redness or ulceration, and underclothing is examined for urine or other stains.

Bladder The bladder is not normally palpable but may be felt if it is overdistended. With the person supine, gently palpate the area just above the symphysis pubis; the distended bladder feels smooth and firm. When the bladder is distended, it is also possible to note a change in note on percussion. Palpation and percussion of a distended bladder causes increased discomfort for the patient.

Assessment of functional status The person's mobility, manual dexterity and communication skills are determined.

Box 19.6 lists the basic skills required by an individual to achieve control of micturition. The nurse and patient collectively identify which of these basic skills the patient possesses, where difficulties are encountered in the course of daily activities, and what measures and techniques the patient uses to compensate for these deficits and their effectiveness.

Analysis of medical and nursing assessments may demonstrate the need for further evaluation by members of the multidisciplinary team such as the continence nurse adviser, occupational therapist or speech therapist. Early referral to the continence nurse adviser may assist in the appropriate management of the incontinence, the supply of appliances or aids, and liaison with community services in anticipation of discharge to ensure continuity of care. The occupational therapist will evaluate the home environment and toilet facilities in relation to the patient's mobility, dexterity and awareness. Difficulties manipulating clothing are also identified. The speech therapist will assess communication skills and recommend means by which the patient can communicate needs. The role of nursing staff and relatives in contributing to the patient's incontinence is also assessed, especially in the institutionalized, the elderly and the disabled. An expectation of incontinence will probably result in incontinence: it becomes a self-fulfilling prophecy. Assistance to allow a schedule of regular voiding may be lacking, resulting in incontinence. Staff and family attitudes and relationships with the patient can be changed by helping them define expectations, set goals and develop strategies for dealing with the individual problem.

Clinical diagnostic measurements

Urine tests A random or midstream urine (MSU) specimen may be sent to the laboratory for routine and microscopic analysis.

Residual urine determination To identify overflow incontinence associated with urinary retention, an in-and-out catheterization is performed immediately after voiding. The amount of urine that remained in the bladder after the person voided is measured and recorded.

Urodynamic investigations These studies provide information on bladder sensation and detrusor muscle and urethral sphincter function. The tests consist of:

1 urine flow studies
2 pressure studies of both bladder and urethra (filling and voiding cystometry, urethral pressure profile)
3 video studies.

Uroflowmetry involves urine flow studies that measure the rate and volume of urine passed and usually include determination of the amount of residual urine in the bladder following voiding. This is a non-invasive procedure and it may need repeating to collect a series of results for comparison. *Cystometry* is a method of recording the bladder's responses to increasing distension. The investigation takes approximately 30 minutes and involves filling the bladder with normal saline whilst measuring the pressure changes in the abdomen and bladder. Synchronous video pressure flow cystourethrography or *videourodynamics* provides information not only on the pressure but also on the appearance of the bladder during the micturition cycle and is considered to be the gold standard for urodynamic investigation (Colley and Pomfret 2001). Patients can find these studies very embarrassing owing to the intimate nature of the procedure

---

Box 19.6 Basic skills required to achieve urinary continence

- The ability to initiate micturition voluntarily at an appropriate time
- The ability to delay, temporarily, the onset of micturition
- Perception of the urge to urinate well in advance of reflex voiding
- Awareness of socially acceptable places and/or circumstances to urinate
- The ability to communicate needs and interpret oral directions and written signs to get necessary assistance or locate the toilet
- The physical mobility and manual dexterity to reach the toilet, to assume and maintain body posture during micturition, adjust clothing, deal with doors, locks, flushing systems, seats and washing facilities.

and lack of privacy leading to severe anxiety (Shaw et al 2000).

Incontinence voiding record or diary

Documentation of the person's ability to void and episodes of incontinence may be obtained in the form of a patient diary or record kept by the individual, carers or nurse. The data are collected for several days to 2 weeks to enable analysis of the frequency of the incontinence and its relationship to fluid intake and physical and social activities and events. This record is useful in helping to develop a management programme appropriate to the needs of the individual.

Management

Interventions to reduce or manage urinary incontinence include:

- drug therapy
- pelvic floor exercises
- behavioural interventions
- protective pads and appliances
- surgery.

There are also a number of general measures that should be used in conjunction with these interventions to alleviate any contributing factors. These are listed in Box 19.7.

Medication

Anticholinergic agents such as tolterodine decrease smooth muscle activity of a hypertonic bladder and may be used to treat urge incontinence related to neurogenic impairment and detrusor muscle instability. For some patients treatment of their cough will solve the problem of their stress incontinence and therefore the medications used in management of problems of the respiratory system can ultimately solve the problem of stress incontinence in some cases.

Box 19.7 General measures directed to the alleviation of contributing factors to urinary incontinence

1 Weight reduction if the person is overweight.

2 Maintaining a fluid intake of at least 2000 mL/day.

3 Decreasing fluid intake if it has been excessive.

4 Review of medication for possible contributing factors and adjustment of these medications if necessary.

5 Adjustment of any diuretic therapy so that the action of the drugs occurs during the day.

6 Decrease in alcohol intake.

7 Institution of measures to suppress a chronic cough.

8 Treatment of any underlying urinary tract infections.

9 Increase in daily physical activity.

10 Prevention or treatment of constipation.

Pelvic floor exercises

Kegel exercises increase the tone of muscles involved in micturition. They may be taught to control stress incontinence in women. The person sits with the feet on the floor and knees apart and is instructed to tighten the perineal muscles, as if stopping the flow of urine, and to hold the muscle contraction and then relax. This involves the contraction and relaxation of the levator ani muscle. This exercise is repeated several times every 2–4 hours throughout the day. A feedback device may be used for patients who lack sensory input as it provides them with pressure readings, demonstrating the effectiveness of the muscle contractions. Some women may be offered vaginal cones to use in addition to the pelvic floor exercises. These are inserted into the vagina for up to 30 minutes twice a day and require pelvic floor contraction to keep them in place (Williams 2004).

Behavioural interventions

A *bladder training programme* is developed whenever possible with the active participation of the patient and family. A detailed chart or diary of urine frequency and volume, fluid intake, the times of fluid intake and voiding, and the circumstances surrounding incidents of incontinence is kept for several days. From this information, the nurse and patient can develop a voiding schedule and a plan that considers the person's needs and daily activities. Voiding normally occurs on arising in the morning, before or after meals, and before retiring in the evening. The voiding schedule may begin by having the person void every 1 or 2 hours, with the intervals increased gradually as control is acquired. The person's level of awareness and perception of the urge to void influence the degree of personal control that can be expected. When a patient is confused and disoriented, it is necessary for others to prompt the patient to follow the schedule and to provide assistance in tasks such as getting to the toilet and manipulating clothing.

Fluid intake of at least 2000 mL daily is maintained throughout the programme to avoid the risks of dehydration and urinary tract infection. Physical activity is increased.

Toilet facilities, a commode chair, bedpan or urinal should be within reach of the person, and privacy provided. An assessment of the home environment is done and recommendations made if necessary for modifications to the home or the purchase or loan of a commode chair or bedpan. A night light should be provided. Voiding should always take place in the usual sitting posture for females and standing posture for males, with the nurse or a relative providing the necessary assistance.

For those with flaccid, hypotonic bladders, *Credé's manoeuvre* is taught. The hands are placed flat over the abdomen below the umbilicus. Manual pressure is exerted over the bladder to initiate flow of urine. Suprapubic tapping or stroking of the thighs may also be used to stimulate reflex voiding when incontinence is the result of neurogenic dysfunction (reflex incontinence).

Suggestions are provided for adapting clothing for the person with impaired manual dexterity or the individual who has minimal time between the sensation or urge to void and the act of voiding (urge incontinence). The person may need instruction and practice with the manipulation of zippers, buttons or other aspects of clothing.

Positive reinforcement or contingency management is a behavioural approach using positive verbal and social reinforcement to establish continent behaviours. *Prompted voiding* and socialization are behavioural techniques that have been used effectively with female nursing home residents to decrease episodes of incontinence. The technique involves asking residents whether they need to void and, if so, assisting them with toileting. The schedule for prompting must be established for each individual in relation to their voiding pattern and activities.

Biofeedback, used alone or in combination with bladder training and positive reinforcement, has been shown to be effective in the treatment of stress and urge incontinence. This procedure provides the person with information about bladder and abdominal pressures which is useful in learning to inhibit bladder contractions voluntarily. This method is most effective when used with cognitively aware individuals.

Protective pads and appliances Various aids are used in the management of incontinence. Self-control of continence cannot be achieved for every patient. Some may continuously require protective measures. Others may require protective measures during assessment and treatment or during periods of illness. Many protective devices and aids are available.

Protective pants and pads Underpads may be used on bedlinen or furniture, or pads are available to be worn by the person. Various types of waterproof pants and pads are also available. Each type is designed to meet a specific need and the absorbency of the various pads varies. The marsupial pants (Kanga pants) are designed with a waterproof pouch to hold the pad in place. Most products are available in a variety of sizes and styles, and some are disposable while others are washable. Use and selection of pants and pads must be individualized and requires the individual's interest and cooperation. Protection of clothing allows the patient to dress normally and participate in social functions. The use of pads or plastic pants for adults may be demeaning and serve to promote feelings of dependence and withdrawal if their use is not discussed and agreed with the person. Sanitary towels are not designed to contain urine and are inappropriate, ineffective and an expensive means of containing incontinence. Patients should be assessed carefully because a wide range of aids exists and it is important to find the right product for each individual.

External urinary drainage devices A condom with an attached drainage bag is useful for men. It may be worn only at night or during the day under clothing; care must be taken to select an appropriately sized condom. The penis is checked frequently for oedema, redness or excoriation. Colley and Pomfret (2001) summarize the value of penile sheaths and urinary collection devices as follows:

C   Cost effective
O   Odour-proof method of management
N   Non-invasive
D   Disposable and discreet
O   On prescription
M   Male image
S   Sexuality preserving

A female external urine collecting device is available. It has an adhesive plate similar to a stoma wafer with an integral pouch which can be attached to a collecting bag. Wear times achieved by this device vary and mobility can be restricted. In order to achieve adherence, the skin around the external genitalia is shaved and a skin-protective gel is applied.

Catheter Catheterization as a means of controlling incontinence is not considered until other alternatives have been tried. An indwelling catheter may be used in some instances to permit increased independence for the patient. For long-term use the catheter should be made of silicone or coated with silicone-elastomer or hydrogel as this produces less tissue inflammation. The smallest size possible should always be used (see p. 640 for a further discussion relating to catheterization).

Intermittent catheterization is an alternative to an indwelling catheter; the person or carer is taught to perform the procedure. The risk of infection is reduced with intermittent catheterization as opposed to an indwelling catheter. It is performed on a regular schedule which is determined in a similar manner to the bladder training schedule.

Electrical devices Electrical stimulators are receiving moderate attention as a means of increasing the tone of pelvic muscles. They create continuous contraction of the pelvic muscles which is relieved by releasing the electrical stimulation to facilitate voiding when desired.

Occlusive devices These are not satisfactory for long-term use. Penile clamps and an inflatable pad which applies pressure against the perineum to close the penile urethra are available for men.

Occlusive devices for females are vaginal tampons and an inflatable vaginal balloon which elevate the bladder neck and apply pressure on the urethra through the vagina and may be useful for minor stress incontinence or during periods of physical activity.

Surgery
Surgical intervention for incontinence is directed to the correction of anatomical defects that contribute to the incontinence (e.g. correction of obstructions in the urinary tract, repair of a cystocele, or uterine prolapse, or prostatic hypertrophy). Urethrovesical resuspension may be performed in women with severe stress incontinence. This procedure increases the support for the bladder and restores the closure of the bladder outlet. Sometimes urinary diversion is performed for uncontrollable incontinence. This is occasionally necessary following radiotherapy for bladder cancer, where the bladder becomes atrophied with a small capacity,

or for congenital malformations of the bladder (e.g. ectopic vesicae), or in spina bifida.

Artificial urethral sphincters can be implanted in men and women. Various types of devices are available but they generally consist of a cuff filled with fluid and a mechanism for diversion of the fluid when voiding is desired.

Nursing intervention

Effective management of urinary incontinence usually involves the collaborative efforts of a multidisciplinary team and the active participation of the individual and carers. The nurse is an important member of this team and is often in the best position to initiate and coordinate activities (Case Study 19.2).

CASE Betty Jarvis is a 76-year-old woman who was admitted to hospital for a total knee replacement. After the operation, the nursing staff noted that she was requesting the bedpan frequently and was often incontinent by the time they got to her.

Mrs Jarvis had a 10-year history of problems with urgency, frequency and incontinence of urine. She had had bladder surgery 8 years ago but this was effective only for the first year. When her symptoms returned she consulted her doctor who told her there was nothing further to be done and she would have to learn to live with it.

Assessment

Bladder. A post-voiding residual volume was requested to determine how well Mrs Jarvis was emptying her bladder. A toileting routine was instituted for the next 48 hours to assess the amount and frequency of voiding. Mrs Jarvis voided 50–75 mL every 2 hours and the frequency increased in direct relation to her intake. In the initial postoperative phase she had an intravenous infusion at 100 mL per hour and was voiding every half hour; once the infusion was stopped this decreased to every 2 hours.

Bowel. Mrs Jarvis stated that her bowels had not moved since before the operation 5 days previously. An abdominal assessment and rectal examination were done. Her abdomen was distended, with bowel sounds present, and was firm on palpation. The rectum was full of very hard, constipated stool.

Once the assessment was complete, it was determined that Mrs Jarvis was voiding small amounts frequently with a normal post-voiding residual volume and was considered to have detrusor instability. The instability was being further exacerbated by her faecal impaction.

Intervention

Mrs Jarvis was put on a bowel programme to resolve the constipation. She was also started on an anticholinergic medication to reduce the irritability of her bladder, thus allowing an increase in voided volumes and the time between voiding. A post-voiding residual volume was determined 5 and 10 days after the start of the anticholinergic treatment to ensure that she was not in retention.

Evaluation

Mrs Jarvis was discharged home 3 weeks after operation and was delighted to have regained her continence after so many years.

Assessment

Assessment is the key to identification of the problem and to determining accurately the type of incontinence and the contributing factors. The nurse plays a vital role in the assessment process in identifying individuals at risk for or with incontinence and in promoting recognition that a problem exists. The nurse is able to document the person's patterns of urinary elimination over a period of time and identify factors associated with the in-continent episodes. The nurse assumes responsibility for ongoing patient assessment and thus reassesses the need for indwelling catheters and ensures that they are removed as early as possible once the reason for their insertion is resolved.

Development of the patient plan of care

The nurse should collaborate with the person and family to develop an effective plan to manage the person's urinary incontinence. Patient and family input is necessary to establish realistic goals and to develop a plan to meet the needs, activities and lifestyle of the patient and family members.

Self-concept

Urinary incontinence has a negative impact on the individual's self-esteem and self-concept. Studies of the prevalence of incontinence recognize that many cases are hidden. They are not identified because the person is reluctant to disclose the information. One of the more constructive interventions the nurse can perform is to get the person and family to talk about the problem and to recognize that in-continence is not a normal consequence of ageing or childbirth and that something can be done to help them. Plans for managing the incontinence should consider the impact of the problem on the person's social activities and include strategies for increased socialization.

Patient and family teaching

Patients and families generally lack information about the nature of urinary incontinence and its management. Patients and families need help to develop self-care skills related to the numerous products and appliances used to control the incontinence. Not all patients want to learn or are capable of learning about their incontinence and its management. Assessment of learning needs should be ongoing to identify when and whether the patient is ready for further information.

URINARY RETENTION

Urinary retention means the person is unable to empty his or her bladder fully. It is characterized by a distended bladder and a sensation of bladder fullness. The person may be unable to void when fluid intake has been adequate, may experience difficulty with starting a stream of urine, or bladder emptying may be incomplete. The person may void frequent small amounts of urine and may experience dribbling. It may be described as a type of incontinence (urinary incontinence with overflow).

Retention may be related to obstructive disease of the bladder or urethra (usually due to enlargement of the prostate gland with ageing in men; see below), surgical intervention or neurogenic disease (Box 19.8).

Benign prostatic hypertrophy

Obstructive disease of the bladder is caused by benign prostatic hypertrophy (BPH), a common condition in later life which affects a high proportion of men. As the prostate gland enlarges it interferes with normal urinary outflow from the bladder. The condition is insidious in onset with the person becoming aware of increasing difficulty in passing urine; dribbling and frequency may develop. In time, chronic retention may occur where the person has a large residual volume of urine in the bladder which then becomes prone to infection. Alternatively, acute retention may intervene; in this situation the patient will have a distended lower abdomen and be in acute pain and distress as he is unable to pass any urine.

It is important, therefore, in assessing any man aged over 50 years, to enquire carefully about any changes in micturition, remembering the possible embarrassment this may cause the patient. This is an area where the nurse has a vital role in the early detection of symptoms and referral for medical treatment in addition to having a strong health education role.

The surgical treatment of BPH involves *transurethral resection of the prostate* (TURP), whereby a cutting diathermy instrument is introduced via a cystoscope and under direct vision the hypertrophied prostate is tunnelled through to enlarge the opening from the bladder and allow normal urinary drainage. Postoperative care is concerned with ensuring that drainage from the catheter is kept free and not blocked by any clots that may form and lead to clot retention. Bladder irrigation using a two-way catheter is therefore required and care must be given to ensuring that the patient regains normal bladder control when the catheter is removed (pp. 645, 646). A more detailed discussion about BPH and the significance of PSA testing can be found on p. 775.

Assessment

The time of last voiding, the volume of fluid intake and the volume of urinary output are determined. Fluid loss by channels other than urinary is also considered. The patient's lower abdomen is examined for distension of the bladder. The patient may complain of low abdominal pain or the distress of feeling the need to void but being unable to initiate voiding.

Nursing intervention

The *goal* is that the patient will establish and maintain a flow of urine from the bladder (see Case Study 19.3).

CASE Frances Lee is an 80-year-old woman who was admitted to hospital in a diabetic crisis in an effort to stabilize her blood sugar level. She was incontinent of large amounts of urine over the first 24 hours and the nursing staff requested an indwelling catheter. They were concerned that prolonged incontinence would put her at risk for skin breakdown and increase the number of linen changes that would be required.

Mrs Lee complained of an ongoing problem with incontinence that had started several years before but had worsened in the past few months.

Assessment

Bladder. Inserting an indwelling catheter at this point would simply postpone the problem of determining the cause of her incontinence and the appropriate treatment. Instead, a postvoiding residual was done to determine the extent to which Mrs Lee was able to empty her bladder completely.

Mrs Lee voided 100 mL and was catheterized for a residual volume of 1000 mL. She did not even seem to be aware that she had to void or that her bladder was so overdistended.

Bowel. An abdominal assessment and rectal examination determined that she was having difficulty emptying her bowels and was in fact constipated.

Mrs Lee was in urinary retention secondary to three factors: diabetic neuropathy which reduced her sensation of filling; faecal impaction which was partially obstructing her urethra; and immobility which made it very difficult for her to get to the bathroom so she often lost the urge to void or ignored it.

Intervention

Mrs Lee was started on a programme of intermittent catheterization four times a day until her residual volumes reduced to 350 mL, when catheterization was reduced to

---

Box 19.8 Causes and characteristics of urinary retention

Causes
- Obstructive disease of the bladder or urethra
- Surgical intervention
- Neurological disease
- Embarrassment or fear
- Constipation.

Clinical characteristics
- Frequent voiding of small amounts (overflow)
- Absence of voiding in 8–10 hours with adequate fluid intake
- Bladder distension
- Urgency and persistent desire to void
- Restlessness
- Pain and discomfort in the region of the bladder and/or kidney.

three times a day. As her bladder tone returned, she began voiding again and her residuals were reduced to twice daily.

The faecal impaction was initially treated with a series of enemas and, once resolved, Mrs Lee continued on a regular bowel programme.

Evaluation

Mrs Lee's condition stabilized over the next few days and she was then transferred to a rehabilitation setting to improve her mobility and evaluate her ability to look after herself. Her urinary retention resolved slowly and she was still on daily residuals when discharged. These were done by the district nurse for further 2 weeks before they were low enough to be discontinued.

Promotion of spontaneous voiding   Nursing measures used to induce voiding include increasing the fluid intake (unless contraindicated), providing privacy, pouring warm water over the perineum, letting the patient hear running water and, unless contraindicated, assisting the patient to assume the normal position for voiding. Women are encouraged to use a commode at the bedside; men may stand beside the bed. A warm bath may prove effective with some patients.

Urinary retention in a postoperative patient may result from incisional pain and discomfort or be associated with embarrassment at the lack of privacy. Analgesics are administered before offering the patient a bedpan or urinal or assisting them to a sitting position, commode chair or to the bathroom. Privacy should be maintained at all times.

Urethral catheterization   Emptying of the bladder by the insertion of a catheter into the urethra and bladder may be done on an intermittent or continuous basis. Urinary catheterization may be performed for reasons other than urinary retention; it may be necessary to assess urinary output accurately in a critically ill patient, to instill certain drugs, to promote healing following surgery, or to measure the volume of residual urine remaining in the bladder following micturition. Before inserting a catheter, the need for it should be thoroughly assessed and documented. Because of the increased risk of infection, as well as the patient's discomfort and loss of dignity, the catheter should be removed as soon as possible.

The procedure and the purpose for it are explained to the patient and privacy is provided throughout the procedure. Precautions are taken to avoid the introduction of organisms and trauma of the mucosa; sterile gloves are worn, and strict aseptic technique is observed throughout the procedure. Sterile anaesthetizing gel should be introduced into the urethra at least 2 minutes before the catheter. The use of anaesthetic antiseptic lubricating gel before catheterization has been shown to, make the procedure as pain free as possible, dilate the urethra facilitating easier insertion, reduce trauma to the urethra and assist with the maintenance of asepsis (Bardsley 2005). The catheter is handled with great care in order to minimize trauma.

If the retention has been acute and severe, not more than 1000 mL of urine are removed initially. The sudden, complete emptying of an overdistended bladder may result in an atonic bladder wall. The sudden release of pressure on the blood vessels in the bladder region causes a sudden inflow of blood, and sometimes capillary bleeding may occur. Rarely, the patient may experience faintness. The catheter is removed or may be clamped after 1000–1500 mL has been drained, and then reopened to allow further drainage at a later time.

Management of an indwelling urethral catheter   A closed drainage system is used to maintain a continuous urinary flow and decrease the potential for the entry of organisms into the system. The catheter is attached to tubing and a collecting bag with a drainage valve, or to a leg bag that contains a valve to prevent backflow of urine into the bladder. The leg bag or regular drainage bag is kept below the level of the bladder and attached to a hanger or hook on the side of the patient's bed or chair. A leg bag is used for the patient who is mobile because it is less cumbersome and can be worn under clothing. The drainage system should not be disconnected unnecessarily for fear of introducing infection to what should be a closed, sterile system.

The drainage system is assessed frequently for patency; kinks in the tubing and tension on the catheter and tubing are avoided. In women, the catheter is taped to the inner thigh; in men, the catheter is taped laterally to the upper thigh or abdomen to prevent pressure on the penile-scrotal angle. The latter is an important preventive measure as erosion of tissue at the penile-scrotal angle may develop if tension is applied to the catheter, and the resulting fistula can be corrected only by plastic surgery.

Indwelling urethral catheters are changed at varying intervals and may be left in place for 4–6 weeks depending on the type of material used in the catheter; information is usually available on the catheter package. Collecting tubing and drainage bags are changed every 2–7 days. Urethral catheters are inconvenient for the patient, but should not interfere with the performance of usual daily activities. Showers are generally permitted.

Measures to prevent the development of urinary tract infections from catheter use are discussed on p. 642.

Patient teaching   Individuals requiring retention catheters during periods of hospitalization require information about the purpose of the catheter and general principles of care and the importance of preventing infections. They are taught to keep the drainage bag below the level of the bladder, to prevent tension on the catheter and to maintain a closed system.

The person requiring intermittent or continuous catheterization at home requires detailed instruction about the supply and care of equipment, and the performance of the procedure if necessary. Infection in long-term catheterized patients is inevitable. It appears that a biofilm consisting of microorganisms and their extracellular products forms and adheres to the catheter and drainage bag.

Referrals are made to the community nurse or continence adviser to assist the person and family in managing the catheter. At home, the drainage tubing and bag required for night use may be cleaned with soap and water and stored dry during the day before reconnection at night. With intermittent self-catheterization it is also possible to wash through the catheter and store it in a clean dry place until required again. Good clean technique is necessary whatever system is adopted and the catheter should be cleaned and stored according to the manufacturer's instructions.

Management of the person after removal of the catheter An indwelling catheter is removed as soon as possible to lessen the trauma to urethral sphincters and the loss of muscle tone that ensues and to reduce the chance of infection. After the catheter is removed, the person is encouraged to pass urine hourly for a few hours and the time and amount of each voiding are recorded, as well as the fluid intake. The patient is assessed for any discomfort, dribbling of urine due to dilatation of the sphincter by the catheter, sensation of urgency or stress incontinence. If the person is unable to void in 6–8 hours and has had an adequate fluid intake, intermittent catheterization may be necessary. If only small amounts of urine are voided, catheterization may be done to measure the amount of residual urine. A bladder training programme may be instituted if difficulties persist after a few days.

Suprapubic catheterization The insertion of a catheter into the bladder through the suprapubic area is a surgical procedure and requires local or general anaesthesia. Nursing care of the patient with a suprapubic catheter and closed drainage system is similar to that of the patient with an indwelling urethral catheter. The suprapubic catheter is sutured in place and then taped to the abdomen to prevent tension on the catheter. The exit site is cared for as a surgical incision. Stomahesive can be used to protect the skin around the insertion site or a transparent, sealed dressing is used.

LOWER URINARY TRACT INFECTION

Lower urinary tract infection (UTI) refers to an acute or chronic infection and inflammation of the bladder (*cystitis*) and the urethra (*urethritis*). About half of all women will experience cystitis at some time during their lifetime (Patient UK 2006). The incidence is less in men but increases after 65 years of age, probably as a result of obstructive disorders and the loss of bactericidal activity of prostatic secretions.

Causes

Lower UTI is most often due to infection caused by the ascent of organisms by way of the urethra, but may also be associated with the administration of certain drugs (e.g. cyclophosphamide) and radiation therapy of the lower abdomen. Predisposing factors are the use of indwelling catheters, trauma of the tissues, stagnation of the urine, and distortion or compression of the bladder by an enlarged neighbouring organ. The latter condition is a factor in cystitis that not infrequently develops in the pregnant woman, especially in the last trimester; the enlarging uterus compresses the bladder. The higher incidence in females is attributed to the shorter urethra of a relatively wide calibre. Sexual intercourse and the type of contraception are precipitating factors. Poor bladder emptying is a precipitating factor in older women. Organisms from rectal and vaginal discharge can enter readily. In the male, it is usually secondary to prostatic hyperplasia or infection or to congenital malformation (e.g. hypospadias).

Clinical characteristics

Frequency, urgency, dysuria and abnormal urine constituents are the primary characteristics of a UTI. The inflammation is generally confined to the mucosa and submucosa, which are hyperaemic and oedematous. Scattered haemorrhagic areas are present, and small ulcerative lesions may develop as a result of sloughing of the lining tissue of the bladder. The urine contains blood cells, pus, bacteria and mucus. If the UTI becomes chronic, the inflammation may extend into the detrusor muscle. Fibrosis of the tissues occurs with persisting inflammation, which reduces the bladder capacity and increases the problem of frequency.

Treatment

In some instances, a UTI is of brief duration, being resolved spontaneously. There is always the danger that the infection may ascend via the ureters and cause pyelonephritis. In uncomplicated cases involving women, a short, 3-day course of trimethoprim is usually adequate. A urine specimen obtained before any antimicrobial drug is given may be cultured to determine the infective organism and its drug sensitivity. Potassium citrate may help by reducing the acidity of the urine. Warm baths may reduce bladder spasm and provide relief. The person is encouraged to drink liberal amounts of fluids, which should include citrus fruit juices.

If the condition persists, the UTI is suspected of being secondary. The patient is then investigated for a primary condition which might be pyelonephritis, a bladder calculus, urethral stricture or, in the case of the male, an enlarged prostate.

As UTI is frequently the result of an ascending infection and occurs readily in females, good personal hygiene and efficient cleansing of the perineum, especially after defaecation, are extremely important and require emphasis in health teaching. Adequate cleansing is often very difficult for the ill person who is weak or handicapped and confined to bed. It becomes the nurse's responsibility to see that the patient is cleansed thoroughly.

Prevention of urinary tract infections

The nurse has responsibilities for health promotion and patient teaching to decrease the development or recurrence of UTI in individuals at risk and to prevent and/or decrease episodes of catheter- or therapy-induced UTI.

Patient teaching

Handwashing and personal hygiene As most UTIs result from bacteria that originate in the gastrointestinal tract, frequent handwashing, especially after defaecation, is an important preventive measure. Women should be taught to wipe the perineal area from the front to the back and then dispose of the tissue. This avoids contamination from the rectal area and should be practised after each bowel movement.

Sexual intercourse This is a contributing factor in the development of UTI in women. For women who experience repeated UTI associated with sexual intercourse, both partners should wash their genitals before intercourse and the female should empty her bladder just before and again after intercourse. She should be taught to drink lots of fluids to keep the urine dilute. The use of condoms should be discussed.

Treatment of altered patterns of urinary elimination Elimination disorders that result in retention and stasis of urine predispose the individual to UTI. If complete emptying of the bladder is not possible, a programme of intermittent catheterization may be indicated. It is important to identify and treat persons with urinary incontinence and retention.

Catheter-induced urinary tract infections

Use of urinary catheters Catheters are a major cause of UTI (Tew et al 2005). They allow entry of microorganisms to the bladder, they offer a surface for the organisms to grow, they are a foreign body and therefore interfere with the body's immune responses, and they may cause chemically induced inflammation of the urethral and bladder mucosa. Catheters also stretch the urethral orifice and injure the tissues. Obstruction of a catheter produces increased intravesicular pressure, promoting the spread of organisms across the mucosa and up into the ureters.

Because of the risk associated with urinary catheters, the following precautions should be taken:

- The need for catheterization, either intermittent or indwelling, should be assessed and documented before the procedure. A catheter should be used only if essential
- Indwelling urinary catheters should be removed as soon as possible
- External urinary devices, such as condom catheters for men, should be used in place of urinary catheters whenever feasible
- Intermittent self-catheterization may be used in preference to indwelling catheters, especially where spinal cord injury is causing bladder dysfunction
- Select the smallest gauge to allow free flow of urine
- Use a lubricant to insert the catheter
- Use a 10 mL balloon for adults and a 3–5 mL balloon for children.

In hospitals or other institutions, strict aseptic technique is required when inserting any catheter. Patients can be taught intermittent self-catheterization, to be performed at home using clean, non-sterile technique.

Care and management of urinary catheters
- When an indwelling catheter is in place, a closed system should be maintained to decrease infection
- Urine specimens should be obtained from the designated port of a closed catheter system using an aseptic technique and syringe with a small-bore needle. The system should not be opened to obtain a specimen
- Wash hands and wear gloves before and after handling the catheter system and teach patients to wash their hands before touching the catheter and attached drainage receptacles
- When emptying the drainage bag ensure that the tap does not come into contact with other surfaces, thereby reducing the risk of infection
- Ensure that the drainage bag is allowed to drain by gravity at all times
- The site of the catheter insertion at the urethral opening provides a port for the entry of organisms. Many topical antiseptic agents and cleansing procedures have been tested to decrease contamination of the urinary meatus. There is no evidence to warrant the adoption of any of these protocols in clinical practice, although daily meatal hygiene with soap and water is recommended (Tew et al 2005)
- Catheters and drainage systems should be changed according to manufacturers' instructions and should not be disconnected except for good clinical reasons.

Tew et al (2005) point out that there is no evidence to support the use of prophylactic antibiotics, the instillation of antiseptics into the collection bag or the use of antiseptic ointments around the meatus. The morbidity associated with the development of UTIs and the potential for mortality makes the care of patients with an indwelling catheter an exceptionally important nursing action. It is important to review the need for a catheter regularly and to maintain vigilance with asepsis and hygiene at all times.

BLADDER INJURY

Accidental injury of the urinary bladder, causing perforation and ensuing extravasation of the urine (escape of urine from the bladder), is not uncommon. It may occur when the pelvis is fractured or as a result of direct blows to the lower abdomen. If the bladder is full and distended at the time of accident, it is more vulnerable.

If the laceration occurs in the upper portion, the rupture is intraperitoneal. Urine escapes into the peritoneal cavity and produces peritonitis. The patient becomes shocked and experiences abdominal pain and tenderness, with a rigid distended abdomen and usually a paralytic ileus.

Rupture of the lower part of the bladder is usually extraperitoneal; urine escapes into the surrounding tissues, and infection, cellulitis and necrosis of tissue may ensue. Occasionally an abdominal or perineal fistula develops.

When there is a history of an injury or blow to the lower abdomen followed by pain and tenderness, injury to the bladder is suspected. A urine specimen is obtained promptly, either by having the patient void or passing a catheter, to determine whether there is haematuria. If blood is present in the urine, cystography may be done to confirm the diagnosis and locate the laceration.

Treatment

The injury is a serious threat to life and requires prompt treatment. The shock and haemorrhage are treated with a blood transfusion and intravenous infusions. An indwelling catheter is inserted into the bladder, and the patient is prepared for abdominal surgery. The site of injury is repaired and a temporary cystostomy (incision of the bladder and introduction of a suprapubic catheter) is carried out to establish urinary drainage and prevent the possibility of pressure on the repair suture line. If the rupture was intra-peritoneal, the extravasated fluid is aspirated before closure.

After surgery the patient is observed closely for signs of infection. Antibiotics may be administered immediately. An accurate record of the fluid intake and all drainage is very important. (See section on nursing care of the patient having had a cystostomy, p. 000. For the care of the patient with peritonitis and paralytic ileus, see Ch. ***.)

TUMOUR OF THE BLADDER

Tumours in the bladder may develop at any age but occur more frequently after the age of 50 years and are twice as common in males as females. Cancer Research UK (2006b) state that bladder cancer accounts for 4800 deaths per year and that 10 200 people are newly diagnosed with the condition annually. The majority arise from the epithelial lining (transitional cell) as papillomas and may be benign or malignant. Those that are benign and recur tend to become malignant eventually. Others appear as ulcers which are usually malignant and are more invasive of deeper tissue layers.

Risk factors

Prolonged occupational exposure to aniline dyes is recognized as a predisposing factor. It is recommended that the period of working with these chemicals should be limited to 3 years and that during this period such persons should have urinary examinations for malignant cells. Workers are also advised of the importance of prompt reporting of any blood in the urine or slight bladder irritation. Smoking has also been cited as a predisposing cause of bladder cancer.

Clinical characteristics

The first symptom is usually intermittent painless haematuria, or cystitis may be the initial factor that prompts the person to seek help. The lesion may encroach on the urethral orifice, giving rise to hesitancy and a decreased force and calibre of the urinary stream. Suprapubic pain and a palpable mass generally indicate that the condition is in an advanced stage. The person may experience pain in the flank region if the growth obstructs a ureteral orifice which causes hydronephrosis. The lesion ulcerates, which accounts for the haematuria, and readily becomes infected. If the infection is severe and anaemia has developed, the patient manifests weakness and loss of weight.

Diagnostic tests

Diagnostic procedures include the following:

- cystoscopy and biopsy
- urine specimen for cytology and midstream specimen for culture and sensitivity
- intravenous urography to identify obstruction or defects of the urinary system
- computed tomography to identify invasion of other organs by tumour.

Treatment

The treatment used depends upon whether the neoplasm is benign or malignant and, in the case of malignancy, upon the stage and the depth of the tissue involved. Surgery, radiation, chemotherapy, or a combination of these, may be used. Small papillomatous growths may be treated by tran-surethral resection followed by electrocoagulation of the base tissue. An indwelling catheter may or may not be inserted in the bladder on completion of the operation. The urinary drainage is observed frequently for possible bleeding. Bladder spasm and irritability may cause considerable discomfort which may be reduced by a warm bath. The patient is encouraged to take a minimum of 2000 mL of fluids daily.

As papillomas, benign as well as malignant, tend to recur, these patients are followed closely for 5–6 years. They are advised to report any bleeding or bladder irritability promptly. A cystoscopic examination is usually done every 3 months during the first year after the resection, every 6 months during the second year, and then annually for 3 or 4 years.

If the neoplasm is malignant, a partial resection of the bladder or total cystectomy (removal of the bladder) may be done.

Partial cystectomy   A partial cystectomy is used only if the cancer is in the upper part of the bladder, well above the urethral orifices. At operation, a tube or catheter is placed in the bladder and brought out through the incision, and an indwelling catheter is also introduced through the urethra. Removal of a part of the bladder obviously reduces its capacity. Adequate drainage in the postoperative period is necessary to prevent distension and possible disruption of the suture line. The tube in the incision may be connected to gentle intermittent suction. The length of time it remains in the bladder will depend on the rate of healing.

The urethral catheter usually remains in place for approximately 2–4 weeks. On its removal, frequency becomes a problem for the patient because of the reduced bladder capacity. This may lead to discouragement and depression; consequently, understanding support from the nurse is essential. Any attempt to reduce the frequency by cutting down fluid intake must be guarded against. The importance of a minimum fluid intake of 2000 mL to prevent dehydration, and the spacing of the fluids so that the intervals between voiding may be increased during certain periods (e.g. at night), should be discussed with the patient. The traumatized bladder gradually becomes less irritable and increases its capacity.

Cystectomy

A total cystectomy with ureteric transplantation for permanent urinary diversion is used when the tumour is situated in the lower part of the bladder or is quite extensive. Permanent urinary diversion may be achieved by continent ileal urinary pouch or the formation of an ileal conduit (Fig. 19.9).

Continent ileal urinary pouch

Several surgical procedures (e.g. Koch, Camay, Mitrofanoff, Indiana) are being done to create a continent ileal or internal reservoir from an isolated segment of ileum which is then connected to the abdominal wall. A nipple-like valve is created to allow insertion of a catheter to drain urine. The internal pouch replaces the external urine collecting bags worn by persons without the built-in reservoir.

Ileal conduit (ureteroileostomy)

This involves removal of a segment of the ileum with its mesentery and blood supply. The open ends of the ileum left by the resection are anastomosed to re-establish intestinal continuity. One end of the resected ileal section is closed. The open end is brought through the abdominal wall to the skin surface and secured. The detached ends of the ureters are implanted in the ileal segment near its closed end. See p. 647 for more detail regarding urinary diversion.

Radiation

Internal or external radiation may be used in treating cancer of the bladder. External radiotherapy may be used to treat the tumour as an adjunct to surgery, or prophylactically to reduce pressure symptoms or tumour mass. During treatment, the individual is likely to experience gastrointestinal disturbance (nausea, vomiting and diarrhoea) and cystitis. This should be discussed with the person before commencing therapy. Information booklets may be useful in reinforcing verbal information. Long-term side-effects of radiotherapy include chronic urinary disturbance, telangiectasia of the bladder mucosa with chronic haematuria, and usually loss of erectile function in men and decreased orgasmic sensation in women.

Intracavity radiation may be achieved by the enclosure of a radioisotope (e.g. ^{60}Co, ^{198}Au) in a catheter balloon which is placed within the bladder. The catheter is connected to a drainage receptacle, and all urine is saved and sent to the radioisotope department. In some instances, radon seeds or radiotantalum (^{182}Ta) needles may be implanted around the lesion. Safety precautions are necessary in the handling of these radioactive materials. Internal radiation causes cystitis, and the patient usually experiences considerable bladder spasm and discomfort. Fluids are given freely and analgesics may be necessary. The application of heat over the bladder region may provide some relief.

In advanced carcinoma of the bladder, and when metastases are suspected, chemotherapy may be used as well as surgery and irradiation. Local or intravesical chemotherapy can be used for the control of some bladder cancers. This can be performed on an inpatient or outpatient basis. The management of this procedure is often performed by nurses, and safety precautions in relation to the handling of cytotoxic drugs should be observed (see Ch. 11).

BLADDER SURGERY

Operative procedures used in the treatment of bladder disease may be transurethral or by open surgery. Transurethral operative procedures may be performed to obtain a biopsy, remove a neoplasm or calculus, or resect the prostate gland. The resectoscope, which is used to resect tissue, is similar to a cystoscope but has insulated walls and is equipped with a wire loop which is activated by a high-frequency current to cut tissue and control haemorrhage by electrocoagulation (diathermy). A lithotrite, which is a special crushing instrument, is used to remove a stone, and the procedure is called *litholapaxy*.

Open surgery on the bladder may be undertaken for repair of a perforation or laceration, the removal of a neoplasm, calculus or the prostate gland, or a segmental resection or removal of the bladder. The open operative procedures include *cystotomy* (an incision into the bladder and closure without a drainage tube), *cystostomy* (an incision into the bladder and the insertion of a drainage tube which is brought out on to the abdominal surface), *segmental resection* (the removal of a section of the bladder) and *total cystectomy* (the removal of the bladder, involving urethral transplantation and urinary diversion). A suprapubic approach is most commonly used in open bladder surgery, with the bladder being opened below the peritoneum.

Nursing care of the patient having bladder surgery

Preoperative preparation

Unless the bladder is injured or there is acute retention that cannot be relieved by urethral catheterization, the patient

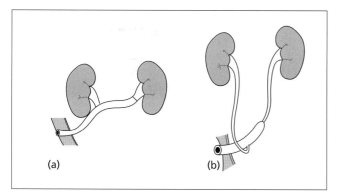

Figure 19.9   Methods of permanent urinary diversion. (a) Ileal conduit. (b) Ileal urinary pouch.

who is to have bladder surgery usually undergoes investigation and preparation. Kidney function is assessed and certain blood chemistry levels are determined (e.g. urea, creatinine, potassium, sodium, chloride, calcium). The urine is examined microscopically and, if infection is present, a urinary antiseptic or an antibiotic is prescribed. The patient is encouraged to take 2500–3000 mL of fluid daily unless a large amount of fluid is contraindicated by cardiac or renal insufficiency. The fluid intake and output are recorded and the balance noted. The patient's nutritional status frequently requires attention. Many of these patients are elderly and the existing condition may have contributed to their lack of interest in food, resulting in deficiencies. In encouraging the patient to take nourishment, its importance in recovery is explained. Dietary adjustments and supplements may be necessary to meet nutritional needs.

During the preparatory period, an indwelling catheter may be used to provide adequate drainage and reduce the residual urine. The patient is usually encouraged to remain ambulatory.

Psychological support in the preoperative phase is equally as important as physical care. Opportunities should be provided for the discussion of feelings and concerns, and for the patient to ask questions. The patient and family are advised as to what may be expected after the operation. If the patient is to have a partial cystectomy, this explanation will include a discussion of the frequency of voiding that will be experienced when the tubes are removed because of the reduced capacity of the bladder. Reassurance is given that this gradually becomes less troublesome.

The immediate preparation for open bladder surgery is similar to that for any patient having abdominal surgery (see Ch. 15).

Postoperative nursing intervention

Preparation to receive the patient after operation includes the assembling of sterile tubing and drainage receptacles ready for prompt connection to an indwelling urethral catheter and a cystostomy tube. A tray of sterile equipment and solution for irrigating the catheters in the event of obstruction by clots should be readily available. Goals for the patient following a cystotomy, cystostomy or segmental bladder resection are listed in Table 19.4.

Maintenance of urinary elimination The patient returns from the operating theatre with an indwelling urethral catheter which is secured to the upper thigh to prevent traction. It is connected to sterile tubing leading to a closed sterile drainage receptacle. The length of the tube should allow for turning and moving the patient without tension being exerted on the catheter.

If there is a cystostomy as well, a tube is anchored in the bladder by a suture at the time of operation. The cystostomy tube is attached to a sterile tube and receptacle.

Both drainage systems are checked frequently (at least hourly for the first 36–48 hours) for patency. The characteristics (colour, consistency, and content or sediment) of the drainage are noted at the same time. The urine will be blood-stained for the first 2–3 hours, gradually becoming lighter. The drainage is best examined in the plastic connecting tubes before it becomes mixed with what is already in the receptacles.

The cystostomy tube, urethral catheter or tubing may become obstructed by a blood clot. The drainage system is checked for patency. If blockage of the tubing is indicated, it may be 'milked' or changed. If the obstruction is within the catheter tube in the bladder, an order may be given to irrigate with sterile normal saline. Some 50–75 mL of the fluid are introduced; if the initial fluid does not return, no more fluid is instilled and the surgeon is consulted. Adequate postoperative drainage is very important to prevent bladder distension and pressure on the suture line.

Bladder irrigation systems are available that may be used to prevent clots blocking the catheter. Specially made-up sterile bags of sterile irrigation fluid may be run into the bladder under gravity and then allowed to drain. It is important to ensure that fluid instilled is drained off before any further fluid is run into the bladder, for reasons discussed

Table 19.4 Identification of problems relevant to the patient who has just had a cystotomy, cystostomy or segmental bladder resection

Patient problem	Goals
1. Altered pattern of urinary elimination related to bladder incision, urethral catheter and cystostomy tube.	Patient will achieve fluid balance
2. Ineffective airway clearance related to anaesthesia and decreased mobility.	Patient will show normal respiratory function
3. Impairment of skin integrity related to surgery and possible leakage of urine.	Wound will heal without complications
4. Pain related to surgical intervention and bladder spasms.	Patient will be free of pain
5. Alteration in nutritional and fluid balance related to surgery and discomfort.	Patient will maintain nutritional status
6. Altered bowel elimination related to surgery and discomfort.	Patient will have normal bowel actions
7. Lack of knowledge concerning fluid intake, catheter care and health supervision.	Patient will show understanding of condition and requirements after discharge

above. This procedure is particularly important after TURP.

The drainage from each system is measured and recorded every 4 hours. Care of the tubing and drainage bag varies with local policy. It may be replaced daily with a fresh sterile set or changed every second day or twice weekly.

The cystostomy tube usually remains in place from 4 to 7 days, depending on the patient's healing. The urethral catheter is generally left for a few days longer or until the incisional opening in the bladder heals. When the cystostomy tube is removed, some urine will escape on to the dressing for a few days until the fistula heals over.

After removal of the urethral catheter, a close check is made of the patient's frequency of voiding and the volume of the daily output for several days. The ambulant patient should be encouraged to record the necessary information. When a urethral catheter that has been in place for several days is removed, dribbling is a frequent problem because the bladder-urethral sphincters have been continuously dilated for a period of time. Frequent perineal exercises, which consist of contracting the abdominal, gluteal and perineal muscles while continuing to breathe normally, may help the sphincters recover their tone and control. Occasionally, a patient may not be able to void and catheterization may be performed if voiding has not occurred within 8 hours.

A permanent cystostomy is sometimes done as a palliative measure for a patient who has an inoperable obstruction of the urethra (e.g. advanced carcinoma of the urethra, bladder neck or prostate). A urethral catheter is not inserted in this patient; bladder drainage is entirely dependent upon the cystostomy tube.

Assessment   As well as frequent checking of the drainage system(s), the patient's blood pressure, pulse, colour and level of consciousness are noted and recorded at frequent intervals, which are gradually lengthened if the vital signs are satisfactory. Haemorrhage and shock are possible complications following either transurethral resection or open bladder surgery. Bleeding may be evident in the drainage, but the dressing, surrounding skin areas and groins are also examined.

The daily fluid intake and output are recorded for a longer period than with most surgical patients. The ratio of the intake to the output is examined by the nurse so that he or she is alert to possible renal insufficiency or retention of urine. The characteristics of the urine are noted for a period of 10–14 days. The appearance of sediment, blood, shreds of mucus-like material, cloudiness or the presence of an unusual odour is reported. Sloughing and ensuing bleeding may occur 8–10 days after the removal of a lesion.

Maintenance of airway clearance   The reader is referred to Chapter 13 for a discussion of the importance of avoiding respiratory and cardiovascular complications in the post-operative period.

Impairment of skin integrity   Compared with other abdominal surgery, the dressing is changed earlier and more frequently for patients who have had open bladder surgery.

There is almost certain to be some leakage of urine through the incision and around the tube. The skin is cleansed of urine frequently and is kept as dry as possible to prevent excoriation and infection. The application of a skin protection preparation may aid in preventing excoriation. If excoriation occurs, the use of stoma or hydrocolloid dressing wafers may help in preventing further skin breakdown and encourage healing. Early referral to the stoma care nurse or wound care specialist nurse (if available) may help obviate problems.

The lower back, buttocks, groin, inner thighs and perineum are examined each time the dressing is changed. If any areas are moist with urine drainage, they are washed and dried thoroughly to prevent excoriation. The bedding is changed as often as is necessary to ensure dryness and comfort.

Control of pain   Bladder trauma and irritation cause bladder spasms which are very painful, and the patient may also experience the desire to void frequently, even though the bladder is emptied by tube drainage. In the case of the sensation of frequency, it may be necessary to explain to the patient that the bladder is empty and that trying to void only increases bladder spasms and pain. An analgesic such as pethidine is usually necessary at regular intervals during the first 48 hours. If the pain and discomfort are not relieved, the surgeon is consulted. Either the catheter or cystostomy tube may require adjusting to relieve the pressure of its tip on the bladder wall.

Maintenance of fluid balance and nutrition   A daily fluid intake of at least 2500–3000 mL (unless contraindicated by other co-existing disease) is necessary to ensure adequate irrigation of the bladder as well as to maintain satisfactory hydration. Most of it usually has to be administered by intravenous infusion during the first day or two. A soft diet is given and is progressively increased to a regular diet as tolerated.

Maintenance of bowel elimination   The patient may be given a mild laxative after 2 days, or an enema may be given. Constipation and straining at stool should be avoided as they tend to increase the patient's pain.

Patient education   Most patients who have had a cystotomy or cystostomy remain in the hospital until the wound is healed and normal micturition is re-established. The nurse should discuss the resumption of their previous activities with them and explain any restrictions indicated by the doctor. They are advised to continue taking a minimum of 2000–2500 mL of fluid daily. Some may require reassurance that no special care of the wound is necessary and that they may resume baths.

If the cystostomy is permanent or a urethral catheter is to remain in place, the patient and a family member are given detailed instruction about the necessary care. This instruction is given over several days and should be completed soon enough for the patient to demonstrate satisfactory self-care before going home. This gives confidence and provides the opportunity to clarify certain points. Verbal and written instructions will include an explanation of the necessary equipment, its use and maintenance, how it may be acquired, and any precautions to be observed in its use. An inconspicuous plastic leg bag that can be strapped to the thigh may be required by the patient if an indwelling catheter is to be used. The lower end of the bag has a valve that permits emptying of the bag into the toilet at necessary intervals. The importance of thorough washing of the hands with soap and running water before connecting or disconnecting the equipment is stressed to reduce the possibility of ascending infection. The patient and a relative are also taught how to anchor the tube that is in the patient to the abdomen or thigh to prevent traction on it.

The patient is reminded of the need to continue taking at least 2000–2500 mL of fluid daily to provide adequate bladder irrigation. Odour is likely to be less of a problem with more dilute urine, and there is less danger of infection with constant washing out of the bladder.

A referral may be made to the district nurse for assistance and supervision when the patient goes home. This is likely to be needed when the patient is elderly and finds it difficult to cope with the necessary care. The patient and family are advised how often the catheter needs to be changed and should be referred to the community continence adviser where possible.

Evaluation

On discharge from hospital, the patient should be able to perform usual daily activities with minimal discomfort and only temporary changes in activity tolerance. The patient and family should be aware of expectations for self-care and community resources available. They should be able to describe plans for follow-up health supervision.

URINARY DIVERSION

Complete removal of the bladder necessitates establishing a new urinary outlet; this may be achieved by ileal conduit (ureteroileostomy) or an internal continent ileal pouch.

After operation, the patient who undergoes a cystectomy and ureteral transplant is seriously ill. The amount of surgery usually involved predisposes the patient to shock. Frequently, considerable surrounding tissue is resected with the bladder (e.g. lymphatics, prostate gland), and if the ileal conduit procedure or internal ileal pouch is used an intestinal resection and anastomosis are done. The patient will have a large vertical or transverse incision through which the bladder is removed, the ureters are freed for transplant, and the intestine is resected. The stoma through which the urine will drain is made separately in the abdominal wall and an internal pouch may be created. Care of the patient requires consideration of the needs incurred by the cystectomy, the intestinal surgery, the ureteric transplantation and urinary diversion, as well as the individual patient's psychological and physiological responses to such radical surgery.

Preoperative preparation

The operative procedure and the permanent change in urinary drainage that will ensue should be explained to the patient and family by the surgeon and stoma therapist. This is likely to produce considerable anxiety and despair and will prompt many questions. The nurse needs to show acceptance of these understandable concerns and provide opportunities for the patient and family members to express their feelings and ask questions and, when they are ready, the necessary adjustments and care associated with urinary diversion are outlined in simple terms. They are told that a relatively normal, active life is possible. This may be reinforced by having a person who has had a permanent urinary diversion and has made a successful adjustment talk with them. If such a person is not available, someone with an ileostomy may prove helpful. The nurse who is willing to take time to talk freely with the patient, discussing future plans, and is patient in repeating answers and reinforcing what has probably already been said can provide immeasurable support. A rapport can be developed that contributes to acceptance of the situation and the development of positive attitudes on the part of the patient and family.

The sexual implications of the surgery should be discussed with the individual and partner, together with the treatment options available should difficulties arise after operation. Whenever sexual issues are discussed, sensitivity and tact are of the utmost importance because of the personal nature of this subject and the potential threat to self-image and self-esteem. Many men and women who undergo surgery of this type fear rejection and abandonment by their partners or, if single, believe they will never have a physical relationship again. The following changes can result from radical bladder surgery: in men, sexual desire and genital sensation is often normal, orgasm intensity may be reduced, ejaculation dry, and erectile dysfunction may be present; women may experience dyspareunia and reduced vaginal secretion but orgasm normally remains the same. Treatment options for men include intercavernosal self-injection technique, penile prosthesis, or use of vacuum devices. Women who experience painful intercourse may wish to try different positions for lovemaking, extended foreplay, or the use of lubricants (e.g. water-soluble gel). Vaginal dilators may be useful to dilate the vagina. Some women respond to hormone replacement therapy.

As part of the physical preparation for surgery, kidney function is assessed and the blood levels of nitrogenous wastes, potassium, sodium and chloride are determined. The patient usually receives a blood transfusion during and probably after the operation, so typing and cross-matching are necessary. At least 2500 mL of fluid daily are given unless contraindicated by cardiac insufficiency or urinary obstruction.

If the intestine is to be entered, the patient may receive a low-residue diet for 3 or 4 days, then clear fluids only for 2 days before operation to reduce the faecal content. The reasons for these restrictions are explained in order to gain the patient's cooperation and acceptance. Laxatives and enemas are also used for cleansing purposes, and a course of an antimicrobial drug that is poorly absorbed from the gastrointestinal tract is given orally to destroy intestinal organisms (e.g. neomycin). A nasogastric tube is passed at operation to provide drainage of secretions and prevent intestinal distension after the surgery. The remainder of the preparation is similar to that for any major abdominal surgery (see Ch. 15).

The operation is a lengthy procedure; relatives should be informed about when they may call to enquire about the person's condition and/or visit.

Management of the patient with a urinary diversion

A large part of the required care is essentially the same as that for any patient having an intestinal resection (see Ch.15). Table 19.5 lists goals relevant to the patient with a urinary diversion.

Maintenance of urinary elimination

On completion of the operation, a disposable clean plastic ileostomy bag is secured to the skin around the stoma. This allows for visualization of the stoma and drainage. Ileostomy bags have a valve system to prevent reflux over the stoma and leakage and they can be connected to larger-volume bags, which reduce the frequency of emptying. A cessation of drainage may indicate occlusion of the stoma by mucus or by swelling and oedema of the tissues, and the surgeon is notified immediately. A sterile catheter may be inserted periodically to determine whether there is residual urine.

Maintenance of integrity of stoma and peristomal skin

The appliance should be removed gently to prevent trauma to the peristomal skin. A tissue or wipe can be used to cover the stoma to collect urine. The skin is gently washed with mild soap and water, and dried. Barrier creams, adhesive preparations and skin sealants may be used on intact skin. A new appliance is applied carefully, ensuring correct fit around the stoma. Transient erythema is usual on appliance removal but this should rapidly resolve. Any persistent redness, broken skin, complaints of discomfort or allergic reactions should be investigated and rapidly treated. The stoma should be monitored for signs of oedema, bleeding, excoriation, ulceration, unusual drainage or discolouration (see Care of the individual with faecal diversion, Ch. 15).

Odour control may be a problem for some individuals. Advice should be given concerning the avoidance of foods that produce strong odours in urine. Introduction of a few drops of vinegar or commercial deodorizer into the appliance via the outlet spout may reduce stale urine odours.

Abdominal pain, distension or rigidity, nausea, vomiting or fever is reported promptly. Any of these symptoms may indicate peritonitis, resulting from the escape of intestinal content from the site of the intestinal anastomosis or from a leakage of urine from the ileal conduit or ureters into the peritoneal cavity.

Maintenance of mobility and physical function

When the ileal conduit opens on to the right side of the abdomen, more complete drainage occurs when the patient is on the right side or back with the trunk elevated. With each change of position, the bag and tubing are checked for any kinks or compression.

Early ambulation is encouraged to foster adequate drainage and prevent complications.

Good pain relief is essential and the nurse carries the main responsibility for ensuring the patient is pain-free in the postoperative period.

Maintenance of nutritional status and fluid balance

The nasogastric tube remains in place for 3–4 days and the patient is given intravenous fluids. The patient is observed for any signs of distension. Once bowel sounds indicate the

Table 19.5 Identification of problems relevant to the patient with a urinary diversion

Patient problem	Goals
1. Altered pattern of urinary elimination related to formation of a ureteroileal conduit.	The patient will maintain urinary elimination
2. Potential impairment of skin integrity (stoma and peristomal skin) due to surgical intervention and irritation.	The integrity of stoma and peristomal skin will be preserved Infection will not occur
3. Alteration in mobility related to surgical intervention and pain.	The patient will be pain-free Normal mobility will be regained
4. Alteration in nutrition and fluid balance related to surgery on intestine, bladder and ureters.	The patient will maintain nutritional status and fluid balance
5. Disturbance in body image related to the urinary diversion and creation of the abdominal stoma	The patient will demonstrate a healthy body image
6. Disturbance in sexual functioning related to damage to nerves, surgical excision of tissue, and trauma to reproductive.	The patient will demonstrate understanding of potential alterations in sexual functioning system
7. Lack of knowledge about self-care of the urinary diversion and follow-up care.	The patient will show knowledge, skills and resources to manage healthcare regimen

re-establishment of peristalsis, and there is no distension, the nasogastric tube is removed. The intake of clear fluids is gradually increased and the diet progresses through soft foods to a light solid diet. Gas-forming foods are avoided for 4–6 weeks and then added gradually as tolerated.

Promotion of a healthy body image

The person with a urinary diversion must deal with the altered body structure of an abdominal stoma that is initially red, swollen and tender, the loss of control of urine, and the perceived effects on social interactions and sexual activity. Acceptance of body image changes takes place slowly. It is important that the nurse encourages the patient to talk through concerns and discuss them with both partner and family.

Initially patients are often uncomfortable looking at the stoma. The nurse can support them in looking and talking about it as care procedures are being performed. The person will need support to touch the stoma and gradually to assume self-care activities. Some patients benefit from talking with others who have learned to manage their urinary diversions and sharing experiences related to care and the resumption of social activities. Information regarding self-help groups should be offered. Before discharge, patient concerns related to sexual function should be assessed and addressed. If the actual or perceived concerns are beyond the scope of the nurse, plans may be made for further assistance from specialists or resources in the community or hospital.

Patient and family education

The patient and a family member are taught the care of the stoma, skin and appliance following the same plan as that outlined for the ileostomy patient in Chapter 15. Emphasis is placed on the precautionary measures necessary to prevent infection. Once the oedema subsides and the stoma shrinks, the stoma is measured for a permanent appliance (approximately 7 days). The patient is taught to measure the stoma in order to adjust the size of the appliance as healing continues to take place.

If a continent internal pouch has been constructed, the individual is taught to insert a catheter through the valve to drain the urine. The nurse helps the person to develop a schedule and to adapt it to usual daily activities as control is established. During this period, the importance of continuing a daily intake of 2500–3000 mL to keep the ureters and ileal conduit patent should be emphasized. The patient and family are cautioned that the doctor is to be consulted immediately if there is a decrease in urinary drainage, abnormal constituents such as blood in urine, fever, pain in the back or abdomen, severe skin excoriation or general malaise. Mucus from an ileal conduit or internal pouch is normally present in the urine. This should be explained to avoid distress or concern. The patient is followed closely after hospital discharge. A referral may be made to the district nurse and community stoma care nurse, and the patient is seen at regular intervals at the clinic or by the general practitioner. These visits may be frequent at first, and the intervals are gradually increased if the patient's progress is satisfactory.

Urinary diversion: summary

Factors to be considered in caring for a patient who undergoes permanent urinary diversion, regardless of the method used, include the following:

- The individual's psychological reaction to a change in body image and normal pattern of function requires thoughtful understanding on the part of the nurse, with sincere efforts to reduce the patient's despair and promote acceptance and adaptation
- Preoperative cleansing and 'sterilization' of the bowel are necessary if the operative procedure involves resection of or entry into the intestine
- Maintenance of continuous, adequate urinary drainage from the ureters after operation is essential to prevent renal complications
- Drainage of urine through an opening on to the skin necessitates special skin care to prevent excoriation and maceration
- A daily fluid intake of 2500–3000 mL of fluid is important to provide good internal irrigation of the renal pelvis and ureters
- A planned programme of teaching the care of the stoma, skin and appliance or drainage of the pouch is given to the patient and a relative. It should take place over a period of time that will allow them to acquire a satisfactory understanding and competence by the time the patient leaves the hospital. The instruction includes an explanation of the need for ample fluids and prompt reporting of decreased urinary drainage and significant symptoms
- Information about the person's previous employment is obtained, and consideration is given as to whether it is possible for previous employment to be resumed or whether a referral to a social worker would be of assistance in finding other employment
- The person requires close follow-up. Frequent home visits by a district nurse, especially during the first few weeks after leaving the hospital, can provide assistance and considerable support to the patient and family. Regular visits to a clinic or the general practitioner are necessary.

SUMMARY

This chapter provides an overview of the structure and function of the kidneys, the formation and composition of urine, and the mechanisms of urinary elimination. The nursing management of persons with acute and chronic disorders of renal function is discussed.

Urinary incontinence is a prevalent health problem, especially in elderly women. Comprehensive assessment of the person with urinary incontinence is essential to define accurately the type of incontinence and the contributing factors. The nurse plays an important role in the assessment process and in promoting effective patient management. Participation of the patient and family in the care process enables the development of a relevant and realistic management programme and facilitates acceptance of the plan of care. Urinary catheters are identified as the major cause of nosocomial infection. The nurse has a responsibility to prevent urinary tract infections from being acquired as a result of catheter use. Permanent urinary diversions cause a disturbance in self-image and necessitate skilled patient and family teaching by the nurse.

Throughout this chapter, emphasis is placed on the impact of renal disorders and altered urinary function on the quality of life of the person and the resulting effects on the family. The nurse plays a vital role in identifying the impact of the disorder on the patient and family, in teaching them self-management skills and in helping them to develop appropriate coping patterns.

REFERENCES

Bardsley A (2005) Use of lubricant gels in urinary catheterization. Nursing Standard 20(8): 41–46.

Bevan M (2000) The older person with renal failure. Nursing Standard 14(32): 48–52.

Brittain K, Perry S, Williams K (2001) Triggers that prompt people with urinary symptoms to seek help. British Journal of Nursing 10(2): 74–86.

Cancer Research UK (2004) Advanced kidney cancer. Online. Available: http://www.cancerhelp.org.uk/help/default.asp?page=4044#biol [Accessed 21.04.2006].

Cancer Research UK (2006a) UK Kidney cancer statistics. Online. Available: http://info.cancerresearchuk.org/cancerstats/types/kidney/incidence/?a=5441 [Accessed 19.04.2006].

Cancer Research UK (2006b) UK Bladder cancer statistics. Online. Available: http://info.cancerresearchuk.org/cancerstats/types/bladder/?a=5441 [Accessed 19.04.2006].

Cheater F (1995) Promoting urinary continence. Nursing Standard 9(39): 33–37.

Colley W, Pomfret I (2001) Continence. In: Crumbie A and Lawrence J, eds. Living with a chronic condition: a practitioner's guide to providing care. Oxford: Butterworth Heinemann, p 121–140.

Department of Health (2004) National Service Framework for Renal Services: Part One – Dialysis and transplantation. London: DoH.

Department of Health (2005) National Service Framework for Renal Services – Part Two: Chronic kidney disease, acute renal failure and end of life care. London: DoH.

Dorey G (2000) Male patients with lower urinary tract symptoms. 2: Treatment. British Journal of Nursing 9(9): 553–558.

Dyer P (2000) Kidney transplantation for Asian people; does biology discriminate? Nursing Times 96(23): 39–40.

Garrett B (1995) The nutritional management of acute renal failure. Journal of Clinical Nursing 4: 377–382.

Haslett C, Chilvers E, Hunter J, Boon N (1999) Davidson's principles and practice of medicine, 18th edn. Edinburgh: Churchill Livingstone.

Hasselder A (1999) Renal transplant; long term effects of immunosuppression. Professional Nurse 14(11): 771–776.

McCann K, Boore J (2000) Fatigue in persons with renal failure who require maintenance haemodialysis. Journal of Advanced Nursing 32(5): 1132–1142.

National Kidney Federation (2001) What are the practical risks and benefits for both donors and recipients? Online. Available: http://www.kidney.org.uk/living-donor/livdon07.html [Accessed 21.04.2006].

National Kidney Federation (2002) Anaemia in kidney failure. Online. Available: http://www.kidney.org.uk/Medical-Info/anaemia/index.html [Accessed 21.04.2006].

NHS Direct (2006) Organ donation. Online. Available: http://www.nhsdirect.nhs.uk/articles/article.aspx?printPage=1&articleId=562 [Accessed 21.04.2006].

Patient UK (2006) Recurrent cystitis in women. Online. Available: www.patient.co.uk/showdoc/23068975 [Accessed 21.04.2006].

Redmond A, Doherty E (2005) Peritoneal dialysis. Nursing Standard 19(40): 55–65.

Renal Association (2006) Chronic Kidney Disease in Adults: UK Guidelines for Identification, Management and Referral of Adults. Online. Available: http://www.renal.org/eGFR/about.html [Accessed 21.04.2006].

Royal College of Radiologists (2003) Diagnostic Radiology Leaflets. Online. Available: http://www.rcr.ac.uk/index.asp?PageID=323 [Accessed 20.04.2006].

Shaw C, Williams K, Assassa P, Jackson C (2000) Patient satisfaction with urodynamics; a qualitative study. Journal of Advanced Nursing 32(6): 1356–1363.

Sheppard A (2000) Monitoring fluid balance in acutely ill patients. Nursing Times 96(21): 39–40.

TalkTransplant (2006) Waiting lists. Online. Available: www.talktransplant.com/Waiting_Lists.aspx [Accessed 27.07.2006].

Tew L, Pomfret I, King D (2005) Infection risks associated with urinary catheters Nursing Standard 20(7): 55–61.

UK Transplant (2005a) UK Transplant activity report 2004–2005. Online. Available: http://www.uktransplant.org.uk/ukt/statistics/transplant_activity_report/transplant_activity_report.jsp [Accessed 20.04.2006].

UK Transplant (2005b) Statistics. Online. Available: http://www.uktransplant.org.uk/ukt/statistics/statistics.jsp [Accessed 21.04.2006].

UK Transplant (2005c) History of the organ donor register. Online. Available: http://www.uktransplant.org.uk/ukt/newsroom/fact_sheets/nhs_organ_donor_register_a_history.jsp [Accessed 21.04.2006].

UK Transplant (2006) Transplant list criteria for potential renal transplant patients. Online. Available: www.uktransplant.org.uk [Accessed 20.04.2006].

UK Renal Registry (2003) UK Renal Registry Report 2003. Bristol: UK Renal Registry.

Williams K (2004) Stress urinary incontinence treatment and support. Nursing Standard 18(31): 45–52.

Wilson LA (2005) Urinalysis. Nursing Standard 19(35): 51–54.

Whyte A (2000) Organ recital. Nursing Times 96(23): 28–29.

FURTHER READING AND USEFUL WEBSITES

Higgins C (2000) Understanding laboratory investigations. Oxford: Blackwell Publishing.

An extremely useful book to have available in clinical practice. It explains all the blood tests that can be carried out and explores why they may be indicated and what normal and abnormal findings mean for the patient.

O'Callaghan C (2006) The renal system at a glance, 2nd edn. Oxford: Blackwell Publishing.

An excellent introduction to renal physiology, pharmacology and pathophysiology. There are clear diagrams with each chapter with clear explanations and descriptions of renal function and disease. This is a book which is aimed at medical students but it will also be of use to nurses who wish to explore this area of clinical practice further.

Association for Continence Advice	www.aca.uk.com
Incontact	www.incontact.org
The Continence Foundation	www.continence-foundation.org.uk
Renal Association	www.renal.org
Royal College of Radiologists Diagnostic Radiology Leaflets	www.rcr.ac.uk
National Kidney Foundation	www.kidney.org.uk
UK Transplant	www.uktransplant.org.uk
British Kidney Patient Association	www.britishkidney-pa.co.uk
National Kidney Federation	www.kidney.org.uk
TalkTransplant	www.talktransplant.com

20 Caring for the patient with a disorder of the nervous system

Claire Mavin

INTRODUCTION

Neuroscience nursing is concerned with caring for those with a disorder of or trauma to the nervous system. As a result, many clients will display neurological impairments and the nurse will encounter these in differing situations, ranging from the seriously head-injured patient requiring emergency surgery and intensive care to control raised intracranial pressure (ICP) to the client with a chronic neurological disorder being cared for and supported in the community.

THE NERVOUS SYSTEM

The nervous system is an integrated, multipurpose system made up of many parts. It contains the higher human functions such as memory and reasoning, controls and coordinates all parts of the body, and provides a complex communication system between the body's internal and external environments.

CLASSIFICATION

The nervous system can be divided into discrete parts for the purpose of description, as outlined in Figure 20.1. However, in reality, the activities of each division are interrelated to harmonize the many complex functions of the whole system.

Structurally, the nervous system is composed of two parts: the central nervous system (CNS) and the *peripheral nervous system*. The CNS consists of the brain and the spinal cord, whereas the peripheral system consists of the spinal and cranial nerves. The two functional divisions of the nervous system are the somatic or voluntary nervous system and the autonomic or involuntary nervous system. The *somatic system* is concerned primarily with the transmission of impulses to and from the non-visceral parts of the body such as the skeletal muscles, bones, joints, ligaments, skin, eyes and ears. Its activities are usually conscious and willed responses. The autonomic system is concerned with regulation of the activities of visceral muscles and glands.

Neurone

The neurone, or nerve cell, is the structural and functional unit of the nervous system (Fig. 20.2). The cell body contains a nucleus and other structures and masses concerned with cell maintenance and activity. The cytoplasmic processes include a single axon and one or more dendrites.

The *axon* is a tubular process that conducts nerve impulses away from the cell body, out to the dendrites of other neurones or to muscles and glands. Near its end, the axon divides into numerous fine branches, each of which has a specialized

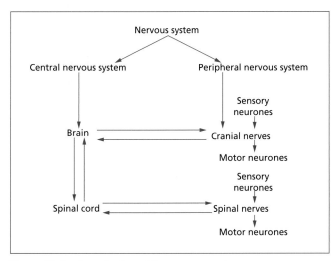

Figure 20.1 Organization of the nervous system.

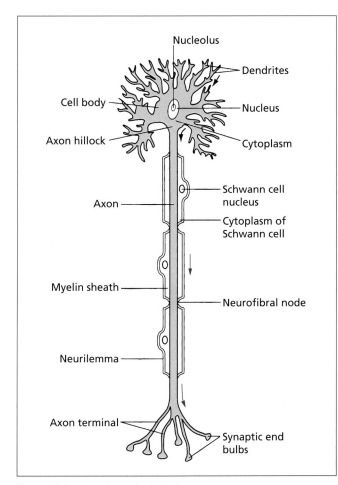

Figure 20.2 Structure of a typical neurone.

ending called the *presynaptic terminal*. *Dendrites* are short, thin projections that receive stimuli and carry impulses generated by the stimuli toward the nerve cell body. Most stimuli affecting nerve cells are chemical messengers (neurotransmitters) that are secreted from one neurone to an adjacent neurone. The profuse branches of dendrites increase the surface area over which impulses may be picked up.

Neurones are classified according to their function into three types:

- motor (efferent or effector) neurones
- sensory (afferent or receptor) neurones
- connecting (internuncial) neurones.

The axons of *motor* neurones transmit impulses from the CNS to stimulate muscle or glandular tissue. Axons of *sensory* neurones transmit impulses to areas of the brain or spinal cord from the periphery. *Connecting* neurones, which occur only in the grey matter of the brain and spinal cord, convey incoming stimuli to neurones of various integrating centres of the CNS. The connecting neurones form the association areas in the cerebral cortex. They have an important role in the CNS because they 'decide' the responses to the sensory impulses and promote the initiation of the appropriate motor neurone response.

Neurones are designed to initiate, receive and react to stimuli, transmit impulses, process and store information. Neuronal activity results in a wide variety of responses ranging from a simple reflex to complex behaviour requiring central coordination.

Unlike most body cells, neurones lose their ability to undergo mitosis early in life. They lose their viability if denied a supply of oxygen or glucose for more than a few minutes. When neurones are destroyed in the peripheral system, neuronal processes may be replaced under favourable conditions. However, in the CNS neurones are not replaced. These unique properties of nerve tissue have important implications for the nursing care of patients with neurological dysfunction.

Nerve impulses

The functions of the nerve cells are to receive, initiate and conduct 'messages' known as nerve impulses. An impulse is a combination of physical and chemical processes which are initiated at the point of stimulation. It occurs as the result of a mechanical, chemical or electrical change at some point in the immediate environment of the neurone. This change temporarily alters the permeability of the cell membrane at that point and is referred to as the *stimulus*. The series of events that result from the change in the membrane permeability produces an electrical current (Fig. 20.3).

When a normal neurone is in a resting state, the outer surface of its membrane is positively charged and the inner surface is negatively charged. As a result, it is described as being *polarized*. This electrical polarity is attributed to the selective action of the cell membrane by which a higher concentration of sodium ions is maintained outside the cell. The positive sodium ions, which are normally attracted to the negative ions within the cell, are not allowed to cross the membrane; if they do so, they are ejected by the cell membrane. The negative electrical charge within the cell is mainly due to the non-diffusable protein anions and retained

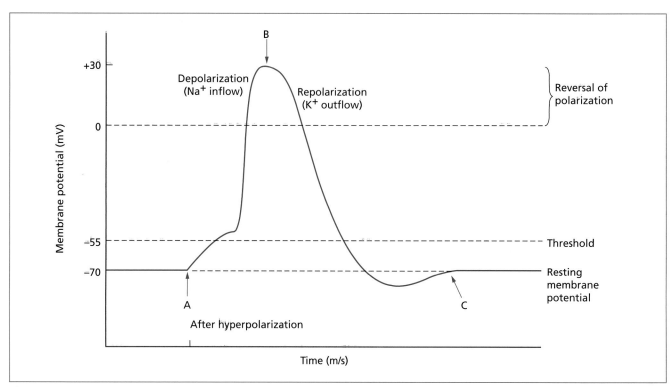

Figure 20.3   Action potential in neurones.

chlorine ions and measures −70 mV (point A, Fig. 20.3). This is known as the *resting membrane potential*. When a stimulus occurs, i.e. one that is sufficient to achieve a threshold of −55 mV, the membrane becomes permeable to sodium. The influx of cations depolarizes the membrane; a reversal of the electrical potential develops as the outer surface of the membrane becomes negatively charged and the inner surface becomes positively charged at +30 mV. This change alters the electrical relationship of the excited area to the adjacent portions; the shift of ions acts as a stimulus and a wave of depolarization passes along the length of the neuronal process (point B, Fig. 20.3). In a fraction of a second, following depolarization, the membrane recovers its normal permeability by the outward flow of potassium and the resting electrical polarity is restored, i.e. *repolarization* (point C, Fig. 20.3).

The velocity of impulse transmission is determined by the diameter of the neuronal process (nerve fibre) and the presence or absence of a myelin sheath, a white lipid and protein insulating cover. Nerve fibres enclosed in a myelin sheath are referred to as *myelinated*. Larger myelinated fibres (A fibres) conduct more quickly than smaller myelinated ones (B fibres) while unmyelinated fibres (C fibres) are slowest of all. Neural impulses travel at a maximum of 130 metres per second in A fibres but can only reach 2 metres/ second in C fibres. This point is crucial to understanding the Gate Control theory of pain explained on p. 124.

Synapses

A synapse is the junction between the axon of one neurone and the dendrite of another (Fig. 20.4). A release of chem-icals at the synapse provides for the transmission of impulses from neurone to neurone. The termination of a nerve fibre in a muscle cell is called a *neuromuscular junction*. This is basically similar to the synapse between two neurones. The synapse of each axon terminal of a motor neurone on a voluntary muscle cell is referred to as a *motor endplate*.

Chemicals released from the terminal portion of the axon may have an excitatory or an inhibitory effect on the transmission of impulses across a synapse and are called *neurotransmitters*. There is evidence that about 30 different neurotransmitter substances exist and new ones are being discovered all the time (Table 20.1). The latest discoveries in the last decade have been the endocannabinoids which are a new family of brain neurotransmitters involved in the regulation of pain, anxiety and hunger. They seem to exert their effect by inhibiting the GABA neurotransmitter system and are the subject of intensive research. The active ingredient in cannabis (delta 9 tetrahydrocannabinol or THC) has a very similar molecular structure which explains that drug's ability to affect mood and emotion (Nicol and Alger 2004).

Reflexes

A reflex is an involuntary, stereotypic response mediated by the nervous system. This means that an abnormal reflex, demonstrated on testing, indicates significant abnormality of the nervous system, hence the importance of testing reflexes as part of the physical exam carried out by doctors and advanced nurse practitioners. Reflexes serve as a defence mechanism and may involve the contraction of muscle tissue or the secretion of a gland. Although reflexes occur without

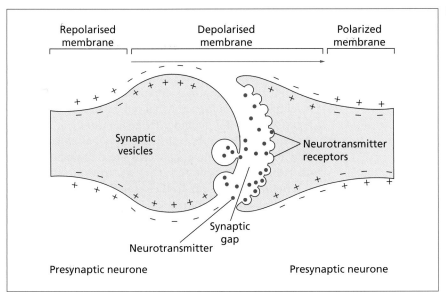

Figure 20.4   A synapse.

Repolarised membrane | Depolarised membrane | Polarized membrane

Synaptic vesicles

Neurotransmitter receptors

Neurotransmitter

Synaptic gap

Presynaptic neurone

Presynaptic neurone

Table 20.1   Principle neurotransmitters

	Action
Acetylcholine	Usually excitatory but can have an inhibitory effect on some of the parasympathetic nervous system
Serotonin	Inhibitor of pain pathway in the spinal cord. Has role in control of mood and sleep
Noradrenaline	Usually excitatory although sometimes inhibitory. Located in the brainstem
Dopamine	Found in the midbrain and usually inhibitory
γ-Aminobutyric acid (GABA)	The most common inhibitory neurotransmitter found in the brain
Glutamate	Excitatory effect found in the brain
Glycine	Inhibitory effect found in the spinal cord
Encephalin	Excitatory to systems that inhibit pain
Endorphin	Excitatory to systems that inhibit pain
Substance P	Excitatory effect found in sensory nerves, spinal cord pathways and parts of the brain associated with pain transmission
Endocannabinoids	Affect pain, anxiety and appetite by regulating the inhibitory actions of GABA

voluntary or willed initiation, the person usually becomes conscious of the reflex activity because the impulses reach the cerebral cortex and are interpreted as sensation. The pathway over which nerve impulses pass is called a *reflex arc* (Fig. 20.5). The arc is comprised of receptors, an afferent pathway (sensory nerve fibres), CNS connections, motor neurones, efferent pathway (motor nerve fibres) and effector organ (muscle fibres or glandular cells). The simplest reflex arc consists of two neurones: a sensory and a motor neurone. The patellar reflex ('knee jerk') which is elicited by tapping the tendon of the quadriceps femoris muscle is an example of this type of reflex.

A *receptor* consists of bare nerve endings or specialized structures sensitive to specific stimuli. An *effector* is muscular or glandular tissue. When a receptor is stimulated by a change in its environment (e.g. pressure, temperature, chemical, stretching), it evokes an impulse in the nerve fibres. The impulse is carried through the cell body of the sensory neurone and along its axon into the CNS. Here, it may pass through one, several or many connecting neurones before it excites a motor neurone whose axon (efferent or motor fibre) carries the impulse out of the CNS to the effector tissue or organ. Ascending axons within the spinal cord convey the message to the brain so that we become aware of

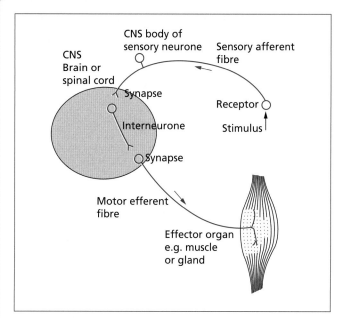

Figure 20.5 Component structures of a reflex arc.

what has happened. The terminal portion of the efferent fibre releases a chemical at its junction with the effector, initiating its response. For example, this response is contraction in the case of muscle, and is secretion if it is a gland that is innervated.

Reflex responses are either protective or postural. Protective reflexes are produced in response to irritating or painful stimuli. Examples include the closing of the eyelid when the cornea is touched lightly (blink reflex) and the rapid withdrawal of a hand from a hot stove (withdrawal reflex).

Postural reflexes maintain an appropriate degree of muscle tone which is essential in supporting the body against gravity and maintaining an upright position. The body can stay upright because muscles exert a continual pull on bones in the opposite direction to gravitational forces. Reflex mechanisms that regulate the muscle contraction necessary to oppose gravity are the stretch reflex and impulses originating in the inner ear (see p. 732).

There are four groups of clinically important reflexes:

1 *Superficial (or skin and mucous membrane) reflexes* – these include the sneeze reflex, the gag reflex, the abdominal reflex and the plantar reflex.
2 *Deep (or myotatic) reflexes* in which receptors are located in deeper tissue such as tendons. An example is the biceps reflex, which produces flexion at the elbow when the biceps tendon is struck.
3 *Visceral (or organic) reflexes* – such as the pupillary reflexes.
4 *Pathological (or abnormal) reflexes* – these are usually elicited only when neurological disease is present. Primitive defence responses, normally suppressed by cerebral inhibitory influences, are frequently present in these reflexes.

Neuroglia

Neuroglial cells occupy 50% of the volume of the CNS and provide a range of support functions for neurones. There are several different types of neuroglial cells; some form the myelin sheath around the axons of peripheral neurones (Schwann cells) and others are involved in the production of cerebrospinal fluid (ependymal cells) while others form a support structure for neurones (oligodendrocytes).

As strong intracellular substances such as collagen and elastin are lacking in neuroglial cells, fresh brain and spinal cord tissue appears soft and jelly-like. In contrast to neurones, neuroglial cells retain their mitotic abilities throughout the lifespan of the individual. From a clinical viewpoint, neuroglial cells are important because they are the most common source of primary tumours in the nervous system.

THE CENTRAL NERVOUS SYSTEM

Meninges

The brain is protected by the skull and three layers of connective tissue membranes known as the meninges. There are three meninges called, from the outer layer inward:

1 the dura mater
2 the arachnoid mater
3 the pia mater.

The dura mater

This is a thick, inelastic, collagenous double membrane. One layer is attached to the skull and the other is adjacent to the arachnoid. Two potential spaces associated with the dura are the *extradural space* between the cranium and the periosteal layer of the dura, and the *subdural space* between the dura and the arachnoid. This latter is said to contain a thin film of fluid.

The tentorium cerebelli separates the superior surface of the cerebellum from the occipital lobes, defining the *supratentorial* and *infratentorial cranial compartments*. The opening in the tentorium through which the brainstem passes is known as the *tentorial notch* or *tentorial incisura*. The notch is of clinical significance when intracranial pressure increases.

The arachnoid

The arachnoid ('spider-web-like') is a thin, avascular, delicate membrane. It conforms to the general shape of the brain. A *subarachnoid space*, filled with CSF, is located between the arachnoid and pia mater.

The pia mater

The pia mater is a thin, vascular, elastic membrane that adheres closely to the brain and spinal cord, following every sulcus and gyrus. The choroid plexuses arise from the vascular structure of the pia mater.

Brain

The human brain is the organ concerned with thought, memory and consciousness. It is also concerned with a range of sensory experiences, with motor activity, with the regulation of visceral, endocrine and somatic functions, and with the use of symbols and signs that underlie communication. For descriptive purposes, the brain may be subdivided into the cerebrum, basal ganglia, thalami, hypothalamus, midbrain, pons, medulla oblongata (known collectively as the brainstem) and cerebellum.

Cerebrum

The cerebrum accounts for 80% of the total weight of the brain. It is divided into two hemispheres by the *longitudinal fissure*. The two hemispheres are joined at their bases by bands of neuronal fibres collectively forming the *corpus callosum*. It is believed that the corpus callosum transfers information from one hemisphere to the other (Fig. 20.6).

In selected higher functions, one cerebral hemisphere appears to be the 'leading' one and is referred to as the *dominant hemisphere*. Cerebral dominance tends to be most complete in relation to the complex aspects of language. Handedness also is related to cerebral dominance, although its relationship is less clearcut than previously believed. In true right-handed persons, it is nearly always the left hemisphere that is dominant and governs language, but the converse of this is not necessarily true. Each hemisphere, independently, contains the ability to learn but the right hemisphere has a superior role in intuitive and creative responses and in spatial perception.

The brain contains areas of grey and white matter. The *grey matter* is a collection of neuronal bodies and unmyelinated processes. *White matter* consists primarily of myelinated fibres coming off cell bodies (axons). Grey matter, which forms the surface of the cerebrum, is called the *cerebral*

cortex. The cortex is believed to contain about 100 billion neurones. It is 2–5 mm thick and is arranged in a series of convolutions or coil-like elevations called *gyri*. Shallow crevices between the gyri are called *sulci*. The folding into gyri and sulci has the effect of increasing the surface area of the brain. Sulci that are particularly deep are called *fissures*.

The cerebral cortex of each hemisphere is made up of primary sensory areas, primary motor areas and association areas. Primary sensory areas are receptive areas for incoming impulses. Primary motor areas are concerned with dispatching outgoing impulses to prompt action responses in peripheral structures.

The motor area that initiates all voluntary movements of the body occupies the strip of the frontal lobe immediately anterior to the central fissure. In general, the motor area in one hemisphere controls the movements on the opposite side of the body. The size of the cortical area representing the body parts is proportional to the complexity and functional importance of the part.

The sensory impulses that enter the cerebral cortex are transmitted to specific areas of the cortex, depending on their origin. Impulses concerned with the somataesthetic senses such as touch, pressure, temperature, pain, and the sense of body position and its parts are transmitted to the parietal lobe immediately posterior to the central fissure.

The primary receptive area for vision is located in the posterior part of the occipital lobe. The primary auditory receptive areas or centres for hearing are located in the superior parts of the temporal lobes.

The frontal lobes contain the motor area. Other areas in the frontal lobes are the premotor cortex, the prefrontal areas and Broca's area. The premotor cortex is also known

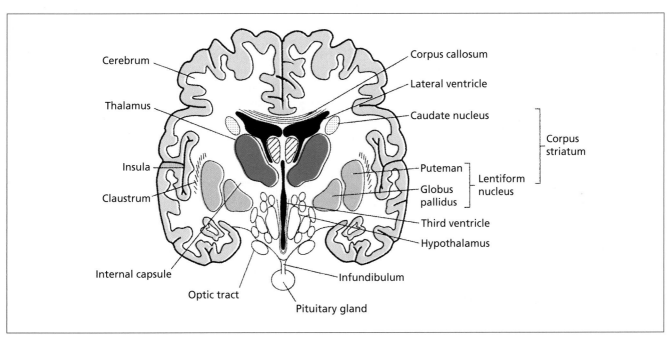

Figure 20.6 Frontal view of the brain.

as the motor association or secondary motor area. The prefrontal areas of the frontal lobe are concerned with memory and ability to concentrate, and ability to think in abstract terms. They are also concerned with personality, emotional reactions, initiative and sense of responsibility for socially acceptable standards. *Broca's area* is categorized as an association area because it aids in the formulation of words.

Beneath the grey cerebral cortex, the cerebrum is composed mainly of white matter. Myelinated neuronal processes are arranged in functionally related bundles called tracts. These are classified as commissural, association and projection tracts:

- *Commissural tracts* transmit impulses between the two hemispheres
- *Association tracts* carry impulses from one area of the cortex to another in the same hemisphere
- *Projection tracts* are ascending and descending pathways from one level of the central nervous system to another. One of the most important of these is the *internal capsule*, a massive bundle of efferent and afferent nerve fibres connecting the various subdivisions of the brain and spinal cord.

Basal ganglia (nuclei)
Basal ganglia are groups of nerve cell bodies deeply embedded within the white matter of each cerebral hemisphere. The functions of the basal ganglia are complex and not clearly understood. The system operates, along with the motor cortex and cerebellum, as a total unit, and individual functions cannot be ascribed solely to the various parts of the system. One of the general functions of the basal ganglia is inhibition of muscle tone throughout the body.

Thalami
The thalami are a pair of egg-shaped masses of grey matter at the base of each hemisphere. Each mass is referred to as a thalamus and forms part of the lateral walls of the third ventricle. The thalami form the main relay centre for sensory impulses and cerebellar and basal ganglia projections to the cerebral cortex.

Hypothalamus
This is an important grey mass that lies beneath the thalamus. It forms the floor and part of the wall of the third ventricle. It contains nuclei of the autonomic nervous system for the control of most of the body's involuntary functions as well as many aspects of emotional behaviour. There are neuronal links between the hypothalamus and the posterior pituitary gland (see p. 551). The hypothalamus is also concerned with gastrointestinal and feeding regulation. Hunger centres and a satiety centre have been identified in this grey mass. In addition, it activates feeding reflexes such as licking the lips and swallowing. It is also known to affect responses such as pleasure and fear.

Brainstem
The brainstem is composed of the midbrain, pons varolii and medulla oblongata. The *midbrain* forms the upper portion and is the location of the nuclei of origin of cranial nerves III and IV. The *pons varolii* is located between the midbrain and medulla. It consists of numerous tracts that link various parts of the brain and serve as conduction pathways.

The *medulla oblongata* lies between the pons and the spinal cord. It is composed of ascending and descending conduction pathways. Autonomic centres that regulate such vital functions as breathing, cardiac rate and vasomotor tone as well as centres for vomiting, gagging, coughing and sneezing reflex behaviours are located in the medulla.

Reticular activating system This is a diffuse system of motor and sensory fibres and nerve cells that forms the central core of the brainstem. It has widespread afferent connections, receiving sensory impulses from all over the body. The cerebral cortex can stimulate this system. It is known to be associated with initiation and maintenance of wakefulness and alertness.

Cerebellum
This lies beneath the posterior portion of the cerebrum, posterior to the pons and medulla. It is separated from the cerebrum by a fold of meningeal membrane (dura mater) called the tentorium cerebelli. Direct input is received from the spinal cord and brainstem and conveyed to the deep cerebellar nuclei and cerebral cortex.

The cerebellum is integrated into many connective pathways throughout the brain for the provision of muscle coordination in the body. All sensations are relayed through the cerebellum, thus providing information about muscle activity. The functions of the cerebellum are essentially to control fine movements and balance, to control coordination of movement and maintain feedback loops to correct movement, and to coordinate the action of muscle groups. Dysfunction of the cerebellum can result in gait disturbance, equilibrium ataxia (overstability or understability) and tremors.

Blood supply to the brain
The ever-active brain receives about one-fifth of the blood pumped by the heart and consumes about 20% of the oxygen utilized by the body. The brain requires a continuous flow of blood because it can store only minute quantities of glucose and oxygen, and derives its energy almost exclusively from the metabolism of glucose delivered by the blood. Its blood requirement is the same whether one is mentally active or sleeping.

Brain cells are extremely sensitive to hypoxia, particularly those of the cerebral cortex. Interruption of blood supply to the brain produces loss of consciousness in seconds. Irreversible brain damage occurs if the blood supply is interrupted for 2–4 minutes. Brainstem neurones are less sensitive to hypoxia than cortical cells; individuals experiencing prolonged hypoxia may survive because the vital centres in the medulla are more resistant and recover, but irreversible cortical damage persists. The arterial blood supply to the brain is derived from two internal carotid arteries and two vertebral arteries. The vertebral arteries unite to form the basilar artery. The internal carotid arteries supply blood, via the anterior and middle cerebral arteries, to most of the hemispheres excluding the occipital lobes, the basal ganglia, and the upper two-thirds of the diencephalon.

Although the vertebral basilar arterial tree and the internal carotid arterial tree are essentially independent, some anastomotic connections between the two systems exist. Small posterior communicating arteries connect the two systems to form an arterial crown known as the cerebral arterial circle of Willis. The anterior communicating artery that connects the two anterior cerebral arteries completes the circle. It allows blood to reach all parts of the brain even after one or more of the four supplying vessels is obstructed. Most venous blood drains into the internal jugular veins at the base of the skull.

Blood-brain barrier This term refers to the very tight junctions that exist between the epithelial cells of capillary walls in the brain and the fact that neuroglial cells are wrapped around the outside of the capillaries making an impenetrable barrier for substances in the blood. The only way to cross this blood–brain barrier is for a molecule to be lipid soluble and so able to pass through the lipid bilayer cell walls as nothing can squeeze between the cells. This barrier phenomenon effectively keeps microorganisms out of the brain. However, it is equally effective in keeping most antibiotics out, as they are not lipid soluble, thus complicating therapy for intracranial infections. This is a key point in developing drugs that are to act on the brain such as general anaesthetics.

Ventricles and cerebrospinal fluid

The ventricular system is a series of cavities within the brain (Fig. 20.7). Each cerebral hemisphere contains a lateral ventricle, which communicates with the third ventricle by means of an intraventricular foramen. The third ventricle is a slit-like space between the thalami and is continuous with the fourth ventricle through a narrow channel called the cerebral aqueduct. The medial opening of the fourth ventricle allows CSF to circulate around the spinal cord. Two lateral openings channel fluid around the brain. This distribution of CSF provides a protective cushion for the brain and cord.

The ventricular system is filled with CSF. Each ventricle contains a *choroid plexus,* which is a rich network of blood vessels covered by a layer of ependymal cells that secrete

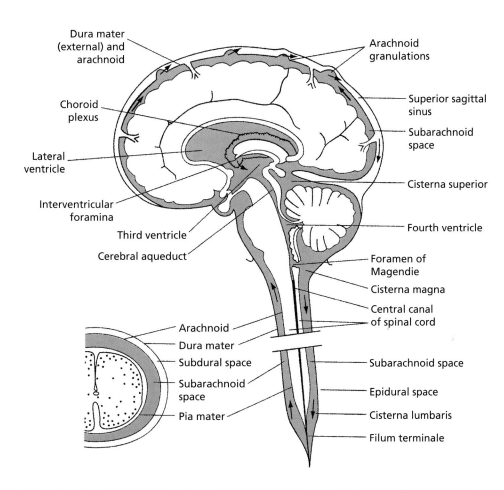

Figure 20.7   Path of flow of cerebrospinal fluid. (Based on an illustration by RJ Demarest, In: Noback CR (1967) The human nervous system. New York: McGraw-Hill.)

CSF continuously. The CSF is a clear, colourless, water-like fluid with a specific gravity of 1.007. It contains occasional lymphocytes and traces of the minerals and organic materials found in blood. The glucose concentration is normally 2.8–4.5 mmol/L and protein concentration is 0.1–0.4 g/L at the lumbar level. The total volume of CSF in the adult ranges from 125 to 150 mL. Normal pressure is 40–180 mmH$_2$O.

The CSF circulates through the ventricular system and around the brain and cord in the subarachnoid space. It is steadily reabsorbed into the arachnoid villi, which are projections from the subarachnoid space into the venous sinuses of the brain. Any interruption within the CSF circuit results in an excessive accumulation of fluid within the ventricles. The condition is referred to as *hydrocephalus*. The brain tissue becomes compressed between the skull and the expanding volume of fluid resulting in increased intracranial pressure.

Spinal cord

The spinal cord is a long, cylindrical structure of grey and white matter within the vertebral column. It is continuous with the medulla oblongata, originating at the foramen magnum of the skull and extending to the first or second lumbar vertebrae. It tapers off into a fine, non-neural cord called the *cauda equina*, which continues inferiorly (caudally) to its attachments in the coccyx. A small canal (central canal) extends the full length of the cord; it contains CSF, and the upper end opens into the fourth ventricle. The cord is surrounded by the three meninges, which are continuous with those encapsulating the brain. The meninges extend to the level of the fifth lumbar vertebra.

The grey matter (cell bodies) in the spinal cord is concentrated in its interior, roughly in the form of an H. White matter, composed of nerve tracts and fibres, surrounds the H-shaped grey matter (Fig. 20.8). Afferent impulses are received by neurones in the posterior columns or horns of grey matter. Efferent impulses are discharged by neurones in the anterior columns or horns of the grey matter. The grey matter also contains neurones that may transmit impulses from one lateral half of the cord to the other, from posterior to anterior and to other levels of the CNS.

Nerve fibres emerge from the spinal cord in uninterrupted series of posterior (sensory or afferent) and anterior (motor or efferent) rootlets which unite to form 31 pairs of posterior and anterior roots. In the area of an intervertebral foramen, a posterior and an anterior root meet to form a *spinal nerve* (Fig. 20.9) which supplies innervation to a segment of the body. The cord has two enlargements: cervical and lumbar. The cervical enlargement (plexus) is associated with nerve roots that innervate the upper limbs, and the lumbar enlargement (plexus) innervates the lower limbs.

The spinal cord has three major functions:

1 It carries impulses via sensory nerves through ascending tracts up to the brain.
2 It carries impulses from the brain via motor nerves through descending tracts to nerves supplying effector organs (muscle and glands).
3 It functions as a centre for reflex actions.

Nerves and tracts

Nerves are bundles of neuronal processes that extend beyond the CNS, whereas tracts are bundles of processes within the CNS. Nerves consisting only of afferent fibres, which transmit impulses from the periphery to the CNS, are called sensory nerves. Motor nerves are composed entirely of efferent fibres, which transmit impulses from the CNS out into the periphery. Many nerves (e.g. all spinal nerves) contain both efferent and afferent fibres and are known as *mixed nerves*.

Structurally, three types of nerve fibres or processes occur:

1 Myelinated or medullated fibres are enclosed in a lipoprotein sheath (myelin) and an outer membranous sheath called the neurilemma (sheath of Schwann).
2 Non-myelinated (non-medullated) fibres have no myelin sheath but do have a neurilemma. Most non-myelinated

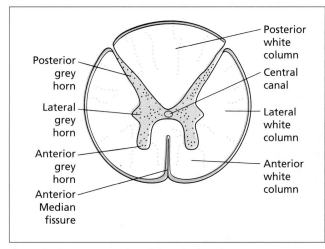

Figure 20.8 Cross-section of the spinal cord.

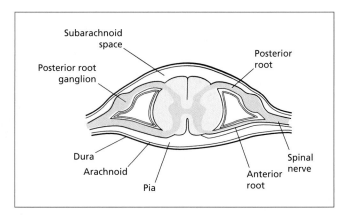

Figure 20.9 The spinal nerve: its posterior root ganglion, posterior root and anterior root.

fibres belong to the autonomic nervous system, which is concerned with visceral activity.

3 A third type has a myelin sheath but lacks the neurilemma. All fibres within the CNS, as well as the optic and auditory nerves, are of this type. Neuronal processes lacking the neurilemma cannot regenerate following injury.

Nerve tracts transmit impulses that are usually similar in origin, termination and function. The origin and destination may be determined from the name of the tract. For example, the corticospinal tract carries impulses originating in the cerebral cortex to the spinal cord; the spinothalamic tract transmits sensory impulses from the spinal cord to the thalamus.

THE PERIPHERAL NERVOUS SYSTEM

The peripheral nervous system is composed of nerves and ganglia. The nerves may be divided into two main groups, *cranial* and *spinal* nerves, according to whether they emerge from the CNS at the cranial or spinal level.

Cranial nerves

There are 12 pairs of cranial nerves that are considered to be part of the peripheral nervous system. They emerge from the undersurface of the brain and are named according to their function or distribution. The origin and functions of cranial nerves are described in Table 20.2.

Spinal nerves

A total of 31 pairs of nerves arise from the spinal cord. They are numbered and named according to the order in which they arise and the vertebral level at which they emerge. There are 8 cervical, 12 thoracic, 5 lumbar, 5 sacral pairs and 1 coccygeal pair.

All spinal nerves are mixed (sensory and motor) and each has two origins which are referred to as anterior and posterior roots (Fig. 20.9). The anterior roots carry two types of motor fibres:

1 The *general somatic efferent fibres* which have axons originating from lower motor neurones (anterior horn cells in the spinal cord) and which innervate voluntary striated muscles.

Table 20.2 Name and functions of the cranial nerves (12 pairs)

Number	Name	Function
I	Olfactory	Olfactory sense (sense of smell)
II	Optic	Vision
III	Oculomotor	Movements of the eyeball and upper eyelid; size of the pupil of iris; control of ciliary muscle to regulate degree of refraction by the lens
IV	Trochlear	Movement of eyeball by superior oblique muscles
V	Trigeminal largest cranial nerve has three sensory divisions: ophthalmic, maxillary, mandibular	Motor function: mastication Sensory function: sensations (pain, touch, temperature) of the face, nose, teeth and mouth
VI	Abducens	Movement of the eyeball by lateral rectus muscle
VII	Facial	Motor function: contraction of facial and scalp muscles (facial expression); secretion of saliva by submaxillary and sublingual glands Sensory function: taste (from anterior two-thirds of tongue)
VIII	Vestibulocochlear Has two divisions: vestibular, cochlear	Sensory function: vestibular branch: equilibrium (position, balance) cochlear division: sense of hearing
IX	Glossopharyngeal	Motor function: swallowing reflex, control of blood pressure through connection with carotid baroreceptors; salivary secretion by parotid glands Sensory functions: taste and oral and pharyngeal sensations
X	Vagus has very wide distribution	Motor function: muscles of pharynx, larynx, thoracic and abdominal viscera (e.g. regulates gastrointestinal motility of peristalsis; influences cardiac rate); secretion by gastric, intestinal and pancreatic glands Sensory function: sensations in pharynx, larynx and thoracic
XI	Accessory	Movement of shoulder and head by trapezius and sternocleidomastoid muscles
XII	Hypoglossal	Movements of the tongue

2 The *general visceral efferent fibres* (autonomic nerves) which innervate visceral and cardiac muscle, and regulate glandular secretions.

The posterior roots convey sensory input via two types of sensory fibre:

1 The *general somatic afferent fibres* which carry impulses for pain, temperature, touch and proprioception from the body wall, tendons and joints into the CNS.
2 The *general visceral afferent fibres* which carry sensory impulses from the viscera into the CNS.

After emerging from the vertebral canal, each spinal nerve divides into two major branches: the anterior and posterior rami. The branches of the anterior rami tend to form intricate networks of interlacing nerve branches before proceeding to the structures they innervate. These networks are referred to as *plexuses*. Spinal nerves lose their individuality after passing through a plexus and they emerge as peripheral nerves. Four major plexuses are formed by the anterior rami of spinal nerves: the cervical, brachial, lumbar and sacral plexuses. The *cervical plexus* gives rise to peripheral nerve branches that innervate muscles of the neck and shoulders. It also gives rise to the phrenic nerve which supplies the diaphragm. Important peripheral nerves that arise from the *brachial plexus* are the musculocutaneous, median, radial and ulnar nerves, all of which supply the upper limbs. The *lumbar plexus* generates the femoral, saphenous and obturator nerves which innervate the lower abdominal wall, external genitalia and parts of the thigh and leg. The nerves leaving the *sacral plexus* supply the buttocks, perineum and lower extremities. The most important nerve derived from this plexus is the sciatic, the longest and largest nerve in the body.

Ganglia

A ganglion is a group of nerve cell bodies located outside the CNS. The ganglia that form the posterior or sensory roots of the spinal nerves lie just outside the spinal cord within the vertebral column. These are the spinal or posterior root ganglia. Other ganglia are associated with the autonomic nervous system and mostly lie adjacent to the vertebral column.

AUTONOMIC NERVOUS SYSTEM

The autonomic nervous system controls the visceral functions of the body. This system helps to control such phenomena as arterial blood pressure, gastrointestinal motility and secretion, urinary bladder emptying, sweating and body temperature. It carries only efferent impulses and the responses are involuntary.

The autonomic system is largely activated by centres located in the spinal cord, brainstem and hypothalamus. In addition, parts of the cerebral cortex can transmit impulses to the lower centres and in this way influence the autonomic system. Often, the autonomic system operates by means of visceral reflexes. That is, sensory signals enter the centres in the CNS and these in turn transmit appropriate reflex re-

sponses back to the organs via the autonomic system to control their activities.

The autonomic nervous system is divided into the *parasympathetic* and *sympathetic* systems. Most viscera have a nerve supply from each division; impulses delivered from one system excite visceral activity, and those originating with the other division inhibit activity (Table 20.3).

Parasympathetic nervous system

The parasympathetic fibres leave the CNS through several cranial nerves (75% are in the vagus or tenth cranial nerve as it is otherwise known) and through the pelvic nerves. The responses to parasympathetic stimulation are localized and specific for parts of the body.

Generally, parasympathetic innervation promotes a normal state; it is concerned with the restoration and conservation of body energy and elimination of body wastes (Table 20.3).

Sympathetic nervous system

The sympathetic nerves originate in the thoracic and lumbar regions of the spinal cord. The sympathetic nerves leave the spinal cord via the anterior roots and form the white communicating rami of the thoracic and lumbar nerves. Through these, nerves reach the trunk ganglia of the sympathetic chain.

The sympathetic system produces generalized physiological responses rather than specific, localized ones. It responds to stress, strong emotions, severe pain, cold, or any threat. The purpose of the responses induced is to mobilize the body's resources for defensive action ('fight or flight') (Table 20.3).

Stimulation of the sympathetic nervous system results in stimulation of the adrenal medullae. Increase in secretion of adrenaline and noradrenaline results and this augments the body defence responses mediated by the sympathetic nervous system.

Chemical mediators

In both the sympathetic and parasympathetic nervous systems, the transmission of impulses from the preganglionic fibres to the ganglia is dependent upon the release of acetylcholine by the preganglionic axon terminals. Acetylcholine is rapidly deactivated by cholinesterase. The postganglionic fibres of the parasympathetic system also release acetylcholine at their junction with the effector organs to facilitate the transmission of their impulses. The neurotransmitter that is released by the postganglionic nerve terminals in the sympathetic system is noradrenaline, which is deactivated by enzymes (e.g. monoamine oxidase) or taken up again by the nerve terminals.

MOTOR AND SENSORY SYSTEMS

Contraction of skeletal muscles normally results only from impulses discharged by motor neurones within the CNS and transmitted along peripheral nerve fibres to the muscle. As the motor centres lie within the cerebral cortex, contractions

Table 20.3 Autonomic effects on various organs of the body

Organ	Effect of sympathetic stimulation	Effect of parasympathetic stimulation
Eye:		
Pupil	Dilated	Constricted
Ciliary muscle	Slight relaxation	Contracted
Glands:		
Nasal lacrimal	Vasoconstriction and slight secretion	Stimulation of thin, copious secretion (containing many
Parotid		enzyme-secreting glands)
Submaxillary		
Gastric		
Pancreatic		
Sweat glands	Copious sweating (cholinergic)	None
Apocrine glands	Thick, odoriferous secretion	None
Heart:		
Muscle	Increased rate	Slowed rate
	Increased force of contraction	Decreased force of atrial contraction
Coronary arteries	Dilated (β_2): constricted (α)	Dilated
Lungs:		
Bronchi	Dilated	Constricted
Blood vessels	Mildly constricted	Dilated
Gut:		
Lumen	Decreased peristalsis and tone	Increased peristalsis and tone
Sphincter	Increased tone	Relaxed
Liver	Glucose released	Slight glycogen synthesis
Gallbladder and bile ducts	Relaxed	Constricted
Kidney	Decreased output	None
Bladder:		
Detrusor muscle	Relaxed	Excited
Trigone	Excited	Relaxed
Penis	Ejaculation	Erection
Systemic blood vessels:		
Abdominal	Constricted	None
Muscle	Constricted (adrenergic α)	None
	Dilated (adrenergic β)	
	Dilated (cholinergic)	
Skin	Constricted	None
Blood:		
Coagulation	Increased	None
Glucose	Increased	None
Basal metabolism	Increased up to 100%	None
Adrenal cortical secretion	Increased	None
Mental activity	Increased	None
Piloerector muscles	Excited	None
Skeletal muscle	Increased glycogenolysis	None
	Increased strength	

are usually produced voluntarily. Involuntary contractions occur in the form of reflex responses.

The process whereby a nerve impulse is converted into muscle action is referred to as *neuromuscular transmission*. Each nerve fibre terminates at a specialized region of the muscle fibre, called the *neuromuscular junction* or *motor endplate*. The endplate is a localized specialization of the sarcolemma. Essentially, the release of acetylcholine at the endplate and its rapid destruction by the enzyme cholinesterase is at the basis of electrical and chemical reactions and the release of mechanical and heat energy in the contraction of muscle fibres.

Voluntary movement

Normal voluntary movements are the result of controlled contraction and relaxation of groups of muscles. All willed movements depend upon excitation of neurones within the cerebral cortex (upper motor neurones) as well as at a lower level (lower motor neurones). Those at a lower level may be the motor components of cranial nerve nuclei in the brainstem or they may be in the spinal cord. Two major neuronal pathways in the CNS are involved in voluntary muscle activity: the *pyramidal tract* and the *extrapyramidal system*.

Pyramidal tract (corticospinal tract)

The pyramidal tract arises in the sensorimotor cortex of the cerebrum and is one of the major pathways whereby motor signals are transmitted from all the motor areas of the cortex to the anterior motor neurones of the spinal cord.

Voluntary movement begins with the stimulation of a discrete area of neurones in the motor area of the cerebral cortex. If the movement applies only to muscles on one side of the body, then only the motor area of the cerebral hemisphere on the opposite side will be involved. The motor fibres pass downward through the brainstem, and in the lower medulla approximately 90% decussate (cross-over) to form the pyramids of the medulla. These fibres descend in the lateral corticospinal tract of the cord and terminate in posterior horns of cord grey matter. Fibres that did not decussate earlier continue on the same side (ipsilaterally) in the anterior corticospinal tracts and cross over further down the cord.

At various levels in the cord, the fibres synapse with neurones in the anterior horns of grey matter. The axons of these neurones form the motor fibres of the peripheral nerves whereby the impulses are delivered to muscle fibres. Some fibres in the tract may synapse in the brainstem with nuclei of cranial nerves. The impulses are then carried out to a muscle by motor fibres of a peripheral cranial nerve.

The neurones of the cerebral cortical motor area are referred to as the *upper motor neurones*. Those with which the axons of upper motor neurones synapse are called *lower motor neurones*. The cell bodies of lower motor neurones reside within the CNS and their axons carry the impulses to skeletal muscles in the periphery.

Extrapyramidal system (extrapyramidal tracts)

This system includes all the tracts exclusive of the pyramidal tract which transmits motor signals from the brain to the spinal cord. Unlike the pyramidal tract, which is a direct link from the cerebral cortex to the spinal cord, the extrapyramidal system conveys its influences to the cord via multineuronal and multisynaptic linkages involving the cortex, basal ganglia, thalami, cerebellum, brain-stem and related structures. Extrapyramidal impulses are initiated in several areas of the brain below conscious level and all are transmitted by reticulospinal tracts to lower motor neurones. The lower motor neurones provide the final common pathway for all the afferent impulses (both pyramidal and extrapyramidal) to skeletal muscles. Inhibition, facilitation and coordination essential for smooth, precise muscle activity is normally provided by the extrapyramidal system.

An imbalance in the interactions within the complex circuitry of the extrapyramidal system occurs with malfunction of various nuclear complexes. The motor disorders resulting from the improper functioning of the extrapyramidal system and associated nuclei include various abnormal movements such as paralysis agitans, athetosis and chorea.

Voluntary muscle activity involves the pyramidal and extrapyramidal tracts in concert. The pyramidal tract transmits the impulses that are consciously initiated to produce a given movement. The other essential components of the movement such as reciprocal relaxation of certain muscles, correlation, stabilization and adjustment in posture are automatically contributed by the extrapyramidal system.

The complex interrelationship of the nervous system means that when considering disorders this cannot be done in isolation. A patient with a head injury may survive the initial trauma but may die from infection or sustain epilepsy as a complication. For the purpose of explanation, the disorders that can affect the nervous system are described as follows:

- trauma including traumatic brain injury (head injury) and spinal cord injury
- cerebrovascular disorders including stroke and cerebral aneurysm
- neoplasms
- epilepsy, both as a disorder and as a symptom of other disorders
- meningitis
- degenerative disorders including acquired immune deficiency syndrome (AIDS), dementia, multiple sclerosis, Parkinson's disease and motor neurone disease.

This is not an exhaustive list of disorders but is representative of those that patients are most likely to present with.

ASSESSMENT OF NEUROLOGICAL FUNCTION

Accurate assessment such as monitoring level of consciousness will inform effective nursing interventions and clinical management. More complex diagnostic investigations such as angiography necessitate neuroradiological intervention using specialist technology.

ASSESSMENT OF COGNITIVE STATUS

The neurological examination is the part of the physical examination that evaluates the function of the cerebrum and the cranial nerves as well as the motor and sensory status, reflex status and the status of the autonomic nervous system.

Cerebral function

Evaluation of cerebral function includes information obtained from observing the patient, evoking responses and questioning family and friends. It relates to the appropriateness of the individual's appearance, behaviour, level of consciousness, mood, attitude and flow of speech. Cognitive functions such as orientation, speech comprehension, general intelligence, attention and concentration, memory retention and immediate recall, vocabulary, judgement and abstract reasoning are also evaluated. Deterioration in one or more of these functions commonly occurs with cerebral dysfunction.

Disease involving the CNS may affect the patient in many ways. The patient's family may report a change in appearance, particularly facial expression, posture and personal grooming. Disordered emotional reactions may be evident in the patient's fluctuating attitudes. There may be inappropriate laughing, crying, irritability or unprovoked expressions of anger. Sharp mood swings may occur; the patient who is withdrawn and depressed or anxious may suddenly become excited or euphoric. Impaired reasoning, unjustified fears, distortion in perception and loss of memory may occur. The attention span may be abnormally short and there may be inability to do very simple calculations or to identify normally familiar objects or sounds. Confusion or disorientation as to time, place or person may occur with a cerebral lesion. The patient's response to stimuli may vary from a coherent verbal response to no response of any sort, even to painful stimuli.

Speech dysfunctions which occur with cerebral lesions vary with the location, size and nature of the lesion. Aphasia, dysphasia, agnosia and apraxia are examples of speech disorders that may occur.

Aphasia refers to the loss of ability to understand words or to use them to communicate. Difficulty in using words to communicate due to lack of coordination and ability to put words in order occurs more commonly and is referred to as *dysphasia*. Aphasia may be classified as *motor* (*expressive, Broca's*) or *sensory* (*receptive*). Motor aphasia implies that the person understands spoken and written words and knows what he or she wants to say but cannot speak the words. Motor aphasias include any loss of communication by writing, speaking or making signs. Sensory aphasia implies that the comprehension of written and spoken words is affected. A patient may suffer auditory aphasia (word deafness) which is the inability to make sense of sound because of an inability to comprehend symbolic communication associated with sound. Some may experience visual aphasia ('word blindness') which means loss of ability to understand the symbolic content of written words or figures and, even though they can see them, they cannot read them. In many instances of aphasia, elements of both expressive and receptive communication are lost.

Certain areas of the cerebral cortex are essential to the recognition of objects by sight, sound, feeling, smell and taste. Cerebral dysfunction may result in the inability to recognize objects through any of the senses and is referred to as *agnosia*. Agnosia may be visual, auditory or tactile. A cerebral lesion may also result in *apraxia*, which is the inability to carry out purposeful, useful or skilled acts in the absence of paralysis, or use objects correctly. *Dyslexia* means inability to comprehend written words.

Cranial nerves

Cranial nerves are referred to by specific name or number (Table 20.2). Most arise from the brainstem, and much information can be obtained by testing cranial nerve function. Evaluation of cranial nerve function involves the following test procedures.

Olfactory (I) nerve

The patient is asked to close the eyes and identify a series of odorous substances such as coffee, peppermint or oil of cloves. Each nostril is tested separately. Inability to identify the substances (in the absence of a cold or allergy) may suggest a lesion in the frontal lobe such as a tumour of the olfactory groove.

Optic (II) nerve

This is tested using ophthalmoscopic examination and evaluation of visual acuity and visual fields. Visual acuity may be grossly evaluated by asking the person to read from a printed page or distant sign both with and without corrective lenses if such are used. (See assessment in Chapter 21.)

Ophthalmoscopic examination may reveal papilloedema, which is oedema of the area where the optic nerve and blood vessels enter and leave the eyeball, and is a classical sign of increased intracranial pressure.

Oculomotor (III), trochlear (IV) and abducens (VI) nerves

These nerves are usually tested together because they are all involved in the muscles that rotate the eyeball, constrict the pupils and elevate the eyelids. On examination, pupils should be round and equal in size and shape. Each pupil is tested, in a darkened room, for the direct light reflex. A light is directed into each pupil and the response observed. The normal pupil constricts briskly in response to light stimulus. The consensual light reflex is also tested. This is a slightly weaker constriction of one pupil when the other is stimulated by light.

Accommodation is tested by asking the person to look at a distant spot and then follow the examiner's finger to within 15 cm of the person's nose. Visualization of a distant object causes pupillary dilatation, whereas viewing a near object produces constriction and convergence. Abnormal pupillary responses suggest neurological dysfunction.

The range of ocular movements is evaluated by asking the person to follow the examiner's finger as it moves up, down, medially and laterally. Inability to move the eye-ball in a particular direction may result in *diplopia* (double vision). Normal eyes move conjugately (track together). Disconjugate movement implies failure of function of one or more of the eye muscles. Abnormal eye movements can result from injury to the nerves themselves or their nuclei in the midbrain and pons. During examination of ocular movements, observations for *nystagmus* are made. This is an involuntary rhythmic movement of one or both eyes in a lateral or vertical direction. It may occur in normal persons with severe myopia or fatigue or it may occur with neurological disease. *Ptosis* (drooping) of the eyelid may occur with paralysis of the levator palpebrae muscle due to damage of cranial nerve III.

Trigeminal (V) nerve

The trigeminal nerve has sensory and motor components. The sensory function is assessed by testing both sides of the face and mouth for touch, temperature and pain sensations while the person's eyes are closed. The motor function is evaluated by having the person make chewing and biting movements. The ophthalmic branch of the trigeminal nerve controls the corneal reflex. If this reflex is intact, the person blinks briskly when the cornea of each eye is lightly touched with a wisp of cotton wool. The corneal reflex is one of the last to disappear when the patient's condition is deteriorating.

Facial (VII) nerve

The facial nerve has a sensory and motor component. The sensory component is tested by seeing whether the person can recognize the taste of sweet and salty substances when applied to the anterior part of the tongue. The motor divisions are tested by asking the person to use the facial muscles in such expressions as smiling, frowning, closing the eyes tightly and puckering the lips.

Vestibulocochlear (VIII) nerve

This nerve has two divisions: the cochlear nerve and the vestibular nerve. The cochlear nerve is tested for hearing acuity by whispering in one ear from a distance of 30–60 seconds (the words 'football' and 'rugby' are commonly used, a different word for each ear). Further tests such as the Rinne and Weber tests are discussed on p. 735. Loss of hearing or reports by the patient of constant or abnormal recurring sounds described as roaring, ringing, buzzing or swishing should be recorded and reported. The vestibular nerve, concerned with equilibrium reflexes, is tested by rotating the patient and performing the caloric test. Dizziness and loss of position balance (equilibrium) may occur with disturbance in the semicircular canals of the internal ear, of the vestibular part of the auditory nerve, or pathway within the brain.

Glossopharyngeal (IX) and vagus (X) nerves

These nerves are usually examined simultaneously because of their overlapping innervation of the pharynx. In response to touching of the pharynx with a tongue depressor, a brisk gag reaction should be elicited. Ability to swallow water is assessed and the posterior third of the tongue may be tested for taste. Absence of the gag or swallowing reflex occurs in neurological damage and renders the person vulnerable to aspiration. To assess the vagus nerve, the ability to speak and to cough is evaluated. Ineffectual cough and a weak, hoarse voice suggest possible vagal involvement.

Accessory (XI) nerve

This nerve is tested by inspecting the sternocleidomastoid muscle and the upper portion of the trapezius muscle for symmetry, atrophy and strength. The person is asked to elevate the shoulders with and without resistance from the examiner's hand, and to rotate the head to each side against the pull of the chin to the midline by the examiner's hand.

Hypoglossal (XII) nerve

This nerve is assessed by observing various movements of the tongue and examining it for symmetry, atrophy and tremor when protruded.

Motor function

This is evaluated by examining muscle symmetry, size, shape, tone and movement. Muscle function, balance accuracy and muscle strength are assessed. Inspection and comparison of muscles on both sides of the body, palpation and measuring the circumferences of areas with a tape measure provides information about size and shape and can reveal abnormalities such as atrophy or hypertrophy. Muscle tone is assessed by palpating muscles at rest and noting the resistance to passive movement. Excessive resistance (*spasticity*), a constant state of resistance (*rigidity*) and decreased muscle tone (*flaccidity or hypotonia*) are examples of abnormal muscle tone.

Movements are examined for 'fine' and 'gross' abnormalities. Fine muscle abnormalities are *fasciculations* which are involuntary ripples, or twitches, that occur when the person is relaxed. They suggest lower motor neurone disease. Gross abnormal movements may indicate extrapyramidal disease and include athetoid, choreiform and dystonic movements, spasms, myoclonus, tics and tremors.

Athetoid movements

These are involuntary, repetitive, slow and writhing. They may be unilateral or bilateral and follow a definite pattern in the individual patient, ceasing only during sleep. Athetosis is commonly seen in persons with cerebral palsy.

Choreiform movements

These are involuntary, rapid, rhythmic and jerky. They begin abruptly, are variable in pattern and distribution, and may occur during sleep. The limbs, face and tongue are most often involved, and difficulty in speaking, chewing and swallowing may be present. The forcefulness of the movements may lead to injury unless protection is provided.

Spasms or cramps

These are sudden, violent, involuntary contractions of a muscle or muscle groups which result in pain, interference with function and voluntary movement. Muscles of the limbs and neck are most frequently affected. The cause may be a lesion within the CNS, such as degenerative changes in the extrapyramidal system, a deficient blood supply to the muscle(s), overstretching and injury of the muscle fibres or a blood calcium or sodium deficiency.

Dystonic movements

These involve spasms in portions of the limbs as well as the trunk. The result is usually slow, grotesque, twisting movements and abnormal posture.

Myoclonus

This is shock-like contractions of a portion of a muscle, an entire muscle or group of muscles restricted to one area of the body or appearing synchronously or asynchronously in several areas (seen most commonly in epilepsy).

Tics

Tics are frequently of psychogenic origin. They are stereotyped, repetitious, purposeless movements that vary from individual to individual. Twitching of a cheek is an example of a tic.

Tremors

These are involuntary shaky movements, particularly of the limbs, which may have a physical or psychological aetiology. A fine, rapid tremor, particularly of the hands, may be associated with anxiety, fatigue or toxic conditions such as thyrotoxicosis, uraemia and alcoholism. *Intention tremor* occurs when a voluntary movement is initiated and progressively intensifies, especially with precision movements. *A resting tremor* is one that diminishes with voluntary movement and disappears during sleep.

Muscles are further evaluated by putting all the joints through a full range of passive movement. Pain, contractures and muscle resistance are abnormal findings.

Muscle strength may be assessed by flexion and extension and other movements, first without resistance and then with the examiner offering resistance. In addition, the person may be asked to hold the arms straight in front with the palms up and the eyes closed for 20–30 seconds. If one arm moves downward or one hand begins to pronate, a *drift* is said to be present, suggesting muscle weakness in that arm. Drift can be tested in the lower limbs by asking the person to raise both legs off the bed while in a supine position.

Coordination, balance and accuracy of muscle function is mediated largely by the cerebellum. These attributes may be assessed by point-to-point tests (e.g. with the eyes open, then repeated with the eyes closed, the person repeatedly touches the examiner's finger and then his or her own nose). Coordination and balance may also be assessed by observing the person's gait while the eyes are open and again when closed. Locomotion depends upon a normal degree of tone, close integration and coordination of the involved muscles of the lower limbs and trunk. These factors are primarily dependent upon normal innervation.

Various abnormal gaits may be observed in the presence of neurological dysfunction:

- The *ataxic gait* is an unsteady, uncoordinated walk. With the feet placed far apart to provide a wide base for support, each foot is lifted abnormally high and slapped down with each step. The steps are unsure, unevenly spaced and may deviate to one side. Ataxic gait is associated with a loss of proprioceptive sense and a lack of coordination of muscle action. It tends to be more pronounced in the dark, as visual influences diminish
- The *stepping gait* (foot-drop gait) is characterized by foot drop due to paralysis of the anterior tibial muscles, usually secondary to lower motor neurone disease. The person looks as though he or she is walking upstairs, because the advancing leg is lifted abnormally high to avoid dragging the foot and stumbling
- *Cerebellar ataxia* is staggering, unsteady and wide based. Turns are made with difficulty. The person is unable to stand steadily with the feet together, whether the eyes are open or closed. It is associated with damage in the cerebellum or related tracts
- *Parkinson's gait* is characteristic of patients with the basal ganglia defects of Parkinson's disease. With this gait, the trunk is stooped forward, the knees are slightly flexed, steps are short and often shuffling and the speed of walking progressively accelerates.

Paralysis or loss of motor function is a common occurrence in neurological disease or injury. Paralysis may be partial and exhibited by weakness (paresis) or complete and may be classified according to the extent of the involvement:

- Monoplegia refers to paralysis of one limb
- Hemiplegia means paralysis of one side of the body. There is loss of muscle power in the limbs and the muscles of the face on the same side. If the side of the face opposite to that of the paralysed limbs is affected, the term alternate hemiplegia may be used
- Paraplegia denotes paralysis of the legs or the lower half of the body
- Quadriplegia or tetraplegia refers to paralysis of the trunk and all four extremities.

Isolated paralysis indicates the loss of the contractile ability of one muscle of a group. It is frequently associated with peripheral nerve damage and is usually accompanied by loss of sensation in the area supplied by the injured nerve.

Paralysis may also be classified as that due to an upper or lower motor neurone lesion. Damage to the motor areas of the cerebral cortex or their projection pathways (corticospinal or pyramidal tracts) produces paralysis due to an upper motor neurone lesion or what may also be termed spastic paralysis. As the lower motor neurones and reflex arc are intact, the affected muscles are still capable of reflex movements and exhibit hypertonicity (spasticity) as well as exaggerated reflexes. There is increased activity of postural (stretch) and protective reflexes. Paralysis resulting from injury of the motor neurones in the nuclei of cranial nerves or in the anterior horns or columns of grey matter in the spinal cord or damage to their axons in the periphery may be referred to as that due to a lower motor neurone lesion or as flaccid paralysis. Flaccidity occurs because the reflex arc is interrupted: there is a lack of reflex innervation and responses.

Serious abnormal postures that may develop with some cerebral and brainstem disorders are decerebrate rigidity and decorticate rigidity (Fig. 20.10). Normally, primitive reflex spinal mechanisms that initiate involuntary muscular responses are kept inactive by cerebral control. These primitive involuntary responses may be referred to as spinal automatisms. When control from the higher centres is abolished, sustained rigid posturing develops.

Sensory function

This includes assessment of the visual, auditory, olfactory, gustatory, touch, proprioceptive, pain and temperature senses. Most of these have been discussed in conjunction with assessment of the cranial nerves. The body areas usually tested for touch, pain and temperature are the face, hands, arms, trunk, thighs, feet, perineal and perianal regions. The patient is asked to close the eyes and each side of the body is compared with the other. Sensitivity to touch (monofilament), superficial pain (a pin prick), deep pressure pain, heat and cold, vibration and position is tested. In addition, the patient is asked to differentiate among various textures.

Sensory tests are often difficult to evaluate and a great deal depends upon the cooperation of the patient. Neurological lesions more often result in a diminution of sensation than in total anaesthesia. A sensory disturbance may be localized in one particular area of the body because of the different sensory pathways being associated with different parts. Hyposensitivity or hypersensitivity in the area may provide information about the location of a lesion.

Reflex status

Evaluation of reflexes provides valuable information about the nature, location and progression of neurological disorders in both the conscious and unconscious patient. Exaggeration or diminished responses of normal reflexes and the presence of pathological reflexes are frequently among the

earliest indications of neurological disturbance. Reflexes most commonly tested are the deep tendon or muscle stretch reflexes, superficial reflexes and pathological reflexes. The part of the body tested should be relaxed and the stimulus applied with the same intensity to each side of the body. Rapidity and strength of the muscle contractions are noted.

The *deep reflexes* are tested by tapping briskly over the relevant tendon, evoking an instantaneous stretching of certain muscles and their resulting contraction. The biceps, brachioradialis, triceps, patellar and Achilles (ankle) reflexes are the most common reflexes to be tested. *Superficial reflexes* are elicited by light, rapid stroking of a particular area of the skin or mucous membrane with an object. The corneal and pupillary reflexes, the pharyngeal or gag reflex, abdominal and plantar reflexes are the common superficial reflexes tested. Diminished superficial reflex responses occur on the opposite side of the body when lesions are present above the decussation of the corticospinal tract. Loss of these reflexes occurs on the same side as the lesion when the lesion is below the corticospinal tract decussation.

The *Babinski reflex* is a useful pathological reflex suggestive of neurological disease, particularly of the pyramidal tract. In response to firm pressure from something like a wooden spatula, stroking of the lateral aspect of the sole of the foot and across the base of the toes, the toes normally curve downwards (plantarflexion). Plantarflexion of the big toe (curling upwards) is the abnormal response indicating pathology of the pyramidal tract. This is called a positive Babinski's reflex.

Consciousness

Consciousness is defined as the complete awareness of self and environment, with appropriate responsiveness to stimuli. It is a dynamic experience involving a series of different elements whose relationship changes incessantly. The precise limits are hard to define as consciousness is inferred from a person's appearance and behaviour.

Two physiological components affect conscious behaviour. These are *content* and *arousal*. Mental activities involve the contents of sensation, perception, attention, memory and volition. Analysis and synthesis of information, along with emotional implications, also occur. The content aspects generally refer to those mental functions carried out in the cerebral cortex. The arousal aspects are reflected in the person's appearance of wakefulness. Cognitive functions are not possible without some degree of arousal. Arousal can exist without the emotional and thinking components of content.

The system of consciousness is driven by an arousal mechanism. Full consciousness depends upon the interaction between the cerebral cortex and the reticular activating system. Neurones in the reticular activating system receive collateral nerve fibres from all sensory pathways that enter the brain via the upper spinal cord or cranial nerves. If the sensory pathways are blocked impulses travel by the collaterals to the reticular activating system, then to the thalamus and on to innervate the cortex. This activation of

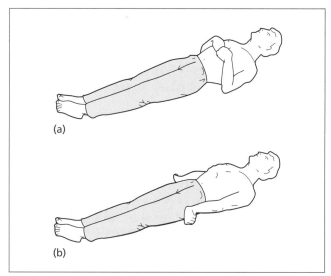

Figure 20.10 (a) Decorticate rigidity (spastic flexion). (b) Decerebrate rigidity (spastic extension).

the cortex produces a state of alertness. Further, it has been postulated that impulses are conducted via a feedback loop back to the reticular activating system, which in turn stimulates the cortex. This continuous circuitry of arousal maintains the state of readiness of the cortex to receive and interpret incoming sensory impulses. A further function of the reticular activating system is to screen and modulate incoming messages so that the cortex is able to process significant information.

Sleep

Normal sleep is a periodic depression of the physiological function of the parts of the brain concerned with consciousness from which a person can be aroused to awareness. Sleep occurs in two ways: first, as a result of decreased activity in the reticular activating system, which produces *slow-wave* or *normal sleep*. This is a restful type of sleep during which the respiratory and pulse rates and blood pressure fall, the pupils constrict and react more slowly to light, the eyes deviate upwards and tendon reflexes are abolished.

The second way by which sleep occurs results from the abnormal channelling of brain signals and is referred to as *paradoxical* or *desynchronized sleep*. Short episodes of paradoxical sleep usually occur about every 90 minutes throughout a night. Heart and respiratory rates and blood pressure alter, cerebral blood flow increases, clonic jerks may occur and rapid eye movements (REM) take place. Most dreams occur during paradoxical sleep.

During normal sleep, activity of the reticular activating system is decreased, whereas in paradoxical sleep some cerebral areas are active while others are suppressed. During sleep, a person may be easily aroused to wakefulness or consciousness by cerebral arousal through stimuli such as pain or unaccustomed noise. The return to wakefulness shows that the reticular activating system is still functioning and capable of screening and discrimination.

CONTINUOUS INTRACRANIAL PRESSURE MONITORING

Direct measurement of intracranial pressure (ICP) is possible with the placement of a pressure-sensitive probe within the intracranial cavity. The pressure-sensitive probe measures the physical pressure at the selected location and this is converted, with the aid of a transducer, into an electrical signal. The result is a reading displayed as numerical data on a monitor or as a pressure waveform.

ICP monitoring is most commonly used following head injury, especially in patients with evidence of raised ICP but who do not have a focal lesion. ICP monitoring is more fully described on p. 687.

DIAGNOSTIC TESTS

Neurodiagnostic procedures supplement and add precision to clinical data. As with any procedure, the patient needs both physical and psychological preparation to promote confidence in unfamiliar personnel and procedures. A routine test to the nurse can be a bewildering and frightening experience for the patient.

Neurodiagnostic tests can be classified as invasive or non-invasive, although this can be slightly misleading; for example, computed tomography is considered non-invasive but some patients may be given an intravenous contrast to enhance the image. Psychological care and patient teaching are very important, as ever. The aim is to reduce any stress that the patient may experience. Patient teaching is the key to achieving this, and the information for each test should include the following:

- use of the test's proper name avoiding the use of abbreviations
- an explanation as to why the test has been ordered
- who will perform the test and when and where it will be performed
- the length of time that the test normally takes
- the preparation procedure for the test, particularly that which is required of the patient
- an explanation of what will happen during the test
- information on whether, if appropriate, the patient will experience any discomfort or pain
- the aftercare routine and why this is necessary.

Some of this information may duplicate information given by medical staff to the patient during the process of obtaining consent. An additional factor to consider is that, with some neurological disorders, the patient's ability to understand explanations may be impaired. This needs to be assessed and taken into consideration when explanations are provided.

Additional precautions are required before tests are performed. It is necessary to ascertain whether the patient has an allergy to iodine if contrast is to be used and, if female, whether there is any possibility of pregnancy. This information should be documented and reported to medical staff where appropriate.

Non-invasive neurodiagnostic procedures

Non-invasive procedures pose minimal risks to the patient but may still provoke a high level of anxiety. This level of anxiety can be decreased following the advice given in the introduction above. This can be done using various media including charts, diagrams, pamphlets and audiovisual materials. Once the material is reviewed, patients should be encouraged to ask questions in order to clarify any misconceptions. A signed consent is not usually required before the test, but if a contrast medium is injected intravenously during the procedure a signed consent will be required.

Neuroradiography

Conventional radiographs of the skull and spine are frequently the first investigation in neurological disease. A wide spectrum of abnormalities may be demonstrated, including fractures, bone destruction, calcification and congenital lesions which may give specific clues to the nature of the underlying problem.

Computed tomography

In *computed tomography (CT)* the scanner circles the patient's head taking multiple radiographs which a computer translates into cross-sectional brain images. These images are based on tissue density and can detect a range of intracranial lesions including contusions; atrophy; hydrocephaly; inflammation; space-occupying lesions such as tumours, haematomas, oedema and abscesses; and haemorrhages. An intravenous contrast may be administered to enhance the image of certain lesions.

An intravenous iodinated water-soluble contrast medium may be used if a plain scan reveals an abnormality or if specific lesions are thought to exist. These would include arteriovenous malformation, acoustic neuroma or intracerebral abscess. The intravenous contrast will show areas with increased vascularity or with impairment of the blood-brain barrier. Intrathecal water-soluble contrast medium combined with CT will outline the basal cisterns, the spinal cord and the lumbosacral nerve roots. Three-dimensional reconstructed images are now possible with sophisticated computer programs and can be rotated on a monitor screen. This is known as dynamic CT.

Magnetic resonance imaging

During scanning, the patients should not have any metal objects on them as this will interfere with the procedure. Magnetic resonance imaging (MRI) has several advantages over CT, notably in investigating the posterior cranial fossa and the spinal cord. It also more clearly demonstrates certain brain lesions, such as the demyelinating plaques of multiple sclerosis. Obtaining images can be a slow process in comparison with CT – taking up to 1 hour to complete. The test requires patients to be enclosed in a long cylindrical tube, often giving a sensation of claustrophobia.

Carotid Doppler ultrasonography

This non-invasive diagnostic study is used to assess the blood flow through the carotid arteries and the extent of sclerotic vascular change that may be partially or completely obstructing the normal flow of blood to the brain. The study may be done on persons who are considered at risk of stroke because of attendant signs and symptoms (e.g. transient ischaemic attacks).

The study involves the placing of a probe over the carotid area. The probe gives off ultrasound waves and receives them back as they rebound from erythrocytes flowing through the carotid arteries.

Single-photon emission computed tomography

This is a form of imaging using compounds labelled with radioactive tracers. A two-dimensional image is produced depicting the radioactivity emitted. The most popular tracer used rapidly diffuses across the blood-brain barrier and thus presents a picture of cerebral blood flow. Single-photon emission computed tomography (SPECT) can be used for detection of early ischaemia, blood flow changes in dementia and evaluation of patients with intractable epilepsy.

Another form of radionucleotide imaging is positron emission tomography (PET). In this, the radioactive emissions (positrons) of the tracer are picked up by sensitive detectors around the head as it distributes in the brain. PET provides safe, rapid scanning of blood flow in the brain, as well as biochemical mapping. It can be used to study diseases related to chemical changes in the brain and to localize the area of action in the brain.

Electroencephalography

The electroencephalography (EEG) is a recording of the brain's electrical activity. Several small electrodes are placed superficially on the scalp in standard positions. The electrodes are attached to an amplifier and recorder. The electrical activity of neuronal dendrites of the superficial layers of the brain are responsible for the low-voltage electrical waves. If the patient has been prescribed an anticonvulsant drug it is usually withheld for 24 hours or more before the test. The patient needs assurance that an electric shock will not occur during the test and that the machine cannot 'read the mind'. The technician cleans the scalp and applies the electrodes with collodion. In some instances needle electrodes are inserted into the scalp, which necessitates cleansing the scalp before the needles are inserted. The patient lies or sits in a quiet, dimly lit room. In order to evoke or accentuate certain abnormal wave patterns the patient may be asked to hyperventilate, or the technician may flash bright lights before the eyes. Some abnormalities become evident only during sleep; therefore, a sedative may be prescribed and recordings made before, during and after sleep.

The EEG may take up to an hour to complete. After the test the patient may need assistance in using acetone to remove the collodion from the hair and scalp. The EEG is particularly useful in evaluating seizure disorders and it may help to localize tumours.

An ambulatory EEG may be performed over a 24-hour period, using a portable recorder attached to the patient's waist. This is used to diagnose petit mal, temporal lobe epilepsy or seizures of unknown origin.

EEG telemetry is frequently used as with this method the patient can be observed with a video camera, while at the same time the EEG tracing can be seen and recorded. This method gives essential information on seizure type and patients' behaviour.

Electromyography

This is a record of the electrical currents produced by skeletal muscles. Small needle electrodes are inserted into a muscle and the electrical currents are recorded with the muscle at rest and during activity. The test is useful to monitor changes in peripheral nerve dysfunction, to determine types of primary muscle disease and to identify defective transmission at the myoneural junction. The patient usually experiences some discomfort when the needle electrodes are inserted, and if many muscles are tested some discomfort may persist.

Neuropsychological tests

These tests are done when deficits in adaptive abilities are suspected. Motor, perceptual, language, visual-spatial, cognitive and other abilities can be assessed to determine the extent of impairment in brain functions. The tests measure deficits in coping skills by evaluating these skills directly rather than indirectly. They require several hours to complete and may result in recommendations concerning educational and vocational placement.

Invasive neurodiagnostic procedures

Invasive procedures carry a greater risk for the patient, thus preparation, both physically and in terms of information giving, is crucial. Signed consent is required for all these procedures.

Lumbar puncture

This involves the insertion of a spinal needle into the lumbar subarachnoid space of the spinal canal. The needle is passed through the intervertebral space between the third and fourth or fourth and fifth vertebrae. Indications include the measurement of lumbar CSF pressure, to obtain specimens of CSF for analysis or to inject drugs such as anaesthetics or antibiotics. Only drugs specifically manufactured for intrathecal injection are used. The patient lies in the lateral recumbent position, with the back on the edge of the bed, and flexes the knees to the chest so that they touch the chin, in order to widen the interspinous spaces. The nurse should be prepared to support the patient behind the neck and knees. The skin is prepared, local anaesthetic injected and a spinal needle is inserted using an aseptic technique. The needle is advanced until the tip is in the subarachnoid space

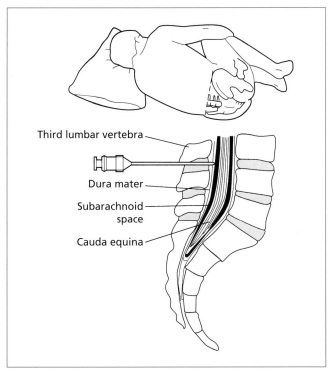

Third lumbar vertebra

Dura mater

Subarachnoid space

Cauda equina

Figure 20.11 Lumbar puncture.

and CSF is obtained (Fig. 20.11). If required, a manometer is attached and the lumbar pressure measured (normal pressure 40–180 mmH$_2$O). Specimens of CSF are collected in the appropriate container as required. When collection is complete, the needle is removed and a small sterile dressing applied once it has been ascertained that there is no leakage of CSF.

The advantage of this procedure is that it permits direct observation of CSF and withdrawal of fluid for examination, thus aiding diagnosis. It is contraindicated in the patient with raised ICP. Removal of CSF may cause herniation of the brain leading to damage affecting the brainstem as medial brain structures are forced through the tentorial notch in response to the increased pressure gradient. After the procedure the patient may experience a transient difficulty with voiding urine; temperature increase due to meningeal irritation; pain, oedema or haematoma at the site of the puncture, and headache may also occur.

There are some specific nursing interventions to implement. Historically, patients were placed on bedrest following the procedure, this is no longer the case and patients are now encouraged to mobilize as symptoms allow. Complications such as difficulty with voiding, raised temperature and headache are dealt with as they arise. Mild analgesia, cold compress and bedrest may relieve the headache.

Cisternal puncture

This is done if a lumbar puncture (LP) is contraindicated or if there is a block in the spinal subarachnoid space. A short needle is inserted into the cisterna magna (a small sac of CSF between the cerebellum and medulla) just beneath the occipital bone. Because this puncture is close to the brain and the patient's cooperation is necessary, anxiety-reducing and supportive measures are essential. The nape of the neck is shaved, the patient is positioned on the side and the head is flexed forward and held firmly by the nurse, or the patient may be sat upright, resting the arms on pillows on a bed-table. Observation is necessary for signs of respiration difficulty, which may suggest that the needle has made contact with the medulla. Usually the patient resumes normal activity soon after the procedure.

Cerebral angiography

This is performed by injecting radio-opaque material into the carotid and vertebral arteries. While this can be done by a direct puncture of the vessel, the method of choice is by a catheter, manipulated into the origin of the vessel via the femoral artery. Under local anaesthesia and using sterile technique, a suitably shaped catheter is passed retrogradely up to the aorta over a guidewire. Selective catheterization of the carotid and vertebral arteries can be undertaken as indicated. During the injection, radiographs are obtained in rapid sequence. After removal of the needle, a sterile gauze pad is applied over the injection site and firm pressure is applied for 5–10 minutes to prevent haemorrhage and haematoma formation.

Following angiography the patient remains on bedrest for at least 6 hours. Neurological observations are carried out frequently and the puncture site is checked for bleeding. A cold compress or ice-bag may be applied to the injection site to control oedema and discomfort and to reduce the possibility of bleeding. If a limb was used for the puncture site (e.g. femoral artery), the distal part is checked for colour, temperature and presence of a pulse. Vasospasm, thrombosis or formation of a haematoma can occur, obstructing the blood supply to the distal portion.

Rarely, cerebral angiography may precipitate a stroke, seizure, allergic reaction to the contrast substance, or other serious complications. Any signs of deterioration in the patient's condition must be reported to the doctor immediately.

Myelography

This is an X-ray examination of the spinal cord and vertebral canal following injection of a radio-opaque contrast substance into the spinal subarachnoid space. It is used to detect and localize lesions that may be compressing the spinal cord or nerves. This procedure is now rarely carried out due to the advances in scanning techniques. When carried out, water-soluble, non-ionic contrast medium is injected into the CSF surrounding the spinal cord and emerging nerve roots.

After the procedure, the patient rests supine in bed, with the head and trunk at 45° and is encouraged to drink plenty of fluid. This position minimizes the volume of contrast that enters the CSF surrounding the brain. Serious complications of myelography are fortunately rare, particularly with the use of the new non-ionic contrast media. However, the neurological status of the patient should be kept under review after the procedure; persistent headache, pain and/or the development of neck stiffness should be reported.

THE PERSON WITH A NEUROLOGICAL DISORDER

The highly complex nature of the nervous system is revealed through its numerous and diverse disorders. The dysfunctions that result depend primarily on the area(s) of the nervous system affected, the extent of the lesion and, to a lesser degree, the nature of the pathological process. For this reason, it is difficult for healthcare professionals to predict outcomes and thereby develop outcome criteria. The focus of nursing activity includes disease stabilization, health promotion and prevention. The family is an integral part of patient care and members are encouraged to participate in all aspects of care, including decision-making, to the degree that they are able. Pathology of the CNS often compromises intellectual and reasoning process, hence the added importance of family involvement and the need for nurses to be aware of concepts such as maintenance of dignity and need for advocacy. There are recurrent legal and ethical issues inherent in the care of patients with neurological dysfunction. Issues such as brain death, persistent vegetative state and surrogate decision-making are only some examples where nurses face ethical dilemmas.

The following sections will consider the common disorders most often encountered in nursing practice.

THE PERSON WITH A CEREBROVASCULAR DISORDER

Cerebrovascular disorders are among the most common of all neurological disorders. The greater number may be classified as ischaemic or haemorrhagic. Either may cause a cerebrovascular infarction, which is commonly known as a stroke.

STROKE

Incidence

Every year in the UK over 150 000 people experience a stroke, most people are over 65 years of age but it can happen to people of any age, even babies (Stroke Association 2006). Strokes are a leading cause of death and disability and more than 250 000 people in the UK live with disabilities that have been caused by strokes.

A stroke involves an interruption of the blood supply to a part of the brain and the development of neurological deficits. If the ischaemia persists, necrosis of the deprived area follows, the infarcted area eventually liquefies and is absorbed, and the neurological deficits remain. The cause of the stroke may be atherosclerosis, cerebral thrombosis or embolism, or intracranial haemorrhage. The artery that ruptures is usually vulnerable due to degenerative vascular changes (atherosclerosis) or the presence of an aneurysm. A haemorrhagic stroke may be precipitated by increased blood pressure and is usually associated with some physical or emotional stress.

According to the rate of development and permanence of the neurological effects, a stroke may be categorized as a transient ischaemic attack, stroke in evolution or completed stroke. Gradual development of stroke symptoms over a period of several hours or days is usually associated with a cerebral thrombosis or slow leak in a cerebral artery. This type of stroke is referred to as a stroke in evolution. A stroke is classified as a completed stroke when the neurological deficits remain longer than 3 or 4 days.

Cerebral atherosclerosis

This is a chronic degenerative process of the cerebral arteries in which the intimal layer gradually develops atheromas (fibrous fatty plaques). These narrow the vascular lumen, damage the underlying layer of tunica media and tend to undergo calcification, ulceration with overlying thrombosis and intraplaque haemorrhage, which worsen the luminal narrowing or cause total occlusion. These degenerative changes result in interference with cerebral perfusion. Although the brain represents only about 2% of the body's weight, it consumes 20% of its oxygen. As the brain cannot store energy nor temporarily exist by anaerobic metabolism, deprivation of oxygenated blood for even a very few minutes leads to neuronal death.

Atherosclerosis affects the larger vessels at the base of the brain first, particularly at the points of vessel branching, and tends to develop silently. The incidence increases with increasing age. Its presence is manifested when it is well advanced by the following signs and symptoms:

1 the development of ischaemia of vital organs (e.g. deterioration of mental faculties)
2 episodes of local neurological dysfunction, which are referred to as transient ischaemic attacks
3 predisposition to thrombosis, which may give rise to emboli
4 weakening of an arterial wall resulting in an aneurysm.

Occasionally, on routine physical examination, a noise or bruit may be heard through a stethoscope placed over the carotid artery when there is turbulent blood flow due to irregularities in the vessel wall.

Cerebral thrombosis and embolism

This is the most common cause of stroke and is usually due to atherosclerosis of the carotid, vertebral or larger cerebral arteries. Embolic material, which may be a thrombus or atherosclerotic plaque that becomes free in the bloodstream, lodges in a cerebral artery, occluding the vessel and resulting in a cerebral infarction (stroke). The middle cerebral artery is the most frequent location. The occlusion occurs suddenly; there is no warning or time for the development of collateral circulation.

This diagnosis can promote much anxiety and uncertainty in the patient and family, who will consequently require information about risk factors, such as smoking, cholesterol and obesity, and a discussion about possible changes in lifestyle that will decrease the level of risk. Risk factors that are the target of educational interventions include:

- diets high in saturated fat but low in fruit and vegetables
- excessive salt intake
- hypercholesterolaemia
- hypertension
- cigarette smoking
- lack of exercise
- obesity
- excessive alcohol consumption.

Control of hypertension and smoking cessation are critical to improving the prognosis and preventing further strokes. The Royal College of Physicians (2004) state that all patients with ischaemic stroke should be prescribed an antiplatelet medication (e.g. aspirin or clopidogrel) unless they are on anticoagulation therapy. If patients have persistent atrial fibrillation, they will be treated with an anticoagulant (e.g. warfarin) rather than antiplatelet therapy. All patients should also be considered for lipid lowering medication if their total cholesterol is >3.5 mmol/L.

Surgical therapy for atherosclerosis causing cerebral ischaemia involves a carotid endarterectomy or cerebral artery bypass.

Transient ischaemic attacks

A large proportion of patients with an atherothrombotic stroke have a history of transient ischaemic attacks. These episodes of local neurological dysfunction last for under 24 hours, most only for 5–10 minutes, and leave no neurological deficit. These transient attacks are due to focal ischaemia incurred by temporary occlusion of an artery by vasospasm, microemboli or insufficient blood supply. They are usually associated with atherosclerosis.

Transient attacks are warning signs of impending complete stroke. One-third of patients with a TIA will have a complete stroke within 5 years while 80% of patients who have had a thrombotic CVA will have a history of previous TIAs (Nowak and Handford 2004). Manifestations include transient paresis or hemiplegia, visual deficits (decreased vision in one eye), difficulty in or loss of speech, difficulty in comprehension, dizziness, unsteadiness and sudden falls.

It is a nursing responsibility to assess the patient's understanding of the episodes and to urge prompt medical attention. Timely admission and investigation (such as carotid Doppler studies) can lead to surgical (e.g. carotid endarterectomy) or pharmacological interventions which will reduce the risk of a disastrous stroke in the near future (Filbin et al 2002). The primary care based therapeutic regimen should involve management of the risk factors for stroke listed above including where appropriate, control of hypertension, weight loss, smoking cessation and prescription of an antiplatelet drug such as aspirin, clopidogrel or dipyridamole.

Endarterectomy

Endarterectomy of the internal carotid artery involves the removal of the atheroma from the intima. A venous graft or Dacron prosthesis may be necessary to reinforce the vascular area from which the plaques are removed.

Not all patients with atherosclerosis or experiencing transient ischaemic attacks are candidates for surgery; those who are very elderly and have extensive vascular disease, or who have serious heart or renal problems, are a high risk.

Nursing intervention Preoperative preparation of the patient for an endarterectomy follows that for neurosurgery outlined later (see p. 714). A specific directive may be received concerning skin preparation.

Postoperative nursing care follows that for the neurosurgical patient. Additional interventions include:

- *frequent monitoring of blood pressure* – an increase may place stress on the operative site and cause severe haemorrhage. Hypotension predisposes to thrombus formation within the artery at the surgical site
- *frequent observation of the operative site* for evidence of bleeding or oedema in the area.

The neck circumference is observed frequently for swelling due to internal bleeding. Respiratory distress is reported promptly: swelling due to oedema or clot formation may compress the trachea and interfere with respirations.

Assessment of neurological function may follow that outlined in Table 20.4.

The patient is kept at rest and quiet with a minimum of stimuli during the first 12 hours; all exertion is avoided. After this period, the patient is gradually mobilized if vital signs are satisfactory and stable.

Cerebral artery bypass

Cerebral artery bypass surgery may be performed on patients who have lesions in the smaller arteries inside the skull that cannot be corrected by endarterectomy. Using microsurgical techniques and a craniotomy just above the ear, a large scalp artery (e.g. superficial temporal) is anastomosed to a blocked artery in order to supply blood beyond the stenosis.

Nursing intervention   Nursing care after operation is similar to that outlined for endarterectomy.

The major complications following bypass surgery include interruption of blood flow through the graft, stroke and subdural haematoma due to bleeding at the surgical site. The patient is positioned off the operative side with the head of the bed elevated 30°. Long-term benefits and indications for cerebral bypass have not been firmly established but there is some evidence of decreased stroke rate and

Table 20.4   Organization of a functionally oriented nursing neurological evaluation

Functional category	Examples of specific function which may be tested
Consciousness	
Arousing (reticular activating system)	Arousability, response to verbal and tactile stimuli
Mentation	
Thinking (general cortical function plus specific regional functions)	Educational level
	Content of conversation
	Orientation
	Fund of information
	Insight, judgement, planning
Feeling (affective)	Mood and affect
	Perception and reaction to ability, disability
Language	Content and quantity of speech
	Ability to name objects
	Ability to repeat phrases
	Ability to read, write, copy
Remembering	Attention span
	Recent and remote memory
Motor function	
Seeing (cranial nerves, II, III, IV, VI)	Acuity
	Visual fields
	Extraocular movement
	Pupil size, shape, reactivity
	Presence or absence of diplopia, nystagmus
Eating (cranial nerves, V, IX, X, XII)	Chewing
	Swallowing
	Gag (if swallowing impaired)
Expressing (facially) (cranial nerve VII)	Symmetry of smile, frown
Speaking (cranial nerves VII, IX, X, XII)	Clarity, presence or absence of nasality
Moving (motor and cerebellar systems)	Muscle tone, mass, strength
	Presence or absence of involuntary movements
	Coordination: heel-to-toe walk, observing during dressing
	Posture, gait, position
Sensory function	
Smelling (cranial nerve I)	Ability to detect odours
Blinking (cranial nerve V)	Corneal reflex
Hearing (cranial nerve VII)	Acuity, presence or absence of unusual sounds
Feeling (sensory pathways)	Pain – pinprick
	Touch, stereognosis
	Temperature – warm, cold

improvement in the quality of life of patients who have had a bypass.

Cerebral aneurysm

An aneurysm is a saccular dilatation of an arterial wall, thought to be caused most often by the congenital absence of muscular and elastic tissue in the wall of that area of the vessel. It may also develop as a result of degenerative vascular changes. The most common cerebral aneurysm is referred to as a *berry aneurysm* because it is a rounded outpouching on a stem. The majority occur at the base of the brain in the circle of Willis at points of bifurcation. The lesion does not always produce symptoms and may be single, or there may be several (Fig. 20.12).

Aneurysms are the cause of death in over 50% of all fatal cerebrovascular lesions in persons under the age of 45 years. Although the weakness in the arterial wall is congenital, actual distension of the vessel occurs much later in life. The distension may produce localizing symptoms by pressure on adjacent structures (e.g. paralysis due to pressure on cranial nerves). Rupture of the artery is the most serious consequence. It may be preceded by a series of small leaks over several weeks manifested by headache and stiffness of the neck, but more often, the rupture occurs without any warning. The most vulnerable persons are those aged 40–60 years and those with hypertension or polycystic disease of the kidneys. Rupture may be precipitated by physical or emotional exertion and the bleeding may occur into the subarachnoid space, cerebral substance or both those areas.

Assessment
Clinical characteristics   Rupture of a cerebral aneurysm forces blood under arterial pressure into the brain tissue and subarachnoid space giving rise to an explosive headache, nausea, vomiting and, in some, rapid loss of consciousness. Symptoms of meningeal irritation will also be present, which include pain and neck rigidity, positive Kernig's sign (inability to extend the knees without pain while in supine position with hips flexed), positive Brudzinski's sign (person in supine position bends the knees to avoid pain when the neck is flexed), photophobia, blurred vision, irritability, restlessness and possible temperature increase. The presence and severity of symptoms are determined by the location and extent of the bleeding.

Investigation   If a patient is suspected of having had a subarachnoid haemorrhage, the investigative approach will differ depending upon the presence of coma or focal signs. If the patient is obeying commands with no focal signs and access to a CT scanner is not possible, lumbar puncture will be performed. If the CSF is clear, no further investigation will occur. Uniformly blood-stained CSF or xanthochromia (straw-coloured supernatant due to the breakdown products of haemoglobin) is indicative that a subarachnoid haemorrhage has occurred. The patient would now be referred for an urgent neurosurgical opinion. The patient showing signs of coma or focal neurological signs will not have a lumbar puncture performed because of the risk of herniation due to raised ICP. Instead, CT is indicated along with an urgent neurosurgical referral. Cerebral angiography or computer tomography angiogram (CTA) is carried out at the earliest opportunity, although in some instances this may have to be delayed because of the patient's condition. CT will confirm the diagnosis of subarachnoid haemorrhage, identify other associated lesions (e.g. hydrocephalus) and help in the identification of the site of the aneurysm

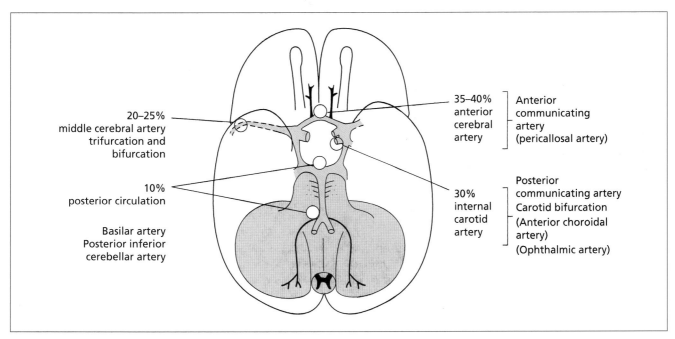

Figure 20.12   Circle of Willis and sites of saccular aneurysms.

rupture. These investigations will assist in determining the grade of the haemorrhage as this is important in relation to outcome. A number of grading systems exist; an example of one incorporating the Glasgow Coma Score is included in Table 20.5.

Prognosis Predicting prognosis following subarachnoid haemorrhage depends on a number of factors. The natural history of ruptured aneurysm shows that, of 100 people with aneurysmal subarachnoid haemorrhage treated conservatively, 15 will die before reaching hospital. Of the remaining 85, a further 15 will die within the next 24 hours. This pattern repeats itself until, at the end of 2 years, only 25 patients are still alive from the original 100. This is described as a high initial mortality rate that gradually declines with time. Neurosurgical intervention can have an impact on these figures. Of patients surviving the initial bleed and admitted within 3 days to a neurosurgical unit, a third die within the following 3 months. Almost half make a good recovery and regain former employment, although, in a proportion, minor personality change and intellectual deficit persist. Factors that provide a prognostic guide include age of the patient, loss of consciousness, clinical condition on admission, and the presence of pre-existing hypertension or arterial disease.

The intracranial complications of subarachnoid haemorrhage are as follows:

- *Re-bleeding* – the patient may experience re-bleeding, approximately 30% of patients rebleed. The risk of death following re-bleeding is twice that of the initial bleed

- *Cerebral ischaemia/infarction* – this most frequently occurs between the day 4 and day 12 after the bleed. It is a serious complication in that 25% of the patients who develop it die. The aetiology is complex and not fully understood, although it is known that vasospasm (arterial constriction) is a major factor. The clinical effects of cerebral ischaemia/infarction may be widespread and devastating, including the development of incontinence, confusion, dysphasia and hemiplegia depending upon the area of the brain affected

- *Hydrocephalus* – drainage of CSF may be impaired by the presence of blood clots, this occurs in about 20% of patients

- *Intracranial haematoma* – the development of a haematoma as the result of the initial bleed may be exaggerated by the presence of brain swelling

- *Epilepsy* – can occur at any stage and adopt either a generalized or partial (focal) format.

Medical management

If surgery is indicated, the patient will be assessed carefully for risk factors. If conservative treatment is considered appropriate this will include bedrest until asymptomatic, analgesia for headache, and control of other symptoms (e.g. nausea) as they arise.

The purpose of the operation is to avoid re-bleeding. Clipping the neck of the aneurysm is the only certain method of preventing a re-bleed. This can be done in a number of ways. Direct clipping using a metal, self-closing

Table 20.5 Grading of subarachnoid haemorrhage

Grade	Glasgow	Coma score
I	15[a]	Neurologically intact (except for cranial nerve palsy)
II	15	Neurologically intact (except for cranial nerve palsy) with neck stiffness, headache or both
III	13–14	(a) Without focal neurological deficit
		(b) With focal neurological deficit
IV	8–12	With or without focal neurological deficit
V	3–7	Unresponsive coma with or without abnormal posturing

[a]Glasgow Coma Scale scoring is calculated as follows:

Eye opening	Spontaneous	4 points
	To speech	3 points
	To pain	2 points
	None	1 point
Motor response	Obeys commands	6 points
	Localizes	5 points
	Flexion	4 points
	Abnormal flexion	3 points
	Extension	2 points
	None	1 point
Verbal response	Oriented	5 points
	Confused	4 points
	Inappropriate words	3 points
	Incomprehensible sounds	2 points
	None	1 point

spring-clip following careful dissection of arachnoid tissue around the neck is the most common. Wrapping the fundus of the aneurysm with muslin gauze is an alternative option if clipping proves difficult.

Coil embolization has become the treatment of choice for most aneurysms. This involves inserting single or multiple helical platinum coils into the aneurysm sac via angiography to introduce thrombosis.

The timing of surgery has been much debated over the years. Traditionally, it was noted that the longer the delay, the better the results from surgery; however, a long delay also increases the patient's chance of dying from re-bleeding. Therefore, surgery was planned to take place between 6 and 14 days after the initial bleed. Operating within 72 hours has the advantage of avoiding the risk from re-bleeding but increases the operative mortality rate. However, it is now suggested that grade I patients should be operated on sooner rather than later as the risk of dying from re-bleeding is greater than the small additional risk of early operation.

Antifibrinolytic agents may be used before operation. These include tranexamic acid and e-aminocaproic acid. The aim is to prevent re-bleeding by delaying clot dissolution around the fundus of the aneurysm.

Nursing care

Assessment Vital signs and neurological status are assessed at frequent intervals during the acute stage. A decrease in the level of consciousness, disorientation and other neurological changes are recorded and reported promptly to the doctor. The blood pressure is followed very closely because a rise may increase the bleeding or precipitate re-bleeding.

Patient problems The problems of the patient treated *conservatively* include:

- Potential for continued intracranial bleeding or for recurrence of bleeding
- Loss of self-care abilities
- Headache
- Anxiety and ineffective coping. Fear of the circumstances and concern for the outcome
- Potential for injury secondary to altered level of awareness, disorientation and immobility
- Alteration in food and fluid intake due to nausea, vomiting and restricted fluid intake
- Alteration in urinary and bowel elimination secondary to reduced level of awareness, decreased intake and enforced immobility
- Potential for complications – re-bleeding, hydrocephalus and vasospasm
- Potential for residual mental and/or physical impairment resulting in need for rehabilitation.

Goals Patient goals are to avoid the complications associated with the above problems and to achieve maximum independence and self-care.

Nursing intervention If the patient's level of consciousness is decreased, the measures already discussed are implemented as part of nursing care.

Observe for bleeding or a re-bleed The patient is kept on bedrest and the bed elevated to about 30° to promote venous drainage and prevent increased intracranial pressure, although in some instances enforced bedrest heightens the patient's anxiety. The blood pressure is monitored frequently; it is important that it remains within the extreme low range of normal. Certain restrictions may be placed on visitors; these should be limited and cautioned against being too lively.

Because self-care requires exertion, which increases the blood pressure predisposing to re-bleeding, assistance is provided with activities such as bathing. However, to maintain dignity, patients who are able can perform some of these tasks for themselves (e.g. eating meals). In change of position, the patient is cautioned against physical effort.

The essential immobility predisposes to venous stasis and thrombophlebitis; the application of antiembolic stockings to the lower limbs is recommended.

Vomiting and coughing are controlled because they increase the intracranial pressure. If the patient is nauseous and vomiting, oral fluids and food are withheld and an antiemetic prescribed. Deep breathing is encouraged at regular intervals to promote pulmonary ventilation.

Alteration in comfort The severe headache that the patient experiences causes restlessness, nausea and vomiting. Nursing measures include keeping the patient at rest and as quiet as possible. Cold applications to the head may help and a mild analgesic (e.g. codeine) is usually prescribed.

Anxiety and ineffective coping The patient will probably be very fearful and concerned for the future. It is important, therefore, to allow and encourage the patient to talk about these fears and answer questions openly. If the patient is alert, it will be helpful to explain the serial assessments, procedures, enforced immobility and restrictions. A calm, reassuring approach can be therapeutic.

The family's perception of the illness, their expectations and coping patterns are assessed. Their role in keeping the patient quiet and at rest is explained to them. They are kept informed as to the patient's progress, and opportunities are provided for the expression of feelings and for questions. Tests and procedures are explained to them.

Potential for injury Impairment of awareness may occur resulting in disorientation. If so, cot sides may be required and frequent close observation made for confusion and restlessness; a mild sedative may be necessary. It may be necessary to have someone remain constantly with the patient to avoid personal injury.

When the comatose patient regains consciousness, frequent orientation to place and circumstances is necessary as well as reassurance as to care and progress.

Potential pressure sores The regular assessment of pressure areas and an appropriate regimen of prevention is necessary.

Fluid and food intake When tolerated, the patient receives a soft diet initially. The fluid intake may be limited to a specific volume per 24 hours to promote a reduction in cerebral oedema and in intracranial pressure. This varies from unit to unit. Some units have a policy of a 3-L minimum intake in 24 hours. An accurate record of the fluid intake and output is maintained.

Urinary and bowel elimination Voiding urine in the supine position may be problematic. Rather than exert the patient by attempting to use a bedpan, it is easier for the patient to get out of bed and go to the toilet – provided they are able to do so safely.

A mild laxative or stool softener may be prescribed to prevent constipation and straining at stool. Enemas are contraindicated.

Potential complications The complications previously outlined will manifest themselves as changes in level of consciousness and vital signs, together with the symptoms of paresis, paralysis or speech impairment. If the spasm persists, infarction of the brain tissue occurs, causing serious neurological deficits.

Treatment of secondary hydrocephalus may involve a cranial burr-hole and the placing of a tube in a ventricle (ventriculostomy) for external drainage of the CSF. If the hydrocephalus persists, a permanent ventriculoatrial or ventriculoperitoneal shunt may be done to drain the CSF.

Residual impairment The patient may recover and be left with brain damage that results in reduced physical and/or mental capacity. This clearly has long-term social and psychological implications for the patient and family which must be addressed realistically and with the support of a wide range of agencies.

The patient treated by surgery The care outlined in the sections on preoperative and postoperative care should be referred to (see p. 714).

Effects of a stroke on the patient

Whether the stroke was due to atherosclerosis, thrombosis, embolism or a ruptured cerebral artery, it may produce a wide range of severe effects, leading to the following range of problems:

- alteration in level of consciousness
- headache and vomiting
- neuromuscular deficits
- incontinence
- eye changes
- impairment of speech
- mental impairment
- unfavourable vital signs.

Alteration in level of consciousness

The patient may experience only a decrease in responsiveness to stimuli, confusion or clouding of consciousness, whereas other patients may suddenly or gradually become unconscious. The coma may last a few hours to days; the gravity of prognosis tends to increase if the coma extends beyond 36 hours.

Headache and vomiting

If remaining conscious, the patient may complain of severe headache as a result of increased intracranial pressure. Vomiting frequently occurs with the initial onset and may be recurring in the conscious patient.

Neuromuscular deficits

The immediate onset may be accompanied by convulsive movements which may be local or general. The effects of the impairment of neuromuscular control by stroke vary from only a muscular weakness to complete paralysis. Hemiplegia (paralysis of one side of the body) is one of the most common effects of a stroke and indicates interruption of motor pathways. The axons of motor neurones which initiate willed movements in each hemisphere converge into the internal capsule. The motor fibres from each hemisphere cross over in the medulla; as a result, paralysis of one side of the body indicates that the cerebral lesion is on the other side; that is, a stroke in the right side of the brain causes paralysis of the left arm and leg. For a few days, there is a marked loss of tone in the affected muscles and an absence of normal reflexes. Even if the patient is in coma, a greater loss of tone in the affected limbs is recognizable (when flexed the limb falls more quickly in a limp, lifeless manner). Later this flaccidity is replaced by spasticity.

One side of the face may be paralysed, which causes the alternating abnormal distension and retraction with each respiration. The mouth is also drawn to one side.

When conscious, the patient may experience difficulty in swallowing (dysphagia), indicating some paralysis of the swallowing muscles.

Incontinence

Urinary and bowel incontinence are common in the early stage. The bladder is atonic and the patient does not experience the desire to void. Later, tone returns and the bladder may become spastic and the patient experiences frequency and urgency. Unless the cerebral damage is extensive, involving both hemispheres, bladder control may be re-established with training. The patient may be insensitive to the defaecation reflex, resulting in incontinence.

Eye changes

The pupils may be unequal in size; the larger of the two is on the side of the lesion. The eyes as well as the head tend to turn to the side of the lesion in the early stage; later the deviations may be reversed. Hemianopia (loss of vision in half of the visual field) occurs and may be temporary. In the unconscious patient, the corneal and pupillary reflexes may be absent and the fundus may reveal papilloedema due to increased intracranial pressure or hypertension.

Impairment of speech

There may be complete or partial loss of the ability to communicate. The speech centre is in the dominant cerebral hemisphere; if the stroke occurs on that side, aphasia is likely to occur. The left hemisphere is dominant in the majority of persons. The patient may not only be unable to communicate verbally but may manifest some impairment of comprehension of either or both written or verbal communication.

The aphasia may take various forms (Box 20.1). In motor or expressive aphasia, the person understands and knows what he or she wants to say but cannot utter the words. In receptive aphasia, the person does not comprehend either written or spoken words. If there is total loss of speech and communication it is referred to as global aphasia and indicates a serious, massive lesion.

Mental impairment

A stroke may impair the patient's memory, comprehension and the ability to reason and make judgements. There may be inability to recognize previously familiar objects or sensory impressions (agnosia) and to use objects correctly (apraxia).

Emotional lability is common: the patient may cry or laugh inappropriately.

Vital signs

The respirations are usually slow and stertorous or may be Cheyne–Stokes. The pulse is usually slow, full and bounding in the initial phase. The temperature may be normal during the first few hours and then become raised. Hyperpyrexia is an unfavourable sign.

Diagnostic procedures

When a stroke occurs, procedures may be carried out to identify the underlying cause because the therapy for an ischaemic stroke differs from that for a haemorrhagic stroke. Diagnostic procedures also may reveal the extent and location of involvement. The main diagnostic tool used is CT

which can show a collection of blood, cerebral oedema or an infarcted area.

Recent advances in the management of patients with non-haemorrhagic stroke include the use of thrombolytic drugs. Patients with witnessed onset of stroke should be assessed urgently by a specialist in stroke medicine. If the patient has a confirmed non-haemorrhagic stroke on CT scan, and fulfil treatment criteria they may be considered for thrombolysis. This treatment must be given within three hours of onset of stroke.

Ongoing assessment

An initial assessment of the vital signs and neurological status establishes a base for ongoing evaluations and prompt recognition of changes. During the acute phase, vital signs, level of consciousness, and motor and sensory functions are monitored at frequent intervals.

After the acute stage, the patient's motor functions and level of awareness are assessed daily. Some improvement may occur day to day as the cerebral oedema and pressure are reduced and collateral circulation is established. The regaining of function tends to follow a pattern in which the facial and swallowing muscles recover first, then those of the lower limbs. Usually, speech and arm functions return more slowly and less completely. Observations are made frequently for early signs of complications such as contractures and pressure sores.

Patient problems include:

- Coma
- Alteration in respiratory process:
  - ineffective breathing pattern
  - ineffective airway clearance
  - impaired gas exchange
- Potential increased intracranial pressure secondary to cerebral oedema and haemorrhage
- Headache and vomiting due to increased intracranial pressure
- Alteration in elimination processes:
  - possible urinary retention with overflow
  - incontinence
  - potential constipation, faecal impaction and bowel incontinence
- Alteration in fluid and food intake: deficit due to coma, vomiting and/or dysphagia. The taking of food may also be influenced by difficulty with mastication as well as swallowing
- Potential for injury secondary to neurological deficits, confusion or fits
- Potential pressure sores related to immobility and incontinence
- Self-care deficits due to coma, paralysis, impaired cognition and awareness
- Impaired verbal communication – aphasia
- Impairment of mobility – occurs in varying degrees, ranging from weakness to complete paralysis

---

Box 20.1   Common types of aphasia

- Auditory aphasia – inability to comprehend the spoken word. May be referred to as word deafness

- Expressive aphasia – individual understands spoken and written words and knows what he or she wants to say but cannot speak the words. Also referred to as motor or Broca's aphasia

- Global aphasia – complete aphasia involving both sensory and motor functions that provide all forms of communication

- Receptive aphasia – inability to comprehend spoken, written or tactile symbols. Also referred to as sensory aphasia

---

- Cognitive dysfunction – impaired awareness, confusion, loss of memory, reasoning and judgement
- Emotional lability – inappropriate responses, for example inappropriate outbursts of anger, crying and laughing. If awareness is not impaired, the patient often manifests the characteristics of the grieving process (denial, anger, depression, gradual acceptance and resolution) (see p. 63)
- Lack of knowledge about rehabilitation and home management.

Goals

In the acute phase, the goals are that the patient will not develop complications related to the problems stated above, while in the convalescent and rehabilitative phase additional goals involve the recovery of maximum independence and adaptation to reduced function.

Nursing intervention

A great deal of patience is needed to support both family and patient in striving to meet these goals. Nurses in both hospital (acute and community hospitals) and primary care (such as the District Nurse) will be heavily involved and good communication between them is essential.

The degree of recovery after a stroke is determined by the size of the haemorrhage and infarction, and is influenced by the patient's age, available rehabilitation programmes, and the individual's personality and behavioural responses. Improvement can occur but deficits that are present after 6 months are usually permanent. Early, sustained and intensive therapy for the highly motivated patient with strong professional and family support frequently results in independence and a very satisfying recovery and quality of life.

Treatment and nursing care of a patient with a thrombotic stroke will differ somewhat to that of a haemorrhagic stroke and, of course, it varies with the degree of cerebral damage and ensuing neurological deficits. In the case of a thrombotic stroke, in evolution, an anticoagulant such as heparin may be administered and efforts are directed to maintaining a normal level of blood pressure. The patient is kept on bedrest with minimal disturbance and environmental stimuli to reduce the potential for haemorrhage. Surgical removal of the thrombus may be undertaken. When the stroke is due to a cerebral haemorrhage, therapy and nursing involve efforts directed towards relief of the increased intracranial pressure, life support measures, relief of hypertension to prevent further bleeding and the prevention of complications.

The care required by the stroke patient during the acute phase following the initial onset differs from that required during the convalescent and rehabilitative phase. The care will also vary with the severity of the stroke and extent of brain damage. During the acute phase, intervention is directed principally towards maintaining life and preventing increased neurological deficits and complications.

Much of the nursing care surrounding problems such as diminished level of consciousness, altered respiratory processes, headache, elimination, personal hygiene and pressure care has already been discussed. Care must be taken with nutrition.

When consciousness is regained, the swallow reflex is tested before giving any fluids orally. If the patient can swallow, a soft diet is given and increased progressively to a full balanced diet as tolerated. The hemiplegic patient may have to be fed at first if the dominant arm is affected but, with the necessary assistance, is encouraged to feed unaided as soon as possible to establish independence.

If one side of the face is paralysed, food is placed in the opposite side of the mouth. Mouth care is then given following each meal to remove retained food particles from the affected side to prevent aspiration and the development of ulcers.

Protection from injury is necessary because of the motor deficits and possible seizures. Contractures and deformities may develop as flexor muscles take over and loss of range of joint movement occurs. Limbs are supported in a natural position. Passive movements of all joints are carried out at regular intervals, for example when changing the patient's position.

Sensory function may also be impaired; as well as a reduced sensitivity to pressure, pain and temperature, there may be loss of the ability to know the location of parts of the body in space (impaired spatial perception). Cot sides may be required; the patient may be disoriented and also, if turning in bed, may not have the normal reflexive muscular responses that would maintain balance and prevent the patient falling from the bed. When allowed up, precautions are taken to prevent falls and accidents (sufficient assistance, hand-rails, walking frames or sticks).

As soon as the condition has stabilized, opportunity is provided for the patient to regain as much independence as possible as active assistance is gradually withdrawn while giving support and encouragement. The call light or buzzer, water, toilet articles and other needed items are placed within the patient's reach. The nurse should encourage the patient to be aware of and to use the affected side if possible.

Patients will be prescribed antiplatelet therapy such as aspirin, clopidogrel or dipyridamole. If they also have atrial fibrillation, they may be prescribed anticoagulant therapy rather than antiplatelet drugs. In addition, the patient's blood pressure will be monitored and their lipid levels will be assessed. They may be treated with antihypertensive medication and lipid lowering drugs in an effort to avoid further strokes.

Family assessment   Once a family assessment has been carried out and problems or concerns are identified, the family will require assistance in developing both short- and long-term plans. Questions may arise about community resources, self-help groups, rehabilitative facilities, home adaptations such as converting a downstairs room to a bedroom, social security payments and possibly employment prospects, to name but a few of the areas of long-term concern for the patient and family.

Rehabilitative phase following stroke

Rehabilitation really commences with the initial onset and acute phase: certain aspects of the care received in the early stage of the illness play an important role in the patient's rehabilitation. As soon as the patient is well enough, an assessment is made of residual disabilities and remaining capacities. A multidisciplinary team then becomes involved in plans to assist the patient to develop maximum potential and independence, and to assist the family with the necessary adjustments. Both patient and family should participate in setting achievable goals. Attainment of the goals usually requires months of perseverance and patience. The patient and family naturally experience periods of frustration, depression and pessimism. Activities are taken in steps so that achievement is experienced. Complete restoration to previous functional ability may not be possible but much can be done to restore the patient to a degree of independence that makes life more tolerable, while supporting key family members who will be giving a great deal of their time in caring for the person. They may have to come to terms with the need for admission of their loved one to a nursing home if the work involved becomes too great or their own health deteriorates. The carer should be supported through this difficult decision as they may have lived in the same house with their spouse for 40 years or more and feel guilty about the reality of admitting their spouse to a care home.

Impaired communication   The aphasia associated with a stroke is usually expressive in type, although variants do occur. The sudden loss of the ability to communicate creates fear and frustration in the patient; feelings of isolation, insecurity and loneliness develop. The nurse endeavours to allay some of the anxiety by anticipating the patient's needs as much as possible, acknowledging the difficulty and concern and indicating time and willingness to work through the problem. The patient is likely to benefit psychologically from knowing that someone understands and will help. Many aphasic patients recover the ability to communicate to some degree. It is not possible to predict this at the onset; speech is usually recovered very gradually and slowly and requires the assistance of those around the patient. The nurse avoids conveying what may be false optimism at first but reassures the patient and family that special assistance will be given to minimize speech and other neurological deficits. In the early stage, gestures to indicate needs and wishes may be encouraged but should not be accepted indefinitely as established use of them inhibit efforts to speak.

If the services of a speech therapist are available, a re-training programme is planned. In many situations, the nurse will be mainly responsible for helping the patient recover the ability to communicate. It is necessary, as soon as possible, to determine whether the patient can express ideas verbally or by the written word, and whether the spoken and written word is understood. Comprehension may be limited to short simple phrases or single words. Rarely, intellectual impairment occurs (e.g. receptive aphasia) that precludes speech rehabilitation. It is important to talk normally and with ease to the patient; auditory stimulation and socialization can play important roles and are considered as valuable as structured remedial drills.

Loss of speech is no indication that intelligence, comprehension and hearing are impaired. The patient should be included in conversation at all times. Short simple sentences, kept at a functional level relating to present and immediate needs and environment, are used if there is evidence of difficulty in comprehension. When encouraging the patient to try, emphasis is placed on nouns and simple responses such as 'yes' and 'no' at first; then progression through verbs and adjectives to short sentences is made. The necessary re-training in many instances is much the same as the process used with the young child learning to communicate. The use of several sensory avenues is usually more effective than the use of just one at a time. Hearing words in direct association with the objects and the printed words that represent them contributes to recovery.

During speech therapy, the patient should be rested and relaxed and in a quiet undistracting setting. The periods of instruction are kept brief as the patient may tire easily and have a short attention span. Emphasis on exact pronunciation is unnecessary and may lead only to frustration and discouragement.

Early in the illness, the family members and others are helped in understanding the patient's communication problems and their role in the recovery of speech. The importance of conversing normally with the patient, expecting a response, making every effort to understand and giving plenty of time to respond should be emphasized to the family, who should be fully involved in speech therapy. At least one member should be given the opportunity to observe a teaching session carried out in the hospital or rehabilitation unit. The need for patience and the need for providing opportunities for the patient to practise and use what speech he or she has are stressed. The family is advised that progress may be slow and is cautioned against making excessive demands on the patient. Progress should be acknowledged because it encourages and prompts motivation for continued effort.

Impaired mobility   The muscles of affected limbs are flaccid for a few days after stroke, then become spastic. The paralysed arm becomes adducted and flexion occurs at the elbow, wrist, fingers and thumb joints. The lower limb assumes a position of external rotation at the hip, flexion of the thigh and leg, and plantar flexion of the foot. With **immobility**, muscles atrophy and the collagen fibres of the connective tissue of the tendons, ligaments and joint capsules tend to shorten and become dense and firm. The process may be hastened by circulatory stasis, oedema and trauma. As a result, if the affected limbs are permitted to remain immobile in the positions they automatically assume, contractures and reduced range of joint motion may become permanent. Deformities are created which actually increase the person's disability and make rehabilitation difficult. Liaison with the physiotherapist is essential when caring for the stroke patient.

Maintenance of joint motion, support to prevent the pull of gravity on joints and subsequent subluxation, and positioning to prevent contractures and maintain good alignment are essential from the onset of the stroke.

When lying on the unaffected side, the patient's unaffected shoulder is brought slightly forward and the arm should lie straight, in line with the trunk. The unaffected leg should be straight. A pillow is placed under the affected arm, which is straightened at the elbow; the hand is straightened, with the fingers spread over the upper part of the pillow. The affected leg is flexed at the knee and hip, with a pillow underneath for support. A pillow is placed along the back of the patient for support.

When the patient is lying on the affected side, a reverse, similar position is adopted, except that the unaffected arm is flexed at the elbow, with the hand towards the edge of the bed. The affected leg is flexed slightly at the knee. Pillows are this time placed under the unaffected, not the affected, limbs for support and to prevent friction and pressure. A pillow at the back should support the patient.

Marked spasticity of the affected hand may necessitate the application of a padded splint, especially at night, to prevent flexure contractures of the wrist and fingers. A support may be provided to prevent foot drop.

The limbs are passively moved through a full range of movements two or three times daily. While the patient is dependent and confined to bed, the position is changed and passive movements are carried out regularly.

The stroke patient is usually assisted out of bed for progressively increasing periods as soon as the condition has stabilized. Balance should be assessed and improved (if possible) before walking is commenced. Being up reduces the possibility of complications and may help to promote a more positive attitude on the part of the patient towards the future. When the patient is up, support of the affected arm in a sling may sometimes be necessary to prevent subluxation of the shoulder joint. A pillow may be used to support the arm when sitting in a chair.

Most hemiplegic patients fortunately experience extensor spasm of the affected knee and hip muscles with weight-bearing, which stabilizes the leg as the unaffected leg is carried through a forward step. Some patients do experience spasm of flexor rather than extensor muscle in the affected leg and as a result, when the patient attempts to walk, the knee and hip flex and do not support him or her. This necessitates the application of a leg brace for stabilization. When assisting the patient who is walking, the nurse or family member provides support from the affected side. An aid, such as a walking frame, may be required to help regain independence. When plantar flexion and toe-dragging interfere with walking, a drop-foot splint may be used. A few hemiplegic patients suffer ataxia and loss of balance which may prevent walking and confine the patient to a wheelchair.

The re-training for self-care is begun as soon as possible. Re-training carried out by the occupational therapist and the nurse includes the simple useful functions on which every person is dependent in normal living. Examples are dressing and undressing, opening doors, using the telephone, writing and the handling of various articles (e.g. cutlery). The hemiplegic patient is taught how to change position in bed (turn, sit up, transfer to a chair, stand up). The bed is lowered and made stationary when transfer techniques are carried out. A schedule of exercises is established to strengthen the trunk and unaffected limb muscles. The programme includes the affected limbs; if the muscles are weak, active assistive and active exercises are used. If the muscles are unresponsive, passive movements are carried out to prevent contractures and ankylosis.

Sensory deficits The patient is assessed for possible impairment of sensory functions such as pain, pressure and temperature. There may also be loss of the ability to know the location of parts of the body in space (proprioception deficit) making the judging of distances and movements more difficult. The patient's vision may also be impaired by the loss of function in the corresponding halves of the visual fields (homonymous hemianopia) in both eyes. The inability to recognize objects by touch, sight or hearing may be manifested. The necessary precautions are established to prevent accidents such as falls and burns, and become an important part of the rehabilitation programme.

Patient teaching The patient should receive information about all the medication they will be taking and it should be impressed upon them that they should not stop the medication unless instructed to do so. They should also be informed that ongoing blood pressure monitoring and cholesterol checks will be important for the rest of their lives. A balanced diet with less fat and salt content may be recommended and a dietary plan reviewed with the patient and family that will meet caloric needs according to weight and energy expenditure. The patient is strongly advised against smoking and should be assisted to stop if they feel able to do so. Women should be advised that they should not take contraceptive pills and patients should be advised against drinking excessive amounts of alcohol.

Pre-discharge planning The total care and rehabilitation programme should be fully discussed with a member of the family. The importance of encouraging and permitting the patient to do things unaided is emphasized. Family and friends find it difficult to stand back while the patient struggles and perseveres with activities. Before discharge, the patient may be encouraged to spend 1 or 2 days at home (e.g. at the weekend) and a home assessment may be carried out by appropriate personnel.

After discharge from hospital, both patient and family still require considerable support and assistance; referrals should be made to appropriate support and community services. Modifications of the home may be necessary to facilitate the development of independence and prevent accidents. Handrails in the bathroom, placement of articles for ready accessibility, and making the bed stationary are a few examples of adjustments that may be made, but they usually cost money and financial assistance will often be required

The assistance of social services may be necessary to help solve the problems imposed by the illness and residual disabilities. The family should be taught to recognize signs of resentment at loss of independence by the patient. By listening to their points of view, by explaining the patient's condition and unusual patterns of behaviour, and by helping the family to organize themselves so that all share in the increased responsibility, complete rejection of the patient may be prevented.

Social contact The patient is encouraged to develop interests and worthwhile hobbies and gradually to assume responsibility for domestic tasks as far as possible. The performance of some useful tasks promotes the patient's morale and greater harmony within the family.

Friends are encouraged to visit and the patient should be included in the social activities of the family. Domestic arrangements may, however, be less than ideal. The patient may live alone in a large house with no close family or live in a small flat in considerable poverty. Elderly patients may have several concurrent medical problems as well as social problems to contend with. Whatever the difficulties, nurses should not be judgemental about families who refuse to have an elderly relative to live with them after a stroke; this will serve no useful purpose for the patient, and antagonism between family and hospital staff is in nobody's interests. The patient may now have to face leaving a home they have lived in for many decades, losing their independence in the process, although this is to be avoided if at all possible – hence the importance of community care.

CASE Susan is a healthy 40-year-old Caucasian woman, divorced and living with two teenage daughters. Her husband was American and now lives back in the USA. Her parents are both dead but she has a brother who lives nearby. She was at an exercise class with friends when she experienced a sudden severe headache and vomited. She then collapsed and developed a right-sided weakness. After she arrived at the hospital, her condition continued to deteriorate and she required intubation to maintain her airway.

On examination in the medical admissions unit, her pupils were equal but sluggishly reactive to light and she reacted only to painful stimulus. Her GCS was 8. Initial vital signs revealed a heart rate of 47 bpm and a blood pressure of 210/98 mmHg. She was also pyrexial at 37.9°C.

The combination of reduced conscious level, hemiplegia and headache suggests a serious illness affecting the nervous system.

As the nurse attending this patient on admission what would your initial impression be? What do you think could be wrong with her? What immediate nursing care would this patient require?

Although various conditions are characterized by a history of headache (e.g. migraine, meningitis, viral illness), the sudden onset of the condition with associated right-sided hemiplegia and reduced conscious level suggests an acute insult to the left side of the brain. A CT scan confirmed that the patient had suffered a subarachnoid haemorrhage.

Your care should include neurological observations, monitoring of vital signs, pulse oximetry (if not admitted to the ICU) and care of the patient's airway including administration of oxygen. Tracheal suctioning may also be required to clear secretions. Fluids (i.v.) will be required to maintain optimum blood volume to the brain and help prevent cerebral vasospasm. Accurate fluid balance charting is critical. Adequate analgesia and anti-emetic medication must be given to prevent pain and emesis. Admission to an intensive care or high dependency unit may be needed for close observation and maintenance of the patient's airway.

Think ahead, what problems do her family face? It is impossible to predict the course of Susan's illness. Nursing care will be directed at managing the acute situation and then assisting with her rehabilitation as her condition allows. Her family and friends will need as much information as you can give them. Advice will need to be realistic with no false reassurance. Susan's recovery will be assisted by the multidisciplinary team and emotional and psychological support during this time will be essential.

THE PERSON WITH TRAUMA OF THE NERVOUS SYSTEM

HEAD INJURIES

Accidents on the roads, in industry and sports, and violence on the streets and in the home (often alcohol related) are the major causes of head injury, which ranks high on the list of causes of morbidity, mortality and permanent disabilities, particularly in young adults. Frequently, head injury is only one of the major problems seen in the traumatized patient and priorities of care are established on the basis of the assessment of the patient as a whole person.

The classification of head injury is underpinned by the pathological processes that have occurred as a result of injury (e.g. a skull fracture). However, all these processes are influenced in one way or another by the level of intracranial pressure (ICP) and cerebral perfusion pressure (CPP).

Intracranial pressure

This is defined as the measurable pressure exerted by the CSF within the ventricles of the brain. It is a phenomenon that constantly changes with transient rises during sneezing and coughing. Raised ICP or intracranial hypertension is when the pressure is increased as the result of trauma or disease and remains so for a period of time. It can be a very serious – sometimes fatal – complication of traumatic brain injury as a result of haemorrhage, brain swelling and/or oedema. These complications can also occur in disorders such as neoplasm where a tumour can act as a space-occupying lesion.

The normal ICP is 0–15 mmHg. This is dependent on normal functioning of the brain, CSF and cerebral blood volume within the rigid bony skull. An increase in the volume of any one of these (brain, blood or CSF) causes an increase in the ICP and a comparable decrease in the volume of one or both of the other contents. The response may be:

1 displacement of CSF
2 a compromise in cerebral blood supply which causes cerebral ischaemia. The latter leads to hypoxia, hypercapnia and acidosis at cellular level, resulting in interruption of cell metabolism
3 displacement of brain tissue (herniation).

As ICP begins to rise, compensatory mechanisms come into play. These include the removal of CSF from the intracranial cavity into the distensible spinal sac; reduction of cerebral blood flow by constriction of the cerebral blood vessels (autoregulation); and shifting of brain tissue to produce internal herniation. The volume–pressure curve (Fig. 20.13) demonstrates this phenomenon. The flattened part of the curve represents the compensatory mechanisms, while the steepened part of the curve represents their exhaustion in a process known as decompression. The timescale over which this occurs will vary. In a patient with a severe head injury, it may only be minutes, whereas for the patient with a slow growing tumour it may be years.

Cerebral perfusion pressure is the pressure required to maintain perfusion of the sensitive nervous tissue. This is necessary to maintain adequate oxygenation of the brain and the provision of essential glucose. Normal CPP is in the range 70–100 mmHg, and reductions below this level in the neurologically impaired patient can have a deleterious effect on brain functioning.

If pressure is distributed unequally between two compartments, tissue will move from the area of higher pressure to the lower one. This is known as herniation or coning, and occurs in several stages (Fig. 20.14). Initially there is a shift of tissue across the brain from the side where the space-occupying lesion is located. This results in the displacement of structures found in the midline. These include the lateral ventricles and the falx cerebri; thus, this is termed a subfalcine herniation. This is referred to as a right to left or left to right midline shift, as appropriate. Once the pressure in the supratentorial compartment has equalized, it is greater than that in the posterior fossa below, thus downward herniation follows. This is termed tentorial herniation and may occur on one or both sides. One consequence of this is that pressure is now applied directly to the third cranial nerve (oculomotor nerve). This controls constriction of the pupil; thus, when the nerve is compressed it no longer functions and the pupil becomes fixed and possibly dilated. Pressure is now beginning to build on the brainstem where the vital centres are located. Changes seen at this late stage would include a widening pulse pressure, a slowing of the heart rate and a reduction in the respiratory rate and possibly apnoea.

Another type of herniation may occur, known as *tonsillar herniation*. A space-occupying lesion in the posterior fossa compressing the cerebellum may force the cerebellar tonsils to herniate downwards with a similar effect on the brainstem.

Causes of increased ICP are swelling of the brain, increased CSF volume and increased blood volume. Swelling of the brain may be due to haemorrhage following trauma, a tumour (increased mass of tissue cells), abscess, inflammatory exudate or cerebral oedema. An increase in the cranial volume of CSF is usually associated with a disturbance in the absorption or outflow of the fluid; it accumulates in the ventricles, compressing brain tissue and blood

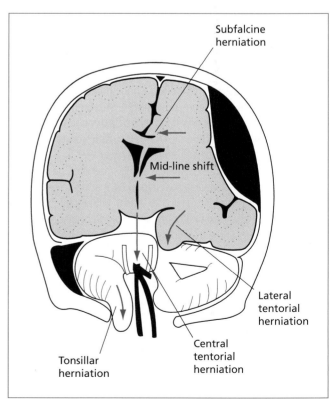

Figure 20.14 Herniation of brain tissue.

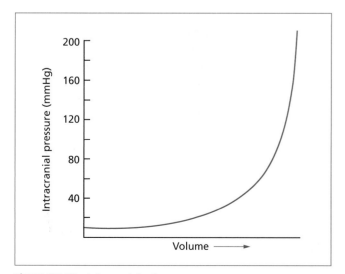

Figure 20.13 Intracranial volume–pressure curve.

vessels. An increase in the intracranial blood volume may be due to compression of the venous sinuses or jugular veins, vasodilatation of the cerebral vessels or be associated with trauma.

Classification of head injury

Head injuries may be classified as open or closed, coup or contrecoup, and primary or secondary:

1 *Closed head injury* refers to injury in which there is no break in the tissues (scalp and skull) that separate the intracranial cavity from the external environment (e.g. subdural haematoma).

2 *Open head injury* means that a break exists in the tissues that separate the intracranial contents from the external environment (e.g. perforating skull fracture).

3 *Coup and contrecoup injuries* result from direct trauma to the head in which the sequence of intracranial events resembles an acceleration-deceleration phenomenon:

   a) *Coup* refers to bruising of the brain tissue that directly underlies the site of impact and that rebounds against that portion of the cranium.

   b) *Contrecoup* is brain injury on the side opposite the site of impact. It is due to the wave of pressure created by the impact, compressing the brain substance against the bony ridges and opposite wall of the cranium. For example, a fall on to the back of the head may cause injury to the frontal and temporal cerebral lobes. Injury to the nerve fibres and blood vessels in the brainstem results from the stress of shearing forces.

The mechanisms of head injury are described in Fig. 20.15.

Primary head injuries
Fracture of the skull

A skull fracture is particularly significant if there is communication between the intracranial contents and the outside (open head injury), or there is depression of a piece of skull, compressing the brain below. If the fracture involves the base of the skull, CSF leakage occurs and there is potential communication between the oropharynx and the meninges, leading to the risk of infection entering the meninges, known as *meningitis*.

No specific treatment is used for a simple linear or comminuted skull fracture, but the patient is kept at rest and under close observation because of potential bleeding and haematoma. Meningeal blood vessels may have been torn and incur extradural, subdural or subarachnoid haemorrhage. Concussion or contusion of the brain is a frequent result.

Early surgical exploration is indicated when a depressed fracture occurs. Skull fragments are elevated and splinters and debris removed. Severe fragmentation and depression may necessitate removal of that area of the skull. Later, a cranioplasty may be done: a plate of inert material (e.g. titanium) is inserted to protect the brain and improve the patient's appearance.

Brain injury

Injury to the brain may result from a blow to the head and may or may not be associated with a fracture of the skull. A head injury may cause concussion, cerebral contusion or laceration, haemorrhage and/or compression.

A brain injury may be mild and reversible or may be severe and irreversible, leaving residual neurological deficits

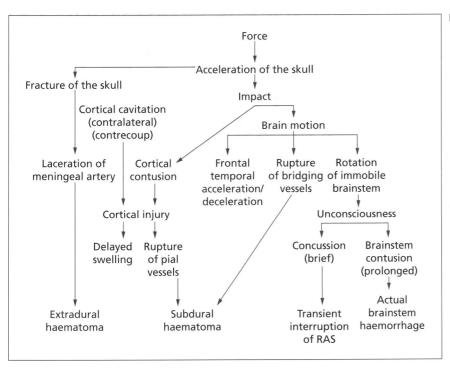

Figure 20.15   Mechanisms of head injury.

if the patient survives. Oedema of the brain and intracranial haemorrhage increase intracranial pressure which, if severe, may compress the brainstem and its vital centres (supratentorial herniation). Initially, *every head injury is considered serious*. It must be emphasized that, regardless of outward appearance, the person requires close observation for evidence of developing secondary brain damage that could result in permanent disability or death.

Concussion   Concussion is characterized by a brief period of unconsciousness due to jarring of the brain and its sudden forceful contact with the rigid skull. The period of unconsciousness is usually at most only a few minutes, depending on the severity of the injury. When the patient regains consciousness, he or she may be confused, dazed and restless, and be unable to recall events that preceded the accident. Headache is a common complaint. If there is no haemorrhage or brain tissue damage, no abnormal neurological findings are present: normal reflexes and muscle tone return.

Nursing intervention   This includes observation for evidence of neurological deterioration if the patient is admitted and, if discharged, ensuring that a reliable person is available. The responsible person is instructed to remain with the patient. If the patient becomes increasingly drowsy or difficult to rouse, or if he or she experiences headache, vomiting, visual disturbances, seizures or a reduction in limb strength, the patient should be brought back to hospital by ambulance immediately. It is advisable to provide instructions in writing for the responsible person because anxiety may affect the ability to recall what has been said. Recovery following an uncomplicated concussion occurs within a short period of time, although some side-effects may persist for weeks.

Cerebral contusion and laceration   Cerebral contusion and laceration refers to bruising and tearing of superficial brain tissue. The multiple areas of tissue damage may give rise to a wide variety of patient responses. It must be emphasized that a patient with a head injury may have significant trauma and still be alert initially. Lesions of the brainstem are usually the most serious. Level of consciousness may be altered for several hours or weeks. A variety of other neurological abnormalities is usually present on both sides of the body. If neurological signs are present on one side of the body, it is probable that a secondary event such as the development of a haematoma has occurred. The tissue injury is usually accompanied by brain swelling and oedema. Recovery may be a lengthy process; permanent tissue damage and scarring may result in permanent disability if the patient survives.

Secondary events following head injury
Intracranial haemorrhage
Haemorrhage within the cranium and the formation of a haematoma following a head injury frequently leads to a

rapid deterioration in the patient's condition. The bleeding may be extradural, subdural, subarachnoid or intracerebral. The clinical characteristics presented are due to increased intracranial pressure and compression of areas of the brain.

Extradural haematoma   An extradural haematoma is an accumulation of blood between the dura and skull (Fig. 20.16) and is a serious complication. As the meningeal artery is frequently torn, extradural bleeding is at arterial pressure. The brain is compressed and displaced, and the ICP rises rapidly. The patient may be comatose for a brief period, regain consciousness, then gradually develop serious neurological symptoms (disturbed vision, dilated pupil and loss of reflex to light in the eye on the affected side, severe headache, confusion, decreased motor and sensory function, seizure, vomiting) and loss of consciousness. Prompt treatment is essential. If an extradural haemorrhage is not recognized and promptly treated, the rapidly increasing ICP may cause tentorial herniation, pressure on vital centres and death within a few hours.

Subdural haemorrhage   Subdural haemorrhage is another possible complication of head injury. Blood accumulates in the subdural space (Fig. 20.16), gradually forming a haematoma which compresses the brain and increases intracranial pressure. The bleeding may occur following a seemingly minor head injury. As the bleeding is usually at venous pressure, the development of symptoms may be delayed and vague but progressively worsen and, eventually, increasing ICP and brain compression lead to coma.

All head injuries should therefore be treated initially as serious and a potential threat to life.

Subdural haemorrhage may be subacute or chronic in patients of advanced age or with cortical atrophy. In these patients, evidence of increased ICP usually appears very gradually and intermittently.

Subarachnoid haemorrhage   Subarachnoid haemorrhage is bleeding of cerebral vessels into the space between the arachnoid and pia mater. The clinical characteristics are similar to those presented by the patient with a subdural haemorrhage and depend on the area of the brain involved. This is rarely seen in trauma and is much more likely to be due to a cerebral aneurysm.

Intracerebral haemorrhage   Intracerebral haemorrhage is bleeding resulting from a torn or diseased vessel within the cerebrum. It may occur as a result of contrecoup injury, a penetrating wound such as a gun-shot or stabbing, or a stroke. The symptoms depend on the particular vessel and cerebral area (Fig. 20.16).

Medical management
The head-injured patient with raised ICP can present in a number of different ways. They may be fully alert and oriented walking into the health centre with a history of injury accompanied by very mild and transient symptoms, or they may arrive in A&E with full paramedical support

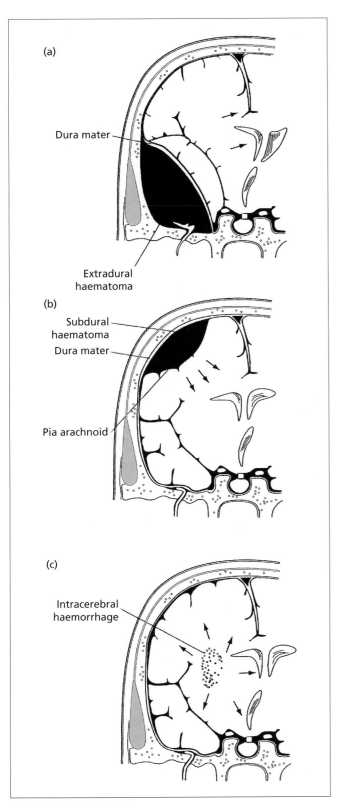

(a)

Dura mater

Extradural
haematoma

(b)

Subdural
haematoma
Dura mater

Pia arachnoid

(c)

Intracerebral
haemorrhage

Figure 20.16 Cranial haematomas. (a) Extradural haematoma. (b) Subdural haematoma. (c) Intracerebral haemorrhage.

deeply unconscious. Neurological deficits can usually be found, for example alteration of conscious level, occurrence of a seizure or onset of confusion. Depending on the severity of injury, the initial assessment will be aided if the following information can be ascertained (Lindsay and Bone 2004):

- *Period of loss of consciousness* – relates to the severity of diffuse brain damage (i.e. the longer the patient is unconscious, the more severe the damage)
- *Period of post-traumatic amnesia (PTA)* – the period of permanent amnesia that occurs after head injury; it is an indicator of the severity of brain damage (i.e. the longer the period of PTA, the worse the brain damage)
- *Cause and circumstances of the injury* – this may indicate whether other extracranial injuries exist
- *Presence of headache or vomiting* – these would indicate the possibility of intracranial haemorrhage.

Table 20.6 lists the signs and symptoms of raised ICP.

A head-injured patient should initially be assessed and managed according to clear principles and standards as embodied in the Advanced Trauma Life Support (ATLS) system and, for children, the Advanced Paediatric Life Support (PALS) system (Scottish Intercollegiate Guidelines Network 2000). Clinical assessment will include seeking evidence of injury including basal skull fracture signs, assessment of conscious level, pupil response, limb weakness and eye movements.

Investigations include skull radiography (to demonstrate fractures), computed tomography (CT) and magnetic resonance imaging (MRI) (may demonstrate cerebral contusions or lacerations and/or an intracranial haematoma) (Hickey 2002).

Intracranial pressure monitoring

A typical system comprises a fibreoptic transducer-tipped catheter, which can be placed in the lateral ventricle, subdural space or extradural space. Less emphasis is now placed on the data obtained from ICP monitoring. It is suggested that the maintenance of CPP is more important (CPP = mean BP-ICP) than just treating raised ICP. This is because it has been shown that patients with a high ICP, low blood pressure and therefore low CPP make a poorer recovery. Measures to reduce ICP must not be used indiscriminately and several guidelines have been issued on this. It is suggested that ICP and CPP monitoring are most relevant for the patient with a flexion response (or worse) to painful stimuli, but this policy will vary depending on a number of factors. The aim is to maintain CPP at more than 70 mmHg.

A number of approaches may be adopted in the management of the patient, and these can be regarded as a menu from which some or all are selected to treat a particular individual depending upon the circumstances. They include the use of hyperosmolar agents, controlled hyperventilation, fluid management, sedatives and surgical intervention.

Table 20.6   Signs and symptoms of raised intracranial pressure

Sign/symptom	Reasons
Early	
Deterioration in conscious level	The most highly specialized cells of the brain are the most sensitive to the oxygen deprivation that occurs with raised ICP. The response to this is that the patient becomes more drowsy
Pupillary dysfunction	Compression of the third cranial nerve (oculomotor) as a result of herniation causes pupillary dilatation, usually on the same side as the space-occupying lesion causing the rise in ICP
Motor weakness	A weakness (hemiparesis) on one side can occur, usually on the opposite side to the space-occupying lesion
Headache	This is initially mild and is thought to occur because the pain-sensitive structures at the base of the brain are distorted. It is usually described as being worse in the morning and improves as the day proceeds. This is because it is known that ICP rises during REM sleep
Papilloedema	Caused by raised ICP when the optic nerve becomes swollen and congested. May be present as an early sign in the patient with a slowly progressing rise in ICP
Later	
Continuing deterioration in the level of consciousness	As ICP continues to rise the patient becomes drowsier and eventually comatose
Vomiting	Thought to be caused by direct pressure on the vomiting centre and is unusual in adults. The mechanism is not fully understood. When it does occur, it tends to be projectile and is not accompanied by nausea
Hemiplegia, decerebration, decortication	This is a later stage to the process described in motor weakness above. Hemiplegia is paralysis of the limbs on one side of the body
Alterations in vital signs	With pressure on the brainstem increasing, changes in blood pressure and pulse become evident. In an attempt to ensure that the brain remains adequately perfused in the face of a rising ICP, blood pressure rises also and eventually the pulse pressure (i.e. the difference between the systolic and diastolic pressures) begins to widen. This is referred to *Cushing's response*. For similar reasons, the pulse becomes full and bounding, and becomes slower
Respiratory irregularities	The brain's attempt to boost the supply of oxygen in response to a rising ICP results in a rise in the respiratory rate quickly followed by a reduction until eventually apnoea supervenes
Papilloedema	May be late finding in some patients when the ICP is markedly increased
Impaired brainstem reflexes	In the latest stages, sustained pressure on the brainstem as a result of herniation results in dysfunction of brainstem reflexes. The testing of these reflexes forms the basis of brainstem death testing

Hyperosmolar agents   These act by establishing an osmotic gradient between the plasma and brain tissue, thus removing water from the oedematous brain tissue to the blood. An intravenous infusion of 100 mL of 20% mannitol over 15 min is a typical adult dose. This will 'buy' time to allow the patient to be prepared for transfer to a specialist unit or for operation. However, repeated doses have progressively less effect and may lead to hypervolaemia with resultant increase in ICP or electrolyte imbalance (Watkins 2000).

Controlled hyperventilation   To achieve this, the patient needs to be paralysed, intubated and mechanically ventilated. Vasoconstriction is achieved as the result of reducing the arterial partial pressure of carbon dioxide ($PaCO_2$), which in turn reduces cerebral blood volume and ICP. It is suggested by Lindsay and Bone (2004) that the resultant reduction in cerebral blood flow may itself cause brain damage. Maintaining the blood pressure and CPP appears to be as important, if not more so, than lowering ICP. It is necessary to measure the amount of oxygen extracted from the brain using a jugular bulb catheter to determine whether or not the brain can withstand further vasoconstriction.

Fluid management   This approach to treatment has been the subject of much debate over time. Some advocate restricting fluid in order to induce slight dehydration. By controlling intake, the extracellular fluid, including that of the brain, is decreased thus reducing ICP. The intake may be set at 1–2.5 L/24 hours. However, some now advocate achieving normovolaemia or increasing fluids. Doing this increases cerebral blood flow and thus improves oxygen delivery to the brain.

Sedatives   Traditionally patients with a head injury were never sedated for fear of masking important signs relating to conscious level. However, there are now special circumstances under which sedation might be used. If ICP fails to respond to standard measures then sedation may help under carefully controlled conditions (Lindsay and Bone 2004). Drugs that may be used include propofol and etomidate, although each has associated ill effects that must be countered. Propofol causes vasodilatation that may need to be counteracted to prevent blood pressure from falling and a reduction in cerebral perfusion. Etomidate inhibits steroid synthesis, and so steroid cover is required.

Surgical intervention Surgery may be performed to remove a focal mass lesion such as an expanding haematoma, and this may be combined with decompression. Withdrawal of small aliquots of CSF via a ventricular catheter results in a reduction of ICP but this provides only temporary relief. To be effective, drainage would require to be continuous, but this is often impractical.

Nursing assessment: altered consciousness

The priority in nursing assessment following head injury is assessment of conscious level.

Interruption of impulses from the reticular activating system, or failure of the cerebral cortical neurones to respond to incoming impulses, produces a loss of consciousness. Other than destruction of the cortical or cortical activating cells (reticular formation) by trauma, the basic factors contributing to unconsciousness are considered to be oxygen and glucose deprivation. Neurones require a constant supply of both of these substances for cellular activity. A deficiency of oxygen for even a few seconds decreases neuronal metabolism to a point at which unconsciousness ensues. Figure 20.17 describes the effects of alterations in level of consciousness from a state of normal awareness to coma or unconsciousness.

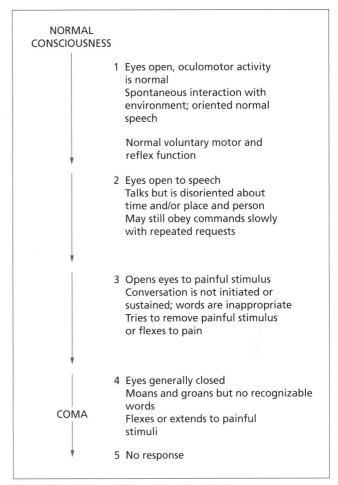

NORMAL CONSCIOUSNESS

1 Eyes open, oculomotor activity is normal
Spontaneous interaction with environment; oriented normal speech

Normal voluntary motor and reflex function

2 Eyes open to speech
Talks but is disoriented about time and/or place and person
May still obey commands slowly with repeated requests

3 Opens eyes to painful stimulus
Conversation is not initiated or sustained; words are inappropriate
Tries to remove painful stimulus or flexes to pain

4 Eyes generally closed
Moans and groans but no recognizable words
Flexes or extends to painful stimuli

COMA

5 No response

Figure 20.17 Signs of altered consciousness.

Causes

The patient's level of consciousness may be depressed due to the effects of abnormal metabolic processes or disease, including trauma, involving the brain or brainstem:

1 Processes that may interfere with the *metabolism* of the brainstem and cerebral cortex:
   a) hypoglycaemia or diabetic ketoacidosis, which produces a deficiency of glucose that is essential for cerebral neuronal functioning
   b) respiratory failure, which produces cerebral hypoxia
   c) renal and hepatic failure, which cause an accumulation of metabolic wastes
   d) electrolyte imbalance
   e) infections and autoimmune disorders
   f) drug overdose.
   Patients' manifestations resulting from altered metabolism show symmetrical changes in motor function.

2 *Space-occupying lesions* affecting the brain may alter the level of consciousness, and include cerebral haemorrhage from vascular diseases and trauma, tumours, abscess and haematoma from skull injuries. Manifestations are usually unequal on each side and may include hemiplegia and small reactive pupils which later become fixed.

3 *Brainstem lesions* that may cause unconsciousness include cerebral haemorrhage and brainstem infarction, tumours and abscesses, as well as trauma that produces direct pressure on the reticular formation tissue in the brainstem. Symptoms include loss of reflexes and pupillary reactions. Patients with trauma or metabolic disturbance will show signs of generalized brain dysfunction rather than focal signs; it is important to assess overall brain function and vital signs frequently.

Assessment of level of consciousness

Decrease in responsiveness to stimuli indicates progressive deterioration in brain function. The chance of complete recovery decreases with increase in the duration of impaired consciousness; decrease in responsiveness to stimuli must be reported immediately in order that measures can be implemented to reduce the risk of irreversible neurological dysfunction or death.

A standardized approach to the measurement of conscious level is essential for improved patient care. Use of a standardized system eliminates confusing language in the description of conscious level and permits efficient transfer of information from one observer to another. An approach that takes this into account is the Glasgow Coma Scale (GCS).

Glasgow coma scale   The GCS provides for evaluation of eye opening and the best verbal and motor responses. Within each of these three parameters, there is a variety of responses which are arranged in scales of increasing dysfunction, as outlined in Figure 20.18. Each aspect is assessed independently of the others.

Eye opening:

- *Spontaneous opening* (4). The nurse approaches the patient's bedside and notes whether the eyes are open or closed. Spontaneous opening of the eyes indicates that the arousal mechanism in the reticular activating system of the brainstem is functioning
- *Opening to speech* (3). If the patient's eyes are closed, the observer speaks, addressing the patient by name. If there is no response to a normal speaking voice, the volume should be increased

- *Opening to pain* (2). Physical stimulation, in the form of the trapezium squeeze (see below), is applied. It is important that observers use the same method of applying physical stimulation to ensure consistent, accurate findings
- *No eye opening* (1). If no response is demonstrated in either eye to increased pain stimuli, there is depression of the arousal system.

The patient may be sufficiently alert to respond by opening his or her eyes, but is restricted by swelling of the eyelids. If the eyelids are swollen shut, the observer records this as a 'C'.

Best verbal response   The patient's ability to speak and to understand the language spoken are determined. If the patient is intubated or has a tracheostomy, verbal response cannot be observed and 'T' is recorded. Speech is first used to stimulate a verbal response by asking the patient simple, direct questions. If there is no response, a painful stimulus is applied. The recommended method for this is the trapezium squeeze. This involves pinching and twisting 2 inches of the trapezius muscle using the thumb and two fingers. Be

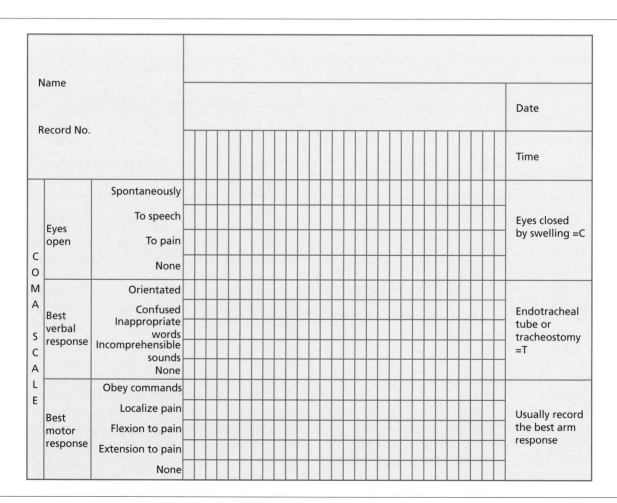

Figure 20.18   Glasgow Coma Scale record sheet.

careful not to injure the patient in the process. The patient's responses are rated as follows:

- *Oriented* (5). The patient is able to respond as to who he or she is, where he or she is, and can give the year, month and day
- *Confused* (4). The patient is not fully oriented to time, place and person
- *Inappropriate* (3). The patient utters words in a disorganized way, swears or does not engage in meaningful conversation
- *Incomprehensible* (2). Responses are limited to moaning, groaning or mumbling sounds with no recognizable words
- *No response* (1). No sounds are made in response to noxious stimuli.

Best motor response   The best possible motor response in either arm is observed and recorded. The patient is asked to raise the arms and hold them outstretched for 10 seconds. It is important to note that some clinical areas breakdown the assessment of motor function to flexion and abnormal flexion, whilst others omit abnormal flexion, this continues to be a source of debate. The ratings in order of decreasing levels of function include the following:

- *Obeys commands* (6). The patient understands verbal, written instructions or gestures and performs the requested movement
- *Localization to pain* (5). There is no response to command. When a painful stimulus is applied, such as trapezium squeeze, the patient moves a limb in an attempt to locate and remove the stimulus
- *Flexion to pain* (4). The arms bends at the elbow in response to trapezium squeeze. Leg flexion is not a reliable gauge because, with brain death, a spinal reflex may be present causing the legs to flex in response to localized pain
- *Abnormal flexion* (3). The arm flexes at the elbow and sometimes pronates, making a fist
- *Extension to pain* (2). The elbow straightens and the arm abducts (usually with internal rotation) in response to pain administered via trapezium squeeze
- *No response* (1). No detectable movement or change in the tone of the limbs is observed in response to repeated and varied stimuli.

Abnormal flexion, extension and no response are all abnormal.

Other neurological parameters   Assessment of pupil responses and limb movements provides information and assists in localizing lesions; for example, if the pupil starts to dilate, pressure on the third cranial nerve is present, and neighbouring parasympathetic fibres that control pupillary constriction are affected. This may indicate coning or herniation of brain tissue through the tentorial hiatus.

Pupils   Each pupil is examined for size and reaction. Normally, the pupils are round in shape, equal in size, and constrict in response to direct light. The *size* of each pupil is measured by comparing it with the pupil scale, as illustrated in Figure 20.19. Pupil *reaction* is measured in response to light; the beam of a pentorch is brought in from the patient's side and directed on one eye at a time.

The surroundings should be dimly lit and the light beam of adequate intensity to obtain accurate results.

Limb movement   Verbal commands are used to elicit movement in each limb. When the patient does not respond to commands, painful stimuli are applied to the nailbed of a finger or great toe. Responses in order of decreasing function are recorded as:

- *Normal power* – the limb movements are appropriate to the normal muscle strength for the patient
- *Mild weakness* – one limb shows normal strength but its opposite is weaker
- *Severe weakness* – the difference between two limbs is very much marked
- *Spastic flexion* – there is slow, stiff movement of the arm with the flexed forearm and hand held against the body
- *Extension* – the elbow or knee are straightened in response to painful stimulation
- *No response* – painful stimulation produces no movement and the limb remains limp.

It is important to compare each side and to record differences between right and left limbs and changes in the responses of an individual limb.

Vital signs   Changes in the pulse rate and rhythm and in blood pressure provide information about possible increased ICP, internal bleeding or shock. A decrease in the respiratory rate indicates pressure in the respiratory centre in the brainstem as a result of raised ICP.

It should be remembered that any changes in the patient's cerebral condition will manifest first as changes in level of consciousness, hence the importance of frequent and accurate observation, using the Glasgow Coma Scale.

The symptoms are summarized in Box 20.2. It should be remembered that a decreased level of consciousness is the first warning of an expanding brain lesion.

Emergency care

Priorities require to be established as follows:

1 Assessment of respiratory status and correction of deficits (airway and breathing).
2 Assessment of conscious level and other neurological parameters including the risk of neck injury.
3 Assessment of other injuries.

Patient problems

The following is a list of some of the main problems encountered in the early stages of recovery from brain injury:

- Respiratory dysfunction secondary to:
  - loss of patency of airway

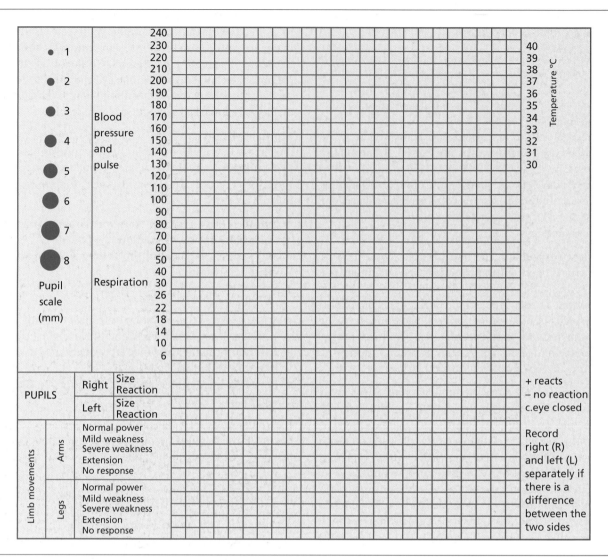

Figure 20.19 Record sheet for other neurological parameters.

Box 20.2   Signs and symptoms of head injury

- Loss of consciousness, which may develop at the time of injury and last for a varying length of time
- Recurrence of unconsciousness following a lucid interval
- Drowsiness and stupor progressing to coma
- Severe headache or dizziness
- Disturbed vision
- Dilatation and failure to react to light of one or both pupils
- Motor and sensory deficits, seizures, nuchal rigidity, speech impairment, disorientation, changes in vital signs indicative of increasing intracranial pressure (see p. 687)
- The escape of CSF from the ear or nose.

- injury to or compression of the respiratory centre in the brainstem
- Alteration in level of consciousness
- Alteration in comfort when conscious – mild to severe headache
- Motor and sensory deficits due to brain compression and damage
- Alteration in level of awareness of self and environment
- Potential for injury related to reduced level of consciousness, confusion, motor and sensory deficits or seizures
- Impairment of skin integrity secondary to scalp wound or immobility (pressure sores)
- Alteration in fluid and food intake secondary to comatose state, fluid intake restrictions per 24 hours, or anxiety
- Alteration in elimination patterns:
  - urinary (incontinence, retention)
  - bowel (constipation and potential impaction)

- Self-care deficits affecting personal hygiene secondary to unconsciousness, enforced immobility or motor deficits
- Anxiety related to confusion and loss of memory of previous events
- Lack of knowledge about diagnostic and therapeutic procedures, condition, hospitalization and post-hospital care.

Goals

The fundamental goal is that the patient will regain consciousness with no long-term deficits. This involves a series of short-term goals, such as a normal breathing pattern and patent airway, avoiding further injury and the complications of having a decreased level of consciousness leading to confusion and immobility. Goals relating to normal body function such as fluid intake and output should also be set.

Nursing intervention

The special considerations previously described for nursing the patient with an altered conscious level, raised ICP, and preoperative and postoperative care are applicable to the head-injured patient.

The head-injured patient is at risk of infection if an open scalp wound is present; the wound is cleansed, debrided if necessary, and sutured. A tetanus vaccine may be required if the patient has not achieved full immunity against tetanus.

Loss of the corneal reflexes, periorbital oedema and ecchymoses are common problems with a head injury. If the corneal reflex is absent, the eyelid may be taped shut with non-allergic tape to protect the cornea from drying and abrasions. The tape is removed every 2 hours and the eye irrigated with normal saline and artificial tears instilled before re-taping. If the eyelids are swollen, it may be necessary for a second nurse to hold the lids open while pupillary reflexes are assessed. If the lids cannot be opened, the doctor is notified; it is important that pupillary changes be detected in sufficient time to institute treatment.

Hyperthermia may develop following head injury due to a disturbance of the temperature control centre in the hypothalamus leading to temperatures of 40°C or more. Vigorous interventions are required to reduce such extremely high temperatures.

Nursing interventions following head injury will be determined by the extent and circumstances of the patient's injury. Interventions can be considered as those required in the acute or emergency phase immediately after the injury, in the ongoing phase immediately following the acute one, and finally discharge/rehabilitation requirements. The timespan over which this continuum extends can be as little as a few days to several months. Within the continuum there are four significant care events that may be required. These include:

1 caring for the patient with raised ICP
2 caring for the unconscious patient
3 caring for the patient requiring neurosurgical interventions and/or intensive care
4 meeting the needs of the head-injured patient, including those required to achieve an optimal outcome.

Caring for the patient with raised intracranial pressure following head injury Head-injured patients with raised ICP may appear to have sustained no injury initially but can become drowsy or confused, or develop speech problems or limb deficits. The immediate nursing aim is to prevent further damaging rises in ICP. The care plan (Table 20.7) outlines the principal interventions and their rationale. The presence of other injuries can alter the management of the patient depending upon the initial survey in the acute phase.

For the patient with increased ICP, treatment may be medical, surgical or a combination of both. Surgical intervention usually deals with the specific cause and may involve ventricular drainage. Medical treatment includes the intravenous administration of osmotic diuretics (e.g. mannitol) and the corticosteroid dexamethasone to try to reduce cerebral oedema.

Assessment The effects of rising ICP on the patient will vary with the speed at which pressure is rising and hence the nature of the lesion itself. The pressure may increase very rapidly, as with an extradural haemorrhage, or it may increase very gradually, as with a slow-growing tumour.

Early symptoms include headache that progressively becomes more severe, drowsiness, slowing of responses and vomiting, which may not be preceded by nausea. It is important that the nurse obtains information from the family about the patient's normal behaviour as a baseline against which to compare current functioning. With further development there is decreasing consciousness, an increase in the systolic blood pressure with a widening pulse pressure, change in respiratory pattern, eye changes (pupillary dilatation, loss of reflex to light stimulus), papilloedema and bradycardia (Table 20.6).

The patient's vital signs and neurological status are assessed to provide a baseline against which any signs of deterioration may be detected. Assessment of the patient's neurological status also includes observations for involuntary movements (twitching, tremors or convulsion), restlessness, rigidity and posturing (decerebrate or decorticate rigidity) (Fig. 20.10).

It is important to assess the patient's level of understanding of the current situation and communication skills, and how the family is reacting to the situation.

The physical assessment should include a careful check on the patient's skin to assess for signs of dehydration and pressure area breakdown.

Patient problems The following is a list of potential problems frequently encountered by patients suffering raised ICP.

- Alteration in respiratory function related to:
  - ineffective clearance of airway
  - injury or compression of the respiratory centre
  - obstruction of the airway by the tongue or aspirate, if unconscious

Table 20.7 Care plan for patient with raised intracranial pressure

Area of care	Nursing interventions	Rationale
Neurological status	Assess baseline neurological observations including conscious level and reassess as determined by patient's status. Assess vital signs particularly temperature. If raised, institute measures to reduce to normal	Changes in neurological status, no matter how subtle, can herald rising ICP and thus risk of brain damage if not detected. A raised temperature will create greater demand for oxygenation, thus raising ICP
Respiratory status	Assess rate, depth and pattern of respirations. Check breath sounds. Monitor arterial blood gases. Suction as required for maximum of 15 seconds. Preoxygenate for up to 1 minute before suctioning with 100% oxygen. Manage assisted ventilation (if required). Provide tracheostomy care (if required)	Patients with raised ICP require adequate oxygenation to ensure that brain is properly perfused. Attention to factors that may impede this will ensure that ICP is not raised further and the outcome from injury will be better
Avoiding increased ICP due to poor positioning or activities	Nurse patient in a 30° head-up tilt. Prone position and extreme hip flexion are contraindicated. Maintain head in a neutral position with sandbags if required. Ensure patient's head does not fall to one side or that tracheostomy tapes are not too tight around the neck. If patient conscious, ask to exhale when turning in bed. Instruct patient not to press down with hands on the bed when moving. Plan nursing activities to avoid clustering of these. Re-position patient regularly and provide skin care	Elevating head of bed and achieving neutral head position ensures adequate venous drainage from head, thus avoiding raises in ICP. Exhaling on turning avoids Valsalva's manoeuvre which raises ICP. Pushing down produces isometric contraction which will result in raised ICP due to initiation of Valsalva's manoeuvre. Clustering of nursing activities have been shown to raise ICP
Elimination	Monitor volume and specific gravity of urine. Monitor stools. No enemas	Indicates diuresis and dilution. Diabetes insipidus indicated by a falling specific gravity and increased output may occur following injury and require treatment. Avoiding constipation prevents initiation of Valsalva's manoeuvre, which can occur when straining at stool or as the result of an enema
Ventricular drainage	Manage ventricular drainage system. Note correct position of drainage bag. Maintain strict asepsis. Maintain closed system	Correct position of bag will result in optimal drainage of CSF. If bag too low, too much CSF will drain resulting in brain herniation; too high means that drainage will not take place thus increasing ICP
ICP monitoring	Manage system. Record data. Maintain asepsis	Recording and reporting data will result in appropriate interventions to avoid further rises in ICP
Seizures management	Maintain seizure precautions	Avoids further rises in ICP. Avoids patient injury

- Potential for injury due to disorientation and impaired awareness, restlessness, seizures
- Severe headache
- Potential hyperthermia
- Alteration in cardiac function secondary to compression and ischaemia of vital centres in the medulla
- Potential for skin breakdown due to immobility and possible restlessness and hyperthermia
- Potential fluid imbalance due to osmotic diuretic, inadequate intake and vomiting
- Nutritional deficit due to inadequate intake and increased metabolic rate with hyperthermia and injury
- Alteration in elimination – bowel and urinary
- Self-care deficit in personal hygiene due to reduced level of consciousness and motor and sensory changes.

Goals The goals for the patient revolve around being free from any of the complications outlined in the above list of problems, having the maximum possible insight into the situation and a satisfactory standard of personal hygiene and comfort.

Nursing intervention

Ineffective respiration If the patient with raised ICP has impaired respiration, then less oxygen is available to perfuse the brain. It is therefore important to ensure optimal respiratory status. The patient may require full artificial ventilatory support. Assessment will include the rate, depth and pattern of respiration. A respiratory rate below 14 or above 24 breaths/minute would give cause for concern. Irregularities in the rate and/or rhythm are indicative of a rising ICP. Assessment might also include pulse oximetry and monitoring of arterial blood gases.

Based on the assessment, appropriate interventions are identified from a menu of activities. These include:

- *Positioning* – normally semiprone with a 30° head-up tilt unless contraindicated. The head-up tilt also assists with minimizing rises in ICP by encouraging venous drainage
- *Use of respiratory aids* – If artificial ventilation is indicated, endotracheal intubation will be required. This requires additional specialized nursing care
- *Suctioning* – oropharyngeal and tracheal suctioning is applied only as required to remove secretions. Excessive suctioning raises ICP. Suctioning is limited to 10–15 seconds per pass and the patient is allowed to recover between suctioning. Pre-oxygenation with 100% oxygen prior to suctioning may be considered to prevent a buildup of carbon dioxide
- *Oxygen administration* – this is administered as prescribed via the appropriate route.

Potential for injury

Increased intracranial pressure Planning and implementation of care must take into consideration the prevention of further increase in the intracranial pressure as well as the reduction of the existing increased intracranial pressure.

Positions and activities that raise the ICP are avoided. The head of the bed is usually elevated to about 30°; the patient with potential or actual increased ICP is never placed in a head-low position but is positioned to prevent any impediment of cerebral venous return. The head is aligned with the spine; flexion and twisting of the head, anything tight around the neck that might compress the jugular veins, and extreme hip flexion are avoided. When moving or changing position, the conscious patient is instructed not to push with the feet or to push or pull with the arms, and to breathe out through the mouth. The latter prevents the Valsalva manoeuvre, which quickly raises the ICP. Clustering of nursing activities should be avoided to minimize rises in ICP.

The corticosteroid dexamethasone may be used to help reduce ICP. The patient receiving dexamethasone is observed for possible side-effects and complications, because corticosteroids suppress the immune response making the patient more susceptible to infection and may also cause gastrointestinal bleeding. An H2 blocking drug such as ranitidine is prescribed to reduce stomach acidity and prevent peptic ulceration.

Disorientation and impaired cognitive function The patient's orientation, judgement, level of consciousness and mobility may change quickly. Protection from injury is necessary. Cot sides may be required unless someone stays at the bedside with the patient. Following an intracranial disorder and increased ICP, patients are frequently subject to spells of dizziness or lapses of orientation, or may be slow in regaining their postural reflexes.

Restlessness This may be due to cerebral hypoxia or increasing rise in the ICP, but restlessness may also be associated with retention of urine, pain, an uncomfortable position, the regaining of consciousness, or fear and concern about the situation. Efforts are made to determine the cause if the patient is restless and to eliminate it if possible. If there are neurological symptoms and changes in vital signs that indicate a further increase in the ICP, they are reported promptly so that further treatment may be undertaken. If the restlessness occurs with the regaining of consciousness, the patient is reoriented to the situation; if the cause of the restlessness is thought to be the patient's anxiety, explanations and reassurance are necessary.

Nursing measures such as position change and staying with the patient and encouraging expression of concerns may promote comfort and reduce restlessness. The environment should be quiet and the lighting subdued. In extreme restlessness, a mild sedative may be prescribed to prevent exhaustion.

The patient with reduced consciousness may be able to hear and comprehend, although not be able to respond. It is important that those caring for the patient continue to communicate with the patient and guard against inappropriate conversation. Verbal communication provides cerebral stimulation and information; it can be comforting and reassuring to the patient. Non-verbal communication by touch and presence is also reassuring to both patient and family. Family members are advised of the possibility of the patient hearing and are encouraged to communicate with the patient even though unresponsive.

Headache The patient usually experiences headache with the onset of increased ICP which progressively becomes more severe as the pressure rises. A mild non-narcotic analgesic such as paracetamol may be prescribed. The patient may find that cold applications provide some relief. As the ICP increases and the patient loses consciousness, pain perception diminishes. A quiet room, subdued lighting and a minimum of environmental stimuli are important, and sudden movements should be avoided.

Alteration in body temperature Compression of the temperature-regulating centre as a result of increased ICP may result in a marked increase in the temperature and, at the same time, the normal physiological heat-dissipating mechanisms are suppressed (dilatation of superficial blood vessels and perspiration). The metabolic rate is increased in proportion to the fever: with a temperature of 40.5°C, there is an increase in metabolism of approximately 50% leading to a major increase in oxygen demand and carbon dioxide output.

The room is preferably kept cool and a light cotton sheet used to cover the patient. If the temperature is raised, the sheet is arranged to cover only the lower half of the body. The patient should not be cooled too quickly; shivering must be prevented because it increases metabolism, oxygen consumption and the production of carbon dioxide and other metabolites that increase ICP.

Alteration in cardiac function   The compression and ischaemia caused by increased ICP may seriously affect the cardiac and vasomotor centres. Close monitoring of the pulse for irregularity and changes in the rate and volume is necessary. A decrease in cardiac output reduces cerebral perfusion to a greater degree, resulting in ischaemia, increased PCO_2 and vasodilatation, and an ensuing increase in ICP. Continuous cardiac monitoring may be established and an antiarrhythmic drug prescribed if necessary. The excessive loss of body fluid as a result of osmotic diuretic therapy may cause a reduction in intravascular volume and a corresponding reduction in cardiac output. Cardiac failure is more likely to occur if the patient has a pre-existing cardiac problem.

Potential for skin breakdown   Maintenance of skin integrity requires special attention because of the patient's immobility and possible restlessness and hyperthermia. The patient's position is changed from side to back (only if conscious) to side every 2 hours unless contraindicated by the location of the patient's intracranial lesion or surgery. For example, if a relatively large space-occupying lesion has been removed, the patient is not permitted to lie on the operative side to prevent a shifting of the brain into the remaining space.

Pressure area care is discussed fully in Chapter 25.

Potential fluid imbalance   The fluid intake is usually restricted to a stated volume distributed over 24 hours to maintain slight dehydration which reduces the extracellular volume and ICP. Intravenous fluids are infused slowly and must be monitored closely; rapid infusion could cause a serious, rapid rise in the ICP.

An osmotic diuretic may be prescribed to dehydrate ('shrink') the brain; the drugs administered for this purpose are principally hyperosmolar solutions which are given intravenously (e.g. mannitol). They promote the transfer of fluid from the brain tissue into the vascular compartment by osmosis and increase the urinary output.

Intravenous infusion is usually necessary owing to an inability to take sufficient fluid orally because of nausea, vomiting or coma.

Nutritional deficit   The headache, nausea, vomiting or loss of consciousness results in the patient's inability to take adequate food, which is reflected in changes in strength and muscle mass. Continuous nasogastric feeding may be given to provide necessary fluid and calories. If the patient is febrile, the increased metabolic rate requires more calories; if the caloric requirement is not met, the patient becomes seriously debilitated.

Alteration in elimination

Bowel elimination   The patient is discouraged from straining to defaecate because the effort involved raises ICP. A mild bulk laxative or stool softener may be given, or a bisacodyl (Dulcolax) suppository may be used as faecal impaction must be avoided.

Urinary elimination   If the patient is unresponsive, incontinence is a problem, making a retention catheter necessary so that an accurate assessment can be made of the output, as well as to maintain skin integrity. The output is noted every hour to evaluate the effectiveness of the osmotic diuretic.

The fluid intake and output are monitored for oliguria and water retention or an excessive volume of urine with a low specific gravity. The excessive output may develop as a result of a disturbance in the secretion of antidiuretic hormone (ADH) by the posterior pituitary lobe. An increase in ADH causes decreased urine formation, whereas a deficiency of ADH causes large volumes of urine to be excreted, necessitating the administration of vasopressin (Pitressin).

The catheter is removed as soon as possible because of the risk of urinary tract infection. For this reason, the use of a condom-type catheter is preferable.

Self-care deficit in personal hygiene   The nurse provides the personal care that the patient would normally carry out unaided, such as bathing, cleaning of teeth and mouth, combing of the hair and feeding. Nursing care should be carried out with undisturbed intervals between to permit adequate rest. If the eye reflexes are absent, the eyes may be irrigated with sterile normal saline and hypromellose drops (artificial tears) instilled three or four times daily to keep the surface of the eye clean and moist. If one or both eyes remain open, a protective shield is applied.

If permitted, the limbs are moved slowly and gently through their range of motion to preserve joint movements.

Ventricular drainage in increased intracranial pressure   A ventricular puncture may be done via a burr-hole in the skull and a tube inserted into a ventricle to establish drainage of CSF to lower the ICP. Externally, the tube is attached to a sterile closed system. The level at which the tubing and bag are placed is prescribed by the doctor. The rate of drainage is monitored very closely; too rapid drainage is to be avoided and blockage of the tube is to be reported promptly. Strict asepsis must be observed in handling the tubes and the dressing at the burr-hole. If the patient complains of severe headache or a neurological disturbance (e.g. disturbed vision) develops that was not experienced before the ventricular puncture, the doctor is notified.

The person with altered level of consciousness

Patient problems   Problems relevant to the patient with an altered level of consciousness are:

- alteration in sensation – visual, auditory, kinaesthesic, gustatory, tactile and olfactory
- alteration in thought processes
- ineffective airway clearance
- impaired physical mobility
- potential for injury
- potential impairment of skin integrity
- nutrition at intake less than body requirements
- incontinence of urine
- incontinence of faeces
- inability to maintain self-care – feeding, bathing/hygiene, dressing, grooming and toileting.

Goals   These principal problems lead to a set of patient goals which involve the patient avoiding harmful complications, maximizing independence and adapting to altered functioning in the above areas.

Nursing Intervention

Identification of changes in neurological function   Monitoring of the patient's level of consciousness, pupillary responses, limb movements and vital signs is carried out continuously. If the patient's condition is changing, data are recorded every 15 minutes. When the patient's neurological status stabilizes, recordings are gradually made less often. Early signs of increasing ICP should be reported promptly to ensure immediate action to prevent cerebral coning. The first sign of increasing ICP is a decrease in the level of consciousness, as measured on the Glasgow Coma Scale – hence the importance of these observations.

Maintenance of a patent airway   The first priority in caring for an unconscious patient is the establishment of a patent airway. As the patient's level of consciousness decreases, the ability to maintain a clear airway is limited. The cause may be obstruction of the airway by the tongue when the jaw and tongue relax, vomit, blood or other inhaled foreign material such as dentures. Ineffective ventilation may occur due to depression of the respiratory centre, accumulation of secretions and foreign material, as a result of depression of the cough reflex, and immobility and weakness of respiratory muscles.

The unconscious patient is placed in a lateral or semi-prone position (unless contraindicated by a chest or spinal injury), with the neck aligned with the spine. If the patient is unconscious as a result of a head injury, a spinal injury should be assumed to be present until proven otherwise (see p. 704 for movement of spinally injury patients. Either position facilitates the drainage of mucus and vomit, and prevents obstruction of the airway by the relaxed tongue and jaw. If mucus collects in the oropharyngeal cavity, frequent suctioning with a flexible catheter is necessary. The catheter is moistened with water before insertion and is handled gently during insertion and on withdrawal to avoid trauma to the delicate tracheal mucous membranes.

If the patient has lost the gag reflex, an artificial airway will be needed. A nasal airway or an endotracheal tube may be inserted to maintain the airway and facilitate the removal of secretions by suctioning.

Oxygen may be administered by nasal cannulae or mask, or mechanical ventilation may be instituted. If the patient is able to follow instructions, deep breathing is practised hourly. Hard, sustained coughing is contraindicated because it causes an increase in ICP. If coughing is necessary to remove secretions and the patient is able to do so, staged coughing is taught. This involves the patient taking a deep breath while relaxing the abdominal muscles, holding the breath, and then exhaling in short, staged intervals involving four or five expirations.

The patient's position should be changed every 2 hours to prevent pressure sore formation and facilitate the removal of secretions from the lungs. Observations are made following each change of position to determine the effect on respirations. Chest expansion is observed and the rate and rhythm of respirations are noted, as well as the patient's colour and general status.

Care of the eyes   Loss of the corneal reflex and depression of lacrimal secretion may result in prolonged exposure, drying and injury to the cornea which may lead to ulceration. The eyes should be examined regularly for signs of inflammation or injury. Contact lenses are removed. Ophthalmic solutions may be prescribed to irrigate the eyes three or four times a day. The eyes may be covered with dressings to protect them.

Care of the mouth   Dentures should be removed only if they pose a danger to the airway. The mouth is cleansed several times a day and teeth are cleaned by brushing when possible. The lips are moistened with a water-soluble ointment or cream. The mouth should be inspected daily for signs of crusting or ulceration of the mucosa.

Positioning   When the patient is placed in the lateral or semiprone position, attention is given to good body alignment and to the prevention of contractures, foot and wrist drop, muscle strain, joint injury, and interference with circulation and chest expansion. The head should be positioned so that the neck is aligned with the spine. The arm that is uppermost is flexed at the elbow and rested on a pillow to prevent drag on the shoulder and wrist drop. The arm that is down is drawn slightly forward, flexed at the elbow, and lies on the bed parallel with the neck and head. The lower limb that is uppermost is flexed at the hip and knee, and supported on a firm pillow; the other lower limb is slightly flexed. The feet are positioned at a 90° angle to the leg and care is taken that *no* pressure is applied by firm objects placed against the feet.

Joint movement   The extremities are passively moved through their normal range of motion at least twice daily to preserve joint function and prevent circulatory stasis. Active exercises are initiated as soon as the patient is able to follow instructions.

Protection from injury   The cot sides of the bed are always maintained in the up position when the patient is unconscious unless someone is in constant attendance on the patient. It may be necessary for someone to be in constant attendance if the patient is restless and thrashing about as a very agitated patient may climb over cot sides and suffer serious injury from the ensuing fall. Placing mittens on the hands may be necessary if the patient is restless, scratches, or pulls on the nasogastric or intravenous tube or the urethral catheter. The mittens are removed every 4 hours; the hands are bathed, the nails are kept clean and short, and the fingers put through their normal range of motion by passive exercise.

The nurse should not attempt to force resisting extremities (such as in spastic flexion or extension) to assume a different position. Forcing a rigid extremity into a different position could result in a fracture of that limb. The use of depressant drugs to control agitation is contraindicated as they may further depress the arousal system.

When the patient is ambulatory but has some impairment of awareness, a safe environment should be provided. Scatter rugs and objects are removed from the patient's path to prevent falling. Sharp objects are removed from the immediate environment.

Fluids and nutrition   The patient is assessed for a gag reflex; as soon as it is present, and the patient is conscious, oral feeds are initiated. When the patient is unconscious or the gag reflex is absent, the patient's nutrition may be sustained by intravenous infusion or feeds given via a nasogastric feeding tube. The liquid feed given by tube contains the essential food elements and the amount is individually calculated to provide adequate caloric intake for the patient's size and metabolic activity. The dietician should be consulted for advice. Frequency of feeding varies from slow continuous to every 4 hours. If there is any regurgitation (fluid welling up around the tube into the mouth), the volume given at one time is decreased and the frequency of the feeds is increased. If the patient's condition permits, it is helpful to elevate the head of the bed slightly during the feeding and for a brief period afterwards. The tube is rinsed with water after each feeding.

The presence of the tube in a nostril tends to irritate the mucous membrane and stimulate mucus secretion. The area is cleansed twice daily with applicators that have been moistened with normal saline, and is then also lubricated lightly. The tube should be secured loosely enough so that it does not press continuously on any one area of the nostril.

Elimination   The unconscious patient has urinary incontinence. An indwelling **catheter** is inserted initially only if it is necessary to facilitate accurate monitoring of output or

if retention of urine occurs. The catheter is removed as soon as possible to prevent complications and promote the return of normal bladder functioning. Condom drainage is established with the male patient as soon as his condition is stable. While the catheter is in place, it is taped to the thigh to prevent undue traction.

If a catheter is not used, frequent attention is necessary to protect the skin. Incontinence pads are used to absorb the urine and are changed promptly after voiding. The skin is washed after each voiding and dried thoroughly. A barrier cream may be applied to the skin. The bed linen is changed as necessary.

The patient may be incontinent of faeces, particularly if receiving tube feedings. Prompt cleansing and changing of soiled pads and bedding are necessary.

Skin care   The unconscious patient is predisposed to the rapid development of pressure ulcers (see p. 889 for preventive measures).

Care should be taken to maintain daily personal hygiene. This includes hair and face washing and shaving. Families should be encouraged to help in these activities if they feel comfortable about it. It is important for families to be included as part of the caring team.

Maintenance or restoration of sensation, perception and awareness   Fluctuations in consciousness affect the patient's ability to receive a stimulus, interpret its meaning and respond with appropriate behaviour. The arousal mechanism may be affected so that repeated stimulation may be required to elicit a response. Sensory stimulation is an important aspect of the care of every patient experiencing alterations in the level of consciousness. The type of stimulation, how it is structured and presented, and its complexity must be planned for each individual according to the level of consciousness, the cause of the decreased consciousness, and the relevance and meaning of the stimulus to this particular individual.

Types of stimuli include auditory, olfactory, visual, tactile, kinaesthetic, vestibular and oral. The nurse should always speak to the patient by name and explain what is being done, and the patient should be informed before procedures such as feeding and turning occur. Touch is used as much as possible. Environmental noise is decreased and night orientation is practised to provide rest. Multisensory stimuli sessions may be carried out three or four times a day. Each method of stimulation is introduced one at a time in a form that is meaningful to the patient.

Caring for the patient requiring neurosurgical interventions and/or intensive care   Following neurosurgery the overall goals of care for patients are:

● continuous assessment of the patient's neurological status
● instituting measures to avoid secondary brain damage
● administration of appropriate therapies.

The main complications of neurosurgery are outlined in Table 20.8.

Preoperative nursing care

Assessment If the preoperative period extends over several days, the patient is observed for possible neurological changes from day to day which may indicate a worsening of the condition. The vital signs are followed closely; pupils are checked regularly for size, equality and reaction to light, and the patient's alertness, orientation, sensory perception, motor ability and strength of limbs are noted.

Vital signs and neurological observations are recorded to provide a baseline for measuring progress in the postoperative period.

Patient problems The patient faces all the usual problems associated with surgery, plus the following problems which are unique to intracranial surgery:

- anxiety related to the intracranial surgery and the outcome
- fluid deficit due to the administration of an osmotic diuretic because of increased ICP
- potential increased ICP
- potential for respiratory depression and thrombophlebitis
- embarrassment and concern related to disfigurement of the head.

Goals Patient goals involve avoiding the potential problems outlined above and being able to talk freely about fears and anxieties.

Nursing intervention

Anxiety Any impending surgery is perceived as a threat to the person and generates anxiety, but that involving the brain is even more threatening. The alert patient and the family are usually very fearful of a fatal outcome or permanent changes, disability, and a loss of intellect and competence. Expression of doubts and concerns is encouraged; time and opportunities for questions and answers are provided. The patient is not left alone for long periods; contact with others interrupts concentration on the operation and provides the opportunity to express fears. Visits are limited to family members and friends who can control their anxiety and show a quiet, reassuring presence with the patient.

It is necessary to explain to the patient and family the need for the operation, the nature of the procedure, the risks and possible outcome. The nurse should be able to answer questions, clarify misconceptions and refer, if appropriate, any special problems to others. The sort of information the family requires is that the patient may have temporary oedema and discoloration of the face and eyes, and possible neurological deficits such as facial paralysis and aphasia after the operation. The fact that these signs are common after surgery will help to reduce the anxiety they generate.

Fluid deficit There is usually concern if a preoperative patient manifests dehydration, and efforts are made to re-establish normal hydration. A fluid deficit in the patient who is to have intracranial surgery may be an important therapeutic measure. A restricted fluid intake may be necessary to control ICP, or an osmotic diuretic such as mannitol to reduce increased ICP may be given.

No attempt is made to increase the fluid intake without a specific directive. The patient may have water up to 4 or 5 hours before the operation unless otherwise indicated.

Common intracranial surgical procedures Intracranial surgery necessitates an opening in the skull. The size and location of the opening depend upon the nature and site of the lesion and the amount of exposure needed for the operation. If the lesion is in the cerebrum, it is referred to as being *supratentorial* and the incision is well above the hairline. If it is in the cerebellar or brainstem regions, it is designated as *infratentorial* and the incision is usually in the occipital region.

The surgical procedures include the following:

- *Burr-hole*. This is a small circular opening into the cranium made with a bone drill. The purpose may be to obtain

Table 20.8 Complications of neurosurgery

Complication	Cause	Interventions
Altered conscious level	Increased ICP due to cerebral haemorrhage/oedema	Frequent assessment of neurological status
Limb weaknesses	Increased ICP due to cerebral haemorrhage/oedema	Frequent assessment of limb movements
Speech problems	Increased ICP due to cerebral haemorrhage/oedema	Frequent assessment of verbal responses
Respiratory problems	Increased ICP due to cerebral haemorrhage/oedema	Frequent assessment of respiratory status
Loss of swallowing reflex	Increased ICP due to cerebral haemorrhage/oedema	Frequent assessment of swallowing reflex
Onset of seizures	Cerebral irritation	Observation of seizures. Interventions to ensure patient safety
Loss of corneal reflex	Increased ICP due to cerebral haemorrhage/oedema	Frequent assessment of corneal reflex
Periorbital oedema	Direct result of surgery	Observe for swollen/bruised periorbital tissues

tissue for a biopsy, aspirate CSF from a ventricle, or relieve pressure caused by swelling and oedema of the brain or a tumour

- *Craniotomy*. In this procedure a scalp incision and two or more burr-holes are made over the area to be explored. The bone between the burr-holes is incised, allowing elevation of a bone flap to provide access to the brain. The opening is curved so that the scalp and bone flap can be folded back to expose the affected brain area
- *Craniectomy*. This involves excision of a portion of the skull and may vary from a small burr-hole to a sizeable area of several square centimetres. The craniectomy may be done to remove shattered bone or to relieve pressure by expanding cranial contents
- *Cranioplasty*. This is a replacement of a section of the cranium with a synthetic material such as titanium to re-establish the contour and integrity of the skull. In some instances, the bone flap that was initially separated from the skull is replaced; this is referred to as an *osteoplastic craniotomy*.

Postoperative nursing care   As all patients suffer some increase in ICP following brain surgery, the nursing care described for increased ICP as well as the care of the unconscious patient are applicable in the postoperative phase.

Assessment   Vital signs and neurological status are determined when the patient is returned from the operating theatre as a baseline against which progress can be assessed. If the patient is conscious, alertness, orientation, speech and ability to move the limbs are checked. The required frequency of these observations may be indicated by the neurosurgeon but usually begins with 15–30-minute intervals which are gradually lengthened to 1 hour, then to 4 hours if the evaluations indicate stability. Care should be taken to assess for pain, headache or other discomfort, as well as for signs of fear and anxiety.

Assessment of the patient's status includes observations for involuntary movements: twitching, tremor, seizure, restlessness, rigidity and posturing (decerebrate rigidity or decorticate rigidity).

If a head dressing is used it is examined for security, for moistness suggesting leakage of CSF, and for evidence of bleeding. There may be a drain attached to a gentle negative-pressure system; if so, the amount and type of drainage should be noted as a baseline.

Patient problems   After intracranial surgery, much of the care cited for the patient with increased ICP and for the unconscious patient is applicable, together with care applicable to any patient after operation. Consideration is also given to the following problems:

- The potential for further increased ICP due to the reaction to the trauma imposed by the operation
- Potential for injury (risk of injury due to malpositioning or disorientation)

- Potential for infection due to open wound and lowered resistance
- Hyperthermia secondary to the disturbance of the temperature-regulating centre
- Knowledge deficit – the patient and family require assistance in making necessary adjustments and planning home management.

Goals   The principal patient goal is a safe recovery from surgery, avoiding the potential problems outlined above and the other general problems related to any postoperative patient or person with reduced consciousness.

Nursing intervention

Potential for increased intracranial pressure   All patients experience some increase in ICP following brain surgery because of the oedema and swelling that result from the trauma and inflammation incurred by surgery. Frequent vital signs and neurological evaluations are necessary to recognize significant changes indicating increased ICP.

The head of the bed may be elevated about 30° to promote cerebral venous return unless contraindicated by shock or a specific directive from the surgeon. A small pillow may be necessary under the head to maintain good neck alignment, which promotes cerebral venous return.

The fluid intake is usually restricted to a stated volume, distributed over 24 hours to maintain slight dehydration which reduces extracellular fluid and ICP. Intravenous fluids are infused slowly and monitored closely; rapid infusion could cause a rapid rise in ICP. An osmotic diuretic may be prescribed to dehydrate the brain.

Potential for injury   After intracranial surgery, the patient is at risk of injury from malpositioning. The required position depends on the patient's level of consciousness and the location and nature of the operation.

While unconscious, the patient is positioned to promote cerebral venous return as well as to prevent obstruction of the airway and aspiration of secretions. The limbs are positioned and supported in the normal way for an unconscious patient. The head of the bed may be elevated 25–30° and the head aligned with the spine. The patient with potential or actual increase in ICP is never placed in a head-low or prone position. Flexion or twisting of the head and extreme hip flexion are avoided because this may increase ICP.

The position is changed at regular intervals (e.g. every 2 hours) from side to side to back to side unless contraindicated. If a relatively large space-occupying lesion has been removed, the patient is not permitted to lie on the operative side in order to prevent a shifting of the brain into the remaining space. Following infratentorial surgery, the patient lies on either side using a small pillow under the head to maintain alignment. Keeping the patient off the back for 2–3 days prevents pressure on the incision, as well as possible forward flexion on the incision. A specific directive as to positioning may be given by the surgeon. When repositioned, the patient is turned slowly with adequate support for the head, so that the head and trunk are turned as if they were one unit. Sudden movement and jarring are avoided at all times.

Trauma to the brainstem may depress the gag and swallowing reflexes, predisposing to aspiration. When oral fluids are permitted, only a very small amount is given at first to test the swallowing reflex.

Potential for infection   Following intracranial surgery the risk of **infection** arises from the open wound, from the patient's lowered resistance as a result of the illness and its related stresses, and from the possible administration of a steroid preparation (e.g. dexamethasone). As infectious processes increase the rate of metabolism, waste products such as carbon dioxide and lactic acid are produced in greater amounts. Waste products in increased amounts cause cerebral vasodilatation, which increases intracranial blood volume and pressure. Strict asepsis is essential when the head dressing is changed. The wound is inspected for redness, swelling, offensive odour and drainage; signs of infection are reported promptly and a swab of the wound drainage is taken for culture purposes. Immediate treatment to prevent meningitis, encephalitis or brain abscess is essential; an antibiotic is prescribed.

Hyperthermia   The patient may develop an increased temperature. To counteract this tendency, the room temperature is kept at 18–20°C and only a cotton sheet and bedspread are used as covers. An antipyretic (e.g. acetylsalicylic acid) is prescribed and administered by rectum.

Decreased intellectual function   In some instances, there may be some residual neurological deficit following an intracranial surgical procedure. A rehabilitation programme is planned and instituted as soon as possible with the goal of restoring the patient to independent useful living within his or her potential. This may involve the physiotherapist, speech therapist, occupational therapist and social worker as well as the doctor and nurse. The patient may have to relearn the performance of ordinary daily activities, and progress from the simple to the more complex much as a child learns. It is frequently a slow process and both the patient and family are likely to have periods of depression and discouragement. The nurse assists them in making their plans for home management and the necessary activities and exercises. A referral is made to appropriate support services so that support and guidance are continued.

Rehabilitation: meeting the needs of the head-injured patient   Rehabilitation forms a crucial part of the recovery process. The aim is to maintain and promote function, improve or prevent further deterioration, and also to prevent further complications from occurring. The challenge in this process is to overcome the neurological deficits that can impede progress during the rehabilitation process. These include motor and sensory impairment, communication disability, psychological disability, social disability, and educational or vocational disability.

Not all patients will respond to rehabilitation, or their condition is so severe that rehabilitation is impossible. The patient's needs are assessed by the multidisciplinary team along with the family, with a view to identifying and providing the optimal care and support to achieve an optimal outcome. Often, the patient's role within the family changes. He or she may previously have been the provider within a family, and now have to revert to being dependent on others. For some, a return to work is impossible as their ability to undertake their normal work may be impaired. Some employers provide assisted support to enable such employees to return to different work or reduced hours. Employment difficulties can have long-term financial implications for the family. An alteration to the patient's personality may affect relationships within a family, resulting in much stress and disagreement. Some families will report that the person has completely changed and is now different from the person they knew before. A family support programme to assist families of head-injured survivors is described by Acorn (1995).

Often, repeated explanations of the patient's change in behaviour toward the family are required, as family members find this change distressing. The reaction of the family can range from apparent calm acceptance to rudeness and verbal aggression towards nursing staff. As the time for discharge approaches, many patients and their families are particularly anxious. Much of this anxiety can be allayed if adequate preparation and reassurance are provided, along with an effective plan for discharge. The residual problems that may persist vary widely, ranging from headache to major behavioural changes with or without neurological deficits. The degree of residual difficulty will determine what action is required in the discharge plan. Other influences may include whether the patient requires further surgery or other therapies, necessitating attendance at a hospital or rehabilitation centre. Brief pre-discharge visits home may be considered and will help to identify potential problems.

It is not usually until the patient is at home that the family fully appreciates the difficulties that may be encountered. At this time, maximum support is needed and the District Nurse will play a key role in helping the family care for their relative. Some of the home routine may need to be adjusted and, while this may be easy in the early stages, it becomes more difficult to accept in the long term. Other members of the family often view the disruption to their personal lives negatively and eventually much of the early support gradually disappears. If the patient is still at a stage in which support is required, this withdrawal can be catastrophic. Very often, the patient's partner is left to shoulder the burden alone, and in this situation a support group such as 'Headway' may help (www.headway.org.uk). This organization seeks to provide help and assistance to the patient and family. Regular meetings and other special outings are arranged, along with helpful literature. Relatives can be provided with a forum for discussion of the problems that they face, and many appreciate sharing their problems with others who are similarly placed. Some families have to acknowledge a sense of failure should the patient have to be admitted for institutional care in either the short or long term. They may feel that they have let the patient down and do not like to admit that they are unable to cope.

SPINE AND SPINAL CORD INJURY

Spinal cord injury is a major cause of serious disability, particularly in males aged between 15 and 30 years. Motor vehicle accidents continue to be a major cause of spinal injuries, and frequently alcohol and drugs are involved. Other causes are falls, diving accidents and sports injuries, particularly horse riding and rugby.

Types of injury

A spinal injury may or may not involve injury to the spinal cord. Fracture of one or more vertebrae may occur with no displacement of fragments, resulting in the cord escaping injury. However, rupture of the ligaments holding the vertebrae in alignment may allow displacement of the vertebral column, leading to serious cord injury, even if no fracture occurs. Injury may be the result of:

- sudden forceful angulation of the spine (hyperextension, hyperflexion or hyperextension-hyperflexion) with or without rotational forces
- excessive force applied along the axis of the spine causing burst fractures and vertical compression (e.g. landing on the feet or buttocks from a height)
- a direct blow to the area of the spine.

Effects of spinal injuries

Injuries to the vertebrae may result in spinal cord contusion, laceration and compression. Bleeding into the tissues and oedema occur, causing swelling and compression of nerve tracts. The damage may be slight and completely reversible or it may leave a minor degree of residual impairment. Oedema and bleeding in the cervical cord area is very serious; compression may interrupt innervation of the diaphragm incurring respiratory failure. A laceration that transects the cord or causes severe compression may result in complete, irreversible interruption of ascending or descending tracts. Destruction of the cord resulting in interruption of its tracts is not always due to transection. Injury may incur haemorrhage, circulatory stasis, extravasation of fluid and blood cells, ischaemia and necrosis of the tissue. Interruption of ascending tracts causes loss of sensation below the site of injury. This means that pain, pressure and temperature sensation may be dulled or lost and the patient may be unable to appreciate the position of affected limbs due to interference with proprioception impulse pathways. Interruption of descending tracts results in paralysis of the parts deriving their innervation from the cord below the level of the lesion. Flaccid paralysis and an absence of reflexes occur first and are usually followed by spastic paralysis and exaggerated tendon reflexes. Bladder, bowel and autonomic nervous functions are disturbed.

When the spinal cord is suddenly transected, a phenomenon known as *spinal shock* develops in which all cord functions including involuntary reflex responses are depressed; there is the sudden loss of all motor, sensory, reflex and autonomic responses below the site of cord injury. This occurs due to the sudden interruption of the initiating and regulatory impulses between the higher centres and the cord below the site of injury; that is, impulses are no longer being passed to or from neurones below the lesion. The result is loss of muscular tone (flaccid paralysis), an absence of reflexes and loss of sensation below the lesion. Cord reflexes for voiding and defaecation are suppressed, and retention and overflow incontinence occur. Vasomotor tone is lost and the blood pressure falls. Body temperature control is affected because there is no perspiration below the lesion; hyperthermia may develop. Spinal shock may subside in a few days or may persist for a much longer period. The loss of autonomic impulses and tone in the intestine may cause distension and paralytic ileus. Occasionally, recovery of reflex activity following spinal shock is characterized by hypersensitivity of the spinal neurones; for example, spasticity of the muscles develops and the bladder becomes hypertonic, resulting in diminished capacity and frequent reflex voiding.

The victim with injury to the spine without cord involvement retains motor and sensory functions and complains of pain at the site of the trauma and in parts innervated by that area. Later this may change; bleeding into the tissue and oedema may occur, causing swelling and compression of the cord. Initial management of spine-injured patients is on the basis of preventing potential cord damage.

The spinal cord and its tracts are not capable of regeneration, but regeneration of the nerve roots (outside the cord) can occur if the neurilemma is not severely damaged. Some recovery of function may occur in the first few weeks as oedema subsides and neurones that were compressed but not destroyed resume activity.

The paralysis that occurs with spinal cord injury may be complete or partial (paresis) and may be paraplegia or quadriplegia. If quadriplegia is complete, there may be no voluntary control of function below the neck and very little potential for independence in self-care. With incomplete quadriplegia, voluntary control of selected muscles in the upper limbs may be restored and independence in many areas of self-care may be possible. Respiratory insufficiency or failure is a major concern in quadriplegia as there is usually some involvement of the nerve supply to the diaphragm and intercostal muscles (Fig. 20.20).

Care of the patient with spinal injury

Care of the spine-injured patient involves three phases: the emergency, acute and rehabilitative phases.

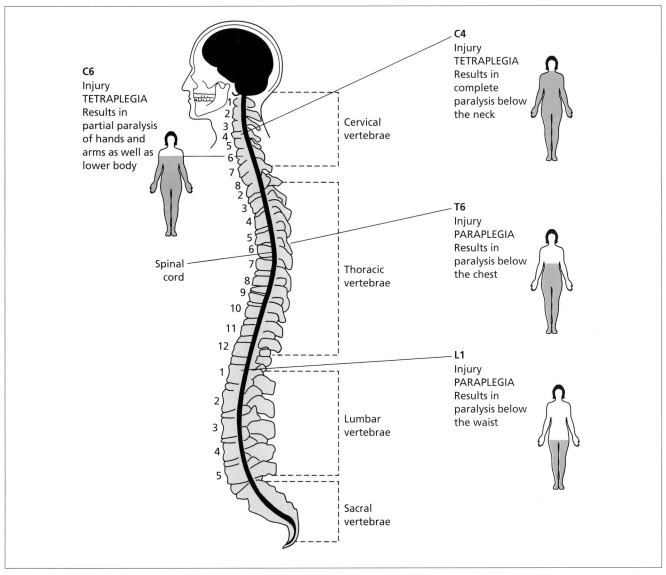

Figure 20.20 Level of injury and extent of paralysis.

Emergency care at the scene of an accident

The principal problem is the potential for further cord damage to occur and the goal is therefore that the patient will suffer no further cord damage.

Intervention Spinal cord injury and permanent disability may be minimized with accurate assessment and appropriate care immediately after the accident. Injury to the spinal cord is suspected if the victim is unable to move any limbs, if numbness or peculiar sensations are present, if there is unexplained shock or if the person is unconscious after a head injury. The victim may also be having difficulty breathing if the injury is cervical. Wounds about the head or shoulders, pain, tenderness or deformity adjacent to the vertebral column also suggest spinal cord injury. If there is doubt regarding the presence of cord injury, the patient should be managed as if one were present.

Usually the spinal-cord-injured victim is conscious. The patient should be kept flat to permit free diaphragmatic breathing and should be advised to keep the head still; neck flexion or side-to-side rotation could seriously aggravate an injured cervical spine. A quick assessment is made for other injuries using the ABCD checklist (Airway, Breathing, Circulation, Disability). Airway obstruction and inadequate ventilation have first priority but, in establishing an airway or in providing assistance, extension of the neck must be avoided. If the patient is unconscious, the modified jaw thrust may be used to open the airway; two fingers are placed at the angle of the lower jaw to lift it forward. With cervical cord injury, the chest wall muscles may be paralysed and entire respiratory function is dependent on the diaphragm; respiratory assistance and suctioning may be necessary.

The patient should not be moved, except for life-saving purposes, until the Ambulance Service is present. Ambulances carry special equipment for moving such patients with the minimum disturbance and paramedics are well trained in the safe handling of such patients. All movements should be smooth and well coordinated. Immobilization of the head and neck using head blocks is carried out. A firm cervical collar or sand bags taped to each side of the head may be used if available.

Care during the acute phase (hospital)
Assessment

1 A brief history of the accident is obtained from the victim or person who was at the site.

2 An immediate assessment is made of the vital signs and continuous monitoring established if necessary.

3 If the patient's condition permits, or a family member is available, a brief review is made of the health history so that significant factors such as allergies, pre-existing disorders and medications being taken are identified.

4 The patient is examined for other injuries and a neurological evaluation is made to identify spinal cord damage. An assessment is made of:
   a) level of consciousness
   b) orientation
   c) motor and sensory functions (e.g. movement of the limbs; levels of sensation)
   d) reflexes (e.g. patellar, abdominal)
   e) condition of the skin – cold or warm, moist or dry all over or above or below a certain level.

5 The patient's understanding of the situation should be ascertained together with his or her feelings.

Patient problems

- Potential for further cord injury
- Anxiety due to fear of paralysis
- Complications of actual cord injury (e.g. spinal shock, respiratory failure, urinary retention or incontinence, pressure sores).

Goals The goals are that no further injury will occur, complications of actual injury will be avoided and the patient will talk about fears and anxieties.

Nursing intervention The treatment of the spine-injured patient depends on:

- whether there is cord injury and neurological deficits or not
- the level of the injury
- the nature of the injury (e.g. fracture fragments compressing the cord, laceration of the cord).

Immediate efforts are directed towards sustaining life and preventing cord damage or, where it has occurred, preventing further injury. The spinal lesion is treated by immobilization of the spine. Realignment of vertebrae and relief of pressure on the cord or spinal roots may be achieved by traction. In some instances, surgery (decompression laminectomy) is undertaken to relieve pressure on the cord, remove vertebral fragments that are hazardous to the cord or to realign dislocated vertebrae that do not respond to traction or hyperextension. The operation may include spinal fusion (Table 20.9) or wiring of the spinous processes to stabilize the spine.

Cervical spine injury Head blocks will be applied as a first-aid measure and should be left in place. When there is a fracture–dislocation with or without neurological deficit, skeletal traction is applied by means of tongs, a halo traction device or a halter.

Tongs are inserted into the skull at approximately the mid-lateral line, a short distance above the ears. The areas are prepared for the insertion by shaving, cleansing and the injection of a local anaesthetic. A very small incision is made in the scalp and small holes are made in the skull with a drill to accommodate the tongs. The scalp may require sutures before a dressing is applied. The sites of insertion of the tongs are inspected daily for signs of infection, the areas are cleansed and an antiseptic spray is applied. Traction of 4.5–13.2 kg may be applied and is achieved by a rope that overlies a pulley; one end is affixed to the tongs and the other hangs free with the prescribed weight attached. The prescribed weight depends on the size of the patient and the amount of displacement. It is usually heavy at first and altered as indicated by radiography or clinical progress, and is reduced as realignment of the vertebrae or fragments occurs.

The patient may be placed on a turning bed (e.g. Egerton electrical turning and tilting bed) that is fitted with a pivoting device; this permits turning without interference to the traction. An ordinary bed with a fracture board, if necessary, beneath the mattress and the headboard removed to allow clearance for traction may be used. The head of the bed is elevated to enable the body to act as countertraction for the weights and to prevent the patient from sliding towards the head of the bed. When realignment of the vertebrae or fragments and sufficient healing are achieved, the patient is fitted with a plastic collar or neck brace to provide cervical immobilization and support, and is gradually ambulated.

The halo traction device involves the application of a metal ring to the head which is secured to the skull by the insertion of four pins (similar to the application of tongs). The sites of insertion into the skull are anterior, posterior and lateral. The ring is firmly anchored to a body cast or special vest by metal rods. This form of cervical immobilization and traction allows the patient to be ambulatory (Fig. 20.21).

If only slight traction is required, a halter-like arrangement may be used in place of the tongs. The halter is arranged to place traction under the chin and occipital area. Prolonged continuous application usually causes considerable discomfort and skin irritation for the patient as a result of the pressure and pull, especially under the chin. Careful monitoring of neurological status and breathing are essential,

Table 20.9 Spinal surgical procedures

Procedure	Conditions in which used
Laminectomy Partial or complete removal of the vertebral arch by the two laminae; precedes other spinal operations to provide access to the canal	Chronic low back pain (disc problems). Spinal fracture (to remove fragments). Cord decompression. Removal of a neoplasm
Discectomy Excision of an intervertebral disc	Ruptured or herniated disc. Chronic low back pain
Spinal fusion Application of bone grafts to two or more adjoining vertebrae to ankylose them	Ruptured or herniated disc. Relief of nerve or cord compression
Rhizotomy Division of transection of a nerve root either outside or within the spinal cord	Chronic pain
Cordotomy Division of the pain-conducting pathways (spinothalamic anterolateral tracts) in the spinal cord Percutaneous cordotomy involves the insertion of a needle (under radiographic guidance) into the spinal cord	Intractable pain (usually associated with malignant disease)

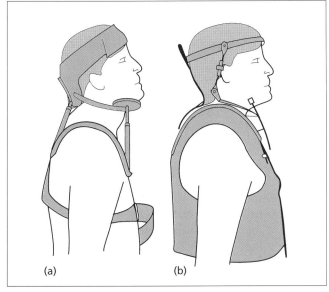

(a) (b)

Figure 20.21 Halo traction as used in cervical vertebral fracture. (a) Four-poster brace. (b) Halo jacket.

together with meticulous pressure care. The patient's personal hygiene is also crucial.

A great deal of psychological support is needed. It is not possible to say in the first few days after injury how much recovery will occur. The nurse should therefore be honest in talking to the patient and family and say it is just too soon to know the extent of possible recovery. A truthful answer is better than avoiding the question or giving false hope to the patient.

Thoracic or lumbar spinal fracture Where there is a fracture of the spine in the thoracic or lumbar region without dislocation and compression of the spinal cord, the patient may be placed flat on a firm mattress on a bed with a firm base, or on a fracture board on an ordinary bed, or on a turning bed for several weeks. If the ordinary bed is used, specific directions are received as to whether the patient must remain on their back at all times. If turning is permitted, precautions are taken to ensure good alignment and avoidance of movement and displacement of the fragments ('log-rolling'). When there is sufficient healing, the patient is gradually ambulated. A brace, plaster jacket or firm corset may be necessary for several months to provide support and immobility of the spine.

A fracture dislocation of thoracic or lumbar vertebrae may be treated by hyperextension of the spine, which may be achieved by various methods. One method is the placing of a firm roll or sandbag across the bed under the mattress to provide the required angulation. Fracture boards are placed on the bed if it has a sprung base, and a very firm mattress is used on which a sponge rubber mattress is placed, because the patient must remain in the supine position.

Long-term care of the patient with spinal cord injury
After the initial stage of admission and stabilization, the patient faces a long road to recovery with the possibility of severe residual disability. Continuous assessment of progress is essential to monitor the effectiveness of care and to detect any of the potential complications of cord injury and immobility. Psychological care is of paramount importance in this period, together with an awareness of how the family might be affected.

Patient problems

- Alteration in breathing pattern – respiratory insufficiency due to interruption of normal innervation of the diaphragm and/or intercostal muscles
- Potential for pressure sores as a result of immobility and impaired tissue perfusion
- Alteration in urinary elimination – retention with overflow or incontinence, due to disturbed innervation
- Alteration in bowel elimination – distension, constipation, incontinence secondary to spinal shock and immobility
- Alteration in food and fluid intake secondary to gastrointestinal distension, anxiety and difficulty in eating caused by immobility and position
- Self-care hygiene deficits due to paralysis and enforced immobility
- Alteration in comfort – pain and spasticity
- Potential for infection
- Potential for muscle contractures, deformities, osteoporosis and thrombophlebitis
- Inability to control body temperature due to dysfunction of the autonomic nervous system
- Disturbance in sleep pattern due to impact of accident, dependency and permanent disability
- Patient and family reactions to change in patient's role, loss of mobility and independence
- Potential for injury due to paralysis, immobility, muscle spasm, loss of sensation
- Sexual dysfunction
- Lack of knowledge and depression due to loss of mobility, independence and roles.

Goals   The patient's goals are to avoid the potential problems listed above and to adapt to altered levels of functioning whilst regaining maximum independence.

Nursing intervention

Respiratory dysfunction   In the acute phase, the patient with cervical or high thoracic cord injury is at risk of respiratory failure, reduced gas exchange and ineffective airway clearance. Initially, diaphragmatic function may appear to be adequate, but during the first 48 hours, oedema develops in the area of the injury. Its progress in the patient with a cervical injury may compromise vital centres in the medulla; respiratory failure develops as well as hypotension and weakening of the pulse. Chest trauma or pre-existing respiratory disease seriously complicates respiratory function.

Endotracheal intubation or a tracheostomy and oxygen administration may be necessary. If ventilatory muscle function is not adequate to maintain blood gas levels, mechanical respiratory assistance is provided. Chest physiotherapy and increased humidity of inspired air and oxygen are provided to mobilize the secretions.

When the patient recovers sufficiently and the blood gas analyses indicate satisfactory levels, mechanical respiratory assistance is discontinued and a regimen of deep breathing and coughing is established.

The patient continues to be at risk of respiratory insufficiency and complications in the postacute phase. Abdominal muscle function may be weak or lacking, and, as a result, the cough is weak in the paraplegic and absent in the quadriplegic patient. Suction equipment should be readily available and intensive physiotherapy provided to help the patient develop an effective cough if possible, as well as to mobilize secretions. During the period during which they must remain flat while the spine heals and stabilizes, spinal-cord-injured patients are predisposed to bronchopneumonia and atelectasis.

Potential for pressure sores   The changes in vasomotor tone and the resulting impairment of tissue perfusion, the enforced immobility and the loss of cutaneous sensation contribute to tissue breakdown. If a pressure sores occur, healing is difficult in patients with spinal cord injury and rehabilitation is delayed.

The patient needs to understand the importance of keeping the skin intact and his or her role in maintaining its integrity. After the period of immobilization to stabilize the spine, as the patient begins to assume the self-care within his or her potential, the importance of shifting of pressure is explained and the patient is taught how to change position at frequent regular intervals in bed and in a wheelchair. The patient is taught to inspect the vulnerable areas at least once daily using a mirror.

Most patients with paraplegia or quadriplegia are eventually mobilized by lightweight wheelchairs. The patient is taught to transfer from bed to chair and from chair to toilet, and that at regular intervals the body weight must be shifted. The patient learns to lift the trunk by pushing with the arms and hands on the chair arms or seat in order to relieve constant pressure on the buttocks and sacral region.

Alteration in urinary elimination   During the spinal shock, the bladder is atonic and there is retention of urine with overflow. The stasis of urine predisposes to infection and the distension may cause fissures or areas of pressure necrosis in the bladder wall. Ureteral openings are dilated, allowing reflux of urine into the kidneys. An indwelling catheter or intermittent catheterization is introduced soon after admission to prevent overdistension of the atonic bladder. The prevention of incontinence also assists in protecting the skin from irritation and breakdown. If continuous catheter drainage is required, a sterile closed-drainage system is used; precautions must be strictly observed to prevent infection. Renal complications (e.g. pyelonephritis) leading to renal failure are a major cause of death in cord-injured persons. The atony of the bladder remains for a varying length of time before hyperreflexia takes over and the bladder becomes hypertonic, resulting in frequent automatic emptying of small volumes. To counteract the hypertonicity and diminished bladder capacity, an indwelling catheter is used or, if intermittent catheterization is used, the intervals are gradually increased. Catheter use is discontinued as soon as possible because of the risk of infection and a bladder training programme is initiated. The reflex emptying of the bladder and incontinence are very distressing to the patient, who may resist an adequate fluid intake with the thought that it may at least lessen the frequency of involuntary voiding. This is dangerous because it predisposes to infection and the formation of calculi. Some patients become dependent on catheter use on a permanent basis, and may have to be taught intermittent self-catheterization.

Ideally, a bladder training programme should be introduced as soon as possible to avoid dependency on a catheter. The patient is taught to initiate the reflexive emptying of the bladder by the Credé manoeuvre or the Valsalva manoeuvre. With some patients, stretching of the anal sphincter by the insertion of a gloved finger into the anal canal in combination with the Valsalva manoeuvre is more effective. The bladder may not empty completely and stasis of urine predisposes to infection. Periodic catheterization may be done to determine residual volume; less than 75–100 mL is usually acceptable. A specimen of urine is submitted for analysis at regular intervals and also if the urine has an offensive odour, is cloudy or there is blood or sediment.

Alteration in bowel elimination   With spinal shock, the gastrointestinal tract becomes atonic; severe distension and vomiting without effort may develop. Gastrointestinal aspiration via a nasogastric tube may become necessary until peristalsis is re-established; abdominal distension causes respiratory embarrassment by pressure on the diaphragm.

The spinal cord injury interrupts impulses from the higher centres of awareness and control. The sensation of the need to defaecate is lost and the rectal and anal sphincters function reflexly (automatic spinal cord response). Because of the immobility and dietary changes the patient experiences constipation, and impaction develops readily. When bowel sounds are present, a mild laxative or suppository (glycerine or bisacodyl) may be used to evacuate the bowel at first, then, as the patient's condition improves and a more normal diet is taken, involuntary defaecation occurs. A diet high in fibre is usually necessary to prevent constipation. The diet is adjusted to the stool consistency and frequency. As soon as the patient is able to sit in a chair, training for bowel elimination by conditioned reflex begins. A regular hour for bowel elimination may be established; the morning is the normal time for most patients. The procedure involves a warm beverage, followed in 30 minutes by the insertion of a glycerine or bisacodyl (Dulcolax) suppository and stimulation by inserting a lubricated gloved finger every 10–15 minutes until defaecation occurs. Once a pattern of regular reflex evacuation has been established, the patient may find that digital stimulation alone or the use of a device to massage the anal canal may be effective.

The patient is assisted to a commode or toilet at the same time each day or every other day. Privacy should be provided. A member of the patient's family or carer should be involved in the bowel training programme as part of the preparation for home management.

Alteration in food and fluid intake   During the initial phase, oral food and fluid are withheld. Some degree of paralytic ileus develops in most spinal-cord-injured patients due to spinal shock. Fluids are administered by intravenous infusion to maintain hydration. A nasogastric tube may be inserted and aspiration established to relieve gastric and intestinal dilatation. When peristalsis is re-established, fluids are administered orally and, if tolerated, solid foods are added. A high-calorie, high-protein diet is important to combat the tendency toward a negative nitrogen balance which is commonly associated with immobility. An adequate nutritional intake also plays a role in promoting tissue healing and resistance to breakdown (e.g. pressure sores) and provides energy for exercises and the rehabilitative programme. Adequate dietary intake is made more difficult by the patient's positioning. Dietary supplements between meals may be necessary. Later, calorie intake may have to be reduced to prevent obesity, which complicates rehabilitation and increases the risk of complications. Bulk and roughage are necessary in the diet to promote bowel elimination.

Calcium intake (milk and milk products) may be restricted to prevent urinary calculi which may develop as calcium moves out of immobilized bones. A fluid intake of at least 3000 mL a day is encouraged to prevent concentration and stasis of urine. Grape and apple juices are preferable to citrus fruit juices; they produce an acid urine which reduces the precipitation of calcium and the formation of calculi as well as reducing the risk of infection. Organisms are less likely to grow in an acid environment.

Some cord-injured patients develop stress ulcers (gastric or duodenal). The aetiology has yet to be fully determined; hyperacidity due to histamine release following the trauma, or mucosal ischaemia, are among the leading theories at present. Ranitidine may be prescribed as a prophylactic measure.

Food must be placed readily within reach and the patient encouraged to feed unaided as soon as the condition permits. Initially those with quadriplegia will require assistance with feeding until appropriate assistive devices are available. Swallowing may be difficult in the recumbent position and inhalation may occur. The patient is encouraged to take only small amounts at a time and swallow frequently. Suction equipment should be readily available in the event of inhalation.

If the partial quadriplegic patient has motor function in the triceps and biceps muscles, self-feeding may be accomplished. With flexion at the elbow and the fitting over the hand of a wide elastic band with a pocket, self-feeding may be achieved. Special utensils such as a spoon fit into the pocket.

Self-care hygiene deficits   The patient will become increasingly aware of limitations and dependency; personal care must be provided with sensitivity to the patient's feelings. It is difficult to convince the patient in the early stages that it is possible that considerable independence will eventually be regained.

In order to regain even minimal independence in self-care, the individual must be able to move about and be able to have some grasp in at least one hand. Paraplegic persons do have the distinct advantage of having the use of both hands and are capable of achieving self-care. The quadriplegic is dependent on head movements, assistive devices and care provided by others.

Alteration in comfort   The patient with a spinal cord injury may experience pain that radiates along the spinal nerves that originate at the level of injury. Spasticity of the muscles below the level of the cord injury is also a source of severe discomfort in paraplegia and quadriplegia, and may lead to contractures and deformities. The pain is severe and fatiguing and may be embarrassing at times for the patient. It may retard rehabilitation. The muscle spasms are hypersensitive reflexes that develop after spinal shock subsides. The stimulus may not even be obvious. Examples of stimuli that may initiate the spastic response include light touching of the skin, jarring of the bed, turning, cold, fatigue, a distended bladder and emotional reactions. Regular passive moving of the limbs through their range of motion is beneficial, especially when done under water. Rarely, severe painful spasticity is treated by surgery; various procedures have been used, including severing of tendons, transection of a nerve root (rhizotomy) and neurotomy (cutting of nerves).

Opioid analgesics are not used with the patient with high cervical injury because of the depressing effect on respiration.

Potential for infection   There is a risk of urinary and respiratory tract infections as discussed earlier in this chapter. Nursing interventions can minimize these risks.

Potential for complications   Complications include muscle contractures, deformities, osteoporosis and thrombophlebitis.

Patients with spinal cord injury and the resulting paralysis develop muscle and tendon contractures and ankylosis of the joints unless preventive measures are observed. The shortening of the muscles and tendons may cause serious deformities that restrict rehabilitation. For example, a flexure contracture of the thigh at the hip joint may inhibit the patient's use of a wheelchair. Wrist drop and foot drop develop readily in paralysed limbs unless preventive measures are instituted. Immobility, muscle spasticity and poor alignment in positioning the patient are contributing factors. Preventive measures include frequent change of position and maintenance of good body alignment using sand bags, and pillows if necessary, regular passive range-of-movement exercises and a physiotherapy programme as soon as the patient's condition permits.

The health of bones normally depends on stress due to muscle pull and weight-bearing. When these are lacking, as with paralysis and prolonged immobilization, bone demin-

eralization and osteoporosis occurs. Therefore, weight-bearing is started as soon as possible to stimulate osteoblastic activity and prevent demineralization. The head of the bed is gradually elevated as tolerated and, when safe, the patient is positioned upright on a tilt table. Weight-bearing for at least a few minutes each day may also help to prevent contractures, particularly in the hips.

Regardless of intervention, eventually atrophy of paralysed muscles does occur to some degree. This is due primarily to absence of nerve impulses to the muscle.

Thrombophlebitis is a common problem in a paralysed patient, particularly in the first 3 months following injury. Absence of the pumping action of contracting muscle and poor skeletal muscle tone which results from paralysis and immobility leads to pooling of blood in the lower viscera and extremities and a reduced venous return. This predisposes to thrombophlebitis. Localized oedema, redness, warmth, tenderness and red streaks of an extremity suggest thrombophlebitis. Deep venous thrombosis may also occur.

Because of loss of sensation, pain and tenderness are not perceived. Assessment for venous thrombosis, done daily, includes calf observation, gentle palpation for calf firmness and measurement of the circumference of the thigh and calf. The tape measure is placed at the same level above and below the knee each time.

Management to prevent thrombosis includes a regular schedule of range of movement and exercises (these activities act as a mechanical pump to increase circulation), frequent change of position, elevation of the legs 15° for stated periods and the wearing of antiembolic stockings while in bed. Subcutaneous heparin, 5000 units twice daily, is often prescribed for the first 3 months following paraplegia.

Inability to control body temperature   This is a common problem for patients with a spinal cord injury. Dysfunction of the autonomic nervous system occurs and there is decreased ability to lose or conserve heat in the paralysed parts of the body. Room temperature is controlled to meet the patient's need because he or she is mainly dependent on environmental temperature for the avoidance of hypothermia.

Disturbance in sleep pattern   This is a common problem as a result of the psychological impact of the traumatic event and enforced immobility and dependency. The cord-injured patient may experience frightening dreams in which the accident is relived. Discomfort and the necessary frequent repositioning as well as a high level of anxiety may disrupt the patient's sleep.

Lack of adequate rest and **sleep** depletes the person's energy and endurance, which are essential for healing and rehabilitation.

Nursing care involves the provision of a quiet environment, comfort measures such as position change, warm drinks and remaining with the patient, encouraging the discussion of anxieties and feelings and to provide reassurance that he or she is not alone. Regular rest periods are scheduled to prevent exhaustion.

Sexual dysfunction The potential for sexual fulfilment is a major concern of the patient with permanent disability. Some patients may express this concern directly but more often concern is present long before it is expressed. If the patient brings up the topic of sexuality, a free and open discussion should be encouraged.

The cord-injured patient needs to know that meaningful and satisfying relationships are still attainable and that, even though he or she may no longer be able to function sexually in the same ways as before the injury, new ways of giving and receiving sexual satisfaction can be learned. The patient needs to understand that the sexuality of an individual involves the total person and that self-image is an important dimension in the resocialization process in disability.

The question of fertility and ability to procreate may also be raised by patients with a spinal cord injury. Male infertility is not uncommon following a cord injury because of testicular atrophy, decreased production of sperm and infrequency of ejaculation. The female with cord injury is usually able to conceive and deliver a child with few adaptations being necessary. As there is a vast body of knowledge specific to sexuality in disability, it is appropriate to discuss other resources of information with the patient. Referral to a qualified counsellor or agency may be advisable.

Patient and family reactions Spinal injury that results in paralysis is a very traumatic psychological experience. Suddenly, the victim is changed from an independent person to one who is dependent on others for even very personal care. Responses and adjustment to the loss of body functions usually parallel the grief reaction, with feelings of anger and despair mixing with frustration and depression.

Initially, shock and denial of reality help the victim to maintain self-control and survive. Consistent, high-quality nursing care is supportive in this phase. Gradually, as awareness develops, the patient may respond with anger and resentment. The nurse needs to listen and try to understand the patient's responses; support at this time may help to strengthen the patient's tenuous grasp of reality.

Anger may be followed by a period of despair and depression in which the patient may eat or drink very little and does not manifest any interest in rehabilitation, family or others. Close observation of reactions and comments indicate to the nurse when to encourage conversation or when presence alone is preferable to the patient. The patient may raise questions that relate to concerns such as independence, financial support and sexuality in the future. Anxiety may escalate in proportion to the unknown; anxiety depletes energy and tends to distort reality. The patient should be assured that everything possible will be done to help regain the ability to do some things unaided. Reassurance should be realistic; offering false hope must be avoided.

It will be some time before the patient begins to see things realistically and explore possibilities for the future. In this reorganization phase, learning to cope with body changes predominates. Assimilation of the changes in body image and pattern of life takes considerable time; periods of withdrawal and depression are to be expected from time to time. Such reactions should be accepted as being part of the process that the patient is going through. Thinking is directed to the positive, and as soon as possible the patient is encouraged and expected to do the things that the functional motor capacity allows. The acknowledgement of improvement and achievement helps to sustain motivation. The development of a sense of worthiness and self-esteem essential for resocialization depend greatly on the positive attitude, appreciation and reliance conveyed by professionals and significant others.

The victim's injury and the possible implications of disability are difficult for family members to accept. As well as concern for the patient, the situation may involve a complete change of lifestyle for them. They may be faced with financial hardships and a disruption of home management. Role functions change, responsibilities are shifted, and plans and goals may be shattered.

Family bonds may become greater as family members face the situation together; new strengths, capabilities and determination to cope with their problems may be revealed. In other instances, the reaction of some family members after the patient's acute phase may be resentment for the individual whose accident has altered their life. The patient can be rejected and feelings of loneliness, fear and depression are increased. There may also be profound feelings of guilt if a family member was in some way responsible for the original accident.

The nurse takes time to talk with the family; they are kept informed of the patient's progress and of the therapeutic and rehabilitative programmes. Their role in supporting the patient is discussed. Time is given to discussing family problems and suggestions are made that assist them in planning and resolution.

Family and friends are encouraged to spend time with the patient to provide support and reinforce the impression that they are not rejecting the patient as useless. Encouraging and letting the patient do things unaided are emphasized. A major multidisciplinary effort will be needed to provide the long-term community care the patient needs.

Potential for injury Limited sensation in the paralysed parts, limited mobility, muscle spasm and dependency place the paralysed patient at risk of injury and complications. It is necessary for the patient to develop the necessary strength in the unaffected parts to mobilize and control the affected parts in order to prevent complications incurred by immobilization and falls. The bones in paralyzed limbs are easily fractured as a result of osteoporosis. A waist strap is used while the patient is in a chair until he or she is strong enough to control the trunk. Consistent use of wheelchair brakes during transfers is essential for safety.

Any local heat application is used judiciously; loss of cutaneous sensation predisposes to burns. The skin is inspected daily for abrasions, bruises, pressure ischaemia and irritated areas.

Rehabilitation As soon as the patient is well enough, an active rehabilitation programme is planned and instituted. The patient and family participate in the planning and scheduling of the programme to meet their knowledge needs and adjustments. Family members should be involved in order to support the patient and maintain consistent care. Rehabilitation begins with simple self-care activities, progressing to more complex activities as skill is achieved. Planned periods of rest and diversion are necessary to offset intensive exercises and prevent exhaustion. The family is cautioned against fostering dependence by doing things that the patient has the capacity to do or learn to do alone.

A major component of rehabilitation concerns work. Some patients may be able to manage to return to their previous employment, but many will not. Re-training may be possible and every effort should be made to allow the patient to regain meaningful employment as this will be beneficial to morale, self-concept, and also the patient's finances.

CASE Andrew is a 37-year-old married construction worker who was at work on a building site 5 days previously, when he experienced pain in his lower back radiating down his left leg whilst lifting a concrete slab. Over the past 5 days despite analgesia, he has experienced increasing back pain, 'pins and needles' sensation in both legs and progressive numbness to his sacral area.

He attended the A&E department, after being referred by his GP, with increasing immobility, and an inability to pass urine since the night before. On examination, his vital signs revealed a heart rate of 100 bpm and a blood pressure of 170/82 mmHg; he was apyrexial and had a respiratory rate of 20. A neurological assessment showed severe weakness of his left leg and mild weakness of his right leg. He had reduced anal tone and an examination of his abdomen showed he was in retention of urine.

The combination of pain, limb weakness and urinary retention suggests a serious illness affecting the spinal nerves.

What immediate care would this patient require?

Your care should include insertion of a urinary catheter and accurate fluid balance. How rapidly would you drain his bladder and why might you do it in stages rather than all at once? (See Ch. 19.) Monitoring of limb power, movement and sacral sensation (including bowel activity) are essential. The patient may be required to be nursed on a special spinal bed until the cause of spinal cord pressure can be determined and treated. This may also mean that the patient may need to be log-rolled to assure spinal alignment.

Adequate analgesia is essential. The patient should also be commenced on a bowel regime as soon as possible. He will probably be distressed and anxious therefore psychological support is essential. You must also keep his wife fully informed and offer her support. Rehearse how you would explain what is probably wrong with him to his wife. It is likely that Andrew is experiencing spinal cord compression related to trauma. The sudden onset makes a tumour unlikely.

Nursing the patient treated by spinal surgery
Spinal surgery may be performed to: remove a neoplasm, a herniated or ruptured disc or bony fragments following an injury; reduce a fractured vertebra; decompress the spinal cord following an injury; relieve intractable pain or spasticity; or suppress involuntary movements.

The care following spinal surgery varies with the operation, the patient's response to it and the surgeon's preferences. For example, some patients are immobilized for weeks, whereas others are ambulated a day or two after the procedure. An understanding of what was done and specific directives are necessary in planning care, especially in relation to positioning and movement. The major principles to be observed with all patients in moving and positioning are the maintenance of proper spinal alignment, the avoidance of any twisting, angulation and jerky movements of the spine and the prevention of strain on the back muscles.

Assessment The patient's vital signs and responses are recorded as a baseline against which any changes in condition will become apparent.

When the surgery is below the thoracic region, assessment includes an evaluation of sensation and motor ability in the lower limbs. The colour and temperature of the limbs and leg and foot pulses may be checked as vascular problems may develop. If the operation was cervical or high thoracic, close observation of the person's respiratory pattern is necessary as well as sensorimotor responses of the arms. Hoarseness of the voice and ineffective cough may develop as a result of injury to the recurrent laryngeal nerve.

Wound area(s) are checked for possible haemorrhage, leakage of CSF and contamination. The patient's sensation of pain should be carefully assessed, together with the standard postoperative parameters of urine output, wound drainage, skin condition, etc.

Patient problems
- Potential for spinal injury – even slight angulation or tension or jerky movements may injure the spine and cause nerve or cord damage
- Potential for respiratory insufficiency due to cord and nerve compression in cervical spinal surgery, immobility and shallow respirations because of the pain
- Pain due to oedema in the operative area, irritation and trauma of nerves at the time of operation and muscle spasm
- Alteration in elimination pattern – retention of urine, paralytic ileus, constipation
- Potential for wound haemorrhage or infection
- Alteration in food and fluid intake
- Potential impairment of skin integrity due to immobility and later due to the wearing of a brace or corset

- Impairment of mobility – enforced immobility and maintenance of spinal alignment
- Lack of knowledge – information is required to prevent recurrence of the back problem, and assistance is needed in planning the necessary adjustments in the resumption of activity and management at home.

Goals Patient goals are similar to those set in the post-operative care of any general surgical patient. In addition, the patient should not suffer any complications related specifically to the spinal surgery.

Nursing intervention The patient should be nursed in accordance with the same principles as a general surgical patient but also taking into account the nursing interventions specifically designed to deal with spinal problems, which were discussed earlier in this section.

THE PERSON WITH A NEOPLASM OF THE NERVOUS SYSTEM

INTRACRANIAL NEOPLASMS

Intracranial tumours may be primary or secondary (metastatic), and may occur at any age and in any part of the brain.

- *Primary* neoplasms may be benign or malignant and commonly arise from the neuroglial tissue, meninges, cerebral blood vessels, hypophysis and nerve fibres, and are named according to their tissue origin (Table 20.10). Most primary intracranial tumours are gliomas. Unlike neoplasms elsewhere in the body, primary neoplasms of the brain rarely metastasize
- *Secondary* intracranial tumours commonly originate in the lungs or breast.

Brain tumours vary in size, location and pattern of growth. The glioblastomas are highly malignant and invasive, whereas others, such as the meningiomas, are generally benign and compressive. This accounts for the great variability in the development of symptoms and in the prognosis after operation. Most brain tumours in the adult tend to occur in the supratentorial compartment (above the brainstem and cerebellum).

Effects on the patient

Any intracranial neoplasm is a space-occupying lesion; as it grows, intracranial content and pressure increase within the rigid cranium. The effects of rising intracranial pressure (ICP) have already been discussed. The manifestations reflect the location: neurological deficits (sensory and/or motor) and behavioural changes appear as the tumour involves specific cerebral areas, some deficiency in mental capacity may develop and seizures may occur due to alterations in the electrical potential of cells. Hydrocephalus may develop if there is interference of the normal flow and absorption of CSF, and endocrine imbalances may occur associated with the compression or invasion of the pituitary gland.

Medical management

Investigation will involve the use of imaging techniques such as CT and MRI. Both will localize and usually identify the lesion. Contrast enhancement may be used in conjunction with CT.

Additional investigations may be indicated depending on the type of tumour. These will include endocrine studies, audiometric testing, visual field testing, chest radiography and determination of the erythrocyte sedimentation rate.

For some patients, a burr-hole biopsy may be indicated. A small piece of the tumour tissue is removed for pathological examination. The success of this technique relies greatly on the skill of the operator removing a specimen of tissue that reflects the true extent and pathology of the lesion.

Nursing the patient with a brain tumour

Caring for the person with a brain tumour can be a difficult and challenging situation for the nurse and the patient's family. The continuum of care can be divided into the care required before and during confirmation of the diagnosis, during treatment and, where applicable, during palliation.

Assessment

An initial evaluation is made and recorded of the patient's motor and sensory functions, speech ability, orientation, behavioural responses, pupillary reactions and any complaints of headache, dizziness, and tingling or numbness. It is important to obtain information about the patient's normal behaviour before the development of the tumour. Assessment is an ongoing process through successive contacts so that changes and newly developed symptoms may be recognized promptly. The nurse's recognition and recording of physical and behavioural changes may play an important role in the diagnosis and localization of the intracranial tumour. Knowing that a space-occupying lesion is suspect, the nurse is especially alert for signs of increasing intracranial pressure. It is crucial to discuss the patient's and family's understanding of the condition in order to plan how they may be assisted and supported. Anxieties and fears, together with the patient's level of knowledge and any coping mechanisms being employed, should all be ascertained.

Patient problems

The patient faces the whole range of potential problems associated with immobility and raised ICP (see preceding sections). In addition there is the very real fear of death itself – understandably leading to severe anxiety and depression as well as seriously stressing family networks.

Goals

Patient goals revolve around avoiding the complications of immobility and raised ICP in general, and specifically in adapting to the fact that the illness may prove fatal.

Nursing intervention

Awaiting results from investigations is an extremely anxious and worrying time for the patient and their relatives. It is important that the nurse establishes the basis of the patient's understanding of these fears and anxieties, and provides

Table 20.10 Classification of brain tumours

Tumour	Origin	Usual sites	Incidence of total (%)	Comments
Tumours of epithelial origin				
Astrocytoma grade I	Astrocytes	Frontal lobes followed by temporal and parietal lobes	} 10	Well-differentiated, insidiously invasive, relatively benign
Intermediate astrocytoma grade II and III	Astrocytes	As above		Less well-differentiated than grade I
Glioblastoma multiforme grade IV	Undifferentiated glial cells	As above	18	Rapidly growing, highly malignant. Extensively invasive
Oligodendroglioma	Oligodendrocytes	Cerebral hemispheres	4	Rare, slow growing
Ependymoma	Ependymal cells of the ventricles and aqueducts	Fourth ventricle but could be in other areas	5	Rare, undifferentiated, slow growing. Seen in childhood and young adulthood
Optic nerve glioma	Cells of the optic nerve	Optic nerve and chiasma	4	Occurs in young adulthood
Medulloblastoma	Undifferentiated glial cells	Cerebellum and roof of fourth ventricle	3	Rapidly growing, malignant tumour of childhood. Development of hydrocephalus is common
Tumours of nerve sheath cells				
Schwannoma	Schwann cells	Cranial nerves VIII, V, and VII within the cerebellopontine angle	} 10	Well encapsulated, slow growing, benign. Complex familial disorder
Neuroma	Schwann cells	Neurilemma of nerves, e.g. VIII cranial nerve		Occurs in young adulthood
Tumours of meningeal and related tissue				
Meningioma	Meninges	Intracranial venous sinuses	15	Benign. Slow growing. Predilection for females

continued

Table 20.10 *Cont'd*

Tumour	Origin	Usual sites	Incidence of total (%)	Comments
Tumours of blood vessel origin				
Haemangioblastoma	Blood vessels	Cerebellar hemisphere	2	Slow growing. May be multiple. May be familial
Germ cell tumour				
Teratoma	Pineal parenchymal cells	Pineal gland		Rare childhood tumour
Malformative tumours				
Craniopharyngioma	Embryological remnants	Rathke's pouch	3	
Dermoid cyst	Ectodermal	Posterior fossa		Fluid-filled cyst containing some solid material (e.g. hair)
Colloid cyst of the third ventricle	Choroid plexus	Third ventricle		Rounded cystic tumour
Vascular malformations				
Angiomas	Blood vessels	Cerebral cortex		Arterial and/or venous anomaly comprising enlarged and tortuous vessels
Angioblastoma	Angioblasts	Cerebellum		
Pituitary tumours				
Pituitary adenoma	Cells of the pituitary	Anterior lobe of the pituitary gland	8	Benign, slow growing and well encapsulated. Classified by clinical syndrome, e.g. prolactin secreting (prolactinoma); excess growth hormone (acromegaly); ACTH-secreting (Cushing's disease)
Metastatic tumours				
Metastatic tumour		Can occur anywhere in cerebrum or cerebellum	12	Well-defined; usually multiple secondaries from breast or lung

information and support when appropriate. Having information and understanding empowers the patient and family and enhances their coping.

Assessment should include observation for increasing ICP (see section on Head injuries, p. 689) and the increased likelihood of seizures. The occurrence of raised ICP and/or seizures are the events most likely to be troublesome for the patient. Each will produce potentially distressing symptoms for the patient such as severe headache, vomiting and other neurological deficits along with the anxiety and distress associated with seizures. Each patient's experience will vary according to the size, location and type of tumour, and for many in the initial stages life will continue almost as normal.

A range of interventions is available for treatment, and nursing management will depend on those selected. These may include steroids, surgery and radiotherapy.

Steroids Steroids are often prescribed once a tumour is suspected, and routinely on diagnosis. Dexamethasone is the most common choice. It reduces swelling around the tumour, decreasing the overall mass of the brain and there-

fore ICP. The effect is rapid and the patient can feel better within 24 hours, experiencing relief from headache, nausea and vomiting, and from the improvement of neurological deficits. However, the side-effects of steroids are well known (such as gastric irritation, diabetes and adrenal insufficiency) and should be checked for regularly.

Surgery Biopsy, partial removal of the tumour with internal decompression, and complete removal are the surgical options. The appropriate approach is determined by the nature of the tumour and its site. In many instances, this will constitute major neurosurgery entailing a lengthy operation and subsequent intensive nursing care. Table 20.11 has further details.

Radiotherapy Treatment may involve irradiation, either on its own or as an adjunct to surgery.

A tumour may be inoperable owing to inaccessibility or because of its type and size. It could be that surgery would involve great risk of postoperative neurological deficits. The patient's condition may be very poor and the doctor may advise the family that the condition will not improve. It then becomes necessary to reconsider the plan of care with a

Table 20.11 Care plan for patient undergoing neurosurgery

Area care	Nursing interventions	Rationale
Preoperative phase		
Physical preparation for operation	Ensure preoperative investigations are complete including appropriate blood tests. Full physical nursing assessment. Immediate preoperative checklist prior to surgery complete	Ensuring that the patient is in an optimal physical condition for surgery will reduce postoperative risks
Psychological preparation for operation	Assess patient's understanding of operation. Evaluate extent of patient's anxiety and coping mechanism in relation to undergoing surgery. Evaluate concerns that family may have. Identify and implement appropriate interventions to alleviate anxieties including the use of a preoperative teaching plan	Reduction of patient anxiety and concerns of the family will result in better recovery
Immediate and early postoperative stage		
Respiratory care	Implement interventions to avoid ineffective airway clearance including a full respiratory assessment and use of appropriate interventions such as oxygenation and suctioning. Some patients will be ventilated requiring additional care	Achievement of a patent airway and adequate ventilation will ensure optimal oxygenation of the brain thus improving outcome from surgery
Neurological status	Monitor conscious level and other neurological parameters for signs of deterioration indicating a rise in ICP. Implement measures to avoid exacerbating rises in ICP due to noxious stimuli. Assess risk of injury due to loss of consciousness or seizure activity	Early detection of complications will enable appropriate interventions to be applied to minimize risk of ill-effects
Pain	Assess for signs and symptoms of pain and initiate interventions to alleviate	Ensuring that the patient is pain free will result in comfort and reduction of anxiety
Fluid balance	Assess fluid intake and output. Administer fluids as per prescription	Achievement of the prescribed fluid balance will avoid development of cerebral oedema
Elimination	Monitor urinary output hourly. Administer catheter care (if appropriate). Avoid constipation	Ensuring optimal fluid balance will avoid development of cerebral oedema

change in emphasis from active treatment to eventual palliation.

THE PERSON WITH A DEGENERATIVE DISORDER

Commonly occurring degenerative disorders of the nervous system include Alzheimer's disease, multiple sclerosis, Parkinson's disease, myasthenia gravis and motor neurone disease. In addition, patients with AIDS will also suffer chronic neurological disease.

The diagnosis of a chronic neurological problem can affect a patient's self-esteem and feeling of confidence, as well as generating fear for the future. These feelings can be manifested as symptoms of anger, denial, powerlessness and depression. The nurse, especially in caring for the family and the patient in the community, has to be aware of the difficulties in adaptation the patient may have at any given time. There are periods of stability, both emotional and physical, together with periods of increased stress when the illness exacerbates.

An explanation of the disorder and the prescribed therapy is made to the patient and family. Opportunities are provided for discussions in which they can ask questions and express their feelings and concerns. They are assisted in planning how to maintain a satisfactory lifestyle, role functions and socialization. The patient is encouraged to be independent and carry out self-care activities. Those around are advised that the patient's intellectual ability is unimpaired; it should be emphasized that he or she needs to be treated normally, to socialize and to do things unaided even though it may take much longer. The environment should be cheerful and free of haste and confusion.

The general *goals* of the patient and family in cases of degenerative neurological disorder are that they will:

1 have knowledge of the disease process and potential complications
2 have knowledge of the healthcare system and available support systems
3 be aware of interventions that maintain optimal functioning.

AIDS
The brain, spinal cord and peripheral nerves are all commonly involved in HIV infection, either as a direct result of the HIV or the depletion of the CD4 cells which occurs (see p. 000). The person may present with a neurological infection such as meningitis, neuropathy or the symptoms of a space occupying lesion. Alternatively, the symptoms may be very similar to those seen in a range of mental illnesses (Haslett et al 2002). Opportunistic infections of the brain include viral infections such as cytomegalovirus, herpes simplex, adenovirus, varicella zoster virus and papovavirus. The most common bacterial infections include cryptococcosis

and toxoplasmosis, which respond well to drug therapy, but this must be continued for the patient's lifetime.

The most frequent problem affecting the spinal cord is a condition known as *vascular myelopathy*, a degenerative condition that presents as difficulty walking, numbness in the feet and paraplegia. There is currently no treatment for this condition.

HIV can also directly invade brain tissue, resulting in a condition known as *AIDS dementia complex* (ADC) or AIDS encephalopathy. ADC has an insidious onset, with impairment in memory and concentration and subtle changes in personality being early signs. The condition may advance to motor difficulties, with ataxia being present, or to psychiatric manifestations such as psychosis or hallucinations. The patient often becomes depressed, resulting in social withdrawal and apathy. It is often difficult to differentiate between psychological symptoms of the illness and neurological changes.

Early and ongoing nursing assessment of neurological change is crucial. Questions relating to memory, concentration, orientation and judgement need to be asked in a safe, non-threatening environment. Safety issues must be continually examined, with the patients often requiring orientation cues and written instruction. Eyesight may be impaired by cytomegalovirus retinitis.

Alzheimer's disease
Alzheimer's disease is a presenile dementia of unknown aetiology and is the most common degenerative brain disorder. A history of familial incidence is considered to play a role in the development of the disease, which is incurable at present. The age of onset is between 45 and 65 years. Both males and females are equally affected. The frontal and temporal lobes are most affected but gradual progressive atrophy of the entire brain occurs. Microscopically, there is widespread loss of nerve cells.

Effects on the patient
In the progress of the disease, three stages may be identified. The *first stage* lasts for 2–4 years and is characterized by subtle changes which may be dismissed as inattention or carelessness. Eventually, there are recognizable changes in personality, loss of memory for recent and remote events, apathy, loss of spontaneity and initiative, neglect of personal hygiene and appearance, and a suspiciousness of other's motives with a tendency to blame them for one's incapacities. Loss of spatial orientation is seen in the inability to put on a garment without confusion as to top and bottom and sleeve and neck. Weakness, muscular twitching or seizures may occur, and motor aphasia (the person cannot recall words he or she wishes to say) and speech slurring may become evident. Indifference to social customs and graces develops.

In the *second stage* of the disease, the changes of the first stage intensify. Disorientation is complete; emotional lability increases and there may be restlessness at night.

Memory loss becomes so severe that even close friends and relatives are not recognized and the patient may not recognize himself or herself in the mirror. Movements are slow, and simple writing, reading, mathematical skills and reasoning deteriorate seriously. Other deficiencies such as inability to recognize objects by way of the senses become obvious. Motor dysfunction may progress from unsteady gait to inability to stand or walk. The person loses weight due to poor nutrition and shows no interest in meals.

In the *final stage* of the disease, movements become stereotyped, there is inability to use language, urinary and bowel incontinence, abnormal reflexes and muscular rigidity develop and, eventually, there is flexion of the lower extremities and the individual becomes bedridden and totally helpless. There is a marked tendency to grasp objects and put them to the mouth. The disease may last for several years before death occurs, often as a result of broncho-pneumonia.

Nursing care

Assessment

The patient assessment involves paying particular attention to nutritional and fluid balance status, skin condition, general personal hygiene and appearance, and elimination patterns. The patient's level of understanding, memory and orientation are key parts of the assessment, and social and family circumstances must also be explored.

Patient problems

The patient's carers may be the focal point of nursing interventions. The age, the health and support systems of the caregivers are important considerations when a patient remains at home. The following is a list of core problems; many more individual problems are possible:

- ineffective coping because of altered cognitive functioning
- potential for injury due to loss of memory, impaired motor and cognitive functioning
- self-care deficits in relation to adequate rest, nutrition and personal hygiene
- alteration in elimination patterns – urinary and bowel incontinence
- potential for social isolation due to loss of interest, initiative and memory (friends and relatives not recognized)
- potential for complications:
  - respiratory dysfunction due to inactivity and lowered resistance to infection
  - impairment of skin integrity due to immobility, incontinence, malnutrition and injury
- knowledge deficit relating to disease progression and alterations in social functioning.

Nursing intervention

Ineffective coping In the early stage, the patient and particularly the family require considerable counselling. Expectations of the patient's abilities should be lowered. The patient needs to be understood and accepted as he or she is, because memory cannot be restored nor behaviour changed. A written outline of daily routines to be carried out may prove helpful. For example, if the person is to carry out a job away from home, it may be useful to refer to a written note.

Each day, the patient identifies a few essential tasks on which to focus, as coping with more than these is too difficult.

Potential for injury The environment is kept free of hazards and stress as much as possible. As disorientation develops and body movements become increasingly more awkward, the risk of falls increases. The patient may forget that a cigarette is burning or that a gas stove has been turned on. With progressive loss of memory, the person requires close supervision. It is important that he or she carries identification in case of wandering off and becoming lost and exposed to the elements. It should be remembered that restlessness and disorientation are likely to be worse at night when sensory stimuli are minimal and there is some decrease in cerebral perfusion.

The patient can usually manage for a longer period and be capable of doing more if in the familiar surroundings of home, where an automatic routine is established.

Self-care deficits Regular periods of rest are planned for the person: fatigue tends to aggravate the manifestations of deterioration. Some patients respond to relaxation therapy tapes. The daily food and fluid intake are noted and the patient is weighed at regular intervals. In the early stage of Alzheimer's disease, the patient gradually loses the appreciation of nutritional needs. The person becomes unable to shop and prepare food, and eventually skips meals. Prompting and assistance with meals and in-between snacks are necessary to ensure that the patient has sufficient nutrition. High-calorie foods and supplements are used when necessary. Plans are made to provide hygienic care as neglect becomes obvious. Provision is made for bathing, grooming, dressing and frequent change of washable clothing.

Alteration in elimination pattern With progression of Alzheimer's disease, the patient develops urinary and bowel incontinence. A schedule for prompting the patient to go to the toilet at intervals determined by customary elimination frequency may help in avoiding incontinence. Constipation may be a problem due to the immobility and reduced food intake. The roughage content of the diet may be increased and a mild laxative (bulk producing or stool softener) may be administered. If the constipation is not recognized and corrected, faecal impaction develops readily.

Potential for social isolation The patient tends to avoid social situations as cognitive and communicative skills diminish. Efforts should be made for exposure to human interaction and for socialization just as long as they have even the slightest meaning. Including the person in short social events and in small-group affairs could be helpful. If a daycare centre is available, the patient will be able to get out of the home and participate in structured social activity.

Potential for complications Because of inactivity and malnutrition, the patient is predisposed to respiratory infection. An exercise programme, walking, deep breathing and coughing, adequate nutrition as well as protection from exposure to those with an infection contribute to the prevention of respiratory infection.

As the immobility, helplessness and malnutrition worsen, the patient becomes more and more predisposed to pressure sores. Regular bathing, careful observation and protection of vulnerable areas, repositioning at regular intervals and prompt changing of clothing or bedding following incontinence are necessary.

Knowledge deficit relating to disease progression and alterations in social functioning Some major adjustments in the lifestyle and relationships of the family, as well as those of the patient, are necessary as the disease advances. Planning for these at an early stage of the disorder facilitates the change process as it becomes necessary. A major effort involving social workers and various members of the community care team is needed to support the family in caring for the patient at home. Although the lifespan of the person with Alzheimer's disease cannot be protracted, the quality of the life of all concerned may be enhanced through early professional intervention, counselling and effective planning. It is helpful to introduce the family to the local branch of the Alzheimer's Society. The association provides family support through meetings, pamphlets and community referrals. The Society also provides education for the general public.

In the early stages, the family is advised of ways to help the patient maintain independence and carry on at home. The family is informed of signs of progression of the disorder and how members can best cope with increasing dependency of the patient. They are alerted to the hazards that may develop with the increasing dementia. When the affected person is no longer productive, roles and relationships must change. It is particularly difficult when a formerly responsible and productive person becomes dependent upon others for decision-making and personal care. The process of adjustment is slow and requires understanding and acceptance of the patient's condition. The family's reactions may indicate the need for a referral for professional counselling.

In the later stages of the disorder, management focuses on helping the family to cope with extremely difficult situations. The family may consist of one person or several people. Anticipatory planning for institutional care has to be encouraged so that, when it becomes necessary, it is part of a rational decision-making process. The family may need considerable persuasion and support in making this decision. Unfortunately, there is no effective treatment for this disorder, although NICE (2001) have recommended that drugs which inhibit the enzyme acetylcholinesterase and so improve synaptic functioning in the brain (e.g. donepezil, rivastigmine and galantamine) can be used by specialist clinicians under particular circumstances. These drugs can delay the degenerative process in some people (British National Formulary 2005, Birks and Harvey 2006).

MULTIPLE SCLEROSIS (DISSEMINATED SCLEROSIS)

Multiple sclerosis (MS) is a chronic, progressive, degenerative disease characterized by patches of demyelination throughout the brain and spinal cord. Myelin is the lipoprotein sheath surrounding the axons of the neurones and enables impulses to travel much faster along the fibre than is possible in unmyelinated fibres. The destruction of areas of myelin is followed by a proliferation of neuroglial cells. Scar tissue forms as hardened (sclerotic) white elevations known as plaque. Nerve fibres (axons) eventually degenerate; there is loss of impulse transmission, and focal deficits occur which in some instances may be permanent. The optic nerves and the cervical spinal cord tend to be most vulnerable to this degenerative demyelinating process in the initial episodes.

Incidence and population at risk

MS has a worldwide distribution and affects 40–60 people per 100 000 population. People are twice as likely to be stricken if they live in cold, damp climates. The UK has been recognized as a high-risk zone; in north-east Scotland and Ulster, the incidence is 100 per 100 000 population, and in the Shetlands and Orkney it is 300 per 100 000. The onset of the disease is highest amongst persons aged 20–40 years, with a slightly higher incidence in women. A familial tendency has been recognized but a definite genetic pattern has not been identified.

Aetiology

The specific cause of MS continues to elude scientists; current evidence suggests that genetic factors, environmental factors, viruses and the individual's immune system may be collectively implicated. The view that viral infection and an immunological abnormality interact to induce the CNS damage is particularly favoured.

Effects on the patient

MS is characterized by remissions and relapses. The course and the effects vary widely from one person to another and are unpredictable. Spontaneous remissions of varying lengths are common particularly in the early years of the disease, and in some instances appear to be permanent. Rarely, MS takes a fulminating, malignant course in which a combination of cerebral brainstem and cord manifestations develops suddenly; the patient becomes comatose, there is no remission and death may occur within a few weeks.

Most patients survive more than 20 years after the initial onset and lead active productive lives for many of those years. A lesser number experience a steady progression of the disease with frequently recurring relapses leading to a chronic incapacitated state, dependency and complications.

The initial onset of symptoms of MS usually develops suddenly (within a day or two) but, with some, may develop slowly over several weeks. The initial onset of exacerbation usually coincides with a stressful experience such as anxiety, trauma, infection, excessive fatigue, exposure to an extreme of temperature and pregnancy.

As the location and extent of the demyelination are so variable, the clinical characteristics are also highly variable from one patient to another. They may include the following:

- extreme fatigue
- visual dysfunction (e.g. diplopia, blurring of vision, nystagmus)
- transient tingling sensations or numbness (paraesthesia) or loss of sensation
- intention tremor
- ataxia
- muscular weakness in one or both arms and legs
- paraparesis
- bladder and bowel dysfunction
- impairment of speech (scanning)
- emotional lability – alternating periods of euphoria, depression and irritability
- personality changes
- cognitive dysfunction – loss of memory and confusion.

Deficits that persist beyond 3 months are usually permanent. Weakness of the respiratory muscles and cough reflex may develop, predisposing the patient to pulmonary complications.

There is no cure for MS; the treatment is symptomatic and supportive, and increases in amount and complexity as the patient's disease progresses. Corticosteroids are now used for severe relapses; a dose of methylprednisolone 1 G daily for 3 days i.v. is the accepted regimen, followed by a reducing dose of oral prednisolone.

Recent research suggests that MS is triggered when the immune system attacks the protein sheath of nerve cells. This led scientists to test beta interferon, a substance which inhibits certain white blood cells, to treat the disease. Studies showed β-interferon can reduce the number and severity of attacks and brain abnormalities in some patients (Bogglid and Ford 2004).

There is no consensus on the role of any specific dietary measures. Physiotherapy is prescribed for most patients to promote activity and independence as long as possible.

Assessment

Assessment should focus on the current neurological problems being experienced by the patient, together with the degree of insight the patient has into the illness. Fears, anxieties and other feelings such as frustration should be gently explored, together with the social and family circumstances of the patient.

Patient problems

The following is a list of the more commonly found problems associated with MS; it should be remembered that many other individual problems are also possible:

- Inadequate or inaccurate knowledge about the disorder, health maintenance and management of a remission
- Alteration in self-image and fear due to the potential change in lifestyle, disability and dependence
- Potential remissions and exacerbations; adjustments in activities to maintain health
- Impaired mobility secondary to muscular weakness, fatigue, ataxia and/or paralysis
- Potential for injury because of difficulty in walking
- Potential sensory deficits – abnormal vision and diminished cutaneous sensation may occur
- Alteration in pattern of elimination:
  – urinary frequency, urgency or incontinence
  – constipation
- Alteration in nutritional status due to loss of appetite secondary to anxiety and depression, weakened mastication and swallowing muscles, and/or inability to prepare meals
- Self-care deficits due to muscular weakness or paralysis, immobility and depression
- Impairment of verbal communication secondary to weakness or paralysis of the muscles involved in producing speech
  Potential for complications:
  – impairment of skin integrity
  – respiratory insufficiency and infection.

Goals

The patient's goals can be summarized as avoiding the complications listed in the above problems and adapting lifestyle to the progressive deterioration in function that occurs. A key goal is to maintain maximum independence for as long as possible.

Nursing intervention

Good counselling and care may contribute to the prevention of relapses as well as help in keeping the patient active and independent for as long as possible. Hospital care usually becomes necessary during acute exacerbations or when complete dependence has been reached.

Inadequate knowledge The patient and family are informed about MS, the nature of the disease, its effects, the fact that relapses of varying length occur and the potential precipitating factors in relapses. They are advised that it is not possible to predict the course of the disorder. Management is discussed in detail with emphasis on continuing former activities and gainful employment, and the necessary modifications in lifestyle to avoid factors known to contribute to a recurrence of symptoms. Important factors in the prevention of potential injuries and complications are outlined.

Community resources for assistance are made known to the patient and family. These include the Multiple Sclerosis Society (www.mssociety.org.uk), social services and community nurses. During relapses, or as the disorder progresses leaving residual disability, assistive devices (e.g. wheelchair), assistance with physical care and/or home management, financial assistance, and support and encouragement may become necessary. The local branch of the Multiple Sclerosis Society is an excellent source of information and assistance. For example, it helps in securing assistive devices, transporting patients to the physiotherapy department or clinic, and contacting other resources for assistance (e.g. social services department) if necessary. The Multiple Sclerosis Society also has voluntary workers who make home visits and arrange occupational and recreational programmes for patients with MS. If the patient's former occupation is too strenuous or stressful, vocational re-training may be appropriate so that the person can return to gainful employment during remissions.

Alteration in self-image and fears   The changes in body function and capacity and increasing loss of independence alter the patient's image of self. Feelings of uncertainty may arise because the outcomes are unclear and planning may be difficult. Roles and relationships change, counselling around sexuality may be helpful, and responsibilities shift. Sensory and motor deficits that occur with MS frequently lead to impaired sexual functioning, which may affect relationships. Fear of the long-term consequences of the disease, increasing dependency and the reactions of others are threatening.

Both patient and family are likely to experience the stages of grief reaction as they come to grips with the realities of the situation. Nursing care involves acceptance of their reactions, supportive understanding and open discussion of concerns. Providing information about the illness, the symptoms and the potential therapy helps to decrease the uncertainty and promote realistic expectations. Anxiety and depression on the part of the patient and family may delay the process of acceptance of the diagnosis, and counselling may be helpful. The patient and family should be allowed to make decisions and be part of the planning for the future.

Maintenance of health   In early remissions when the residual effects are likely to be minimal, the patient is encouraged to resume his or her usual pattern of life, modifying it as necessary to avoid overfatigue, emotional stress and infections as these may precipitate a relapse. Regular and adequate rest, a well-balanced diet, and learning to accept what cannot be readily changed to avoid emotional stress, reduce the risk of an exacerbation.

In the case of the female patient, menstruation and fertility are unaffected but the woman is advised of the increased risk of a relapse incurred by pregnancy. In addition, delivery may be complicated by spasms of the hip adductor muscles. Contraceptive pills may aggravate symptoms of MS.

Impaired mobility   Muscle spasticity and weakness, especially in the lower limbs, are common disabling factors in MS. A carefully controlled physiotherapy programme is instituted within the patient's tolerance to keep the patient active and prevent muscle contractures and atrophy.

Exercises in a warm pool reduce the spasticity. Close observation is made for signs of excessive fatigue and a rest period should follow the exercise period.

A walking stick or crutches may be necessary to assist the patient in maintaining mobility. Walking between parallel bars may be helpful. When walking becomes impossible, a wheelchair is provided and the patient is taught to transfer from bed to chair and from chair to toilet unaided if there is sufficient strength in the arms.

Family members require instructions on how to transfer the patient from the wheelchair to the bed, and vice versa, if the patient is experiencing weakness or motor deficit in the upper limbs.

Spasticity may become a painful problem in the disabled limbs. Passive movements of the affected limbs and the use of drugs that act by impairing nerve impulse transmission at spinal muscle level, e.g. baclofen may reduce the spasticity and prevent contractures. Baclofen is, however, contraindicated in the presence of peptic ulceration (British National Formulary 2005).

Potential for injury   The patient is at risk of injury especially as walking becomes increasingly more difficult. To prevent falls, floors are kept clear of scatter rugs, stools, electrical flexes and other articles over which the patient might trip. Hand-rails in appropriate places facilitate safer mobility. Shoes that provide firm support and have non-slip soles are worn.

Potential sensory deficits   Sensory deficits such as impaired vision and diminished temperature and pressure sensations increase the patient's potential for injury. If a portion of the visual field is affected, the patient learns to turn the head in order to bring objects into the range of vision. Diplopia may be relieved by wearing an eye patch on one eye and then periodically placing it on the other eye. The patient and family are taught safety measures to prevent burns, for example control of the temperature of food and beverages as well as bath water. Areas of diminished sensation are inspected daily for irritation and injury.

Alteration in pattern of elimination   Urinary frequency and urgency are common problems for the patient with MS. Later, as the disease progresses, loss of sphincter control and incontinence may develop. Also, drug therapy to aid detrusor stability, e.g. oxybutynin may be used. The patient is advised to set up a regular schedule for going to the toilet to avoid the distress caused by urgency and dribbling or incontinence. If the patient's mobility is impaired, a prompt response to the patient's request for assistance is necessary.

Some patients experience urinary retention or may not completely empty the bladder when voiding. The use of catheterization is avoided if possible because of the risk of ascending urinary tract infection. If catheterization becomes necessary, strict asepsis is observed, a high fluid intake is encouraged (3000 mL daily) and regular assessment is made for infection (temperature, culture of urine).

Constipation is a frequent problem as a result of the reduced mobility, and should be dealt with by standard methods (high-fibre diet, etc.) where possible.

Alteration in nutritional status The patient's weight is recorded at regular intervals as the food intake is frequently reduced owing to a poor appetite which develops as a result of the patient's anxiety, immobility, weakness in mastication and swallowing, or the patient's inability to shop and prepare meals.

Well-balanced meals that are easily digested are necessary; the food intake is monitored. High-calorie drinks may be necessary in order to meet the patient's requirements for energy and tissue maintenance. If the patient is overweight, a decreased caloric intake is prescribed to reduce the burden on weakened muscles.

Self-care deficits in hygiene Nursing care includes repeated assessments of the patient's ability to complete self-care, which may become increasingly difficult as the disease progresses and care provision increases. For example, muscular weakness or paralysis of the arms may prevent the patient from cleaning the teeth and combing the hair. Food particles and mucus may accumulate in the mouth if swallowing is difficult, necessitating mouth care after each meal.

Impairment of verbal communication The speech may progressively become slower and more difficult as muscular weakness increases, creating frustration for both the patient and carers. Referral to a speech therapist may be helpful. Nursing care includes support and reinforcement of the therapy, talking with the patient, encouraging verbal responses and acknowledging even slight achievement without, however, being patronizing.

Potential for complications As mobility and sensory perception deteriorate, the potential for skin breakdown increases; meticulous pressure care is therefore required.

PARKINSON'S DISEASE (PARALYSIS AGITANS)

Parkinson's disease is a complex clinical syndrome associated with a decreased concentration of the chemical dopamine and its major metabolite. Dopamine is essential for normal neurotransmission and functioning of the basal ganglia. It is produced by the substantia nigra, a nucleus of highly pigmented cells in the midbrain which function as a part of the extrapyramidal system. Dopamine exerts an inhibitory effect on movements by opposing or lessening the stimulating effect of acetylcholine. When a deficiency of dopamine occurs, tremors, rigidity, slowness and limited voluntary movement become evident.

Types, aetiology and incidence
The cause of the illness is unknown and it may be that the clinical picture of parkinsonism merely represents a common end stage for several different disease pathways. Parkinson's disease affects one person out of 500 in the UK. About 10 000 people are newly diagnosed each year and one person in every 20 of these will be below the age of 40 (Parkinson's Disease Society 2006).

Effects on the patient
The disease produces increasing physical disability as it progresses. At first, tremor and muscular rigidity develop insidiously and disappear with voluntary movement and sleep, although becoming more pronounced with fatigue and stress. The tremor initially usually develops in the fingers and thumb, producing the characteristic pill-rolling movement. The arms are adducted and semiflexed and the normal arm swing associated with walking is absent. Movements are slowed and a monotone becomes evident in the speech.

As the disease progresses the trunk and head are flexed forward, the patient may have difficulty in starting to walk and in turning, and the gait is slow and shuffling. Rigidity of the facial muscles and unblinking eyes produces a mask-like inexpressive appearance.

With further deterioration, the patient becomes more stooped and when walking there is a progressive acceleration of steps, producing what is known as a *festination gait*, making stopping difficult and predisposing to falls. There is difficulty in changing position and the patient has difficulty with tasks involving finger movements.

Drooling occurs due to the decrease in automatic swallowing of saliva. Disturbances in autonomic innervation may develop; there may be excessive, or an absence of, perspiration, and disordered temperature regulation. Excessive lacrimation, ptosis and/or pupillary constriction may develop. Gastrointestinal activity may be slowed, causing constipation.

Pain and fatigue are experienced because of the continuously increased traction of muscles on their attachments. Speech becomes weak, slurred and devoid of any inflections as the muscles concerned with articulation become more involved.

In the final stages, the patient becomes disabled to a greater degree because of the inability to initiate voluntary movement. Speech becomes incoherent and difficulty in mastication and swallowing develops. The respiratory volumes are reduced and the ability to cough is diminished, predisposing to respiratory complications.

Up to now, the patient's intellectual functioning was unaffected, but at this later stage, dementia may become evident in some patients.

Assessment
Assessment of the patient should focus on the degree of disability and any techniques the patient may use to help cope with such disability. The effects on family and the social circumstances should be investigated, together with the patient's feelings about the condition.

Patient problems
- Inadequate or inaccurate knowledge about the parkinsonian syndrome, its characteristics, prescribed treatment and management

- Muscular dysfunction due to impairment of extrapyramidal control – tremor, rigidity, slowness and lack of coordination
- Potential for injury due to muscular dysfunction
- Altered body image and loss of self-esteem secondary to incapacity, change in role, appearance and dependency
- Nutritional deficit due to difficulty in eating, mastication and swallowing, anorexia and nausea caused by the prescribed medication
- Impairment in communication – speech difficulty secondary to the rigidity of the muscles involved in speech and reduced pulmonary volumes
- Potential for complications:
  - respiratory complications due to respiratory muscle dysfunction, causing reduced pulmonary volumes and the inability to cough to remove secretions
  - break in skin due to immobility and falls
  - impairment of eye function due to diplopia or to drying and injury of the cornea caused by a reduction in blinking and moistening of the surface of the eye
  - potential medication reaction; medication withdrawal leading to parkinsonian crisis.

Goals

The goals are that the patient and family will accept and adjust to the situation and the patient will maintain independence, accustomed role and a relatively normal lifestyle for as long as the condition permits.

Nursing intervention

The patient with Parkinson's disease is managed at home on a drug programme until the advanced stage of the disorder causes marked disability and dependency. The community nurse assumes the major role in assessing the patient's needs and providing the necessary counselling and guidance for the patient and family at the onset and through successive months and years. It is important that the nurse recognizes the emotional, physical and socioeconomic problems incurred by the disease. The fact that the patient's intellect is unimpaired must be kept in mind as well as a tendency to become very self-conscious, depressed and withdrawn because of the appearance and limitations enforced on the patient by the disease.

The patient is advised to contact the national Parkinson's Disease Society (www.parkinsons.org.uk). Socialization in structured groups of persons with similar problems can be helpful.

Difficulty in movement requires care to be taken to avoid hazards that may cause falls and also emphasizes the need for teaching about pressure care. Encouragement with a physiotherapy programme is essential to promote inability for as long as possible.

Loss of normal smooth, coordinated mobility, change in appearance, loss of the capacity for gainful employment and self-care, and loss of accustomed social interaction result in the patient's altered self-image, loss of self-esteem and depression. The patient is encouraged to express his or her feelings and to take an active role in setting realistic goals and planning management. The patient may develop an acute sense of humiliation leading to withdrawal and isolation.

The patient's strengths and potential capacity should be emphasized and independence encouraged in order that socialization and group activities may be promoted. Every effort should be made to try to encourage the patient's self-esteem.

The expertise of other professionals will be required to provide counselling, motivation, guidance and support. Involvement in the local branch of the Parkinson's Disease Society may be useful for some patients.

The quality and quantity of food taken by the patient and body weight are followed closely. Only a small amount of food may be taken because of fatigue and depression. The patient should be encouraged to be as independent as possible in feeding. The patient may be less self-conscious and eat more if privacy is ensured and ample time is allocated for each meal. Sensitive provision of protection for clothing at meal times is essential to preserve the patient's fragile self-esteem.

Constipation is a common occurrence because of the decreased activity, decreased food (bulk) intake and decreased fluid in the gastrointestinal tract due to an inadequate intake and the loss of saliva (drooling). The drug therapy may also contribute to the problem.

The fluid, roughage and bulk intake are increased. A stool softener or bulk-producing laxative (e.g. bisacodyl) may be necessary to prevent faecal impaction. The patient is encouraged to establish a regular time for defaecation; a raised toilet seat will make defaecation easier.

Urinary dribbling and incontinence may occur; the cause may be the inability of the patient to reach the toilet soon enough. A regular toileting schedule is arranged and the patient prompted and assisted if necessary. A commode or urinal is kept readily available for use at night.

The patient experiences the discomfort of continually contracted muscles and readily becomes fatigued. Physiotherapy, avoidance of prolonged periods in one position and planned rest periods contribute to comfort.

As a result of disturbed autonomic nervous system control, excessive perspiration may occur. Daily bathing and frequent change of clothing may be needed to promote comfort and to control body odour.

The rigidity of the muscles involved in speech and the reduced pulmonary volumes that may develop interfere with the patient's enunciation and volume of speech. Deep breathing with slow exhalation, singing and speech classes in groups help to improve speech. Facial exercises such as smiling, blowing out, grimacing, eye movements and neck extension performed before a mirror may lessen facial rigidity.

The patient may experience prolonged exposure and drying of the surface of the eye due to a reduction in the normal frequency of blinking. This may lead to corneal irritation. The instillation of artificial tears may be prescribed and the patient and/or a family member is taught how to instil the solution. Diplopia may become a problem. A patch on one eye may help.

The patient is observed for any reaction to prescribed medication. Carbidopa is commonly given as co-careldopa to promote the entrance of levodopa, the precursor of dopamine, into the brain. Long-term side-effects include memory loss, mood swings and behaviour change. Dopamine receptor agonist drugs such as bromocriptine are usually started before levodopa therapy. Anticholinergic drugs such as benzhexol (Artane) may be used to try to reduce muscle tone, but they too have side-effects such as blurring of vision, retention of urine and palpitations. An assessment is made for positive responses as well as for undesirable side-effects, for example: Is the tremor less? Has the patient's gait improved? If side-effects develop, the doctor is notified; an adjustment in dosage may be necessary or another drug prescribed.

Sudden withdrawal of an anti-parkinsonian drug or severe emotional disturbance may precipitate a reaction referred to as a *parkinsonian crisis*. This is characterized by a marked aggravation of tremors, rigidity and akinesia. Tachycardia, increased respirations, acute anxiety and diaphoresis also occur.

The reaction is a medical emergency requiring prompt treatment. Treatment includes respiratory and cardiac support, the administration of an anti-parkinsonian preparation and the parenteral administration of a sedative such as phenobarbitone may be necessary.

HUNTINGTON'S DISEASE (CORTICOSTRIATONIGRAL DEGENERATION)

In the UK, between 6500 and 8000 people live with Huntington's Disease (BBC 2005). It occurs in all racial groups. This condition was first described by George Huntington, a New York physician, in 1872 as an inherited condition of chorea and dementia in a group of families on Long Island. Early in the seventeenth century, many English people migrated to America for religious and political reasons. Three men from the Suffolk village of Bures landed in Boston in 1630. Some 300 years later, a researcher was able to trace the transmission of many cases of Huntington's disease, via 1000 affected descendants, back to these men.

Inheritance

The disease is transmitted by a dominant gene which, when present, will always produce Huntington's disease. Both sexes are equally affected and each child of an affected parent has a 50% chance of developing the disease in later life.

Pathology

It has been shown biochemically that the concentration of γ-aminobutyric acid (GABA), an inhibitory neurotransmitter, is greatly reduced in the substantia nigra, with a resultant fall in the activity of the enzyme glutamic acid decarboxylase (GAD). It therefore appears that there is death of the nerve cells producing GABA. Experiments suggest that GABA pathways exist between the basal ganglia and the substantia nigra.

Huntington's disease appearing before the age of 20 years is passed from the father in 80% of cases; in cases of very late onset, the abnormal gene is more commonly transmitted by the mother. The nature, course and prognosis of the disease should be explained very carefully to the family, and they should be offered genetic counselling. For some families, contact with the Huntington's Disease Association may be helpful (www.hda.org.uk).

Treatment and nursing care

There is little to offer the patient in the way of treatment. Phenothiazines, haloperidol or tetrabenzine may control the chorea in the preliminary stages of the disease. The patient will ultimately require long-term care. The choreic movements may make eating and drinking difficult. Swallowing can be difficult and it is important to ensure that the patient receives adequate nutrition. A high-calorie diet with frequent glucose drinks between meals is helpful. Eventually the patient will need to be tube fed. Constipation can be a problem and is dealt with using an aperient and suppositories. Speech will deteriorate to loud grunting noises which others may find distressing. Occasionally there will be outbursts of aggression arising from the sheer frustration of not being able to communicate. Devising alternative methods of communication becomes a challenge and often the carers can help with this.

The patient will eventually become totally dependent, emaciated and immobile. Limbs become rigid, producing an abnormal posture. Prevention of skin breakdown becomes a priority. The aim of care should be the relief of symptoms as they develop to ensure the patient maintains his or her dignity and a peaceful death. The family will also require constant support and encouragement.

MOTOR NEURONE DISEASE (AMYOTROPHIC LATERAL SCLEROSIS)

This is a progressive chronic disease in which there is a degeneration of motor neurones in the spine (anterior horn cells), brainstem and/or cortical motor areas.

The cause of motor neurone disease is unknown. The onset of the disorder occurs most often between the ages of 40 and 60 years. The muscles innervated by the affected neurones lose their ability to contract, and therefore they atrophy.

Effects on the patient

The first symptom is usually weakness of the hands and arms; finer movements are lost and articles are dropped. Twitching and hyperreflexia develop along with the spasticity and weakness of the lower limbs. As the disorder progresses, speech, swallowing and respiration are impaired as motor neurones at higher levels are involved. The diagnosis is made on the patient's symptoms and their progressive nature. Electromyographic studies are done to confirm the loss of innervation to the muscles. The course is usually progressively retrograde; rarely is there a remission.

Treatment and nursing care

There is no specific treatment for motor neurone disease. When the disease is diagnosed, the patient and family are advised by the doctor of the expected progression and fatal outcome of the disorder. They require support, opportunities to express their feelings and ask questions, explanations and assistance in planning home management. The nurse can advise them to contact the Motor Neurone Disease Society. The patient is encouraged to remain active within the potential muscular ability and every effort should be made to encourage independence despite increasing disability. It should be kept in mind that in motor neurone disease the cognitive ability remains unaffected. Obviously home management must be individualized because of the variability of symptoms and stages of the disease in patients. Progression of the disease and increasing dependency eventually necessitate the use of a wheelchair.

The speech therapist has a vital role to play in the management of swallowing and speech. He or she should be introduced to the patient early on in the illness and will monitor progression and introduce communication aids at the appropriate stages.

Dysarthria and dysphagia are very distressing features in the later stages of the illness. The patient may become very embarrassed by the speech and the constant drooling of secretions. Privacy at meal times is very important, and the patient should be given small meals and nourishing drinks frequently. A portable tracheal suction machine can be supplied for home use and it is important that the patient and family are taught the correct way to use it. It may become necessary in the later stages to feed the patient via a nasogastric tube, or a gastrotomy tube may be inserted under radiographic control. These are very distressing procedures to both patient and family, and much time must be taken with them to explain and teach them how to use the tubes.

MYASTHENIA GRAVIS

Myasthenia gravis is not a degenerative condition but is included here because of its chronic, progressive nature. It is a neuromuscular disorder characterized by weakness and easy fatiguability of voluntary muscles due to interference with impulse condition at the neuromuscular junction.

The condition occurs as a consequence of an autoimmune destruction of the postsynaptic receptors for acetylcholine at the neuromuscular junction. An immunological basis is felt to be the cause due to an increased incidence of autoimmune disorders in patients and first degree relatives, and the association of the disease with certain histocompatability antigens.

Incidence

It is not a common disorder. The incidence is highest between 20 and 30 years of age, and women are affected more frequently than men at this age. In later years, men and women are equally affected.

Effects on the patient

The onset of myasthenia gravis may be insidious with the symptoms of fatigue and weakness being associated with muscular activity. Initially, only the extrinsic ocular and levator palpebrae muscles may be involved, resulting in ptosis of the eyelids and diplopia. This may be referred to as *ocular myasthenia*. More generalized muscle involvement (generalized myasthenia) with progression of the disease produces the following manifestations:

- an expressionless appearance due to weakness of facial muscles
- difficulty with mastication and swallowing
- nasal voice tone that loses volume as the patient talks
- limb weakness, which becomes evident with the patient experiencing difficulty with self-care management (e.g. bathing, brushing the teeth, combing the hair)
- respiratory difficulty
- loss of control of bladder and rectal sphincters.

Muscle weakness is most noticeable at the end of the day and after exercise. Some recovery of strength is evident upon rising in the morning or following a period of rest. Mild atrophy may occur in the affected muscles and some aching may be present. Usually, sensation is unchanged.

There is great variability in the course of the disease; spontaneous remissions may occur. Factors that may aggravate symptoms include infection, temperature extreme, exposure to sunlight, emotional stress and physical exertion. Weakness of the diaphragm and intercostal muscles is serious; respiratory insufficiency and complications may be fatal.

Medical management

There is no known cure for myasthenia gravis. Treatment includes the administration of drugs, plasmapheresis and surgery. The drug most commonly used is an acetylcholinesterase antagonist preparation such as neostigmine or pyridostigmine. This decreases the activity of acetylcholinesterase, the enzyme responsible for degrading acetylcholine at the neuromuscular junction. Response to such a drug is used as a diagnostic test during medical investigations for myasthenia gravis. The patient is usually hospitalized and observed for reactions to the drug. If the patient does not respond, the corticosteroid prednisone may be given for its antibody suppressant effect, on the basis that the disorder is an abnormal immune response.

Surgical therapy involves thymectomy (the removal of the thymus gland). Hyperplasia occurs in many of the patients, or a thymic tumour may be present, and removal of the gland results in a marked improvement in some and complete remission in others. Surgery is used mainly in younger patients in the early stages of the disease.

Problems and goals

The patient faces lengthy periods of remission and progressively deteriorating exacerbations of the illness. The familiar problems of progressive disability have to be faced (see p. 723), with most of the patient's care taking place in the community.

Nursing intervention

Most patients with myasthenia gravis are managed in the home. Hospitalization may be necessary for evaluation, establishing the required medication dosage, exacerbation of symptoms, respiratory failure or myasthenic crisis. Nursing management is primarily concerned with maintenance of muscle strength and the prevention of complications especially the potentially fatal respiratory failure and muscle atrophy.

The reader is referred to preceding pages in this chapter for a discussion of the general care required for patients with a neurological disorder.

A major potential problem unique to myasthenia gravis which may occur involves a crisis reaction to drugs. The patient who requires high doses of an anticholinesterase drug is at risk of developing a *cholinergic crisis*. This is a life-threatening reaction resulting from overmedication necessitating prompt emergency treatment. A dramatic increase in myasthenic symptoms occurs in about 1 hour, the patient experiences extreme weakness, blurred vision, nausea, vomiting, intestinal cramping, diarrhoea, increased salivation and bronchial secretions, respiratory insufficiency, bradycardia, constricted pupils and increased perspiration.

Treatment involves withholding the anticholinesterase. Endotracheal intubation, mechanical respiratory assistance and frequent suction are necessary to prevent severe respiratory failure, hypoxia and death. Atropine sulfate may be prescribed to lessen the secretions. Following the cholinergic crisis, regular dosage of the anticholinesterase is decreased.

A crisis may also develop due to undermedication, and is referred to as *myasthenic crisis*. The symptoms are similar to those that occur in a cholinergic crisis but develop 3 hours or more after taking the anticholinesterase drug. An anticholinesterase preparation, e.g. neostigmine is given as well as supportive treatment as indicated (e.g. respiratory assistance). The regular dosage of the anticholinesterase is increased.

THE PERSON WITH A SEIZURE DISORDER

A seizure is the manifestation of abnormal, rapid and uncontrolled neuronal electrical discharges within the brain. It is characterized by sensory, motor and autonomic disturbances, and changes in level of consciousness. The term ***epilepsy*** refers to a chronic tendency to have recurring seizures of unknown cause and is therefore not strictly a disease. In the normal brain, a certain stability exists between excitation and inhibition. When a seizure occurs, the ability to suppress abnormal neural activity may be impaired or lost, or there may be increased excitation within the neurones. The abnormal activity may occur in a small group of neurones and remain relatively localized or may spread to involve extensive areas of neurones. In some seizures, no focal origin (i.e. localized area) of abnormal electrical discharges can be identified; large areas of the brain appear to be involved simultaneously.

INCIDENCE AND CAUSE

The disorder characterized by recurring seizures and commonly referred to as epilepsy represents one of the most common neurological problems affecting individuals irrespective of geographical location, sex and race. About 5% of the population has a seizure of some type during life, and in the population at large about 0.5% has epilepsy (recurrent seizures). In the UK, around 440 000 people have active epilepsy and over half of these will have developed epilepsy before the age of 15 years (Epilepsy Action 2006).

Epilepsy may be idiopathic (without known cause) or symptomatic (a symptom of another disorder). The latter type of seizure is secondary and may be caused by almost any intracranial pathological condition and by many general systemic disorders. Symptomatic seizures may occur with increased intracranial pressure or brain damage associated with a head injury, cerebral oedema or an intracranial space-occupying lesion, haemorrhage or infection. They may be a sequel to brain injury or infection that has resulted in brain damage and scar tissue formation. General systemic conditions in which seizures most commonly occur include hypoglycaemia, hypocalcaemia (tetany), renal insufficiency (uraemia), hypoxia, high fever (especially in children), toxaemia of pregnancy and chemical poisoning (e.g. alcohol, strychnine, amphetamine, lead, some insecticides).

There is no known specific cause of primary (idiopathic) epilepsy but an inherited predisposition to hypersensitivity and dysrhythmia of the neurones is considered to play a role.

CLASSIFICATION OF EPILEPSY

Seizures are classified according to whether their onset is *focal* (partial) or *generalized*. Partial seizures are further subdivided according to whether consciousness is retained throughout the seizure (*simple* partial seizure) or impaired at some point (*complex* partial seizure). A partial seizure can progress to a generalized one.

DESCRIPTION OF SEIZURES

Simple partial seizures

A focus within a particular part of the brain, usually the motor strip, is irritated resulting in a disturbance in function of the affected area. Typically, a focal seizure comprises of a twitching of the thumb or side of the face. The patient does not lose consciousness. If the twitching spreads to affect other parts of the body, it is referred to as a *Jacksonian seizure*. For example, the twitching may start in the thumb and then spread to affect the hand and arm, and possibly include the affected side of the body.

Complex partial seizures

These seizures, which normally originate in the temporal lobe, are usually preceded by an aura or warning. This is then followed by an episode of altered behaviour in which the patient performs a series of repeated movements. *Automatism*, in which the patient may continually rub his or her hands or pluck at the clothes, may be demonstrated. The patient may also describe a sensory experience; for example, he or she may describe a particular smell, and some describe experiencing familiarity with an unfamiliar situation (i.e. *déjà vu*).

Absence seizures

As the name implies, in an absence seizure there is a brief alteration in consciousness which onlookers often do not notice. It typically occurs in childhood and is often noticed only as the child falls further behind with school work. In complex absences, automatism, as previously described, accompanies the brief alteration in consciousness.

Myoclonic seizures

These involve sudden, repeated jerking movements of one or more of the limbs during which there is a momentary loss of consciousness. They can occur repeatedly over a number of hours and are most frequently seen within 1 hour of waking from sleep. If standing, the person would fall to the ground.

Tonic clonic seizures

These occur in several distinct stages. First, the patient may experience an aura. This often takes the form of a strange taste in the mouth or feeling but does not occur in everyone with this type of seizure. It can act as an early warning which, once recognized by the patient, can allow them to move to a safe place. This is followed by a loss of consciousness which heralds the start of the seizure proper. Should the patient be standing, he or she will fall to the ground. The tonic phase is signalled by a stiffening of the body. The jaw closes tight shut and the patient may utter a cry as the thoracic muscles contract and air is forcefully ejected via the vocal chords. As apnoea intervenes, the patient becomes cyanosed and is often incontinent of urine or faeces.

After a period of time, the patient will start to breathe stertorously, accompanied by rhythmic jerking of the limbs. Frothing of the mouth occurs as a result of excessive production of saliva. The patient is usually tachycardic and sweating. Once the jerking movements begin to subside, coma supervenes. Most patients fall into a deep sleep for a number of hours and are usually amnesic once they waken, and display episodes of drowsiness and confusion.

Status epilepticus

Status epilepticus is a serious form of epilepsy in which seizures occur in such rapid succession that recovery of consciousness between the episodes does not occur. Hyperpyrexia develops, coma deepens and permanent brain damage occurs due to anoxia. Complete exhaustion and death occur, if the patient is not treated.

The most common cause of status epilepticus is considered to be abrupt discontinuation of an anticonvulsant drug. Untreated or inadequately treated seizures may also lead to this emergency condition.

In status epilepticus, initial control of the seizures is by the use of intravenous diazepam. If this and other anticonvulsant drugs fail, the patient is given muscle relaxants, intubated and ventilated.

ASSESSMENT

A tonic clonic seizure is a sudden emergency that will be over very quickly. It is important that the nurse can give a clear account of the fit to medical personnel when required, so close observation is essential.

Patient problems

- Potential for injury due to the loss of consciousness and uncontrolled strong muscular contractures
- Potential lack of knowledge about the disorder, the treatment and necessary modifications in lifestyle that may be necessary
- Alteration in self-image due to anxiety and the stigma that a segment of society attaches to epilepsy

Goals

The goals are that the patient will suffer no harm as a result of the seizure and also be aware of the needs for long-term self-care in avoiding further fits.

Nursing intervention

Potential for injury

When a patient has a seizure, the most important function is to protect the patient from injury.

During a seizure, the nurse stays with the patient; safety, and the observations and recording of events are paramount. A seizure cannot be stopped once it has begun; it is self-limiting and no immediate treatment will shorten it. If the patient is in bed, the pillow is removed and the top bedding turned down so that the patient's responses can be observed. If the patient is up, and has not already fallen, he or she is eased to a semiprone position and a folded blanket or towel placed under the head to prevent injury during the clonic phase. Restrictive clothing at the neck is loosened and the immediate area cleared of anything that might contribute to injury (e.g. furniture, electric fan, lamp). No attempt is made to insert anything between the teeth as the teeth are clenched and there would be a risk of pushing the tongue into the oropharynx, obstructing the airway. In addition, injury to the teeth and soft tissue may occur; aspiration of blood or a broken tooth may become a possibility. As soon as the clonic phase begins to subside, the patient is turned on the side to promote drainage of secretions and prevent aspiration. Suction may be necessary. The patient is protected as much as possible from exposure to others.

During the seizure, the following observations are made:

- How long did the seizure last? As soon as you know the patient is fitting, glance at your watch and make a note of the time
- The mode of onset – did the patient indicate an aura? Was there a cry? Is there deviation of the head and eyes; if so, to what side? In what part of the body did the initial phase start?
- Are the seizure movements localized or generalized? If generalized, are they symmetrical or asymmetrical?
- Is the patient cyanosed?
- Are the teeth clenched and is there frothing at the mouth?
- Is there incontinence of urine or faeces?

Following the seizure, the patient will be drowsy and disoriented for some time; close observation is therefore essential for the patient's safety. When the patient wakens, reorientation may be necessary as well as an explanation of the event.

In the interest of safety and the prevention of injury for self and others, the person with epilepsy may not be allowed to drive a motor vehicle, operate certain machines, or work at heights or where there is loud noise or flashing lights. The patient may be advised against swimming, climbing, riding, cycling and participation in contact sports. Decisions regarding activities are based on the type, frequency and severity of seizures and the patient's response to the prescribed drug.

Family members are taught what to do when a seizure occurs so that they can respond effectively.

Knowledge deficit

No one anticonvulsant drug has been demonstrated to be superior to another, but they do have different side-effect profiles. It is therefore a matter of finding the drug and dose that works best with minimal side-effects for each individual. NICE (2004a,b) have issued guidance on the use of antiepileptic medication. Patients need to be well educated about their medication, its side-effects and possible interactions with other medications. Phenytoin in particular interacts with many drugs from oral contraceptives to antibiotics. This illustrates why it is essential to obtain a thorough previous medical history before safe prescribing can occur. It is emphasized that the drugs must be taken at the prescribed frequency, even though there are no seizures; effective blood levels of the drug must be maintained by adherence to the prescribed dosage and frequency, and alcohol should be avoided. Sudden withdrawal of medication can trigger rebound seizures and therefore the patient must be informed of the dangers of suddenly ceasing their medication. Drug doses must not be altered except with the appropriately qualified clinician's approval; the drug is prescribed on an individual basis according to the type, severity and frequency of the seizures and the individual's response. The patient is cautioned against the taking of any non-prescription drugs.

The importance of regular follow-up visits is emphasized. The patient taking phenytoin may require assessment of blood plasma level monitoring for optimal dose adjustment although ongoing monitoring is not recommended. Due to the potential side-effect of many of the drugs used, full blood count, liver function tests and folic acid should be evaluated regularly.

The patient and family are requested to keep a record of seizures which includes antecedent events or any known or suspected precipitating factor(s). Information about the British Epilepsy Association (www.epilepsy.org.uk) may be very useful. The mutual support offered to the patient and family by groups such as this can be invaluable. A Medic Alert identification bracelet or pendant should be worn so that appropriate care can be given during a fit or an emergency. The patient should always carry the names, addresses and telephone numbers of persons to be contacted.

Alteration in self-image

Patients express anxiety and embarrassment and see themselves as being different and inferior, having to adjust to potentially disruptive seizures and dependency on medication. Acceptance of the diagnosis is difficult for the patient, who may respond with denial, anger, resentment and despair before acceptance and adaptation. Fears and anxieties that are unexpressed and unrelieved may result in ineffective coping. A thorough evaluation of the patient's attitude toward epilepsy and expectations concerning health maintenance is essential. The attitudes and expectations of family members should also be evaluated because their understanding and support is crucial to the patient's ability to adjust to his condition which can have major employment implications. Patients with epilepsy may only drive a private car if they have been seizure-free for a year and are not allowed to drive an HGV or public service vehicle such as a bus (further details are available at: www.dvla.gov.uk).

Epilepsy is not yet clearly understood and there is no known cure. Because of this, and the historical context, fear of the disorder is widespread. At one time, the disorder was thought to be caused by the possession of a person by devils and, even today, myths, misunderstandings and social stigma still exist. As a result, the patient may fear rejection by peers and employers and refuse to disclose the health problem even though it would be wiser to do so. Concerns about the person's intellectual abilities, psychological stability and ability to perform efficiently on the job have been expressed by educators and employers. It is important for the nurse to be aware of potential prejudices that may be encountered by the patient and his or her family. The fact that mental capacity and abilities are as varied among people with epilepsy as in any cross-section of society and that epilepsy is not synonymous with learning disability or psychosis requires emphasis.

Some controversy exists concerning genetic predisposition to epilepsy. It is considered by some authorities to be greatest when epilepsy develops early in childhood and when both parents suffer epilepsy. Genetic counselling may therefore be advisable for a person with epilepsy who is contemplating having children. In addition, women who are on antiepileptic medication need specialist advice when they are planning a pregnancy and they also specialist advice regarding forms of contraception.

THE PERSON WITH AN INFECTION OF THE NERVOUS SYSTEM

There is a range of infective conditions that may affect the nervous system, for example encephalitis (infection of the brain), cerebral abscess, poliomyelitis and rabies. Fortunately, these conditions are very rare, as is tetanus, a condition in which the nervous system is attacked by the exotoxins of the *Clostridium tetani* organism. Tetanus may be fatal due to effects of the exotoxin on the nerves controlling respiration – hence the importance of tetanus prophylaxis.

MENINGITIS

Meningitis is an acute inflammation of the pia and arachnoid meningeal membranes of the brain or spinal cord. The cause is usually a bacterium or virus. Almost any bacterium can cause meningitis, but the most common are the meningococcus, the pneumococcus and *Haemophilus influenzae*. Meningitis is frequently secondary to infection of the sinuses, ears or respiratory tract. The meningococcus can produce meningococcal septicaemia – a severe life-threatening condition associated with meningitis. This may involve a characteristic rash, shock, renal failure and intravascular coagulation, amongst other complications.

Effects on the patient

The onset of meningitis is insidious when caused by a virus. The bacterial type is more sudden and acute, manifested by rash, headache, irritability, nausea, vomiting, back pain, chills and fever and symptoms of meningeal irritation. Photophobia is a common complaint. The classical signs of meningeal irritation include neck rigidity (stiffness of the neck and severe pain with forceful flexion), positive Kernig's sign (inability to straighten the knee when the hip is flexed), and positive Brudzinski's sign (hip and knee flexion in response to forward flexion of the neck). Signs of increased intracranial pressure such as raised blood pressure, pupillary changes, changes in respiratory patterns, seizures, bradycardia, confusion, drowsiness and coma may develop. Focal neurological signs rarely occur.

The medical diagnosis of meningitis is made on the basis of clinical signs and symptoms and is confirmed by isolating the organism from the CSF. The CSF is under increased pressure, is cloudy or purulent, and has an increased leucocyte count, a high protein content and a reduced concentration of glucose. Blood, nose and throat cultures are done to assist in identifying the organism, and radiographs may be taken of the chest, skull and sinuses to detect areas of inflammation.

Meningitis requires emergency treatment, as delay may result in cerebral damage and disability or death. It includes administration of intravenous penicillin initially and other antibiotics as appropriate after sensitivity of the infecting organism has been determined. Prophylactic treatment with a 2-day course of oral rifampicin for close contacts may be ordered. There is no specific treatment for viral meningitis.

Assessment

A full assessment of the patient along the lines discussed earlier in the chapter is essential, paying particular attention to the level of consciousness and other neurological parameters.

Patient problems

A wide range of problems associated with immobility, a severe infection and a diminished level of consciousness may be encountered by the patient. They are summarized below; other individual problems may also coexist:

- Alteration in comfort due to the headache, back pain and fever
- Potential for increased intracranial pressure secondary to the intracranial inflammatory process
- Fluid and nutritional deficit due to nausea, vomiting, headache, fever, confusion and decreased awareness
- Potential for injury due to seizures, disorientation or coma
- Potential spread of infection to others, particularly if the causative organism is the meningococcus
- Self-care deficits secondary to discomfort, reduced awareness, weakness or coma
- Potential for inadequate knowledge about management of the convalescent period and residual disabilities.

Goals

Patient goals will be the avoidance of complications and potential problems as outlined above while making a full recovery without any long-term deficits.

Nursing intervention

Much of the care required has already been discussed in this chapter; the following special points should, however, be noted:

- A major problem of the patient with meningitis is discomfort due to headache, back pain, fever, photophobia and anxiety. Nursing care includes the provision of emotional support, reassurance that help is available and an explanation of all nursing activities. Irritability due to increased reaction to sensory stimuli is minimized by maintaining a cool, quiet, darkened environment, by approaching the patient gently with a soft, calm voice and by keeping communication simple and direct.
- The possible spread of the patient's infection to others must be considered. The hospital infection control department is consulted; it may be necessary to use isolation procedures.
- After meningitis the patient is usually debilitated and readily fatigued, and may have some residual neurological

deficits. Several weeks or months may be needed for the patient's convalescence and rehabilitation. The family and patient should be forewarned of this and given support and encouragement throughout this difficult period. After the initial acute phase, a highly nutritious diet is encouraged and a regimen of range-of-movement exercises is established to prevent weakness, contractures and joint ankylosis, and to promote circulation.

● Minor disabilities may resolve with time, whereas others may be residual and require detailed evaluation and an intensive rehabilitation programme. The nurse plays a role in supporting the patient and interpreting the rehabilitation programme to the family, and in assisting them to make plans for adjustments and home management.

THE PERSON WITH A PERIPHERAL NERVE DISORDER

Disorders of the cranial nerves may be secondary to other diseases but a few are primary to specific nerves. The more common of these are trigeminal neuralgia and Bell's palsy. Peripheral nerve dysfunction may be incurred by direct local trauma (pressure, severance, infection and inflammation) or may be secondary to a variety of general conditions such as malnutrition, alcoholism and chemical poisoning.

TRIGEMINAL NEURALGIA (*TIC DOULOUREUX*)

Trigeminal neuralgia is a very painful disorder of the sensory fibres of the trigeminal (fifth cranial) nerve. It is characterized by recurring episodes of excruciating pain along the distribution of one or more divisions of the nerve. The attack is brief, lasting from seconds to 2 or 3 minutes.

The episodes recur frequently, day or night for several weeks at a time. The onset of an episode may occur spontaneously or may coincide with touching or movement of the face or exposure to cold or a draught. The patient may relate the precipitation of pain to eating, talking, cleaning the teeth, or washing or shaving the face. The recurring incapacitating pain has been known to cause severe depression and even suicide. The cause of the neuralgia is unknown.

The patient may be treated by medication or surgery. There is no specific drug for the disorder. Anticonvulsant agents such as carbamazepine or gabapentin (if carbamazepine is not tolerated) may suppress or shorten the painful episodes. These drugs may produce side-effects (Table 20.12). An analgesic may be prescribed. For some patients drug therapy is not effective and if this occurs, they should be referred to specialist neurosurgical services for further advice and assessment. The patient may be considered for microvascular decompression or percutaneous radiofrequency thermocoagulation. This procedure, permits destruction of the pain sensory fibres by use of an electrode and leaves the neurones and fibres concerned with other areas and the corneal reflex intact.

BELL'S PALSY (PERIPHERAL FACIAL PARALYSIS)

Bell's palsy is a disorder of the motor component of one of the facial (seventh cranial) nerves and is characterized by loss of the ability to move the muscles on one side of the face.

The condition is most common in persons aged between 20 and 40 years. The patient may experience pain behind the ear or in the face for a day or two before the onset of paralysis. When paralysis occurs, a drawing sensation on the affected side is experienced. There is flaccidity, drooping of the mouth, drooling, flattening of the nasolabial fold,

Table 20.12 Principal antiepileptic drugs

Drug	Indications	Side-effects
Carbamazepine	Complex partial seizures, tonic clonic and simple partial	Dizziness, double vision, unsteadiness, nausea and vomiting
Diazepam	Status epilepticus, absence attacks and myoclonus	Sedation
Lamotrigine	Partial or generalized seizures	Mild sedation, blurred vision, ataxia, nausea and vomiting, headache, diplopia
Phenobarbital	Tonic, clonic and partial seizures	Drowsiness, unsteadiness, tolerance, habituation, withdrawal seizures
Phenytoin	Tonic clonic, simple and complex partial seizures	Drowsiness, unsteadiness, slurred speech, with prolonged use, gingival hypertrophy, acne, coarsening of facial features
Primidone	Tonic clonic and partial seizures	Drowsiness, unsteadiness, toleration, habituation, withdrawal seizures
Sodium valproate	Idiopathic generalized epilepsies	Tremor, irritability, restlessness, occasionally confusion
Vigabatrin	Partial epilepsy	Visual field defects

widening of the palpebral fissure and inability to close the eye completely on the affected side. There may be watering of the eye. The individual is unable to smile, whistle or grimace. The taste sensation is lost over the anterior two-thirds of the tongue on the respective side. Herpes lesions may appear on or in the corresponding ear. In 80% of the victims, muscle tone begins to return in a few weeks and movement is usually restored over a period of months.

The treatment of Bell's Palsy is controversial. Steroid tablets may be prescribed for 1–2 weeks, although the condition often resolves without any medication. Patients should be advised about eye protection and they may need to wear a pad or goggles for a while.

POLYNEURITIS (MULTIPLE PERIPHERAL NEURITIS)

Although the term neuritis implies inflammation, it is more often applied to any neuropathy where there is dysfunction and pain of peripheral nerves from any cause. Polyneuritis is a disorder in which there is pain and impaired function along the distribution of many peripheral nerves. It is usually symmetrical and both motor and sensory disturbances occur.

Effects on the patient

The symptoms generally start in the parts innervated by the distal portions of the nerves and spread proximally. The patient first experiences pain, pins and needles, tingling and weakness in hands and feet ('glove and stocking' effect), then a progressive loss of sensation, diminished tendon reflexes and inability to perform finer movements. The areas are tender and sore when subjected even to light pressure.

The causes include toxicity, nutritional deficiencies (especially vitamin B complex), metabolic disorder and cell-mediated immunological response. In some instances, the cause is not identified.

Some of the more common polyneuropathies are diabetic polyneuritis, vitamin deficiency polyneuritis associated with alcoholism, arsenic or lead polyneuritis, malnutrition polyneuritis and acute idiopathic polyneuritis (Guillain–Barré syndrome).

GUILLAIN–BARRÉ SYNDROME (ACUTE INFECTIVE POLYNEUROPATHY)

The Guillain–Barré syndrome is an inflammatory disease of the spinal nerve roots within the dural sheath, of the peripheral nerves and may also involve the cranial nerves. The loss of nerve impulse conduction that occurs is due to compression, demyelination and nerve degeneration as a result of the inflammation and oedema.

Incidence and aetiology

It may occur at any age but the incidence is greater in persons 30–40 years of age. Men and women are equally affected. The cause of the disorder is unknown but viral infection and immunological reaction are both suspect.

Frequently, the patients give a history of having 'just had' an upper respiratory infection or a gastrointestinal disturbance.

Effects on the patient

The onset of Guillain–Barré syndrome is usually abrupt. Bilateral muscle weakness, beginning in the legs, may ascend to involve the trunk, arms and cranial nerves. Paraesthesia may precede the weakness. Within a few days, the weakness is followed by flaccid motor paralysis with weakness of the respiratory muscles. If the cranial nerves become involved, inability to swallow, talk or even close the eyes develops. Muscle tenderness or sensitivity of the nerves to pressure may be experienced. Autonomic changes include sinus tachycardia and hypertension in the acute phase followed by hypotension.

Guillain–Barré syndrome is life-threatening due to potential respiratory and vasomotor failure if mechanical ventilation and vasopressor drugs are not promptly available. The mortality rate is estimated at 10–20%; death may result from a superimposed infection. Complete spontaneous recovery within weeks or months is usually anticipated in the survivors.

In some instances, steroids may be used to counteract the inflammation. Treatment is mainly supportive and intensive nursing care along the lines discussed in this chapter is needed to help the patient survive the acute episode.

CASE Kenny is a 44-year-old nurse who made an appointment to see his GP, with a history of viral illness within the previous 2 weeks. He is married to a school teacher and has two teenage children. On awakening this morning he found both his legs to be weak when stepping out of bed and complained of tingling in his arms and legs. General lethargy accompanied these symptoms.

His GP arranged admission to the medical observation ward where over the next 24–48 hours the weakness ascended to include his trunk and upper arms. He also complained of difficulty when breathing, and his respiratory effort was noted to be laboured.

The neurologist was asked to review Kenny and a diagnosis of Guillain–Barré Syndrome was confirmed.

What immediate nursing care do you think Kenny would require over the next few days?

Immediate care should include monitoring of vital signs; including respiratory rate, FiO$_2$ and Forced Vital Capacity (FVC). Care of the patient's airway including administration of oxygen/ventilation and tracheal suctioning if required. Admission to an Intensive Care Unit or High Dependency Unit may be required if the patient requires mechanical ventilation. Plasmapheresis and immunoglobulin therapy may also be indicated. Accurate monitoring of limb power is essential and limbs showing weakness must be carefully positioned and supported. Psychological support is essential as he may be very anxious due to his knowledge of the possible outcome of the condition.

Prior to discharge what would be the priorities in his care and what problems might he face after discharge?

This is a long-term disorder with patients taking up to 6 months to recover and approximately one-third of patients will be left with significant long-term neurological deficit. Prior to discharge, therefore, there would be emphasis on physiotherapy to build up his strength, mobility and respiratory function. Careful assessment of his abilities and home circumstances are essential pre-discharge. Key issues would be whether he needed any aids to allow him to manage at home, as it would be very difficult for his wife, given her job, to look after him. There would also be concerns about when and if he could resume his own employment with potential psychological implications such as anxiety and depression as a result. The primary healthcare team responsible for him after discharge will need to be fully informed of his progress and there must be follow-up out patient arrangements in place.

SUMMARY

The critical importance to human functioning of the nervous system cannot be overemphasized and the features unique to this system must be borne in mind at all times. Health problems may affect a person at any age and be potentially devastating in impact, leaving major long-term deficits. The nursing care of patients whose central nervous system has been impaired by trauma or disease is challenging and demanding, requiring patience, understanding and long-term commitment.

REFERENCES

Acorn S (1995) Assisting families of head injured survivors through a family support programme. Journal of Advanced Nursing 21(5): 872–877.

Birks J and Harvey RJ (2006) Donepezil for dementia due to Alzheimer's Disease (Cochrane Review) The Cochrane Library Issue 1. Chichester, UK: John Wiley and Sons.

BBC (2005) Huntington's Disease. Online. Available: www.bbc.co.uk/health/conditions/huntingtons1.shtml [Accessed 20.04.2006].

British National Formulary (BNF) (2005) British National Formulary 49; March. London: BMA/RPSGB.

Bogglid M, Ford H (2004) Multiple sclerosis. In: Clinical Evidence 11. London: BMJ Publishing. p. 322–324.

Epilepsy Action (2006) The role of primary care in epilepsy management 2. Epilepsy Action: Leeds.

Filbin M, Tsien C, Caughey A (2002) Clinical cases in emergency medicine. Malden: Blackwell Science.

Haslett C, Chilvers E, Boon N, Colledge N (2002) Davidson's principles and practice of medicine, 19th edn. Edinburgh: Elsevier.

Hickey JV (2002) The clinical practice of neurological and neurosurgical nursing, 4th edn. Philadelphia: Lippincott.

Lindsay K, Bone I (2004) Neurology and neurosurgery illustrated, 3rd edn. Edinburgh: Churchill Livingstone.

National Institute of Clinical Excellence (2001) Alzheimer's disease – donepezil, rivastigmine and galantamine (No. 19).

Online. Available: www.nice.org.UK/page.aspx?o=TA019 [Accessed 20.04.2006].

National Institute of Clinical Excellence (2004a) Technology appraisal No.76. Newer drugs for epilepsy in adults. London: NICE. Online. Available: www.nice.org.UK/pdf/TA076

National Institute of Clinical Excellence (2004b) Technology appraisal No.79. Newer drugs for epilepsy in children. London: NICE. Online. Available: www.nice.org.UK/pdf/TA079

Nicoll R, Alger B (2004) The brain's own marijuana. Scientific American 291(6): 44–51.

Noback CR (1967) The human nervous system. New York: McGraw Hill.

Nowak T, Handford G (2004) Pathophysiology, 3rd edn. Boston: McGraw Hill.

Parkinson's Disease Society (2006) Who gets Parkinson's? Online. Available: www.parkinsons.org.uk/Templates/ Internal.asp?NodeID=89606 [Accessed 20.04.2006].

Royal College of Physicians (2004) Primary care concise guidelines for stroke. Online. Available: www.rcplondon.ac.uk [Accessed 20.04.2006].

Scottish Intercollegiate Guidelines Network (2000) Early management of patients with a head injury. Edinburgh: SIGN.

Stroke Association (2006) Information. Online. Available: www.stroke.org.uk [Accessed 14.04.2006].

Watkins L (2000) Head injuries: General principles and management. Surgery 128(2): 219–224.

FURTHER READING AND USEFUL WEBSITES

Hickey JV (2002) The clinical practice of neurological and neurosurgical nursing, 4th edn. Philadelphia: Lippincott.
An invaluable textbook covering all aspects of neuroscience nursing practice. Provides in-depth information on all the major areas of practice with a clear explanation of the underpinning skills and knowledge. Comprehensively referenced and clearly written.

Gerrero D (1998) Neuro-oncology for nurses. London: Whurr.
Useful textbook providing insightful knowledge of the multiple problems facing patients with tumours of the nervous system. Written from a multidisciplinary perspective it provides guidance on the care required by these patients.

Landstaff D, Christie J (2000) Trauma care: a team approach. Oxford: Butterworth Heinemann.
A helpful text emphasizing the team approach to the care of trauma patients. Although it deals with all types of trauma the threads woven through the book make it useful reading for nurses dealing with patients with trauma to the nervous system.

McLean C (2001) Moving and positioning patients with altered intracranial haemodynamics. Nursing in Critical Care 6(5): 239.
Helpful up-to-date article on nursing patients with raised ICP. Reviews the research previously carried out and places this in the context of modern day nursing practice.

Alzheimer's Association	www.alzheimers.org.uk
British Epilepsy Association	www.epilepsy.org.uk
British Vascular Foundation	www.bvf.org.uk
Brain Injury Association	www.headway.org.uk
Huntington's Disease Association	www.hda.org.uk
Multiple Sclerosis Society	www.mssociety.org.uk
Parkinson's Disease Society	www.parkinsons.org.uk
Stroke Association	www.stroke.org.uk
Trigeminal Neuralgia Association UK	www.tna-uk.org.uk

21 Caring for the patient with a disorder of the senses

Mike Walsh

INTRODUCTION

Usually, people are able to interpret the world and communicate with it by using five special senses. These are sight, hearing, taste, touch and smell.

The senses all work in a similar way: sensory receptor cells in the relevant organ are stimulated, and the sensory impulse produced is transmitted to the relevant part of the brain via the cranial or the spinal nerves. Different parts of the brain are responsible for receiving and interpreting sensory impulses from different parts of the body.

Sensory impulses for sight, hearing, taste and smell are all transmitted via the cranial nerves, whereas sensory impulses for touch are carried by general somatic afferent nerve fibres via the spinal cord to the brain. (For a fuller discussion of the nervous system, refer to Ch. 20.)

It can be seen from Figure 21.1 that there are many potential areas for problems to arise in the sensory pathway. The first occurs when a stimulus fails to reach the receptor cell. This happens if you have a heavy cold – even a strong smell cannot reach the sensory receptor cells for smell, which lie high up in the nose. The second potential failure is if something fails within the organ, preventing the receptor cells from functioning. For example, the receptor cells on a detached retina cannot hope to function correctly. The next possible problem area is within the transmission system of nerves that link the sensory organ with the brain. Finally, there may be problems within the brain itself, which prevent correct reception and interpretation of the incoming sensory impulses. In some rare cases, this leads to a situation where different senses become blended so that the person may feel a taste or see colours when they listen to certain sounds. Many cases have been reliably documented such as seeing blue when listening to a C-sharp note played on a piano or experiencing a bitter taste in response to touch sensation of the hands. This is known as *synesthesia* and is believed to happen when activation of one sensory area of the brain inadvertently activates a different sensory area at

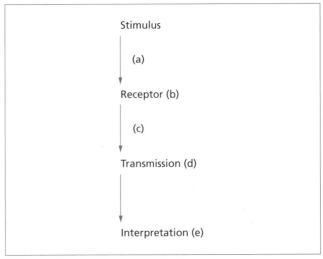

Figure 21.1 Problems in the sensory pathway. (a) The stimulus fails to reach the receptor cells (e.g. glue ear, heavy cold). (b) The receptor cells fail to receive the stimulus (e.g. detached retina). (c) The receptor cells fail to trigger the sensory nerve. (d) The nerve pathway is injured. (e) Brain injury or a congenital problem prevents reception of interpretation of sensory impulses.

the same time, due to abnormal neural structures within the brain (Ramachandran and Hubbard 2005).

This chapter focuses on problems associated with the ear, nose and eye, and the care required by people with these disorders. There is much still to learn about how our senses work, as the example of synesthesia illustrates.

STRUCTURE AND FUNCTIONS OF THE EAR

The **ear** is concerned with the special sense of hearing as well as with the maintenance of balance and equilibrium. Figure 21.2 shows the principle components. It has three divisions: the external and middle ears for the collection and conduction of sound waves, and the inner ear, which converts sound waves into auditory nerve impulses which proceed to the brain. The inner ear also plays a crucial role in balance and equilibrium. The eighth cranial nerve provides the afferent nerve pathway and is divided into the cochlear branch which carries impulses to the interpretive centres for sound in the temporal lobes, and the vestibular branch which transmits impulses to areas of the brainstem and cerebellum associated with control of body posture.

EXTERNAL EAR

The **outer ear** consists of the *auricle* (*pinna*) and the external auditory meatus. The auricle consists largely of cartilage and leads to the external auditory meatus. This ends at the tympanic membrane (eardrum), which separates the external and middle ears. The skin lining of the canal is covered with fine hairs near the opening and has special glands which produce a sticky, waxy secretion called *cerumen* which helps prevent small foreign bodies entering the auditory

canal. The *tympanic membrane* is a thin, semitransparent membrane covered externally with skin and internally with mucous membrane, which is continuous with that which lines the middle ear cavity. The middle layer is composed of thin elastic and fibrous tissue.

MIDDLE EAR

This portion of the ear is contained within a small cavity in the temporal bone. The cavity communicates with the nasopharynx by means of the *auditory* or *Eustachian tube*, and with the mastoid cells. The auditory tube permits the entrance of air into the **middle ear**; this equalizes the pressure on the internal surface of the eardrum with atmospheric pressure. The cavity is lined with mucous membrane which is continuous with that of the auditory tube and mastoid cells. The *mastoid cells* are small air spaces within the posterior portion of the temporal bone, just behind the middle ear.

The middle ear cavity contains three small bones called the auditory ossicles, which are movable for the purpose of transmitting and amplifying sound vibrations. The first ossicle, the *malleus*, is attached to the eardrum and articulates with the second ossicle, the *incus*. The incus articulates with the third ossicle, the *stapes*, which is attached to the membranous oval window (fenestra ovalis) that leads into the inner ear. The middle ear also has two small muscles; one, the tensor tympani, is inserted on the malleus and the other, the stapedius, is inserted on the footplate of the stapes. Contraction of these muscles reduces the amplitude of the sound waves entering the middle ear and cochlea and therefore protects the inner ear from damage due to loud noise.

INNER EAR (LABYRINTH)

The **inner ear** consists of a system of irregularly shaped cavities containing fluid and complex membranous structures that initiate nerve impulses in cranial nerve VIII as a result of sound waves (cochlear branch) or change of position (vestibular branch). The *bony (osseous) labyrinth* contains the *membranous labyrinth*, which conforms fairly closely to the shape of the bony-walled cavities, and is divided into a series of channels: the cochlea, vestibule and semicircular canals (Fig. 21.3):

- The *cochlea* is a complex snail-shaped structure (Fig. 21.4). Auditory nerve impulses are produced by receptor cells within the organ of Corti (special cells with hair-like projections on the surface of the basilar membrane) when stimulated by vibrations of the basilar membrane (Fig. 21.5)
- The *vestibule* lies between the cochlea and the semicircular canals. Within the cavities of the vestibule are hair-like projections and calcium carbonate concretions (*otoliths*) which respond to movements of the head by giving rise to neural impulses concerned with the maintenance of equilibrium

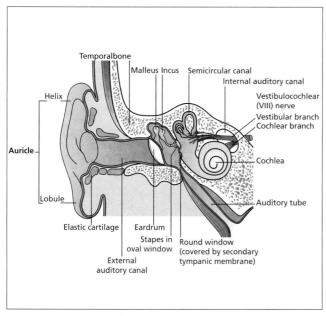

Figure 21.2 Main structures of the ear. (Based on Tortora and Grabowski 2003, p. 545.)

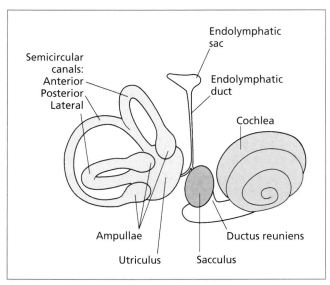

Figure 21.3   The membranous labyrinth of the ear.

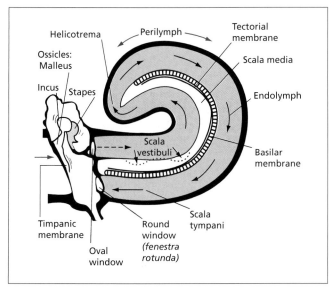

Figure 21.4   Schematic drawing of the cochlea.

● The *semicircular canals* are hollowed out of the temporal bone at right angles to each other. Each membranous semicircular canal has a dilated portion at one end, called the *ampulla*, which contains special sensory hair cells, forming the *crista acustica*, or crista ampullaris. The crista is sensitive to movement of the endolymph within the ampulla and initiates neural impulses concerned with balance and position. These are transmitted by the vestibular branch of cranial nerve VIII to the central nervous system.

AUDITORY PATHWAY

Sound waves passing into the external ear strike the tympanic membrane, causing it to vibrate with the same frequency as the sound waves. This in turn results in vibrations

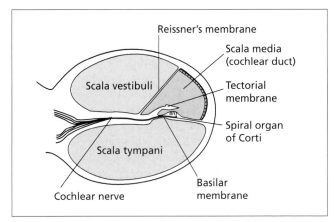

Figure 21.5   Cross-section of the cochlea.

of the ossicles in the middle ear. The stapes, being attached to the oval window, causes its membrane to move in and out. This mechanism amplifies the vibrations of the oval window by a factor of 20 compared with the tympanic membrane but, if the amplitude of the waves is excessive (i.e. the sound is very loud), the vibrations may be modified by contraction of the tensor tympani and the stapedius muscles. The vibrations caused by the sound waves are transferred through the endolymph to the basilar membrane. Movements of the endolymph and basilar membrane stimulate the receptor cells of the organ of Corti, initiating neural impulses which are transmitted via the cochlear branch of cranial nerve VIII. The impulses are then transmitted through the thalami and eventually reach a cortical area of the temporal lobe (auditory centre) where they are interpreted as sound. Each ear delivers impulses to both auditory centres.

PITCH AND INTENSITY OF SOUND

The pitch of a sound depends upon the frequency of the vibrations (number of cycles per second). Frequency is measured in units called hertz (Hz) and one cycle per second equals 1 Hz. The pitch of sound is therefore measured in Hz. The fibres of the basilar membrane vary in length. It is thought that different frequencies stimulate selective areas of fibres and cells of the membrane, that is, each place on the basilar membrane is sensitive to sound waves of a certain frequency.

The intensity, or loudness, of a sound depends upon the amplitude or height of the soundwaves which control the vibrations or displacements of the delicate middle and inner ear structures. Loudness is measured in decibels (dB) which is a logarithmic scale. An increase in 10 dB from say 50–60 dB therefore corresponds to a 10-fold increase in loudness. A whisper measures 30 dB, normal speech 60 dB, shouting 80 dB, a nearby motorcycle 90 dB. The volume reached at large rock concerts is regularly 110 dB or more and some headphones can also be played at this volume. Hearing damage develops with repeated exposure to sounds over 90 dB (Tortora and Grabowski 2003).

EQUILIBRIUM AND BALANCE

When the head moves, neural impulses originate in the semicircular canals and the utricle and saccula, and are transmitted by the vestibular branch of the cranial nerve VIII. The vestibular nerve fibres pass to groups of neurones (vestibular nuclei) in the brainstem from which impulses may be delivered to the cerebellum, reticular formation, down the vestibulospinal tracts to motor neurones that innervate skeletal muscle, the oculomotor centre and the thalami. The principal purpose of these impulses is to orient the person in space, and to stimulate muscles in a reflex action so that s/he may assume an upright position or maintain the position that has been assumed against gravity.

THE PERSON WITH A DISORDER OF THE EAR

The ear is concerned with the special sense of hearing and with the maintenance of equilibrium. There are several places where the mechanisms involved can be disturbed. These are shown in Figure 21.6. The principal problems for people with disorders of the ear are related to loss (or potential loss) of hearing. The examinations, characteristics and tests used to determine the cause and severity of hearing loss are therefore given in detail here. Any specific tests for other conditions are given in the section on common disorders of the ear.

ASSESSMENT

The aim of the assessment of a person presenting with a problem relating to hearing or equilibrium maintenance is to determine the point at which the auditory mechanism is disturbed and with what severity. Any alteration in hearing or balance has an effect on normal living which is assessed in order to document change over time and to judge the effectiveness of any treatment or aids provided.

HEALTH HISTORY

As with any illness, the person's health history is noted, paying particular attention to previous ear disease, injuries or surgery, current and past occupations, family history of ear problems, current and past medications that might be relevant. The details of the present disorder (including the use of any hearing aids) are noted and any relevant changes in social or psychological behaviour described.

PHYSICAL EXAMINATION

The ear is inspected inside and outside. The pinna (auricle) is examined for size, position, symmetry and lesions, and the entrance of the ear canal is inspected for presence of debris or pus. The mastoid process is palpated, especially if infection of the middle ear is suspected and the tragus is palpated if infection of the external canal is suspected. It is also valuable to palpate the pre and postauricular lymph nodes for tenderness and swelling. The ear should then be inspected with an auriscope (otoscope) which has a magnifying lens in addition to a light. (See Fig. 21.7 for correct technique.) The canal is inspected for lesions, foreign bodies, and the amount and characteristics of the cerumen (wax). The tympanic membrane is viewed and the colour and tension noted (normal: a shiny light pearl-grey with a clear cone of reflected light). It is examined for retraction or bulging, increased vascularity and perforation.

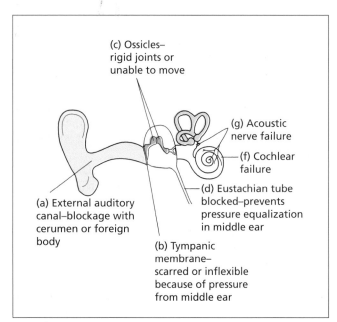

(c) Ossicles– rigid joints or unable to move

(g) Acoustic nerve failure

(f) Cochlear failure

(d) Eustachian tube blocked–prevents pressure equalization in middle ear

(a) External auditory canal–blockage with cerumen or foreign body

(b) Tympanic membrane– scarred or inflexible because of pressure from middle ear

Figure 21.6 Potential hearing loss problems.

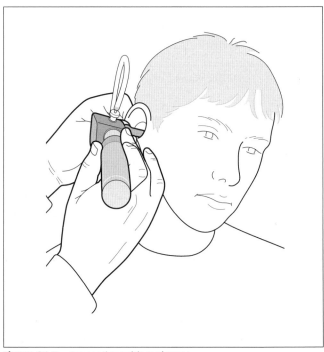

Figure 21.7 Inspection with auriscope.

Hearing evaluation

In hearing evaluation, the examiner assesses the degree of hearing loss and establishes whether it is due to conductive or nerve impairment. Conductive deafness results from failure of the conducting mechanism to transmit sound impulses from the external ear to the inner ear. Neural deafness can be a result of disease of the sensor organ (the cochlea), auditory nerve or auditory cerebral centre.

Hearing screening

A quick evaluation of hearing acuity can be made using whispered and spoken voice tests. Auditory acuity can be tested by first exhaling and then whispering a word or sequence of numbers softly towards one ear from a distance equal to arms length whilst the other ear is occluded. This is repeated for the other ear using a different word or sequence and the results are compared. The accuracy of this test has been scrutinized by Pirozzo et al (2004) in a systematic review of the literature and they concluded it is accurate for detecting hearing impairment in children and adults. More sophisticated testing of hearing loss involves audiometry. A specialist makes measurements with sophisticated equipment in a sound proof booth across a range of frequencies. Normal hearing is defined as having over 80% of the acuity that would be expected for a person of that age (Black and Hawks 2005).

Tuning fork tests

These are used to differentiate the type of deafness. A tuning fork with a frequency of 512 or 1024 Hz should be used. The tests should be made in a room free of noise:

The Rinne test. The Rinne test measures air and bone conduction. A tuning fork of 512 Hz is struck and held 2.5–5.0 cm in front of the patient's external auditory canal. It is then placed firmly on the mastoid process and the patient is asked to state whether it is heard better by air conduction (AC) or bone conduction (BC).

Further information can be obtained by placing the fork on the mastoid and asking the patient to state when the vibrations can no longer be heard, noting the time interval involved. The tuning fork is then quickly moved to be placed just at the entrance of the ear canal and the length of time the patient can still hear the sound is also noted. Normally air conduction will be longer than bone conduction and the record in the patient's notes is AC>BC (positive Rinne). Conversely, if the tuning fork can be heard longer by bone conduction than air conduction, bone conduction is better than air conduction – a negative Rinne test result.

In the normal ear, air conduction is better than bone (i.e. positive Rinne test result).

Weber's test. This test is used to assess whether there is conductive hearing loss in one ear compared with another. The tuning fork is set in vibration; the stem is held against the middle of the forehead and the patient is asked whether the sound is heard better in one ear than the other. Normally, the sound appears to be in the midline, being heard equally by both ears. If unilateral *conductive* deafness is present, the sound is greater in the affected ear. In lateralized, *sensorineural* loss of hearing (see below), the sound is heard in the normal ear.

CLASSIFICATION AND CAUSES OF HEARING LOSS

A hearing deficit may be congenital or acquired and may be classified as conductive, sensorineural, central or combined.

- In a *conductive hearing loss*, sound waves fail to reach the internal ear as a result of some disturbance in the external ear, middle ear or the oval window. The person with conductive deafness tends to speak softly as he or she can hear himself or herself
- In *sensorineural deafness*, which may also be called *nerve* or *perceptive deafness*, the disorder is located in the organ of Corti, cochlear branch cranial nerve VIII or auditory impulse pathway or centre within the brain. The person with nerve deafness cannot hear anything, so tends to shout, hoping to hear
- *Central hearing loss* denotes a hearing deficit resulting from disturbances within the brain, principally the auditory centre in the temporal lobe
- *Combined hearing loss* occurs because of impairment within both the conductive and neural auditory mechanisms
- *Congenital loss of hearing* may be due to a prenatal malformation or lack of development of a part of the auditory apparatus. Heredity may play a role, or it may be the result of a viral infection in the mother during the first trimester of the pregnancy, the effect of a toxic drug taken by the mother during pregnancy, hypoxia or a birth injury
- *Acquired impairment of hearing* may be caused by obstruction of the external auditory canal by a foreign body or impacted cerumen, infection (e.g. otitis media), a neoplasm (e.g. acoustic neuroma), an ototoxic drug (e.g. streptomycin), trauma associated with a skull fracture or excessively loud noise, or obstruction of the Eustachian tube. Degenerative changes in the auditory pathway are frequently associated with the ageing process (presbykousis) and may also cause acquired hearing loss.

The problems of loss of hearing depend on the degree of deficit and on the age at which it developed. In the case of a child with a congenital loss of hearing causing total deafness, all communication will need to be visual and tactile, so affecting the child's whole life and producing behavioural, socioeconomic and emotional changes for the entire family. A partial hearing loss in an adult does not have the same impact.

The clinical characteristics of loss of hearing can be described in relation to:

- direct effects of impaired hearing (e.g. communication difficulties)
- direct behavioural response to impaired hearing
- indirect psychosocial response to impaired hearing.

Box 21.1   Clinical characteristics of loss of hearing

Direct effects

- Failure to perceive a threatening situation
- Failure to respond when addressed
- Frequent requests for repetition
- Misinterpretation
- Changes in speech such as low volume or lack of inflection

Behavioural responses

- Turning the head to direct the 'good' ear towards the sound
- Strained, confused expression
- Short attention span
- Lack of interest
- Irritability
- Fatigue due to the effort of trying to hear

Psychosocial responses

- Withdrawal from group activities (hearing is more difficult in a group)
- Avoidance of noisy places and situations
- Some people respond by talking continuously, to avoid the situation of someone else speaking and being unable to hear
- Some pretend they can hear, and assume a permanent smile or responsive look, often inappropriately
- Changes in normal activities (such as watching TV, going to the cinema, etc.) may produce anger, boredom, loneliness, etc.

These are described in Box 21.1.

The *goals* of nursing care are to assist the patient to:

1 preserve or maintain hearing
2 identify factors contributing to hearing loss
3 maintain or develop ability to communicate with others
4 recognize and develop strategies to counteract psychosocial changes.

NURSING INTERVENTION

Preservation of hearing

Nurses, especially those working with industrial workers and schoolchildren, have an important role in the prevention of hearing loss. The public requires education about the causes and early signs of impaired hearing and about significant preventive measures.

Good prenatal care and the avoidance of contact with persons with measles or other viral infections are important in preventing congenital deafness. Immunization against measles should be promoted and is most effective when part of the combined triple MMR vaccine. Prompt treatment of respiratory infection and infectious diseases may allay the complication of otitis media. Prompt medical treatment and follow-up are urged for persons with an ear disorder. The nurse caring for a patient receiving any of the aminoglycoside antibiotics (e.g. neomycin, gentamicin) must be alert for early signs of damage to hearing, as this is a well known dose-related side-effect of this class of drugs (British National Formulary 2005).

The danger of introducing foreign objects into the external ear canal should be emphasized to patients. Cleansing the ear with applicators or hairpins is dangerous, as accidental perforation of the eardrum may occur.

The occupational health nurse, especially in an industry in which there is prolonged, intense noise in the work environment, must be aware of the possibility of noise-induced hearing loss. Frequently the employees tend to accept noise simply as a necessary part of the occupation and do not realize that hearing damage may be developing insidiously. Gradual loss of hearing usually involves, first, failure of response to high-frequency sounds. Later, areas of the cochlea that respond to lower frequencies become damaged. In order to protect persons exposed to noise that endangers hearing, protective devices in the form of ear defenders should be provided. Employees should receive regular hearing tests and be exposed to an active educational programme.

High-intensity music such as rock music is another source of noise pollution. Public education about the effects of noise pollution and the importance of the use of ear defenders to decrease the intensity of the noise is necessary and should be directed to high-risk groups.

Advice

Suggestions of strategies that can sometimes help in interactions with someone who is hard of hearing are listed in Box 21.2.

Hearing aids

Some people with a hearing deficit may be helped by using a hearing aid, which is a small, battery-operated instrument that amplifies sounds. Aids are helpful to people who have reduced conduction of sound waves into the inner ear. Few of those with sensorineural loss of hearing receive help from hearing aids; amplification of sound does not assist with the distortion and impaired discrimination resulting from impairment of the neural elements of the auditory apparatus. Before purchasing a hearing aid, the person with a hearing deficit should be examined by a doctor for evaluation of the residual hearing and identification of the type of hearing loss. The selection of the aid is based on the patient's particular type of hearing loss. If an aid is recommended, it should be worn for a trial period to determine whether it does help.

Box 21.2 Suggestions to improve communication with a person who is hard of hearing

For those speaking to a person who is hard of hearing

- Use touch to attract attention

- Avoid a noisy environment

- Do not speak until you have the person's attention. The speaker's face should be in full view of the listener so that lip movement may be observed

- Determine which is the better ear and go to that side if possible

- Speak slowly, enunciate clearly and avoid raising the pitch of the voice. Increase the volume but do not shout. Guard against running words together. Use the natural form of conversation rather than broken and incomplete sentences

- Exaggerated lip movements will only confuse the listener

- If repetition is necessary, rephrase the communication if possible. Remember that vowels are heard more readily than consonants

- Always check that important communications have been understood

- Increase the use of touch to express emotion and comfort

- Patience, tact and understanding are needed. Avoid any irritation or annoyance; such reactions only discourage the listener

- Do not prolong a conversation unnecessarily

- If a hearing aid is used, give the listener time to adjust to it

- If a misinterpretation occurs, do not ridicule it or treat it as a joke

- When a person hard of hearing enters a room, make an effort to draw him or her into the group. Advise them of the topic of conversation and encourage them to participate

- If it is not possible to communicate verbally, write the message down

- If a patient is totally deaf and does not lip-read, pictures or symbols that represent objects may be helpful to orient the patient and for use during hospitalization

For those who are hard of hearing

- Look directly at the speaker (preferably in a good light), as observation of lip movements proves helpful

- Concentrate on the speaker

- Observe the total situation, as this may give a lead to the topic of conversation

- Acknowledge your hearing deficit; do not guess at things rather than ask for repetition

- Indicate understanding of the speaker

- Tell people you need to communicate with that you are hard of hearing

- Ask for written information where possible, or ask where you can get it

- Limit stressful situations to avoid fatigue

- If your attention is wandering, ask for a short break

- Try to develop interests that do not involve a lot of listening or verbal interaction.

Auditory and speech training

Auditory training is intended to help the individual utilize residual hearing effectively and improve communication skills. The process helps the patient develop good listening skills and increases his or her awareness of sounds and other clues.

Lip-reading or *speech reading* is the process of interpreting spoken words through the study of lip movements, facial expressions, body movements and gestures used in speech. Training helps the individual to use these cues consciously and effectively.

Speech training is provided to maintain existing speech skills, which deteriorate when the usual monitoring mechanism of hearing is lost. Hearing is necessary to assess loudness, clarity, tone and rate of speech. The congenitally deaf child requires a different type of programme to develop speech and language skills.

Community resources

Those who are deaf or hard of hearing and their families should be familiar with the Royal National Institute for the Deaf and Hard of Hearing. Assistance may be provided in the form of procuring medical examination and treatment, counselling as to the type of hearing aid that would be helpful, obtaining vocational training and employment, arranging for special classes (e.g. speech) and obtaining printed advice in pamphlets.

COMMON DISORDERS OF THE EAR

Impacted cerumen

The normal secretion of the external auditory canal (cerumen) may accumulate and become hard and dry. The retention may be due to abnormal narrowness of the canal, dryness of the skin or excess hair in the canal, or misguided attempts to clean the ear with cotton-wool buds. It may also be associated with the person's occupation; it is a common problem for those working in a dusty or dry environment.

Symptoms develop with the obstruction of the canal; the person may experience a sense of fullness, noises, loss of hearing, irritation or, rarely, a cough. The latter is a reflex response to stimulation of the vagus nerve. Examination of the ear with an otoscope reveals a firm yellow or dark mass.

Ear syringing is the traditional method of removing the wax. Although there is widespread consensus that this is effective, there are no RCTs to support this technique and there are many reported complications such as perforation of the ear drum, otitis externa, tinnitus, pain and vertigo (Browning 2004). An alternative is to try and use a wax softener (arachis or olive oil) but again the evidence is lacking as to how effective the different preparations are.

Otitis externa

This is a generalized inflammation of the external ear. The cause is frequently bacterial, but in some instances may be a fungus, or the inflammation may be associated with eczema or an allergic reaction. An infection is more likely to develop in a warm moist atmosphere or if the person swims frequently. It may be secondary to trauma inflicted by efforts to remove wax. External otitis may also be due to allergic dermatitis.

Characteristics

Pain, discharge from the external auditory meatus and tenderness are common. The patient may complain of pruritus or have raised temperature. Upon inspection, the ear canal may show signs of inflammation and swelling.

Treatment

Paracetamol may be necessary for pain relief. Thorough cleansing of the ear may be sufficient to encourage recovery or a wick soaked in aluminium acetate solution may be packed into the ear. If infection is present, a topical preparation of neomycin based ear-drops (which may include a steroid) can be prescribed. Van Balen et al (2003) present strong evidence for the use of steroids with either, antibacterial ear drops, or acetic acid drops. Their RCT covered 47 general practices and measured patients' self reported symptoms. They showed that the presence of steroids in either type of drops reduced the period until self reported cure by a mean of one day. As with all antibiotics, the use of antibiotic ear drops is used after a careful assessment of the pros and cons of treatment. Avoiding the overuse of antibiotics, even in ear drops, can help to prevent the problem of bacterial resistance and the potential for untreatable infections in the future.

Acute otitis media

This is an inflammation of the middle ear and is frequently a complication of an upper respiratory tract infection or an infectious disease, as in measles. Often the organisms gain access through the auditory tube and, less frequently, through a perforation in the tympanic membrane. The disorder is usually acute but may become chronic. Young children frequently present in A&E or in primary care with this condition, frequently being under 3 years of age.

The initial inflammatory response causes congestion and swelling of the mucous membrane lining of the middle ear, and the cavity fills with exudate. The tympanic membrane bulges externally and, unless the infection is checked, the exudate generally becomes purulent. If the cavity is not drained, the tympanic membrane may rupture spontaneously.

Characteristics

The patient with otitis media experiences a sensation of fullness in the ear and dullness of hearing at first, then severe pain, and increasing loss of hearing because of failure of the conduction of sound waves through the middle ear. The temperature and leucocyte count are raised and the patient feels generally ill. Examination of the eardrum by means of an auriscope reveals redness, hyperaemia and external bulging due to the pressure of the collection of exudate in the middle ear, or rupture and discharge in the advanced stage.

Treatment

As the causative agent is frequently viral, analgesia (paracetamol or ibuprofen) may be the only medication required. In 80% of children with acute otitis media (AOM) the condition will have resolved within 3 days. In children without systemic features, the British National Formulary (2005) recommends that a broad spectrum antibacterial may be started if their condition has not resolved after 3 days. However, O'Neil and Roberts (2004) report that 97% of under 3 year olds attending their GP with AOM in the UK receive antibacterial treatment, so there is something of a discrepancy between what is recommended and practiced. If bacteria are cultured from any discharge an appropriate systemic antibiotic is required together with analgesia. The eardrum may occasionally be surgically opened to permit drainage if the exudate is producing excessive pressure on the eardrum and there is danger of spontaneous rupture. The operative procedure is referred to as a *myringotomy*. Delayed treatment of acute otitis media may predispose to mastoiditis, chronic otitis media and permanent hearing loss.

The patient having a myringotomy receives a local anaesthetic. Fluid is aspirated from the middle ear cavity through the incision, and a culture is taken. The patient is encouraged to lie on the affected side to promote drainage. A persistent increase in temperature, pain and deep tenderness in the region of the mastoid, headache, drowsiness or disorientation is reported to the doctor. These may indicate the onset of a serious complication such as mastoiditis, meningitis or brain abscess.

Chronic otitis media

This chronic inflammatory disorder is associated with a permanent perforation of the tympanic membrane. It is usually a result of repeated episodes of AOM that were not treated or were caused by virulent or antibiotic-resistant organisms. The perforation may also be the result of mechanical trauma or blast injury.

The location of the perforation is an important factor in the severity of the disease. If it is central, or at least does not involve the margin of the eardrum, the perforation is less serious and can be treated more effectively. This type of perforation is categorized as *tubotympanic*. If the perforation involves the tympanic margin in the posterior-superior area, it is called an *attic or marginal perforation*.

Characteristics

The otitis media associated with a central perforation is manifested by purulent discharge through the perforation in the eardrum with an offensive odour (otorrhoea). The discharge may be greatly increased during periods of acute upper respiratory infections or if water gets into the ear during bathing or swimming. Over a period of time, middle ear structures are damaged by the infection and necrosis. There is usually some impairment of hearing, which worsens during exacerbations.

Treatment

The initial treatment of the patients with a *tubotympanic perforation* is directed towards eliminating any upper respiratory tract infection as well as that in the ear. An antibiotic is administered orally or parenterally. The ear is cleansed by suction and dry mopping, followed by the instillation of an antimicrobial solution. If the exudate is excessive, it may be removed by daily aspiration by the doctor.

When the infection is cleared up, the perforated area very occasionally fills in with scar tissue. If the perforation persists, a tympanoplasty may be done to improve the patient's hearing and reduce the risk of reinfection by establishing a barrier between external and middle ears. Tympanoplastic surgery is undertaken only if infection is controlled.

In *marginal (attic) perforations* the disease involves the bony rim of the tympanic membrane and the mastoid cells as well as the middle ear structures. An invasive *cholesteatoma* may develop; this is a mass that forms in the middle ear as a result of the growth of epithelial tissue implanted in the middle ear from the collapsed parts of the eardrum when it perforates. The mass compresses middle ear structures and mastoid cells, causing necrosis and bone erosion. The presence of the cholesteatoma predisposes to the serious complications of labyrinthitis and brain abscess.

Marginal perforation and the development of a cholesteatoma are treated by radical surgery. A mastoidectomy is done, the cholesteatoma and middle ear debris are removed and reconstruction is undertaken to provide a conductive channel. The operation is done in two stages. The first operation removes the cholesteatoma and clears out the infected and necrotic tissue. The patient receives antibiotic therapy and, when the area is free of infection and there is no drainage, the reconstructive plastic surgery is undertaken.

Mastoiditis

The small spaces (air cells) in the mastoid communicate with the middle ear cavity and are lined with mucous membrane which is continuous with that of the middle ear. As a result, infection may spread readily to the mastoid in acute or chronic otitis media. The patient experiences tenderness over the mastoid process, headache and fever. Mastoid radiographs show a cloudiness in the mastoid cells.

Treatment and nursing intervention

The patient is often in severe pain with the presence of otorrhoea. Urgent treatment is necessary including hospital admission, powerful analgesia and intravenous antibacterial therapy (Reynolds 2004). If the infection is neglected or is virulent and unresponsive to the antibiotic given, bone tissue of the mastoid may become infected, necessitating surgery. A myringotomy and a simple mastoidectomy are done. A simple mastoidectomy involves an incision behind the auricle and the removal of the diseased bone by curettage.

If the patient develops chronic otitis media and chronic mastoiditis, more extensive surgery may be undertaken. A radical mastoidectomy involves the removal of the diseased mastoid tissue and the incus, malleus and remainder of the tympanic membrane, leaving the mastoid and middle ear as one large cavity. This operation on the middle ear results in loss of hearing.

Patients who have had surgery on the tympanic membrane should be informed that they may experience intermittent sharp pains for up to 3 weeks after operation due to the Eustachian tubes opening, allowing air to enter the middle ear. The external auditory canal will be packed immediately after operation and it is important that no water be allowed to enter the canal for up to 6 weeks after surgery.

The patient is observed closely for any sign of facial paralysis. Facial paralysis is a threat in mastoidectomy because of the proximity of the facial (seventh cranial) nerve to the operative site. Vertigo is another potential complication because of the proximity of the semicircular canals to the area being operated on. The patient is generally allowed up on the evening of surgery or the following morning; someone remains at first in case of dizziness and nausea which may develop as a result of labyrinth disturbance, especially following a radical mastoidectomy.

Otosclerosis

This is a chronic ear disease in which the stapes becomes immobilized because of progressive growth of bone tissue over the oval window and fixation of the stapes, interfering with the transmission of vibrations into the inner ear. Both ears are affected eventually.

The disease appears to be hereditary and has a higher incidence in females. The ability of the stapes to vibrate decreases progressively, and the loss of hearing usually becomes apparent in the teens or twenties, and during pregnancy. The person may complain of tinnitus as the deafness becomes more marked. The testing of hearing with a tuning fork reveals that the person has good bone conduction of sound but none by air.

Treatment

A hearing aid may be of some help for a period of time, but a stapedectomy has proved to be the treatment of choice at present. By means of a surgical microscope, the surgeon works through the external auditory canal and the middle ear. The stapes is removed, and a prosthesis introduced to transfer the vibrations of the incus through the oval window into the inner ear. The oval window niche is sealed using a free graft of fat or vein, and protected with Gelfoam. Only one ear is done at a time.

After operation, dizziness and nausea may be troublesome because of the disturbance of the labyrinth. A specific directive is received from the surgeon about the position in which the head is to be maintained as practices vary in different hospitals. The patient is instructed not to blow the nose to prevent air from being forced through the Eustachian tube to the middle ear. The patient is cautioned to move slowly and not to stoop over. If vertigo is experienced, ambulation may have to be delayed. The patient requires assurance that the dizziness is temporary. The patient should be observed closely for nystagmus or any sign of facial palsy.

Tinnitus

Tinnitus or ringing in the ears may be unilateral or bilateral and constant or intermittent. It may be of high or low pitch and vary in quality from a humming, buzzing, hissing, roaring, popping or pulsating sound. The sound sensation experienced by the patient is without a relevant external stimulus. It is heard only by the patient and not by others. Tinnitus is not a disease but a symptom. It may be a symptom of any abnormal condition of the ear, may be associated with deafness, or it may be drug related. In many cases there is no treatment for tinnitus and the patient has to learn self help measures to live with the condition. Simple measures such as putting a radio under the pillow in bed at night can help to drown out the noise and prevent the patient from concentrating on the disturbing sound of the tinnitus.

Vertigo and vestibular dysfunction

Vertigo is a disturbance of equilibrium characterized by a sensation of movement or rotation of self or of the surroundings. The patient experiences feelings of dizziness, lightheadedness, falling or spinning. It may be accompanied by staggering or falling, clumsiness, nausea, vomiting or nystagmus which produces blurring of vision. Vertigo may occur suddenly, be transient in nature, or recur as with Ménière's syndrome. Disorders of the labyrinth are the most common cause. Disturbances in the pathways in the central nervous system may also produce vertigo.

Disorder of the vestibular system or lesions of the brain stem/cerebellum are the most common of many possible causes of nystagmus (Haslett et al 2002). Nystagmus occurs when the systems that control eye movement are ineffective. As a result, the eyes wander off target and repeated corrections are necessary to bring the eyes back on to the target object. Typically, the eyes drift slowly in one direction and then move rapidly back to the correct orientation giving a to-and-fro movement.

Ménière's disease or syndrome

This is a disorder of the internal ear characterized by recurrent attacks of severe vertigo, nausea, vomiting, tinnitus and a progressive loss of hearing. The cause is not known but an excess of endolymph (endolymphatic hydrops) develops, resulting in increased pressure and dilatation of the canals. Vascular spasm and allergic reaction have been suggested as possible aetiological factors. The disorder usually makes its appearance between the ages of 40 and 60 years, and occurs more often in males.

The episodes have a sudden onset, and the patient is generally prostrated by the dizziness and nausea. Attacks last from hours to days and may occur in clusters. Treatment is symptomatic and the patient should remain in bed in a quiet environment with precautions taken on movement because of the vertigo that accompanies the disorder. Medications such as prochlorperazine or betahistine may relieve the dizziness.

STRUCTURE AND FUNCTIONS OF THE NOSE

The nose is concerned with the special sense of smell as well as being the first organ of the respiratory system. Any alteration to the function or structure of the nose can affect the sense of **smell**. Air breathed in through the nose is warmed, filtered and moistened before entering the lower respiratory passages and the lungs.

Figure 21.8   The nasal cavity.

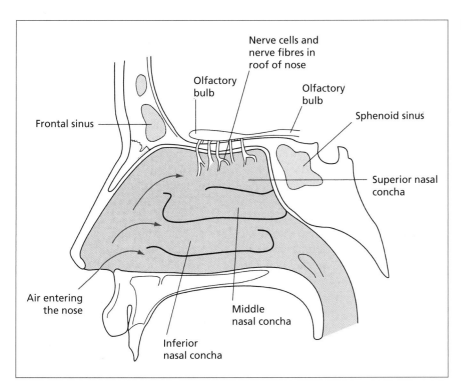

Nerve cells and
nerve fibres in
roof of nose

Olfactory
bulb

Olfactory
bulb

Sphenoid sinus

Frontal sinus

Superior nasal
concha

Air entering
the nose

Middle
nasal concha

Inferior
nasal concha

NASAL STRUCTURE

The two anterior nares (nostrils) form the openings into the nasal cavities, which are separated from each other by the nasal septum formed of cartilage and bone (Fig. 21.8). The roof of the nose is formed by the base of the skull. The floor is formed by the roof of the mouth and is composed of the maxillary bones, the palatine bones and the soft palate. The lateral walls of the nose are formed by bone of the maxilla and the ethmoid bone. Three bony ridges – the inferior, middle and superior conchae (or turbinates) – project from the outer wall of each nasal cavity partially to divide it into three passages. At the back of the nose these passages lead to the pharynx. The interior of the nose is lined with mucous membrane. Most of this membrane is covered with minute hair-like projections called *cilia*. Moving in waves, these cilia filter the air passing through the nasal passages and sweep the debris out of the cavity, together with nasal mucus. The mucous membrane also acts to warm and moisten the inhaled air and is therefore a very vascular tissue.

The nasal cavities have connections with the middle ears by the pharyngotympanic (Eustachian) tubes, and with the eye region by the nasolacrimal ducts. The adenoids, two small areas of lymphatic tissue, can be found on the wall of the nasopharynx, behind the nose.

The olfactory region

The first cranial (olfactory) nerve provides the afferent sensory impulse pathway. The nerve endings, the olfactory receptors, are located in two pea-sized areas high in the interior of the nasal cavity.

Molecules of the odorous material are carried into the nose with inhaled air where they stimulate molecular receptor sites on the olfactory hairs, tiny cilia which project from the dendrites of the first order neurones making up the olfactory pathway. When an individual is exposed continuously to an odour, perception of the odour decreases and eventually ceases. This loss of perception affects only that specific odour. The sense of smell may be diminished or lost entirely as a result of nasal obstruction or infection or trauma to the nasal tissue or the olfactory nerve. The complete absence of the sense of smell is called *anosmia*. We may distinguish up to 10 000 different odours (Tortora and Grabowski 2003).

The sense of smell deteriorates with aging and also as a result of smoking. Hyposmia means a reduced ability to smell and affects over half the population who are over 65 years of age.

The two senses of smell and taste are inextricably linked. Taste registers only five qualities: salt, sour, bitter, sweet and *unami* (a Japanese word meaning savoury). Other qualities of taste depend on smell. The sense of smell may affect the appetite positively or adversely, depending on whether the smell is pleasant or unpleasant.

The paranasal sinuses

The paranasal sinuses are commonly referred to as nasal sinuses, or simply as 'the sinuses'. They are the eight cavities in the skull that are connected with the nasal cavity. They are arranged in four pairs, with members of each pair placed symmetrically on each side of the head:

- the *maxillary* sinuses in the maxillae
- the *frontal* sinuses in the frontal bone
- the *sphenoid* sinuses in the sphenoid bone behind the nasal cavity

● the *ethmoid* sinuses in the ethmoid bone behind and below the frontal sinuses.

The function of the sinuses is not clearly understood but it is thought that they may help with the warming and moistening of inhaled air and provide a resonating chamber for the voice. Being air-filled chambers, they make the skull lighter than it would otherwise be.

The sinuses, all lined with mucous membrane, are each connected with the nasal cavity. One of the functions of the nose is to drain fluids discharged from the paranasal sinuses.

THE PERSON WITH A DISORDER OF THE NOSE OR NASAL SINUSES

ASSESSMENT

Health history

A nursing assessment of a patient with a disorder of the nose or nasal sinuses involves collecting information about any previous trauma or surgery that may have affected the anatomy of the region. Any history of previous, associated symptoms should also be recorded. Past medical history of hayfever, asthma or eczema is relevant in the assessment of a patient with a disorder of the nose as is a family history of each of these. A family or personal history of atopic type conditions (hayfever, asthma or eczema) can point to a possible allergic cause for the patient's symptoms. Smoking history is also important.

Information is obtained about the drugs being taken for the current problem, which may include inhalations and decongestants, as well as other medications.

The reason for seeking health care is identified. The manifestations, the duration, the timing and severity of the symptoms are determined.

Physical examination

The nose is examined both inside and out. The external nose is examined for asymmetry and lesions. The nostrils are examined for the presence of debris or discharge. The inside of the nasal cavity may be examined with nasal speculae and a light source for lesions and foreign bodies, and to determine the amount and characteristics of the nasal mucus. Any oedema or congestion of the mucous membranes will be noted. Air entry via each nostril is assessed by occluding the other. The patient may be asked to sniff to aid this assessment.

COMMON DISORDERS OF THE NOSE AND NASAL SINUSES

Acute coryza (common cold)

Most adults experience, on average, two to four attacks of acute coryza per year. The mucous membranes of the nose become swollen and there is a nasal discharge. Some types are accompanied by fever, muscle aches and general discomfort with sneezing and running eyes. Breathing through the nose may become difficult or impossible. Coryza is often accompanied by inflammation of the throat and sinuses.

Acute coryza is caused by a rhinovirus but may be complicated by a bacterial infection. The best treatment for the common cold is rest, preferably in bed, a well-balanced diet and sufficient liquid intake. Mild analgesia may be taken to relieve headache or fevers. It must be remembered that the common cold is highly contagious, both by direct contact with the virus (e.g. on a handkerchief) and by droplet inhalation (transmitted when coughing or sneezing).

Allergic rhinitis

Allergic rhinitis involves similar symptoms to the common cold of a running, congested nose and sneezing. However, it is an allergic response which may be seasonal in nature and caused by pollen (hay fever) or be caused by another non-seasonal allergen such as house dust or animal dander. There may be a similar response from irritants such as various chemicals or extreme cold, but this is not an allergic rhinitis. The symptoms can be treated in the first instance by steroid nasal sprays and avoidance of the trigger in the environment. Some patients also need to take an antihistamine when symptoms become particularly troublesome.

Epistaxis (nosebleed)

Epistaxis is usually due to the rupture of small blood vessels overlying the anterior part of the cartilaginous nasal septum. A minor nosebleed may be caused by a blow on the nose, irritation from foreign bodies (or fingers), or vigorous nose blowing. Treatment involves sitting the person up with head tilted forward to prevent the swallowing of blood, which is a gastric irritant. Pressure should be applied to the soft portion of the nose by grasping it between the thumb and forefinger. Pressure may need to be applied for up to 15 minutes. Once the bleeding has been arrested, the person should rest quietly for 1 hour or so, and avoid stooping or lifting for several hours. If bleeding persists, medical help should be sought as it may be necessary to pack the nose or cauterize the bleeding vessel.

Sometimes nosebleeds have serious underlying causes such as arteriosclerosis, polyps or other growths in the nose, hypertension or vitamin deficiencies. Anyone who experiences frequent or profuse nosebleeds should therefore seek medical advice. It is possible to lose a great deal of blood through a nose bleed and therefore if patients present to A&E with uncontrolled bleeding from the nose the nurse must be vigilant in taking regular blood pressure and pulse readings and assessing for hypovolaemic shock.

Surgery to the nose

Nasal surgery is indicated in a variety of conditions ranging from removal of a foreign body (usually in children) to the correction of a deviation of the nasal septum (caused by irregular growth or injury). Removal of polyps or other growths may be performed to restore normal nasal breathing, as may adenoidectomy in children. Cosmetic plastic surgery to correct disfiguring nasal anatomy is a common operation.

Any operation on the nose may result in swelling and bruising which may last for up to 6 weeks, so the success of the operation cannot be assessed immediately. The patient needs to be aware of this before the operation.

After operation, the most common complication is bleeding. Excessive bleeding is indicated if the patient becomes restless, swallows repeatedly or spits up blood. Nasal packing or a splint may be left in the nose to prevent the formation of a haematoma. These are usually removed by the surgeon or at the surgeon's direction. If severe swelling or bleeding are expected, ice compresses may be used to reduce these.

Most nasal surgery results in some mild discomfort. This is partly due to the swelling and bruising but also to the presence of crusts of dried blood and mucus in the nose. The patient must be discouraged from attempting to dislodge these by nose blowing or picking. Lubricants or humidification may be used to help soften crusts, but no swabs or other objects should be inserted into the nose. Mild analgesia may be given to reduce the discomfort.

Sinusitis

Sinusitis is the inflammation of one or more of the paranasal sinuses. It tends to occur when an upper respiratory tract infection spreads from the nose to the sinuses but may be associated with allergies, air pollution, diving or swimming. Any alteration to normal nasal breathing, such as that caused by a deviated nasal septum or polyps, may lead to sinusitis. As the inflammation of the mucous membranes lining the sinuses increases, swelling occurs and partially or totally occludes the ostium (opening into the nasal cavity), preventing the exudate from draining. Mucus then accumulates and becomes infected, creating pressure within the sinus. Thus the symptoms of sinusitis are pain located in and around the affected sinus, headaches, nasal discharge, fever and general malaise.

Radiological confirmation of the diagnosis can be undertaken, and this helps to identify any underlying problem such as polyps or deviated septum.

The treatment of acute sinusitis is with antibacterials (amoxicillin) and decongestants, with the inhalation of steam to help encourage drainage. Analgesia is given to relieve the discomfort. However, a review by Ah-See (2004) reported two randomised controlled trials (RCTs) which showed amoxicillin made no difference in symptoms compared with a placebo in patients with clinically diagnosed sinusitis. The evidence base for treating sinusitis with antibacterial drugs is therefore absent.

Chronic sinusitis occurs when the mucous membranes become thickened and obstruct the ostium, even when infection is not present. This prevents normal drainage from the sinus so that build-up of mucus occurs and frequent infections exacerbate the condition.

Treatment involves the identification and treatment of any underlying pathology, such as polyps or a deviated nasal septum. Changing the quality and humidity of the air in the home or workplace by using air-conditioners or filters and humidifiers may reduce the number and severity of the attacks. Failing this, drainage of the sinus may be performed surgically. Chronic sinusitis may lead to complications due to the proximity of other structures, such as the bones of the middle ear, the mastoid process and the brain, and for this reason it needs to be treated aggressively.

Disturbance in the sense of smell

While any of the above disorders can produce a disturbance or absence of the sense of smell, this condition (*anosmia*) is not life-threatening. The greatest impact is in the potential failure to smell burning or toxic chemicals, and the reduction in pleasure obtainable from the enjoyment of the taste and smell of foods, drinks and perfume.

STRUCTURE AND FUNCTIONS OF THE EYES

Vision, like all other sensory mechanisms, requires receptors, an afferent pathway to carry the impulses into the central nervous system and an interpretive centre. The **eyes** serve as receptors which are sensitive to light rays, the pathway is formed by the optic nerves and tracts within the brain, and the interpretive centres are composed of groups of neurones localized in the cortex of the cerebral occipital lobes (visual centres). In addition, the visual apparatus includes intrinsic and extrinsic muscles which play an important role in vision. There are also several accessory structures that function to protect the eyes. The main structures in the eye are shown in Figure 21.9.

LOCATION OF THE EYE

Each eyeball rests in a cone-shaped cavity (the *orbit*) in the skull. The orbit is covered posteriorly by a fibrous sac lined with a smooth moist membrane which promotes smooth movement of the eye in its socket. The space between the intraorbital structures contains fatty tissue, which serves as a cushion for the eyeball.

The accessory structures include the eyelids, lacrimal system and extrinsic ocular muscles.

EYELIDS (PALPEBRAE)

The upper and lower eyelids serve as protective coverings. The space between them is referred to as the *palpebral fissure;* the angles or corners where the lids meet are known as the *inner* (medial) and *outer* (lateral) *canthi*. Each eyelid has an outer layer of skin, a layer of firm fibrous tissue (*tarsal plate*), sebaceous-like glands (*meibomian glands*) which secrete an oily substance on to the free margins of the lids, and a mucous membrane lining called the *conjunctiva*. The conjunctiva is reflected over the anterior portion of the eyeball forming the bulbar conjunctiva, and is continuous with the corneal epithelium. The secretion of the meibomian glands prevents adherence of the lids when the

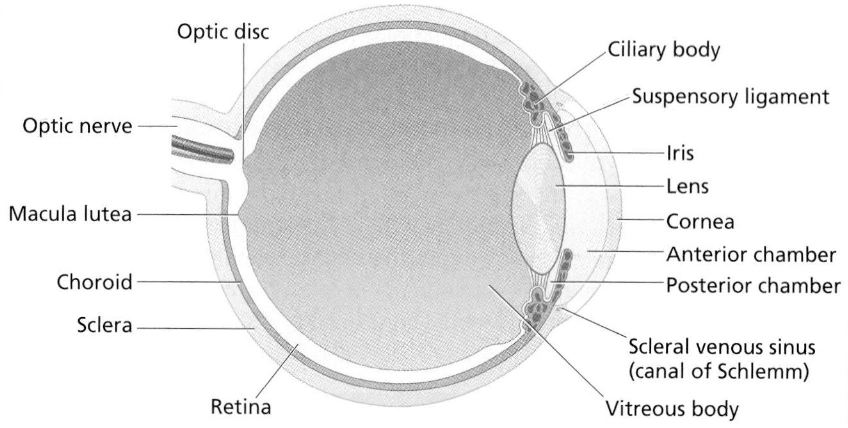
Optic disc
Ciliary body
Suspensory ligament
Optic nerve
Iris
Lens
Macula lutea
Cornea
Anterior chamber
Choroid
Posterior chamber
Sclera
Scleral venous sinus
(canal of Schlemm)
Retina
Vitreous body

Figure 21.9 Main structures of the eye. (Based on Tortora and Grabowski 2003, p. 535.)

eyes are closed and also prevents the overflow of normal amounts of lacrimal secretion. The eyelashes emerge from the free borders of the eyelids to protect the eye from dust and perspiration.

LACRIMAL SYSTEM

The **lacrimal apparatus** protects the eye by continuously secreting a fluid that 'washes' over the anterior surface of the eyeball, keeping it moistened and cleansed. The system of each eye consists of a gland, ducts and a drainage system. The lacrimal gland lies in a slight depression in the outer superior portion of the orbit. The secreted fluid eventually drains through two small openings (puncta) in the medial canthus into two short canals (lacrimal canaliculi). The canals drain via the nasolacrimal duct into the nasal cavity. Increased lacrimal secretion (lacrimation) occurs in response to irritation of the conjunctiva or to certain emotions.

EXTRINSIC OCULAR MUSCLES

Several external muscles have their origin in orbital structures and insert on the eyeball to provide movement of the eye within its socket. There are four *recti muscles* which move the eye up, down, medially and laterally, and two *oblique muscles* which provide rotation of the eye and modify the straight movements of the recti muscles. For most movements various combinations of recti and oblique muscle action are necessary.

The levator palpebrae superioris muscle inserts in the upper eyelid and is responsible for raising the upper eyelid (opening the eye).

EYEBALL

The **eyeball** is spherical with a slight anterior bulge. It is composed of three layers of tissue which enclose the iris and special transparent, refracting structures. The tough, outer coat forms the *sclera* and *cornea*. Underlying and attached to the sclera is a thin, heavily pigmented, vascular coat, the *choroid*, which prevents reflection of light rays.

The *ciliary body* consists mainly of muscle tissue that holds the lens in position. The action of the ciliary muscle influences the curvature, and thus the refractive power, of the lens.

The second layer of the eyeball continues forward and inward beyond the ciliary muscle to form the iris. The *iris* is composed of circular and radial muscles and pigmented cells, and is perforated centrally, creating the opening referred to as the *pupil*. The iris, ciliary body and choroid are known as the uvea or uveal tract.

The *retina* is the innermost coat of the eyeball; it consists of two layers, one of which is pigmented with melanin and the other consists of the light sensitive receptors which give rise to nerve cells required for vision. Melanin is a pigment that absorbs light and so prevents scattering of stray light rays within the eye which would interfere with vision. This explains why the pupil of the eye looks so dark as the viewer is seeing this melanin rich layer within the eye. Melanin also explains the differences that occur in eye colour. The more melanin there is in the iris the darker the iris while if there is less melanin, the green and blues dominate.

There are two types of receptor cells in the neural layer of the retina:

- The *rods* have a lower response threshold, making them more sensitive to lower levels of illumination (such as moonlight) but only operating in shades of grey
- The *cones* have a higher response threshold and, as a result, function in bright light and provide colour and detailed vision.

In the centre of the retina, a small area occurs in which the inner layers of cells are absent and only cones are concentrated. Light rays falling on this site strike the cones directly and produce the greatest visual acuity. This area is referred to as the *fovea centralis*. Near this area is a pale area called the *optic disc*, or *fundus oculi*, where the optic nerve and the central retinal vein and artery leave and enter the eyeball. The disc is a blind spot, because the area is devoid of rods and cones.

The *lens* is elastic and is the only transparent tissue in the body. It achieves this remarkable property by a process of apoptosis (pre-programmed cell death) which stops just short of the actual death of the cells making up the lens. The result is viable cells that are completely transparent (Dahm 2004). The lens is suspended just behind the iris by ligaments that attach to the ciliary body. Its shape varies with age; it is spherical in infancy, gradually flattening to a disc shape with age. In the elderly, the lens tends to flatten and becomes less elastic.

Divisions of the interior of the eyeball

The interior of the eyeball is divided into the anterior and posterior cavities. The *anterior cavity* is the space between the cornea and lens and is subdivided into the anterior and posterior chambers. The anterior chamber lies in front of the iris. The posterior chamber is situated behind the iris but in front of the lens. The content of the two chambers is *aqueous humour*.

The *posterior cavity* lies posterior to the lens. It is filled with the *vitreous humour*, or *vitreous body*.

Fluid system of the eye and intraocular pressure

The interior of the eyeball is filled by the aqueous and vitreous humours and the crystalline lens. The vitreous humour is a clear, jelly-like mass enclosed in a hyaloid membrane. It fills out the larger and posterior portion of the eyeball that lies behind the lens.

There is a continuous flow of aqueous humor into and out of the eye. The fluid originates from capillaries contained in processes of the ciliary body. After circulating around the posterior chamber, it flows through the pupil into the anterior chamber. From here, a small amount of the aqueous humour continuously drains into the canal of Schlemm, from which it is carried into the venous circulation. The aqueous humour carries nutrients to the lens and cornea, and removes waste products. This is necessary because both structures are avascular; the presence of blood vessels would alter their transparent nature. The production of aqueous humour and its drainage are constant in order to maintain a normal intraocular pressure, which is 16–21 mmHg. Any interference with normal drainage of the fluid from the anterior chamber raises the pressure, leading to decreased blood supply, pain and impaired vision.

VISUAL IMPULSE PATHWAY

Impulses generated by the rods and cones synapse through several neurones and ganglions to the optic disc where they unite to form the optic nerve. At the base of the brain, the nerve fibres from the medial half of the retina of each eye cross, going to the opposite sides of the brain. The fibres from the lateral halves of the retinae do not cross but continue on to the corresponding side of the brain. This arrangement forms the *optic chiasma* (Fig. 21.10). Within the brain, visual impulses are transmitted to the visual centre in the occipital cerebral cortex, where they are interpreted as sensations of light, colour and form. Other cerebral areas are necessary for normal vision; correlation with information stored as memory has to occur in order to give meaning to what is seen.

EYE REFLEXES

Some fibres of each optic tract terminate in a group of neurones referred to as the *superior colliculus* in the midbrain. From here, efferent impulses originate, resulting in blinking of the eyelids, movement of the head, or dilatation or constriction of the pupil.

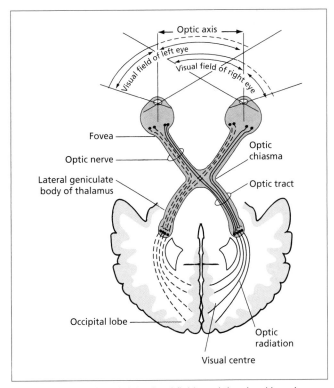

Figure 21.10 Left and right visual fields and the visual impulse.

The pupils are normally round and of equal size. They adjust to light by constricting, and to darkness or dim light by dilating. A second reflex that may be noted is the *accommodation reflex*. The normal response is constriction of the pupils as the person's gaze is shifted from a distant to a near object such as the nurse's finger held 10 cm from the end of the patient's nose. This reduction in size of the pupil allows a sharper focussing of close objects. The normal reflexes are summarized therefore as pupils equal and reacting to light and accommodation (PERLA).

THE MECHANISMS OF FOCUS

Several processes may be necessary to focus the light rays on the retina in order to form a clear image.

Refraction

The cornea and lens are the principal refractive media in the eye; the lens is particularly significant in that its curvature and degree of refraction can be varied by the ciliary body, according to the amount required to focus the light rays on the retina. However, about 75% of the refractive power of the eye comes from the cornea, 25% from the lens. Various errors of refraction occur that interfere with the ability of the eye to focus light rays on the retina, resulting in impaired vision.

Emmetropia implies normal refraction.

Short-sightedness, called *myopia*, is the result of light rays from an object at 6 m or more being focused at a point in front of the retina. Close objects can be seen, but distant objects are blurred. Correction may be made by use of a concave lens, which produces divergence of light rays (Fig. 21.11).

Long-sightedness (*hypermetropia*) is due to insufficient refraction and, as a result, light rays from an object at 6 m or less are focused at a point behind the retina. The person sees distant objects more clearly than close ones. Correction may be made by use of a convex lens, which focuses light rays by convergence (Fig. 21.11). In the later years of life, as part of the ageing process, the lens loses its elasticity and becomes thinner and flatter. This lessens the normal degree of refraction and the person becomes far-sighted, a refractive error referred to as *presbyopia*.

In some persons, the horizontal and vertical curvatures of the cornea are uneven, producing differences in the degree of refraction. This results in different focal points; some light rays may be focused on the retina, but others may fall short or be carried to a point beyond the retina. This type of refractive error is known as *astigmatism*.

Accommodation

This is the process by which the degree of refraction by the lens is changed in order to focus rays from objects at various distances. This is made possible by the elastic nature of the lens and the action of the ciliary muscles on the suspensory ligaments (Fig. 21.12).

Pupillary modification

The pupillary aperture is varied to control the amount of light entering the eye. For clear vision of near objects, the iris constricts the pupil of each eye to prevent divergent rays from entering. The opening is also reduced to restrict the entrance of excessively bright light, which may harm the retina. The iris constricts the pupil through parasympathetic innervation; sympathetic nervous stimulation produces dilatation of the pupil. In dim light and when focusing on a distant, wider visual field, the iris dilates the pupil to admit more light rays.

Convergence

Although light rays from the same object(s) fall on both retinae, only single vision is experienced. This is due to light rays from the object falling on corresponding points of the two retinae. This is brought about by convergence, which involves the extrinsic muscles (recti and oblique). The movements of the two eyes must be coordinated accurately. As an object is brought closer to the eyes, convergence of their axes occurs as they turn inward. For distant objects, convergence is not necessary; the eyes remain parallel.

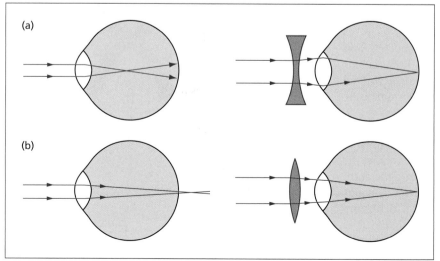

(a)

(b)

Figure 21.11 Diagram showing the use of lenses to correct common eye problems. (a) Myopia and correction by concave lens. (b) Hypermetropia and correction by convex lens.

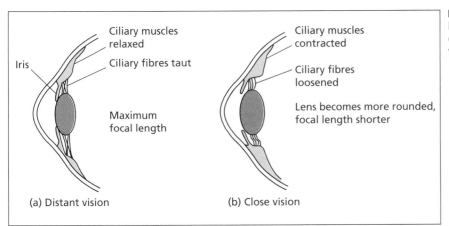

Figure 21.12 Diagram showing the ciliary body, suspensory ligaments and lens, and the changes in accommodation for (a) distant vision and (b) close vision.

Strabismus (squint) is a defect that interferes with coordination of the eye movements, and the light rays do not fall on corresponding points of the two retinae. It is usually due to an abnormal extrinsic muscle, or to an undiagnosed refractive error. Two images result and the person 'sees double'; this is termed *diplopia*.

LIGHT AND DARK ADAPTATION

Light adaptation

When exposed to intense light, adaptation takes place by constriction of the pupils and lowering the eyebrows, eyelids and head; the visual purple (rhodopsin) within the rods is bleached, which reduces their sensitivity and responses.

Dark adaptation

When a person goes from a light to a dark area, there is a period when nothing is seen, followed by the outlines of objects gradually becoming visible. This vision in dim light is due to an increased sensitivity of the rods as they produce a chemical pigment, visual purple or rhodopsin. Vitamin A is essential for the formation of the chemical; if it is deficient, the person experiences night blindness. At the same time that the rods increase their sensitivity, the pupils dilate to admit more light.

THE PERSON WITH HEALTH PROBLEMS RELATED TO VISION

ASSESSMENT

It is necessary, in most instances, to carry out a thorough assessment before a diagnosis is made and, if appropriate, treatment prescribed. (*Immediate* action would be required if the patient's eye was damaged by trauma such as the accidental instillation of chemicals.) This includes a history of the patient's ocular disorder, general health and lifestyle, and an examination of the eyes. The latter involves inspection, palpation and the use of special equipment.

Health history

- *Age*. The age of the person in relation to developmental changes and effects of ageing on the eyes is important
- *Occupation and lifestyle*. Information is obtained as to the demands for visual acuity, potential for eye injury and the use of protective devices. Sporting activity such as playing squash should be checked together with occupational hazards including the use of VDU screens
- *Family history*. As many eye disorders are inherited, it is significant to learn of any family history of eye disorders, diabetes mellitus, cardiovascular disease and thyroid disease
- *Past health*. Any childhood and adult illnesses, injuries and previous eye problems should be noted and the treatment and responses elicited. Ocular changes may be secondary to a disorder such as hypertension, diabetes mellitus, renal disease, hyperthyroidism and brain injury or tumour. Degenerative disease in the elderly is frequently the cause of loss of vision.

The use of corrective lenses should be ascertained together with the date of the last eye examination.

Current symptoms

The presenting complaint should be noted. Some common symptoms are listed in Box 21.3.

The PQRST symptom analysis tool may be used to assess the presenting complaint in a systematic way (see p. 128). Information concerning the nature of the complaint, duration, factors that provoke or relieve the symptom may be ascertained by use of this tool (Walsh 2006).

Examination of the eyes
Macroscopic examination

Tests for eye movement and measurement of visual acuity are usually performed before the examination of internal structures of the eye or tests that involve the touching of normally sensitive eye structures.

Initial observations of the eyes include noting: general appearance, symmetry of visual axes and physical features,

> **Box 21.3** Common symptoms related to problems with vision
>
> - Changes in visual acuity
> - Blurring of vision
> - Halos
> - Flashes of light
> - Spots before the eyes (floaters)
> - Excessive lacrimation or epiphora
> - Double vision (diplopia)
> - Light sensitivity (photophobia)
> - Night blindness
> - Recurring headache
> - Discomfort, burning sensation or itching of the eyes.

any discharge and its characteristics, excessive or deficient lacrimal secretion, swelling or discolouration of extraocular structures or surrounding tissues, and the presence of a foreign body. The size and equality of the pupils are recorded. The medial canthi are examined for swelling and redness and *gently* palpated for tenderness.

The eyelids, lashes and brows are inspected for:

- redness or any discolouration
- crusting
- eversion or inversion of the lids
- complete and equal opening and closing of the lids
- swollen areas or oedema.

The areas are very gently palpated for tenderness and nodules. The colour of the conjunctiva of the lids is noted, as are any swollen or raised areas.

Assessment of extraocular muscle function

The patient sits facing the examiner, holding the head in a fixed position. The neuromuscular balance or straightness of the eyes is assessed by shining a light directly on the patient's eyes. The patient is asked to look at the light, which should be reflected in corresponding positions in the pupillary corneas. If there is deviation of one eye, asymmetrical reflection occurs.

When the light is moved, the movements of both eyes should be coordinated and symmetrical. The patient should be asked to follow the light with their eyes without moving their head. The examiner should test the movement of the eyes to the extreme positions by drawing an imaginary large H in the air with the light. At the extremes of movement, the eyes should be observed for nystagmus. Abnormal response in movement may indicate paralysis of one or more extraocular muscles, muscular imbalance or injury.

Assessment of eye reflexes

Pupillary reflexes are observed in a dimly lit room by shining a light from the side on to the pupil of one eye at a time. Both pupils are observed; the normal response is constriction of both pupils when the light is shone in one. This is referred to as *consensual pupil reaction*.

The accommodation reflex is elicited by having the patient focus on a light held about 50 cm from the nose. As the light is brought to within 10 cm of the patient, the eyes normally converge and the pupils constrict.

Measurement of visual acuity

Visual acuity is the ability to distinguish details of objects and reflects ocular function. Each eye is tested separately; the eye not being examined is completely covered, but without any pressure being applied directly to the eye. A well-lit standard wall chart (Snellen chart) with rows of letters of gradually decreasing size is used, placed 6 m from the patient. The person is asked to read the chart through to the line of smallest letters that can be seen.

The distance from which the normal eye can read each line is known. The top line of the Snellen chart is perceived by the normal eye at 60 m, the second line at 36 m, the third at 24 m, the fourth at 18 m, the fifth at 12 m, the sixth at 9 m, the seventh at 6 m, and the eighth line at 4 m. Visual acuity is expressed as a fraction; the numerator represents the distance between the chart and the patient, and the denominator is the distance from which a person with normal vision could read the same line. Visual acuity recorded as 6/6 means normal vision. If the patient 6 m from the chart can only read the line that the normal eye could read at 12 m, the visual acuity is expressed at 6/12. The larger the denominator recorded, the poorer is the vision. In a person with severe impairment who can only see a hand moving in front of the face, the visual acuity may be recorded as HM (hand movements). If the person can distinguish only between light and dark, the recording is PL (perception of light), and if there is no light perception it is expressed as NPL (no perception of light). A recording of 3/60 or less in the better eye when wearing glasses or contact lenses indicates that the person is legally blind.

Near vision is assessed by having the individual hold a card about 32 cm from the eyes. The print on the card is sized proportionately to the 6 m.

Visual field measurement (perimetry)

A semicircular instrument, called a perimeter, which is marked in degrees, is used to determine whether the patient's visual fields are normal or restricted. Defects in the visual fields are frequently associated with intracranial lesions, retinal damage or damage to an optic nerve.

Estimation of the visual field may also be made by the confrontation test. An object is moved slowly from beyond the patient's (and the examiner's) peripheral vision towards the central line of vision. The patient is asked to indicate when the object first comes into view and this is compared with when it was first seen by the examiner. The difference is recorded, taking for granted the examiner's vision is normal. The test is made using lateral, upper and lower fields.

Measurement of intraocular pressure

The detection of increased intraocular pressure is important; an excessive pressure may be very painful and progressively causes permanent damage within the eye, leading to loss of vision. The pressure is measured with an instrument called a tonometer. A few drops of a local anaesthetic (e.g. tetracaine (amethocaine) 0.5–1%, oxybuprocaine 0.3%) are instilled in each eye. The tonometer is then placed on the corneal surface, causing indentation; the extent of the indentation reflects the intraocular pressure. If the pressure is high, the cornea resists indentation. The normal intraocular pressure is approximately 16–21 mmHg. A second instrument that is now generally employed to measure the ocular tension is the applanometer. This is an electronic device that is considered to provide a more accurate measurement of the intraocular pressure.

The patient with raised intraocular pressure is at risk of serious impairment of vision due to ischaemic neuropathy.

Slit-lamp microscopy (biomicroscopy)

A more detailed examination of the internal structures of the eye can be made by the use of slit-lamp microscope. It is helpful in locating foreign bodies in the eye and identifying ulcer erosion as well as degenerative and inflammatory conditions.

Fluorescein staining

A fluorescein strip, which is a sterile strip of paper that has been impregnated with a solution of sodium fluorescein, is moistened at one end and lightly applied to the lower conjunctival sac. A single-drop, disposable dispenser may be used as an alternative. The dye flows over the eye, and abrasions and corneal ulcers readily stain a yellowish-green.

After the examination, the eye is irrigated with a sterile saline solution to remove the dye.

Ophthalmoscopic examination

With an ophthalmoscope, the posterior, internal surface (fundus) of each eye is magnified 15 times and observed. The lens, vitreous body, blood vessels, retina, optic nerve and disc are viewed. To obtain a wider view, the pupil may be dilated by the instillation of a mydriatic such as tropicamide 0.5–1%. Ophthalmoscopy is valuable in the recognition of some systemic disorders, as well as in the assessment of ocular function. Nurse practitioners are increasingly carrying out ophthalmoscopic examination of the eye. As a result, they may detect disorders such as hypertension, renal disease or diabetes which produce characteristic changes in the eye visible only on ophthalmoscopy.

Electroretinography may be done to record the extent of the electrical response made by the retina to light stimulation and gonioscopy may be carried out to examination of the angle of the anterior chamber by means of an optical instrument (gonioscope).

CLINICAL CHARACTERISTICS

Impairment of vision

The development of significant signs and symptoms of impaired visual function varies greatly. The onset of changes may be insidious in some cases, but in others, the onset may occur suddenly and be acute. One or both eyes may be involved. The manifestations may be principally subjective or may be objective only, with the abnormal structure or function being noted by an observer. In some instances, manifestations may be recognized without tests or the aid of instruments.

The signs and symptoms of eye disorders include the following characteristics.

Subjective manifestations

1 Difficulty in reading and seeing objects clearly, blurred vision or headaches when reading or doing close work. These symptoms may be caused by simple refractive errors or by cataract, glaucoma, inflammation of the cornea (keratitis) and ulceration leading to scarring and opacity, degenerative changes, detachment of the retina or a systemic disease such as hypertension, diabetes mellitus or arteriosclerosis.

2 Photophobia (sensitivity to light) may be associated with inflammation of the conjunctiva, cornea or iris.

3 Excessive tear flow may indicate trauma, chemical irritation, allergy, inflammation of ocular tissue or obstruction of the tear duct.

4 Dryness of the conjunctival surface due to decreased lacrimal secretion which may be due to severe dehydration or cerebral trauma or disease (e.g. rheumatoid arthritis). It is frequently a problem in an abnormally dry environment and in the elderly. Some drugs may suppress lacrimal secretion.

5 Ocular pain may be due to irritation from a foreign body, infection, inflammation of eye tissues or accessory structures, or increased intraocular pressure (glaucoma).

6 Diplopia (double vision) is most frequently experienced by patients with a head injury or cerebral disorder (e.g. brain tumour) that incurs a paralysis or functional imbalance of the extraocular muscles.

7 Spots before or floaters in the eyes, single and occasional, are common and of no clinical significance. Frequent or sudden development of numerous spots or floaters may signify an intraocular haemorrhage or threatening haemorrhage of the retina. In the latter, the patient may experience flashing lights followed by a clouding across the eye.

8 Scotoma or blind spot develops as a result of damage to an area of the retina or optic nerve. It may be caused by an inflammatory disease process within the eye or a degenerative disorder. If the scotoma occurs in the same area in each eye, the aetiology may be intracranial, affecting the fibres in the visual pathway.

9 Halos around lights are usually associated with increased intraocular pressure and glaucoma.

10 Extensive loss of visual acuity of 3/60 or less in the better eye with correction, or a restriction of the visual field to 20° or less, indicates blindness according to the legal definition.

Objective manifestations

1 The person is observed holding reading material or an object nearer than 30 cm to the face or beyond the distance of approximately 40 cm.

2 A strained expression or scowl may be noted when an effort to see is being made.

3 The younger person may fail to develop at a normal rate or make normal progress at school.

4 Errors are made because of misread information or directions.

5 Deviation of one eye (the visual axis of one eye differs from that of the other eye) indicates impaired extraocular muscle structure or function. The latter may be due to a disorder involving the oculomotor (third cranial) nerve.

6 Discolouration of the eyelid or surrounding tissue. Redness of the eyelids suggests infection, allergy or injury. Redness of the exposed area of the eye may be caused by conjunctival irritation by a foreign body, infection or trauma, or may be incurred by a subconjunctival haemorrhage associated with trauma, hypertension or inflammatory disease of intraocular structures. Discolouration of surrounding tissue may be the result of extravasation of blood related to an eye or facial injury.

7 Discharge (serous or purulent) or crusting may indicate infection, chemical irritation, allergy or trauma of the eyelid or eye.

8 Swelling or oedema may develop with local trauma, infection or cyst, or may be associated with renal or cardiac failure, a cerebral disorder or head injury.

9 Abnormal pupillary shape or reaction. Constriction, asymmetry or failure of normal reaction to light is most often due to some cerebral disorder or iris collapse. A greyish white colour of the pupil suggests an opacity of the lens (cataract).

10 Exophthalmos or proptosis (prominence or bulging of the eyes) is usually caused by hyperthyroidism.

11 Ptosis or a lag in the closing of eyelid may indicate some oculomotor (third cranial) nerve involvement. The drooping of both eyelids is also characteristic of myasthenia gravis.

THE PERSON WITH VISUAL IMPAIRMENT

Then latest prevalence data for visual impairment is from the 1997 census in which 354 153 people were registered blind or partially sighted in the UK and a total of 1 066 740 were classed as visually impaired, of whom 75% were aged 75 years or over (Royal National Institute for the Blind 2001). Visual impairment is therefore a major problem, particularly amongst elderly people. People are very dependent upon their sense of vision, as most of our knowledge of the environment is obtained through our eyes. The eyes are also used in expressing emotions. Any impairment or loss of vision is a serious threat. In many instances, the ability to freely move about safely and the privilege of enjoying colour, form, depth, beauty and distance are lost. Loss of vision results in reduced sensory input and stimulation; this may lead to boredom and reduced responsiveness and disorientation to time and place on the part of the person unless stimuli by other channels (e.g. hearing and touch) are increased and the person's interest is maintained.

The nurse should appreciate the incalculable value of sight and the natural anxiety and concern of the patient when it is threatened. Reduced vision affects the patient's whole way of life – socially, physically, economically and emotionally. Effective nursing care can be planned only if the nurse has an understanding of the causes of visual impairment as this will allow the identification of appropriate goals for the individual. The majority of people with visual impairment are over 65. A range of important factors associated with aging such as impaired balance and mobility are therefore going to interact with visual impairment to increase the problems faced by the older person.

Causes

Visual impairment may be due to a primary eye disorder or may be secondary to a neurological or systemic disorder. The causes include:

- structural or functional defect in the eye or extraocular structures (e.g. malfunction of the extraocular muscles causing deviation of one or both eyes)
- ageing (e.g. the lens becomes less spherical with age, may become opaque and the nucleus hardens)
- infection
- trauma – chemical or mechanical
- new growth
- impaired innervation of the eyes due to a neurological disorder (e.g. brain tumour or injury)
- systemic disease (e.g. hypertension, diabetes mellitus, cardiovascular disease)
- inadequate knowledge about the factors that contribute to the preservation of good vision (e.g. nutritional requirements, protection of eyes in potentially hazardous situations).

Goals

Patient-centred goals common to most patients with visual impairment are:

1 Vision will be preserved
2 Factors contributing to visual impairment will be identified
3 The patient will receive meaningful sensory input
4 The patient will remain oriented
5 Injury or complications will not occur
6 If visual impairment is permanent, the patient will learn to be as self-caring as possible, retaining maximum independence.

Preservation of vision

The maintenance of vision and prevention of loss of sight includes consideration of the following:

Good general health

There is a tendency to consider vision as being independent of general health. It remains good in some serious bodily disorders, whereas others may have a serious effect on visual acuity.

Optimum diet

Vitamins A, B complex and C are considered important; a deficiency of vitamin A may cause drying and changes of the cornea and conjunctiva and a decreased production of the retinal pigment, rhodopsin, leading to night blindness. A deficiency in the vitamin B complex may predispose to retinal changes. Vitamin C plays a role in resistance to infection.

Protection of eyes

Occupational health nurses have a very important role to play in preventing eye injury by ensuring that staff wear protective goggles. Welders need to wear goggles that will protect their eyes from ultra-violet radiation. Office workers also need to be aware of hazards to their eyesight resulting from inadequate lighting and overuse of VDUs.

Regular periodical eye examination

Some eye diseases and changes develop insidiously without markedly reducing vision or causing pain until they are well advanced. Regular eye examination may reveal early signs, and a serious disease may be checked before it progresses to loss of vision and blindness. If glasses are necessary, only those that have been properly prescribed should be used. Lenses are individually ground for each eye according to the testing and examination findings. Box 21.4 lists the terms used in eye examinations and to describe errors of refraction.

Care and use of glasses and contact lenses

If glasses are worn, the importance of protecting the lens from scratches and maintaining good alignment is stressed. If glasses are not straight or if the distance between the eyes and lenses is not equal, the degree of refraction is altered. Lenses in spectacles are safer if made of impact-resistant material.

When the patient receives a contact lens, detailed instructions and demonstrations are necessary. A contact lens is a thin plastic disc shaped to fit the anterior surface of the eye. The outer surface is ground to meet the patient's visual need. The patient is taught the daily procedure of putting in and removing the lens, the cleansing and care of it, and the prevention of complications. Meticulous care is necessary to

Box 21.4	Terminology and abbreviations used during eye examinations
RE	Right eye
LE	Left eye
BE	Both eyes
Emmetropia	Normal vision (normal refraction)
Myopia (M)	Short-sightedness
Hypermetropia (hyperopia; H)	Long-sightedness
Presbyopia	Reduced accommodation associated with the ageing process
Astigmatism	Uneven curvature of the cornea; results in different focal points
Diplopia	Perception of two images of a single object (double vision)
Hemianopia	Loss of vision in one-half of the visual field
Entropion	Turning in of the eyelid
Ectropion	Turning out of the eyelid
Ptosis	Drooping of the upper eyelid
Aphakia	Absence of the lens of an eye
Hyphaema	Haemorrhage into the anterior chamber of the eye
Hypopyon	White blood cells in the anterior chamber
Photophobia	Hypersensitivity to light
Ophthalmologist (oculist)	A doctor who specializes in the treatment of eye disorders
Optometrist	A person who examines the eyes to assess vision and prescribes corrective spectacles or lenses
Optician	A specialist who prepares spectacles or lenses according to prescription
Mydriasis	Dilatation of the pupil
Mydriatic	Drug that dilates the pupil
Miosis	Contraction of the pupil of the eye
Miotic	Drug that contracts the pupil
Proptosis (exophthalmos)	Bulging forward of the eyes
Epiphora	Excessive lacrimal secretion (tears)

prevent complications such as infection, which are painful and could ultimately cause loss of vision. Washing the hands thoroughly with soap under running water before handling the lens is emphasized. If worn in both eyes, on removal each lens is stored separately in containers marked for right and left; the correction in one may be quite different to that of the other. Directions for cleansing are provided in writing. Before applying the lenses, they are rinsed free of any chemical that may have been used for cleansing and a wetting solution may be used. Solutions must be fresh and are not re-used.

The patient is advised to use the lens for brief periods at first, progressively increasing the length of time until the eye is comfortable with it. Unless the lenses are of the extended-wear type, they are removed at the end of each day; they are *not* worn during sleep. If the eye is inflamed or painful or if there is excessive lacrimal secretion (tearing), the lens is not applied. The most common complications that develop are conjunctivitis, corneal abrasion and keratitis.

Prevention of trauma

The loss of vision due to exposure to chemicals, dust, wind, ultraviolet light or direct sun rays, and eye injury by mechanical objects (e.g. flying pieces of metal or wood), is preventable in most instances by the use of standard safety measures and devices. The use of legislated safety helmets, shatterproof goggles or shields in potentially hazardous situations should be observed. Sunglasses may be necessary to protect the eyes from ultraviolet radiation in bright sunshine (e.g. when skiing or using a sun bed). Welders should use protective eye shielding for the same reason, to avoid ultraviolet radiation causing very painful damage to the outer layers of the corneal epithelium, known as 'arc eye'. The use of adequate protective equipment as well as observance of established safety rules in sports such as squash, where there is a potential for injury, should be promoted.

Rubbing of the eyes should be avoided because of the possibility of trauma and the introduction of infection, especially if wearing contact lenses. Cautious use of sprays and caustic solutions and the wearing of protective goggles when exposed to caustic substances should be emphasized.

First aid and prompt treatment

In the event of an accident, no 'eyedrops' or ointment should be instilled in the eyes. The eye should be gently irrigated with copious amounts of water which will frequently remove any foreign body. If the foreign body cannot be easily removed in this way or if there are signs of inflammation or any other disturbance in an eye, early medical treatment is required. Foreign bodies frequently end up adhering to the undersurface of the eyelid (conjunctiva) where they may be seen only by everting the eyelid. In this position, they are known as subtarsal foreign bodies. If a chemical spray or irritating solution accidentally gets into the eye, immediate and extended irrigation with water or saline is recommended and urgent medical treatment sought to avoid potential ulceration and blindness.

Principles to be observed in eye-care procedures

1 The patient receives a full explanation of the procedure and is advised that it is important that the head is held steady.

2 Hands are washed thoroughly before and after doing any eye procedure.

3 Precautions are used to protect the unaffected eye from possible injury and cross-infection from one eye to another. Irrigation solution or eye drops being used in the affected eye must not be permitted to enter the unaffected eye. Similarly, dressings from the affected eye should not touch the unaffected eye. Dressings and swabs are used only once.

4 Pressure on the eyeball is avoided.

5 When irrigating the eye, the solution is directed on to the nasal side of the eyeball. The eye is gently wiped from the inner canthus to the outer canthus.

6 Solutions and drugs should always be fresh; they are dated as to preparation and expiry.

7 Frequent, regular assessment of the eye and the patient's vision is made. The eye is examined before and after each procedure; alteration in comfort, change in colour, discharge, dryness, oedema or swelling is brought to the attention of the doctor.

8 If both eyes are involved, separate sterile equipment and solutions are used for each eye. In the case of infection, the eye manifesting less inflammation and discharge is treated before the other eye. These precautions are aimed at reducing the risk of cross-infection.

9 A separate sterile eye-dropper is employed for each drug used in the eye.

10 If the eyelid does not close, precautions are necessary when handling articles such as bed-linen, towels and clothing to avoid abrasions and injury of the conjunctiva and cornea. An exposed (open) eye may become dry and susceptible to ulceration; the instillation of artificial tears may be prescribed as a prophylactic measure, as may ointment applied to the exposed conjunctiva.

11 It is important that the patient is warned of any effect the eye drops may have; some will paralyze the muscles of accommodation and cause blurring of vision.

12 Eye dressings are normally applied to protect the eye, to absorb lacrimal secretions or exudate, or to apply pressure. The skin around the eye should always be supported gently when the dressing is removed.

13 Drops are instilled at the *lateral* aspect of the inner lower lid, with the patient looking up, so that direct corneal contact is avoided and reflex squeezing of the eye prevented.

14 In order to keep the affected eye at rest, the unaffected eye may be covered. Adaptation to light is resumed gradually; the unaffected eye may first be exposed by wearing a shield with a small central opening. This minimizes eye movement. A similar shield may also be used later on the affected eye; however, it is more usual for the patient to wear dark glasses. Extreme gentleness is

used when changing a dressing or doing any treatment; caution is used to avoid pressure on the eyeball.

15 Great care should be taken to prevent the eye opening under the dressing as this can cause corneal abrasion. The dressing should be secured firmly.

CARE OF THE VISUALLY HANDICAPPED PATIENT

Maintenance of orientation and reduction of anxiety

Impairment and threatened loss of vision arouse considerable fear, insecurity and emotional reactions. All the implications that impaired vision may have in the present and future 'crowd in' on the patient and he or she may become panicky and lose control. Behavioural responses must be assessed frequently; with reduced or no vision, the patient (especially if elderly) may become disoriented, particularly if not in a familiar environment.

Individuals deprived of visual input become more dependent on other senses such as hearing and touch. The understanding of the nurse as to what the patient may be experiencing, the provision of emotional support and the use of communication techniques that promote the use of other senses contribute greatly to the care of this patient.

Factors that help to reduce the patient's anxiety include the following suggestions. The patient is carefully oriented to any new environment; if confined to bed, the orientation is by a verbal description. If allowed up, the verbal description is combined with helping the person to explore the ward environment. An explanation is made of how usual daily needs will be met.

The patient is given the opportunity and encouragement to express concerns and to ask questions. The person who cannot see is spoken to while being approached and is advised who is speaking. Any treatment or investigative procedure should be well described in advance. It means a great deal to the patient to have the call-button always within reach; this means that help is always at hand. The patient should not be left alone for long periods for, although a lot of physical care may not be needed, support and contacts are still required. The nurse should take time to talk to the patient and, as required, indicate the time and describe the place and current situation and details of the environment. The patient may have visual memory from which it is possible to recall sufficiently to form a mental picture of what is being described. Some appropriate form of diversion, such as a radio and visitors to chat with or read to the patient, is encouraged to provide sensory input. Noisy, confusing situations are avoided; the visually handicapped patient is usually more sensitive to sounds and voice inflections. An effort is made to anticipate the patient's needs.

Maintenance of a safe environment

Adequate orientation and frequent observations are important to prevent accidents when the patient's vision is seriously impaired. If the patient is disoriented, it may be necessary to have someone present to ensure patient safety.

The environment must be checked carefully for any hazards for the unseeing, ambulatory person. He or she should be escorted around the area until familiar with it and encouraged to move about alone. Stools, rugs or other such articles should be removed. Furniture is not moved from its original position when possible, and doors are kept closed or wide open. The person is cautioned about nearby stairs and radiators. All members of the staff should be made aware of the individual's degree of visual handicap.

Continuous assessment

Prompt recognition of change in the eye, visual acuity and orientation is very important, as failure to do so can lead to an increase in the amount of impairment. The nurse is required to be familiar with any specific observations that are important in certain eye disorders. Generally, significant factors that should be brought promptly to the doctor's attention include increased temperature, discharge, unrelieved pain, headache, any evidence of disturbance in the unaffected eye, and signs of bleeding, infection or inflammation in the anterior segment.

Positioning and activity

Patient positioning varies with different conditions and is usually indicated by the doctor. Prolonged restriction of activity is relatively rare; patients worry less and have fewer complications when allowed up as soon as possible. If the patient is required to remain in bed, lying flat with the head immobilized, the arms and lower limbs are moved through a range of motion, and active exercises of the legs are begun as soon as the doctor permits.

Eating and drinking

The patient frequently experiences anorexia due to anxiety and because of the difficulty with taking food when vision is impaired. The necessary assistance is provided and, when feeding, the food is described; only small amounts are offered to avoid choking and coughing, because coughing raises the intraocular pressure. As soon as the patient is well enough, self-care and independence are major considerations; however, assistance is withdrawn gradually, not all at once.

The position of different foods on the plate may be described using the clock analogy. Aids such as plate-guards and non-slide mats may also be useful.

Some visually handicapped patients are reluctant to socialize at mealtimes in case they cause embarrassment; the use of aids can help them overcome this. Drinks should be offered regularly and poured out if necessary; it is often difficult for the patient to do this – and they may just not drink. Aids are available to help with pouring drinks.

Communication

Verbal communication should be clear and concise and may need frequent repetition. Touch and tone are very important, as they offer a form of non-verbal and verbal reinforcement of which the patient can be aware.

Rehabilitation of the blind

There are two official categories of visual handicap in the UK:

1 *Blindness*:
   a) so blind as to be unable to perform *any* work for which eyesight is essential
   b) visual acuity of below 3/60
   c) visual acuity of 6/60 and below if there is considerable contraction of the visual field.
2 *Partial sight*: a visual acuity of 6/60 or less, the individual being substantially or permanently handicapped by defective vision. The category to which the person is assigned (according to the amount of visual impairment) dictates eligibility for help.

The patient with marked visual impairment or with total loss of vision needs a great deal of assistance in adjusting to the situation. The individual needs to realize that life still has meaning and potential. Emphasis is placed on what is possible given that the person still has visual memory of form, colour and space, and can learn that other senses may be put to greater use.

The development of independence is started as soon as possible, beginning with self-care (feeding, bathing, dressing and hair). Assistance is given with moving about the room and then from room to room, locating furniture and necessary articles by touch. The environment is organized to provide safety.

Anyone walking with a blind person allows the individual to take an arm rather than grasping the person and pushing. Writing is practised, beginning with the person's signature. Differentiation by touch is also tested and practised. The person learns to tell the time by using a specially designed watch.

Various forms of diversion and recreation are introduced (e.g. tapes/CDs of books and music). The patient is referred to the social services and the Royal National Institute for the Blind, which provide vocational training, assistance in learning Braille and in finding a job, recreation, transportation and financial assistance when necessary. The use of the white cane is introduced and the necessary guidance given on excursions beyond the house until the person is capable of safely getting around alone. Other people may prefer the use of a guide-dog – it is a matter of personal choice.

The patient and family are advised of the financial assistance available for the registered blind or registered partially sighted, and are assisted in making an application for it. The family may require help in accepting the blind patient and in organizing the home environment in the interest of safety and independence.

COMMON EYE DISORDERS

Refractive errors

Various errors of **refraction** occur which interfere with the ability of the eye to focus light rays on the retina, normally resulting in impaired vision (see p. 746 for a discussion of short-sightedness, long-sightedness, presbyopia and astigmatism).

Blepharitis

This is an inflammation of the eyelid; it is usually bilateral and affects the marginal area of the lids.

Characteristics

The patient may complain of itching or irritation. The margins of the lids are reddened and develop crusts or scales. It may be associated with seborrhoea (excessive sebaceous gland secretion) of the scalp and eyebrows or be staphylococcal in origin.

Treatment

Therapeutic measures include gentle removal of the crusts once or twice daily with warm water and the application of the prescribed antibacterial ointment; if the cause is seborrhoea, washing with an antiseborrhoeic shampoo may help.

Conjunctivitis

Inflammation of the conjunctiva may be caused by bacteria, viruses, chemicals or an allergic reaction, and may be acute or chronic. Sources of eye infection include foreign bodies, dust, hands, infected neighbouring structures (nose, face, sinus) or contaminated equipment or solutions used in treatment. Viral infections are a very contagious form of conjunctivitis and prompt therapeutic measures are necessary to prevent its rapid spread to other people. Infection may begin in the conjunctival lining of the eyelids and spread, or remain confined to that area.

Characteristics

The inflammation is manifested by irritation, feeling of grittiness, pain, redness, encrustations, and excessive lacrimation or serous and purulent discharge. The patient may complain of photophobia. When infection is present, a culture may be made from a swab of the discharge for identification of the invading organism; this should be carried out before instilling an antimicrobial agent.

Treatment

Frequent gentle cleansing of the lid margins is necessary to prevent encrustations. Precautions must be observed to treat each eye separately so that infection is not transferred from one to the other. The patient is usually more comfortable in dim light or darkness, and dark glasses ease the discomfort in the early stages. Chloramphenicol ointment or drops are the most frequently prescribed treatments but other antibacterial agents such as gentamicin, fusidic acid or ciprofloxacin may be used. If the patient does not respond, this indicates a viral cause. The patient is advised to keep the hands away from the eyes and, if responsible for instilling medications, the patient must be cautioned to wash the hands thoroughly under running water before starting and after completing the medication procedure.

If the conjunctivitis is due to allergy, efforts are made to identify the allergen so that it can be avoided if possible; it may be air-borne or transferred by the person's hands or by towels. A topical antihistamine such as antazoline or azelastine or an anti-inflammatory preparation such as sodium cromoglycate may be instilled as eye drops (British National Formulary 2005).

Hordeolum (stye)

A hordeolum, or stye, is a small abscess that develops within a marginal sebaceous gland or hair follicle of an eyelash. A small, red, swollen tender area appears. Spontaneous drainage of pus may be hastened by a topical broad-spectrum antibiotic such as chloramphenicol ointment, which should be instilled regularly.

Chalazion

A chalazion is a cyst that forms in a meibomian (sebaceous) gland. It may remain as a small, firm, painless swelling in the lid for a long period. Eventually, it may become infected and irritate the palpebral conjunctiva. Application of chloramphenicol ointment is usually prescribed. Recurrence frequently necessitates a small incision for drainage and curettage.

Glaucoma

This disorder is characterized by an increase in the intraocular pressure above the normal, which causes damage to the optic disc and visual field loss. It is one of the leading causes of blindness in the world. Normal intraocular pressure is generally maintained by a balance between the production of aqueous humour by the ciliary body and its drainage from the anterior chamber via the canal of Schlemm. If an imbalance occurs between production and drainage, the pressure increases, compressing the retina and the blood vessels within the eye. Permanent optic nerve damage leading to blindness results unless there is early recognition and treatment of the disease.

Glaucoma is usually due to some interference with the outflow of aqueous humour from the anterior chamber into the canal of Schlemm. It may be classified as primary, secondary or congenital. The primary acute form may be referred to as *acute angle-closure glaucoma*; the primary chronic type is called *open-angle* or *simple chronic glaucoma*.

Secondary glaucoma may be associated with infection, inflammation, trauma or a tumour within the eye.

Open-angle (chronic) glaucoma

This chronic and more common type develops very gradually; the cause is not understood but the frequency of familial incidence points to hereditary aetiology that results in degenerative changes. It is one of the leading causes of blindness worldwide (Kass et al 2002). It is usually bilateral and has a higher incidence in persons over the age of 40 years; this emphasizes the importance of regular eye examinations that include the measurement of intraocular pressure. A pressure of between 24 and 32 mmHg is a major indicator for prompt referral and treatment.

Characteristics

Because of the insidious onset of open-angle glaucoma, the central field of vision is not lost for some time. The disorder is frequently well advanced before the person seeks assistance. The visual field diminishes progressively, and the individual may become aware that something is wrong when discovering objects on either side that have been 'missed', or if halos are persistently seen around artificial lights. The condition may be discovered during a routine examination. As the condition progresses, the person may complain of some pain in the eye(s), especially in the morning on awakening. If chronic glaucoma is not recognized and treated in the early stage, the person eventually goes blind.

Treatment

Treatment is aimed at reducing intraocular pressure. Latanoprost (0.005%) eye drops will increase uveoscleral outflow of aqueous humor and drugs such as dorzolamide will assist by reducing aqueous humor production (British National Formulary 2005). Additionally a miotic such as pilocarpine is prescribed up to four times a day. This opens up the inefficient drainage channels in the trabecular meshwork, thereby increasing drainage of the aqueous humour. Miotics cause constriction of the pupil as a side-effect. Laser surgery may be used to create an opening in the anterior chamber angle to improve the drainage of aqueous humor (Watkinson 2005).

Teaching the patient with glaucoma

Because glaucoma accounts for such a large proportion of blindness, more effort has been directed toward informing the general public about the disease and the significance of early recognition. The Royal College of Ophthalmologists' website (http://www.rcophth.ac.uk) has a series of patient education handbooks which may be downloaded covering a whole range of conditions including glaucoma.

Glaucoma cannot be cured, but blindness can be prevented by continuous use of a miotic as prescribed, by operation and by medical supervision, if it is begun early in the disease.

An important nursing responsibility is to alert the patient to activities and situations that predispose to a rise in intraocular pressure. The condition is explained to the patient and family, and emphasis is placed on the need for some precautions to prevent visual damage. Emotional and stressful situations are avoided as much as possible; the patient must learn to tolerate and live with what cannot be changed.

The patient and family must appreciate the importance of regularly scheduled visits to the ophthalmologist for measurement of the intraocular pressure and visual field and acuity testing. They are taught the correct method of instilling the prescribed miotic, and cautioned against the use of any solution or medication that is not prescribed by the doctor. An identification card or Medic Alert pendant indicating that the person suffers from glaucoma is recommended. Some job modification or change may be made by encouraging the patient to consult with the employer and occupational health department, but every effort should be made to continue employment.

Acute angle-closure glaucoma

This form of glaucoma is characterized by rapid marked increase in intraocular pressure as a result of a complete block in the outflow of the aqueous humour. The iris appears to have been pushed forward, narrowing the peripheral angle between it and the cornea (Fig. 21.13) and, with dilatation of the pupil and the concomitant thickening of the iris, the openings in the filtration angle that lead into the canal of Schlemm become occluded. The condition demands prompt emergency care because rapid compression of the retinal blood vessels develops, and destruction of the optic nerve cells and fibres occurs, with resultant loss of vision. It is therefore an emergency condition needing immediate intervention to prevent loss of sight.

Characteristics

The patient with acute glaucoma experiences severe pain, nausea and vomiting, halos or rainbows around artificial lights, and sudden reduction in vision such that hand movements only may be seen. On examination, the pupil is seen to be semi-dilated and fixed, and there is evidence of congestion with a marked increase in intraocular pressure. The cornea becomes oedematous and hazy losing its lustre and transparency. Intraocular pressure can be as high as 60 mmHg.

Carbonic anhydrase inhibitors such as acetazolamide are the drugs of first choice as they reduce aqueous humour production. They should be given stat. intravenously and combined with immediate administration of a topical beta-blocker such as timolol eye-drops and an alpha-adrenergic agonist (e.g. apraclonidine eye-drops) for emergency management. Dexamethasone 0.1% and hypromellose 0.5% eye drops are then instilled every 15 minutes for 1 hour to reduce inflammation and congestion of the eyes. Once intraocular pressure has been brought under control, a miotic such as pilocarpine can be given to open the closed angle. Intravenous mannitol may be used if the patient's intraocular pressure does not respond to this regime (Watkinson 2005). A quiet environment is provided and the patient is helped to relax, positioned with the head and shoulders elevated; analgesia is prescribed to relieve the pain.

The definitive treatment is usually surgical involving *laser iridotomy*, where an opening is made in the iris using a laser beam.

Cataract

A cataract is a clouding of the crystalline lens, resulting in opacity. It may be classified as a *degenerative* or *developmental* (congenital or juvenile) cataract; the latter type of cataract occurs most often in infants whose mothers have a history of a viral infection (e.g. German measles) during the first trimester of pregnancy, or is associated with a genetic defect that, for example, causes an inborn error of metabolism.

The degenerative cataract has a higher incidence in persons over 50 years of age. As the lens cells are effectively dead, they have no repair or regeneration mechanisms. Consequently, minor damage accumulates over a lifetime to cause cataracts in many people. Dahm (2004) points out that exposure to highly reactive molecules such as free radicals and ultraviolet radiation are two such mechanisms while exposure to high blood sugar levels seen in diabetes mellitus is another cause. The impact of cataract and age-related degeneration (yellowing) of the lens is most strikingly seen when comparing the paintings of the great French Impressionist artist, Claude Monet in the 1890s with

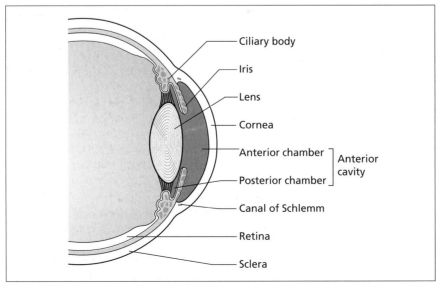

Figure 21.13 Diagram showing how a disturbance in the balance of fluid within the eyeball increases pressure in the eye and can result in glaucoma. Solid arrow indicates normal direction of fluid movement. Broken arrow indicates abnormal movement in glaucoma.

Ciliary body

Iris

Lens

Cornea

Anterior chamber ⎤
                  ⎬ Anterior
Posterior chamber ⎦ cavity

Canal of Schlemm

Retina

Sclera

his paintings of the same scenes 30 years later. Other known causes of degeneration include exposure to ionizing radiation or after prolonged steroid usage.

Characteristics

The opacity develops very gradually (unless caused by trauma) and may be localized to the centre of the lens, incurring early impairment of vision, or it may start in the periphery. A cataract, even in its early stage, is readily recognized through the pupil, using an ophthalmoscope. As it matures, the examiner is not able to visualize the fundus or optic disc and the pupillary area appears grey or whitish because of the opaque lens behind it.

The loss of the normal refractive ability of the lens prevents light rays from being focused on the retina. Vision becomes blurred, objects may appear distorted and colour perception decreases. Visual loss is very gradual and is directly proportional to the degree of opacity of the lens. Cataract may be unilateral or bilateral; if bilateral, the opacity does not usually develop at the same rate in both lenses.

Treatment

Cataract is irreversible but, as loss of transparency of the lens develops, visual acuity and distant vision can usually be improved by increasing the correction of lens in the person's spectacles. Eventually, the opacity increases to the point that no light rays pass through the lens to reach the retina.

When the person's visual impairment becomes a handicap and interferes with usual lifestyle and activities, surgical treatment is undertaken to insert a small plastic intra-ocular lens (IOL).

The anterior portion of the capsule and the lens content may be removed, or the procedure may involve phacoemulsification. Phacoemulsification involves the introduction of an instrument into the eye through a small incision and ultrasonic vibrations fragment the lens content, which prepares it for aspiration. The extracapsular extraction leaves the posterior part of the capsule intact and the vitreous body undisturbed.

If an IOL cannot be inserted, *intracapsular cataract extraction* is performed. The lens is removed, complete with its capsule, usually by cryoextraction in which a probe-like instrument is introduced so that it lies against the lens and is cooled to 230–235°C. The lens and its capsule freeze to the probe, and are removed when the probe is withdrawn.

Usually cataract extraction is done in only one eye at a time; if both eyes are affected, they are treated (in most cases) in separate operations.

Care of a person with a progressive cataract

During the period through which the lens is progressively losing its transparency, a nurse usually has contact with the patient only at the clinic, the surgery or on home visits that are for some other purpose. However, if the patient is a nursing home resident they will be in contact with nursing staff continuously. Assessment of visual impairment should be ongoing.

Potential patient problems
- Anxiety due to the visual impairment and fear of blindness and dependency
- Potential for injury
- Decreased mobility, usually due to a fear of moving about, especially outside the immediate familiar environment
- Alteration in self-image.

Anxiety   The nurse explains to the patient and family what cataracts are and reassures them that it is a common problem. They should be advised that vision can be improved by corrective lenses in glasses for a period of time and that eventually the cataract can be treated by surgery. Details should then be given about what this will entail.

Potential for injury   Advice should be given to the patient and family about adjustments within the patient's environment that may be necessary to prevent accidents. Improved lighting may help and other aids, such as stair rails, can be installed. Direct vision into sunlight and bright lights is avoided. Driving should be discussed with the patient and the advice of the ophthalmologist sought.

Decreased mobility   Because of the fear of falling, or of making errors and being unable to read signs, price tags, etc., the patient becomes reluctant to venture beyond immediate familiar environments and activity may gradually decrease. Socialization decreases. The patient should be encouraged to go out with family members and friends, not to hesitate to ask for assistance when alone, and to turn the head to obtain a direct view of an object if peripheral vision is poor. The patient and family are informed that books in large print are available in public libraries. They are also advised of the services of the local branch of the Royal National Institute for the Blind. Registration as blind or partially sighted will make certain benefits and allowances available.

Alteration in self-image   The person with loss of vision may become depressed and lose self-esteem as activity and participation progressively become restricted and dependence upon others increases. The positive aspects of life should be emphasized and accessible forms of diversion discussed. Unless there is some existing complication that contraindicates surgery, the patient is reassured that this is a temporary problem that will be relieved by the operation.

Postoperative care of patients following intraocular surgery   An operation for the treatment of cataracts is one of the most common intraocular operations. The care outlined in the following section applies to all intraocular surgery as well as that specifically for cataracts.

The period of bedrest and hospitalization following eye surgery is now reduced to a minimum, with day-case surgery becoming more common. The problems of bedrest and immobility are therefore much reduced.

The major concerns following eye surgery are potential eye injury and complications such as infection. The nursing care for each potential problem is outlined below.

Pain The patient may experience some burning or smarting sensation which can be relieved by a mild analgesic. Severe pain, particularly if it develops suddenly, or a feeling of pressure within the eye, can be an indication of haemorrhage and so must be identified promptly and reported to the surgeon.

Potential for eye injury related to surgery The main potential problems are intraocular haemorrhage, increased intraocular pressure and rupture of an incision line. To avoid these, the surgeon may request restrictions in activity and positioning, in which case the head may need to be supported by a nurse when transferring from trolley to bed, and when moving in bed. These restrictions must be understood by the patient and relatives.

Any increase in pressure on the eye is to be avoided. Possible causes include straining at stool, vomiting or retching, coughing, sudden movements and bending or leaning over the side of the bed. Nursing care is directed to avoid these situations, so a high-fibre diet is given, with plenty of fluids and a stool softener if necessary; antiemetics are given as necessary; the patient is shown how to cough with the mouth open, if coughing is unavoidable and instruction on permitted activity is given.

Any prescribed dressings and drugs (including eyedrops) are given and a protective eye shield may be used at night for additional protection.

Any pain that is severe or of sudden onset is reported to the surgeon.

Potential for infection The length of time a dressing is kept on depends on the operation, the surgeon and the treatments required. Whenever a dressing is touched, strict asepsis is observed and the eye is inspected for inflammation or discharge.

Prophylactic antibiotic drops may be prescribed, with the addition of systemic therapy if infection is suspected. Any discharge is swabbed for culture and sensitivity.

Topical corticosteroids may be prescribed to reduce the effects of inflammation on intraocular structures.

Potential for injury related to sensory deprivation or disorientation When vision is severely impaired either by the operation, swelling or dressings, or because the room is darkened, the patient will need additional care and support to reduce the fear and anxiety associated with loss of sight, even if it is only temporary.

On return from theatre, the patient will need to be oriented to location, staff and time, and this should be repeated whenever a person enters the patient's vicinity. The call button must be ready and within reach, and the patient should not be left alone for long periods; frequent communication reduces the potential for sensory deprivation.

When ambulatory, the patient is assisted until familiar with the environment. Footstools, loose rugs and other hazards should be removed, and the furniture kept in a specific position where possible. Doors should all be either kept open or kept closed.

If the patient becomes confused, sedation may be prescribed. If possible, a friend or family member should stay with the confused patient to ensure his or her safety.

Inadequate nutrition Self-care in eating and drinking may not be possible if vision is impaired after operation. A fluid intake and output chart should be kept until a normal intake is achieved. Help should be given to pour drinks and with feeding, and appropriate foods chosen and aids used to help independence.

Nausea and vomiting should be avoided (to prevent increase in intraorbital pressure) and antiemetics given as necessary.

A high-fibre diet should be provided (to prevent straining at stool) and a stool softener given if necessary.

Inadequate knowledge of care and rehabilitation The patient's home situation should be assessed and the patient and family assisted to make appropriate changes.

The restrictions on normal activities required to avoid an increase in intraocular pressure must be understood. These restrictions include bending over, pushing, avoidance of falls and bumps, and sexual activity. Information must be given as to how long these restrictions are likely to be needed.

The patient and/or family must understand and learn the care of the eye, eye socket or artificial eye, such as cleaning and dressing it, the instillation of drops or ointment and the avoidance of rubbing or friction on the eye. They must also be aware of the symptoms that indicate the need to contact the ward or surgeon (pain, inflammation, discharge or loss of vision).

The care and appropriate use of any glasses or contact lenses must be understood. Restrictions on reading or watching television may be imposed on the patient to avoid straining the eye, and restrictions on driving may be needed for a period prescribed by the surgeon. These need to be understood. Any further appointments or follow-up care must be given to the patient.

Specific postoperative care following cataract surgery

Contact lenses When the dressing is removed, dark glasses are worn because the patient may experience discomfort in the eye with exposure to light; gradual adaptation is necessary. If an intraocular lens has not been implanted at the time of the operation, the patient may be fitted with a contact lens some weeks after surgery. The lens may be of the type that has to be removed each night, or an extended-wear type that can be left in the eye for several weeks. With the latter, the patient returns to the clinic or ophthalmologist at regular intervals (approximately 90–120 days) to have the lens removed, cleansed and replaced.

Complications Complications that may occur following cataract extraction include the following:

- *Haemorrhage* into the anterior chamber (hyphaema) is a serious complication that may occur in the early postoperative period. The patient experiences sharp pain in the eye and, on examination, blood can be seen in the eye. The patient is placed at rest, the head is elevated and the ophthalmologist is notified immediately. A mydriatic preparation is usually ordered to dilate the pupil and rest the eye

- *Wound rupture and iris prolapse* occurs rarely and is manifested by a misshapen iris and bulging in the incision area. It requires prompt surgical treatment to avoid serious visual impairment. Mydriatics must not be instilled if a prolapse is suspected as this can worsen the condition
- *Infection* may develop as an acute bacterial endophthalmitis leading to pain, loss of vision and inflammation. A severe infection may manifest itself as a *hypopyon* – white cells in the anterior chamber and corneal haze. It is treated by topical and parenteral antibiotics
- *Retinal detachment* occurs rarely as a result of the formation of adhesions within the eye, usually between the retina and the vitreous (see treatment of retinal detachment below)
- *Glaucoma* may also develop as a result of adhesions forming between the iris and the cornea, blocking the filtration angle.

Age-related macular degeneration

This degenerative disorder of the macula is the leading cause of blindness in people over 65 in the UK, affecting approximately 220 000 people (Owen et al 2003). In most cases, degeneration of the retinal epithelium cells responsible for supporting the macula and removing waste products of metabolism from its cells lies at the root of the problem. As a result, there is an accumulation of metabolic waste products in the retina, macula cells degenerate and the central part of the visual field deteriorates although peripheral vision may be unaffected. The deterioration in vision is very slow unlike an alternative form of macular degeneration characterized by the growth of abnormal blood vessels in the macula which can lead to loss of sight in a few months (Watkinson 2005). This condition can have a familial tendency and unfortunately, there is no cure. Laser treatment (photodynamic therapy) may assist by limiting further loss of vision, but it cannot restore vision already lost.

Diabetic retinopathy

This disease involves degeneration of small retinal blood vessels leading to bleeding and growth of new blood vessels within the eye. It is secondary to diabetes mellitus (see p. 557) and is most likely to occur in people with poorly controlled diabetes. NICE (2005) estimate that 20 years after the onset of type 2 Diabetes, 60% of people will have diabetic retinopathy leading to visual loss. Laser surgery is the main treatment, however, it cannot be emphasized enough that effective, tight control of diabetes is the best option as it may prevent the problem in the first place. NICE (2005) guidelines encourage indirect ophthalmoscopy and digital photography as the best screening tools for the early detec-

tion of this condition. Screening should significantly reduce the incidence of visual impairment.

Detachment of the retina

Retinal detachment is separation of the pigmented epithelium of the **retina** from the layer of rods and cones; the pigmented layer remains attached to the choroid. The separation occurs as a result of tears or holes in the retina. These openings permit fluid from within the eye to leak through and accumulate in the retina, causing the separation.

The cause may be degenerative retinal changes associated with the ageing process, aphakia (absence of the lens), trauma or tumour. The trauma may be directly to the eye (e.g. penetrating foreign body) or may be associated with a head injury. Retinal detachment may occur as a complication following cataract extraction or an inflammatory intraocular disorder. There is a higher incidence in those who have myopia and are over 50 years of age. The damaged areas are usually toward the periphery of the retina but may occur in the area of the macula, causing severe visual impairment.

Characteristics

Manifestations of a detached retina appear suddenly and are preceded by flashes of light, blurred vision, floating particles in the line of vision before the sensation of a curtain coming in front of a part of the eye, restricted visual field and eventual loss of vision occurs.

Treatment

The patient is placed at rest and both eyes may be covered. A mydriatic and cycloplegic drug such as cyclopentolate hydrochloride (Mydrilate) may be prescribed for instillation to dilate the pupils and arrest accommodation by depressing ciliary action. The ophthalmologist indicates the position the patient is to assume: left or right lateral, or on the back (never prone). The position is such that the detached area of the retina will approximate the underlying layers. A sedative or tranquillizer may be prescribed to reduce the patient's fear and apprehension, and promote immobility. The patient is advised of the importance of maintaining the recommended position and of avoiding sudden movements, bending over, coughing, sneezing and rubbing the eye. The patient should be informed that assistance is close at hand and how it may be summoned.

Surgical intervention is usually undertaken fairly early. Various procedures are used, but the underlying principle is scarring of the area. As the scar tissue forms, it fills in the retinal hole and provides attachment to the underlying sclera.

Vitrectomy is fast becoming a common surgical method of treating complicated retinal detachments. The retina is reapposed to the underlying pigment epithelium by removing vitreous humour and replacing this with liquid gas or oil. This method requires strict positioning for 2–3 days after operation.

After the operation, a patch is placed over the eye for 24 hours. Dilating and antimicrobial eye-drops may then be ordered. The patient is instructed to ask for assistance when ambulating and not to bend or strain. The light in the room is kept low to decrease light sensitivity when the patch is removed and dark glasses may be worn. Because of the amount of oedema within a confined space (the orbit), pain can be a problem and may be for 6–8 weeks after the operation. A full explanation of the cause of pain and regular analgesia may be given. Analgesia to take home should also be prescribed.

Before discharge, the patient is taught to instill the eye drops and is given written instructions about activity limitations. No heavy lifting or heavy work is undertaken for a period of at least 5–6 weeks. Appointments are made for follow-up care. The patient must be cautioned against bumping the head, rapid eye movements, reading and close work.

Uveitis

Inflammation due to injury or infection may develop in the uveal tract, which includes the choroid, iris and ciliary body. It may also be associated with collagen disease (e.g. rheumatoid arthritis, sarcoidosis).

Characteristics

The eye is reddened and the patient complains of pain, photophobia and impaired vision in the affected eye. The pupil usually remains constricted.

Treatment

Treatment may include rest of the eyes, the application of heat and the administration of an antimicrobial drug if infection is suspected as being the cause. A mydriatic (e.g. atropine, cyclopentolate, tropicamide) is instilled to dilate the pupil and prevent adhesions from developing between the iris and the lens. A corticoid preparation may be given systemically and also instilled in the eye(s) to arrest the inflammatory process and scar formation; scar formation is likely to cause loss of vision.

Keratitis

This term is used for inflammation of the cornea, which is a serious condition. It may be due to infection or trauma and is likely to lead to ulceration and scarring. The affected areas lose their transparency, diminishing the light rays entering the eye.

Debilitated persons and those with vitamin A deficiency and allergies develop corneal ulceration more readily with an eye infection or trauma. The inflammation may be superficial or deep and in some instances becomes chronic.

Characteristics

Keratitis is manifested by irritation, discharge if the cause is infection, redness of the eye due to injection of the peripheral areas of the cornea by blood vessels, photophobia and lacrimation. Ulcerated areas may be identified by the instillation of fluorescein, which outlines the lesions.

Treatment

Prompt medical treatment is necessary to prevent perforation of the cornea and serious visual damage. Keratitis

frequently may be prevented by early removal of foreign bodies as well as early treatment of injuries and infection.

Treatment includes rest, the use of antimicrobial drugs, the instillation of a mydriatic and the administration of systemic analgesia to relieve pain. The eyes may be covered to protect them from light and to limit eye movement. If ulcers develop and are complicated by corneal perforation, the aqueous humour escapes, the anterior chamber collapses and there may be intraocular bleeding. The patient is placed on complete bedrest, a mydriatic is instilled in the affected eye to dilate the pupil, and a pressure dressing is applied. Sometimes a soft contact lens called a protective membrane or bandage lens is applied.

If a cornea appears to be in danger of perforating, the lids may be closed over it, either by closure by tape or actually sutured shut, a tarsorrhaphy. In severe cases, surgery to the cornea (keratoplasty) may be required.

Vitreous haemorrhage

The most common cause of vitreous opacity is bleeding from adjacent papillary, retinal or ciliary vessels. With minimal bleeding, the patient may be conscious of floaters or 'small black dots'; more serious bleeding causes a sudden flood of floaters and subsequent loss of visual acuity so that the patient is only able to perceive light.

The haemorrhage may be associated with trauma, retinal tears and detachment, hypertension or diabetes mellitus. Many people with diabetes develop diabetic retinopathy, which is a common cause of blindness; increased vascular permeability, microaneurysms and atheroma (fatty plaques in the walls of the arteries) develop in the ocular blood vessels in diabetic retinopathy. Fragile vessels in the vitreous frequently bleed.

Loss of vitreous transparency may also be caused by uveitis in which the inflammatory exudate and debris are carried into the vitreous and cause opacity.

Minor haemorrhages into the vitreous resolve fairly quickly. In more severe bleeding, which causes a serious visual impairment or where there is a loss of vitreous transparency due to other aetiological factors, a *vitrectomy* may be undertaken. This involves the removal of vitreous content and opacities with a special instrument to which there is a fibreoptic light attached. The vitreous is replaced with a liquid or gas.

Keratoconus

This is a rare degenerative disorder of the cornea that is seen in young persons, usually young men. There is a degenerative thinning and protrusion of the central cornea, usually of both eyes. Severe astigmatism develops, causing visual impairment.

An excessive amount of fluid collects posterior to the protruding cornea, and scar tissue develops as a result of the damage to tissue by stretching and rupture. The person experiences blurring of vision in the early stages but progressive changes may eventually lead to complete loss of vision. The patient may be helped at first by the wearing of hard contact lenses but may finally require keratoplasty.

Keratoplasty (cornea transplantation)

Loss of vision due to destruction of the cornea, keratoconus or loss of transparency may be corrected by a cornea transplantation. The central portion of the affected cornea is removed and replaced with a cornea obtained from a cadaver. The period between death and removal of the graft should not exceed 6–8 hours, and the transplant must be performed within 24–48 hours. Corneal tissue can now be preserved for up to 2 weeks as corneal buttons and still remain viable, which has reduced the need for the majority of patients to be sent for urgently, and this operation can now be planned for. During the interval following enucleation, the donor eye is refrigerated at 4°C to minimize degenerative changes. Rejection is less of a problem with corneal transplantation than with other types of organ transplantation. It is suggested that this is due to the avascularity of the cornea. In the absence of blood vessels, donor tissue antigens do not get into the recipient's blood to initiate the formation of antibodies and sensitized lymphocytes.

Preoperative preparation

A detailed discussion of all that is involved in a keratoplasty occurs between the surgeon and the patient and family. The patient is informed that several weeks will elapse following the transplant before the results can be evaluated.

The immediate preoperative period is now a planned admission. Blood specimens are collected for the usual preoperative blood studies, and the surgeon usually prescribes the instillation of a miotic (e.g. pilocarpine 2–4%) in the affected eye to constrict the pupil so that the lens is protected during operation. Acetazolamide may be prescribed to reduce the intraocular fluid volume and tension.

Types of keratoplasty

The operative procedure may be a penetrating keratoplasty or a lamellar transplant. The *penetrating transplant* involves a full-thickness removal of the central portion of the affected cornea and replacement with an equivalent full-thickness section of the donor cornea. In a *lamellar keratoplasty*, a partial-thickness piece of the donor cornea replaces superficial layers of the recipient's cornea.

Postoperative management

The patient experiences some pain and a mild analgesic may be prescribed. The main cause of discomfort is the presence of the sutures giving a continuous 'foreign body' sensation. The sutures stay in for 3–9 months, but the eyes usually become more comfortable as the epithelium grows over the sutures.

The patient is allowed up as much as he or she wishes after recovery from the anaesthetic.

The eye is protected by a dressing. Sunglasses are worn during the day; at night, a shield (usually of plastic) is applied.

Topical medications prescribed for instillation for a period of time may include, in addition to a mydriatic such as cyclopentolate (Mydrilate), a corticosteroid preparation to suppress inflammation which would reduce the clearness and transparency of the cornea. A prophylactic topical antibiotic may also be used for a few days. When instilling ointments or drops, as always, precautions are observed to avoid any pressure on the eye and to avoid having the dropper or the tube applicator touch the eye.

During the weeks and months after the transplantation, the patient may have alternating periods of optimism and discouragement. It is important for the patient to be informed before leaving the hospital that healing will be slow because a transparent cornea does not have blood vessels.

A family member and the patient receive demonstrations and instructions in the care of the eye and the instilling of medications in preparation for leaving the hospital. If a family member or the patient is not able to undertake the care safely, a referral may be made to the district nurse. The patient is followed closely by frequent visits to the clinic or surgeon.

Injury to the eye

An eye may be traumatized by a foreign body, laceration or chemical agent. The patient may experience the discomfort associated with 'something in the eye' excessive lacrimation, pain, redness and sensitivity to light. Persisting pain, loss of vision and bleeding usually manifest a serious injury. With any type of injury, contact lenses should be removed promptly.

A *foreign body* may lodge on the conjunctiva or may be embedded in the conjunctival or corneal tissue, causing inflammation and possible ulceration. In some accidents, the injury may penetrate the lens or even the retina. If a foreign body is not washed out easily, the patient is promptly referred to an ophthalmologist or accident and emergency department. Fluorescein dye may be used in the eye during the assessment to localize the foreign body. Deep metal foreign bodies may be removed with a strong electromagnet. If the foreign body has caused an abrasion or was penetrating, an antibiotic ointment is instilled and a dressing may be applied.

Lacerations of the eyeball seriously threaten vision because of the formation of scar tissue in healing and by predisposing the eye to infection. Prompt treatment and strict asepsis are very important.

Various *chemicals*, acids and alkalis (such as cement or mortar) may cause serious irritation or burns of the conjunctiva and cornea. Emergency treatment consists of washing the eye with copious amounts of water or saline. The lids must be wide open and assistance may have to be provided in order to keep the eye open during the flushing. The person should be taken to an A&E department as quickly as possible where they should receive high priority in whatever triage system is in use. A local anaesthetic may be instilled to provide relief and facilitate examination of the eye(s). Both eyes are covered to limit eye movement.

Strabismus (squint)

Normally, both eyes perform an equal range of movement and assume corresponding lines of position when focusing on an object. Strabismus ('cross eyes') is characterized by the deviation of one eye from the position of the other. One eye (the normal or fixing eye) focuses directly on the object, but the other one (the deviating eye) appears to be focused on a different object or area.

The inequality in the movement of the eyes is due to an imbalance in the function of one or more extrinsic ocular muscles. The defect may result in the eye being turned medially, producing a convergent strabismus (*esotropia*). If the eye is turned laterally, the condition is referred to as divergent strabismus (*exotropia*). The result of the unequal movement and two points of focus is double vision (*diplopia*). Two images are formed on the retinae and the visual centres in the brain receive two sets of impulses, each producing a separate picture.

Strabismus may also be classified as being non-paralytic or paralytic. *Non-paralytic strabismus* (the more common) is the result of a congenital abnormality. The defect is in the central nervous system mechanism that coordinates the movements of the eyes in order to bring them into the positions that will focus the light rays from an object on corresponding areas of the two retinae. The person may be able to focus the right eye on an object of attention but the left deviates, presenting a second image.

The person with strabismus develops single vision over a period of time, seeing only what the fixing or non-deviating eye perceives by involuntarily suppressing the confusing image presented by the deviating eye. Non-paralytic strabismus is generally recognized in early childhood.

Paralytic strabismus is due to the inability of the extra-ocular muscles to move the eye into the position corresponding to that of the other eye. As a result, the person experiences diplopia. The cause of paralytic strabismus may be a defect in the muscle itself or a disturbance in the muscle innervation. The condition may be a manifestation of a disorder within the brain or orbit that interferes with the transmission of impulses by the third (oculomotor), fourth (trochlear) or sixth (abducens) cranial nerve.

Treatment

Strabismus requires medical treatment; unfortunately, in some instances parents think it will correct itself as the child becomes older. A delay may result in permanent damage; constant suppression of the image presented by the deviating eye may lead to loss of vision in that eye (amblyopia). The form of treatment will depend on the cause and severity of the strabismus. Obviously, if it is secondary to a lesion that is interrupting nerve impulses, the primary condition is surgically treated, if possible. Strabismus in the child may be corrected by the wearing of prescribed glasses. The unaffected eye may be covered for periods to enforce the use of the deviating (or so-called 'lazy') eye. Special eye exercises may be ordered (*orthoptics*).

If the condition does not respond to these conservative forms of treatment, surgical correction may then be undertaken. The procedure may involve shortening or lengthening of one or more extrinsic eye muscles. After the operation,

exercise and the wearing of glasses may still be necessary for a period of time. The patient requires continual medical supervision.

Neoplasms of the eye and accessory structures

Tumours that develop in the skin on other parts of the body may also occur on the skin of the eyelids. Neoplasms of the external structures are usually discovered in the early stages because they are visible.

Neoplasms of the eye may be benign or malignant and the latter may be primary or secondary. Secondary malignancies in the eye are rare. A biopsy is done if the neoplasm is accessible. Malignant melanoma is the most common intraocular tumour. It usually originates in the choroid, ciliary body or iris. Retinoblastoma which develops in both eyes is attributed to a genetic defect that is considered to be hereditary.

Early symptoms of an intraocular neoplasm depend on its location. As it enlarges and spreads, pain is experienced because of the increased intraocular pressure; retinal detachment, intraocular haemorrhage and loss of vision occur. Primary malignant tumours may be treated by radiotherapy, local excision or enucleation.

Enucleation

Enucleation is the removal of an eyeball and may be necessary because of a malignant neoplasm, deep infection, severe trauma or persisting pain in a blind eye. Rarely, an enucleation is done to remove a disfiguring blind eye. When an eyeball is removed, the extrinsic muscles are severed close to their insertion, and may be arranged around a plastic ball to provide support and movement for an artificial eye. A plastic shell is inserted as soon as possible to maintain lid tone and prevent adhesions from developing between the layers of conjunctiva which would make the fitting of a prosthesis difficult. The prosthesis is made as soon as the incision has healed and the oedema has subsided.

The patient should not be discharged until able to clean the socket and handle the shell proficiently. A district nurse may be asked to visit.

Occasionally, the operation performed is an evisceration in which the contents of the eyeball are removed, leaving the sclera. This is more usually performed when infection is present, to prevent spread to the brain.

A more radical procedure may be necessary in malignancy or severe trauma. The operation performed is called *exenteration* and involves the removal of the eyeball and the surrounding structures. These operations can be psychologically very distressing as they alter the individual's body image. The patient should be given time to express feelings.

Sympathetic ophthalmia

After an eye injury, especially a deep penetrating one, the patient may develop panophthalmitis (inflammation of the ciliary body, choroid and iris) in the uninjured eye. This response is not understood; it has been suggested that it may be an allergic reaction to the pigment released by the damaged eye. Any redness or tearing of the uninjured eye and any complaint of photophobia, pain or loss of vision must be reported promptly. The condition may develop soon after the injury or several months or years later. Unless the inflammatory reaction is checked promptly, loss of vision results. Corticoid preparations are used locally and systemically. Rarely, the injured eye is removed to prevent sympathetic ophthalmitis from developing.

SUMMARY

The importance of all the senses to normal human functioning and independence is apparent. The psychological trauma of any threat to a person's senses, particularly vision, hearing or touch must always be considered, whatever the setting they are in. There must be a greater awareness of the importance of good communication and education of patients threatened with the loss of one of their senses.

REFERENCES

Ah-See K (2004) Effects of treatment in people with clinically diagnosed acute sinusitis. Clinical Evidence 12: 792.

Black J, Hawks J (2005) Medical surgical nursing, 7th edn. St Louis: Elsevier/Saunders.

British National Formulary (BNF) (2005) British National Formulary 49. London: British Medical Association/Royal Pharmaceutical Society of Great Britain.

Browning G (2004) Effects of methods to remove symptomatic earwax. Clinical Evidence 12: 730–31.

Dahm R (2004) Dying to see. Scientific American October: 82–89.

Kass MA, Heuer DK, Higginbotham EJ et al (2002) The Ocular Hypertension Treatment Study: a randomised trial determines that topical hypotensive medication delays or prevents the onset of primary open-angle glaucoma. Archives of Ophthalmology 120(6): 701–713.

Haslett C, Chilvers E, Boon N, Colledge N (2002) Davidson's principles and practice of medicine, 19th edn. Edinburgh: Churchill Livingstone.

National Institute for Clinical Excellence (NICE) (2005) Management of Type 2 diabetes – retinopathy: Early management and screening. Guideline E. Online. Available: www.nice.org.uk/page/.aspx?o=27967

O'Neil P, Roberts A (2004) Acute otitis media; effects of treatment. Clinical Evidence 12: 327–332.

Owen C, Fletcher A, Donoghue M, Rudnicka R (2003) How big is the burden of visual loss caused by age related macular degeneration in the UK. British Journal of Ophthalmology 87: 312–317.

Pirozzo S, Papinczak T, Glasziou P (2004) Review: the whispered voice test is accurate for detecting hearing impairment in children and adults. Evidence Based Nursing 7(2): 56.

Ramachandran V, Hubbard E (2005) Hearing colors, tasting shapes. Scientific American Mind 16(3): 16–23.

Royal National Institute for the Blind (2001) The prevalence of visual impairment in the UK. A review of the literature. Online. Available: www.rnib.org.uk [Accessed 23.02.2006].

Reynolds T (2004) Ear, nose and throat problems in Accident and Emergency. Nursing Standard 18(26): 47–53.

Tortora G, Grabowski S (2003) Principles of anatomy and physiology, 10th edn. New York: Wiley.

Van Balen F, Smit W, Zuithoff N (2003) Clinical efficacy of three common treatments in otitis externa in primary care: randomised controlled trial. British Medical Journal 327: 1201–1205.

Walsh M (2006) Nurse practitioners; clinical skills and professional issues, 2nd edn. Oxford: Butterworth-Heinemann.

Watkinson S (2005) Visual impairment in older people: the nurse's role. Nursing Standard 19(17): 45–52.

USEFUL WEBSITES

Clinical Evidence	www.clinicalevidence.com
International Glaucoma Association	www.iga.org.uk
Macular Disease Society	www.maculardisease.org
Royal College of Ophthalmologists	www.rcophth.ac.uk
Royal National Institute for the Blind	www.rnib.org.uk

Caring for the patient with a disorder of the male reproductive system

Mike Walsh

INTRODUCTION

Great attention has been paid to women's health as a subject in its own right, and men's health has been rather neglected in comparison. The men's health agenda is huge but this chapter concentrates only on the male reproductive system. You should recognize, however, that men's health encompasses issues such as cardiovascular disease, mental health, suicide risk, alcohol abuse, trauma and violence, all of which are more prevalent in the male half of the population. A man's self-concept and self-esteem are closely linked to his sexual health. Many individuals will have a partner whose views and feelings must also be taken into account; the partner may also have to adapt to significant changes in the patient as a result of illness and treatment.

SUMMARY OF PHYSIOLOGY

IN UTERO DEVELOPMENT

The adult **male reproductive system** consists of the paired testes, epididymis, vas deferens, common ejaculatory ducts, urethra, penis and scrotum. The accessory organs are the seminal vesicles, prostate gland and the bulbourethral glands (Fig. 22.1). Sex itself is determined at the time of fertilization by the inclusion of the XX chromosomal pair of the female or the XY genotype of the male. In this early period of human development, sex differentiation can be determined microscopically by the presence or absence of Barr bodies in a cell nucleus that has been taken from the embryo. As the embryo grows, an internal genital ridge develops but remains undifferentiated in either sex until the seventh week of intrauterine life.

While internal development proceeds, the external genitalia are also becoming differentiated – so much so that by the 16th week of embryological life the sex of the infant can be determined externally. At this time the testes are not present in the scrotum but are in the abdomen. As the fetal testes begin to produce testosterone, in about the 7th month of fetal life, descent occurs, and they pass through the inguinal canal and the external inguinal ring to enter the scrotum by the 9th month. After descent, the testis shows a decline in its production of testosterone until puberty. As in all processes, descent may not occur or may occur imperfectly. This may result in undescended testes.

THE TESTES

Each lobe of the testis contains a seminiferous tubule surrounded by tissue that produces the male hormones, of which testosterone is the most prominent. At puberty, under the complex control of the hypothalamus and pituitary glands, the testes are stimulated to produce male hormones. Under the influence of these androgens, the body begins the process of puberty. The external organs of reproduction grow and develop. The distribution of body hair changes to that of the adult male. The larynx and musculoskeletal systems develop and change. Concurrently, the testes begin to produce sperm. Puberty ends with the sexual and reproductive maturity of the individual.

Spermatogenesis

Spermatogenesis begins in the seminiferous tubule and, when growth is complete, the sperm is released into the lumen of the seminiferous tubule, rapidly transported to the epididymis and thence through the duct system. Although sperm may appear to be mature at the time of release into

Figure 22.1 The male reproductive system.

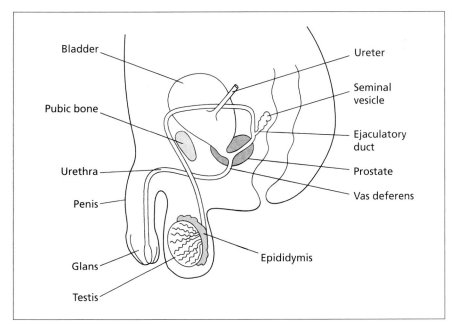

the tubule, they undergo further maturation, increasing in fertility and vigour as they progress through the ducts.

Spermatogenesis is also sensitive to heat, and occurs at a temperature a few degrees lower than body temperature. It is for this reason that the testes are suspended in the scrotum, allowing the temperature of the testes to be regulated by the body.

A feedback mechanism controls the production of sperm and testosterone. The anterior pituitary gland, when stimulated by the gonadotrophin-releasing hormone (GnRH) of the hypothalamus, releases two hormones: follicle-stimulating hormone (FSH) and luteinizing hormone (LH). FSH stimulates the seminiferous tubule to begin spermatogenesis.

Luteinizing hormone stimulates the interstitial cells of the testes to produce testosterone, which maintains and completes spermatogenesis. Testosterone is necessary to complete the step from spermatocyte to fertile spermatozoa.

High levels of testosterone exert an inhibitory effect on the hypothalamus. When testosterone reaches a low level, it no longer exerts this inhibitory effect and more GnRH is released, repeating the cycle.

DUCT SYSTEM AND ACCESSORY GLANDS

The viable sperm must be transported from the testis to the penis and thence to the female reproductive tract so that fertilization may take place. Here the duct system and the **accessory glands** play a major role. As a secretory organ, the *seminal vesicle* does not store sperm but rather produces an alkaline fluid that is rich in nutrients and prostaglandins. These nutrients provide for the sperm until fertilization. The prostaglandins are believed to aid fertilization by reacting with cervical mucus to make it more penetrable by sperm and to induce contractions in the uterus and tubes which help sperm to reach the ovum.

The *prostate gland*, which is fused to the neck of the bladder, surrounds the urethra. It develops in puberty and is easily palpable on rectal examination. During the years of sexual maturity the prostate secretes a thin, milky-looking fluid which is alkaline. This, together with the alkaline seminal vesicle secretions, reduces the acidity of seminal fluid and vaginal secretions. This is an important reproductive function, as the motility and viability of sperm are greatly reduced in an acid solution.

Further alkaline fluid is added to the semen by the *bulbourethral glands*. These paired glands lie posterior to the urethra and discharge their fluid into it when they contract at ejaculation. This fluid seems to function merely as a lubricant and fluid medium for the sperm.

Semen is an alkaline, viscous fluid varying at one ejaculation from 2 to 6 mL in quantity and containing nutrients to support the sperm. The normal sperm count is about $60–100 \times 10^6$ sperm per mL. A sperm count of below 20×10^6 per mL indicates probable infertility. The *sperm*, which are actively motile by lashing their tails, move rapidly up through the uterus into the outer third of the fallopian tube where fertilization usually takes place.

SEXUALITY

Sexuality is broadly defined as the becoming and being of a man or a woman. As such, adult sexuality has four major divisions, as shown in Figure 22.2:

1 **Biological sex.** Biological sex refers to the individual's physical attributes. In men, this is based in the genotype XY, and includes internal and external genitalia with the corresponding underlying hormonal, neural, vascular and physical components.

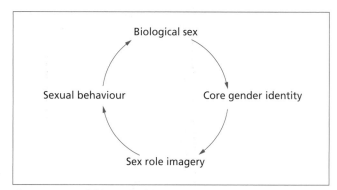

Figure 22.2   Divisions of adult sexuality.

2 *Core gender identity.* This refers to one's inner sense of being a man or a woman and is established early in life, usually by 3 years of age. At this age, the child knows he is a boy. In most cases, the core gender identity corresponds to the physical attributes of the individual.

3 *Sex role imagery.* This refers to the learned behaviour that the particular society ascribes to its men and women. Sex or gender role imagery is complex because it includes the myriad beliefs about what is often labelled feminine or masculine by a society. It also conveys the image of appropriate sexual conduct for particular social groups. Sex role imagery represents much of the learned behaviour that influences human choice and lifestyle. Much stereotyping of human behaviour has resulted from the need for society to set up expectations by which to guide and judge sex role behaviour. These roles can be used to set the parameters of a culture's moral agenda. The learning of sex role imagery begins in infancy and continues throughout most of life. This learned behaviour, combined with personal experience, is internalized and becomes the individual's personal belief about sexuality. If the nurse is to demonstrate cultural competence, s/he must be aware of the differences that exist between cultures in regard of sex roles and behaviours whilst balancing this against the basic human rights of people regardless of gender.

4 *Sexual behaviour.* This refers to sexual expression and is the acting out of sexual feelings and beliefs. It includes a broad spectrum of human behaviour including sexual lifestyles ranging from celibacy, monogamy, multiple sexual partners, same sex partners or participation in group sex.

Sexual behaviour involves both health and psychosocial risk taking and therefore cannot be excluded from nursing's public health agenda. We know the risks include possibly contracting a fatal disease (HIV), social dislocation (breakdown of relationships) or isolation (due to homophobia). Humans have always taken risks in their every day lives and we should not expect sex to be exempt from such risk taking behaviour (Price 2005). This is a key fact to remember in supporting patients and carrying out health education work. Price (2005) argues that sex is not only a physical activity between people but

is also any behaviour that has a major subjective element involving attitudes, beliefs, feelings, self concept and emotions. Being a man and sex are therefore bound together. We need to include both sexual fantasy and sexual reality in our understanding of sex. This applies to both men and women and we will return to these issues several times in this chapter.

These four aspects of sexuality are interrelated and reinforcing. Biological make-up and learning promote a core gender identity which influences acceptance of specific sex roles. Sexual expression reflects biology, gender identity, sex role and behaviour.

PHYSIOLOGICAL ASPECTS OF SEXUAL RESPONSE

Human **sexual response** occurs as a result of stimulation. This varies from purely mental images such as fantasy, dreams or remembered events to stimulation received through the senses. Touch is probably the most important source of stimulation and certain areas of the body appear to be more sensitive as stimulators of sexual arousal than others. These areas vary for each individual but the penis in the man and clitoris, labia and vagina in the woman are usually the most sensitive of the areas.

Learning modifies the emotional and physiological responses to sexual stimuli. As a result of previous learning or past experience, however, similar sexual stimuli may elicit a wide range of responses.

The response is a total one, but the most noticeable changes are seen in the primary sexual organs. The sexual response cycle has been divided into four progressive phases. The phases do not differ between the sexes and depend in each sex on the same physiological mechanisms:

1 *The excitement phase.* The person becomes sexually aroused in response to any source of stimulation. This phase is quite sensitive to outside influences and, if the stimuli are interrupted or not intense enough, the excitement phase may be prolonged or aborted.

2 *The plateau phase.* Sexual tension is intensified and reaches the pre-orgasmic level. Alteration in stimuli may also cause this phase to be prolonged or to revert to the pre-plateau level of sexual arousal.

3 *Orgasm.* This is the phase of release of sexual tension and is accompanied by ejaculation. It is experienced as an involuntary subjective feeling of pleasure or relief. This feeling is concentrated in the clitoris, vagina and uterus of the woman and in the penis, prostate and seminal vesicles of the male. There is much individual variation in the intensity and duration of orgasm; generally this relates directly to the degree of sexual arousal that preceded the orgasm.

4 *The resolution phase.* Following orgasm, the individual enters the phase during which the body returns to its pre-excitement state. Within this resolution phase the male passes through the refractory period, a time during which

the male cannot be re-stimulated to orgasm. The length of the refractory period varies with sexual episodes and may vary from a few minutes to several hours in the same individual.

Most of the observed responses during sexual excitement and resolution are due to two physiological mechanisms: vasocongestion and myotonia. *Vasocongestion* occurs as the muscular walls of the arterioles relax and expand allowing blood to rush in. This marked influx of blood into the area exceeds the ability of the veins to remove it and a period of vasocongestion occurs. *Myotonia* is increased muscle tension. During sexual activity, both smooth and skeletal muscles are affected.

Vasocongestion is triggered by a nervous impulse. Effective stimulation activates the parasympathetic nervous system and inhibits the sympathetic fibres. The parasympathetic nerve fibres cause the arterioles to relax and expand. Vasocongestion and penile erection result as the corpora cavernosa and corpus spongiosum become engorged with blood. It is the coordination between smooth muscle contraction and relaxation that controls the arterial and venous blood flow responsible for the erection (Vetrosky 2000). At orgasm, the sympathetic fibres are stimulated, causing the bladder sphincter to close and smooth muscles in the wall of the genital ducts to contract rhythmically, producing ejaculation.

Erection of the penis may be partial but it is considered to be functionally erect if vaginal penetration can be achieved before ejaculation. The first phase of ejaculation is called emission and occurs when semen is pooled in the prostatic urethra and the man is aware of impending ejaculation. This is followed by the second stage: expulsion of semen and sperm from the penis via the urethra.

A simple reflex arc also exists in the spinal cord. With genital stimulation, erection and ejaculation will occur after the spinal cord has been severed if the area of spinal nerve damage was above the sacral and lumbar areas governing erection and ejaculation. Because pleasure is experienced via sensory input to the brain, the sexual response is not felt by the individual if the spinal cord is transected.

DISORDERS OF THE MALE REPRODUCTIVE SYSTEM

PRINCIPLES OF ASSESSMENT

Privacy and sensitivity are essential to carry out the assessment, especially given the embarrassment that questions about sexual functioning may cause. As Peate (2005a) has observed, examination of the male genitalia, where relevant, is increasingly being seen as part of a holistic health assessment. A history should be taken before the physical examination and questions should be asked on a need-to-know basis but should not be omitted for fear of embarrassment. The patient's vocabulary may be limited and his language may be considered 'crude'; however, if they are the only words he knows then they should be accepted as part of the non-judgemental approach that should characterize any nurse–patient interaction. Above all, you need to know exactly what, where and for how long the patient has had a problem. Avoid ambiguous phrases such as 'down below' which could mean penis, scrotum, groin or anal area, or 'having sex' which could mean anything (such as masturbation, oral sex, anal sex or full penetrative vaginal intercourse). The man should always be asked for his understanding of the problem and what he considers to be the chief complaint. This should be followed by checking the following in the history (Jarvis 2004):

1 Past medical history with special attention being paid to the reproductive system. Childhood should be included (e.g. undescended testicle) as well as adult life (e.g. vasectomy or previous sexually transmitted infection (STI)). Current or recent medication should be checked because the side-effects of various drugs include impairment of sexual function. Although all histories should include smoking behaviour, this is particularly important in this context as smoking causes erectile dysfunction (approximately 120 000 cases in the UK attributable to smoking) reduction in semen quality, reduced response to fertility management and is associated with fetal malformation (Peate 2005b). If HIV is suspected, intravenous drug use should also be checked.

2 Any significant points in family history such as whether the man has fathered any children. If he has, this indicates he was fertile at that time and this provides useful information for the subsequent assessment.

3 Review of function to identify the cause of concern:
   a) any changes or disturbances in function such as:
      – difficulty in passing urine
      – frequency, hesitancy, straining, urgency or nocturia
      – dysuria (a burning pain on micturition)
      – changes in colour/smell of urine
      – difficulty in obtaining or maintaining erection
      – decreased libido
      – relationship difficulties
   b) the presence of any signs or symptoms of disease. If present they are explored in order to determine their location, character, duration and severity. The common manifestations of disorders are:
      – pain: burning on micturition or a constant painful sensation in the scrotum
      – lesions
      – urethral discharge
      – itching
      – scrotal swelling
      – testicular mass

4 The patient's sexual roles (heterosexual or homosexual) and how the presenting health problem may affect self-concept and relationships with significant others. Other psychosocial factors such as employment and home circumstances should be explored.

The physical examination should follow the following steps (Walsh 2006):

● Inspection of the groin area for a normal distribution of pubic hair and any other obvious abnormalities of the genitalia
● Palpate the groin for any evidence of tenderness or unusual masses (enlarged lymph nodes or herniae)
● Examine the penis for any lesions on the shaft (e.g. genital herpes) and noting whether it has been circumcised
● The glans should be checked to ensure the external urinary meatus is in the correct place (congenital malformations which locate the meatus on the under surface such as hypospadias may have not been corrected). If the male is uncircumcised he should be asked to retract the foreskin to allow examination of the glans which should be covered in a moist film called smegma
● Examine the external urinary meatus by asking the man to press just behind the head of the penis with first finger and thumb to splay the orifice open and shine a pen torch into the area. Pink mucosa should be apparent
● Examine the scrotum which should be darker than other skin with the left testicle lower than the right
● Finally palpate each testes with a gentle rolling motion between thumb and first and second fingers. It should feel smooth and rubbery. Any small lumps (typically the size of a pea) on the front or side indicate a possible testicular tumour and require urgent medical referral

A digital rectal exam to check the size and morphology of the prostate may be needed but this is usually carried out by a medical or advanced nurse practitioner. A careful explanation is needed together with privacy. The assisting nurse should ensure the patient is turned on his left side with knees drawn up towards the chest. Particular care is needed in elderly men who may have arthritic hips and therefore find this a difficult position to adopt. Standing upright and leaning forward may be an easier option. The nurse should ensure the patient is safe (e.g. cot sides *in situ*) and provide psychological support during what can be an uncomfortable and embarrassing procedure. Asking the patient to take a deep breath and breathe out during actual insertion of the gloved finger can reduce anal spasm, making the procedure less traumatic.

PATIENT PROBLEMS

The normal functioning of the reproductive system gives constant reassurance of a man's essential maleness. The distortion or interruption of these processes may prove very disturbing to the individual and family. The man may experience problems in relation to self-image and have fears about future sexual performance. Body parts that contribute to self-esteem and identity have a high psychological investment. The threat posed by disease or loss of these body parts depends on:

● their meaning to the individual
● his stage of development of body image and self

● the reactions of the social group, including the partner, to which the patient belongs.

The person may fear loss of reproductive function. The ability to reproduce is seen by many as a criterion of usefulness and sexuality. The loss of function may be followed by feelings of uselessness or of being only half a person. These feelings can be particularly distressing to the man with erectile dysfunction. The inability to obtain an erection may make him feel less of a man, and he may fear that his partner will also perceive him as being inadequate in some way. Thus, to the fear of loss of reproductive function may be added the fear of loss of a loved one. For some, the fear of loss of libido as well as sexual function may be very frightening and can cause the patient much anguish. In addition to the effects of loss of function there is also the possibility of cancer affecting the genital tract. Cancer is a word that strikes fear into most people and cancer of the testis is predominantly a cancer of younger men. This diagnosis can have a devastating psychological impact. A recent development of concern to the gay community on the West Coast of North America is the growth of cancer of the anus caused by unprotected anal sex (see p. 776).

Most people have been culturally conditioned to the idea that some areas of the body should not be discussed, much less exposed, to examination or discussion. Such experiences may disturb the individual and produce shame that may be enhanced by lack of privacy and exposure of the body in examinations or during care. Others may feel guilt over their illness. Sexually transmitted infection (STI) and cancer arouse guilt feelings in certain individuals which may be expressed as a feeling of 'being punished for past deeds'.

You may be dealing with patients who experience anxiety and fear, shame, guilt, diminished self-esteem or re-awakened anxieties over personal identity. In addition, the long shadow of AIDS is a particular, unspoken fear for many patients.

GOALS

Patient goals may include:

1 resolving dysfunctional sexual problems
2 achieving a sense of self-worth
3 being able to verbalize fears and anxieties
4 showing understanding of health problems and what medical intervention involves
5 adapting to a change in sexual role and/or function
6 being aware of and avoiding risk factors in sexual activity.

NURSING INTERVENTION

These goals may be achieved by the following nursing interventions:

● Assess the degree of threat posed by loss of function or body parts to the individual and plan, give and evaluate nursing care for that individual based on the assessment

- Give physical nursing care that:
  - promotes feelings of dignity and self-worth by attention to personal hygiene and grooming
  - promotes the return of health, control over body functions and independence
- Reduce fear and guilt by:
  - acknowledging and discussing feelings
  - anticipating the need for explanations and interpretations
  - clarifying and correcting misinformation about causes of illness, physiology and the consequences, if any, of treatment on present function
  - maintaining a confident, non-judgemental approach to the patient
  - assisting in acknowledging the loss, if any
  - obtaining appropriate additional sources of spiritual or emotional help for the patient
  - offering information and useful contact addresses/ websites for patients and relatives
- Assist men (and their partners) to think critically about the risks they take and the options available.

EVALUATION

Interventions are successful if behavioural changes have occurred, although these may be difficult to document in areas such as self-concept, anxiety and guilt. The patient may, for example:

- state that he feels better, less frightened, happier or at ease with himself
- take an interest in personal appearance and renew interests in social life, which may also indicate a return to a more positive outlook toward the future
- demonstrate an understanding of the illness, treatments and any residual changes in function to the level of ability or willingness
- demonstrate a knowledge of the risk factors that may lead to a recurrence of the problem and the actions that may reduce or eliminate the risk factors, if appropriate
- discuss alterations in body function and structure with the nurse and so indicate a willingness to begin to deal with the problem or to accept it with appropriate adjustments.

Adjustment to many of these changes requires some time and expectations of resolution and effectiveness of intervention must be realistic.

SEXUAL ISSUES ASSOCIATED WITH GIVING NURSING CARE

Several issues involving sexuality may arise in the course of nurse–patient interactions. They reflect the changing role of the patient and involve confusion over the meaning of nursing or patient actions. The most common arise from the intimate level of care involved in nursing and acting out sexual behaviour by the patient.

Touch

The nurse may feel uncomfortable at having to touch the genitals of patients. The patient may also experience discomfort at being cared for so intimately by the nurse. It reinforces for many adults the dependent child-like role associated with nursing care. On the other hand, touch may be a source of great comfort to patients. Touch should be used only with permission and its purpose should be understood by both patient and nurse.

Male erection

The erections that may occur during the delivery of nursing care are most often the result of the stimulation of the spinal reflex arc. The stimulus from a full bladder or perineal care may produce this non-sexual or non-psychological erection. Should this occur during care it is important for the nurse to remain calm, acknowledge the situation and finish care. A flustered nurse who 'runs away' from the patient may increase his confusion, shame and guilt. The patient also needs to understand the nature of reflex, non-sexual erections.

Sexual acting out

A patient may act out sexually to test sexual image, to gain control of the situation, or to attract attention. Examples of sexual acting out in this context include touching the nurse inappropriately, improper suggestions or gestures toward the nurse or self-exposure. The nurse should address the situation directly and unambiguously. The nurse–patient relationship should be defined and any misconceptions about role and function clarified. Limits are set, clearly defined and enforced. Sexual harassment from *any* source – patient or staff – is unacceptable.

The patient should be helped to explore anxiety and fears. As these are identified and appropriately dealt with, the sexual acting out usually ceases.

VARIATIONS OF SEXUALITY

Variations of sexuality can occur in each of the four areas of sexuality but most are psychosexual in origin. Only a few arise from physical illness and trauma, or congenital error. Most become obvious through difficulties in sexual expression.

Variations in sexual expression are classified by object choice and sexual aim. *Object choice* refers to problems such as paedophilia, incest, animal contacts or fetishism (sexual arousal associated with inanimate objects). Variations in *sexual aim* refer to problems such as voyeurism, exhibitionism and sado-masochism. Variations in sexual aim and object choice can be interrelated.

Gender dysphoria (transsexuality) is where the individual appears to have a gender identity at odds with his or her physical self. The person will usually cross-dress and may seek out gender realignment (sex change) therapy because of a deep need to have a body similar to the gender identity. A limited number of gender dysphoria clinics do exist but usually only take patients with a GP referral. The nurse should know the nearest clinic to where s/he practices (often the GP does not) so she can support the patient in his request for help from the GP. However, transvestism (cross-dressing) itself does not indicate transsexuality. Transvestism covers a whole spectrum of complex behaviours ranging from men who have a fetish about female underwear through those who like dressing fully as a woman, to those who actually wish to be women. Most transvestites are heterosexual, although some may be bisexual or gay. Transvestism might be an unusual behaviour, but it is not a health problem unless it causes significant mental distress through feelings of guilt and anxiety.

Occasionally, a child reaches puberty and is then discovered to be genetically and internally different from the external genitalia. Because the child has been socialized in the sex role defined by the external genitalia, continuation in the sex assigned at birth is usually advised. It is usually more successful to alter the physical state than to attempt to reverse gender identity and several years of gender role learning. Parents of a child born with ambiguous genitalia should understand the necessity to delay sex assignment until careful physical and genetic screening indicates the true sex of the infant.

Sexual concerns

Many persons experience doubts over their inner sexual feelings. This may be more prominent in adolescence when the final development of gender identity takes place, but may recur throughout the individual's life. As sexual identity is considered to be an important component of overall identity, this may stimulate concerns over self-identity. The growing awareness that a young man is gay may cause great psychological distress and may also be the cause of bullying at school with possibly disastrous consequences.

Homophobia is sadly prevalent in society today and a cause of considerable stress and ultimately ill health. A recent public health presentation (that the author attended at the University of British Columbia, in 2005), stressed a range of issues that impact upon gay men such as the fact they have a far higher than average rate of drug misuse and alcohol-related problems. It was suggested this was because they did not tend to settle down early in life like many straight men do when they marry and take on family responsibilities. As a result they 'party' for the next 40 years with predictable consequences. Of particular concern was the effects of homophobia driving men out of small towns where their families resided and into the big city where they became dislocated from main stream society and shared something of the experiences of recent immigrants with resultant harmful effects on their health.

Concerns over expected performance are also prevalent in straight and gay men. The man may doubt whether he has the necessary physical attributes, experience or appeal to attract, satisfy and keep a sexual partner.

Sexual dysfunction

Sexual dysfunction in the male is most frequently associated with the inability to achieve an erection (impotence or erectile dysfunction) and to delay ejaculation until both partners achieve a sense of satisfaction (premature ejaculation). Reliable epidemiological evidence on the prevalence of erectile dysfunction is difficult to find but Webber (2004a) notes that the literature suggests a strong relationship with age and suggests approximately 30 million men in the USA alone are affected.

Erectile dysfunction (ED) can be the result of psychological, interpersonal or physical factors. In the large majority of cases, the root cause is physical but psychological feedback mechanisms are usually at work producing a complex interplay of physical, psychological and interpersonal factors:

- Psychological causes may be anger, depression, anxiety, ignorance, or deeper psychosexual conflicts
- Interpersonal factors involve conflicts with the partner or an inability to establish interpersonal relationships
- Physical causes include diabetes, neurological or endocrine disorders, penile problems such as abnormality of the corpora, alcohol and drug abuse, smoking, renal or liver disease or the side-effects of drugs such as antihypertensives, antidepressants and H_2 antagonists such as cimetidine.

The presentation is usually in primary care and may be as a result of the partner urging the man to (reluctantly) attend the health centre. The history is crucial in diagnosis, a physical examination is also necessary. Many patients will not make a connection between the side-effects of their medication (e.g. antihypertensive drugs) or diseases such as diabetes and their ED.

Key questions in the history suggested by Walsh (2006) are:

- How quickly has the problem developed? (slow onset suggests organic cause)
- Is it situational or partner related? ('yes' indicates a psychological cause)
- Can you obtain an erection at other times, such as on wakening? ('yes' indicates a psychological problem).

During history taking, the patient is asked whether there are any sexual complaints. This makes sexuality an acceptable topic to discuss should the patient have a problem or develop one in the future. If the patient does present with a sexual problem, it is discussed in a frank, open manner, maintaining a broad, objective attitude toward the patient's sexual beliefs and practices. The patient is not urged to disclose more information during a session than he is comfortable in revealing. The patient's sexual concerns are assessed in the context of other problems and in the context of value systems.

Treatment initially concentrates on any potentially reversible factors such as medication the patient may be taking, treating pre-existing diseases such as diabetes, lifestyle modification (smoking, recreational drug use, alcohol consumption) and relationship problems. The administration of an oral erectogenic agent such as sildenafil (Viagra) is extremely effective. This drug is a potent inhibitor of an enzyme (phosphodiesterase 5; PDE-5) which regulates a key intracellular messenger (cyclic guanosine monophosphate; cGMP) involved in triggering smooth muscle relaxation and hence increased arterial inflow and corporeal veno-occlusion. The drug therefore works only if the patient's ED is caused by a disturbance in the normal blood flow involved in obtaining an erection: it is not suitable for all men. With all the recent publicity that has surrounded this drug, it is important in talking to patients and their partners to introduce an element of caution about the appropriateness of sildenafil.

The link to smoking is now obvious due to the arterial damage accumulating from smoking. This is exacerbated by the effects of nicotine on the brain which causes rapid contractions of penile tissue which in turn further reduce penile blood flow (Peate 2005b). Evidence shows that penile blood pressure in 20% of men with erectile dysfunction who smoke is abnormally low. It is estimated that some 50% of male smokers will experience some degree of ED as a result of this problem (Peate 2005b). Smoking cessation therapy carried out in primary care is therefore a very effective nursing intervention which can help many men.

Other therapies include counselling and the use of vacuum constriction devices, which draw blood into the penis by creating a negative pressure around it, and then applying a constrictive ring to the base of the penis. These devices have not been the subject of any large RCT to evaluate their effectiveness. A second-line therapy which may be used if first-line therapies do not succeed consists of intraurethral administration or intracavernosal self-injection of alprostadil.

RAPE TRAUMA SYNDROME

This condition is usually associated with females. Since 1994, male rape has been recognized as a legal assault and Walby and Allen (2004) estimate that 5% of men may become victims of sexual assault at some point in their lives. The subject is largely taboo, which is why a leaflet on male rape produced by 'Victim Support' is very welcome (Dunn 2005). The leaflet dispels some common myths such as it is only strangers who carry out such attacks. As with female rape, the attacker is often known to the victim. Further myths include the notion that women never carry out such attacks and that male rape only occurs in prison. No assumptions can be made about the sexuality of either victim or attacker. The long-term psychological effects, as with female victims can be devastating and lead to suicide attempts.

CONGENITAL ANOMALIES OF THE REPRODUCTIVE SYSTEM

Maldescent of testes

Approximately 4% of newborn males will exhibit some form of maldescent of the testes (Black and Hawks 2005). The majority of testes descend during the first 3 months of extrauterine life. *Cryptorchidism* is the term used to describe the condition in which the descent of the testis is interrupted anywhere along the normal path of descent. This is a major risk factor (1 in 80) for the development of testicular cancer in adult life (Black and Hawks 2005). Because histological changes are observed in the undescended testes as early as 4 years of age, treatment is initiated early to ensure maximum functioning of the testes. *Orchidopexy* (surgical placement and fixation of the testes in the scrotal sac) is the primary method of treatment and should be completed by the age of 1 year.

Should the condition not be diagnosed until after puberty, orchidopexy is indicated even though the man may be sterile. There are two reasons for this. First, the Leydig cells of the testes continue to produce male hormones which will sustain the secondary sex characteristics. Second, such testes have a higher incidence of malignancy than do normally positioned testes (see above) and can be more easily examined yearly for malignancy in the scrotum than in the abdomen. In unilateral conditions, the extrascrotal testis will be removed to reduce the possibility of malignancy further. This leaves the man with one functioning testis as a source of sperm and male hormones.

MALE FERTILITY CONTROL

Condom

The condom is a thin rubber sheath that is placed over the penis before intromission. It prevents pregnancy by acting as a mechanical barrier to the sperm. It is also very effective in preventing infection with a sexually transmitted disease. Proper use includes application before intromission to avoid the possibility of a pre-ejaculatory emission of semen into the vagina and careful withdrawal of the penis and condom following intercourse to be sure that some semen is not lost into the vagina or over the vulva. Spermicidal jelly may be used as a lubricating agent over the condom. This provides additional safety, particularly if the condom should be defective. However, newer methods of manufacture have greatly reduced this hazard. The condom is reasonably priced and is available without prescription. This greatly increases its availability and makes it one of the most widely used methods in the world.

Some couples find the condom objectionable as a method of birth control because it may interrupt sexual foreplay; it can lessen sensation, and its effective use relies heavily on the motivation of the male. These objections can be overcome if it is used by a man who is taking a mature responsibility for his behaviour, especially in view of the risk of contracting AIDS.

Vasectomy

This simple operation can be done on an outpatient basis or at a clinic. Under local anaesthesia a small incision is made slightly to one side of each spermatic cord. The vas deferens is exposed, severed and electrocoagulated. Thus, new sperm are barred from reaching the vagina. Other sperm are still present in the tract above the ligation. For this reason, a man is not considered sterile until he has had two negative sperm counts after operation.

The first sperm count is done after 10 ejaculations and is repeated following a further series of ejaculations until a negative sperm count is obtained.

In the immediate postoperative period, the man may expect some minor bruising and discomfort for 24–72 hours. The discomfort is relieved by a simple analgesic, rest and wearing a scrotal support. Protected intercourse is resumed when he feels comfortable to do so. Few major side-effects, either physical or emotional, are reported following the procedure.

Some cases are recorded of reconstructing the vas deferens. However, the rate of successful reconstruction is low. This is partly due to extravasation of sperm, which causes the development of sperm antibodies following vasectomy. Even though physical reconstruction of the vas deferens might be possible, the antibodies continue to destroy the sperm. Vasovasostomy (repair of the separated vas deferens) produces fertility in only a small minority of men. Thus, the patient should regard a vasectomy as irreversible.

INFECTIONS OF THE MALE REPRODUCTIVE TRACT

Balanitis

Balanitis is an infection of the **glans penis**. Many different organisms may be causative. It is generally associated with poor personal hygiene in the uncircumcised male, especially if he is diabetic, but may be associated with STI. Symptoms include redness, swelling, pain and possibly a purulent discharge. The disease may be chronic and may cause the formation of adhesions and scarring.

Treatment

The infection is treated with the appropriate antimicrobial following culture and sensitivity tests. In severe cases, once the inflammatory process is controlled, circumcision, the excision of the **prepuce**, may be advised.

On return from the operating theatre, the patient has a small petroleum jelly gauze dressing, which is changed following each voiding. The patient may be taught to do this and how to care for the dressing at home.

Should bleeding occur, a pressure dressing is applied. The dressing may make voiding impossible or difficult. Usually the dressing can be removed within a short period of time.

Circumcision may also be indicated as a means of dealing with the following problems.

Phimosis

Phimosis is a condition in which the preputial orifice is too small to permit retraction over the glans. It may be congenital but is most frequently a sequel to infection or trauma.

Paraphimosis

Paraphimosis occurs when a narrowed prepuce is either forced back over the glans or is gradually retracted over it. It then forms a tight, constricting band around the glans; venous return is impaired, and swelling and pain follow. The foreskin may be replaced with the aid of ice packs and lubricating gel but sometimes a general anaesthetic is needed as the condition is so painful. Occasionally the foreskin may have to be incised; a slit is made up the dorsal surface. This is usually followed by circumcision after the treatment of any infection that may have been present.

Prostatitis

Prostatitis is inflammation of the **prostate** gland and may be either acute or chronic, bacterial or non-bacterial in origin. The most common infecting agents are either gastrointestinal bacteria or those responsible for STIs. The presenting patient is usually under 50 but with symptoms suggestive of 'prostatism' (see p. 773).

In the acute stage, fever and chills are accompanied by pain, haematuria, frequency and dysuria. A urethral discharge may be noted. Rectal examination usually reveals an enlarged, tender, 'hot' prostate in acute cases. Infection of the seminal vesicles almost invariably accompanies prostatitis. The patient may require admission for intravenous antimicrobial therapy and adequate pain control. Prostatic massage and instrumentation of the urethra are avoided to prevent possible spread of the infection to the epididymis, bladder and kidney. Exceptions are made only to relieve acute urinary retention, which may be a sequel to the enlarged prostate.

The patient is placed on bedrest. Hydration, analgesics and stool softeners are useful as supportive therapy. Appropriate antimicrobial drug therapy is prescribed in accordance with local protocols and culture and sensitivity results. The patient is in considerable pain. The nurse often sees a tense, anxious and frightened patient who needs reassurance and support. Analgesics and warm baths help to relieve the pain and bladder spasms. The irritable bladder may require special attention, and antispasmodics and bladder sedatives are frequently ordered.

In cases in which treatment is early, excellent results usually follow. However, the acute picture may become chronic. The symptoms are mild and include a low-grade fever and some bacteria and pus in the urine. The chronic infection may stubbornly resist treatment, although the fluoroquinolones or trimethoprim are the antimicrobials most likely to succeed as they penetrate prostatic tissue more effectively than other drugs (British National Formulary 2005).

Epididymitis

This condition is rare before puberty and involves infection of the epididymis. The testes may become involved (epididymo-orchitis). It is usually seen in young men as a result of an STI with *Chlamydia trachomatis* or *Neisseria gonorrhoeae* most commonly implicated. It may occasionally be caused by a gastrointestinal organism such as *E. coli*. Fever, malaise and chills accompany swelling and pain in the scrotum. The patient may be so uncomfortable that he may walk in a waddling fashion. Symptoms of cystitis may be present, and a painless swelling consisting of an accumulation of fluid within the scrotum often develops (hydrocele). The swelling and irritation associated with the inflammation cause congestion of the testes, which impedes the circulation of blood. If necrosis of the tubular epithelium and fibrosis occluding the ducts occurs sterility may follow.

The patient is placed on bedrest. The scrotum is elevated on towel rolls and ice packs may be applied. Constipation should be prevented as attempts at defaecation under these circumstances can be very painful. After the patient is ambulant, a roomy scrotal support is worn. Antimicrobials and analgesics are given. Chronic epididymitis may follow an acute episode and, if the involvement is bilateral, sterility may follow.

Orchitis

Inflammation of the **testes** may follow any infectious disease or may be acquired as an ascending infection from the genital tract. Most commonly it follows mumps parotitis. The mumps virus is excreted in the urine; therefore, the spread to the testes in this case appears to be by descent. The onset is sudden, manifested by pain and swelling of the scrotum followed by fever and prostration. Urinary symptoms are usually not present. A hydrocele may develop, and the involvement may be unilateral or bilateral. Sterility probably follows death of the spermatogenic cells from ischaemia. Bedrest, scrotal support, and local applications of heat or cold are ordered. A padded athletic support may be worn continuously. Antimicrobials are used in some situations but are not of value against the mumps virus.

SEXUALLY TRANSMITTED INFECTIONS

These are on the increase worldwide and young men are the most at risk. The health problem of greatest concern is HIV/AIDS but all these infections pose major health risks for both men and women and are therefore dealt with in some depth in Chapter 9. However, we will briefly consider the male dimension to STI as this is a chapter on male reproductive health.

During 2004, the Health Protection Agency estimated that there were approximately 58 000 people living with HIV, most of whom are male (Health Protection Agency 2005), of whom one-third were unaware they were infected. The highest risk group remains men who have sex with men (MSM) who have an incidence rate of 3%, i.e. three new cases per 100 MSM per year. What is particularly disturbing is that MSM also show the highest rates of syphilis (p. 166) and gonorrhoea infections (p. 164) indicating widespread unprotected casual sex, while 25% of gonorrhoea amongst MSM is resistant to the main antimicrobials of choice (ciprofloxacillin) compared with 14% in the whole population. While there was a welcome overall 11% fall in gonococcal infections in the UK between 2003 and 2004, the rate of infection is not decreasing in MSM. The implications of these statistics for syphilis and gonorrhoea for HIV infections are obvious and there is a need for a major education program targeting younger MSM in particular, to prevent the spread of HIV in countries such as the UK. However, HIV is not confined to MSM, it is a worrying problem in intravenous drug users and is also creeping into the heterosexual population. Some 75% of new heterosexual cases seen in the UK during 2004 were acquired in Africa. The situation in the developing world is all too well known and will be reviewed in Chapter 9.

OTHER DISORDERS OF THE REPRODUCTIVE TRACT

Spermatocele

A spermatocele is a cyst of the spermatic cord which contains sperm in a thin white fluid. It lies above the **testis** and is separate from it. Usually a spermatocele requires no treatment. Sometimes it may become large enough to be confused with hydrocele and to be aggravating to the patient; then it may be excised. The aetiology is unclear.

Varicocele

Varicocele is the dilatation of the venous plexus about the testis. It usually occurs on the left side for anatomical reasons. Its appearance on the right side is unusual and may indicate that a tumour is occluding the vein above the level of the scrotum. Some testicular atrophy may occur if the circulation is impeded for long periods of time. This may result in subfertility. On palpation behind and above the testis, the doctor feels a mass of tortuous veins that empties when the patient lies down.

Treatment may consist of a scrotal support which relieves the dragging sensation. If fertility is an issue or the condition is severe, the internal spermatic vein may be ligated. The results are usually excellent. A scrotal support may be worn for 4–5 days following surgery, as scrotal oedema may be present.

Hydrocele

A hydrocele is a collection of fluid in the tunica vaginalis. It may occur following local injury, infection or a neoplasm, and may be unilateral or bilateral. More often it is chronic and the cause is unknown. In newborn babies the cause is usually a late closure of the processus vaginalis; this frequently closes spontaneously. In some young men a chronic type exists because the processus vaginalis never closes completely, and a connection remains between the peritoneal cavity and the tunica vaginalis.

Treatment is not required unless the testis cannot be palpated to rule out abnormality, circulation to the testis is impaired, or the hydrocele becomes large, unsightly and uncomfortable. Then the hydrocele is aspirated, and a sclerosing drug may be injected. In chronic cases, the tunica vaginalis is excised (hydrocelectomy). After operation, the scrotum is elevated on a pillow or bridge dressing, and a pressure dressing is applied. Depending on the operation, there may or may not be a drain present in the incision. The patient must be observed for haemorrhage, which may be concealed in the hydrocele sac. When ambulatory the patient usually requires a fresh scrotal support daily. Immediately after the operation he may need a larger support than usual.

Torsion of the testis

Torsion of the testis occurs when the testis rotates upon the spermatic cord impairing the blood supply to the testis. Often this is due to spasm of the cremaster muscle combining with incomplete attachment of the testis to the scrotal wall allowing rotation to occur. It typically affects teenage boys and causes sudden, severe pain in the area of the testis that is unrelieved by rest or support. School nurses, A&E, walk-in clinic, and primary care nurses should be very alert for this problem as they are likely the first points of contact. Swelling and discolouration of the scrotum occur (Walsh 2006). The presentation may include nausea and vomiting (a reflex action brought on by the severe pain) and pain referred to the abdomen causing a potential for mis-diagnosis. Because the torsion reduces the blood supply to the testis, testicular atrophy follows rapidly. Surgical intervention is required as a matter of *urgency* to maintain normal testicular function.

Benign hyperplasia of the prostate

It is not known why benign enlargement of the prostate gland occurs with ageing. However, it is estimated that 10–30% of men in their early 70s have symptoms of this disorder (Webber 2004b) which are due to the enlarging prostate interfering with the free flow of urine from the bladder into the urethra.

Effects on the patient

Gradually, the man may experience hesitancy in beginning the flow of urine. The stream of urine is reduced in force and size. Incomplete emptying of the bladder produces residual urine which reduces bladder capacity so that urgency and frequency result. Nocturia occurring three or more times in one night is a good indication of frequency. Often, cystitis occurs as well. In view of these familiar symptoms, a reliable scoring system has been developed to assess the extent to which prostate symptoms are affecting the patient's lifestyle (Table 22.1). This can be used especially in primary care to monitor changes over time. In severe cases, the bladder becomes overdistended, and hypertrophy and small diverticula follow as weakened areas of bladder mucosa bulge out between the bands of muscle fibres. The back-up of urine causes hydroureter or even hydronephrosis. Over long periods of time, renal function may be impaired. Backache and sciatica may also bring the patient to the doctor, as the enlarged prostate exerts pressure on nerves.

Table 22.1   International Prostate Symptom Score*

Symptom	Not at all	< 1 time in 5	< half the time	Half the time	> half the time	Almost always	Your score
Straining	0	1	2	3	4	5	
Weak stream	0	1	2	3	4	5	
Intermittency	0	1	2	3	4	5	
Incomplete emptying	0	1	2	3	4	5	
Frequency	0	1	2	3	4	5	
Urgency	0	1	2	3	4	5	
Nocturia (times per night)	0	1	2	3	4	5	
Total scores: 0-7 mild symptoms; 8*19 moderate; 20-35 severe							

Quality of life scale:

Delighted	0
Pleased	1
Satisfied	2
Mixed	3
Dissatisfied	4
Unhappy	5
Terrible	6

*From Barry et al (1992)

Frequently, the patient does not seek medical attention until acute retention of urine occurs. Alcohol and some medications can be the precipitating factors. The patient is catheterized with the smallest size catheter possible and urine is slowly released from the bladder. This prevents a sudden release of pressure in the abdomen which could cause shock and haemorrhage. Shock follows the rush of blood from vital centres to fill the newly released blood vessels. This sudden filling may cause small blood vessels in the bladder mucosa to rupture. The catheter remains in place for 2–3 days, after which normal voiding patterns usually return. The patient is cautioned to avoid an excessive intake of fluid in a short period of time, as this rapidly distends the bladder, precipitating retention. He should void frequently when he has the urge to do so in order to avoid overdistension of the bladder. If followed, these instructions should help the individual to avoid acute retention. Retention may lead to frequent voiding of small amounts of overflow urine, particularly where the problem has become chronic.

Treatment   Watchful waiting and lifestyle modification combined with drug therapy may be sufficient to manage men with mild to moderate symptoms. Finasteride interferes with testosterone metabolism and therefore reduces the size of the prostate, improving urine flow rates and reducing symptoms. Side-effects include the development of erectile dysfunction and ejaculatory disorders. An alternative approach is through the use of α-blockers which relax smooth muscle in the prostate and therefore improve urine flow (e.g. alfuzosin, doxazosin). This group of drugs has significant cardiovascular side-effects and interactions with other drugs, and the patient needs careful monitoring and education about the medication. There is evidence that the herbal remedy Saw Palmetto is as effective as finasteride, but without the side-effects, for mild to moderate symptoms and this can be readily obtained in most health food shops (Bandolier 2000).

Surgery is indicated to relieve more severe symptoms and to prevent infections of the urinary tract and renal damage. If the amount of residual urine in the bladder is greater than 75–100 mL, the surgeon may feel an operation is necessary even though the symptoms are not severe. Residual urine is estimated in several ways. Immediately after voiding, a catheter may be passed and any remaining urine is drawn off and measured. A radio-opaque contrast medium can be injected into the bladder. The man is then asked to void, and postvoiding films are made. Direct visualization of the bladder may be done by cystoscopy, and any bladder changes noted. Intravenous urography will indicate the extent of ureter and kidney involvement. Renal function tests may be ordered as well.

A period of preoperative preparation may be necessary. Education is an essential part of preoperative preparation, as for any surgical procedure.

Transurethral resection of the prostate   This is the most frequently performed operation. The operation is carried out with a resectoscope, an instrument similar to a cystoscope but equipped with cutting and cauterizing attachments. This slender instrument is inserted up the urethra to the prostatic urethra, and the enlarged prostate is removed in pieces. The capsule remains intact. During the operation, the bladder and urethra are irrigated continuously with a sterile, isotonic, non-conductive, clear fluid. In this manner, debris and blood are washed away.

Immediately after the operation, the catheter drainage is bloody. A closed irrigation system is usually initiated to prevent blockage of the catheter by any clots. The nurse must be alert for signs of haemorrhage by paying close attention to the blood pressure and pulse of the patient, and the amount of drainage. The drainage is watery and blood-tinged for 24–48 hours after operation.

The fluid used to irrigate the bladder during the operation may be absorbed, causing haemodilution. The signs and symptoms of this may be those of sodium deficiency or excessive blood volume. Complaints of headache, nausea, vomiting or muscle weakness should not be ignored by the nurse but must be reported. Hypertension, restlessness, apprehension, shortness of breath or blurred vision likewise should be reported. After the operation, normal saline may be given intravenously. The nurse must observe the patient for signs of pulmonary oedema.

Complaints of spasmodic, intermittent pain by the man, in the suprapubic region or a constant desire to void are related to bladder spasms. In severe cases, he will need medication to obtain relief. The nurse should explain bladder spasms and catheters before operation to the patient and instruct him not to try to void after surgery.

Complaints of persistent pain in the suprapubic area may be due to an overdistended bladder from a catheter that is not draining properly or from haemorrhage into the bladder. Rarely, the bladder may have been perforated during the operation and blood and urine seep into the abdominal cavity. First, the nurse irrigates the catheter and patency is established. The pain should diminish proportionately; if not, other causes must be ruled out. Analgesia may be given to the patient to give pain relief during this period but analgesia alone does not provide relief from an overdistended bladder.

Because haemorrhage remains a threat, even in the later postoperative period, care is taken to prevent its occurrence. The patient is cautioned against straining to pass stool, and a light diet is usually ordered. Enemas are contraindicated during the first postoperative week.

Because of the danger of a urinary tract infection, a prophylactic antimicrobial may be prescribed. The catheter is removed 3–7 days after operation and, for a short period after this, the man is usually instructed to record and measure each voiding. If difficulty in voiding is still present, the catheter may be reinserted. The nurse should watch for signs of incontinence which may follow or signs of urinary retention which may indicate a urethral stricture. Before being discharged the man should be told that an episode of bleeding may occur about the 2nd to 4th week after surgery. In that event, he should contact his doctor. Also, he is warned to avoid any straining, heavy lifting or vigorous exercise for about 1 month after the operation.

The procedure does carry potential risks. Many patients are elderly and have significant other pathology which increases the risks of anaesthesia and the other postoperative risks. In addition, incontinence (due to pelvic floor weakness) erectile dysfunction and dry or retrograde ejaculation (into the bladder) are common complications. Black and Hawks (2005) cite extensive evidence showing that men are greatly helped by regular pelvic floor exercises, especially if commenced before surgery and helped by biofeedback. Weekly training sessions over several weeks (up to five) coupled with daily exercises of 18 strong contractions per day are advocated by Dorey (2005) who also finds strong evidence that in the process, erectile dysfunction is also decreased together with the incidence of post-micturition dribble.

For these reasons, some surgeons prefer to carry out a minimally invasive procedure (less extensive) such as transurethral incision of prostate (TUIP), which is suitable for men with smaller prostates and which produces fewer side-effects.

In view of the risks involved in surgery, it is important that the man is allowed to explore the alternative medical management with appropriate lifestyle modifications. The specialist nurse can fulfil a valuable role by having such discussions and offering support to the patient in whatever decision he comes to.

Other operative procedures   If the prostate is very large or if the procedure is being carried out because there is evidence of malignancy, the surgeon may undertake an open operation to remove the prostate (prostatectomy). Three approaches are used, all of which carry more risk than transurethral resection of the prostate (TURP).

Suprapubic prostatectomy   A small abdominal incision is made above the pubis and directly over the bladder. The bladder is opened and, through another incision into the urethral mucosa, the prostate is excised. The prostatic capsule remains intact. Sometimes only a Penrose drain in the suprapubic incision is all that is judged necessary in the postoperative period. It is usually removed after 36 hours. If a cystostomy tube is present, it is removed 3–4 days after the operation. The indwelling catheter usually stays until the incision is nearly healed. The suprapubic incision may take time to heal. Bladder spasm and leakage of urine from around the cystotomy tube is a frequent difficulty for these patients.

Retropubic prostatectomy   This allows for total removal of the gland in cases of prostate cancer. Urinary results are excellent and potency may be maintained. An abdominal incision is made above the bladder. The bladder is not incised, but the surgeon dissects down between the pubis and the bladder to reach the prostate. The capsule is opened and the tissue is removed.

Perineal prostatectomy   The surgeon excises the prostate through a semicircular incision in the perineal body. The prostatic capsule is opened and the gland is removed, making this a suitable operation in cases of prostatic cancer. Incontinence and erectile dysfunction are common complications.

Carcinoma of the prostate

Carcinoma of the prostate gland is the second most common cause of death in men from malignant disease in Europe and the USA. The lifetime risk of being diagnosed is 1 in 14 for all men (Cancer Research UK 2004). However, far more men are likely to die *with* cancer of the prostate than *from* this disease as it is often very slow growing and asymptomatic for a long period, yet in some men it can metastasize and spread aggressively leading to a rapid death. The tumour most often arises in the posterior prostatic lobe and is usually hormone related, depending upon androgens to retain its integrity. The actual cause of the cancer is unknown.

The tumour causes an increase in levels of a protein called prostate-specific antigen (PSA) above the normal range of 0–4 ng/mL (PSA normally has the function of liquifying the consolidated ejaculate post ejaculation). However, other conditions such as benign hyperplasia of the prostate can produce the same effect on PSA levels. This creates a problem as a prostate cancer that is undetectable by any other means in its early stages shows high PSA levels (PSA-detected cancer) but a high PSA level does not necessarily mean cancer as this may be due to many other causes. As a result of this and other problems, PSA testing at present is lacking both sensitivity (the probability of identifying true positive cases with a disease) and specificity (probability of identifying true negative cases without a disease). Its use in primary care is therefore not justified as a means of early detection. A transrectal ultrasound guided prostate biopsy is needed to take a tissue sample which will allow the diagnosis to be made (Drudge-Coates 2005).

Effects on the patient

The symptoms are essentially those of benign enlargement of the prostate. On rectal examination, the examiner palpates a hard nodule. As the nodule may resemble other conditions, a biopsy is often done. Transrectal ultrasonography may help in locating and staging the malignancy. Needle biopsies can now be done by putting a needle gauge into the ultrasound probe. This has greatly increased the accuracy of biopsies. The patient receives a cleansing enema before the procedure. On discharge the patient is told that blood-stained urine is to be expected for a short time.

Classification

Carcinoma of the prostate is classified into four stages based on the results of rectal examinations, serum acid phosphatase levels, radiography of the skeleton and metastases. Stages T1 and T2 indicate the tumour is contained within the prostate capsule and this is termed localized prostate cancer. In stages T3 and T4, spread has occurred beyond the capsule and these are referred to as advanced stage prostate cancers. Metastatic spread to lymph nodes and distant organs (especially skeletal) now occurs (Black and Hawks 2005).

Treatment and nursing intervention

Various treatment options have been tried over the years. Surgery may consist of radical prostatectomy by the retro-pubic or perineal routes, or minimally invasive TURP. Radiation therapy may be helpful in early lesions and in reducing pain from skeletal metastases in advanced cases. Alternatively, hormone therapy may be tried, aiming to block the production of the androgens that the tumour seems to need for its growth. It will not cure the disease but it may slow down the rate of growth of the tumour (Drudge-Coates 2005). However, the facts at present are that no treatment has been shown to cure prostate cancer, to provide an extension of life or to do the patient more good than harm. It is also true that some patients with the disease live for many years with little significant impact upon their lives, while others become very ill very quickly and die. Again, the reason for these different outcomes remains unknown.

Once the cancer has spread to the lymph nodes and skeleton (metastatic disease), deterioration and death are fairly rapid and 70% of patients will not survive 5 years. It is now true to say most patients will die *from* the disease rather than *with* the disease (Drudge-Coates 2005). In view of the poor state of knowledge about this disease, informed patient choice should be a major consideration in deciding what treatment options to follow. The nurse has a major role to play with medical staff in facilitating informed patient choice in a clinical area such as this.

Carcinoma of the testis

The tumour is usually derived from germ cells (95%). Cryptorchidism or undescended testicle is the major iden-tified risk factor for cancer of the testis increasing the risk to between 5 and 10 times that of the general population. There is also a strong genetic predisposition as rates are five times higher in Caucasian compared with black men, while brothers of men with testicular cancer have up to 10 times the population risk of developing the disease (McCullagh and Lewis 2005). This indicates that the opportunities for primary detection are very limited as the known risk factors are largely predetermined. However, we also know regular testicular self examination can produce early detection with a dramatic impact upon cure and survival rates. There is therefore plenty of scope for primary care nurses to play a key role, through patient teaching and health education, in the early detection and treatment of this cancer.

Half of all cases occur under the age of 35 and approxi-mately 1900 new cases present every year in the UK (Cancer Research UK 2002). As testicular cancer is usually very chemosensitive, there is a potential for a high cure rate and figures as high as 95% are claimed if detected before the cancer metastasizes beyond the testicular region (McCullagh and Lewis 2005). This is further aided by the fact that these

Box 22.1	Procedure for testicular self-examination

- Become familiar with the normal weight, texture and consistency of your testicles by carrying out self-examination every month

- Carry out the procedure after a bath or shower as the scrotum is then relaxed and its contents are easiest to feel

- Roll each testicle gently between your forefinger and thumb to check that the surface is smooth and free of lumps

- Become familiar with the feel of the epididymis which runs at the back of each testis. This is a normal part of the testis and should not be confused with a new lump

- If you detect a lump, make an appointment at once to see your GP.

cancers produce distinct chemical tumour markers which allow recurrence to be detected before any clinical signs (Cook 2000). When these factors are combined with the fact that the organ is palpable and early detection is therefore possible, it is desirable that all men should be taught how to examine the testes (Box 22.1). This is especially important for men with a history of cryptorchism or a family history of cancer of the testis. Detection before metastatic spread is lifesaving yet there is still widespread ignorance amongst young men about testicular self examination.

Although the tumour is rare – and this should be stressed in teaching – each man should be alert to possible changes in his testes. Regular monthly TSE, carried out after a bath or shower when the tissue is relaxed, takes only a couple of minutes and will detect any significant changes early. The early sign is a painless lump about the size of a pea but sometimes there may be a dull ache and a sense of heaviness or dragging in the scrotum if the tumour is more advanced. The man should also be alert to a testis that feels enlarged, is firm, gives the impression of heaviness and, when squeezed, fails to elicit the deep visceral pain that is usually associated with testicular pressure.

Treatment of testicular cancer

Treatment involves removal of the tumour and affected testis and may be followed by chemotherapy and/or radiotherapy depending upon his clinical condition and the tumour. Cytotoxic chemotherapy may be used after operation if the patient had a teratoma or if recurrence occurs as shown by increased levels of the markers α-fetoprotein (AFP) or human chorionic gonadotrophin (HCG).

Cancer of the penis

Malignancies of the penis are essentially malignancies of the skin. The glans and prepuce are nearly always affected. The disease is less frequent among circumcised men. In populations with poor genital hygiene, frequent sex partners, low age at first intercourse and a high incidence of HPV infection, carcinoma of the penis also has a higher incidence. HPV is associated or co-exists in many cases. Treatment is by excision of the affected areas or by partial or total amputation of the **penis**.

Anal carcinoma

This is a rare condition that is usually considered to affect more women than men. Approximately 4000 new cases are seen each year in the USA (Cancer.org 2005) and about 400 in the UK (CancerBACUP 2005). There is evidence, however, that this type of cancer is increasing amongst MSM who do not use condoms for anal sex giving rise to the speculation that it is being caused in MSM by the same mechanism as cervical cancer in women, i.e. human papillomavirus or HPV. Women are likely to develop anal cancer within the anal canal, whilst in cases seen in men it is found around the outer region of the anus. Rates of anal cancer in MSM in cities such as San Francisco and Vancouver which have large gay populations, are now said to rival those of cervical cancer before the introduction of a screening programme. The annual percentage change shows an increase of 2.4% for US men over the period 1975–2002 compared with 1.7% for females, which suggests this may be beginning to develop as another male sexual health problem (National Cancer Institute 2005). Anal cancer is a serious life-threatening disease but with early diagnosis treatments are highly effective. Pain and bleeding per rectum are the main symptoms.

SUMMARY

The area of men's health has been substantially neglected and the various taboos associated with sexuality have ensured that this is particularly so in the case of men's reproductive health. We cannot ignore the fact that men die significantly younger than women in all developed countries and also make much less use of primary health care in these countries. These facts are not unconnected. Nurses have a great opportunity to remedy this poor state of affairs, and low-cost interventions such as health education and allowing men to talk through the treatment options before arriving at an informed therapeutic choice can make a major contribution to improving the health of 50% of the population. There are, of course, major cultural factors such as the 'macho, laddish' image to contend with, which will change only slowly, but that is no reason for not beginning the change process. In addition the scandal of underfunding of research into clinical problems such as prostate cancer needs urgently to be addressed as a matter of public health policy. Above all, the nurse needs to be clear about his or her own sexuality and moral beliefs about sex and reproduction before addressing the needs of the patient. Empathy and sensitivity are essential for good nursing practice in this area, together with a non-judgemental approach.

CASE An anxious looking 30-year-old single man attended the walk in centre where you work, at 11 a.m., complaining of an aching pain in the left side of his scrotum which started suddenly this morning. It was worrying him as he had experienced nothing like this before and it prevented him from going to work. The pain was worse now than when he woke up. He took 2 paracetamol but it had not been relieved. He was particularly concerned because after he had masturbated this morning he noticed some blood in his semen. When he passed urine about an hour previously, there was soreness but 'It was nothing like as bad as when I had gonorrhoea 5 years ago, that was like pissing razor blades', he informs you.

- Carry out a PQRST symptom analysis on his main symptom: his pain.

  When you ask him about any urethral discharge, fevers or chills, nausea, diarrhoea or abdominal pain he answers in the negative.

  When questioned about recent sexual encounters he states he has no regular partner but enjoyed a three-some with a male/female couple about 10 days ago and the condom broke while he was receiving anal sex. He also confirms that he had an HIV test a year ago as 'I like to be adventurous with sex and swing both ways'; fortunately his HIV test was negative.

  His general appearance is clean and tidy, although he looks anxious. Vital signs are normal. There are no rashes or abnormalities about his skin. Genital examination reveals a tender left testicle and erythema on the left side of the scrotum with some oedema and tenderness over the left epididymis. He has a circumcised penis which appears normal and a normal distribution of pubic hair.

  The patient was referred to the acute hospital where Doppler ultrasound showed increased bloodflow to the left testicle consistent with epididymitis. There was no evidence of a torsion testes on the Doppler (decreased blood flow due to arterial occlusion). His urine analysis had revealed traces of blood and bacteria. The final diagnosis was sexually acquired epididymitis due to Chlamydia for which he was prescribed a 7-day course of doxycycline.

  (Adapted from Filbin et al 2002).

And finally ... did you know epididymitis is the most common reason for days lost from military service in the US Army?

REFERENCES

Bandolier (2000) Saw Palmetto and prostatic hypertrophy. Online. Available: www.jr2.ox.ac.uk/bandolier/band73/b73-2.html

Black J, Hawks J (2005) Medical surgical nursing, 7th edn. St Louis: Elsevier.

British National Formulary (BNF) (2005) British National Formulary No. 49. London: British Medical Association/Royal Pharmaceutical Society of Great Britain.

CancerBACUP (2005) Anal cancer. Online. Available: www.cancerBACUP.org/Cancertype/Anal/Analcancer

Cancer.org (2005) Anal cancer. Online. Available: www.cancer.org/docroot/CRI/content

Cancer Research UK (2002) Testicular cancer. London: CRUK.

Cancer Research UK (2004) Cancerstats monograph; cancer incidence, survival and mortality in the UK and EU. London: CRUK.

Cook R (2000) Teaching and promoting testicular self examination. Nursing Standard 14(2): 48–51.

Dorey G (2005) Restoring pelvic floor function in men; review of the RCTs. British Journal of Nursing 14(19): 1014–1021.

Drudge-Coates L (2005) Prostate cancer and the principles of hormone replacement therapy. British Journal of Nursing 14(7): 368–375.

Dunn P (2005) Breaking the silence. Emergency Nurse 13(3): 10–11.

Filbin M, Tsien C, Caughey A (2002) Clinical cases in emergency medicine. Malden, MA: Blackwell.

Health Protection Agency (HPA) (2005) Online. Available: www.hpa.org.uk/publications/hiv_sti_2005

Jarvis C (2004) Physical examination and health assessment. St Louis: Elsevier.

McCullagh J, Lewis G (2005) Testicular cancer; epidemiology, assessment and management. Nursing Standard 19(25): 45–53.

National Cancer Institute (2005) Cancer of the Anu, anal canal and anorectum. Online. Available: www.seer.cancer.gov/statfacts/html/anus

Peate I (2005a) Examining adult male genitalia: providing a guide for the nurse. British Journal of Nursing 14(1): 36–40.

Peate I (2005b) The effects of smoking on the reproductive health of men. British Journal of Nursing 14(7): 362–366.

Price B (2005) Practical guidance on sexual lifestyle and risk. Nursing Standard 19(27): 46–52.

Vetrosky D (2000) Anatomy and pathophysiology of erectile dysfunction. Nurse Practitioner 25(6 Suppl): 6.

Walby S, Allen J (2004) Domestic violence, sexual assault and stalking: findings from the British crime survey. London: Home Office Research, Development and Statistics Directorate.

Walsh M (2006) Nurse practitioners: clinical skills and professional issues. Edinburgh: Elsevier.

Webber R (2004a) Erectile dysfunction. Clinical Evidence 12: 1262–1270.

Webber R (2004b) Benign prostatic hyperplasia. Clinical Evidence 12: 1231–1250.

USEFUL WEBSITES

Cancers of the male genital tract	www.cancerBACUP.org.uk
	www.cancerresearchuk.org
	www.prostate-cancer.org.uk
	www.seer.cancer.gov
Self help	www.patient.co.uk
	www.medic8.com
Epidemiology of sexually transmitted disease	www.hpa.org.uk
Male rape and sexual assault	www.victimsupport.org
Gender dysphoria	www.gender.org.uk/gendys/index.htm
	(or write to Gendys Network, BM Gendys, London WC1N 3XX)

23 Caring for the patient with a disorder of the female reproductive system

Lesley Kyle

INTRODUCTION

Health care for women has never been so important as their average lifespan extends in to their 80s and their role in life changes so radically. Reproduction remains the female's role although this is now happening later for many women due to career choices and freely available contraception. Many women also choose to limit their family size and return to work to potentially provide a better standard of living for their family. Both their physical and psychological health are extremely important and care should be available in accessible clinics based in the community to meet local needs. This is often provided by nurse practitioners or other specialist nurses offering women more choice regarding contraception, advice on menopause and management of breast problems.

This chapter focuses on some of the problems that concern women across the lifespan.

PHYSIOLOGY OF THE FEMALE REPRODUCTIVE TRACT

IN UTERO DEVELOPMENT

The adult female reproductive tract consists of paired ovaries, uterine tubes, a uterus and vagina (Fig. 23.1). Externally, the labia, clitoris and Skene's and Bartholin's glands are part of the reproductive system (Fig. 23.2).

Sex is determined at the time of fertilization by the inclusion of the XX chromosomal pair of the female or the XY genotype of the male. As the embryo grows, an internal genital ridge develops but remains undifferentiated in either sex until the 7th week of intrauterine life. At that time, under the regulation of the Y chromosome, seminiferous tubes and Sertoli cells differentiate. At this time, sex differentiation can be made morphologically because the genital ridges of the embryo have grown and evolved into a rudimentary ovary or testis depending on the sex of the cell (Fig. 23.3).

While internal development proceeds, the external genitalia also become differentiated. During this phase of development, three small protuberances consist of the genital tubercle and, on either side of this tubercle, the genital swellings. The external area may be referred to collectively as the vulva, perineum or pudenda. Generally, perineum refers to the area stretching from the symphysis pubis laterally to the thighs and posteriorly to the tip of the coccyx.

The female genitalia arise from these three ridges. The tubercle becomes the clitoris, and the genital swellings develop into the labia majora and minora. As the labia meet anteriorly, they form a loose-fitting hood like a fold over the clitoris. This fold is similar to the prepuce of the male penis. Posteriorly, the labial folds fuse just before the anus.

By the 16th week of embryological life, the sex of the infant can be determined externally. In early development,

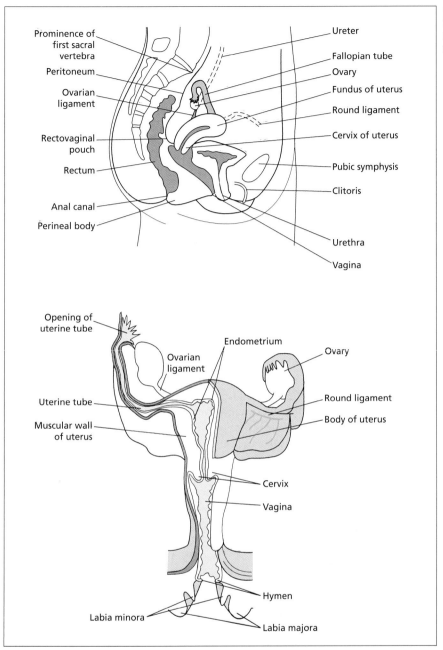

Figure 23.1 (a) Median sagittal section of the female pelvis. (b) Anterior view with some structures cut open to expose internal structure.

the ovaries are abdominal organs. As further growth takes place, the ovaries descend.

The female reproductive system functions to produce the female hormones (oestrogen and progesterone), to ripen ova for fertilization, and for intercourse to fertilize the ova. In addition, the reproductive organs incubate the human conceptus, providing it with safety and nourishment until the fetus is expelled to continue its growth and development externally.

THE OVARY

The ovary is a small almond-shaped organ lying posterior to the broad ligament of the uterus. Cross-sections of the ovary show a cortex and a medulla. The cortex, or outer layer, is composed of connective tissue and cells, among which are scattered the ova and developing follicles. Over this outer layer of the cortex is a thin layer of germinal epithelium. The medulla is composed of connective tissue containing blood vessels and smooth muscle fibres.

The fetal ovary is recognizable very early. By the 4th month of intrauterine life, some cells in the ovary have differentiated sufficiently to be recognizable as primary oocytes. Initially, these oocytes number in the millions, but most degenerate. At birth, fewer than two million are present; at puberty there are about 300 000 and of these only 400–500 will develop to ovulation. By the menopause, few primordial follicles remain, and they soon degenerate. Throughout childhood, some of these oocytes develop but never reach maturity and ovulate. Then, under the influence of the

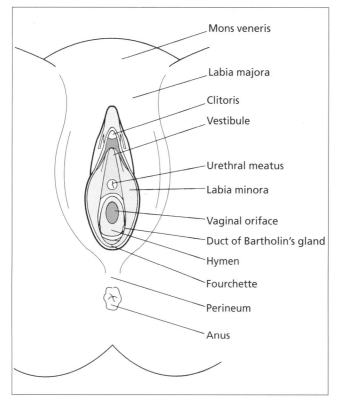

Figure 23.2 Female external genitalia.

Labels:
- Mons veneris
- Labia majora
- Clitoris
- Vestibule
- Urethral meatus
- Labia minora
- Vaginal oriface
- Duct of Bartholin's gland
- Hymen
- Fourchette
- Perineum
- Anus

maturing hypothalamus, which stimulates the anterior lobe of the pituitary to produce gonadotrophins, puberty begins.

The *secondary sex characteristics* then begin to develop. First, there is growth and development of the breast tissue. Pubic hairs appear and the internal and external organs of the reproduction become fully developed and functional. The vagina, under the influence of oestrogens, thickens and develops several layers of squamous epithelium. This makes it more resistant to infection. Previously the vaginal pH was neutral or alkaline; now it becomes acidic. This is largely due to Doderlein's bacillus, which oxidizes the glycogen that has been deposited in the vagina to form lactic acid. Concurrently, the ovaries are developing and menarche, or the beginning of menstruation, occurs. The average age at which menses commence is around 13 years in British girls according to Whincup et al (2001).

As in the male, gonadotrophin-releasing hormone (GnRH) stimulates the anterior pituitary gland to release two hormones: follicle-stimulating hormone (FSH) and luteinizing hormone (LH). FSH and LH are not secreted continuously but in a pulsating manner, with the amplitude and frequency of the pulses varying with the phase of the cycle. Under this hormonal influence, *primordial follicles* in the ovary begin to develop. Each primordial follicle is composed of an oocyte and surrounding granulosa cells. As growth occurs, the oocyte or ovum enlarges and there is an increase in the number of granulosa cells. Growth is eccentric and the ovum comes to lie at one side of the group of granulosa cells. Fluid

rich in oestrogens and inhibin collects between these cells and the ovum. Inhibin is produced by the granulosa cells under the stimulation of FSH. As more inhibin is produced, it exerts an inhibiting effect on the production of FSH, causing the levels to fall. As the follicle grows, cells begin to form around it and are called *thecal cells*. These thecal cells, stimulated by the FSH and LH, produce oestrogens.

In what is known as the *proliferative phase*, many follicles in both ovaries start to ripen but usually only one follicle continues on to ovulation. The others undergo degeneration. The thecal cells surrounding these degenerated follicles continue to produce oestrogens. The mature follicle may now be termed a *Graafian follicle*, after de Graaf who first described it in 1672 (Fig. 23.4).

As the Graafian follicle approaches ovulation, it comes to lie close to the surface of the ovary. The tissue over it becomes thin and taut. Soon the follicle wall ruptures and the ovum is expelled into the abdominal cavity. The time of the rupture is designated as *ovulation* and marks the end of the preovulatory (proliferative or follicular) phase.

The ovary now embarks on the *luteal* (secretory) *phase* of its cycle. Immediately after ovulation, the wall of the follicle collapses inward and some haemorrhage may occur into this cavity. In a few hours, the remaining granulosa cells hypertrophy and begin to show the characteristic yellow of the corpus luteum. These yellow granulosa cells are now called *luteal cells*. The luteal cells are stimulated to become the corpus luteum and to begin producing progesterone. Oestrogen continues to be produced as well. The corpus luteum reaches full maturity by about the ninth day after ovulation. At this time, it is easily recognizable on the surface of the ovary as a raised yellow area and may constitute nearly half the volume of the ovary. Near this time, the corpus luteum may receive a message that the ovum has been fertilized. If it does so, the corpus luteum is maintained and becomes known as the *corpus luteum* of pregnancy. If fertilization does not occur, the luteal site begins to degenerate and progesterone production drops. As the site degenerates, so do the thecal cells. Oestrogen production from this source declines. The luteal site shrinks to form a small mass of whitish scar tissue on the surface of the ovary which is known as the *corpus albicans*.

Hormones and the ovarian cycle

In response to the falling oestrogen and progesterone levels, the hypothalamus signals the anterior pituitary gland to release FSH and LH. Under this stimulus, the follicles begin to develop and the thecal cells produce oestrogen. The rising levels of oestrogen exert a negative feedback effect on the hypothalamus to reduce the amount of GnRH released and hence the amount of FSH and LH. The levels of FSH and LH fall slightly following the initial rise in oestrogen levels (Fig. 23.5). As oestrogen peaks, it is thought to exert a positive feedback effect on the hypothalamic-pituitary axis that results in a surge of LH and, to a lesser extent, of FSH. This surge of LH occurs about 24 hours before ovulation (Fig. 23.6).

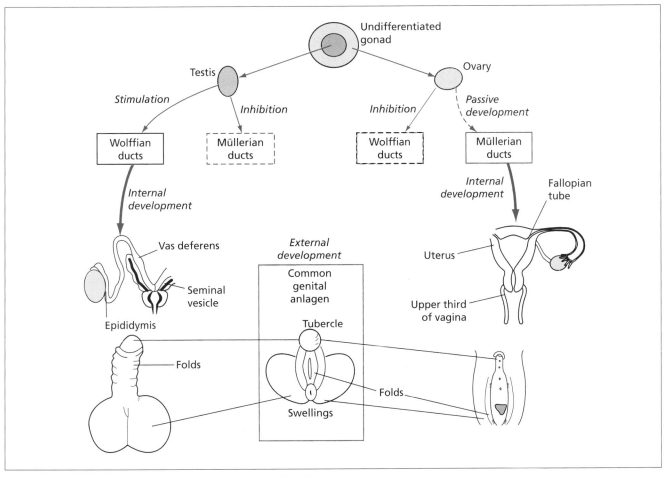

Figure 23.3 Normal sexual development in the male and female.

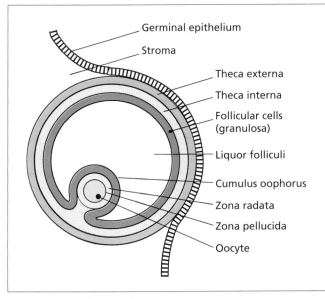

Figure 23.4 Mature Graafian follicle.

In cycles where the LH surge does not occur or is of insufficient magnitude, ovulation fails to occur. Exactly how the LH surge affects ovulation is unclear, except that it is necessary for completion of the cycle. Follicles will grow and develop under FSH stimulation but will fail to ovulate without the surge of LH.

Ovulation occurs in a climate of falling oestrogen, LH and FSH levels and a rising progesterone level, as LH stimulates the follicular site to begin production of progesterone. As the preovulatory cycle is one of high oestrogen level, the postovulatory phase is one of high progesterone level. The other hormones continue to be produced, but at lower levels. These levels of FSH and LH are too low to stimulate the development of new follicles. The cells of the corpus luteum are organized to enlarge, proliferate, secrete and then degenerate. The surge of LH seems to be the main organizing factor for this. This stabilizes the corpus luteum and the length of the postovulatory phase of the cycle. As the 12-day-old corpus luteum degenerates and becomes a corpus albicans, the levels of progesterone and oestrogen drop, signalling the hypothalamus to begin releasing GnRH again, thereby repeating the cycle.

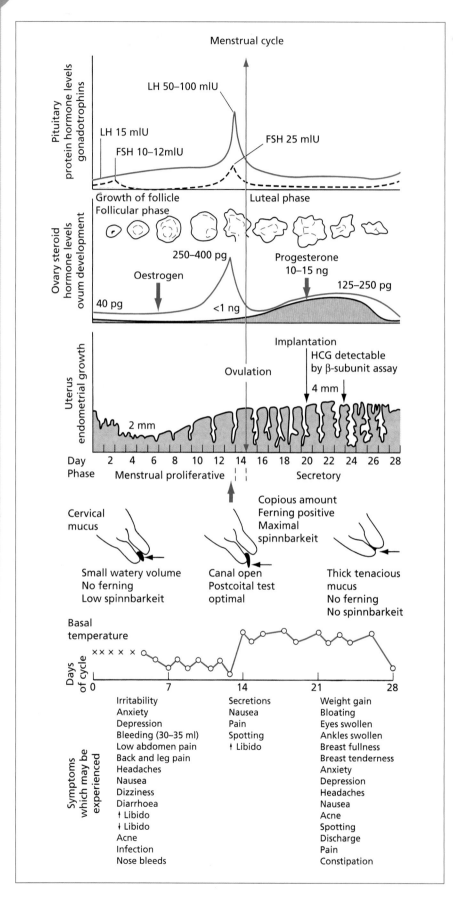

Figure 23.5 Summary of menstrual cycle events. FSH, follicle-stimulating hormone; HCG, human chorionic gonadotrophin; LH, luteinizing hormone; IU, international units.

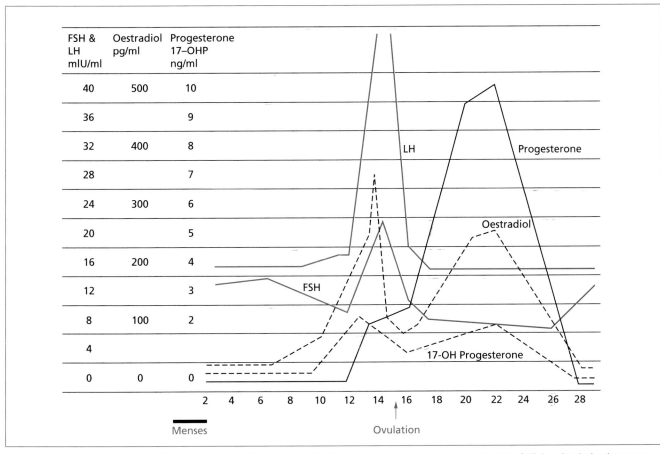

Figure 23.6 Plasma concentrations of gonadotrophins and ovarian hormones during one ovarian cycle. FSH, follicle-stimulating hormone; LH, luteinizing hormone; OHP, hydroxyprogesterone; IU, international units.

THE UTERUS

The uterus is a thick-walled, muscular, pear-shaped organ about 7.5 cm in length in the adult woman. It is held in position by its ligaments and by the pelvic floor. The uterus is composed of three layers:

1 an inner mucous layer, or endometrium
2 an inner muscular layer, or myometrium
3 an outer serous layer which covers the entire body of the uterus except where it is reflected up and over the bladder.

The uterus is divided into two distinct parts, the *body* and the *cervix*. The cervix projects into the vagina. The endometrial lining of the body of the uterus extends downwards, undergoing certain modifications in the cervical canal and terminating just above the external os of the cervix where it meets the stratified squamous epithelium of the vaginal wall.

Uterine cycle

The endometrium is a thin, pink membrane that is attached directly to the underlying muscle layer. It is richly supplied with blood vessels and tissue spaces. At the beginning of the new cycle it is about 0.5 mm thick. In response to the oestrogens of the preovulatory phase of the ovary, the endometrium begins to proliferate and continues to do so throughout the cycle until it reaches a peak of proliferation

and secretion several days after ovulation. In this secretory stage, the endometrium may be 5–6 mm in depth. In short, all is ready for implantation of the fertilized ovum, should it appear. In perfect timing, the endometrium reaches its peak of development approximately 7–8 days after ovulation, or just when the fertilized ovum should appear in the uterine cavity ready for implantation.

If the ovum has been fertilized and the corpus luteum is continuing to secrete progesterone, the endometrium is maintained and implantation may occur successfully. However, should the corpus luteum not receive this message, it begins to degenerate. Oestrogen and progesterone production decline. This decline in hormone level causes the endometrium to retract and degenerate. Vasoconstriction of blood vessels occurs and the uterus becomes ischaemic. Shortly thereafter, the endometrium begins to slough away and menstruation begins. The process of sloughing takes 3–7 days, with each woman usually establishing her own pattern. Menstrual flow is composed of endometrial tissue, mucus and some blood. As the tiny arterioles constrict and relax, bleeding occurs. Usually not more than 30–60 mL of blood is lost per menstrual period. This blood does not clot because of the action of fibrinolytic enzymes released into the uterine cavity during menstruation. Occasionally, a heavy menstrual loss neutralizes the available fibrinolysins and clots occur. At the completion of menstruation the endometrium has returned to its non-proliferative state. It is now ready to respond again to the rising oestrogen levels.

OVULATION

Menstrual cycle

The uterine and ovarian cycles are often referred to as the menstrual cycle. This cycle begins on day one, which is the day on which menstruation begins, and continues until the day before menstruation begins again. Ovulation occurs on or around the 14th day of a 28-day cycle. However, this is subject to many factors, and the timing of ovulation in any one woman is a matter of considerable variation.

The menstrual cycle is divided into two independent sections: the preovulatory and postovulatory phases. The two phases are independent because the length of one does not control the length of the other. Ovulation is the dividing factor signalling the end of one phase and the beginning of the next. Not all cycles are ovulatory and it is known that women may have an anovulatory cycle and still menstruate. The precise mechanism for this phenomenon is not clearly understood. The most common explanation is that a follicle develops but there is a failure of the LH surge and the follicle degenerates. Anovulatory cycles are most common in adolescent girls in whom the first menstrual periods may be anovulatory and in women at the menopause. Follicles do not mature at the same rate each month. This produces a month-to-month variation in the timing of ovulation and the length of the preovulatory phase in any one woman. This variation in timing is evident by variation in the onset of menstruation.

The onset of menstrual flow is controlled by the corpus luteum of the ovary. Once ovulation has occurred, menstruation follows 14 days later; this time relationship is constant. Fluctuations in the length of the cycle arise in the preovulatory phase. These events produce a natural variation in cycle length from month to month. Age is an important physical influence on cycle length in women. The menstrual pattern throughout life is divided into three zones: two of transition and a central period of increasing stability. The two transition periods (post-menarche lasting about 5–7 years, and premenopause lasting 6–8 years) are characterized by variation in cycle length.

As a girl ages, her average cycle length shortens and variation in cycle length reduces. The younger the girl when she experiences menarche, the sooner she begins to develop a more 'regular' cycle. As ageing continues, there is a decrease in the number of follicles that begin to develop. This results in a gradual reduction in hormone levels, particularly inhibin, with corresponding increases in circulating FSH throughout the cycle. Documentation of these high FSH levels is the first laboratory indication of the perimenopausal period. These high FSH levels induce rapid follicular development and a correspondingly shorter preovulatory phase. As the process continues, there is a failure of the LH surge and anovulation follows, contributing to increasing irregularity in the cycle length. Eventually the ovary ceases to respond and menopause occurs.

Cervical, vaginal and tubal cycles

Changes may also occur in the cervix, vagina and fallopian tubes in response to stimuli from the ovary. Oestrogen prompts the endocervical glands to respond by increasing their secretions. Cervical mucus reaches its peak of production at ovulation. The consistency of the mucus changes at ovulation and becomes thinner. These changes demonstrate the timing of the body as the mucus will permit easy entry of the sperm at ovulation – the most logical time. Indeed, it appears that the cervical mucus permits passage of sperm through the cervix only at this particular time.

Changes in the vagina and fallopian tube are minimal compared with the changes in the ovary, uterus and cervix. The vaginal epithelium proliferates and reaches a peak at ovulation time. The fallopian tube secretes fluids that provide nutrients first for the ovum and then for the conceptus until implantation occurs.

PHYSIOLOGICAL ASPECTS OF SEXUAL RESPONSE

The general sexual response cycle consists of four progressive phases which are the same for both sexes (see Ch. 22, p. 765 for a summary of these stages). In the female, Bartholin's glands secrete a fluid that serves to lubricate the vaginal introitus. However, the amount of mucus secreted by these vulvovaginal glands is minimal and most vaginal lubrication arises from the vaginal walls themselves. Very quickly following sexual stimulation, the vaginal walls exhibit a 'sweating'-like appearance as beads of mucoid material appear throughout the rugal folds. Soon the droplets run together to form a complete coat of lubrication over the inner surface of the vagina. The cervix also appears to play a relatively minor role. This seems to be confirmed by the fact that little or no secretory activity of the cervix has been observed during sexual activity. Also, women who have undergone hysterectomy and bilateral salpingo-oophorectomy produce reasonable vaginal lubrication in response to sexual stimulation. Indeed, the same response will develop in artificially constructed vaginas, and the source of lubricating material is presumed to be the same.

The vagina also responds to sexual stimuli by enlarging. The inner two-thirds of the vagina expand and lengthen, forming a basin for the seminal pool that will form in the posterior fornix of the vagina just below the cervical os. The outer-third of the vagina becomes engorged and constricted, serving to assist the vagina to form a reservoir for the semen.

An orgasm may occur as a generalized systemic feeling, with sensation localized in the clitoris, and rhythmic muscular contractions of the outer third of the vagina and the uterus. With orgasm, pelvic engorgement of blood vessels is rapidly resolved. This causes the uterus to return to its normal position, placing the cervix near to or in the seminal pool, thus facilitating movement of sperm through the cervix.

The clitoris seems to be a unique organ in human anatomy. As the primary focus of sensual response, it appears to serve no other function. Made of fibrous tissue with two corpora cavernosa and richly innervated, it undergoes engorgement and enlargement when the female is sexually stimulated either physically or mentally. The tumescent clitoris then retracts against the symphysis pubis and becomes difficult to see or feel.

The subjective experience of orgasm is synchronous with orgasmic platform contractions and the pleasure associated with orgasm is related to their number and intensity. Following orgasm, the woman enters the resolution phase. Unlike the male, a woman, if provided during this phase with sufficient further stimulation, may return to the orgasmic level.

MENOPAUSE

Around 1900, the average age at menopause in the UK was approximately 50 years and female life expectancy was similar. Currently, the average age of menopause has changed little as it is now approximately 52 years. However, mean female life expectancy has lengthened to approximately 81 years. This means that today the average woman can expect to spend almost 30 years of her life in the post-menopausal state. The emotional, physical and medical implications of this relatively recent situation are many, and currently constitute one of the fastest growing areas of female medical research.

The cessation of menstruation is perhaps the most obvious sign of menopause. However, the transitional period is known as the *climacteric* which can take a few months to several years and is the result of altered ovarian function. This fluctuation leads to a variety of menopausal symptoms which may occur intermittently (Menopause Matters 2006). Eventually the menses may become irregular and finally cease. Menopause is complete when the woman has had her last menstruation and the woman is considered to be post menopausal when she has had no menses for at least 1 year. As the perimenopausal woman may ovulate erratically, contraception needs to be continued.

Decreasing oestrogen levels stimulate gonadotrophic hormones (FSH, LH), which show a proportionate rise, but the ovary does not respond fully. The body, previously functioning smoothly under balanced hormonal control, responds to these imbalances with 'hot flushes' in about 70% of women. A hot flush is a sudden feeling of heat in the face, neck and chest associated with patchy flushing of the skin. There is usually profuse perspiration, perhaps palpitations, a generalized feeling of heat and a sensation of acute physical discomfort. Some flushes are accompanied by nausea, dizziness and headache. A hot flush lasts for about 3 minutes. The monitoring of women having hot flushes confirms that an average temperature shift of about 2°C from core to skin occurs. The hot flush is followed by vasoconstriction and shivering as the body attempts to correct the shift in temperature from skin to core.

The exact mechanism is not understood but the same factors that trigger a rise in LH are also thought to trigger a hot flush. Low circulating levels of oestrogen are thought to contribute to this phenomenon. However, these symptoms are unpredictable, hence uncontrollable, and can be embarrassing, anxiety producing and sleep disturbing.

Other physical symptoms include insomnia, headaches, joint pains and urinary symptoms such as frequency and urgency.

Psychological symptoms may be related to changes in hormone levels and include anxiety, loss of concentration, mood swings and irritability. Sexual problems may be related to vaginal dryness and dyspareunia or loss of libido due to lower oestrogen levels. Many women accept these changes with only some minor disturbance, although most appreciate freely available sources of education and reassurance (Menopause Matters 2006).

Assessment and treatment

Women have individual needs and should be assessed by taking a full history of symptoms, lifestyle, past/family history and health beliefs. Information regarding available treatment should be evidence-based, using a risk/benefit analysis of what is most acceptable to them.

Hormone replacement therapy

The principal goals in the management of the menopausal woman are three-fold:

1 To maintain or improve quality of life
2 To increase lifespan
3 To reduce risks factors

The benefits of HRT, although well documented (Box 23.1), continue to remain controversial.

HRT is available in numerous combinations of oestrogen and progestogen or unopposed oestrogen for women who have had a hysterectomy. The administration route is mainly transdermal patches or oral administration.

In all cases, treatment should be a mutual decision between the woman and her healthcare provider. However, this is not always the case and a woman's level of knowledge may play a significant role in determining whether she receives HRT or not. The use of HRT has raised anxieties in relation to increased risks of other pathologies developing. These include thrombosis and cancer. However, the research evidence appears to suggest that risks are minimal provided there are no pre-existing diseases or contraindications from

---

Box 23.1   Documented benefits of HRT

- Relief of menopausal vasomotor symptoms
- Reduced incidence of osteoporosis
- Reduced incidence of hip fractures
- Reduced risk of colonic cancer

family history. The risks and benefits of HRT should be reviewed at least annually with each woman to enable each individual to make a personal assessment of the current evidence.

It should be understood that not all oestrogen production ceases at menopause. The ovaries do not appear to be inert when the woman is postmenopausal, and it is thought that they continue to excrete small amounts of hormone. This is in addition to oestrogens from the adrenal gland. Over the years, oestrogen production declines further and the development of other organ changes occurs. The vulva becomes atrophic and thin as a result of reabsorption of fatty tissue. The uterus decreases in size; the endometrium becomes thin and atrophic. The vaginal epithelium thins out and is more susceptible to injury and infection. Lubrication of the vagina may require supplementation so that dyspareunia (painful sexual intercourse) does not occur. Topical oestrogen creams may relieve these symptoms.

Sexual function can continue with little change in the vast majority of postmenopausal women. The most important factors in the continuance of sexual function appear to be the opportunity for and the frequency of intercourse, so that the changes of menopause themselves do not mean this phase of a woman's life must cease. Indeed, relief from fear of pregnancy may make the experience a more enjoyable one.

CASE Sue is a 49-year-old teacher, married with two children who are now at university. She presented with hot flushes, night sweats and heavy irregular periods for the last 6 months.
On further questioning, she was also experiencing some vaginal dryness but no loss of libido and no urinary symptoms. She had no medical history of note and her family history included her father having angina and hypertension, aged 70.
Sue had never smoked, drinks 10–15 units of alcohol each week, eats a low-fat, high-fibre diet, takes regular exercise by walking daily and has a good relationship with her husband. She has no known allergies and is taking no medication. Her health beliefs involve using natural remedies and to avoid HRT if possible. She had a normal cervical smear last year.
Assessment was made using the Menopause Matters (2006) decision tree with a risk/benefit analysis of possible treatments. Sue was interested in the information provided on this website and wanted to consider alternative therapies. She agreed to keep a diary of her symptoms and to return in 6 weeks for review.

Women who have never needed to take regular medication often feel the need to explore all the possibilities before they make a decision about HRT. Experiences of family and friends may have an impact on some women's choices whilst others will be prepared to rely on the guidance of the healthcare professional with whom they are consulting. This case study highlights a number of issues that would need to be addressed with Sue including her possible ongoing need for contraception and the risks and benefits to her if she decided to start on HRT. Use of the Menopause Matters

website can be very helpful for patients and healthcare professionals alike when dealing with these issues.

DISORDERS OF THE FEMALE REPRODUCTIVE SYSTEM

HISTORY TAKING

This involves the nurse using a framework to collate as much information as possible allowing the woman to 'tell her story' and establishing a therapeutic relationship. This would include the following :

- Chief complaint
- Present illness
- Symptom analysis using PQRST (see p. 128)
- Medical history including any surgery or medical conditions
- History of previous pregnancies
- Current health including current medications
- Family history
- Menstrual history – including menarche, last menstrual period, length of cycle, duration of flow, amount of flow, menopause and last cervical smear test
- Contraception – present method and past methods
- Lifestyle – smoking status, alcohol, diet, work, sleep, relationships, occupation
- Allergies
- Review of systems including an overview of all other aspects of the woman's health.

PHYSICAL EXAMINATION

The physical examination may include a general examination, with inspection and palpation of internal and external genitalia (Figs 23.7, 23.8). The examination is personal and invades body boundaries and there is a sense of exposure, particularly during vaginal examination. The nurse can help to reduce these feelings by a sensitive and supportive approach. The nurse should avoid the expression 'relax' and instead explain how to loosen the pelvic floor muscles. Most women appreciate simple explanations of what to expect as the examination progresses. One of the most critical factors in gaining a woman's confidence is to explain the procedure during the examination.

POTENTIAL ISSUES

The woman with a reproductive problem presents various special concerns. Being female usually provides a woman with an inherent set of behaviours that are culturally and physiologically determined, that may help to guide her actions. The normal functioning of her reproductive system can provide reassurance of her essential 'femininity'. The distortion or interruption of these processes may prove very disturbing to the woman and/or her partner. The woman may experience problems in relation to self-image and have fears about future sexual performance and attractiveness.

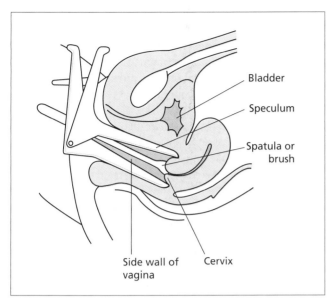

Figure 23.7 Internal vaginal examination demonstrating the position of the speculum and Ayre spatula used to obtain cervical cells for a smear test.

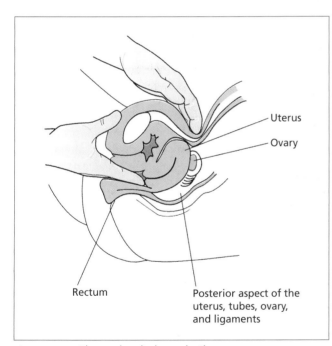

Figure 23.8 Bimanual vaginal examination.

Body parts that contribute to self-esteem and identity have a high psychological investment. The threat posed by loss of these body parts depends on:

- their meaning to the individual
- her stage of development of body image and self
- the reactions of the social group, including the spouse, to which the patient belongs.

Many people have been culturally conditioned to the idea that some areas of the body should not be discussed – much less exposed to examination. Others may feel guilt over their illness. Sexually transmitted infection, abortion and cancer arouse guilt feelings in some individuals. You may be dealing with patients who experience anxiety and fear, shame, guilt, diminished self-esteem or reawakened anxieties over personal identity.

GOALS

A patient's goals may include:

1 resolving dysfunctional sexual problems
2 achieving a sense of self-worth
3 being able to verbalize fears and anxieties
4 showing understanding of health problems and what medical intervention involves
5 adapting to a change in sexual role/and or function
6 being aware of and avoiding risk factors in sexual activity.

NURSING INTERVENTION

These goals may be achieved by the following nursing interventions:

1 Assess the degree of threat posed by loss of function or body parts to the woman; then plan, provide and evaluate nursing care based on that assessment.
2 Provide nursing care that promotes feelings of dignity, self-worth and attractiveness. Encourage the return of health, control over body functions and independent self-care.
3 Reduce fear and lessen potential guilt by:
   a) acknowledging and discussing feelings
   b) anticipating the need for explanations and inter-pretations
   c) clarifying misinformation about causes of illness and the consequences of treatment
   d) maintaining a confident, non-judgemental approach to the patient
   e) assisting in acknowledging the loss, if any
   f) obtaining appropriate additional sources of spiritual or emotional help for the patient
   g) offering information and support for relatives.

EVALUATION

Interventions are successful if behavioural changes have occurred, although behavioural changes may be difficult to document in areas such as self-concept, anxiety and guilt. The patient may, for example:

- state that she feels better or less frightened
- take an interest in personal appearance and renew interests in social life, which may also indicate a return to the more positive outlook toward the future
- demonstrate an understanding of the illness, treatments and any residual changes
- demonstrate a knowledge of the risk factors that may lead to a recurrence of the problem and the actions that may reduce or eliminate the risk factors

● discuss alterations in body function and structure with the nurse and so indicate a willingness to begin to deal with the problem or to accept it with appropriate adjustments.

Adjustment to many of these changes requires some time. Expectations of resolution and the effectiveness of intervention must be realistic.

VARIATIONS OF SEXUALITY

Variations in sexuality can occur in several areas of sexual expression, but most differences are psychosexual in origin. Only a few disorders arise from physical illness and trauma or congenital malformation. Most variations become obvious through difficulties in sexual expression.

During middle adolescence, teenagers begin to adjust and become more comfortable with their changing bodies. The majority of adolescents proceed through this experience fairly easily, although for some it is a time of intense emotional upheaval. Sexual orientation develops during early childhood. One's gender identity is usually firmly established by the age of 2 years. Studies demonstrate that the sense of masculinity or femininity is essentially solidified by age 5 or 6 years.

Homosexual characteristics appear to surface several years before the period of adolescence. Theories about the aetiology of homosexuality include genetic, hormonal, environmental and psychological origins. The young adolescent may experience intense confusion and anxiety as he or she struggles with these personal issues. The nurse must be sensitive and aware of the psychological and medical implications of homosexuality. A trusting, non-judgemental, caring attitude can provide the basis for a therapeutic relationship during this potentially sensitive time.

CONGENITAL ANOMALIES OF THE REPRODUCTIVE SYSTEM

Absence or duplication of organs

The uterus, cervix and vagina can undergo duplication or incomplete fusion. The exact incidence of such anomalies is unknown, as they are largely asymptomatic. Some may cause sterility in women or an increased risk of abortion. Sometimes an organ is completely absent. Some absence (*agenesis*) or maldevelopment of tissue (*dysgenesis*) is determined genetically. *Ovarian agenesis* may be the result of an XO genotype (Turner's syndrome). The patient with this genotype may present a characteristic appearance from birth with a webbed neck, multiple anomalies, low birthweight or irregularities of the hairline. However, in others, the patient may present in adolescence because of failure of the menarche to appear.

Imperforate hymen

Usually this condition is not discovered until adolescence when the girl may present herself because of absence of menstrual flow. Menstruation occurs but the blood is re-

tained behind the closed hymen. The patient may complain of crampy, lower abdominal pain occurring monthly. She may also notice dysuria, frequency and urinary retention as the growing mass of retained menstrual blood accumulates in the vagina, putting increasing pressure on the bladder and urethra. Treatment consists of a cross-shaped incision of the hymen which allows drainage of the debris. This debris is often a thick, chocolate-like material. Because of this old blood, the risk of postoperative infection is greatly increased. The nurse must pay careful attention to good aseptic technique after the operation to reduce the risk of infection further. The nurse must see that adequate drainage is maintained, frequent cleansing of the perineum occurs, and perineal dressings are changed frequently.

The hymen may also be rigid. This is usually discovered when the patient presents with a complaint of dyspareunia. In mild cases, the patient will be instructed to dilate the hymen digitally, usually while sitting in a bath of warm water. If this does not succeed, vaginal dilators may be inserted by the doctor or nurse and later by the patient. In more difficult situations, hymenotomy is performed.

CONTROL OF FERTILITY

Limiting the world population through fertility control has become a political as well as a religious and personal issue. The implications of overpopulation have usually been stated in terms of the developing nations, but have taken on a global context. In addition, contraception is considered to be a matter of personal decision: it can exercise an important liberalizing potential for the family or single person. In the light of these discussions, the health professional has a responsibility to extend the knowledge and availability of contraception to anyone who requests it. With more nurse led family planning clinics available, the nurse has a major role in the control of fertility.

NURSING RESPONSIBILITIES

After an initial interview with the person, and preferably their partner, who is seeking birth control advice the nurse may need to refer the woman to an appropriate clinic. The couple can be assisted in making a decision by the presentation of concise, factual information about the methods available. The woman should choose a method that will be most compatible with her personal circumstances. Most certainly, this should be the one she will use and feel comfortable in using. No method of birth control is effective unless it is used constantly.

The patient or couple will need counselling in the proper use of the method they have chosen and what to expect in the period of initial adjustment. The nurse is responsible for gaining sufficient knowledge of the complex subject of contraception to be able to present factual knowledge to couples and to discuss the advantages and disadvantages of each method. In addition, the nurse will need to understand much of the emotional, social and religious aspects of contraception.

Nurses who are competent in family planning and who have completed the extended and supplementary prescribing course are now able to prescribe the contraceptive pill, Depot-Provera injection as well as emergency contraception (Nurse Prescribers' Formulary 2005). This not only enhances the nurse's role but also provides holistic care for the woman consulting her.

A detailed presentation of family planning is beyond the scope of this work, but a brief outline of the methods follows.

METHODS OF CONTRACEPTION (BOX 23.2)

Condom

The condom is a thin rubber sheath that is placed over the penis before insertion. It prevents pregnancy by acting as a mechanical barrier to the sperm. Some couples find it objectionable as a method of birth control because it may interrupt sexual foreplay, it can lessen sensation, and its effective use relies heavily on the motivation of the male. These objections can be overcome if it is used by a man who is taking a mature responsibility for his behaviour, especially in view of the risk of contracting AIDS and other sexually transmitted infections.

Box 23.2 Methods of contraception

Spermicidal agents
- Foam, gels, jelly, pessaries suitable for use with barrier methods. Not adequate when used alone

Barrier methods
- Condom
- Femidom (female condom)
- Cervical cap
- Diaphragm

Hormonal contraception
- Oral contraceptive pills
- Contraceptive patches
- Depo-Provera injections
- Implant

Intrauterine devices (IUDs)
- Coil
- Gynefix

Intrauterine system (IUS)
- Mirena intrauterine system

Surgical methods
- Tubal ligation
- Vasectomy.

Femidom (female condom)

The female condom is now available in the UK. It is pre-lubricated, but does not contain a spermicide. The female condom is available in over 35 countries and is a female-controlled barrier method for the prevention of pregnancy and infections, including HIV.

Diaphragm

The diaphragm is a thin rubber cap that is inserted into the vagina by the woman and placed over the cervical os. The cap provides a mechanical barrier to the sperm. In addition, a spermicidal jelly is placed on both sides of the cap. When the diaphragm is in place, the spermicidal jelly will be in contact with the cervix and vagina. The diaphragm is not dispensed without a prescription and requires individual fittings initially, after a few months of use, and following pregnancy or miscarriage. The woman also requires careful teaching in the proper insertion and care of the diaphragm. The diaphragm is inserted manually and the position should be checked after each insertion.

In its proper position, the diaphragm cups the cervix with the anterior side behind the pubic bone and its posterior side in the posterior fornix of the vagina. Properly positioned, it is not felt by either partner during intercourse. Removal should not take place before 6 hours following coitus to ensure completion of spermicidal action. The diaphragm can be left in place for up to 24 hours, but should then be removed for cleaning. The diaphragm is not an option for women with a latex sensitivity.

Spermicidal preparations

Spermicidal contraceptives are available in various forms including gels, creams, foams and foam tablets. These preparations are suitable for use with an additional barrier method (i.e. condom or diaphragm). These chemical agents do not give adequate protection when used alone. The spermicidal agent should remain in the vagina for at least 6 hours to be sure that all sperm are dead.

Oral contraceptives

Contraceptive pills are synthetic chemical hormones. The pills are divided into two types: the combined pill and the progestogen pill. The combined pill contains synthetic oestrogen and progesterone hormones in each pill. The high hormone levels depress the hypothalamus, which in turn inhibits the release of pituitary gonadotrophins that stimulate ovulation. Thus, the woman is anovulatory. Protection is established as soon as the woman begins taking the pills, if she starts taking them on day 1 of the menstrual cycle.

The progestogen pill, or 'mini-pill', contains a progestational agent and no oestrogen. Many of a woman's menstrual cycles while on the progestogen pill may be ovulatory. The pill depends on the effects of progestogen to produce changes in cervical mucus, the endometrium and hormonal levels to inhibit fertilization. Because of the reduced oestrogenicity of the pill, it has fewer major side-effects than the combined pill. This makes the low-dose combined pill the pill of choice initially. The risk of pregnancy in both types of pills is minimal if taken as prescribed.

The combined pill is taken once a day for 21 days and no pill, or an inert sugar pill, is taken for the next 7 days, regardless of the woman's menstrual period. Initially the first pill is taken on the first day of the woman's menstrual period. Now the pills will regulate her menstrual cycle and she takes them as prescribed. Progestogen pills are taken every day without omission. This does make it easier for women to follow, for no timing, counting or remembering is required – other than to take the pill. To maintain consistently high hormonal levels in the body, some of the progestogen pills need to be taken at approximately the same time every day although the newer progestogen pill desogestrel (Cerazette) can be taken within 12 hours of the usual daily time.

Withdrawal bleeding is regulated by the combined pill and occurs regularly at some time during the seven hormone-free pill days. This withdrawal bleeding simulates menstruation. With the withdrawal of the high hormone levels, the endometrium sloughs away. However, menstruation is usually scantier and shorter, because the endometrium is thinner.

Much discussion has occurred over the possible side-effects or complications on the use of oral contraceptives (Box 23.3). For many women, adjustment to oral contraceptives may take some months. During that time, the woman may experience nausea, fullness and tingling in her breasts, headache, some spotting between menstrual periods, weight gain, chloasma (hyperpigmentation of localized areas of skin), acne, loss of libido or changes in vaginal discharge. On the other hand, she may feel better, have relief from menstrual cramps and have an increased libido. Sometimes changes in dosages or changes in the type of pills helps.

The missed pill is cause for concern in many women and she should be given clear advice about what to do when she is first issued with the pill. The woman is best directed to the information leaflet in each packet of pills, the Family Planning Association's information which can be accessed at www.fpa.org.uk, or information from Marie Stopes International which can be accessed at www.mariestopes.org.uk. In general, if a combined pill has been missed it should be taken as soon as the woman remembers it and the next pill should be taken at the usual time. This may mean taking two pills in one day. Should more than one pill be missed, then the couple should use an alternative form of birth control for the remainder of that cycle. If several pills are missed, or if the missed pill is adjacent to the pill free interval, the doctor or nurse should be consulted, as the woman may be at risk of ovulation and will need extra advice. The woman should also be taught that oral antibiotics and diarrhoea affect the rate of absorption of the pill; therefore alternative methods of contraception should be used if such problems arise. If the woman is taking a progesterone-only pill, one missed pill puts her at risk of pregnancy. She should take the pill as soon as she remembers it and carry on with the next pill at the usual time but assume that the contraceptive effect has been disrupted and use extra precautions such as a condom for at least the next 2 days (Nurse Prescribers' Formulary 2005).

Major complications of the pill are rare but serious. For some women the hazards of the pill are still less than the hazards of pregnancy or an abortion. Major concern revolves around the increased incidence of diseases of the circulatory system in women using the pill. The major circulatory diseases include thromboembolic disease, coronary artery disease, cerebrovascular accidents and hypertension. The risks rise with age, cigarette smoking, obesity and family history of thromboembolic disease. Thus, the smoking woman who is over 35 years of age is placing herself at considerable risk if she continues to use the pill. Such women should be counselled to give up smoking and, if unable to do so, to consider another method of contraception.

However, medical opinion still supports widespread use of the pill for carefully chosen women, although it may take several months for some women to find an acceptable oral preparation. Some benefits may accrue, however, for a woman who has been taking oral contraceptives. Women who have been taking the pill for longer than 1 year have lower risks of endometrial and ovarian cancer (British National Formulary 2005).

Women on a contraceptive pill should see a medical practitioner or suitably qualified nurse prescriber every 6–12 months to have their blood pressure and weight mon-

---

Box 23.3 Side-effects of oral contraceptives

Oestrogen
- Breakthrough bleeding
- Nausea
- Headaches
- Chloasma
- Increased vaginal discharge
- Cervical erosion
- Cystic breast changes

Progestogen
- Acne
- Depression
- Dry vagina
- Loss of libido

Oestrogen and progestogen
- Weight gain
- Post-pill amenorrhoea
- Increased breast size
- Breast tenderness.

itored, and for an assessment of their general health. A cervical smear test is performed according to the NHS Cancer Screening Programmes (2004) every 3 or 5 years. Women are taught to seek prompt medical care if they experience severe or recurrent abdominal pain, chest pain and shortness of breath, severe headaches, eye problems such as blurred vision or flashing lights, or tenderness and warmth over veins in the legs.

Danger signs associated with oral contraceptives are:

- sudden severe chest pain
- sudden shortness of breath
- severe leg or calf pain
- prolonged headache
- hypertension (blood pressure above 140/100 mmHg)
- sudden vertigo, weakness or motor disturbance
- blurred vision and eye problems.

It is extremely important to note that the use of oral contraceptive agents alone in no way protects the woman from acquiring a sexually transmitted infection. Prevention of such infection through safer sexual behaviour is discussed further below.

Intrauterine device

Long-acting reversible contraception methods are described by NICE (2005) as the intrauterine device (IUD), Depot-Provera injection and Implanon. An IUD is a device that is placed inside the uterus, where it prevents fertilization and inhibits fertilization, although the exact action is not fully understood. Most IUDs used today are made from a flexible plastic with the addition of copper to improve effectiveness.

The device must be inserted and removed by a suitably trained person. Complications of the use of an IUD include increased menstrual loss and cramping. These are the most common side-effects, and some women require removal of the IUD for these reasons.

Pregnancy does occur in about 3% of women using an intrauterine device. The IUD containing 380 mm of copper is licensed for use for 5–10 years and the pregnancy rate is <20/1000 in 5 years (NICE 2005).

The IUD may contribute to the development of pelvic inflammatory disease (PID) which may lead to sterility. The only sign of this infection may be irregular intramenstrual bleeding and complaints of pain. If an infection is suspected, the IUD is removed and the infection treated. The IUD is contraindicated in women with a current pelvic infection or those at a high risk of one.

Intrauterine system

Levonorgestrel is released directly in the uterine cavity from an intrauterine system (IUS) (Mirena). The effects are therefore mainly local and hormonal with menstrual loss being minimal for many women and the return of fertility when the system is removed is rapid and complete. Essentially, the cautions and contraindications are similar as for standard IUDs. Effectiveness continues for 5 years but the beneficial effects of levonorgestrel diminish after 3 years.

The Mirena IUD is licensed for contraception, primary dysmenorrhoea and prevention of endometrial hyperplasia for those women taking oestrogen replacement therapy (British National Formulary 2005).

Depo-Provera

Medroxyprogesterone acetate is a long-acting progestogen given by intramuscular injection. This method of contraception can be used by women desiring short-term as well as long-term contraceptive protection. Long-term contraception is provided by repeat injections every 12 weeks. There are reports of delayed return of fertility and irregular cycles after discontinuation of treatment. Heavy bleeding has been reported in patients given medroxyprogesterone acetate immediately postpartum. A reduction in bone mineral density and osteoporosis has been reported, although this usually occurs in the first 2–3 years of use and then stabilizes (British National Formulary 2005). The Committee on the Safety of Medicines' (CSM) advice is that Depo-Provera should only be used in adolescent girls when other methods are inappropriate. All women should be counselled and risks evaluated after 2 years and it should be avoided in those women already at risk of osteoporosis.

Implant

The levonorgestrel-releasing implant system (Implanon) is more than 99% effective and needs replacement every 3 years (British National Formulary 2005). It is a small tube inserted under the skin which releases the hormone progesterone slowly into the bloodstream. It must be inserted and removed under a local anaesthetic by a qualified health practitioner (NICE 2005).

Sterilization

Sterilization means the termination of reproductive capacity. As the social and emotional barriers to sterilization have altered, it has increased in popularity. When family size is complete, many couples choose sterilization as the method of birth control. In other cases, when the hazards of pregnancy are life-threatening, sterilization may be strongly indicated. In men, this involves the procedure known as vasectomy, which is discussed in Chapter 22.

Tubal ligation

Tubal ligation is the comparable operation to vasectomy in men. It can be done vaginally but is usually performed abdominally via a laparoscope. Under general anaesthesia, two small incisions are made in the abdomen. The fallopian tube is dissected, a loop of tube is lifted up, ligated, and the tube above the ligation is either crushed with a clamp or severed. In some operations, the uterine end of the tube may be turned back and embedded in the posterior wall of the uterus. Tubal coagulations, in conjunction with a laparoscopy, may also be done. In the hands of a skilled operator, the procedure is safe and associated with few side-effects.

As in the male, the tubes can be reconstructed, but the success rate is not high. Thus, the patient should see the operation as irreversible. The operation, although frequently performed as a day case, is not entirely harmless. Rare major postoperative complications are pulmonary embolism and later tubal pregnancy. In addition to the consent for operation, there is a separate consent form for sterilization which must be signed before the operation.

Rhythm method (natural family planning)

This method requires temporary abstinence from coitus during the possible ovulation time of the woman. It is the only method of contraception that is officially sanctioned by all religions. The rationale of the method is based on several assumptions:

- that a woman is fertile only during ovulation
- that ovulation occurs once a month at a predictable time
- that the ovum can survive for approximately 24 hours
- that sperm will survive in the genital tract for 72 hours.

Placing these assumptions together, and allowing 3 days before and after ovulation for the lifespan of the sperm, we arrive at 6 days. As we know that the time of ovulation varies in any one woman, we must allow 1 or 2 days for extra safety on either side. This now gives us a fertile period of approximately 8 days' duration, falling near the middle of the menstrual cycle.

The main problem is the timing of ovulation. Because no anticipatory method of timing ovulation has been discovered, we must rely on a retrospective view of the time of ovulation in any one woman. Under the influence of the rising progesterone levels following ovulation, the basal body temperature in women shows a rise. The rise will be noticeable within the first 24 hours following ovulation. The temperature remains slightly increased for the remainder of the cycle. Also, at the time of ovulation, the cervical mucus changes. There is an increase in amount and reduction in viscosity. Women can be taught to recognize and record these changes. An attempt is made to predict the time of ovulation for the woman after she has; carefully recorded the dates of her menstrual periods, the mucus changes, and has also recorded her temperature taken daily at a uniform time. Depending on the woman or clinic, this may be done for 3–6 months. An average is then calculated from these dates and her individual period of likely fertility should be reviewed at specified intervals. During periods of her life when ovulation is being established or re-established – postpartum, during lactation, menopause and periods of emotional stress – the method is highly unreliable. In women with very regular periods and high motivation, the method has had success. A urine testing kit is now commercially available which indicates when ovulation is due. This increases the reliability of this method.

Other methods not recommended for contraceptive purposes

Breastfeeding

Under the stimulus of regular demand breastfeeding, many women remain anovulatory for several months. Others quickly regain their fertility. Breastfeeding is not suggested as a form of contraception. Women who are breastfeeding should be advised to use a form of contraception that will not interfere with the physiology of lactation. Suggestions are barrier methods or progestogen-only hormonal preparations.

Coitus interruptus

This method consists of the male withdrawing his penis from the vagina before ejaculation occurs. This is a highly unreliable method as some sperm may escape before ejaculation actually occurs. Also, this method may require more control and experience than many couples possess.

Emergency contraception

For some women or couples there is occasionally a need for emergency contraception (EC) (Box 23.4). Progestogen only emergency contraception (POEC) is available in the UK and is now being sold over the counter to women over the age of 16. Two tablets of levonorgestrel 750 µg taken by mouth is a highly effective method or Levonelle one stop is also available as a once only tablet containing 150 µg levonorgestrel.

This needs to be initiated as soon as possible after unprotected intercourse, within 72 hours but is most effective if taken within the first 12 hours.

Women should be advised that if they vomit within 2–3 hours of taking the tablets they will need replacement tablets. She should use a barrier method until her next period and this may be earlier or later than expected. She must return to the clinic if she experiences lower abdominal pain and also in 3–4 weeks if her period is heavy, light or absent. At this time, the nurse will be able to discuss in more detail the various methods of contraception available.

CASE Mika, aged 18, attends the surgery on Monday morning requesting emergency contraception. She went out to a nightclub on Sunday night and met up with a previous boyfriend whom she spent the night with. They had unprotected sexual intercourse approximately 9 hours ago.

Mika has no significant medical history or family history. Her menstrual history includes a regular cycle every 28 days with 4–5 days of bleeding and her last period was 3 weeks ago. She has not been using contraception for 6 months but was previously taking a combined pill. She had never smoked, drinks alcohol at weekends and takes no regular or over the counter medication. She is an art college student and lives at home with her parents. Her blood pressure is 110/70 and body mass index is 23. She states that she has

Box 23.4 Indications for emergency contraception
- Unprotected sex
- Condom rupture
- Diaphragm displacement or misuse
- Potential pill failure
- Sexual assault.

had no other episode of unprotected intercourse since her last period which was normal, regular and on time.

A prescription for Levonelle One Stop 150 µg is given to Mika and she is advised to take it as soon as possible. She is given a leaflet explaining possible side-effects, what to do if she vomits and also if she experiences lower abdominal pain. She is advised to use a barrier method of contraception until her next period and a follow-up appointment is made to ensure the treatment has been effective. Further health promotion advice would be available to Mika at that time.

There is a great deal of information for women and their partners to take in when they attend for emergency contraception and it is essential that nurses take time to discuss their concerns, fears and anxieties. Women often feel guilty and ashamed that they need to attend for such help and the nurse needs to be sensitive to each individual's needs. A young woman such as Mika needs to be encouraged to return for further advice and support once the moment of crisis is over and it is therefore important to maintain an open door and to make her feel welcome to return. The service needs to be delivered in such a way that young people will return for help and the nurse plays an essential role in making young people feel accepted and respected.

DISORDERS OF THE MENSTRUAL CYCLE AND MENSTRUATION

MITTELSCHMERZ

Mittelschmerz is a feeling of lower abdominal pain on one side on or near ovulation time. It is thought to be caused by fluid or blood escaping from the outer ruptured follicle site and causing peritoneal irritation. It occurs in about 25% of women. Occasionally, when the right side is involved, fear of appendicitis may bring the woman to the surgery.

PREMENSTRUAL SYNDROME

Premenstrual syndrome (PMS) is probably experienced by most women in mild forms. However, extreme cases are seen. The symptomatology includes a feeling of fullness or heaviness in the lower abdomen, backache, painful breasts, irritability, headache, weight gain premenstrually, nervousness, depression and insomnia.

No single cause has been identified. What seems clear is that somatic and psychological symptoms exist; they occur but in varying degrees with each cycle. Among the treatments that are usually tried are the combined contraceptive pill, pyridoxine (vitamin B_6) or progestogen. Any of these treatments may help some women. For patients suffering severe psychological symptoms, psychotherapy may be recommended, both to provide support and to distinguish between other emotional disturbances that may be present and masking premenstrual tension.

DYSMENORRHOEA

Dysmenorrhoea is defined as pain with menstruation. Two types, *primary* and *secondary* dysmenorrhoea, are commonly distinguished.

Primary dysmenorrhoea

Primary dysmenorrhoea is a spasmodic type of pain, occurring at the onset of the menstrual period and lasting from 1 to 24 hours. It is most common among young girls, beginning with the menarche and fading away around 24 years of age or after the delivery of a full-term infant. No pathology in pelvic structures is associated with this type of dysmenorrhoea. In addition to the cramps, there may be shivering, a feeling of tension, nausea, vomiting, pallor and syncope.

Prostaglandins are considered to be the cause of the increased myometrial activity and subsequent pain experienced. Excessive quantities of prostaglandins are synthesized during the breakdown of the secretory endometrium in some women. They cause increased muscular contractions and uterine ischaemia, and are also responsible for the symptoms of nausea, vomiting and pallor by their influence on smooth muscle. Other cramps are caused by clots stretching the internal os of the cervix. Dysmenorrhoea is also associated with ovulation, as anovulatory cycles are rarely accompanied by dysmenorrhoea.

Analgesics that are prostaglandin inhibitors (e.g. ibuprofen, mefenamic acid) may be prescribed together with a course of oral contraceptives. This induces anovulatory periods and may be followed by very good results. It may be diagnostic: should dysmenorrhoea continue, the nurse may look for other causes.

Secondary dysmenorrhoea

Secondary dysmenorrhoea is a constant type of pain which often starts 2–3 days before the period and persists well past the first day. It may continue for a day or two after the period. Pain may radiate through the abdomen into the back and down the thighs. It occurs after several years of normal painless menses and is frequently associated with pelvic pathology. The most frequent causes are endometriosis, tumours, inflammatory disease and fixed malpositions of the uterus. It is essentially a symptom of disease. Should the nurse be consulted by a woman describing these symptoms, the woman should be referred to a gynaecologist.

ABNORMAL BLEEDING PATTERNS

Terms used to describe irregular, absent or excessive patterns of bleeding are defined in Box 23.5.

DYSFUNCTIONAL UTERINE BLEEDING

True dysfunctional uterine bleeding refers to that which occurs in the presence of endocrine dysfunction rather than organic disease. It may be seen as chronic epimenorrhagia or even as an episode of acute bleeding. Some episodes of

Box 23.5   Abnormal bleeding patterns

- *Amenorrhoea* – absence of menstruation; may be primary, where the periods fail to start at puberty, or secondary, where periods stop after several months or years of normal menses

- *Menorrhagia* – excessive bleeding at the time of normal menses

- *Polymenorrhoea* – cyclical bleeding that is normal but occurs too frequently

- *Epimenorrhagia* – cyclical bleeding that is both excessive and too frequent

- *Metrorrhagia* – any bleeding that occurs between menstrual periods; any bleeding per vagina at any time other than normal menses is included, even if it amounts to only slight staining.

haemorrhage are caused by high levels of oestrogen in the proliferative phase of the cycle. These high levels depress the hypothalamus-pituitary complex and no ovulation occurs. Because there is no ovulation, no progesterone is produced and the endometrium remains proliferative. As oestrogen levels fall, usually after a 6–8-week period of amenorrhoea, bleeding occurs. This disorder is associated with the older woman.

Other episodes of bleeding are related to fluctuating oestrogen levels produced by an imperfectly functioning hypothalamus-pituitary-ovary feedback mechanism. Follicles are stimulated to partial maturation: some oestrogen is produced but then the level falls, producing intermittent, irregular and possibly prolonged bleeding. The causes are related to immaturity or ageing of the feedback mechanism. In most cases, treatment consists of administering oral contraceptives. They exert a regulating and inhibiting effect on the endometrium and feedback mechanism. Three to six cycles of hormonal therapy are usually required to re-establish the normal menstrual pattern.

ENDOMETRIOSIS

Endometriosis is the location of endometrial tissue outside the uterine cavity. The cause is unknown but risk factors include an early menarche or a late menopause. Symptoms include dysmenorrhoea, dyspareunia, non-cyclical pelvic pain and subfertility. It appears to be associated with retrograde menstruation which involves bleeding into the peritoneal cavity via the fallopian tubes. Farquhar (2002) suggests the incidence is 40–60% in those women with dysmenorrhoea and 20–30% in those with infertility.

The endometrial tissue can be found in the peritoneal cavity, on the broad ligaments, ovaries and in the pouch of Douglas. It responds to the menstrual cycle by proliferating and shedding in response to oestrogen and progesterone.

The blood collects in small scars of bluish-black colour, usually pea sized but sometimes bigger. If the cyst ruptures, the bloody contents will promote the development of adhesions which may distort the position of the uterus and fallopian tubes, leading to infertility (Farquhar 2002).

Symptoms and diagnosis

The patient may have no symptomatology, and the disease may be discovered only incidentally at abdominal surgery. More commonly, the patient complains of pain. Secondary dysmenorrhoea may appear, with pain becoming severe 1–2 days before menstruation. The pain gradually becomes worse and may be described as 'boring'. This is due to the distension and pain of the swollen, shedding areas contained within the fibrous capsule of the cysts. The patient may also complain of backache and dyspareunia of a deep nature localized in the posterior fornix of the vagina. Pain may be acute and localized in the abdomen when a cyst ruptures. Sometimes the adhesions become severe enough to cause a bowel obstruction or painful micturition.

Laparoscopy

The gynaecologist may feel that direct viewing of the pelvic organs is necessary, in which case laparoscopy is used, usually as a day case. Laparoscopy provides direct visualization of the anterior aspect of the tubes and ovaries. The procedure is done under general anaesthesia.

Treatment of endometriosis

This is based on the age of the patient, her desire for more children and the severity of the disease. Pregnancy relieves the symptoms and may be advised if the couple want children. Pseudo-pregnancy may be achieved by the administration of progestogen for varying periods of time, or danazol 200–800 mg daily for 6 months. Danazol is a synthetic androgen which suppresses ovulatory function and inhibits LH and FSH synthesis and release. This produces amenorrhoea and an atrophic endometrium for the duration of therapy. Some women have intermittent spotting during therapy. When therapy is discontinued, the patient usually remains symptom-free for a period.

Treatment may be surgical and is directed at preserving reproductive function. Affected areas are ablated by laser and fixed organs are released. Infertility often ceases after operation. In very severe cases a hysterectomy may be done. Depending on the extent of cystic involvement, oophorectomy may also be performed. The symptoms usually disappear at menopause as ovarian atrophy begins and hormonal stimulation declines.

DISORDERS OF PREGNANCY

ECTOPIC PREGNANCY

Implantation of the fertilized ovum anywhere outside the uterine cavity is considered an ectopic pregnancy. Most frequently, this occurs in the ampullary portion of the fallopian tube, but it may be ovarian, abdominal or cervical. Women with a history of one ectopic pregnancy have an increased risk of having a second one.

An ectopic pregnancy results when the passage of the zygote to the uterine cavity is impeded or slowed. Any blocking of the tube or reduction in tubal peristalsis will cause this. Previous salpingitis, tumours and hormonal imbalances may all play a part. As implantation occurs, the chorionic villi burrow into the thin tubal wall. Eventually, they burrow into a blood vessel and bleeding occurs. If the bleeding is sufficient, the fetus dies – this is the fate of most. The abortus may be retained in the tube as a tubal mole or may be extruded through the end of the fallopian tube as a tubal abortion. Occasionally, the trophoblast burrows through the wall of the tube and out into the peritoneal cavity. This is known as a ruptured tubal pregnancy and often occurs as the result of a pregnancy in the narrow isthmus of the tube. A secondary abdominal pregnancy may follow if the chorionic villi settle elsewhere in the abdominal cavity and begin to grow.

The incidence of ectopic pregnancy has been increasing throughout the Western world in the past 10–15 years. The increase seems to be due to many factors such as an increase in pelvic infection, widespread IUD use, fertility induced by ovulatory agents, reconstructive surgery of fallopian tubes, or better and earlier diagnosis. The condition is a serious one and ectopic pregnancy still contributes significantly to maternal mortality statistics.

Effects on the patient

The woman has a history of the early signs of pregnancy, including amenorrhoea usually of 6–10 weeks' duration. Soon after her first missed period, she may have complaints of a localized pain on one side, probably due to distension of the tube. After that, she may have sharper, intermittent pain in the same area. This may be due to strong peristaltic waves of the tube attempting to pass the embryo or abortus along the tube. At some point, the patient may experience a sharp, severe pain. This is probably synchronous with separation of the embryo and some haemorrhage. The sharp pain may be followed by generalized abdominal discomfort as blood spills into the abdomen. Referred shoulder pain may occur. At this point, many women present for treatment.

Diagnosis usually includes a single pregnancy test, or serial ones, ultrasonography and, if necessary laparoscopy, depending on the urgency of the presenting symptoms. Examination of patients with suspected ectopic pregnancy should be gentle as too vigorous an examination may precipitate an acute rupture before surgery can prevent it.

ACUTE RUPTURED TUBAL PREGNANCY

Sometimes the patient reports no early symptoms but experiences one episode of acute abdominal pain shortly after her missed period. This acute pain is often accompanied by vomiting and fainting. Some vaginal bleeding may be present but appears too minimal to warrant the reaction of the patient. The patient may go rapidly into shock with a drop in blood pressure, rapid weak pulse, pallor, sweating, low temperature and cold extremities. The abdomen is distended with blood and may be tight and tender to touch. A pelvic examination of the patient may be difficult because of the exquisite tenderness. The patient presents as an emergency situation.

When the diagnosis of a ruptured tubal pregnancy is confirmed, a salpingectomy (removal of the fallopian tube) with the removal of the fetus is most often performed. Ectopic pregnancies in other locations are investigated in a similar fashion. Treatment is usually surgical removal of the fetus. However, abdominal pregnancies have been carried to term and have been delivered by laparotomy.

ABORTION

An abortion is the cessation of a pregnancy before the 24th week of pregnancy. It may be induced or occur spontaneously, the lay term for a spontaneous abortion being a 'miscarriage'. The incidence of abortion is difficult to state accurately but between 10 and 20% of all conceptions are thought to abort. A classification of abortion is given in Figure 23.9.

Most known causes can be separated into three major groups: fetal, maternal and faulty environment. Fetal causes are often associated with chromosomal or other abnormalities that are incompatible with life. This has been considered to be as high as 40% of all causes of abortion. Maternal

Figure 23.9 Classification of abortion.

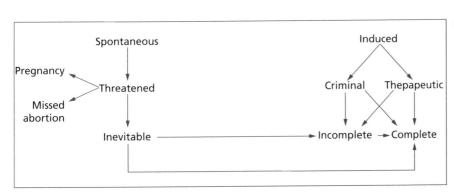

and environmental causes are more varied. For example, severe infection in the mother may lead to endotoxins invading the fetus, usually causing its death and later expulsion. Drugs ingested by the mother may damage the fetus directly or may damage the placenta and hence the nutrition of the fetus. Hormonal imbalances may be the cause of some abortions, especially in cases where the thyroid gland is involved. Lack of progesterone may result in a poorly developed endometrium. As a result, implantation of the fertilized ovum in the endometrium does not occur, or does so ineffectively. Anatomical uterine defects or uterine pathology cause some abortions. Nutritional factors are linked to abortion and premature labour, for adequate nutrition of the woman plays an important role in her reproductive capacity.

In some women with a threatened abortion, the threat to the pregnancy is slight. With care, the woman may carry the pregnancy to term. As any bleeding, however minor, per vagina is abnormal in the pregnant woman, any evidence of such bleeding is taken as a sign of threatened abortion until proven otherwise. In addition, some backache or mild intermittent lower abdominal pain may be present. If the abortion is not immediate, cramping and bleeding continue, cramps become stronger and regular, the cervix dilates and the membranes rupture.

The inevitable abortion becomes the complete abortion when all products of conception are expelled. This usually occurs before the 12th week of gestation. The abortion is incomplete when some of the products of conception are retained. This is usually the placenta and membranes, and is more frequent following the 12th week, when the placenta is more firmly embedded.

A missed abortion is one in which the fetus dies and symptoms of pregnancy cease, if they had been present at all, and the products of conception are retained in the uterus. After this, the uterus is not observed to increase in size. Indeed, it begins to regress slightly as the amniotic fluid is absorbed. No fetal heart is heard. The patient remains amenorrhoeic and the breasts regress. The abortus may be expelled spontaneously or the woman may need surgery to remove retained products of conception.

A woman is considered to be a 'habitual aborter' when she aborts three or more consecutive pregnancies. The causes can be any of the causes of a single abortion but persist through several pregnancies. In addition, an incompetent cervix is frequently associated with loss of pregnancy in the second trimester. Possibly because of inherent problems in the cervix or trauma to the cervix, the cervix dilates easily and will not retain the pregnancy. Loss of the pregnancy usually occurs later, at about 16–20 weeks. Dilatation of the cervix is rapid, with little pain and bleeding. Rupture of the membranes occurs, followed by the expulsion of the fetus.

Treatment and nursing care
Threatened abortion
The treatment of threatened abortion is aimed at preserving the pregnancy. Ideally, every woman should know how to recognize pregnancy and be aware that bleeding is not

normal. In this case, she should notify the midwife or doctor straight away.

There is a growing number of early pregnancy assessment units to which a woman with early pregnancy bleeding may be referred. This allows the woman immediate access to care, which will include ultrasonographic assessment and psychological support for herself and her partner. Admission to hospital has been significantly reduced. Bleeding usually ceases within 24–48 hours. If the cervix is seen to be closed on careful speculum examination, the pregnancy is generally thought to be safe. If the woman is admitted because bleeding persists, observations of vaginal blood loss are essential. All packs and clots should be saved to estimate loss, and tissue sent for histological examination. Other observations of pulse, blood pressure and temperature will be done as the woman's condition dictates.

On discharge home, the patient is instructed to take extra rest and to avoid strenuous exercise, heavy lifting or fatigue. Coitus may be restricted for a period of 2 weeks or longer. Should bleeding recur, the woman generally has access back to the pregnancy assessment unit via her general practitioner or midwife.

Missed abortion
Missed abortion is generally not diagnosed until the woman attends for review or for her first antenatal visit. She may or may not have experienced some brown vaginal loss. There may be a weak pregnancy test result that indicates only the presence of placental tissue. On enquiry, the midwife or nurse may ascertain that the early symptoms of pregnancy diminished earlier than expected. Diagnosis is made by ultrasonography.

If missed abortion is confirmed, the obstetrician is faced with the choice of evacuating the uterus or waiting until it is done spontaneously. Physically there is usually no pressing need, but emotionally it is very distressing to the woman and her family to know that she is carrying a dead fetus.

Inevitable abortion
The treatment of an inevitable abortion is similar to that of a threatened abortion. The patient is placed on bedrest. Blood is taken for estimation of haemoglobin, typing and cross-matching. The amount and character of the bleeding is observed carefully. Blood pressure and pulse may need to be taken every 10 minutes if bleeding is profuse, and the patient must be observed for other signs of shock. Any tissue or suspicious clots are saved to be examined for traces of fetus and placenta. If products of conception are retained, the uterus must be emptied. The two causes of significant bleeding are retained products of conception and spontaneous coagulation of exposed blood vessels, which may occur when the uterus fails to contract. Wherever products of conception remain, the potential for infection is high.

If the abortion has been complete, the woman is treated similarly to the postpartum patient. If the patient has a Rh-negative blood group, she receives Rh_0 (anti-D immunoglobulin) to prevent the formation of antibodies in further pregnancies. A slight lochial discharge is expected and the woman must be advised upon perineal care. Depending on the state of health, she will be discharged home on the same day. To reduce the risk of infection, coitus is contraindicated until lochial discharge has ceased. This usually occurs within 2 weeks.

Emotional response to spontaneous abortion In early abortion, the response to the loss may be surprise, relief, disappointment, grief, guilt and anger in differing proportions depending on the meaning of the loss at that time. The woman who has had several abortions may be experiencing this loss and also the threat of the loss of ability to ever bear a live child.

Most women express surprise at the abortion. They are unprepared for the pain, loss of blood and, if recognizable or noticed, the sight of the fetus. It seems that the concept of a baby is so vague in their minds at this time that such real evidence of a fetus is unexpected. Because of the ambivalence of the first trimester, many feel guilt associated with the negative thoughts they may have had about the pregnancy or its timing. The partner too may have to readjust to his revised status.

In later abortion, the pregnancy has usually been accepted as real and the fetus becomes a baby to the majority of women. Most couples have begun to establish a relationship with the baby, and loss at this stage is usually perceived as the loss of a baby. There may be more desire to see the fetus, to know the sex and weight, and to identify the baby by name even though it may legally be an abortion. Emotional response may be more intense and appear more painful if there is no 'object' to attach the pain to. Seeing the infant or keeping a picture of the baby may assist with the grieving and the resolution of the loss for some parents.

Others will not choose or require such a method of relating to the fetus.

The reactions of parents who have chosen therapeutic abortion for genetic reasons are similar to those of these parents. Guilt may be increased in some. Others are fearful of the censure and disapproval of hospital staff. Immediate nursing interventions are aimed at acknowledging the loss, accepting the feelings and wishes of the parents, and reinforcing reality. This assists in promoting the long-term goal of resolution of normal grieving.

A brief review of the grieving process with the parents is helpful (see Ch. 4) so that they will understand the feelings of grief, irritability and fatigue that may come. The value of rest, sleep and exercise in coping with grieving is stressed. Unequal patterns of grieving and ways of obtaining support are discussed. Follow-up support is a great value to some. One source of support and information is the Miscarriage Association which can be contacted via the web at www.miscarriageassociation.org.uk.

Therapeutic abortion There has been a large increase in the number of therapeutic or induced abortions performed throughout the world, in response to the liberalization of abortion laws. It is estimated that legal abortion for social and medical reasons is now available to over half the world's population, making therapeutic abortion one of the most common medical procedures performed. This raises serious questions about poor contraceptive provision and advice, environmental factors and women's role in society.

In the UK, the Abortion Act 1967 gives indications and restrictions for therapeutic abortion (Box 23.6). All abortions performed outside the limits of the legal conditions are illegal. For these reasons, the nurse should be acquainted

---

Box 23.6   Indications for therapeutic abortion under the Abortion Act 1967

1 The continuance of the pregnancy would involve risk to the pregnant woman greater than if the pregnancy were terminated.

2 The continuance of the pregnancy would involve risk of injury to the physical or mental health of the pregnant woman greater than if the pregnancy were terminated.

3 The continuance of the pregnancy would involve risk of injury to the physical or mental health of the existing child(ren) of the family of the pregnant woman greater than if the pregnancy were terminated.

4 There is substantial risk that if the child were born it would suffer from such physical or mental abnormalities as to be seriously handicapped.

The restrictions

1 That one or more of the above conditions are believed to be present in the opinion of two doctors, who are acting together in good faith and in full knowledge of the facts.

2 That this opinion be notified to the Department of Health (or appropriate authority in Scotland and Northern Ireland).

3 That the operation be carried out in a NHS hospital or an approved establishment.

4 That the doctor carrying out the operation notify the Department of Health (or appropriate authority in Scotland and Northern Ireland).

5 That the consent of the woman be obtained. If the patient is under the age of 16 years, the consent of the parents is also necessary.

with the law pertaining to the area in which he or she practises.

Early abortions

Surgical abortion Some abortions performed before 12–14 weeks of gestation are done by suction, dilatation and curettage (D&C). If done before 8 weeks' gestation, the cervix usually does not require dilatation but it is more difficult to ensure complete evacuation of the products of conception. The procedure is most commonly done on a day-care basis. A general anaesthetic may be given but many abortions, particularly those not requiring cervical dilatation, may be done without anaesthesia or with a local anaesthetic such as a paracervical block. Some surgeons administer intravenous oxytocin (Syntocinon) before suctioning to ensure a strong firm contraction of the uterus; others do not consider this necessary.

The aspirated tissue is caught in a gauze trap to facilitate recovery for immediate inspection and for examination by the pathologist. Immediate identification of fetal tissue is important to confirm the diagnosis of an intrauterine pregnancy that has been completely evacuated. It is necessary to confirm the intrauterine pregnancy to avoid an ectopic pregnancy continuing unnoticed. Immediate inspection and, later, pathology reports may confirm a molar pregnancy which, if left undetected, would deprive the patient of important follow-up care.

Many patients experience some cramping following abortion, which is normal. The cramps are frequently gone by the time the effects of the anaesthetic, either general or paracervical, are over, but may persist for longer. A mild analgesic may be required. The patient is then observed for a few hours more or allowed to go home with instructions, depending upon her condition.

Medical abortion Mifepristone (RU486) is an antiprogesterone agent used as a medical method of inducing abortion. A pregnancy requires progesterone to prevent uterine contraction. Abortion is induced between 36 and 48 hours using a combination of mifepristone and prostaglandin to make the uterus expel the pregnancy under medical supervision. This is most effective in women who are up to 9 weeks' pregnant (Royal College of Obstetricians and Gynaecologists Guideline 2004).

This method can also be used for women who are over 9 weeks pregnant but more prostaglandin may be needed to induce an abortion so this could take longer and the woman needs to be cared for in a clinic or hospital by an experienced nurse or midwife.

Late abortions *Prostaglandins* may be given in an intravenous drip which is carefully regulated by an infusion pump. The dosage is started at very low levels; the responses of the patient, fetus and uterus are carefully monitored. The dose is increased gradually until the uterus is contracting satisfactorily. Labour and delivery or abortion will follow for most patients in 12–24 hours. If the stimulation is not sufficient, additional stimulation with oxytocin may be given.

This is associated with an increased risk of rupture of the cervix and uterus, so the response of the contracting uterus must be monitored carefully. The patient's complaints of discomfort or pain should be heeded. The cervix may be softened by applying a topical prostaglandin preparation.

Nursing care after abortion

Most patients having an abortion are discharged within hours of being aborted, or within 1–2 days. They need clear discharge instructions so that they may take care of themselves in the days that follow. Each patient must be told:

● to resume normal activities gradually
● to expect intermittent menstrual-like discharge for the next week or two, but no heavy, bright-red bleeding
● to use sanitary pads as long as bleeding occurs; the use of tampons is inadvisable
● that some cramping may occur but should not persist or be severe
● to report any fever or unusual discomfort
● that it is wise to limit coitus while the menstrual-like flow continues, to reduce the risk of infection
● 24-hour helpline number to contact immediately if any unusual signs should occur
● follow-up appointment for 2 weeks
● how to obtain support and counselling after discharge as if for a spontaneous abortion
● to expect a menstrual period within 4–5 weeks of the procedure; if this does not occur, it may indicate a continuing intrauterine or extrauterine pregnancy or a new pregnancy. Ovulation occurs as early as 18 days after an abortion and pregnancy is possible immediately. Birth control advice and teaching should be given to the patient as necessary.

While therapeutic abortion is now associated with low maternal morbidity and mortality rates (lower than for pregnancy in many countries), it does carry some serious risks that need to be considered. Psychiatric sequelae are rare but do occur. The main concern appears to be an increased incidence of spontaneous abortion and premature labour in women who have had a previous abortion. The risk is greatest with the older methods of dilatation and curettage, and is greater still when damage to the cervix has been documented. It is important to educate women who are making such choices to seek abortion as early as possible so that the need to dilate the cervix is reduced. Prevention is better than cure, and nursing has an important role to play by providing knowledge of and access to contraception for those who need it (Royal College of Obstetricians and Gynaecologists 2004).

Criminal abortion Criminal abortion is a dangerous procedure. Often women attempt to abort themselves by means of strong douches or instruments which they insert into the uterus. Frequently, the instrument used punctures the posterior fornix of the vagina, the cervix or perforates the uterus. The bowel may be involved should the instrument be inserted far enough. Conditions can be furtive, untrained people frequently officiate, and sterility is not maintained. These patients frequently contract an infection and present a grave situation. The situation is known as a septic abortion. Infection is essentially an endometritis, which may spread to peritonitis or to septicaemia.

INFECTIONS OF THE REPRODUCTIVE TRACT

Bartholinitis

Bartholinitis is an infection of the greater vestibular gland and may or may not be gonorrhoeal in origin. The infection is an ascending one, progressing up the ducts to the gland. Symptoms are usually those of an acute infection: pain, swelling, inflammation and a purulent discharge. Cellulitis of the surrounding tissues aggravates the situation, but the infection may localize and become an abscess. This is usually excised and drained. Sometimes the infection subsides, leaving the duct scarred and occluded. This may be followed by a cyst filled with the secretions of the gland, which cannot now escape. The cyst is usually a painless swelling in the lower third of the labium minus. Treatment is to excise the cyst and gland. Alternatively, a marsupialization (conversion of the duct into a pouch) of the cystic duct may be done. This leaves the functioning gland in place.

Frequent baths are advised, as well as careful drying of the vulva and perineum. The use of a cool hairdryer is preferable to towels to reduce the risk of cross-infection.

PELVIC INFLAMMATORY DISEASE

Pelvic inflammatory disease (PID) has come to mean all ascending pelvic infections once they are beyond the cervix. Many organisms may be responsible for the symptoms. However, among the most frequent are *Neisseria gonorrhoeae*, *Chlamydia* and *Staphylococcus aureus*.

Effects on the patient

The typical picture is one of systemic infection with fever, chills, malaise, anorexia, nausea and vomiting. This is usually accompanied by lower abdominal pain which is either unilateral or bilateral.

In more chronic cases, this pain is increased before and during menstruation. Pain is experienced on movement of the cervix. Leucorrhoea is present. With gonorrhoeal or staphylococcal infections, the discharge is usually heavy and purulent. Spread of infection occurs by two main routes, although a third is possible (Fig. 23.10).

Symptoms depend on which route the infection follows. In route I, the bacteria spread along the surface of the endometrium to the fallopian tubes and into the peritoneum. The consequences of this route may be adhesions or cysts of the tube, with consequent infertility. In more advanced cases, abscesses develop about the ovary. Infection following route II is spread mainly through the lymphatics and produces a pelvic cellulitis, in contrast to the more localized endometritis or salpingitis (infection of the fallopian tube) of route I.

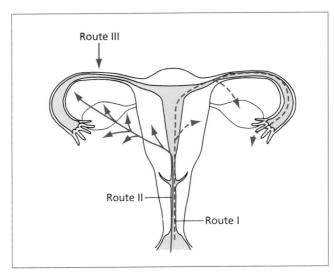

Figure 23.10 Common routes of the spread of pelvic inflammatory disease. Route I, commonly gonococcus and staphylococcus; route II, frequently streptococcus; route III, tuberculosis, usually a descending infection from another source.

Thrombophlebitis may follow this cellulitis. Advanced and virulent infections admitted by either route may become systemic and may show all the signs of septicaemia.

Treatment and nursing care

The patient with an acute episode is usually admitted to hospital. The patient is placed on bedrest in a semirecumbent position to promote drainage of pus into the vagina. Heat to the lower back and abdomen may be soothing. Analgesics and sedation may be ordered. The patient will receive antibiotics following culture and sensitivity studies. In some cases, blood cultures may be obtained. In cases of prolonged, debilitating infection that is resistant to conservative treatment, salpingectomy or hysterectomy may be done. In the long term, women may experience infertility from occluded fallopian tubes or fimbria, or ovaries distorted by adhesions as a result of the infection.

TOXIC SHOCK SYNDROME

Toxic shock syndrome is a rare systemic disease occurring as a result of the circulating toxins produced by the bacterium *Staphylococcus aureus*. The organisms produce two toxins:

- enterotoxin F, which affects the intestinal mucosa causing gastroenteritis
- exotoxin C, which is pyrogenic.

Signs and symptoms occur following the introduction of toxins into the bloodstream. The disease varies from a subclinical form to a severe septicaemia. Clinical characteristics commonly include a high fever, rash, vomiting, diarrhoea, headache, sore throat and muscle pain. Hypotension progressing to shock occurs within 48 hours in severe cases. Laboratory results indicate renal, hepatic and haematological involvement. Diagnosis is confirmed by swabs positive for

S. aureus taken from the patient's nose, throat, vaginal discharge and blood cultures.

The disease is associated with vaginal tampon use but is not caused by them. A significant number of women in the severe state are menstruating and using tampons. It is related to the fact that women have *S. aureus* present in the vagina. Tampons act as a dam to vaginal flow, providing ideal conditions for bacterial growth. Some tampons were found to carry the organisms and have now been withdrawn from the market. Synthetic material tampons aggravate the situation by their greater drying effect. They may create microulcerations in the vaginal mucosa, allowing microorganisms to escape into the bloodstream.

Treatment is supportive, aimed at relieving the symptoms, and curative by eradicating the source of toxin production. If associated with tampon use, the tampons are removed and the vagina cleansed with a disinfecting solution and daily saline douches. The patient receives systemic medication to which the organisms are sensitive. These measures prevent further development of the bacteria but are ineffective against the already circulating toxins.

Box 23.7 outlines general instructions for tampon use.

VAGINAL DISCHARGE

Vaginal discharge may be normal physiological discharge, which is usually clear or white, non-irritating with a pH between 3.8 and 4.2, or it may be a symptom of intravaginal pathology or infection:

- vaginitis – inflammation of the vagina, characterized by increased vaginal discharge containing increased white blood cells
- vaginosis – characterized by increased vaginal discharge without inflammatory cells.

Leucorrhoea

Physiological leucorrhoea is a normal whitish discharge which helps to keep the vagina moist. It is composed of endocervical secretions, leucocytes, desquamated epithelial cells and other normal flora of the vaginal tract. The pH is

---

Box 23.7   General instructions for the use of tampons
• Use only one tampon at a time
• Use a tampon of the absorbency that will control the flow; that is, never use one of super absorbency when a regular one would do. This reduces the chance of vaginal drying with subsequent trauma and ulceration
• Change the tampon frequently (every 4–6 hours)
• Do not forget a tampon; always check by finger insertion in the vagina
• If you suspect an infection, immediately remove the tampon and consult your nurse.

---

normally 4–5 but varies during the life cycle of the woman. At birth, the pH may be as low as 5 under the hormonal stimulus of the mother. As a child it is 6–7. At menarche, the pH becomes acidic again and assumes the adult pH of 4–5. Postmenopausally, oestrogen is withdrawn, and the pH rises to 6–7 again. The quantity of the discharge also varies among women during stages of the menstrual cycle and during pregnancy. An increase is usually noticed at ovulation, during sexual stimulation and during pregnancy.

Monilial vaginitis

Monilial vaginitis (thrush) occurs when the vagina is invaded by the fungus *Candida albicans*. Pregnant women and diabetics are predisposed because of glycosuria and the increased glycogen present in the vagina during pregnancy. A thick, white, curdy vaginal discharge is present which frequently causes pruritus and irritation of the vulva. The vaginal walls are reddened and covered with typical white patches. When the patches are swabbed off, bleeding may occur. Diagnosis is confirmed microscopically from a vaginal swab.

The patient is instructed in perineal care and hand washing to avoid reinfection and spread of the fungus to others, especially children. Clotrimazole vaginal cream or in the form of pessaries achieves good results, and may be given to pregnant women. Some women may choose to treat the infection with oral medication such as a single dose of fluconazole (Nurse Prescribers' Formulary 2005).

SEXUALLY TRANSMITTED INFECTIONS

The health problem of greatest concern is AIDS. This produces a range of effects on the person and has been dealt with as appropriate elsewhere in this text (see p. 157). Other sexually transmitted infections are considered in this section. Sexually transmitted infections (STIs) are an increasingly serious problem, especially in the younger population. Within the UK, the number of diagnoses of genital chlamydia, herpes, gonorrhoea and genital warts has risen steadily over the past 5 years. As with previous years, rises were sharpest in teenage males and females. Risky behaviour for the acquisition of a STI is listed in Box 23.8.

Gonorrhoea diagnoses in England declined in the 1980s but is now on the increase again particularly in men with a rate of 229/100 000 in 2004, 25% of whom are homosexual. The rate of gonorrhoea infections in women was 168/100 000 (Health Protection Agency 2004). Infection is often asymptomatic, particularly in females, but complications can include infertility and ectopic pregnancy.

Diagnoses of chlamydial infection have shown a 6% rise for women aged 16–19 and 12% in men aged 20–24 from 2003–2004. However, those who remain undiagnosed are continuing to spread the infection and as a result the National Chlamydia Screening Programme (Department of Health 2005) has been introduced to monitor opportunistic screening at approximately 80 sites in England. Many cases of chlamydia infection are asymptomatic and thus go

---

Box 23.8   Risky behaviour for STIs

- Early age of sexual intercourse
- Multiple sexual partners
- Sexual abuse or rape
- Sex with a homosexual or bisexual male
- Anal sex
- History of previous sexually transmitted infection
- Alcohol and drug use, intravenous drug use (self and partner)
- Prostitution.

---

undiagnosed. Long-term complications can be severe, especially for females, in whom it can lead to pelvic inflammatory disease, ectopic pregnancy and infertility.

Genital warts are the most common viral sexually transmitted infection and in 2004, there were 76 678 new cases diagnosed in England. Warts are caused by a virus, the human papillomavirus (HPV) and certain types of wart have been associated with cervical cancer.

In the UK, patients with STIs are treated in specialist genitourinary medicine departments on an outpatient basis. In assessing the patient, the history is crucial and should include:

- date of last menstrual period
- current medications
- current symptoms including the time of onset; colour, odour, quantity and consistency of discharge; bleeding; constant or intermittent symptoms; relationship of symptoms to sexual intercourse and menses
- associated symptoms such as fever, abdominal, pelvic or joint pain, nausea, vomiting, diarrhoea, dysuria, haematuria, genital itching, swelling, burning, ulcerations and rash
- social history including age of first sexual activity, frequency of sexual contacts, number of sexual partners, last sexual intercourse and partners over last 3 months, sexual preferences, known contact with STI risk, any partner symptoms, drug use
- past medical history including previous STI, pregnancy history, methods of contraception (oral and barrier methods), recent antibiotic use
- personal hygiene such as tampon use, douches, sprays, menstrual towels.

Common conditions are reviewed below.

Chlamydia trachomatis

A chlamydial infection is a parasitic sexually transmitted infection of the reproductive tract. The woman may present with symptoms of increased vaginal discharge, intermenstrual spotting and vague pelvic pain. Unfortunately, the woman is often asymptomatic and the infection may go unnoticed and untreated for several years. Chlamydia is a common cause of pelvic inflammatory disease as well as an increasing cause of infertility.

Diagnosis is confirmed via an endocervical swab for cells using a *Chlamydia*-specific antigen swab. Doxycycline 100 mg twice daily for 7 days is an effective treatment or an alternative is one 1-g tablet of oral azithromycin, which provides an equally effective cure (British National Formulary 2005). The single oral dose significantly reduces patient error and is a convenient method of treatment for many people who have been diagnosed with Chlamydia. Sexual partners of the woman require treatment as well and advice is needed regarding abstinence from sexual intercourse during the treatment period to avoid reinfection. It is important that women are treated in a specialist genitourinary medicine (GUM) clinic once they have a confirmed diagnosis to enable contact tracing and to ensure that they receive appropriate advice and treatment to meet their individual needs.

Gonorrhoea

The specific organism causing gonorrhoea is *Neisseria gonorrhoeae*, which is transmitted almost exclusively by sexual intercourse.

Symptoms appear 3–7 days after initial contact. Infection can be transmitted to the urethra, anus and cervix, as well as the nasopharynx. As many as 50% of women may be asymptomatic. The most common presentation is vaginal discharge, lower abdominal pain and dyspareunia due to cervicitis. Untreated gonorrhoea can produce systemic infections characterized by joint pain and generalized rash.

Diagnosis is confirmed via endocervical, pharyngeal, rectal or urethral swabs as indicated. Ciprofloxacin plus azithromycin 1 g by mouth provides excellent treatment for gonorrhoea as well as the assumed concomitant Chlamydia infection (British National Formulary 2005). Partner notification and treatment is required.

Trichomoniasis

The most common cause of vaginitis is a flagellated protozoon, known as a trichomonad. Trichomonads may be found in the large bowel and occasionally in the bladder and vestibular glands. They can be sexually transmitted, and in men, trichomonads may be harboured in the urethra, bladder or prostate.

The woman presents with symptoms of a heavy, greenish-yellow frothy discharge which has a foul odour. This heavy discharge may be irritating to the vulva, causing pruritus and excoriation. The vaginal mucosa is reddened and is slightly oedematous. The patient may complain of dyspareunia and, if the bladder is involved, of dysuria and frequency. As the condition becomes chronic, the woman has fewer symptoms. Diagnosis is confirmed when trichomonads are seen microscopically on a vaginal swab.

Men frequently have few symptoms. There may be some urethral itching and a slight discharge. Invasion of the bladder may produce frequency and burning on micturition. Treatment is usually the oral administration of metronidazole 250 mg three times a day for 10 days (British National Formulary 2005). Repeat swabs will then be done, and a repeat course of therapy may be necessary. During treatment, a condom should be worn until both partners are considered cured. The woman may be given vaginal pessaries instead of oral therapy. A pessary is inserted morning and night daily for 4–8 weeks. This is continued throughout the menstrual period, as the menstrual flow is alkaline and provides an excellent medium for growth of the protozoa. Insertion is like that of a vaginal tampon. The patient is instructed to remain flat for about 10 minutes after insertion.

It is important to advise the patient that no alcohol is to be consumed while on metronidazole therapy as severe gastrointestinal upset will occur.

Human papillomavirus infection

Human papillomavirus (HPV) is the causative organism in condylomata acuminata or genital warts. These warts may be confused with those of syphilis, but they are different: they are less flat and more cauliflower-like. Some attain a large size. The viral infection was previously thought to be benign but recently HPV has been associated with several genital cancers in both men and women.

The infection may be silent. No visible warts are present, but a type of HPV-induced cervical dysplasia exists that is seen during colposcopy or as a result of a smear test. In a number of those cases, the dysplasia may progress to cervical neoplasia or, if on the vulva or vagina, to vulvar intraepithelial neoplasia (VIN). Some 90 genotypes of the virus exist, but only a few are associated with malignant changes (Schiffman and Castle 2006). HPV infection is more common in women and during pregnancy but many men also have the infection. The infection appears to go through the stages from infection with visible warts to a spontaneous regression of the warts in a significant number of women. It may then enter a latent phase.

The risk factors for acquiring the virus are early age at first intercourse (<17 years old), multiple sexual partners, a history of sexually transmitted infection, poor personal and sexual hygiene, a sexual partner with a similar history, a history of anal intercourse, and immunosuppression or immunodeficiency for any reason. Sexual intercourse is the major method of transmission.

Those presenting with external warts are screened for other STIs, and if present, they will be treated. A colposcopic examination and smear tests will be done. The partners of infected patients should also be examined and treated if necessary. External warts can be treated with podophyllin 10–25% in tincture of benzoin (British National Formulary 2005). This caustic agent is applied with a cotton applicator, washed off in 4 hours and can be applied by the patient once instructed. The surrounding skin is coated with petroleum jelly before application of the podophyllin. In some clinics, warts are treated with cryotherapy using liquid nitrogen.

Cervical and vaginal warts need to be treated by a suitably qualified nurse or doctor in clinic.

Non-visible warts (small flat warts on the cervix or areas of dysplasia associated with the HPV on vulva or penis) are frequently vaporized with a carbon dioxide laser. Because the virus tends to recur, treatment during pregnancy is delayed until the third trimester. This virus is a stable one and can be transmitted from specula to other patients if instruments are not properly cleaned and sterilized.

Syphilis
Effects on the patient
Incubation varies between 10 and 90 days. In most cases, the disease is spread by sexual intercourse. In the untreated condition, three stages are distinguished. The stages may overlap or be widely separated.

The *primary lesion* is a small, painless chancre or ulcer. It is deep and has indurated edges. Usually this chancre heals spontaneously, giving the false impression that the disease is cured. This primary lesion appears most commonly on the penis of the male. In the female, it may appear on the labia, vagina or cervix.

The *secondary stage* is usually characterized by a rash appearing over the body. This rash may be accompanied by condylomata lata on the female vulva. This is a cauliflower-like collection of flat, grey, vulvar warts. Like all lesions of syphilis, these are teaming with spirochaetes and are highly infectious. The rash is usually accompanied by malaise and fever. In a short period, the rash regresses and the patient enters the latent stages. *Latency* refers to the absence of symptoms in the infected individual. Pregnant women can still infect their fetus *in utero*, thus demonstrating the infectiousness of the blood.

In the *tertiary stage* the bones, heart and central nervous system, including the brain, can be affected. Personality disorders arise and the typical ataxic gait of the tertiary syphilitic appears. A large, ulcerating, necrotic lesion known as a *gumma* now occurs. It is rarely seen in the genital tract, but may occur on the vulva or the testes. At this stage the disease may be arrested, but not reversed.

Diagnosis is made by a careful history, clinical findings, and cultures or biopsies from the lesions. Blood serology is also assessed. As blood serology is not positive for about 4 weeks after the onset of the disease, the early diagnosis is made from scrapings of the lesions. These scrapings are made before antibiotic therapy is initiated so that the diagnosis can be confirmed.

Treatment
Treatment is by antibiotic; penicillin or doxycycline may be used (British National Formulary 2005). The Jarisch–Herxheimer reaction is a local and systemic reaction that may occur after beginning antisyphilitic therapy. Fever, sweating and headache appear 2–12 hours after treatment. The reaction should be differentiated from a penicillin reaction.

Genital herpes

Herpes simplex virus (HSV) enters the body via mucous membranes. After entry, the virus replicates and spreads to sensory nerves. In genital herpes, the virus travels to the dorsal root ganglion. In most cases, approximately 2–4 weeks later, the primary outbreak occurs resulting in the characteristic clinical presentation. These symptoms include multiple painful genital ulcers, headache, fever, swollen lymph nodes, fatigue and 'flu-like' symptoms. Secondary outbreaks present with similar, although less severe symptoms.

Current primary prevention techniques do not appear to be effective as the number of new cases of genital herpes has risen steadily over the past 5 years. One of the difficulties in preventing the spread of HSV is that viral shedding, and thus transmission of the virus, can occur when the host carrier is currently asymptomatic (i.e. has no visible lesions). Condoms appear to be somewhat effective against transmission but, because lesions and viral shedding can occur over skin not covered by the condom, this protection is suspect. Despite the problems associated with safer sex practices and barrier protection, condom use must be strongly advised with each and every act of sexual intercourse.

New research involving the Disabled Infectious Single Cycle (DISC) vaccine is currently in phase II and III clinical trials. This vaccine will disable HSV replication and shows potential promise in limiting the spread of the herpes virus.

Currently, treatment involves antiviral therapy using drugs such as acyclovir 400 mg by mouth three times daily for 7–10 days for primary outbreaks (British National Formulary 2005). Antiviral medicines are also used for episodic and suppressive therapy. It is important to note that these drugs do not cure or prevent the spread of HSV. They are utilized simply to reduce the incidence and severity of symptoms.

Nursing intervention

Most cases of sexually transmitted infection are treated on an outpatient basis, and the person should be taught about the nature and transmission of the disease in order that they may in future protect themselves and others. No immunity develops and reinfection can occur easily. Strict personal and perineal hygiene should be observed. Hand washing following any handling of the genitalia is imperative to prevent cross-infection. For example, the gonococcus can be readily carried to the eye, which quickly becomes infected. Blindness may ensue if treatment is not received. Women who are handling small children need to be especially careful. Sexual intercourse is to be avoided until the doctor notifies the individual that the infection has been treated successfully. All equipment must be sterilized after use, and dressings or swabs are disposed of in a safe way. Syphilis may be transmitted by direct contamination of a laceration with living spirochaetes. For this reason, the routine use of universal body substance precautions will also control inadvertent transmission of this disease to health professionals. Once therapy has been initiated, the patient is usually non-infectious within 48 hours.

Tables 23.1, 23.2 summarize the physical examination findings and follow-up of patients with STIs. Box 23.9 outlines a clinical pathway for diagnosing sexually transmitted infections.

DISPLACEMENTS AND RELAXATIONS OF THE FEMALE GENITAL ORGANS

RETROVERSION AND RETROFLEXION OF THE UTERUS

The normal position of the uterus is one of some anteversion and anteflexion (Fig. 23.11). It is not a fixed organ. The filling of the bladder or bowel may cause a change in uterine position. On occasion the uterus assumes a retroverted or retroflexed position. When retroverted, the fundus points toward the sacrum and the cervix toward the anterior vaginal wall. Retroflexion refers to the position of the fundus of the uterus in relation to the cervix. In retroflexion the fundus bends back over the cervix (Fig. 23.11). Degrees of retroversion and retroflexion are possible, so the case may be mild or extreme.

The aetiology appears to lie in a weakness of the supporting structures which may be either congenital or acquired. The acquired weakness is frequently due to injuries during the maternity cycle. Adhesions and tumours may pull or push the uterus into this position.

The patient may complain of backache, infertility, dyspareunia or dysmenorrhoea, but she is frequently symptomless unless the situation is extreme. Backache and dysmenorrhoea are probably associated with pelvic congestion. Infertility may arise because the cervix does not reach the seminal pool. Frequently, the ovaries prolapse and become congested and enlarged. Because of this, intercourse may be painful.

Treatment

Usually the uterus is replaced manually and a vaginal pessary is inserted to hold the uterus in place. The pessary functions by holding the cervix in a posterior position. This in turn rotates the uterus forward. When the pessary is properly in position, the patient is unaware of its presence and no difficulty is experienced on voiding or during intercourse. The gynaecologist may then give the patient a 6-week trial period without the pessary to see whether she remains free of symptoms. If not, a further trial with the pessary may be given. In other cases, the uterus will be surgically suspended by shortening the round ligaments. This is done when the pessary does not correct the situation.

PROLAPSE, CYSTOCELE AND RECTOCELE

Uterine prolapse refers to the downward displacement of the entire organ. Prolapse (Fig. 23.12) may occur in varying degrees.

Table 23.1   Summary of physical examination findings for sexually transmitted infections

Infection	Incubation period	Patient complaints	Clinical findings
Chlamydia trachomatis	7–21 days	Females: 80% may be asymptomatic Pelvic pain Watery, purulent drainage Postcoital bleeding Males: 50% may be asymptomatic – dysuria with scant thin, grey discharge	Mucopurulent vaginal discharge Friable cervix, positive chandelier sign Bartholinitis, salpingitis Urethritis Pelvic inflammatory disease (PID)
Neisseria gonorrhoeae	3–7 days	Females: 50% may be asymptomatic Labia pain and swelling Purulent vaginal drainage Sore throat Males: scrotal pain with creamy white urethral discharge; 10% asymptomatic	Bartholin abscess Skene abscess Purulent vaginal drainage Inflamed vulva Mucopurulent cervicitis Joint pain with rash Urethritis
Trichomonas vaginalis	7–30 days	Dysuria, vaginal pruritus Frothy green vaginal drainage Foul odour Males: 15–50% asymptomatic	'Strawberry cervix' Friable cervix Frothy, thin, green drainage Vaginal erythema Urethral discharge
Herpes simplex (HSV-2)	2–14 days (long latency period)	Painful ulcerations and vesicles, sores Dysuria, urinary retention Fever malaise Tender groin nodes	Speculum examination may be impossible Tender inguinal lymphadenopathy Multiple, clear, fluid-filled vesicles over perineal, rectal, vaginal area Crusting, ulcerations Febrile Distended suprapubic area
Human papillomavirus (HPV) Highly variable 'Genital warts' Condylomata acuminata	90 days to several years	May be asymptomatic Genital itching, burning Warty growth on genitals Bleeding warty growths Males: may partially obstruct penile meatus	Papillomatous lesions noted on vaginal areas, penis, perineal area Soft, pink, flesh coloured Cervical smear noting Koilocytes
Treponema pallidum Primary syphilis	10–90 days	Often asymptomatic. Painless solitary sore noted on vaginal or oral area	Chancre non-tender with 'punched in' centre and indurated border Non-tender lymphadenopathy Chancre heals spontaneously in 3–10 weeks
Secondary syphilis	30–90 days	Warty growths on genitalia Generalized rash, especially on palms and soles of feet Headache, malaise	Genital condylomata Copper-coloured maculopapular rash Anaemia, alopecia, oral mucous patches

Table 23.2 Summary of follow-up for patients with a STI

Infection	Clinical follow-up
Chlamydia	If no response to treatment or possibility of re-infection Gonorrhoea cultures if not done Consider test of cure 3 weeks after completion of treatment
Gonorrhoea	Test of cure recommended at least 72 hours after treatment completed Chlamydia swab if not previously done
Trichomoniasis	None necessary unless symptoms persist or recur after treatment
Herpes simplex (HSV-2)	As symptoms dictate Follow-up of secondary infections Suspected ocular lesions Follow-up cervical smear
HPV	Weekly for 4–8 weeks during treatment if warts recur Cervical smear every 6 months until normal
Syphilis	Serology tests for syphilis should be done at 3, 6 and 12 months Falling titre should be demonstrated if treatment adequate
Pelvic inflammatory disease (PID)	Re-evaluate outpatient therapy and symptoms within 24 hours, or sooner if symptoms worsen or fail to improve Inflammatory symptoms often secondary to sexually transmitted infections Re-examine after completion of course of medication for pelvic, bimanual exam and review of culture results

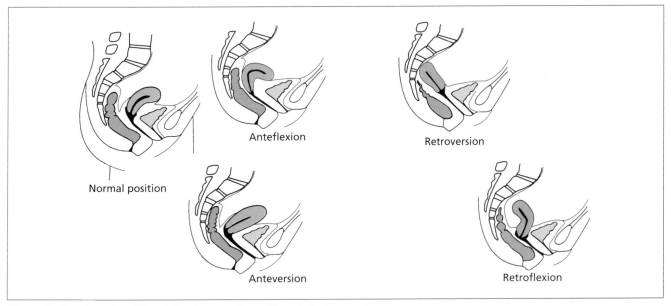

Figure 23.11 Normal position of the uterus and four different displacements.

First-degree prolapse describes the condition existing when the uterus descends within the vagina. Second-degree prolapse occurs when the cervix protrudes through the introitus. Procidentia, or third-degree prolapse, refers to the entire uterus protruding through the introitus with total inversion of the vagina.

Cystocele, urethrocele and enterocele refer to herniations or relaxations of the bladder, urethra, rectum and small bowel into the vagina (Fig. 23.13). They may occur singly or in combinations with some degree of uterine prolapse.

The single most important aetiological factor in the development of these conditions is thought to be injury at childbirth. The pelvic floor and supporting structures may be stretched and torn during the process of delivery and are thereby weakened. Further relaxation results after menopause as the tissues atrophy following oestrogen with-

Box 23.9 Clinical pathway – sexually transmitted infections

Patient presents with vaginitis
↓
History and physical examination
↓
Cervicitis → Yes → Culture for *Neisseria gonorrhoeae* and *Chlamydia*
↓
No
↓
Abnormal physical exam → Yes → Ulcers, lesions, foreign body → Consider biopsy
↓
No
↓
Vaginal discharge → Yes → Clue cells on wet mount → Yes → Initiate treatment for bacterial vaginosis
↓   ↓ (note this is not a sexually transmitted infection)
           No
           Trichomonads on wet mount → Yes → Initiate treatment for *Trichomonas vaginalis*
           ↓
           No
           ↓
           Hyphae on wet mount → Yes → Initiate treatment for thrush
           ↓
           No
           ↓
           Consider additional diagnostic testing
No
↓
Vaginal irritation → Yes → Consider contact or allergic vaginal dermatitis
↓
No
↓
Postmenopausal vaginal atrophy → Yes → Consider HRT

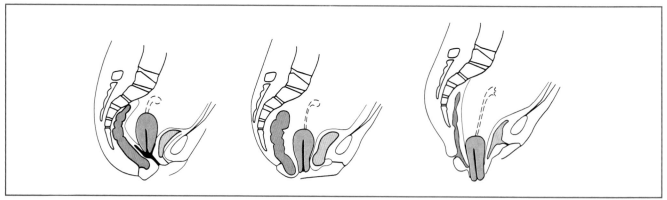

Figure 23.12 Types of uterine prolapse, from left to right: first-degree; second-degree; and third-degree (procidentia) prolapse.

drawal. Large intra-abdominal tumours may also place an added strain on already weakened tissue. In some rare cases, the structures seem to be congenitally weak. Diagnosis is usually confirmed by bimanual and rectal examinations. The patient will be asked to bear down, cough or strain while the doctor estimates the degree of prolapse or herniation.

Treatment and nursing care

The best treatment is prevention. Better care during pregnancy has helped to reduce the incidence of these complications. Exercises should be taught by the physiotherapist and encouraged by the nurse to all patients in the postpartum period; the same exercises may be taught to help

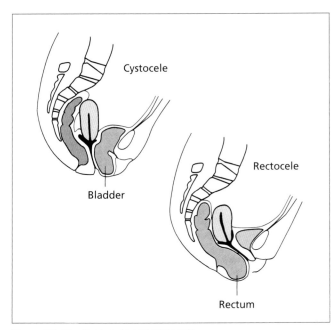

Figure 23.13   Cystocele and rectocele.

relieve mild prolapse. These consist of alternately tightening and relaxing the gluteal and perineal muscle tone. The woman should continue to practise these exercises several times a day for several weeks.

In situations in which surgery is contraindicated, the use of ring pessaries may be employed. A variety is available for different degrees of prolapse. Surgical intervention is frequently necessary to correct the situation. Anterior and posterior colporrhaphy and perineorrhaphy are used to repair a cystocele and a rectocele, respectively.

STRESS INCONTINENCE

Stress incontinence is the involuntary loss of small amounts of urine when a woman coughs, sneezes or otherwise suddenly increases the intra-abdominal pressure. Urge incontinence and frequency are related to abnormal detrusor function. The urge to void and the ability of the bladder to contract are controlled by the detrusor muscle which lines the bladder wall. As the bladder fills, the detrusor muscle is stretched and nerve endings send a message of the need to void to the brain via the spinal cord. Sometimes, an irritable detrusor muscle overreacts, sending a message before the bladder is really full and contracting quite vigorously, sometimes involuntarily. The patient complains of an urgent desire to void, not always reaching the lavatory in time.

Continence is maintained at the junction of the urethra and bladder by continuous spiral muscles from the base of the bladder to the upper urethra. Assistance is also received from the muscles surrounding the urethra, as well as a tight supporting perineal floor. In the continent woman these relationships can be demonstrated radiologically by observing that the angle between the urethra and posterior wall of the bladder is approximately 90° (Fig. 23.14a). Normally this

angle is obliterated only at micturition (Fig. 23.14b), when an increased intra-abdominal pressure combines with a relaxed urethrovesical muscle and perineal floor to lower the base of the bladder. However, in stress incontinence, the slight effort of straining, coughing or sneezing is sufficient to reduce this angle, and an involuntary loss of urine occurs. This explanation is thought to describe about 90% of cases of stress incontinence. A woman may have a cystocele (Fig. 23.14c) and still be continent if the relationships demonstrated by the angle are maintained. However, many women with a cystocele also have accompanying stress incontinence.

Diagnosis is made following a physical examination and a urodynamic evaluation. A pelvic and modified neurological examination is done to diagnose any underlying pelvic or neurological disease. The urodynamic evaluation, which includes a series of tests, helps to distinguish true stress incontinence from other conditions such as unstable bladder or a neurogenic disorder. The series of tests usually requires an outpatient visit. In preparation, the patient is instructed not to void or take self-medication for 6–8 hours before going to the clinic. This provides a full bladder for testing and avoids drug effects on nerve conduction.

Initially the patient is instructed to void into a funnel connected to a flowmeter. This meter is an electronic device that calculates the rate at which urine flows, the time taken to void and the volume voided. The results are printed on a graph. An abnormally high rate of flow is associated with stress incontinence. Immediately after this, the patient is catheterized for residual urine.

This test may be followed by cystometrography, which involves a catheter being passed into the bladder and a transducer into the rectum. The catheter tests for uterine contractibility and measures residual urine, while the rectal transducer measures detrusor activity. The bladder is filled with fluid, usually water, and the patient is asked to tell the operator when she feels a sense of fullness and when her bladder actually feels full. She is told to void and then asked to stop voiding. The transducer meanwhile records on a graph the changes in bladder pressure associated with these events. The operator can assess how the patient perceives and responds to these sensations and requests. Normally bladder pressure increases when voiding, as the bladder relaxes. This may be combined with a urethral pressure profile. Urethral pressure is recorded as the catheter is slowly withdrawn at a constant rate through the urethra.

Treatment

Stress incontinence is aggravated by chronic urinary tract infections, obesity and chronic coughing. Prevention includes the education of women about stress incontinence and the aggravating factors. Any urinary and vaginal tract infections are treated; the obese patient is advised to lose weight and an appropriate diet is discussed to assist her with this. The heavy smoker is advised to reduce or stop smoking as a means of reducing coughing, and is also instructed about stop-smoking programmes designed to help in this. Mild

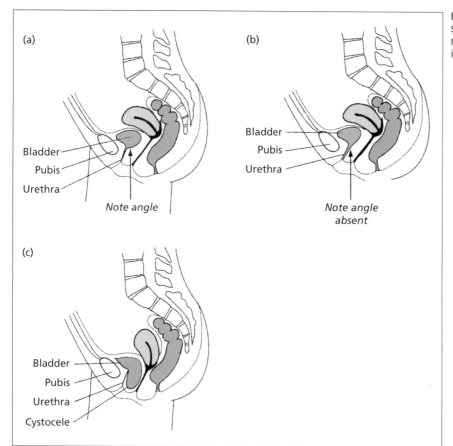

stress incontinence and abnormal detrusor activity are treated similarly. They also frequently coexist. The woman is assisted to re-establish a normal voiding pattern and bladder control. She is usually provided with a bladder drill and exercise regimen.

Bladder drill involves routines related to voiding. The patient is instructed to void every hour by the clock whether she feels the need to or not. When she has kept herself dry in this way for 3 or 4 days, she increases the time interval between voidings by one half-hour every 3 days until she can comfortably hold urine for hours. She is instructed to drink plenty of non-stimulating fluids (e.g. caffeine-free) during the day, to drink nothing for 2 hours before going to bed, and to empty her bladder completely before going to sleep. She is also instructed to empty her bladder before and after sexual intercourse.

The exercises consist of always giving an extra push at the end of voiding to make sure that all urine is expelled. She is also instructed to practise tightening the buttocks and pelvic floor muscles, and to stop and start the stream of urine during micturition. The exercises are practised several times a day. If the patient is unsure whether or not she is practising them correctly, she can be taught to insert two fingers into the vagina and contract the vaginal muscles to grip the fingers as tightly as possible. This provides the patient with a direct measure of her progress. Once she has

learned the technique, it can be practised without inserting her fingers.

BENIGN AND MALIGNANT DISORDERS OF THE REPRODUCTIVE TRACT

POLYPS

Polyps are common benign growths occurring mainly in the endometrium and cervix. The polyp has a characteristic smooth, shiny surface and is pink to deep red in colour. Polyps are small in size and seldom exceed more than 3 cm in length. Their aetiology is unknown. No symptoms are usually present, but occasionally postcoital bleeding occurs. Treatment is by surgical excision of cervical polyps and may be followed by dilatation and curettage to remove endometrial polyps.

Myomas of the uterus

A myoma (fibromyoma, leiomyoma) is a benign tumour of the uterus composed of myometrium and fibrous tissue. Colloquially, myomas are known as 'fibroids'. At least 25% of women over 35 years of age show some evidence of myomas. Myomas occur mainly in the uterine body. According to the position they are classified as subserous, submucous

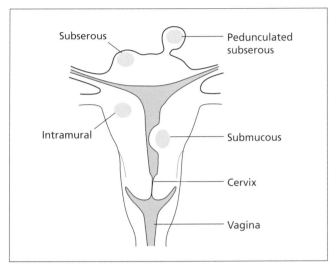

Figure 23.15   Possible positions of uterine myomas.

or intramural (Fig. 23.15) and may become pedunculated. A pedunculated fibroid in the uterine cavity may be referred to as a fibroid polyp. This may be extruded through the cervix and may come to lie in the vagina. Myomas in the broad ligament or cervix are rare. Several fibroids of varying sizes may be present in any one woman. As the fibroids become larger, their blood supply may be reduced, causing some degeneration.

Effects on the patient

Symptoms vary with the size and location of the tumour. Frequently, with small tumours, there are no symptoms. Occasionally hypermenorrhoea occurs. Pain is rarely a symptom but is associated most frequently with torsion of a pedunculated myoma. Sometimes the myoma passing through the cervix causes cramps. Dysmenorrhoea may occur as a result of mechanical interference. Large myomas can cause frequency or retention of urine. Pressure on veins, lymphatics and nerves of the pelvis may cause varicosities, unilateral or bilateral oedema of the lower extremities, or a radiating pain through the thighs. Occasionally, these tumours may be the cause of abortion or infertility.

Treatment

Treatment depends on the age of the woman, her desire for more children and the size of the myoma. In the young woman who wants to have children, a myomectomy is usually done. This is the enucleation of the myoma, but the uterus is retained. Blood loss during the operation may be extensive if the surgeon excises multiple myomas from a large uterus which may not contract efficiently. Persistent oozing of blood may occur after the operation for the same reasons. The nurse should be alert to this possibility and monitor blood pressure closely. In the young woman, myomas are not a contraindication to pregnancy and usually cause no difficulty. Rarely, they may obstruct labour or cause a post-partum haemorrhage.

TUMOURS OF THE OVARY

Tumours of the ovary are many and varied. The aetiology of most is unknown.

Polycystic ovary disease

Polycystic disease of the ovary appears in the late teens and early 20s with variable symptoms. These may include a history of sterility, secondary amenorrhoea, hirsutism and cysts bilaterally in the ovary. The ovary shows some enlargement and presents a glistening white appearance. The symptoms are thought to follow an endocrine imbalance, probably arising in the ovary but affecting the hypothalamus. The ovaries produce an excessive amount of androgens, which inhibit maturation of a follicle with subsequent disturbance of the ovarian-hypothalamic relationships. What triggers the imbalance is unknown.

Carcinoma of the ovary

Ovarian cancer is a major cause of death worldwide and the twelfth most commonly diagnosed cancer in the UK. Each year, around 7000 women in the UK are diagnosed with ovarian cancer (Cancer Research UK 2006a). The two most influential risk factors are advancing age and the presence of certain gene mutations.

Effects on the patient

In its early stages, the ovarian tumour is often symptomless. The symptoms result from the size of the tumour and its position. An increase in girth may be noticed but ignored. Pressure on the bladder causes frequency or a feeling of fullness. Constipation, oedema of the legs, anorexia and a full feeling in the abdomen may be present. Pain may be associated with stretching of the tissues as the tumour enlarges. Ascites may be present, accompanied by difficulty in breathing.

Treatment

Because of the danger of malignant growth, any ovarian mass is observed suspiciously. Conservative treatment may be considered but often other tumours demand biopsy, and a laparotomy is indicated. After diagnosis, the surgeon strives to preserve as much ovarian function as possible. In pre-menopausal women benign growths (if size permits) will be enucleated and ovarian function retained. Malignant growths are treated with total hysterectomy and bilateral salpingo-oophorectomy (removal of the fallopian tubes and ovaries). Surgery is followed by chemotherapy. Unfortunately, many malignancies have metastasized before discovery of the tumour. Prognosis is poor and surgery may be only palliative. Further treatment is directed toward relieving the symptoms of the terminally ill patient. Recurrent ascites may be a problem, and frequent paracentesis may be indicated.

Complications of ovarian tumours

Torsion or twisting of the growth on its stalk frequently occurs. Circulation is impeded and necrosis may follow. The patient usually feels a sudden severe pain in the lower abdomen. Treatment is by an immediate laparotomy and excision of the tumour. The cyst may rupture. Often the 'chocolate cyst' of endometriosis ruptures and drains fluid into the abdomen. Again, the patient may present with an acute abdomen.

Haemorrhage and infection occur in tumours as well. Usually they are more common in the malignant tumour. Postsurgical menopause is the result of bilateral oophorectomy. The symptoms are similar to those of regular menopause. Replacement therapy with oestrogens may begin before the patient leaves the hospital if it is not contraindicated, for example because the malignancy is aggravated by oestrogens.

CARCINOMA OF THE CERVIX

Carcinoma of the cervix is a common malignancy of women. In 2001 there were 2418 new cases recorded (NHS Cancer Screening Programmes 2004). The woman who smokes, has a history of infection with certain strains of HPV, or had an early sex life with several partners is more apt to develop the disease.

Cancer of the cervix is a disease that is preceded by several earlier cervical changes (Fig. 23.16). These changes usually occur at the squamocolumnar junction of the cervix (Fig. 23.17) and initially are evident only on histological examination. They reflect a varied pattern of development. Some cases arise with no known precursor stage, whereas others appear to have gone through all the changes or any combination of them. The earlier changes may be reversible, and so do not always herald cancer. How many of these will reverse is unknown, but about 50% of women with carcinoma in situ are thought to develop invasive cancer; this development takes an average of 10 years. The cervical smear is the best method of early detection of these changes. Combined with treatment of these changes, it is largely responsible for the declining mortality rates associated with cervical cancer.

Because 5-year survival rates are excellent in cases that are discovered early, the NHS Cancer Screening Programmes (2004) in England now recommend that all women who are sexually active and over 25 years of age should have cervical smear tests at least every 3 years and every 5 years for women over 50. Nurses have a role in disseminating this knowledge. Liquid based cytology has been recommended by NICE (2003) as the best method to use as there is increased

sensitivity and specificity. There is also a lower incidence of inadequate samples at 1.4% and the improved efficiency of laboratory samples has reduced waiting times for results. However, it is important to provide information in relation to false-positive and false-negative results. It is imperative that nurses and doctors provide balanced information to women about the range of cervical tissue anomalies and outcomes of subsequent screening and treatment (NHS Cancer Screening Programmes 2004).

Cervical smear grades, cervical intraepithelial neoplasm (CIN) and cervical cancer is divided into stages (Table 23.3). Cervical cancer is divided into the following stages:

- *Stage 0* is carcinoma *in situ*. There is an intact basement membrane containing the malignant cells
- *Stage I* is invasive cancer, which means the basement membrane has been breached and the cells are invading the surrounding tissue
- *Stages IA and IB* refer to degrees of this invasion which is still within the confines of the cervix. Unfortunately, about 20% of patients with stage I disease will already have spread to the lymphatics. A small lesion similar to an erosion may be present on the cervix
- In *stage II* the carcinoma has spread to close adjacent structures and the upper-third of the vagina may be involved
- By *stage III* invasion has reached the pelvic walls and lower vagina

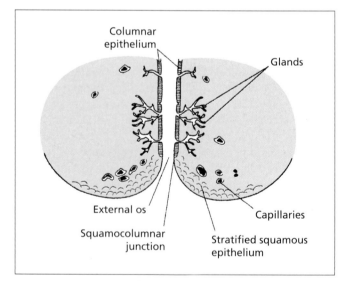

Figure 23.17 Squamocolumnar junction of the cervix.

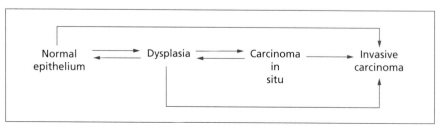

Figure 23.16 Patterns of development of cancer of the cervix.

Table 23.3 Grading of smear test, cervical intraepithelial neoplasm (CIN) grade and cancer stage

Smear	Class	CIN grade	Cancer stage
I	Normal cells	–	–
II	Atypical cells	–	–
IIIA	Mild dysplasia	I	–
III	Moderate dysplasia	II	–
IV	Severe, carcinoma *in situ*	III	0
V	Invasive, below the basement membrane	–	IA, B
–	–	–	II
–	–	–	III

- *Stage IV* is marked by extensive pelvic involvement, including the bladder or bowel, and distant metastases may be present.

Treatment

Treatment is usually guided by the stage assigned to the situation by the gynaecologist. The smear results are organized into five classes. An abnormal smear indicates that there are pre-cancerous changes in some of the cells covering the cervix. In classes I and II, the cells are non-malignant. Class II may have atypical cells suggestive of viral changes possibly due to the herpes virus or HPV. Other infections may contribute and the patient will be treated accordingly. Some of these altered cells may revert back to normal epithelium. Class III is suspicious and arouses concern. The patient is referred to colposcopy clinic and a biopsy is performed. Classes IV and V are positive, indicating that definite changes are present that require biopsy.

Colposcopy

This is organized in an outpatient clinic by a gynaecologist who has received specialist training. The colposcope is a specially designed microscope that provides visualization of the cervix to show the type and extent of any abnormality on the cervix (The Colposcopy Unit 2004).

Normally, the cervix contains glycogen. This is depleted in areas of abnormal cell change. When Lugol's solution (iodine in potassium iodide) is swabbed on the cervix, the normal epithelium stains a dark brown. Glycogen-deficient areas are a pale colour by contrast, and these are the areas requiring biopsy

A *punch biopsy* may be done with special punch biopsy forceps. The biopsy is the size of a pinhead and should not be painful. However, if a larger area is identified it may be necessary to use diathermy excision known as LLETZ (Large Loop Excision of the Transformation Zone) or LEEP (Loop Electrical Excision Procedure). Occasionally, cold coagulation is used but LLETZ is most commonly used. The area of cervical intraepithelial neoplasia (CIN) which are abnormal cells caused by the wart virus (HPV) can be removed using a

local anaesthetic and usually takes less than 15 minutes. There are few complications, although some women can bleed excessively following treatment and women should be advised about this possibility and what to do should this happen. Follow-up involves a 6-month colposcopy and smear test and then annual cervical smear tests for 5 years.

Further treatment may be a *cone biopsy*. This is an operative procedure in which a cone-shaped segment of the central cervix is removed. On examination, the section may contain all of the malignant area. In these cases, the biopsy may be considered sufficient treatment. Preoperative and postoperative care for the patient is similar to that for other vaginal surgery, such as a D&C. The major difference is that these patients face the threat of malignant disease and may be extremely anxious. Considerable skill in providing supportive nursing is demanded of the nurse. Haemorrhage is a threat, and the patient should be warned of this. Bleeding from the biopsy site may occur up to 1 week after the biopsy when the patient is at home. The nurse should inform the patient of this possibility before discharge.

The biopsy results may indicate normal cells, dysplasia or invasive carcinoma. Carcinoma *in situ* may be treated with a cone biopsy. All carcinoma *in situ* must be treated to ensure prevention of invasive carcinoma. Invasive carcinoma of the cervix will be treated according to the stage in which it is classified.

CARCINOMA OF THE ENDOMETRIUM

This is a malignancy which appears to be increasing in incidence worldwide; it is the fifth most common cancer in women in the UK with 6000 cases diagnosed each year (Cancer Research UK 2006b). As it is a disease largely of older women, this increase may be due to a lengthened lifespan. Oestrogens aggravate the tumour and prolonged oestrogen therapy has been implicated as a contributing cause of endometrial cancer.

The first symptom is a painless, bloody, vaginal discharge. Between 30 and 40% of women with postmenopausal bleeding have cancer of the endometrium. Bleeding postmenopausally should therefore never be ignored but investigated immediately. An endometrial biopsy is usually done. The growth is usually in the fundus of the uterus, but may arise in or spread to the isthmus. The thick body of the uterus contains the growth and it metastasizes late in its growth. Survival rates are improving at over 75% (Cancer Research UK 2006b), referral to a gynaecologist is necessary to determine treatment options.

THE WOMAN WITH A DISORDER OF THE BREAST

Breast problems and concerns account for a large number of consultations in general practice, family planning and well-women clinics. Nurses today stand in an excellent position to provide current practical information to these women. Although much controversy continues to surround the importance of breast self-examination, nurses can help women to be breast aware and empower women to make their own health decisions regarding breast self-care.

ANATOMY AND PHYSIOLOGY OF THE BREAST

The breast is a glandular organ that lies over the second to sixth ribs on the chest wall. During puberty, breasts increase in size, connective tissue increases, the ducts lengthen and breast lobules are formed.

The ductal system of the breast extends from the nipple to the lobule (Fig. 23.18). There are approximately 15 to 20 ducts which open on to the nipple. From the lobule, which ends in 100 or so tiny bulbs called acini – where milk is produced – the ducts extend towards the nipple and enlarge, where they are called the lactiferous sinuses. It is these that open on to the nipple for the secretion of milk. The nipple is surrounded by the areola, which may vary in colour from pinkish to dark brown. It contains small elevations known as the tubercles of Montgomery, and these help to lubricate the area during breastfeeding.

Apart from lobules and ducts, the breast contains fat and blood vessels, predominantly from branches of the internal mammary and lateral thoracic arteries. Major lymph drainage is to the axilla and internal mammary chain. The lymph drainage system is thought to be important in relation to the spread of the malignant disease. The breast tissue is held in position by Cooper's ligaments – fibrous bands that run from the fascia between the lobes to the skin and extend up towards the armpit, forming the axillary tail. Two muscles lie beneath the breast: the pectoralis major and the pectoralis minor. Breast structure varies considerably. At the time of menarche, the breast begins to grow rapidly under the influence of sex hormones. Each month, when a woman approaches menstruation, the size of the breasts may fluctuate. This is in preparation for a possible pregnancy. If a pregnancy does occur, then the breast enlarges even more and the acini multiply. By the end of pregnancy, the breast is almost entirely a glandular structure. After pregnancy, these

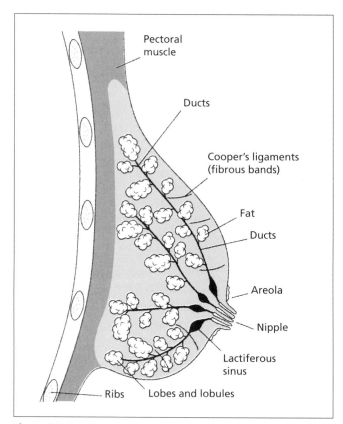

Figure 23.18   Sagittal section of the breast.

changes subside and the breast becomes less glandular. As the woman grows older, the lobules and acini begin to decrease and fatty tissues increase. This is accelerated with the menopause.

Oestrogen and progesterone produced by the ovaries influence the initial growth and subsequent development of the breast. The proliferation and development of the mammary tissue during pregnancy is stimulated by oestrogen and progesterone produced by the corpus luteum and the placenta. Other hormones believed to be involved are prolactin and the adrenal corticosteroids. It has been surmised that the high levels of sex steroids present during pregnancy inhibit the action of prolactin on breast tissue. After separation of the placenta at delivery there is rapid fall in oestrogen and progesterone production, the inhibitory effect is lifted, and milk production is stimulated. Prolactin levels rise rapidly during breastfeeding, thus stimulating additional milk production.

CLINICAL EXAMINATION

This should only be undertaken by nurses who are competent and working within their code of professional conduct (Nursing and Midwifery Council 2004) as well as within local guidelines and protocols. It is very important to take a detailed history before performing a clinical examination. If any of the risk factors mentioned above are present, they must be taken into account. It is important, if the woman is premenopausal, to determine the start of her last period because this may necessitate bringing her back for a further examination at a different time in the cycle as breasts are frequently tender and 'lumpy' premenstrually.

Obviously symptoms noted by the woman herself are important:

- If the patient has found a lump in her breast, has it changed in size, become larger or smaller? Is it tender?
- Has one breast increased or decreased in size? Most women have one breast slightly larger than the other and this sometimes becomes more obvious if the patient has put on weight.
- Has there been any nipple discharge? This is particularly significant if it occurs spontaneously. Was the discharge blood stained? Has there been any nipple change?
- Is there any nodularity or thickening in one area? This can be just as important as a lump.
- Has the woman noticed a dimple or crease, and what position was she in when she noticed this?

Examination of the breasts should always be performed in two parts: observation and palpation. The woman should sit on the side of the couch, facing you, and you should stand back to see whether there is any difference in size or shape. It is common to have one breast slightly larger than the other and the woman may need to be reassured that this is a common occurrence. The woman should then be asked to raise her arms above her head for you to observe any dimples or creases. She should then place her hands on her hips, push in and bring the elbows forward. The woman should then put her hands on the side of the couch, keeping the arms straight and pushing down, and then lean forward. Women feel reassured if you always explain what you are looking for.

These three positions that the woman is asked to adopt – with hands raised, with hands on hips, and leaning forward – are very important when looking for a dimple or crease because they may appear in only one of the three positions. When documenting findings, it is essential that, if a dimple or crease was observed, the position of the woman is stated. If an abnormality has been noted, it is sometimes helpful to mark the area so that when physically examining the patient attention can be paid to this area with regard to identifying any nodularity, thickening or lump that may be associated with the dimple or crease that has previously been observed.

While the woman is in the sitting position, the supra-clavicular fossa can be palpated, either standing in front of the patient or from behind. The infraclavicular area can also be felt by running the hands down from the clavicle to the breast. Then the axilla should be palpated by feeling high up into the axilla with the flats of the fingers and bringing them down towards the axillary tail.

On completion of this part of the examination, the woman should be asked to lie down. Her arm should be raised above her head on the side of the breast that is to be examined first. The clinical examination should be performed with the flat of the fingers and a systematic examination carried out.

If an abnormality is detected, the fingertips are used to determine the consistency, size and mobility. The clinical examination must cover the whole breast and not forget the axillary tail and beneath the nipple. After examining both breasts individually, the patient should turn on to her side in the oblique position, with her arm raised above her head. This positioning allows for a more thorough examination of the outer quadrant of the breast, particularly in the larger-breasted patient; quite often a lump that was not felt with the patient lying on her back is very obvious in this position. Figure 23.19 shows the most common sites for breast cancer.

BREAST AWARENESS AND BREAST CARE ADVICE

Breast awareness

There has been much controversy surrounding the issue of breast self-examination. Nowadays, breast self-examination has been overtaken by the concept of 'breast awareness' which *currently* is what all healthcare professionals should be promoting in their advice to women. The difference between the two is subtle, as women are still being asked to look at and feel their breasts, but not in such a ritualistic way as with breast self-examination. It can be helpful to explain the basic anatomy and physiology of the breasts, so that women understand why their breasts might feel lumpy pre-menstrually – particularly in the upper outer quadrants.

Women should be encouraged to become familiar with how their breasts normally look and feel, and how this can vary at different times of the month:

1. Don't feel the breasts before a period.
2. Use the flat of the fingers and not the fingertips.
3. Don't feel the breasts between thumb and forefinger.
4. Remember that nine out of ten breast lumps are *not* cancer.

There are two distinct parts to being breast aware: *looking* and *feeling*.

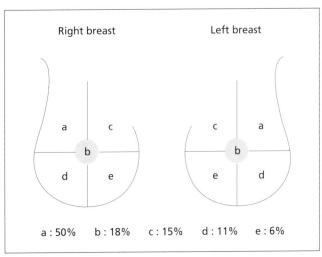

Figure 23.19   Most common sites for breast cancer.

Looking
- Note any change in the shape of the breast, looking down and looking in the mirror
- Note any puckering or dimpling of the skin. A crease in the skin can also be important
- Note any change in the nipple: whether the nipple starts to go in, or points in a different direction; whether the nipple becomes reddened and perhaps moist.

Feeling

The most important aspect of feeling is for women to get to know what is normal for them, and then to notice whether there is any change from this normality. A lump in the breast should never be ignored, and any change in the way the breast normally feels should be followed-up. This is why being breast aware just before a period is due is not sensible, and may give rise to unnecessary anxiety. However, women who are breast aware will appreciate that such changes are normal for them and not be alarmed at pre-menstrual lumpiness and tenderness.

The flat of the fingers should be used when checking the breasts, either in the bath or shower with a soapy hand, or lying on the bed using talcum powder. Starting at the 12 o'clock position, move the fingers, pressing gently down and around the outer circumference of the breast, and then in ever-decreasing circles towards the nipple, making sure that all areas of the breast have been examined. Finally, press gently down on the nipple (Fig. 23.20). If a woman finds anything that is different (e.g. a lump, puckering or nipple change) or is anxious or worried about her breasts, she should be advised to see her nurse or doctor for an examination (Box 23.10).

Breast care advice

Brassières

Women often complain of breast discomfort, particularly pre-menstrually. One of the reasons for this might be an ill-fitting or underwired bra. Women should be advised to be correctly fitted: most large department stores have experienced staff who can measure and give advice on this.

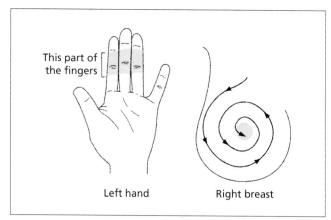

Figure 23.20 Area of fingers to be used in breast awareness and circular method of self-examination.

Intertrigo

A rash in the inframammary fold is common in women with large breasts and is usually due to not drying the area thoroughly after a shower or bath. Excessive perspiration may also cause a rash, and advice about wearing a cotton bra may be helpful.

Inverted nipples

Inverted nipples are very common and may be bilateral or unilateral. They should be kept clean by gently using a cotton-wool bud. Any change in nipple inversion must be reported to the general practitioner.

Breast discomfort (mastalgia)

Breast discomfort may possibly be helped by taking vitamin B_6 50 mg with one multivitamin tablet daily. Evening primrose oil or starflower oil (containing gamolenic acid) might also be helpful; the recommended dosage should be obtained from the packet. Reducing or abstaining from caffeine may also be helpful, as may reducing salt intake in prepared food.

BREAST DISORDERS

Cysts

Cysts are basically fluid-filled sacs which are found most commonly in the 40–60 years age group. They can vary enormously in size, depending upon the amount of fluid in the sac and are usually found in the upper outer quadrant.

On clinical examination, cysts may feel round, soft and mobile and symptoms may include pain and tenderness. Cysts can also fill rapidly, which of course may be very frightening to a patient, but this is something you should explain when discussing breast awareness with your patient. Cysts usually subside or disappear with the menopause unless the woman is taking hormone replacement therapy (HRT) when they may persist.

Investigations and treatment

Mammography may be performed to rule out incidental carcinoma. Ultrasonography, if available, should be performed, although occasionally the turbid contents of the cyst may produce echoes. Needle aspiration of a cyst should

Box 23.10 Breast awareness
Women should be aware of:

Women should be aware of:

- change in the breast shape or size
- any dimpling, puckering or creases in the skin
- any lump or thickening in the breast
- any alteration in the nipple – whether it starts to go in or points in a different direction
- any discharge from the nipple.

be performed if the cyst is causing pain, is very large, or is worrying the patient. The fluid from a cyst can vary tremendously in colour: clear, green, straw-coloured, milky chocolate coloured, or blood stained. After aspiration of the cyst, the patient should be re-examined to determine whether there is any residual mass. If so, repeat needle aspiration should be performed and the cells sent for cytological examination to check for underlying cancer.

Fibroadenomas

Fibroadenomas are the most common benign lumps in younger women and usually occur between the ages of 20 and 30 years. A fibroadenoma is a solid, fibrous nodule which is histologically composed of glandular elements and connective tissue. On clinical examination, a fibroadenoma is usually well circumscribed, firm and mobile and they can be round, disc-shaped or lobular. Methods of diagnosis are clinical examination, ultrasonography and fine-needle aspiration cytology.

Fibroadenomas may increase in size, may stay the same, or may disappear. They can be related to the hormonal influences of the menstrual cycle. If ultrasonography is performed, a measurement can be taken, and when the patient is reassessed at a later date ultrasonography and measurement may be performed again to see whether there is any change in size. If the above tests have been performed and it has been established that the lump is indeed a fibroadenoma, the patient may be given the option of excision or observation. If the above tests are not available, excision is usually performed to exclude malignancy.

Duct papilloma

Duct papillomas are very common and may be single or multiple. They are caused by solitary papillary benign lesions growing in one of the main ducts close to the nipple. Presentation will be with nipple discharge, which may be serous or blood stained. Occasionally a palpable mass may be felt at the areolar margin. Treatment is usually excision of the offending duct – microductectomy.

Duct ectasia

Duct ectasia is due to dilatation of major or minor ducts within the breast which leads to the retention of secretions within them. If the secretion leaks from the duct, it may cause an inflammatory reaction. Symptoms are nipple discharge, nipple retraction and/or a palpable mass. Investigations performed are mammography, clinical examination and fine needle aspiration and, if necessary, excision biopsy.

Lipoma

Lipomas (fatty growths) may be found in the breast and may be mistaken for cysts because, on physical examination, they are mobile and smooth. Ultrasonography and fine needle aspiration will establish a diagnosis.

BREAST IMPLANTS

Approximately 80% of silicone breast implants are placed for cosmetic purposes and about 20% for breast reconstruction after surgery. With regard to breast cancer risk, no epidemiological study so far has found an increased risk of breast cancer in women with breast implants compared with those without.

BREAST CANCER

Breast cancer is the most common malignancy in women. It is currently estimated that in the UK one in nine women will develop this disease at some time during their lives (NHS Cancer Screening Programme 2004). The risk of breast cancer increases with age and in 2002 there were 42 000 new cases of breast cancer diagnosed in the UK (1% of these were in men) (Cancer Research UK 2006c). Breast cancer is the most common cancer in women worldwide and is higher in Western developed countries.

Early detection continues to be the mainstay of successful treatment. In fact, research demonstrates there has been a reduction in the mortality rate from breast cancer since national screening was introduced in the UK in 1988. For women who have positive diagnosis, there is a bewildering range of available treatments which can cause confusion for the woman, her family and other health professionals with whom she may wish to discuss the issues.

Risk factors for breast cancer

Family history

The most common risk factor is a history of breast cancer in a first-degree relative on the maternal side. This risk nearly doubles if the relative was pre-menopausal and almost trebles if the cancer was bilateral, or there was more than one first-degree relative who was pre-menopausal. In certain families, it is clear that breast cancer is hereditary. In 40% of these families there is a mutation in a gene known as *BRCA1* located on chromosome 17 and also a further gene, *BRCA2*, has been isolated (Dixon et al 2002).

The Family History Study (FH01) is a research project evaluating the effectiveness of mammographic surveillance for women under 50 with a family history or breast cancer (NHS Cancer Screening Programmes 2006). There is also a multi-centre trial Magnetic Resonance Imaging for Breast Screening (MARIBS) running for 5 years which will compare mammography with magnetic resonance imaging (MRI) for women at high risk due to their family history.

Menstrual history

An early menarche before 12 years and a late menopause after the age of 55 years increases a woman's risk factors. Women who have had a premenopausal oophorectomy are at a substantially reduced risk of developing breast cancer.

Age

Age is another very important factor, with older women being at a much greater risk than younger women. The increase of risk rises steadily from the age of 40 years and 80% of cases are in post-menopausal women.

Reproductive history

Nulliparous women are at greater risk than those who have had children, but another important risk factor is a woman's age at her first full-term pregnancy. The risk of breast cancer in women who have their first child after the age of 30 years is about twice that of women who had their first child before the age of 20. Women who have their first child after the age of 35 appear to be at even higher risk than nulliparous women (Dixon et al 2002).

Breastfeeding

Results of studies on lactation and breast cancer are confusing, although breastfeeding appears to be protective against the development of breast cancer, particularly in young women. However, the risk decreases with increasing duration of breastfeeding, with breastfeeding each baby for 3 months or longer giving greatest protection.

Oral contraception

Numerous case-controlled studies have been done comparing use of the oral contraceptive pill in breast cancer cases and age-matched controls. It has been established that there is no association between use of oral contraception and breast cancer amongst women in their late 20s and 30s after one or more pregnancies; moreover, oral contraception seems to have a protective effect against benign breast disease (British National Formulary 2005). Cancer Research UK (2006c) states that there is a slight increase in the risk of breast cancer in recent or current users of the contraceptive pill but there is no increase in incidence 10 years after stopping the pill.

Hormone replacement therapy

The benefits of hormone replacement therapy (HRT) are well known, and include protection against osteoporosis and associated fractures as well as an increased quality of life in women suffering from menopausal symptoms. With regard to breast cancer risk, most studies have shown that there is an increased risk in long duration of use. However, it appears that if breast cancer is diagnosed in women who are already taking HRT, it tends to be of a lower grade and be associated with a relatively good prognosis. Unfortunately Cancer Research UK (2006c) point out that HRT reduces the sensitivity of mammography and they state that current users of HRT have a 66% increased risk of breast cancer when compared with women who have never used HRT. Hannaford (2004) presents these statistics in a slightly different way and states that the absolute risk of breast cancer in women treated with HRT equates to an extra 2–6 cases per 1000 over a 5-year period depending upon the patient's age and the length of time she has used the treatment for. It is important to give the woman every opportunity to consider the pros and cons of treatment for her individual situation and to make her own informed decision regarding whether or not to use HRT.

Diet, weight and alcohol

Fat consumption has been investigated and no definite conclusion can be drawn from available data, although it has been shown that obese women are at a greater risk than slim women. Alcohol has been associated with a moderately increased risk of breast cancer, particularly in thin pre-menopausal women.

Breast cancer and men

According to Cancer Research UK (2006c), it is estimated that in the UK, 300 men develop breast cancer every year. Certain aspects of breast cancer in men are controversial. Some of these questions are directed towards risk factors: do men share the same risk factors as women and will men benefit from the same established treatment guidelines? Some studies suggest that breast cancer in men might be more aggressive as it appears that a higher proportion of men actually die from the disease. Many factors come into play when analyzing the data, such as men are usually diagnosed later in the course of the disease. Also aggressive screening programmes are not directed toward men as they, as a whole, are not at increased risk for developing breast disease. Men do, however, share a good portion of risk factors with women. Box 23.11 lists a number of risks *specific* to men.

DIAGNOSTIC INVESTIGATIONS

Mammography (breast X-ray)

Mammography is an X-ray technique used to visualize the internal structures of the breast. The National Breast Screening Programme aims to screen asymptomatic women between the ages of 50 and 70 years by inviting them to attend for mammography. One and a half million women are screened each year. The aim of the NHS breast screening programme is to reduce mortality from breast cancer in the population of women invited to be screened (NHS Breast Screening Programmes 2006).

The recommended views for mammography screening are the mediolateral oblique, as this single view demonstrates the maximum amount of breast tissue and the craniocaudal view to demonstrate where abnormalities are, in relation to the nipple. Most abnormalities are found in

---

Box 23.11 Breast cancer risk factors specific to men

- Exposure to female hormones
- Mumps orchitis
- Undescended testes
- Hyperprolactinaemia
- Gynaecomastia
- Jewish ancestry.

the upper outer quadrant, and such a mammogram demonstrates this area clearly. Both these views are obtained by the breast being compressed between two plates while the exposure is made. The procedure may be uncomfortable but should not be painful. Suspicious mammograms will prompt a recall to the screening unit, causing much anxiety to the woman, but further investigations may show nothing abnormal. It is hoped that taking two mammograms as a routine will reduce the number of recall visits and minimize stress and needless worry.

The practice nurse, as a member of the primary care team, is in an ideal setting for encouraging women in this age group to attend for screening by providing the information and counselling related to all aspects of the programme. Screening is not performed routinely in women under the age of 50 years in the UK. This is due to the poorer sensitivity of X-rays in the more dense breasts of pre-menopausal women, and the fact that breast cancer incidence is lower in younger women. Women over the age of 70 years are not screened routinely but can have mammography on request (NHS Breast Screening Programmes 2006).

Mammographic screening of asymptomatic women may pick up small impalpable tumours and microcalcification, which may be the only indication of early disease such as ductal carcinoma *in situ* (DCIS). In symptomatic women, it is a technique used for problem solving, although it must be remembered that 5–10% of cancers are not detected by mammography because the density of the tumour is less than that of the glandular tissue (NHS Breast Screening Programmes 2006). This can usually be resolved by clinical examination, ultrasonography and fine-needle aspiration.

Ultrasonography

Breast ultrasonography is now widely accepted as a valuable adjunct to mammography and is more useful in younger women. High-frequency sound waves are beamed through the breast using a hand-held 7.5-MHz transducer. Images are built on a screen which are then frozen and a picture can be printed. The use of ultrasound in the clinical area can be very helpful for distinguishing between cystic and solid lesions. If there is any doubt with regard to the interpretation of any abnormality, the woman would be referred for detailed ultrasonographic assessment in a diagnostic imaging unit.

Ultrasonography may also be used when obtaining cells from an impalpable lesion by guided needle aspiration. The lesion is visualized on the screen and a needle is introduced into the breast. The needle is guided into the lesion by watching the screen; cells are withdrawn and sent for cytological examination. This is not a painful procedure and takes only a few minutes.

Cytological investigations (Box 23.12)

Fine-needle aspiration cytology

Fine-needle aspiration cytology (FNAC) has become an accepted diagnostic procedure in outpatient departments and specialist centres. The test should be performed only by staff trained in the procedure. The advantages of the test are

---

Box 23.12   Cytological investigations

Nipple discharge
If a discharge is elicited by gently squeezing the nipple then it should be tested to see whether it is blood stained. A slide should be drawn gently across the nipple to obtain a smear. If two slides are obtained, one is wet-fixed with cytofixative and one is air-dried. This is because of the different staining techniques used.

Cyst aspiration
The fluid obtained from the cyst is discarded, but if the aspiration is blood stained then the contents in the syringe should be emptied into a universal container and sent for cytological examination.

Solid nodule or nodular area
Fine-needle aspiration is performed to obtain cells from the appropriate site for diagnostic purposes. It is now becoming accepted practice in younger women to leave fibroadenomas *in situ* once a diagnosis has been established.

---

that it is simple, quick and relatively painless, and in a rapid diagnostic unit results are obtained while the woman is in the clinic, thereby making further visits to obtain results unnecessary. If a diagnosis of cancer has been made, staging investigations and treatment can be discussed at that visit. If the woman is to have mammography, this should be undertaken before FNAC or cyst aspiration is performed as the oedema or small haematoma caused will obscure detail and give rise to a false-positive diagnosis.

Advanced breast biopsy instrumentation (the ABBI system)

The ABBI system is one of the latest developments in the goal to reduce the invasive nature of breast biopsy. Breast biopsy using the ABBI system has many distinct *advantages* over traditional breast biopsy procedures:

- local anaesthesia as opposed to general anaesthesia
- outpatient procedure
- small resultant scar.

Stereotactic fine-needle aspiration cytology

This is a diagnostic technique used in the X-ray department. A needle is guided into an impalpable lesion or an area of grouped microcalcification under radiographic control and cells are obtained for cytological examination. The advantage of this test is that it avoids unnecessary biopsy. However, the procedure is not available in all breast cancer centres because it requires the cytopathologist to be present and special X-ray equipment in addition to the standard mammography machine.

Tru-cut® biopsy

This test is performed when a histological diagnosis is required. Local anaesthetic is infiltrated into the skin and the breast where the core tissue is to be removed. A small incision is made in the skin and a narrow-bore cutting needle which has been inserted into a mechanical biopsy gun is then inserted through the incision and guided into the area to be sampled. A core of tissue is obtained which is then fixed in formalin. The test should not be painful, but the slight noise of the needle action should be demonstrated first so that the woman is prepared. Firm pressure should be applied over the area for a few minutes afterwards to prevent bleeding, then an occlusive dressing applied.

Problems

Complications that may occur after fine-needle aspiration, although fortunately fairly rare, include the following:

- *Haematoma or bruise*. This can occur if a large vessel is punctured during aspiration – the procedure may have to be abandoned and pressure applied. It may also occur if pressure is not applied correctly after completion of aspiration
- *Pneumothorax*. This is a rare complication and may go undetected if the pneumothorax is small. Subtle clues, such as sharp pain, coughing or a hiss of air on withdrawing the needle without evidence of air in the syringe, may occur (NHS Breast Cancer Screening Programme 2001).

Surgery

There is some controversy surrounding surgical options for breast cancer and there has been a considerable change of opinion over the past few years. The surgeon will recommend the operation that offers the best chance of successful treatment, depending on the type of cancer, as well as the size and location of the lump.

CASE Mary aged 46 attended surgery complaining of a blood stained nipple discharge for the last few days and a tense feeling in her right breast. She had first noticed this during her last period and it had not resolved. She described a swollen area with no pain or nipple discharge and she was unable to feel a lump. She had attended for a cervical smear 3 months earlier and as part of that consultation, breast awareness and how to detect abnormalities were discussed.

Mary had three children aged 18, 15 and 10 and had recently become a grandmother caring for 6-month-old Lucy, as well as working on the family farm.

She had no medical history of note but had a family history of breast cancer in her maternal grandmother, who died aged 55 of the disease.

Mary was an ex-smoker, having stopped 2 years previously and admitted to drinking 1 or 2 bottles of sherry a week to help her to relax. Her diet was low in fibre and high in fat and her body mass index was 22. She took no medication.

On examination, the left breast showed no abnormality, but the right breast was found to have a discrete lump in the upper outer quadrant. This was irregular, fixed, painless and measured approximately 3–4 cm. She also had enlarged axillary lymph glands under her left arm.

According to NHS guidelines and local protocol, Mary was referred to the breast clinic at the hospital under the '2 week

rule' and was assessed within 1 week. She had an ultrasound scan and mammogram followed by fine needle aspiration cytology, which showed malignant cells.

Having discussed her options with her breast care specialist, she then had a mastectomy and axillary clearance with latissimus dorsi reconstruction. This was then followed by a course of chemotherapy for 6 weeks.

Mary's main issue throughout her treatment was how her role within the family had to change so that she had to rely on others to care for her when she had always provided the care for her family. Support was provided by both hospital and general practice team members by good communication and sharing of knowledge.

Mary has been maintained for the last 2 years on tamoxifen and clodronate, has regular reviews with her breast care specialist and is once again caring for her family.

In summarizing the care of women with breast disease, it is obvious that teamwork is an important factor in both screening and treatment. The NHS has issued guidelines for the referral of women with breast problems (Austoker and Mansel 2003). These include detailed guidelines on who to refer depending on clinical history and examination for women who present with breast lump, pain or nipple discharge. There is also a guideline for those women who present with highly suspicious symptoms to ensure they are referred urgently and assessed within 2 weeks whenever possible.

Treatment is now better organized between hospital, screening unit and home, proving less emotionally traumatic for the woman and her family. The research and advances being made into the diagnosis and treatment of breast disorders mean that guidelines are constantly changing, requiring all healthcare professionals to keep up-to-date. The informed nurse can provide support and information, but most importantly can provide continuity of care for the woman undergoing treatment for a breast problem.

SUMMARY

This chapter has introduced the main areas of women's health that the student nurse will encounter in both hospital and primary care environments. Clearly, it is a vast area and the nurse wishing to specialize in this field will find there is much more to learn. You need to be clear about your own sexuality and moral beliefs about sex and reproduction before you can address the needs of your patients. Empathy and sensitivity are essential for good nursing practice in this area as your patient may face some difficult moral and ethical dilemmas in seeking treatment for her health problems, often in the face of a rapidly changing healthcare environment with apparently conflicting research messages. Teamwork and a non-judgemental approach will help you to meet the needs of the patient. The nurse should be the patient's close and trusted companion at all times, as a source of health promotion, support and care.

REFERENCES

Austoker J, Mansel R (2003) Guidelines for referral of patients with breast problems, 2nd edn. (revised). Sheffield: NHS Breast Screening Programme.

British National Formulary (BNF) (2005) British National Formulary. London: British Medical Association/Royal Pharmaceutical Society of Great Britain.

Cancer Research UK (2006a) UK Ovarian cancer statistics. Online. Available: http://info.cancerresearchuk.org/cancerstats/types/ovary [Accessed 31.03.2006].

Cancer Research UK (2006b) UK Uterus cancer statistics. Online. Available: http://info.cancerresearchuk.org/cancerstats/types/uterus/incidence [Accessed 31.03.2006].

Cancer Research UK (2006c) UK Breast cancer statistics. Online. Available: http://info.cancerresearchuk.org/cancerstats/types/breast/incidence [Accessed 31.03.2006].

The Colposcopy Unit (2004) Colposcopy. Online. Available: www.colposcopy.co.uk [Accessed 31.03.2006].

Department of Health (DoH) (2005) The National Chlamydia Screening Programme. Online. Available: http://www.dh.gov.uk/PolicyAndGuidance/HealthAndSocialCareTopics/sexualhealth [Accessed 05.04.2006].

Dixon M, Gregory K, Johnston S, Rodger A (2002) Breast cancer (non-metastatic). Clinical Evidence—Concise 8: 1218.

Farquhar C (2002) Endometriosis. Clinical Evidence 12: 1267.

Hannaford P (2004) HRT: The bottom line. Trends in Urology Gynaecology and Sexual Health January/February: 5–7. Online. Available: www.tugsh.com

Health Protection Agency (2004) Epidemiological data – HIV and sexually transmitted infections. Online. Available: http://www.hpa.org.uk/infections/topics_az/hiv_and_sti/epidemiology/epidemiology.htm [Accessed 05.04.2006].

Menopause Matters (2006) Menopause Matters. Online. Available: www.menopausematters.co.uk [Accessed 30.06.2006].

NHS Breast Screening Programme (2001) Guidelines for non-operative diagnostic procedures and reporting in breast cancer screening. Publication no. 50. Online. Available: http://www.cancerscreening.nhs.uk/breastscreen/publications/qa-08.html [Accessed 05.04.2006].

NHS Breast Screening Programme (2006) Screening for Breast Cancer in England: Past and Future Advisory Committee on Breast cancer Screening. Publication no. 61. Online. Available: http://www.cancerscreening.nhs.uk/breastscreen/publications/nhsbsp61.html

NHS Cancer screening programmes (2004) NHS Cervical screening programme. Online. Available: http://www.cancerscreening.nhs.uk/cervical/index.html [Accessed 04.04.2006].

NHS Cancer Screening Programmes (2006) Key research in breast screening. Online. Available: http://www.cancerscreening.nhs.uk/breastscreen/research.html#family-history [Accessed 31.03.2006].

National Institute for Clinical Excellence (NICE) (2003) Full guidance on the use of liquid-based cytology for cervical screening. Online. Available: http://www.nice.org.uk/page.aspx?o=TA069guidance [Accessed on 06.04.2006].

National Institute for Clinical Excellence (NICE) (2005) New guidelines on long acting contraception promote greater choice for women. Online. Available: http://www.nice.org.uk/page.aspx?o=276552 [Accessed 06.04.2006].

Nursing and Midwifery Council (2004) The NMC Code of Professional Conduct: Standards for Conduct, Performance and Ethics. London: NMC.

Nurse Prescribers' Formulary (NPF) (2005) Nurse Prescribers' Formulary 2005–2007 London: British Medical Association/Royal Pharmaceutical Society of Great Britain.

Royal College of Obstetricians and Gynaecologists (2004) Care of the Woman Requesting Induced Abortion. London: RCOG.

Schiffman M, Castle P (2006) When to test women for human papilloma virus. British Medical Journal 332: 61–2.

Whincup P, Gilg J, Odoki K, Taylor S, Cook D (2001) Age of menarche in contemporary British teenagers: survey of girls born between 1982 and 1986. British Medical Journal 322: 1095–1096.

FURTHER READING AND USEFUL WEBSITES

Bobak I, Duncan Jenson M, Lawdermilk L, Shannon E (2003) Maternity and women's health care, 8th edn. London: Mosby.

Department of Health (2005) The National Chlamydia Screening Programme. Online. Available: http://www.dh.gov.uk/PolicyAndGuidance/HealthAndSocialCareTopics/sexualhealth

Guillebaud J (2004) Contraception: your questions answered, 4th edn. Edinburgh: Elsevier.

Menopause Matters (2006) Menopause Matters. Online. Available: www.menopausematters.co.uk

NHS Breast Screening Programme (2006) Screening for breast cancer in England: Past and Future Advisory Committee on Breast Cancer Screening. Publication no. 61. Online. Available: http://www.cancerscreening.nhs.uk/breastscreen/publications/nhsbsp61.html

NHS Cancer Screening Programmes (2006) Key research in breast screening. Online. Available: http://www.cancerscreening.nhs.uk/breastscreen/research.html#family-history

24 Caring for the patient with a disorder of the musculoskeletal system

Mike Walsh

INTRODUCTION

Pain and loss of mobility, either temporary or permanent, are the most common consequences of musculoskeletal disorder. Both symptoms obviously have a major impact upon the person's independence. Patients often represent opposite ends of the age spectrum – from children through to the most elderly in society. All can suffer trauma or disease and this wide age range is only one of the factors that makes nursing orthopaedic patients such a challenging area of care. A multidisciplinary approach that fully involves the family and patient is essential if the patient is to return to the community with maximum independence.

STRUCTURE AND FUNCTION OF BONES

Bone is a rigid connective tissue consisting of bone cells, calcified collagenous intercellular substance and marrow. Each bone, except at joint surfaces, is covered by a tough, supportive membrane called the *periosteum*. The periosteum is firmly attached to the underlying bone by penetrating fibres, and its blood vessels give off many branches which enter the tissue to provide the essentials for growth, repair and maintenance. The inner layer of the periosteum gives rise to the osteoblasts, which function in the development and replacement of bone. The shaft of the long bones is hollow and is lined with a comparable membrane referred to as the *endosteum*. Although approximately two-thirds of bone tissue is inorganic mineral substance, which gives it the characteristic hardness and inert appearance, bone is viable tissue undergoing constant metabolic processes.

There are three types of bone cell:

- *Osteoblasts* are found beneath the periosteum on the surface of growing bones and in developmental or ossification areas within the bones
- *Osteocytes* are matured osteoblasts that become imprisoned in small spaces by calcification. It is believed that these regulate bone metabolism
- *Osteoclasts* are considered to be responsible for the breaking down and reabsorption of bone tissue.

Normally, there is a constant turnover of the mineral deposits. This continuous breaking down, reabsorption (by osteoclasts) and new bone formation (by osteoblasts) is necessary, because old bone becomes weak and brittle. The mineralization and strength of bone are influenced by the amount of weight bearing and muscle pull to which the bone is subjected. Physically active people have stronger and more resistant bones than non-active persons. One of the complications of hospitalization and prolonged bedrest is the decalcification and weakening of the bones; the calcium is excreted by the kidneys and there is therefore a risk of the formation of renal calculi. In older persons, the bones tend to become brittle and less resistant to stress, increasing the possibility of fractures. This is due to the general decline in cell reproduction which results in a slower rate of production of the collagenous matrix and mineralization as well as of reabsorption.

TYPES OF BONE TISSUE

Each bone is composed of two **types** of tissue: compact and cancellous. Outer layers consist of dense, *compact* tissue (cortical bone), and the interior is of a spongy or porous nature (*cancellous*), which contains the red bone marrow. The thickness of each type of tissue varies in different bones as well as in parts of the same bone.

In the long bones (e.g. humerus, tibia, femur), the ex-tremities have a thin outer layer of compact tissue enclosing a larger mass of cancellous tissue (Fig. 24.1). The shaft is formed mainly of two thick layers of compact bone separated by a small amount of porous tissue. The central hollow portion of the shaft forms the medullary canal, which is filled with *yellow marrow*, consisting largely of fat cells and blood vessels. Flat bones (e.g. skull bones, scapula, ribs) have a thicker layer of cancellous tissue lying between two relatively thin layers of compact tissue. Short and irregular bones such as those of the wrist and ankle have a thin shell of compact tissue enclosing a fair thickness of cancellous tissue.

FUNCTIONS OF BONES AND CONTAINED MARROW

The bones are bound together by ligaments and collectively form the skeleton, which provides a supporting framework for the body and protection for vital structures. They assist in body movement by providing attachment for muscles and leverage for their action. The bones also serve as the body's store of calcium. If the blood calcium concentration falls below the normal level, the deficit may be met by the withdrawal of calcium from the bones. Conversely, much of the excess in the blood is deposited in bone tissue. The role of the red bone marrow in the formation of blood cells is discussed on p. 365.

DEVELOPMENT AND GROWTH OF BONES

The development of the bones begins in approximately the 6th or 7th week of embryonic life and is not normally completed until the late teens or early 20s. Bones are initially

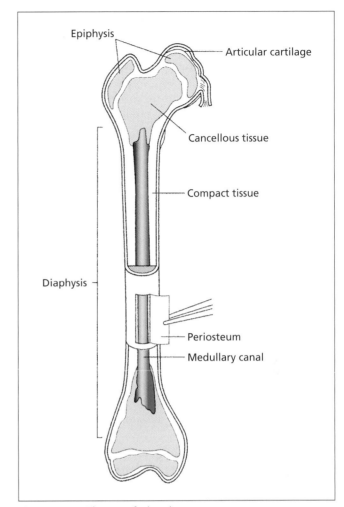

Figure 24.1 Diagram of a long bone.

composed of membranous connective tissue or cartilaginous tissue, which is gradually replaced by bone in the process of ossification.

The bones, which are preformed of cartilage, undergo *intracartilaginous ossification*, which involves removal of the cartilage and its replacement by bone tissue. Osteoblasts, osteoclasts and blood vessels invade internal areas of the cartilage, setting up ossification centres around which cartilage is progressively removed and replaced by bone tissue.

In long bones (Fig. 24.1), an ossification centre appears within the shaft (*diaphysis*) and later, around the time of birth, at each end (*epiphysis*). As ossification proceeds, growth of the cartilage continues, resulting in a persisting thin strip of cartilaginous tissue between each epiphysis and the diaphysis, which is referred to as the *growth or epiphyseal plate*. The bones continue to grow as long as new cartilage develops to maintain this plate. Cessation of growth occurs when it becomes ossified, and the epiphyses are fused with the diaphysis. Bones grow in circumference by the formation of layers of bone (by osteoblasts) beneath the periosteum whilst the medullary canal is progressively widened by the action of osteoclasts to keep the bone dimensions in proportion.

Factors in bone development, growth and repair

Several factors influence the development, growth and maintenance of normal bone structure. They are summarized in Box 24.1.

Bone growth and ossification are also influenced by such hormones as the growth hormone produced by the anterior pituitary gland, thyroxine from the thyroid gland, and parathyroid hormone produced by the parathyroid glands. Bone metabolism is also affected by other hormones such as oestrogen, androgens and calcitonin.

In addition to these factors, the demand placed on the bones by weight bearing and muscle pull plays an important role in the shaping of bone.

STRUCTURE AND FUNCTION OF JOINTS

A **joint** or articulation is a point of contact between bones that permits flexibility in the skeletal system and allows for movement. Joints are classified according to their structure and the kind of movement that they allow. The *structural* classification of joints is based on the kind of tissue that connects the bones and on the presence or absence of a synovial (joint) cavity, while their *functional* classification takes into account the degree of movement they permit.

CLASSIFICATION OF JOINTS

There are three major functional classes of joints:

1 Structurally immovable joints are classified as *fibrous*, with the bones united by fibrous connective tissue. The sutures between the bones of the skull are examples of such joints.

2 Slightly movable joints are referred to as *cartilaginous* because the bones are held together by cartilage – a strong avascular material. The inferior tibiofibular joint and the symphysis pubis (in the pelvis) are examples of slightly movable joints.

3 Freely movable joints have a space between articulating bones called the synovial or joint cavity. These joints are classified structurally as *synovial* and include the hip, knee, shoulder and elbow (Fig. 24.2). As most of the joints in the skeleton fall into this last category, they will be described in detail.

SYNOVIAL JOINTS

Freely movable or **synovial** joints, consisting of articulating bones and the joint cavity, are enclosed in a tough fibrous capsule (the articular capsule) which is continuous with the periosteum of the bones. This arrangement serves to stabilize the joint and keep the bones in normal apposition. The joint may be further reinforced by ligaments extending from one bone to another.

The inner surface of the articular capsule is lined with synovial membrane (synovium), which secretes synovial fluid. This fluid lubricates the joint, reduces friction and provides nourishment for the articular cartilage that covers the articulating surfaces of the bones of the joint. Some freely movable joints also have flat, crescent-shaped pieces of cartilage interposed between the articulating surfaces to cushion and protect the bone surfaces. For example, in the knee joint, semilunar cartilages referred to as *menisci* are located between the condyles of the femur and tibia (Fig. 24.3). Bursae are also situated between some body parts to reduce further the friction created by various movements of the body. These sac-like structures are lined with synovial membrane.

Box 24.1 Factors in bone development, growth and repair

- *Calcium and phosphorus*: needed for ossification and constant formation of new bone

- *Vitamin D*: used in the absorption and utilization of minerals

- *Protein and vitamin C*: acts in formation of collagenous, fibrous, intercellular matrix in which minerals are deposited

- *Vitamin A*: essential to tissue growth

- *Somatotrophic and parathyroid hormones*: play a part in bone growth and ossification

- Oestrogen, androgens and calcitonin: have roles in bone metabolism

- *Weight bearing and muscle stress*: needed for maintenance of bone strength and shaping of bone

---

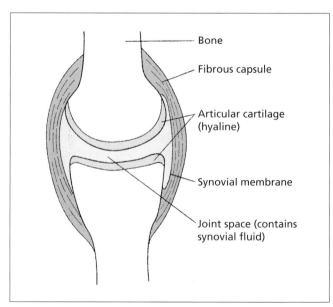

Figure 24.2 A synovial joint in frontal section.

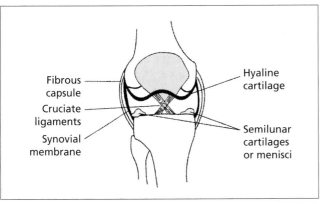

Figure 24.3   Knee joint, showing supporting ligaments and medial lateral menisci.

Freely movable joints are also differentiated by the type of movement they permit. These movements are limited by several factors, including the shape of the articulating bones, the tension of the ligaments, and the arrangement and tension of muscles. Generally, these joints permit one or more of the following movements: flexion, extension, abduction, adduction, rotation, circumduction, eversion, inversion, pronation and supination (Fig. 24.4).

How movement occurs at joints

To enable **movement** to occur, each synovial joint has at least one pair of muscles surrounding it. These work together so that when one is contracting (the *agonist*) the other is relaxing (the *antagonist*). Each muscle is attached to

Figure 24.4   (a–f) Joint movements.

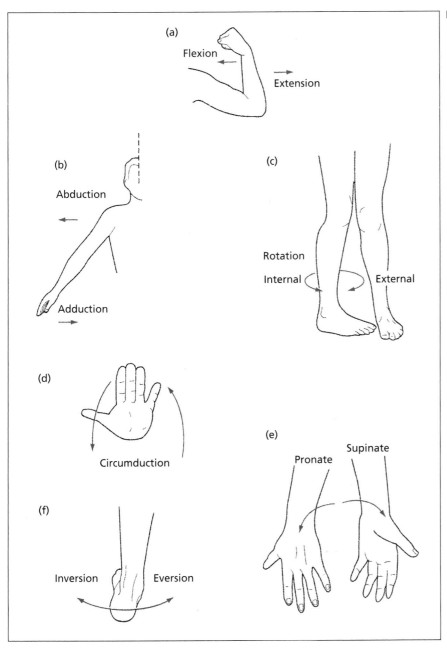

bone by a tendon at either end. The proximal tendon is usually referred to as the *tendon of origin*; the distal tendon is referred to as the *tendon of insertion*. Thus, when the muscle on the inner aspect of the joint contracts, the distal (furthest) bone is brought nearer the body (*flexion*). To allow this movement, the muscle on the outer aspect of the joint must relax. Similarly, when the muscle on the outer aspect of the joint contracts, the joint straightens (*extension*). Examples of this are the contraction of the hamstring muscle group behind the knee which produces flexion of the knee. This can occur only if the quadriceps muscle group relaxes sufficiently to allow flexion. This 'working in pairs' is essential for smooth joint movement.

This brief overview of the musculoskeletal system has set the scene for consideration of the two main groups of disorders that effect this system; trauma (e.g. fractures) and progressive long-term disease (e.g. osetoarthritis or osteoporosis).

TRAUMA ASSESSMENT

The patient who has been injured will have suffered an unpleasant experience which may well have been both frightening and painful. Whether a nurse encounters the patient in a first aid situation, an A&E unit or on the ward, these elements of psychological stress and pain should be considered carefully when assessing the patient.

In all acute trauma situations the priority is to assess the 'ABCDE of resuscitation', i.e. the patency of the person's *a*irway and cervical spine assessment, their *b*reathing, *ci*rculation and any evidence of *d*isability (including level of consciousness) and *e*xposure (undressing). This primary assessment should always precede the secondary assessment, which should then focus on pain and psychological status alongside the main injury itself. Assessment should then move on to consider the rest of the patient, checking for other less obvious injuries, unrelated but coexisting medical conditions (e.g. is the patient also diabetic?) as well as social factors. When women are assessed, the nurse should be aware of the possibility of domestic abuse which can happen to women from *any* social background and non-accidental injury should always be considered when assessing an injured child.

It is important to obtain a history of the injury and the degree of force involved. Certain mechanisms of trauma produce characteristic patterns of injury; knowledge of how the accident happened will therefore focus the nurse's attention on certain possible injuries. For example, a fall on an outstretched hand in an elderly person may produce a fracture of the lower extremity of the radius (Colles' fracture) but less obviously, it may produce an impacted fracture of the upper humerus.

An injured limb should be assessed gently with the minimum amount of movement because of the pain this may cause and also the risk of making the injury worse.

Pain is obviously a key sign of trauma, but is not necessarily always present or related in intensity to the severity of the injury. The cardinal sign of a fracture is localized bony tenderness, i.e. gentle pressure on the fracture site produces a painful response. In assessing a patient this is a key observation for the nurse to make.

The cardiovascular status of the limb must also be assessed as trauma may occlude the arterial blood supply leading to ischaemia, nerve damage and, in extreme cases, loss of the limb itself. The nurse must locate and mark a peripheral pulse, which should be monitored regularly. This is equally important on the ward after treatment such as reduction of a displaced fracture and immobilization in a plaster cast as swelling and arterial compression within the limb may be sufficient to occlude the blood supply. Abnormal sensation or loss of sensation distal to the injury is probably indicative of nerve damage and therefore a key sign that must be reported at once to paramedics in the field or senior staff in A&E.

The limb should also be assessed for evidence of deformity or shortening. Dislocation of a joint will obviously lead to deformity, as may a displaced fracture. Fractures of the femoral neck region characteristically produce shortening of the injured limb by approximately 2 cm and external rotation of the limb.

In assessing the injured limb for localized bony tenderness, pain, neurovascular compromise and deformity, the nurse must not lose sight of the whole person and their psychological status. The person may be very tearful and obviously frightened, or stoically silent. Either way the person has recently had a very unpleasant and probably painful experience which may affect their life for months and even years ahead. A wide range of thoughts and fears may be running through the injured person's head, whether it be in an A&E department or the ward. Quality nursing care requires these thoughts and fears be explored.

An elderly woman living alone may have suffered a fractured wrist which can usually be treated on an outpatient basis once the fracture has been reduced and immobilized in a plaster cast, but how well can that patient manage at home with her arm in plaster? Can she manage to walk safely with her Zimmer frame? What if the plaster becomes wet as a result of washing? Another common injury in elderly women is fracture of the femoral neck. The patient may be terrified of becoming a burden on relatives. She may feel her family will see this as too much of a burden and put her in a home. These are just some of the fears and anxieties that may affect a patient and which the nurse needs to try to discover if help is to be offered.

Patient assessment therefore needs to be a continual process and incorporate far more than the injured limb.

MEDICAL INVESTIGATIONS

Radiography is always considered following injuries to bones and joints. Because a film is a flat surface, at least two different views of each area of interest are taken, at different angles, to provide a three-dimensional guide to structure. This is particularly important when displacement is being identified.

In the acute stage of an injury, care must be taken not to move the patient unnecessarily. Casts, immobilization devices or traction should not be removed while radiographic investigations are performed in order to prevent the risk of displacement of the fractured bone.

Although radiography is used in the A&E department, advances in imaging science allow for various other sophisticated techniques to be used subsequently, such as radioactive bone scans, computed tomography or magnetic resonance imaging.

FRACTURES

A **fracture** is a break in the continuity of a bone, separating it into two or more parts. The soft tissues in the area surrounding the fracture are also involved in the injury.

CAUSES

The majority of fractures are due to violence incurred by falls, blows or rotational stresses. In each case, the force is in excess of the bone's resistance and may have been applied directly or indirectly. In direct violence, the fracture occurs at or near the site of the applied force. When indirect violence is the cause, the force is applied at a point remote from the site of the fracture. For example, in a fall on the outstretched hand, the stress may be transmitted to the radius, ulna, humerus or clavicle. Occasionally, a fracture may be due to a sudden forceful contraction of attached muscles; this is known as an avulsion fracture.

A fracture can occur as the result of disease of the bone which has weakened its structure to the point that it can no longer withstand the normal stresses and strains of everyday life; this is known as a *pathological fracture*. Metastases, primary tumours, osteitis fibrosa cystica due to hyperparathyroidism, osteogenesis imperfecta (a congenital condition affecting the formation of osteoblasts) and most commonly, osteoporosis, are examples of diseased conditions of bone that may lead to spontaneous fracture. Prolonged stress may also cause a fracture in certain bones. This is known as a *stress fracture* and may, for example, affect the fibula in professional sports people such as a cricketer who is a fast bowler.

TYPES OF FRACTURE

The types of fracture are listed in Box 24.2 and illustrated in Figure 24.5. Injury and fracture of the spine and skull are discussed in Chapter 20 as there is often serious neurological involvement.

PHYSIOLOGICAL RESPONSES

Local

A fracture is always accompanied by some degree of damage to the surrounding soft tissues. Blood vessels within the bone, the periosteum and surrounding tissues are torn, resulting in haemorrhage and then the formation of a haematoma. The periosteum at the site may be stripped away from the underlying bone tissue, interrupting the blood supply into the area and thus contributing to the death of bone cells. There may also be haemorrhage into adjacent muscles and joints and damage to ligaments, tendons and nerves. Soon after a fracture occurs, the muscles in the area go into

---

Box 24.2 Terms used to describe types of fracture
• *Traumatic or pathological*: traumatic is the result of violence; pathological is spontaneous or the result of disease
• *Incomplete*: break not all the way through bone (e.g. greenstick fracture in children)
• *Complete*: bone is separated into two distinct parts
• *Closed (simple)*: overlying skin is intact
• *Open (compound)*: a wound exists over the fracture establishing communication between the fracture and the outside air
• *Complicated*: fracture includes injury to adjacent structures (e.g. blood vessels, nerves or organs)
• *Comminuted*: more than one line of fracture and more than two fragments
• *Transverse*: line of fracture is at right angles to the long axis of bone
• *Spiral*: curves in spiral fashion around bone
• *Impacted*: one fragment is driven into another (cancellous bone usually involved)
• *Crush or compression*: fracture occurs in cancellous bone which is compressed beyond limits of tolerance
• *Avulsion*: a ligament or tendon under excessive stress fractures or tears away its bony attachment
• *Depressed*: a segment of cortical bone is depressed below the level of surrounding bone.

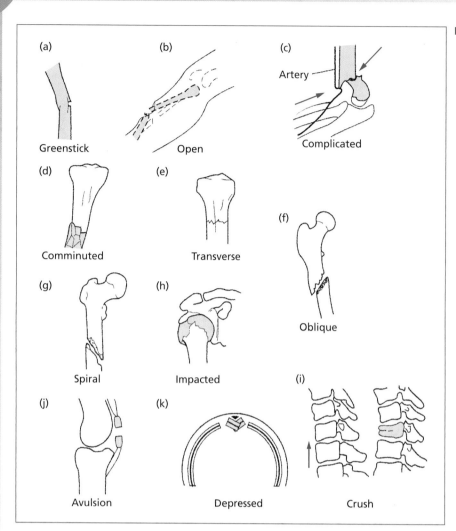

Figure 24.5 (a–k) Types of fracture.

(a) Greenstick

(b) Open

(c) Artery Complicated

(d) Comminuted

(e) Transverse

(f) Oblique

(g) Spiral

(h) Impacted

(i)

(j) Avulsion

(k) Depressed

Crush

spasm, causing severe pain and possible displacement of a fragment due to tendon pull.

Depending on the fracture, visceral injuries may occur, which may threaten the patient's life. Examples of such injuries are rupture of the bladder by a fractured pelvis and rupture of the spleen or perforation of a lung by a fractured rib.

Systemic

The patient suffers some degree of shock which is influenced by the severity of the injury, the amount of soft-tissue damage, associated disorders or multiple injuries, and the patient's age and general condition at the time of injury. A fracture of the femoral shaft results in a blood loss of approximately 1 L and will probably lead to hypovolaemic shock, whereas a fracture of the tibia produces blood loss of approximately 500 mL. Usually a slight increase in temperature and leucocytosis occur in the first 2 or 3 days.

In addition, there is also the psychological dimension to consider as different people respond in different ways to the same injury. The psychological response and degree of motivation shown by the patient may affect recovery time significantly.

Clinical characteristics of fractures and patient assessment

The following discussion is an important guide to assessment and care planning as it highlights potential and actual problems the patient may have. The symptoms of a fracture vary with its location, type, the amount of displacement of the fragments and the degree of damage to soft-tissue structures (Table 24.1). The symptoms also vary with the patient's personality and perception of the injury, coupled with the social norms experienced by the patient.

The patient or an observer usually relates a history of a fall, blow or sudden forcible movement, and the victim may actually say that he or she heard the bone break. Sudden severe pain at the site is experienced which may or may not persist. Frequently, because of injury, nerve function is impaired and pain may be absent for a brief period following the injury. As function returns, muscle spasm in the area, as well as tissue damage, accounts for much of the pain, which becomes worse with any movement. Obvious deformity may be present as a result of displacement of the fragments, and there may be shortening of the affected limb due to contraction of attached muscles; this is particularly apparent in femoral fractures. Impaired mobility and loss of

Table 24.1 Specific problems of a patient with a fracture

Patient problem	Causes
Sudden severe pain at site (may or may not persist)	Injury, impaired nerve function, muscle spasm, tissue damage
Deformity or shortening of limb	Displacement of bone fragments, muscle spasm
Impaired mobility and loss of function	Disruption of bone, nerve compression by bone fragments
Loss of circulation	Arterial compression by bone fragments
Swelling	Bleeding and/or escape of fluid into tissues; after 2–5 days area may become discoloured (ecchymosis)
Crepitation (grating sound)	Movement of bone fragments at fracture end

mechanical support occur, and in the case of long bones, there may be obvious movement in a part that is normally rigid. Complete loss of function may result from nerve compression by displaced fragments; this is usually restored when the fracture is reduced and the fragments are placed in normal apposition and alignment. The blood supply to a limb may be severely impaired if an artery is trapped in the fracture. In severe cases, the limb may be lost due to gangrene if the blood supply is not quickly restored by manipulation of the fracture to restore normal anatomy.

Crepitation (a grating sound produced by movement of the ends of the fragments) may be noted if the patient moves the part. Under no circumstances should any attempt be made to elicit crepitus because of the possibility of further serious damage to soft tissues (e.g. blood vessels and nerves), unnecessary painful displacement of fragments and the possible production of an open fracture. Swelling may develop rapidly over the site of the fracture because of bleeding and the escape of fluid into the tissue. After 2 or 3 days, this area frequently becomes bruised and discoloured (*ecchymosis*).

In the case of the rupture of an organ by a bone fragment, symptoms of impaired function of the damaged organ appear. With rupture of the bladder by a fractured pelvis, extravasation of urine gradually becomes evident, and blood appears in the urine. Although rare, perforation of the intestine is associated with pelvic fracture and causes severe shock and peritonitis; the abdomen becomes distended and board-like. A serious complication of a rib fracture may be puncture of a lung (pneumothorax). The patient may develop shock, respiratory distress, coughing and haemoptysis.

Some fractures, especially those that are incomplete, impacted or of short bones, may produce few signs and symptoms. The fracture may be suspected only on the basis of the history of violence, tenderness on pressure over the site, or the patient's complaint of pain upon use of the part or weight bearing on it. Again, no attempt should be made to elicit symptoms by having the person move or stand. The patient is treated as having a fracture if there is any doubt.

Diagnosis of a fracture is based on the history of the accident, physical examination of the patient and radiographs of the affected part.

FRACTURE HEALING

Bone is different from many of the specialized tissues because of its ability to regenerate and hence restore the continuity that was disrupted by the fracture. Immediately after a fracture, the space between the fragments and around the fracture site is filled with blood and inflammatory exudate. The haematoma and the exudate are invaded by fibroblasts and capillaries from adjacent connective tissue and blood vessels, forming granulation tissue. Simultaneously, osteoblasts proliferate, mainly from the inner surface of the periosteum (and endosteum in a long bone) and invade the granulation tissue. Calcium salts are deposited, forming a loosely woven, bone-like tissue referred to as a *callus*. This forms a 'collar' around the bone at the fracture site, giving it greater thickness than the original bone. The callus unites and helps to stabilize the fragments but is not strong enough to bear weight or withstand stress. If the blood supply is poor, or if it is disturbed by excessive mobility at the fracture site, cartilage may be formed instead of bone. As the osteoblasts increase, the callus is gradually restructured by ossification (production of a collagenous fibrous network that becomes impregnated with mineral salts) to form bone tissue. Remodelling is the final stage of fracture healing. The external bulbous bony area is remodelled by the action of osteoclasts.

In some instances, a fracture is complicated by malunion, delayed healing or non-union:

- *Malunion* implies healing of the fracture in an abnormal position. There may be angulation of the bone or overriding of the fragments which alters the shape and length of the limb. Function may be impaired. The cause is usually ineffective reduction and/or fixation during healing
- *Delayed healing* simply implies that the fracture is not healing as rapidly as is normally expected
- In *non-union*, the granulation tissue that formed between the fragments following the fracture is converted to dense fibrous tissue instead of normal callus and bone tissue. Causes of delayed union or non-union include too wide a gap between the fragments, the interposition of soft

tissues or a foreign body between the fragments, poor blood supply to the site, loss of the initial haematoma by the escape of blood through an open wound or surgical intervention, infection of the bone, malnutrition and disease of bone (e.g. bone metastases).

GENERAL PRINCIPLES AND METHODS OF TREATMENT OF FRACTURES

Emergency care

Emergency treatment of a person with a fracture usually occurs at the site where the injury took place. The patient's general condition and the extent of injuries are quickly assessed (see p. 825) and priorities are set. Respiratory insufficiency, haemorrhage or shock may be evident and take precedence over injured bones.

The first aid treatment is very important; movement of the patient or improper handling may cause serious tissue damage and increased pain, haemorrhage and shock. If a fracture is obvious or suspected, paramedic care at the site of the accident and during transportation to a hospital is directed toward reducing pain and preventing further tissue damage, including to underlying tissues and organs, and a closed fracture becoming open. The patient should receive a minimum of handling (unless there is danger of further injury) until the emergency services arrive. Before moving the patient, the fracture site and the joint above and below are immobilized in order to reduce the risk of further damage and to relieve pain. A splint can be improvised from whatever is available (e.g. a board, two or three thicknesses of cardboard, a folded quilt or blanket, pillows). In the case of a board, the surface applied to the patient must be padded (towels or clothing may be used) to prevent pressure. If the limb is in an abnormal position, it is splinted in that deformed position; no attempt is made to reduce the fracture or restore the limb to a normal position. The easiest splint is the patient's own body: an uninjured leg can act as a splint for an injured leg and the trunk can splint an injured arm. Thus, a lower limb may be immobilized by placing a pillow or folded blanket between the legs and tying them together. In the case of an arm, it may be secured against the trunk by bandages and a sling. If it is an open fracture, the wound is covered with the cleanest material available in order to prevent further contamination and reduce infection risks. If the bone is protruding from the wound, no attempt is made to replace it or reduce the fracture. Nothing is given by mouth in case a general anaesthetic proves necessary.

When the patient arrives at the hospital a quick assessment is made of the general condition and, if there is respiratory insufficiency or shock, appropriate treatment is instituted before the fracture receives attention. When the general condition is satisfactory, radiographs are taken of the fracture area.

The patient may be disoriented, frightened and agitated. An ongoing explanation of what is about to be done and what the patient can do best to assist in care often helps to keep the patient calm. This makes it possible to provide efficient on-the-scene care and prevent further injury.

Treatment

The treatment of a fracture usually involves reduction, fixation of the part, protection while the bone heals, and rehabilitation during and after the healing process to restore normal function. When possible, bone stress is utilized to increase the process of repair. The bone fragments are mechanically fixated to enable immediate use, creating stress at the fracture site which accelerates osteoblastic activity. Some fractures, such as those of distal phalanges of the fingers and toes, may heal without reduction and fixation. However, regular analgesia will be required to maintain mobility.

Reduction

This is the procedure by which fragments are brought into their pre-injury position so that the normal shape and length of the bone are restored and union is promoted. Obviously, reduction is necessary only if there is some displacement of the fragments (Fig. 24.6). It is carried out as soon as possible. A delay makes it more difficult to obtain satisfactory alignment because of the rapid organization of the blood clot and the development of associated muscle spasm. Also, there is likely to be less tissue trauma with early reduction.

A fracture may be reduced by a number of methods, with the use of general or regional anaesthesia or an opioid analgesic. Methods for reducing fractures include closed manipulative reduction, traction applied distal to the fracture, or open (internal) reduction. In *closed reduction*, the clinician manipulates the fragments into position by manual traction,

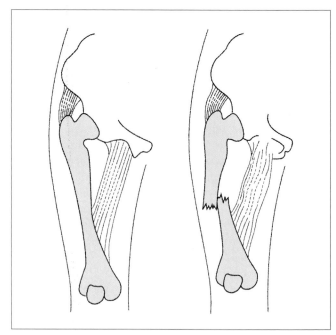

Figure 24.6 Fracture of the femoral shaft. The pull by the adductor muscles causes displacement of the fragments.

pressure and/or rotation. In fractures in which one fragment is overriding the other and there is considerable muscle pull, continuous *traction* may be applied to the distal fragment to bring it into apposition and maintain the alignment. This method of reduction is used most often in fractures of the femur because the pull of the strong thigh muscles tends to displace the fragments and cause overriding. The traction may be applied to the skin (skin traction) or directly to bone (skeletal traction). In some fractures, reduction can be achieved only through an *open surgical incision*.

Fixation

Various methods are used to maintain reduction and hold the fragments in position. They may be categorized as cast splintage (plaster of Paris commonly), external fixation, functional bracing, traction, or internal fixation. The method used depends upon the particular bone (e.g. location – short, long or flat), the type of fracture and the muscles involved.

External fixation   This is most commonly achieved by enclosing the part in a cast (Box 24.3). A *plaster cast* is most widely used and is made by the application and moulding of moist plaster of Paris (POP) bandages to the affected part. A chemical reaction hardens the plaster (and gives off heat) making it rigid. However, it takes more than 24 hours to set fully. An alternative is to use synthetic casting materials which set fully in 30 minutes, and are much lighter, waterproof (unlike POP) and stronger.

Before either cast is applied, the skin is cleansed and examined for any contusions or abrasions. The part is then enclosed in stockinette for skin protection. Extra padding is used over bony prominences or to fill in spaces that might weaken the cast. It is also applied when swelling is anticipated.

A *walking cast* may be applied with stable fractures of the tibia and fibula. A 'rocker' or sole plate incorporated in the base of the plaster enables the patient to be weight bearing. A *bivalve* cast may be removed for brief periods to allow skin or wound care or other treatment; however, this is rarely

used for fracture prior to callus formation because of the danger of loss of position. When swelling of the limb is expected, for example in a recent injury, a plaster back slab may be applied rather than a cylindrical cast. This is made by the application of slabs of plaster of Paris to the posterior of the limb; the slabs are then secured in position with cotton bandages. The rationale is that, if necessary, the cotton bandages can be easily split to prevent circulatory and neurological impairment.

External skeletal fixation   With this method of treatment, the bone fragments are pierced above and below the fracture by screws or pins and these can then be attached to a rigid external metal framework. The pins are then held in proper relation to one another by an external support which either runs parallel to the bone or is circular around the limb. External fixation may be used in the treatment of fractures associated with extensive damage to the soft tissues where the wound needs to be accessible. It may also be used in the management of infected fractures, in multiple fractures (to facilitate the treatment of other fractures), severely disrupted or unstable fractures, and in pelvic fractures. External fixation is designed to hold the fracture without a plaster cast until union, and allow access to any wounds. The disadvantages are the risk of pin-track infections, the loosening of the pins and delayed union, as external callus formation may be suppressed by tissue trauma and rigid immobilization of the fracture. Damage to soft tissues may occur inadvertently during fixation.

Traction   Traction (which may also be employed to correct a deformity, relieve pressure on a spinal nerve or prevent a contracture deformity in cases in which there is muscle spasm) is most commonly used to reduce and maintain reduction in fractures of the limbs by overcoming the effects of gravity and muscle pull. It involves the application of a force along the long axis of the bone distal to the fracture. For this force to be effective, a force in the opposite direction is required (countertraction). Countertraction is necessary and is usually provided by elevating the foot of the bed in the case of a lower limb; the weight of the body on the incline supplies the required countertraction. Traction is now used much less frequently as both internal and external fixation techniques have become more widespread and the importance of early mobilization has been recognized.

An important use of traction is to overcome the deforming muscle pull that is associated with fractures of long bones such as the shaft of femur. This is needed in emergency care environments such as A&E. A fracture of the femur is accompanied by marked displacement of the fragments due to the contracture of the very strong muscles of the thigh and hip. The adductor muscles produce a lateral bowing (Fig. 24.6). Fixed traction is commonly applied via the traditional Thomas' splint or one of the more modern telescopic versions. This is characterized by traction between two fixed points. In a Thomas' splint traction is exerted by either skin extension tapes tied to the distal end of the splint or by pas-

---

> **Box 24.3   Types of cast**
>
> - *Plaster*: a cylinder that encases a fractured limb
> - *Walking*: a weight-bearing wooden heel and sole (rocker) is incorporated into the cast
> - *Body (jacket)*: applied to the trunk
> - *Spica (shoulder/hip)*: applied to the trunk and shoulder or hip
> - *Bivalve*: moulded to trunk or limb and cut down each side when dry. Held in place with Velcro or bandages
> - *Splint*: plaster of Paris, metal, fibreglass thermoplastic or polyurethane material moulded to support the affected limb.

sing a pin through the tibia and pulling directly on the bone. Countertraction is obtained by the thrust of the upper ring of the splint against the ischial tuberosity (Fig. 24.7).

The alternative to fixed traction is balanced (sliding) traction. Here the opposing traction forces are 'balanced' allowing the patient to move about the bed without disturbing the desired line of pull. Traction is applied by the use of a weight and pulley system. A cord passes over the pulley to the weights and is usually attached to a skeletal pin which passes through the patient's bone (skeletal traction) (Figs 24.8, 24.9).

Skeletal traction Skeletal traction is achieved by the insertion of a metal wire (Kirschner wire) or pin (e.g. Steinmann or Denham pin) through the bone distal to the fracture. By this means, traction is applied directly to the skeleton. A special traction stirrup or U loop is fastened to

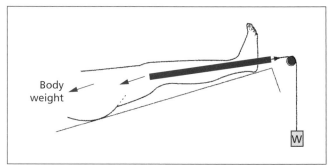

Figure 24.8 Balanced (sliding) traction. *Note* elevation of foot of bed uses patient's own body weight as counter-traction.

Figure 24.7 (a) Fixed traction using skin traction and a Thomas' splint. (b) Fixed traction using a skeletal pin and a Thomas' splint.

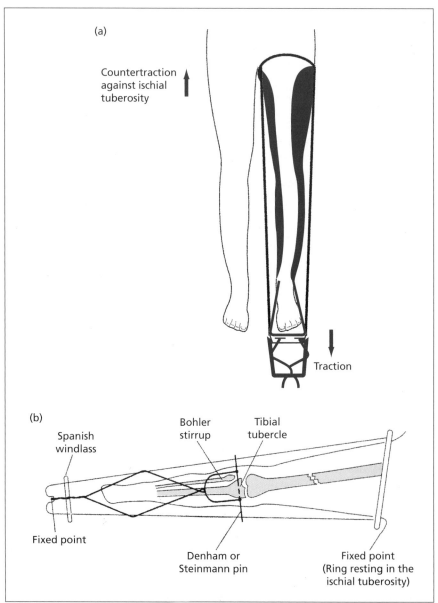

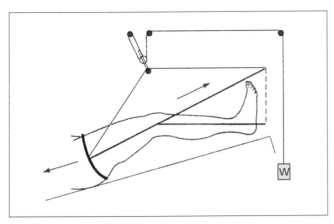

Figure 24.9 Suspension of the Thomas' splint.

the protruding wire or pin (Fig. 24.10); cord is attached to this which leads to a weight and pulley system. Counter-traction is obtained by gravity and the patient's body weight on an inclined bed. The limb in traction is then usually suspended off the bed surface.

Balanced skeletal traction This is commonly used with a half- or full-ring Thomas' splint and with a Pearson's knee flexion piece to obtain reduction of a fracture of a shaft of a femur and to maintain reduction until union occurs.

Firm cotton slings are secured to the upper part of the Thomas' splint to support the thigh and to the Pearson's knee flexion piece to support the leg. The Thomas' splint extends from the groin to beyond the foot in line with the femur. The knee is in 10–20° of flexion to control rotation and prevent stretching of the posterior knee capsule and ligaments, and subsequent joint instability. Some provision may be made to support the foot to prevent footdrop. The skeletal traction is usually applied to the proximal area of the tibia. The pull is exerted in line with the femur by means of a traction cord attached to the bow or stirrup that is fitted to the protruding ends of the pin that passes through the bone. The traction cord passes over a pulley and suspends a weight. The proximal and distal ends of the splint are suspended by separate cords, pulleys and weights. Countertraction is obtained by elevating the foot of the bed. When the patient moves up or down in the bed, the splint moves as well, and traction is maintained. The patient has greater freedom of movement and is usually more comfortable in this system of traction. It also has the advantage of allowing a certain amount of movement in adjacent joints.

Internal fixation Some fractures require internal surgical reduction and fixation. Various types of internal fixation devices are used. These include stainless steel or vitallium wire, screws, plates, intramedullary nails, or banding circumferentially around the bone. The metal may be secured to the sides of the bone, placed through the fragments or passed through the intramedullary cavity of the bone. Internal fixation may be reinforced after the wound is

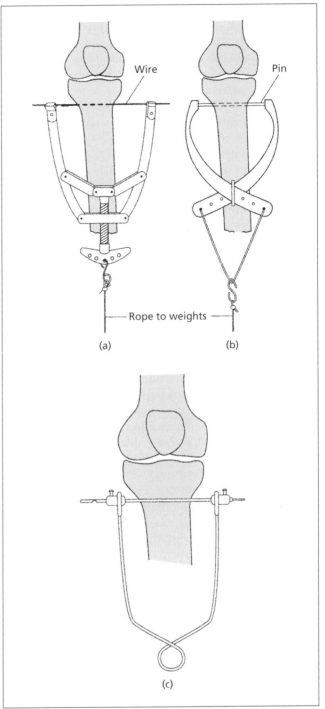

Figure 24.10 Skeletal traction may be applied by (a) a Kirschner wire and traction stirrup; (b) a Steinmann pin and traction stirrup; or (c) a Steinmann pin and Böhler stirrup.

closed by the application of a cast or splint. However, new devices of such strength and design are being made that external splintage is not always required, thus allowing immediate joint freedom, early weight bearing and short-term hospitalization.

Special internal fixation devices are used to immobilize the fragments in a hip fracture or fracture of the femoral neck such as dynamic hip screws or cannulated screws. In patients with an intracapsular fracture through the neck of the femur there is a risk of avascular necrosis of the femoral head (death of bone due to lack of blood supply); in these cases a hemiarthroplasty is performed by replacing the head of the femur with a metallic prosthesis (see p. 840).

Following any method of reduction and fixation, a postoperative/reduction radiograph is vital to ensure that the position is maintained. Radiographs are then taken periodically to determine that healing is occurring and the bone fragments remain in the correct alignment.

Functional bracing This technique for managing leg fractures involves applying two casts to the leg above and below the knee, but leaving the knee joint free. The two casts are connected by hinges to stabilize the limb. The result is increased patient mobility, a limb that can be used for weight bearing, a joint that does not become stiff from disuse and improved fracture healing from the beneficial effects of load bearing. Functional bracing is usually applied 3–6 weeks after the injury when the fracture is beginning to unite (Solomon et al 2005).

Open (compound) fractures
The patient with an open fracture requires special treatment as soon after the accident as possible. The site is potentially infected and there is usually a greater amount of soft-tissue damage and destruction. Bone infection (osteomyelitis) and necrosis impede fracture healing and may result in serious disability. An initial wound assessment takes place in A&E as soon as possible. The wound will be irrigated to remove gross contamination and dressed with saline and iodine soaks. Intravenous opioid analgesia is essential (usually morphine) and the limb should be kept immobile with frequent checks on the distal pulse to ensure there is no neurovascular damage. The patient will be a high priority for theatre, where the surgeon will explore and debride the wound (the removal of foreign material and excision of dead tissue). The repair of severed or torn tendons or nerves may be necessary. The fracture is reduced and then immobilized. If there has been gross contamination, the wound may be packed and left open until the danger of infection is past. Drains are inserted in the wound. Antimicrobial therapy may be prescribed.

Before administration of the anaesthetic, the patient's anti-tetanus status should be checked and if a booster dose is needed, it will be given. If the person is not protected, human tetanus immunoglobulin is given.

CARE OF THE PATIENT IN A CAST

The care of the patient following the application of a cast requires the following considerations.

Drying of the cast
Complete drying of a plaster cast following its application may take several hours or days, depending on the material used, its thickness and the temperature, humidity and circulation of the air. During this period, support of the cast and handling are very important, because the cast is vulnerable to pressure and cracking which could alter its shape and cause indentations that result in undue pressure on an area of the body or make it ineffective. When the part must be lifted, it is supported on the palms of the hands to avoid making indentations by the fingertips. In the case of a body or long leg cast, firm support along the line of the cast is ensured. Pillows with plastic or rubber undercovers are placed under the part encased in plaster so that the cast is not subjected to pressure by the firm mattress. As it is moulded to the contours of the part to which it is applied, support by an extra pillow or folded flannelette sheet may be necessary under such regions as the lumbar or popliteal area.

Drying is promoted by exposure to dry, warm, circulating air which evaporates the moisture from the cast. The bedding is arranged so that the cast is left uncovered. If it is a large or body cast, two or three persons work together to turn the patient and pillows are used to avoid strain on any part of the plaster. A moist cast has a dull grey appearance but, when dry, it appears white and shiny. Casts made from materials other than plaster of Paris usually dry more quickly. A study of the instructions that come with these materials will explain the drying time.

Weight bearing on a walking cast is begun when the cast is thoroughly dry. If POP has been used, this is usually after 48 hours.

Patient problems

Unless the patient experiences complications or requires surgery, the plaster cast will be applied in the A&E department. This greatly reduces the time the nurse has to assess the patient and/or family for their response to, or understanding of, the injury and the care required. Rapid assessment and intervention are necessary.

It is important to assess whether there are any skin lesions (e.g. wounds, pre-existing skin conditions) as these will be enclosed in the cast, possibly for several weeks, leading to the risk of tissue necrosis, suppuration or infection. Swelling should be assessed carefully because of the risk of neurovascular compromise if the limb becomes compressed within the cast. It is important to check that any jewellery has been removed; a ring, for example, could act as a tourniquet around the finger if severe swelling develops in a wrist fracture.

Apart from such physical factors, the nurse should assess the patient's level of comprehension of what is happening. After discharge from A&E, the patient will be responsible for the self-care of the cast and fracture. This requires education concerning swelling and circulation, the condition of the cast, pain control, etc. The nurse needs to assess the patient's grasp of language and intellectual functioning in order to ensure that teaching is delivered in an effective and appropriate way.

The social consequences of injury have already been raised and the nurse has a responsibility to assess whether the patient will have any significant social problems as a result of having a limb in a cast. This is particularly true of groups such as the elderly or lone parents who may find coping alone very difficult in these circumstances.

Table 24.2 gives a summary of some of the principal health problems that assessment may reveal for the patient with a limb in a cast.

Nursing management

Assessment and monitoring of the cast

Assessment of an inpatient with a cast involves neurovascular evaluation of the affected limb every 30 minutes for the first 4 hours and then every 4 hours for several days. The affected extremity is compared with the uninjured one for alterations in colour, temperature, sensation, movement and swelling. Any blanching or the presence of a bluish colour indicates an interruption in circulation to the part. Touching the toes or fingers will identify temperature differences; pressure applied to these extremities will elicit from the patient any differences in sensation; patients should be asked to demonstrate movement of fingers or toes. Pain assessment is ongoing.

The nurse checks the cast with the palm of the hand for any warm or soft areas. Areas of discolouration or changes in discoloured areas are looked for. A musty smell will be present if infection has occurred, so any odour should be noted as part of the nurse's assessment. As odour is a late sign, infection may be suspected before a musty smell is detected due to localized pain, raised temperature, etc. When an opening (window) has been made in a cast to allow for treatment of an incision or wound, the section is removed regularly to assess the status of the wound and surrounding skin. The skin next to the edges of the cast should also be inspected for signs of rubbing, soreness, etc., especially if a resin cast is used.

The mood of the patient should also be assessed; younger patients in particular may become bored and frustrated at their lack of activity.

Nursing intervention

To alleviate and prevent further swelling, the affected limb is elevated above the level of the heart. This is achieved by the use of pillows, and elevating the foot of the bed when a leg is affected. To elevate the arm, a draw sheet (or towel) may be used by folding the sheet in half and placing the flexed elbow on the fold with the fingers towards the sheet ends. Several large safety pins are carefully inserted on either side of the arm and the sheet ends are pinned over an intravenous stand which supports the weight of the arm. Ideally, the hand should be well above the elbow and the elbow off the bed to promote drainage of tissue and reduce swelling. Once the oedema has gone, normal positioning may resume.

If the patient is going home from A&E, detailed printed instructions, reinforced verbally, should be given on care of the cast and limb. Swelling in an injured arm is prevented by the use of a high arm sling. When the lower limb is injured, it should always be elevated above heart level to prevent swelling, when the patient is sitting down.

Care must be taken to avoid getting a plaster cast wet as it will disintegrate with resultant loss of immobilization and fracture position. The cast can be protected when bathing or in inclement weather by plastic bags or some other waterproof material which is sealed around the edges of the cast

Table 24.2	Principal problems for the patient with a limb in a cast
Patient problems	**Goals**
1. Potential problem of further injury related to pressure on soft tissue, nerves or arteries	The patient will: 1. understand the importance of the absence of pain and feeling of pressure, irritation or loss of sensation in the affected limb 2. have normal temperature and colour in the fingers or toes 3. demonstrate movement of the fingers or toes 4. show no sign of skin breakdown.
2. Immobilization due to limitation of movement by the cast	The patient will: 1. demonstrate a safe method of walking and the use of aids such as crutches and walking sticks, when these are being used 2. demonstrate a safe method of transferring from bed to chair or chair to chair when walking is restricted.
3. Potential problem of lack of knowledge due to changes in self-care	The patient and/or family will be able to: 1. describe the care of the cast 2. list risk factors related to potential for further injury or damage to the cast 3. describe the action to undertake if the cast becomes loose 4. describe the activities the person may engage in 5. identify the outpatient clinic for follow-up treatment and where emergency care can be received.

to prevent moisture from seeping under it. Casts of other materials may be allowed to become wet but saturation should be avoided.

To prevent skin irritation, exposed edges of a cast may be padded by folding the stockinette from under the cast over the top and bottom edges of the cast. The use of powder or lotion under a cast should be avoided as these tend to cake and cause more irritation. The patient should be cautioned against inserting objects such as knitting needles under the cast to try to relieve irritation as this may lead to serious skin breakdown and infection.

Patients with leg casts may be taught to use elbow crutches. The nurse will walk with the patient initially to ensure safety. Walking casts should be protected with a boot or other covering.

The patient and/or family are taught to assess the cast and affected limb, the care of the cast and where to report any alterations in sensation, comfort or signs of drainage. Activities that may be undertaken should be discussed and reasons given for any restrictions.

Removal of the cast

When the cast is taken off, the rigid support to joints that have been immobilized for a considerable period of time is removed. The patient is likely to be discouraged by the stiffness, instability and weakness encountered and requires reassurance that with exercise and progressive use, function will be restored.

The cast is removed by special cast cutters or a plaster saw. As this may be frightening, the nurse describes the equipment and the process to the person before removal begins. The limb must be handled gently and with support under the joints. The skin is bathed gently, and an application of oil or lanolin is made to soften the accumulation of dry, scaly skin. Vigorous rubbing is discouraged to avoid skin irritation and abrasions.

Rehabilitation

A regimen of passive and active exercises and massage is established to restore joint and muscle function. Weight-bearing and activities are gradually resumed. When the cast is removed and the limb becomes dependent, oedema and swelling are likely to occur. The patient is advised to elevate the limb when sitting and lying, and an elasticated tubular bandage (Tubigrip) may be applied when walking to control the oedema, which gradually becomes less troublesome as muscle tone improves and there is increasing activity.

CARE OF THE PATIENT WITH EXTERNAL SKELETAL FIXATION

Preoperative preparation

The length of time that elapses between the time of injury and surgery varies and is dependent on the patient's general state of health and associated injuries. The care of the patient in the A&E department and following admission to the ward includes observations of vital signs to detect signs of hae-

morrhage and shock, and observations of colour, temperature, sensation, movement of digits and pulse are made of the injured limb to detect impaired circulation or nerve damage; any abnormal signs are reported to the doctor immediately. Pain as a result of the injury and potential for infection as a result of an open wound are specific problems that need to be addressed between arrival in A&E and transfer to the operating theatre. Analgesics are administered to alleviate pain. Wounds and surrounding skin are cleansed according to the preference of the surgeon and covered with an antiseptic soak and sterile dressings. This reduces the risk of infection and, by keeping the tissue moist, improves its viability, thereby promoting postoperative wound healing.

The likely appearance of the limb post-operatively should be explained to the patient, depending upon how the fracture is to be immobilized (e.g. external skeletal fixation). This will help to alleviate some of the problems, associated with altered body image, that could otherwise occur after surgery. The nurse should be available to the patient and encourage free discussion of fears and anxieties concerning treatment and recovery.

Postoperative care

If an external skeletal fixation system has been applied to a fractured limb, the limb *must* be elevated to help reduce swelling.

In addition to the problems usually experienced after operation, the patient with external fixation has an added potential problem of infection at the pin sites. The nurse checks the external fixation system daily to ensure that the clamps and nuts are tight. This routine is explained to the patient so s/he understands that it is an expected procedure. The pin sites are observed for bleeding or leakage of exudate; they should be dry approximately 48 hours after surgery. Most trauma units have their own protocols for care of pin sites; however, there is a lack of any evidence base to support these protocols. A systematic review by Temple and Santy (2005) revealed only one trial in the whole literature (from 1996) which met the methodological criteria to be considered valid. This trial found *not* cleaning pin sites produced significantly fewer infections than cleaning them! There is an obvious need for some major RCTs to produce evidence about the best approach to pin site care.

Pain, tenderness, erythema, swelling and increased skin temperature at a pin site must lead the nurse to suspect pin-site infection. Any of these clinical features must be reported to the doctor, and a wound swab should be taken and sent for microscopy, culture and sensitivity. Antibiotic therapy is prescribed and the pin may be removed. Any loosening of a pin must also be reported as this increases the risk of pin-track infection; the offending pin is usually removed. Any exposed pin tips must be covered by metal or plastic caps or corks to prevent damage by the sharp-ended pin to the other limb or body or to the nursing staff.

The patient usually requires a strong analgesic at regular intervals during the first 48 hours following surgery. If severe or moderate pain persists after this time, the surgeon must be informed as it may be an indication of infection. The patient is usually confined to bed until bone and skin healing is progressing satisfactorily. Exercises of all joints, including those of the affected limb, are commenced as soon as possible to maintain muscle tone, strength and mass, and to maintain joint movements. The patient with a lower limb fracture is at high risk of the formation of deep vein thrombosis. Foot and leg exercises are commenced on the day after the application of the fixation device and observations are made to detect any signs of this complication.

Some patients may be upset on seeing their injured limb and the fixation system. The nurse needs to show patience and understanding, and should encourage the patient to express any anxieties and fears. By encouraging the patient to participate in the planning of care and to take an interest in the care of the fixation system and the rehabilitation programme, the nurse may assist the patient in coming to terms with an altered body image.

The patient with a lower limb fracture is taught to mobilize with the aid of crutches; weight bearing on the affected limb is not permitted because of the risk of refracture and bone displacement until callus formation is detected by radiography. Once callus has formed, the patient may be taught to bear weight partially through the affected limb.

The external skeletal fixation device is removed once fracture union has occurred, as diagnosed by radiography. After removal of the fixation system (from a lower limb) the patient is generally not permitted to bear weight fully for a further 2 weeks.

CARE OF THE PATIENT IN TRACTION

Assessment

The ongoing nature of assessment is well illustrated in the case of a patient on traction where several weeks may elapse before the traction is discontinued.

Of particular importance is the patient's skin condition due to the high risk of **pressure sore** development. Regular monitoring is therefore essential along with the pin sites to detect any early signs of tissue breakdown or infection. The use of a pressure sore risk calculator such as the Norton or Waterlow scale is strongly recommended.

The patient's normal bowel habits and diet should be assessed due to the risks of **constipation** associated with inactivity. Constipation should be detected early by frequent monitoring rather than at the late stage where the patient is impacted. Hospitalization, immobility and frequent use of opioid analgesics predisposes to constipation and in older patients an accompanying detrimental effect on mental state.

Micturition is difficult in traction, particularly for female patients. Any previous history of retention or incontinence needs to be noted and ongoing assessment of urinary output is essential to prevent the risk of retention developing.

The patient's hobbies and interests should be explored as inactivity and boredom can quickly become major problems. Worries about work, income, housing and family, to name but a few social factors, may develop and the nurse therefore needs to assess how the patient feels about these important areas.

Patient problems

The nurse plans the care of the patient in traction to prevent the potential problems listed in Table 24.3.

Nursing intervention

Infection at the pin sites
See care of pin sites (p. 835). While the pins are in place, they should remain static and the patient pain free. On removal, there should be no sign of infection and the pin sites should heal within a week.

General muscle wasting due to immobility
The following steps should be taken to minimize this problem:

● Encourage the patient to be as self-caring as possible within the confines of the traction. This will promote the

Table 24.3 Principal potential problems for the patient in traction

Potential patient problem	Goals
1. Infection at the pin site	The patient will not develop an infection at the pin sites
2. General muscle wasting due to immobility	The patient will not suffer muscle wasting in the uninjured limb and it will be minimal in the injured limb
3. Skin breakdown due to traction and immobility	The patient will not suffer any break in skin due to traction or immobility
4. Constipation due to immobility	The patient will be able to defaecate normally without feeling discomfort or requiring artificial stimuli
5. Urinary retention	The patient will be able to empty the bladder in comfort when the need is felt
6. Boredom and depression due to enforced immobility	The patient will develop ways of coping with the inevitable boredom and will be able to express any negative feelings that might occur

use of various muscle groups, particularly in the upper body, and may be more appealing to the patient than simply 'doing the exercises'

- Teach the patient to lift himself or herself up the bed on to a bedpan using an overhead monkey pole. This will strengthen the muscles of the arms and chest, which will help the patient to use crutches once mobilizing commences. It also helps to prevent skin breakdown due to friction caused by dragging on the sheets
- Commence a physiotherapy programme to ensure all muscle groups are put through a range of activities daily. The physiotherapist can identify muscles that are particularly at risk of atrophy and teach the patient the required specific exercises. The nurses and physiotherapist should work together with the patient to ensure the patient understands the exercises and the nurse can supervise them in the physiotherapist's absence. The aim is that, when the traction is removed, the patient's general musculature will be in good condition with minimal evidence of muscle wasting, enabling mobilization to commence.

Skin breakdown due to traction and immobility

Pressure sores are not inevitable and can be prevented. Frequent inspection of all vulnerable **skin** areas should be carried out for the first 48 hours.

- *Under the ring of the Thomas' splint.* When this is first applied, the skin is at special risk as the thigh may continue to swell and the circulation in the skin becomes compromised. By gently moving of the skin under the ring, the nurse can see the skin and also relieve any pressure. It is essential that all the skin under the ring is inspected. The patient may find this uncomfortable and unnecessary, and clear explanations are required beforehand. The use of padding under the ring is to be discouraged as it only creates pressure in other areas. If the ring appears to be getting tighter and the skin is in danger, the doctor should be informed and bolt cutters obtained in case the ring needs to be split and removed
- *In the popliteal area where slings may rub and the skin is vulnerable.* When a Pearson knee flexion piece is used, the knee will be partly flexed which increases the likelihood of rubbing. The skin should be protected from the rough sling by padding
- *Over the head of fibula.* Here the skin and peroneal nerve are at risk of pressure from the side of the splint. This is a particular problem if the leg falls into external rotation and rolls outward, resting on the side arm of the Thomas' splint. The patient's leg should be positioned in such a way that it rests centrally and any rotation is corrected by small pads. The use of a foot piece may also correct this malalignment
- *Over the Achilles tendon.* This is superficial and frequently damaged by pressure from the edge of the last sling. If a foot piece is not used and the heel is left free to hang over the edge of the last sling (thus avoiding the heel rubbing), the area that is then at most risk is the skin over

the Achilles tendon. If a sore develops the resultant injury to the Achilles tendon may mean further hospitalization and immobilization long after the original injury has healed

- *The back of the heel of the injured leg.* This should be free of the bed; if it is found to be lying on the bed, the balance weight suspending the Thomas' splint needs increasing, thus elevating the leg (helping to reduce swelling), making it easier for the patient to move and lifting the heel free
- *The back of the heel of the uninjured leg.* This is subject to friction on the bedding, particularly while the patient is learning to lift himself or herself free of the bed. If counterpanes are traditionally used at the bottom of traction beds they should be removed because they are very rough. Occasionally the use of sheepskin bootees may be called for but these are of use only if they are put on when the traction is first applied and if they are maintained in the correct position
- *Buttocks and sacrum.* These areas are at risk due to friction caused by the patient not being lifted properly or not lifting themselves properly. Shearing forces caused by the movement of muscle and bone under the skin may destroy the microcirculation to the skin and reduce the skin's viability. Unrelieved pressure is also a cause of skin breakdown in these areas. When patients are on traction it is very difficult to change their position so that their buttocks and sacrum are free from pressure. Simply asking the patient to lift themselves free of the bed for a short while and then replacing themselves in a slightly different position will help. Specialized mattresses may be used. The potential need should be recognized on admission and the patient either admitted on to the mattress or transferred on to it from theatre.
- *Elbows.* Even in young patients, elbows become quite sore from their use as 'body props'. To prevent this from occurring, patients must be well supported by pillows in a position that is comfortable but allows them access to their locker, books, etc.

After 48 hours the skin will still need to be inspected in all these areas at least twice a day. However, there should be much more patient involvement, with the patient being told exactly what to look for in the early signs of skin breakdown. For some patients, 48 hours is too early to start to take on this responsibility, but many patients are ready and will take a much more active interest in their progress if given this responsibility in these early days.

Constipation due to immobility

The following interventions should be applied to prevent problems with defaecation:

- Dehydration must be avoided; a fluid intake goal of 2 L/day may be set. If the general condition does not allow for this, an intravenous infusion may be required. If the patient is dehydrated in the first 24–48 hours, the faeces will become hard and painful to pass. This will make the patient reluctant to use a bedpan

- The patient must be given some privacy – somewhere where nobody else will be aware of the noises and odours that may result in attempts to defaecate
- Although hospital food is supposed to be high in fibre, the patient might be encouraged to ask any friends or family who visit to bring in fruit, fruit juice or bran-based breakfast cereals, especially in the first few days when the problem of constipation appears to be at its worst
- The nurse should ensure that using a bedpan is not a painful experience. Ideally, analgesia should be kept at an appropriate level from admission so that the patient will not equate moving with pain. If a patient is having difficulty opening the bowels, pain experienced due to being transferred to a bedpan will only make matters worse; the situation may be eased by the use of a slipper bedpan.

Urinary retention

The following interventions should reduce the risk of urinary retention and infection:

- Male patients find the horizontal position they may have to adopt (lying on their back with the foot of the bed elevated) much more difficult to cope with than females. The man should be regularly offered a urinal and told about the need to pass urine. In exceptional circumstances, the doctor may agree to lowering the foot of the bed to see whether that helps the patient to adopt a better position. However, as this may alter the fracture position, it should not be undertaken without written instructions. Occasionally the use of a sedative such as diazepam may be used to relax the patient, facilitating the passing of urine in these unnatural circumstances
- Catheterization should be seen as the last resort and the catheter should be removed straightaway. After a few days, passing urine usually becomes less of a problem, but the patient needs to be reminded to continue drinking to prevent dehydration and the renal complications of calculi and urinary tract infections.

Boredom and depression due to enforced immobility

To reduce the boredom of traction, the following interventions can be used:

- Ensure the patient has sufficient diversions such as books, radio, television, etc., to hand. These may help the patient to keep in touch with usual interests and activities
- The nurse should spend time listening to the patient and concentrate on what the patient is trying to say
- The nurse must recognize that there are times when it is more appropriate to call in other professionals, such as a social worker, counsellor or minister of religion during convalescence and rehabilitation.

Patients may from time to time feel depressed and unhappy but progress may be aided by the free expression of needs and fears. Once the patient begins to mobilize, the patient will probably be surprised and depressed by the weakness, joint stiffness and instability in the limb.

Appropriate passive, active and resistive exercises of the affected limb are introduced. These may be planned and supervised by a physiotherapist, but the nurse must be familiar with the plan so that the necessary assistance is provided when the therapist is not at the bedside. In the case of a lower limb, arm and shoulder exercises are continued to strengthen the upper limbs in preparation for the use of a walking frame or crutches. When weight-bearing is permitted, the person begins to relearn to walk using a walking frame, crutches or a walking stick. Firm, low-heeled, walking shoes, preferably with a non-skid rubber heel, should be worn.

The patient may need prompting to maintain an erect posture (avoid bending forward) and to increase the degree of flexion of the thigh and leg when raising a foot off the floor to take a step in order to overcome the tendency to shuffle. Most patients require a good deal of encouragement and reassurance from the nurse. Physical assistance and support are withdrawn gradually, but the nurse remains with the patient when getting in and out of bed or a chair until it is evident that he or she can safely manage alone.

A home assessment may be carried out before discharge to determine what barriers to access and mobility may exist and whether there is someone who will be at home to assist the patient. If the patient experiences difficulties with self-care or mobilizing, a referral may be made to the primary health team so that assistance and supervision will be available. Resumption of the former occupation and activities will depend on progress in relation to mobility and independence.

CARE OF THE PATIENT WITH INTERNAL (SURGICAL) FIXATION

Preoperative care

Internal fixation greatly speeds the recovery process and avoids many of the problems of immobility and bed rest discussed above. However, there may be complicating health problems associated with such surgery as well as the injuries it is seeking to repair. When the person has suffered fractures of the shaft of femur or pelvis hypovolaemic shock is likely. This should be treated in the A&E department by the use of plasma expanding agents and blood transfusion. By the time the patient is transferred to theatre the condition should be stabilized and the patient pronounced fit for anaesthesia.

How soon after injury the internal fixation occurs depends on factors such as the patient's general condition, the type of fracture, the position of the bone ends and the surgeon's preferences.

During the preoperative period, some temporary form of immobilization is applied to relieve pain or prevent the situation worsening. The injured limb should be handled as little as possible but the patient will need to use a bedpan and pressure area care, so some form of external splintage may be used, such as a vacuum splint, backslab or sandbags. Analgesia will need to be given and its effect monitored.

When elderly patients are awaiting surgery, the nurse must be aware of the psychological effects of the strange environment, the accident, pain, journey to hospital, and perhaps several hours of lying in the A&E department looking at the ceiling. The use of reality orientation should be employed to remind the patient exactly where he or she is, what has happened, and what is going to happen in the near future in order to prevent anxiety and confusion.

Before surgery, most patients will have an intravenous infusion started to correct any evidence of dehydration and provide access for drugs. Blood should be taken for biochemical analysis, grouping and cross-match should a transfusion be needed. A fluid balance chart should be started at the same time and all intake and output recorded. The patient's urine should be tested as soon as possible to detect any abnormalities such as bleeding into the urinary tract, particularly in patients who may have incurred even apparently minor pelvic injuries. Patients will need electrocardiography (ECG) if this was not done in the A&E department in order to ensure their cardiovascular system is fit for general anaesthesia and the stresses of surgery.

Postoperative care

Following internal fixation of fractures, the general principles of postoperative care are applicable, with the following additions.

Where surgery is performed on a limb, it should be elevated immediately. If a plaster cast has been applied, the patient's extremities should be examined for colour, sensation, warmth and movement every 30 minutes, to ensure there is no compromise of the circulation. The digits should be compared with those on the uninjured side and if any difference is observed the nurse in charge should be informed immediately. Sometimes the situation can be relieved by elevating the limb higher, thus reducing the swelling, but more often than not the plaster will need to be split to allow some expansion. If a backslab has been applied the cotton bandages will need cutting down to skin, especially if there has been some haemorrhage, as blood-soaked bandages are notoriously harsh: they do not 'give' and may act as a tourniquet. Any blood staining on a plaster should be outlined after the first couple of hours so that continued bleeding can be monitored.

Where a plaster cast has not been applied, the circulation to and sensation of the limb distal to the operative site should be monitored to ensure no damage was incurred during the operation or before surgery while the limb was splinted.

All wound drains should be inspected regularly and changed as required. The amount of drainage should be entered on the patient's fluid balance chart. Drains are removed when they have stopped draining, usually after 48 hours.

The patient may be allowed out of bed but, in the case of surgery on a lower extremity, there must be clear instructions from the surgeon concerning the period before weight-bearing can commence. Mobility can be facilitated by the use of a wheelchair and crutches. When sitting, provision is made for elevation and support of the affected limb. Precautions against pressure sores and slumping posture are necessary when the patient is allowed up in a chair for long periods. Skin care is provided at regular intervals and patients are taught to shift the weight frequently so that no one area is subjected to continuous pressure. Adjustments may also be necessary to avoid prolonged pressure on the popliteal area of the unaffected, dependent leg and to prevent forward sagging of the shoulders.

Exercises of the affected part are started as soon as the surgeon permits. They may be limited to isometric contractions for a period, followed by the gradual introduction of passive and active movements and resistive exercises. In the case of a lower extremity, weight-bearing is guided by radiographic indications of satisfactory healing. The overambitious patient is cautioned not to attempt standing or walking without the assistance of a physiotherapist or nurse. The patient should have a firm, non-skid pair of shoes and be assisted first to stand. The physiotherapist or nurse stands facing the patient and places the hands to the sides of the patient's lower chest. The patient is encouraged to stand erect, knees extended and head up. When sure of balancing in the upright position, the patient is then assisted with the next step, which may be the use of crutches, a walking frame or simply walking with only the assistance of one person. Support is given to the affected side.

TREATMENT AND NURSING CARE REQUIRED FOR SPECIFIC INJURIES

Below, a brief summary is provided of the more common injuries, their treatment and the nursing care required.

FRACTURES OF THE NECK OF FEMUR

Fracture of the neck of femur occurs most often in elderly women, due in part to hormonal changes and the effect this has on bone reabsorption, leading to osteoporosis (see p. 871). The weakened bone is less able to resist the force of impact should the person fall, especially if they land on the trochanteric region, resulting in a femoral neck fracture. Elderly people are much more likely to fall. Cox and Newton (2005) cite data suggesting in excess of 400 000 older people attend A&E each year in the UK as a result of falls which are the leading cause of mortality due to injury in those over 75. This follows from the fact that falls in older people are estimated to result in a hip fracture in approximately one-quarter of those affected (Minns et al 2004), indicating that preventing falls could also prevent much morbidity and mortality in our ageing population. There are two categories of fractures involving the femoral neck region (Fig. 24.11):

- *Intracapsular fractures* occur through the joint and capsule and include subcapital fractures, transcervical fractures and impacted fractures at the base of the neck of femur

● *Extracapsular fractures* may involve either the greater or lesser trochanter or the intertrochanteric area. These are called intertrochanteric (across the base of the femoral neck) or pertrochanteric (through the trochanter) fractures.

Assessment

The initial assessment in A&E should focus on how much pain the patient is experiencing. The affected leg should be gently and carefully examined. Tenderness around the femoral neck is usually present and there is often shortening and external rotation. Occasionally a patient may continue walking on an *undisplaced* fracture, although in considerable pain. The rest of the patient should be assessed for other injuries sustained at the same time. Such are the effects of ageing that the nurse should also be alert to other pathological processes that may co-exist. It is important therefore to screen for hypothermia (especially in winter), diabetes (possibly undiagnosed) or any signs of cardiovascular disorder. Such information is essential for correct triage and nursing care in A&E.

Other important information concerns the patient's general condition, whether he or she looks well cared for or neglected, and the state of the skin. This is a group of patients at high risk for pressure sore development. Many departments now have a fast track policy aimed at admitting elderly patients with fractures of the neck of femur to a ward bed within 1 hour in recognition of the special problems faced by this group of patients, such as pressure sore development. Vital information about home circumstances is available from the ambulance crew in A&E that may not be available to the ward staff. The patient's orientation and understanding of the situation should also be assessed as confusion may develop speedily.

While the surgeon may carry out a technically correct repair to the fracture site, the patient's long-term prognosis may depend far more on skilled nursing care to prevent complications such as pressure sores, constipation, chest infections or confusion, and on the resolution of social problems.

The patient's nutritional status should be assessed, as poor nutritional status (a common problem in older people) will delay healing and limit recovery.

The principles outlined above, of assessing not only the obvious injury but also the rest of the patient, of checking for co-existing health problems, assessing the patient's psychological status and exploring social factors, apply equally to all A&E patients.

General principles of treatment

Surgical reduction and fixation of the joint is the treatment of choice. Elderly patients cannot survive the complications of prolonged bed rest and immobility and paradoxically, the worse the patient's general health upon admission, the more urgent is the need for surgery due to the adverse effects of immobility. As a student, you may be surprised at surgeons taking very frail and unwell elderly patients to theatre within 24 hours of their fall; however, their condition will only deteriorate further if they are not at least given the chance of surgery. A variety of metal nails, plates and screws may be used for internal fixation.

Intracapsular fractures are highly likely to damage the blood supply to the head of the femur if there is any displacement at the fracture site (Fig. 24.11). If there is no displacement and it is thought the head will survive, two or three cannulated screws are inserted in a relatively simple operation. However, if there is any displacement the femoral head will need to be removed and replaced with a prosthesis. In extracapsular fractures, head viability is not a problem and a fixation device such as a compression screw plate is used to hold the fragments. Older patients with co-existing medical problems may not be fit for a general anaesthetic so surgery may be performed under spinal anaesthesia if necessary.

After 48 hours, following a check radiograph and the removal of any wound drains (provided they have stopped draining), the patient should be able to mobilize. The amount of weight bearing allowed depends on the severity of the fracture, the precision with which the bone fragments are held by the fixation, and the ability of the patient to understand how much weight can be taken by the injured leg.

Nursing care for patients who have had a prosthesis inserted is much the same as that following a total hip replacement. Local protocols designed to prevent hip prosthesis dislocation should always be followed.

Good pain control is essential and patient-controlled analgesia (PCA) is used if the patient is able to manage a PCA pump. Apart from the continuing risk of pressure sore development, other major potential postoperative complications include dehydration, constipation, confusion and deep venous thrombosis.

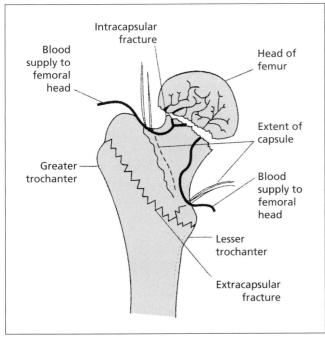

Figure 24.11 Intracapsular and extracapsular fractures of the neck of femur.

Blood supply to femoral head

Intracapsular fracture

Head of femur

Extent of capsule

Greater trochanter

Blood supply to femoral head

Lesser trochanter

Extracapsular fracture

A multidisciplinary rehabilitation process should begin immediately after operation so that the patient has the best chance of maximum recovery. About 50% of patients suffering this injury lose the ability to live independently (Prodigy 2005). A major Canadian study found that increased risk of institutionalization was directly related to poor mental functioning in hospital and that the risk was four times greater in men than women (Cree 2000). This latter finding is an example of the influence of social factors on health. The study also found that each increase in age by 10 years was associated with an increased risk of institutionalization by a factor of 2.5.

Much interest has centred on the use of multidisciplinary care pathways in this group of patients (see p. 10). Choong et al (2000) compared the progress of 55 patients who were on a pathway with 56 who were not. There were no significant differences between the patients initially (e.g. mean age 84 and 82, respectively) but the pathway group had a mean total length of stay of 6.6 days compared with 8 days for the control group. This suggests that an integrated care pathway approach has contributed to reducing inpatient stay by 21%. Commenting on this research, Swanson et al (2000) noted that those patients who benefited most from the pathway approach were the most frail and elderly. However, as they observed, community services have to be fully involved in coping with the accelerated throughput of such elderly patients that may result from pathway use.

A recent study visit (2005) by one of the authors to North America included the opportunity to see such pathways in action at St Paul's Hospital, Vancouver, where they had been designed by Faith Forster (Acute Care Nurse Practitioner) and her colleagues. Patient care was managed by a reference pathway which outlined the daily tasks necessary to reach the required patient outcomes in the following areas:

- treatments
- assessments
- diagnostics
- consults
- nutrition
- activity
- teaching and discharge planning.

The major goals for the pathway are that:

1 the patient returns to their previous levels of functioning (physically, mentally and socially) and if admitted from home, will return to home
2 the acute ward stay will be 6 days before transfer to a rehabilitation unit
3 no pressure ulcers will develop
4 the patient will achieve the activity goals set in the pathway, especially that they will be able to pivot transfer to a chair on postoperative day 1 and will have started physiotherapy by day 2.

The pathway ran from the preoperative admission day to the 6th postoperative day. All the multidisciplinary team use this documentation except the doctors who continue to use their traditional progress notes. Patients and family have their own version of the pathway so they can assess progress and keep informed. A key aspect is variance charting to check whether there are deviations from the pathway and this is focussed on the following care categories:

- pain
- cognition
- elimination
- skin
- nutrition
- activity
- vital signs
- teaching
- any other concerns not documented above.

These care areas are checked and signed for three times daily with clear goals set for patient progress under the areas on each day the patient is on the ward. A combination of this pathway and two excellent acute care nurse practitioners managing it with the cooperation of all members of staff, has certainly produced impressive results for this group of patients, at least as far as can be judged from a 1 day visit.

In view of the high levels of mortality and morbidity associated with hip fractures, there has been much interest recently in the use of hip protectors for older people. They are designed to be worn over the greater trochanter and lessen the impact in the event of a fall. Minns et al (2004) present a detailed account of the use of hip protectors including the results of laboratory trials on a specially designed impact testing rig. Six different commercially available designs were tested and two transmitted such force to the bone that fractures were still possible while the other four pads reduced the transmitted force to an average of 0.5 kN compared with an impact force of 3.5 kN. In other words, a person not wearing a pad would experience approximately seven times the force on impact if they fell compared with a person wearing an effective pad. This degree of protection is lost, however, if the pad is incorrectly placed. The researchers were also concerned by the high interface pressures between skin and pad during wear while lying on the hip and the threat this posed to tissue viability. A skin/mattress interface pressure of 60 mmHg is considered to be the maximum compatible with healthy undamaged skin but most of these pads produced much higher values in the region of 250 mmHg. Over a period of time, therefore, tissue damage is likely. Their use during sleep and bed rest is therefore placing the patient at risk of pressure sore formation in the hip regions.

Given these findings, we should ask what difference do hip protectors make to real people in real life, as opposed to artificial testing in a laboratory? The findings are not encouraging. Parker et al (2004) analyzed data from 14 trials involving 11 018 elderly patients to see if wearing hip protectors made a significant difference to the incidence of hip and pelvic fractures. The trials were split into two groups methodologically and whilst the weaker methodology (five trials) showed a slight improvement in fracture rates which was statistically significant, the second group of nine more rigorous trials showed no statistically significant improvement. This further weakens the arguments in favour of their use and Griffiths (2005) notes that there is little to justify their use except in further carefully controlled, rigorous clinical trials. As Griffiths observes, nurses would do better to concentrate their efforts on preventing falls in older people in the first place. Cox and Newton (2005) offer just such an example in the development of an integrated falls service in a day hospital setting. This service brought together the expertise of physiotherapists and occupational therapists, together with nurses, to tackle the problem from a falls prevention perspective. Cox and Newton report significant improvements in both patient mobility and confidence as a result.

FRACTURES OF THE SHAFT OF FEMUR

The causes of and consequently the group of patients associated, with this type of fracture differ considerably from those suffering a fractured neck of femur. It is caused by high-energy trauma, frequently a road traffic accident, and often involves men in the 16–35-year age group.

Anatomically these fractures range from the subtrochanteric region in the proximal third of the femur, through midshaft fractures, to supracondylar fractures in the distal third. The fractures are often spiral, with at least three fragments, due to a twisting injury, but direct trauma usually results in the more manageable transverse fracture.

Complications

The major complications which may result from fractures of the shaft of femur are the following:

- *Hypovolaemic shock*. Even when there is no obvious sign of haemorrhage a litre of blood can be contained within the thigh from a fracture of the shaft of femur
- *Damage to the femoral artery*, often a tear from a sharp bone fragment
- *Damage to the femoral nerve*, again from a sharp fragment
- Following an open comminuted fracture, *loss of bone fragment* at the scene of the accident. This will lead to a shortening of the limb. Occasionally the fragment may be found and used in the treatment
- *Fat emboli*. Fat embolism refers to a condition seen sometimes after fracture of the femoral shaft. The patient develops confusion, fever, tachycardia and respiratory distress within 72 hours of injury and is found to have multiple fat emboli affecting the lung fields. It is a life-threatening condition and is thought to be associated with a range of other post traumatic respiratory problems. Solomon et al (2005) observes that the source of the fat emboli is most likely to be the marrow of the fractured bone and urges careful monitoring of PO_2 levels as a drop to below 8 kPa is a common finding in these situations. Oxygen therapy

is essential together with corticosteroids and heparin to reduce pulmonary oedema and intravascular clotting, respectively.

Treatment

The treatment for fractured shaft of femur depends on the severity and position of the fracture and how well callus formation takes place. In most cases, the patient is initially nursed in skeletal traction until the callus is seen on radiography and the fracture is in an acceptable position. Intramedullary nailing is then the standard treatment and acts as an internal splint. It is inserted the length of the femur along the medullary canal.

Once the wound drains have been removed and the check radiograph shows a satisfactory position, the patient is usually allowed to commence mobilizing either partially or non-weight-bearing using crutches. The patient will require a programme of exercises, particularly static exercising of the quadriceps, to ensure the retention or building up of the quadriceps muscles. The physiotherapist will also gradually introduce knee flexion, although this may be limited in the early stages of rehabilitation.

Once the patient is confident on crutches, he or she may be discharged, although an appointment will be required for the removal of stitches and follow-up in the outpatient department. Before discharge, patients should be reminded that, if the leg suddenly becomes painful or swollen or the wound becomes red and inflamed, they should telephone the orthopaedic outpatient clinic (giving the name of the consultant concerned) or, if out of clinic hours, attend A&E. All internal fixation carries a risk of infection which should be treated aggressively at the first indication.

FRACTURES OF THE TIBIA

Tibial fractures are classified according to whether they are open or closed, their position, and the degree of displacement at the fracture site. Fractures of the fibula are not considered separately as the treatment is usually in association with that of the tibia. Isolated fractures of the fibula with no tibial involvement are relatively minor and are treated in the A&E department.

Tibial plateau fracture

Although this frequently appears to be a minor fracture, it always involves the articular surface and therefore potentially can cause serious disruption to knee function. Treatment is therefore geared towards function and restoring knee movement.

If the fracture is depressed, the patient will require elevation of the fragment under general anaesthesia to restore the joint surface. Any displacement of the fracture will require internal fixation. After operation, the priority is to encourage a rapid recovery of the normal range of movement of the knee. Until recently, continuous passive movement (CPM) machines have been extensively used. However, Black and Hawks (2005) cite compelling evidence which fails to find any significant advantages in the use of these machines when compared with encouragement towards active exercise and good physiotherapy.

Tibial shaft fractures

These fractures vary from the undisplaced, closed fracture which is treated with an above-knee plaster of Paris cast in the A&E department, to the open, grossly contaminated, displaced comminuted fracture seen following a severe road traffic accident. As tibial fractures, particularly in the middle to lower third, have a reputation for poor healing, if the fracture is open, the problem of infection has to be considered very quickly. The problem of soft-tissue swelling and fracture shape frequently make the use of plaster of Paris unacceptable. The alternatives in regular use are intramedullary nailing, external fixators, which allow nursing access to any wounds while holding the fracture position, open reduction and internal fixation using a compression plate.

Specific patient problems

The specific problems that patients with these fractures may develop include the following:

- *Gross infection.* The patient will require diligent observation of temperature, pulse and respiration 4-hourly, until all the wounds are healed
- *Poor healing rate.* A close observation of pedal pulses must be made to ensure adequate perfusion of the lower leg. Excessive soft-tissue damage may produce swelling, leading to compartment syndrome in which the muscle fasciae of the three compartments in the lower leg come under intense pressure, eventually compromising the major arteries. This situation requires prompt action; usually fasciotomies are performed in theatre to relieve the pressure and restore an adequate blood supply
- *Knee and ankle stiffness.* The physiotherapist and the nurse are responsible for ensuring that the patient's range of movements in these joints are kept at an optimum. Ankle stiffness will add considerably to the patient's mobilization problems when the fracture is united
- *Problems from the pin sites.* These were discussed above (see p. 835).

Fractures of the malleoli

These are usually the result of a twisting injury from stepping on to uneven ground. To understand the mechanism of the injury the nurse needs to know the anatomy of the ankle joint (Fig. 24.12). The talus is held in a box-like structure, with three sides provided by the lateral malleolus of the fibula and the medial and posterior malleoli of the tibia. If the leg is held straight and the foot forced to twist, the displacement of the talus may break off one, two or three of the malleoli. In a more severe injury, two or even all 3 malleoli are involved this is referred to as a bimalleolar or trimalleolar fracture.

If the fracture is displaced, patients are usually admitted for open reduction and internal fixation. Swelling is usually

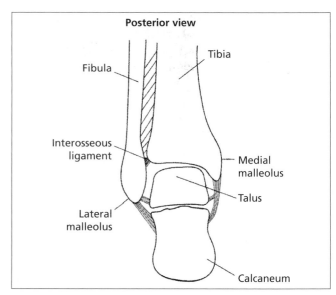

Figure 24.12 The anatomy of the ankle joint.

severe and if the injury is not fixed rapidly, surgery may have to be deferred, until the swelling has subsided several days later, due to skin-closure problems. Internal fixation usually involves the use of screws and possibly a plate to stabilize the fibula if required. After surgery, the lower leg will be immobilized in a cast. An undisplaced single malleolar fracture (usually the lateral malleolus) is managed conservatively in a POP cast. The nature of the injury and its treatment will determine the length of time the cast remains and the delay before partial weight bearing on crutches is allowed.

The Ottawa Ankle Rules (Stiell 1992) are a widely used set of rules which guide the practitioner's decision-making, in light of clinical findings, concerning whether to order radiographs or not (see Case Study 24.1).

CASE Elaine was a 56-year-old office worker, wheeled into the A&E Department in a wheelchair by her son one Sunday morning. She had fallen down the last two steps of the staircase at home at 6 p.m. the previous night after finishing off cleaning the stair with a vacuum cleaner. It had been really painful and when she tried to stand up she could not weight bear. She had hobbled to the settee and sat there with her leg up on some cushions while waiting for her husband and son to come home from a football match. While waiting, she rang her neighbour as it was so painful. She had given her 2 paracetamol and a bag of frozen peas from the freezer to put on her ankle and wanted to dial an ambulance. However, Elaine was having none of it, 'I want to be here when they get home or else David (her husband) will panic', she had said.

Elaine's husband and son eventually arrived home at 7.30 p.m. and wanted to take Elaine to the A&E. However, she was reluctant as she didn't want to cause a fuss and she did not want to be in A&E on a Saturday night because of everything she had heard about violent drunks in A&E. She asked them to leave it until Sunday morning and so they did.

On that Sunday morning, her son Brian duly took her to A&E where she was seen initially by the triage nurse who sent her on to the nurse practitioner for detailed assessment. The NP took a full history of the accident. She carefully established the exact position of the foot, the mechanism of injury and the force involved when Elaine fell. She got Elaine to demonstrate the movement of her foot with her uninjured foot and noted carefully the phrase 'turn inwards' used by Elaine. It looked like there had been a major stress placed on her lateral ligaments which if they had been torn, would lead to instability in the ankle, whether there was a fracture of the lateral malleolus or not. The NP also took a focused medical history which revealed no other serious medical problems or significant family history. Elaine was not on any regular medication and had no allergies that she knew of. She was a non-smoker and a light social drinker consuming around 5–6 units a week.

The physical examination revealed swelling and some bruising around the right ankle and foot. This was all the more obvious when compared with the other ankle as a reference. Her injured ankle also felt warmer than the uninjured ankle, indicating increased blood supply and vasodilation, classic signs of trauma and inflammation. The NP now began to palpate down from the head of the fibula towards the injured area, aiming for the most likely site of the fracture last, to cause minimum distress. The posterior aspect of the lateral malleolus was very tender upon palpation raising the real possibility of a fracture. Elaine confirmed she had had little sleep because of the pain which she now rated as 7 out of 10 and she was still unable to weight-bear.

She was asked to demonstrate her range of active movements on her uninjured ankle (reference) which were normal and then on her injured ankle which were severely restricted. Soft-tissue injury is sufficient to restrict range of movement, in addition to bony injury.

The A&E department used the widely accepted Ottawa ankle rules to determine suitability for X-ray. They state an X-ray should be performed if any one of the following is present:

1 Bony tenderness along the posterior edge of the lower 6 cm of the fibula or tip of the lateral malleolus.
2 Bony tenderness along the posterior edge of the lower 6 cm of the tibia or medial malleolus
3 Inability to weight-bear immediately after injury and in A&E.

Elaine had two out of the three clinical signs and so needed radiography (anteroposterior and lateral views). While she was waiting, she was given paracetamol and an NSAID under a patient group directive to achieve analgesia. The X-ray revealed a transverse fracture through the lateral malleolus but no evidence of disruption of the joint due to ligament rupture. The injury was therefore stable and could be managed conservatively with a non-weight-bearing below knee POP backslab and a referral to see the orthopedic specialist the following morning. Patient teaching concerning the importance of rest and elevation to reduce swelling were given along with a sheet of printed instructions to reinforce the points made. Elaine was also taught about the importance of checking the warmth, sensation and colour of her injured foot compared with the uninjured to ensure their was no neurovascular compromise. The department also checked to ensure she could manage at home and gave her a supply of NSAIDs to go with the paracetamol she had at home.

(This patient is based on a case study presented by Hubble 2005.)

Specific patient problems

The specific problems following surgery to the ankle are the following:

- *Risk of infection.* The patient may have two wounds so the risk of infection is doubled. If the fracture was open, the chances of infection are also increased. If it was initially a closed fracture, it has now effectively been converted to an open fracture
- *Circulatory compromise* due to swelling. On return to the ward, the patient's leg should be elevated well above the level of the heart. Circulatory observations should be performed half-hourly for at least the first 12 hours; these should include pedal pulses if possible. Some surgeons use plaster of Paris following internal fixation, especially in severe fractures where it is considered that the fixation is less than perfect. Sometimes the patient will simply have wool and a crêpe bandage around the wounds. If there is a plaster cast, it should be split to allow for swelling
- *Wound drains*, which require attention to ensure their patency is maintained. These should be changed as required until the wound(s) stop draining. Any drainage stains on the plaster should be outlined 4-hourly so that loss can be monitored.

FRACTURES OF THE CALCANEUM

These fractures are the result of jumping or falling from a height and landing on the feet. Spinal fractures may commonly occur at the same time. In the absence of displacement, the treatment remains admission, high elevation and ice packs to reduce the tremendous swelling that can result. Internal fixation may be required for displaced fractures.

Specific patient problems

This injury is often seen following an unsuccessful attempt to commit suicide. The result is that the patient has both the physical discomfort of two very painful heels and the emotional trauma of still being alive and facing the problems that prompted the suicide attempt, and also having to face the world in the knowledge of the failure of the attempt. The nurse must be able to care for such patients with empathy, being non-judgemental and recognizing the need to bring in other professionals and take their advice on care.

Ankle stiffness is a common problem. As soon as the swelling starts to subside, the physiotherapist and nurse must outline a programme to improve the patient's ankle movement. At first, this may be mainly passive movement but will gradually progress to include more active exercises.

FRACTURES OF THE PELVIS

The pelvis is a ring of bone and fractures that can be broadly classified as those which break that ring potentially causing instability, or those which leave it intact, involving isolated fractures. Fractures of the pelvic ring are more serious, especially if unstable. Such an injury indicates a great deal of energy was involved and raises the real possibility of serious injury to other pelvic organs. Because of the difficulty in making exact diagnoses in some parts of the pelvis, the patient may require a CT scan to augment the radiographs. This should not however delay urgent treatment, as major blood loss may occur. As the function of the pelvis is to protect key internal organs, when it is fractured there is a high risk of damage to the bowel, bladder and urethra. Also in danger are the abdominal aorta and internal iliac arteries.

In displaced, open and complicated fractures, the patient usually requires open reduction and application of an external fixation device. Some parts of the pelvis may also be fixed with a small plate and screws. This can be performed only once the general condition has been stabilized and any bleeding blood vessels repaired.

Undisplaced fractures, such as those sustained by the elderly when they fall and 'sit down', resulting in fractures of the pubic rami, are treated by a short period of bedrest, analgesia and early mobilization. Often, there is little visible damage, but after 2–3 days, the bruising starts to show and the whole of the perineum may turn purple.

Injuries resulting in diastasis at the symphysis pubis may be treated by nursing the patient on slings that cross over the front of the pelvis, pulling the pelvis into shape.

Specific patient problems

The following problems commonly affect patients with fractures of the pelvis:

- *Pin sites.* The care required for these is slightly different as very often, there are more than one inserted in adjacent bone. Instead of a puncture in the skin there may be a slash of 2–4 cm which will require regular dressings to prevent infection
- *Bladder and/or urethral involvement.* All urine passed should be tested for haematuria for at least 24 hours or until it has been clear for 24 hours. A suprapubic catheter may be inserted to keep the bladder empty until it has healed and the risk of chemical peritonitis has subsided
- *Bowel involvement.* Rupture of any part of the intestinal tract introduces the risk of peritonitis from spillage of the bowel contents into the peritoneum. Signs such as abdominal pain, pyrexia and shock indicate this complication may have occurred
- *Implications for childbearing in females.* In females of childbearing age, injuries to the pelvis carry with them the risk of creating the inability to carry a fetus to full term. Thus, every effort must be made to restore the anatomical position of the pelvis. The situation must be discussed with the patient, who should be examined by an obstetrician.

This would be an opportunity for these problems to be aired and may provide the patient with some comfort
- *Neurological problems.* These mainly affect the sacral plexus and the sciatic nerve. Such damage is recognized by absent plantar flexion and ankle jerk. However, the damage is usually only a temporary result of bruising and stretching of the nerves rather than any more permanent damage.

Fractures of the *acetabulum* are technically pelvic fractures though rather different from those discussed so far. They are usually caused by indirect violence driving the head of the femur through the acetabulum such as may occur when a knee strikes the dashboard of a car in a high speed road accident. The head of the femur needs initially to be held out of the acetabulum by traction. Surgical reconstruction of the joint may be needed to try and prevent osteoarthritis developing subsequently, especially in a young patient.

FRACTURES OF THE NECK OF HUMERUS

These injuries are usually seen in older osteoporotic patients who have fallen on an outstretched hand. Extensive bruising develops over the upper arm a day or so later and is a key sign to look for in any older person reporting a fall. Attention tends to focus on the wrist as people assume a Colles fracture; a careful patient history will, however, indicate a painful shoulder and gentle undressing reveal the tell-tale bruising. Impacted fractures with little or no displacement are treated symptomatically, using the support of a collar and cuff sling until the pain starts to subside, and then encouraging movement. Movement should be introduced gradually; this is often limited and follow-up physiotherapy is usually required.

Comminuted and grossly displaced fractures of the neck of humerus (in elderly patients) require surgery and a replacement prosthesis is inserted to replace the head of the humerus due to the risk of avascular necrosis.

Specific patient problems

Patients with undisplaced or minimally displaced fractures are treated in the A&E department. More serious fractures may result in any of the following problems:

- *Injury to the brachial plexus.* As well as circulatory observations, sensation and motor function of the affected hand should be observed because stretching of the nerve plexus at the time of the accident or during operation may occur. Usually this is only temporary; nevertheless it must be monitored in case it is of a more serious nature
- *Avascular necrosis of head of humerus.* This is not common in comminuted fractures
- *Arterial obstruction.* Occasionally, a displaced bone fragment may cause occlusion of the axillary artery. This usually resolves following reduction of the fracture. Circulatory observations of the hand (including a radial pulse) must be performed half-hourly for at least the first 12 hours after operation

- *Maintenance of the position of the hand and arm after surgery.* The patient may have a collar and cuff sling, with or without a body bandage, after operation. The nurse should ensure both are comfortable, not rubbing, and are providing the support required
- *Joint stiffness.* This is a particular problem with the elderly and, left untreated, quickly leads to loss of independence even when the fracture has united. The importance of performing exercises prescribed by the physiotherapist cannot be overemphasized.

FRACTURES OF THE SHAFT OF HUMERUS

Humoral fractures may be the result of indirect violence such as falling on an outstretched hand, or direct violence such as falling on the side. They may be open or closed fractures, although open fractures are mainly found in those involving the middle third of the humerus. Conservative treatment of such fractures involves reduction of the fracture under sedation or general anaesthesia (if necessary) and the application of a hanging 'U' slab as a temporary measure to allow for swelling. The patient will require a broad arm sling under the clothes for support. An above-elbow plaster is subsequently applied with the elbow at right angles, a collar and cuff sling should be applied as the weight of the plaster is designed to act as traction on the fractured shaft. Occasionally internal fixation using an intramedullary nail or plate may be performed.

A particular problem in children is a tendency for the fracture to occur in the supracondylar region of the humerus and this tends to occur most often in the age range 4–8 years. Any child presenting with a history of a fall onto an outstretched hand and a painful elbow should be prioritized for treatment as this injury can cause serious neurovascular complications. The radial pulse should always be assessed to ensure the brachial artery has not been compromised (Platt 2004).

Specific patient problems

The following problems may occur in fractures of the humerus:

- *Radial nerve palsy.* This is recognized by a drop wrist and sensory loss on the back of the hand between the thumb and index finger
- *Non-union due to loss of position.* To prevent this, the nurse must be vigilant in ensuring that the correct sling is worn and that it is providing the correct support. This may be difficult if the patient is unable to get out of bed and sit upright. Careful explanations of the rationale for care should be given to the patient and repeated as frequently as necessary.

FRACTURES OF THE WRIST

Colles fractures are probably one of the most common fractures the nurse is likely to encounter. Most are dealt with in the A&E department. They are usually the result of falling on an outstretched hand, particularly in the elderly. The displacement of the radius leads to the 'dinner fork' deformity when the wrist is viewed laterally. The fracture is often reduced under haematoma block, carried out by infiltration of the fracture haematoma with 1% lignocaine (Summers 2005). A below-elbow backslab is then applied. This is completed when the medical staff are sure that the inevitable swelling is receding and that finger movement is good, usually up to a week later. The Bier's block is an alternative form of regional anaesthesia which may be used to facilitate reduction.

Specific patient problems

The following problems may occur after a Colles fracture:

- *Stiffness and swelling of the fingers.* All jewellery, including wedding rings, should be removed as soon after the accident as possible. Finger exercises should be taught, and a leaflet with a description of the exercises and information on who to contact if the fingers suddenly swell or movement becomes more difficult should be supplied
- *Carpal tunnel syndrome.* This is caused by median nerve compression in the wrist and is recognized by paraesthesia over the anterior aspect of the thumb, index and second finger, and half the ring finger. Surgical decompression is required
- *Loss of independence.* As this fracture frequently occurs in the elderly, the nurse must ensure that the patient will be able to manage alone or has someone to help. For many old people, adapting to changes in circumstances takes a long time and 'young' hospital staff are in danger of dismissing the difficulty that such patients encounter in coping with relatively minor fractures
- *Other complications* include Sudek's atrophy (decalcification of bone and swelling, stiffness of the wrist) mal-union (fracture heals in an abnormal position) and osteoarthritis due to damage of the joint surfaces. (See Case Study 24.2 for an example of a patient who suffers a Colle's fracture)

CASE Shareen is a recently retired 62-year-old teacher who was putting her rubbish out for the dustbin collectors one icy January morning. She slipped on the ice and tried to break her fall by putting out her left hand. She heard a snapping sound and felt immediate severe pain in her wrist. She found herself sitting on the path leaning against a wall and realized she had badly hurt her right wrist. She was able to lift her left wrist with her right hand and place her left arm across her lap. Fortunately, she did not hit her head against anything when she fell. Her next door neighbour had heard her cry out when she fell and quickly came to the scene. She helped Shareen into her own car and drove her to A&E, which was 6 miles away and then helped her into the waiting room. She was triaged as in need of urgent care, because of her severe pain and distress.

What would your priorities be if you were assigned to her care?

Observation of the hand and wrist reveals that the skin is a normal colour and feels the same temperature as the other hand (What is that telling you?). You notice a marked deformity and angulation, strongly suggestive of a Colles' fracture. (What is the immediate significance of the obvious deformity and fracture displacement?)

This is a good time to assess the neurovascular state of her hand, has she has normal capillary refill after blanching (under 2 seconds when the tip of her finger is squeezed)? Can she feel you touching all the fingers on her affected hand? Apart from the pain, are there any other unusual sensations. The deformity, apart from being a potential cause of neurovascular problems, indicates she will probably need reduction of the fracture. This does not usually need a general anaesthetic; however, it is a wise precaution to keep her 'nil by mouth', especially as she may become nauseated in response to the opioid analgesic she will probably receive.

You should be assessing her pain score now, which is 8 on a 10 point scale. So now you need to relieve her pain by:

1 supporting the arm with a broad arm sling and pillow to rest the arm on
2 giving her some Entonox gas as a temporary analgesic, but remember she will need to breathe it steadily for 2–3 minutes to get maximum relief
3 arranging for opioid analgesia such as a carefully titrated dose of i.v. morphine which is administered via an i.v. cannula which is heparinized and secured *in situ*.

Now you need to find out exactly what happened to be sure there are no other injuries such as a head or neck injury. You check whether she has any other serious medical problems such as diabetes or hypertension, fortunately she has not. You should also check who she lives with, as there may be a dependent relative at home. Shareen is actually a widow with two grown up children who live nearby so you should contact one of them. Her daughter Alison is able to come over to the A&E at once. As Shareen lives alone, do check whether the house was secured before she left; fortunately her neighbour locked up for her.

While medical staff are completing the paperwork for wrist radiography you could be doing a base line set of vital signs to make sure they are all within normal limits. Examination of her injured wrist and hand reveals she still has her wedding and engagement rings on her ring finger, which is swelling up considerably. These need to be removed immediately as they may act as a tourniquet and endanger the viability of the digit. Unfortunately, they cannot be removed which leaves staff no choice but to cut them off. This causes Shareen considerable distress for, as she tells you, those rings have never been off that finger for 37 years. Tact and understanding is needed to use the ring cutter swiftly and painlessly, the rings can be secured in her handbag and she can be reassured that a good jeweller will restore the rings completely.

Shareen should then be accompanied to the radiography department; in view of the fact that she has received i.v. opioid analgesia, any signs of respiratory depression should be reported immediately. You return with the radiographs and Shareen. They show a comminuted fracture of the distal radius with dorsal displacement and some radial angulation.

This means the far end of the radius (distal) has fractured into several pieces (comminuted) and the hand is now displaced backwards relative to the forearm if she was standing in the anatomical position (dorsal displacement) with also some shift of the hand towards the radial (thumb) side of the wrist so that it no longer makes the normal straight alignment with the forearm (radial angulation). Clearly, this needs reduction under hematoma block and plastering with a backslab to hold the fracture in position overnight whilst allowing room for further swelling. This should all be carefully explained to Shareen and her consent sought to this procedure. You notice she is very reluctant to agree, remaining tearful and distressed. What should you do?

Stay with her.

Your presence is therapeutic, perhaps enquire if anything else is distressing her besides the pain and shock of the injury. That is when she tells you it is only 3 months since her husband collapsed and died after being admitted through this A&E unit to the coronary care unit upstairs. 'It brings it all back ...' she sobs and you offer her some tissues and lay a gentle hand on her shoulder, while pulling the curtain across the cubicle to giver her grief some privacy.

While the orthopaedic surgeons are preparing to undertake this procedure in A&E, Shareen's daughter Ali arrives and she is very anxious and worried about her mum. She hurries into the cubicle. You ask if they want to be left alone and Shareen says no, 'Please stay, it's comforting, I was just telling her about Bill, she says to her daughter.

Other staff then arrive and take her through to the treatment room, you accompany her and watch the experienced staff administer the haematoma block, wait until it has taken good effect, distract (pull apart the bone ends), correct (reverse the deformity) and manipulate the wrist into slight ulnar deviation to correct for the radial deviation caused by the fracture. A POP backslab is expertly applied and a very relieved Shareen is taken off to radiography again for check radiographs to ensure fracture reduction has been correctly carried out. Your job is to ensure elevation of her hand and observe for good colour, warmth and lack of abnormal sensation.

Arrangements now need to be made for discharge and Shareen is relieved when her daughter says 'Come home with me mum, the kids will enjoy having grandma around for a few days'. The A&E staff are relieved also, as this can be a tricky situation sometimes. Before discharge, however, a careful teaching session is needed to warn Shareen about the possible risks of swelling even with a backslab, a printed sheet is given to her containing the key information including instruction about finger movements and exercises. The arm is elevated in a high arm sling to reduce swelling, an appointment for the orthopaedic clinic the following morning is made and a course of analgesia prescribed. Shareen eventually leaves the department 5 hours later to go home with her daughter.

Smith's fractures are often described as reverse Colles fractures. They are caused by falling on the flexed wrist; radiography confirms the anterior displacement of the distal fragment. It may be possible to manage this fracture after reduction in a cast but internal fixation may be required.

Scaphoid fractures are another common wrist injury occurring from a fall on an outstretched hand. The scaphoid is one of the eight carpal bones that make up the wrist and sits in a strategically important position as its articulation ensures it plays a key role in the complexities of wrist movement and is also aligned with the radius, the major bone of the forearm. This tends to place the greatest loading on the bone during a fall. There is frequently little to see with a scaphoid fracture other than some swelling. The cardinal sign of any fracture however is localized bony tenderness and gentle pressure on the 'anatomical snuff box' usually elicits this sign if a fracture is present. The 'anatomical snuff box' is the slight hollow on the radial side of the wrist from which gentlemen used to sniff their snuff in previous centuries. It is a difficult fracture to locate on X-ray and often it is treated as a fracture (with POP) even if the original radiographs are inconclusive, providing the clinical signs and history are consistent with the injury. Failure to treat properly can have major adverse, long-term implications for wrist function such is the key location of this small bone (Hunter 2005).

The foregoing is not an exhaustive list of fractures but highlights some of the more common fractures a nurse is likely to encounter. For a more detailed account of fracture care, the reader should consult a specialist text.

INJURIES TO JOINTS

Injuries to joints may range from a mild sprain to complete dislocation with associated fractures. The overall aim of care is to allow the joint surface time to recover, in order to reduce the likelihood of secondary osteoarthritis, while keeping the patient as active as possible to overcome muscle wasting around the joint which may lead to permanent joint instability.

SHOULDER DISLOCATION

In this injury, the shoulder is usually dislocated anteriorly as a result of a fall or sports injury. If a direct blow to the shoulder has occurred, a cervical spine injury should be considered a possibility until ruled out by radiography. In the 18–35-year age group it is usually due to a sports or motorcycle accident in which the individual is thrown and lands on an outstretched hand and the body rotates above the hand. It is also quite common in the elderly, usually following a more minor injury due to the lax musculature of the shoulder joint in this age group.

As soon as the injury has been confirmed by radiography, the shoulder should be reduced as the longer it is left, the harder it is to relocate the humeral head. One approach is to give the patient intramuscular analgesia and lie him or her prone on a trolley with the affected arm hanging free over the side. Spontaneous reduction may occur due to gravitational traction and the muscle relaxant effect of the analgesia. However, some patients will find this position suffocating and very difficult to maintain. Alternative techniques, such as Kocher's or the Hippocratic method to reduce the dislocation, are usually successful if combined with intravenous diazepam and an opioid analgesic. Occasionally general anaesthesia is required.

In younger patients, post-reduction care includes a check radiograph, the application of a bandage (including the forearm) to prevent abduction and external rotation (e.g. a vest made from stretchable net such as Netelast). Both these movements predispose to re-dislocation. If recurrence becomes a problem, the patient may eventually require a surgical repair.

In the elderly, recurrence is not such a problem but there is a high risk of stiffness leading to loss of independence; thus mobilization of the shoulder may begin after 1 week.

Specific patient problems
Axillary nerve palsy
This potential problem is caused by compression of axillary nerve by the displaced humerus. It should be tested for in the A&E department by a pin-prick test over the outer aspect of the shoulder. The condition may be severe enough for the patient to lose deltoid function and, although it is usually temporary, months of physiotherapy may be necessary for full recovery.

Rotator cuff tear
The head of the humerus is held in place in the glenoid cavity of the scapula by the tendons of the shoulder joint muscles which fuse and form the rotator cuff. The cuff inserts at points around the greater and lesser tuberosities of the humerus. If it is torn, the most common problem is in abducting the arm. The condition may be helped by physiotherapy but a repair of the tear may eventually be required.

Loss of independence
Use of the shoulder is essential to perform many aspects of self-care and loss of function is a major potential problem in all shoulder injuries, especially in older patients.

HIP DISLOCATION

In adults, this is a high energy injury associated with road traffic accidents and is often accompanied by fractures of the affected leg. Injury may range from incomplete dislocation (subluxation), when the head of the femur is partly out of the acetabulum, to complete dislocation, when the femoral head is lying behind the acetabulum (posterior dislocation). The head of femur may have been driven through the acetabulum (central dislocation and technically a fractured pelvis, see p. 845). The patient will usually be in great pain, have a partially flexed hip joint and the leg will be internally rotated. Once the hip has been reduced, the joint should be rested, usually on skin traction and then 'free in bed' for several weeks, before weight-bearing can take place. The need to fix other injuries may lead to a different course of action. Damage to the sciatic nerve is a common result of this injury. The other main presentation of a dislocated hip is more accurately described as a dislocated hip prosthesis and occurs in elderly patients who have had arthroplasty surgery to the hip (see p. 863). Much lower energy levels are involved in causing this problem, typically just a simple fall.

SOFT-TISSUE INJURIES IN THE KNEE

Meniscal tear injuries usually occur in young people who engage in sports and are the result of rotational stress on the flexed, weight-bearing knee. The medial meniscus is damaged much more often than the lateral due to anatomical reasons. The extent of the tear may vary from being small and undisplaced to one in which the whole of the meniscus is involved and displaced to such an extent there is complete loss of joint function. Arthroscopy may confirm diagnosis and a partial menisectomy may be performed via the arthroscope. The aim of treatment is to leave as much of the meniscus intact as possible.

A major postoperative problem is instability of the knee joint following quadriceps wasting. Static quadriceps exercises are necessary to overcome muscle wasting in the thigh. The physiotherapist will organize an exercise programme but the nurse needs to be able to reinforce the necessity of practising the exercises and ensure they are being performed correctly for maximum benefit.

The other main group of injuries involves damage to the cruciate ligaments or the medial collateral ligament. Adams (2004) presents a detailed discussion of the assessment and management of these injuries and the familiar RICE approach in the initial stages is recommended (Rest, Ice, Compression, Elevation). This deals with the initial swelling and pain. Ice packs need to be applied for at least 10 minutes to be effective but no more than 30 minutes due to the danger of skin damage. The general approach is to manage this group of injuries conservatively with the aid of analgesia, support bandages and crutches, aiming for early mobilization.

SOFT-TISSUE INJURY OF THE ANKLE

These injuries occur most commonly following inversion injuries, usually damaging the lateral ligament. The following classification is widely used (Blenkinsopp and Paxton 2004):

- First-degree: no gross damage to collagen fibres or laxity in the joint
- Second-degree: partial tear of fibres in the ligament leading to some degree of laxity but the ligament is still grossly intact
- Third-degree: complete tear of the ligament with abnormal laxity of the joint.

The patient complains of pain and swelling over the lateral or medial malleolus, although the radiographs are normal.

Initial management should consist of RICE (see above). Following first-degree sprains the patient is often given a support bandage, such as double Tubigrip, and should be advised to rest at home with high elevation of the ankle to reduce the swelling. There is in fact no evidence to show this improves the outcome; however, analgesia and early mobilization will improve the outcome, so the rest period should be short, only 48 hours. Paracetamol or ibuprofen are effective and codeine may be added as a separate prescription to the paracetamol if required. Topical ibuprofen has no evidence to support its use and should be discouraged (Blenkinsopp and Paxton 2004). If weight-bearing is painful, a pair of crutches should be provided.

In third-degree injuries where the lateral ligament is completely torn the patient will require complete immobilization in a below-knee weight-bearing plaster.

Specific patient problems

Specific problems include the following:

- *Loss of independence*. Some patients will need to be admitted overnight, even following relatively minor injuries, until they are safe to mobilize on crutches. This, of course, is particularly true of the elderly individual who lives alone
- Circulatory compromise due to swelling
- In the long term, *ankle instability* may be the result of this injury and the patient will require surgery to reconstruct a stable joint.

AMPUTATION OF A LIMB

War and the widespread use of landmines has left an ongoing legacy of injuries requiring lower-leg amputation in many parts of the developing world. Children and young adults are those most affected. In the developed world amputation is due mostly to the effects of peripheral vascular disease (PVD) and affects mostly those over 55. Atherosclerotic disease of arteries in the lower limb progressively reduces the blood supply to the lower leg. Eventually the supply of oxygen to the muscles is inadequate for walking more than a few hundred metres and ischaemic pain develops forcing the patient to rest (see p. 280). This is the same mechanism that produces angina due to diseased coronary arteries, and is called intermittent claudication. Progression of the disease reduces the distance the person can walk and pain may even develop at rest. Although vascular surgery can improve the situation, gangrene and continuous pain may eventually develop leaving no alternative other than amputation. Amputation of a limb is a very mutilating procedure and an extremely devastating experience for the individual. However, it frequently provides relief from severe intractable pain due to PVD or osteomyelitis and allows a significant improvement in mobility.

In those for whom an amputation is a necessity, the loss of the limb has become less obvious and less disabling nowadays as a result of improved prostheses and rehabilitation programmes.

REASONS FOR AMPUTATION

An amputation is performed to preserve the patient's life or may be undertaken to improve function and usefulness. Conditions that necessitate amputation include:

1 Insufficient blood supply to the part (PVD) and resulting gangrene
2 Severe, uncontrollable infection such as gas gangrene (*Clostridium perfringens* infection) or chronic osteomyelitis in which there is marked bone destruction
3 Malignant neoplasm (e.g. osteosarcoma)
4 An injury that has resulted in irreparable crushing of the limb or laceration of arteries and nerves or blast injury
5 A handicapping deformity (e.g. flail limb).

LEVEL AND TYPES OF AMPUTATION

Occasionally an amputation is an emergency surgical procedure performed because of irreparable traumatic damage to a part. But, when possible, the level of the amputation is decided before operation so that the patient may be informed of the anticipated extent of the loss. The decision as to the level is based on achieving:

● complete removal of the diseased tissue
● viable tissue and an adequate blood supply to the remaining part of the limb
● a stump that will allow for a satisfactory fitting and functional movement of a prosthesis.

Adequate soft tissues (skin, subcutaneous tissue and muscle) are preserved so that the end of the bone is well padded and covered. If possible, the stump should be the optimum length for adequate leverage on the prosthesis. Too long a stump may interfere with the function of the prosthesis joint below. In amputation of the lower extremity, the knee joint is maintained, if at all possible, because mobility and agility are acquired more readily. The prosthesis for the above-knee amputation limits the person, especially if elderly, because of the high energy demands for locomotion.

Two types of operative procedures are used:

1 In the *closed* or *flap type* of procedure, fascia, probably muscle, and full-thickness skin flaps are brought over the end of the bone. In a below-knee or a Syme's amputation, the posterior flap is usually longer, with the suture line situated on the anterior aspect of the stump. This arrangement prevents direct pressure on the scar by the prosthesis in weight-bearing.
2 A *guillotine* or *open amputation* is reserved for emergency cases in which the limb has been severely traumatized and contaminated, or in which an infection such as gas gangrene has already developed. The skin and other soft tissues are severed at the same level as the bone. The wound is left open to promote adequate drainage and closed later when infection has been brought under control. Traction may be applied to the skin while it remains open to prevent retraction of the soft tissues.

Traumatic amputation implies the loss of a whole or part of a limb in an accident. This is frequently a life-threatening situation because of the concomitant haemorrhage. A second problem incurred by such circumstances is contamination of the wound. Immediate emergency care is directed toward arrest of the bleeding and getting the person to where blood replacement may be instituted. Precautions are taken to handle and transport the amputated part with the patient carefully, because efforts may be made to reattach the separated unit.

Disarticulation is the term used when the amputation is at the level of a joint.

PREOPERATIVE NURSING INTERVENTION

Psychological preparation

When the amputation is an elective procedure, the surgeon, nurse and the rehabilitation team work together to inform the patient and family of the need for the operation and the level at which the limb will be removed and what functional restoration can be anticipated. When the patient is first advised of the loss of a part of the body, regardless of how functionally insignificant, the information is still likely to be a shock, causing considerable emotional disturbance. The patient's body image and independence are seriously threatened and encouragement is needed to talk freely about fears and anxieties. Good nurse–patient communication is essential both before and after operation to help the patient resolve these fears and adapt to a change in body image. Reactions vary among patients, depending on culture, personality, life situation and the impact loss of a limb is perceived as having on the individual's social circumstances.

The patient and family receive explanations of how the problems associated with the loss of a limb may be handled through a planned rehabilitation programme. The knowledge that the interest and assistance of specialists in this area are available may help the patient to develop a positive attitude toward overcoming the handicap. Opportunities are provided for questions and discussions about what is likely to take place before and after the operation. The patient may derive support from a visit by someone who has had a similar amputation and has been successfully rehabilitated.

Physical preparation

Normal preoperative preparation is required as for any major operation, but in addition, exercises are introduced that will facilitate postoperative mobilization and rehabilitation. These include active exercises of the unaffected limbs to prevent loss of muscular strength. If the use of walking aids is anticipated, arm strengthening exercises using weight-lifting and push-ups may be introduced to strengthen the shoulder and arm muscles. Overprotection of an affected lower limb usually results in continuous flexion of the hip and knee joints, leading to contractures. This is discouraged by lying the patient in a prone position several times a day.

POSTOPERATIVE NURSING CARE

Assessment

The blood pressure, pulse and respirations are recorded, colour noted and the stump examined at frequent, regular intervals for the first 48 hours for early signs of shock and haemorrhage. The patient is observed for psychological distress following the amputation. Even though he or she was prepared for and consented to the operation, the actual loss of the body part may cause severe depression. The nurse is also alert for any indications of infection such as pyrexia, raised pulse, increased pain, erythema and wound discharge.

Patient problems

Potential patient problems following an amputation are listed in Table 24.4.

Nursing intervention

Promotion of healing

The stump is usually enclosed in a thick soft dressing and elasticated bandages. When a soft dressing is used, any blood staining is reported immediately. If serous drainage soaks through the dressing, it is promptly reinforced and pressure is applied until the bleeding is brought under control, if necessary by the surgeon. Continuous closed wound suction drainage may be established to prevent haematoma formation. The wound dressing, provided it is comfortable, is generally left undisturbed until the wound drain is removed, thus reducing the risk of introduction of infection. The wound drain is removed 2–4 days after operation and the sutures are left in place for 10–12 days for an above-knee amputation and 3–4 weeks for a below-knee wound, in order to ensure firm healing.

Unless the surgeon instructs otherwise, the patient should lie in a supine position with the stump resting flat on the bed. Following an amputation above the knee, the patient must be guarded against shortening of the hip flexors and abductors. In an amputation below the knee, the patient is encouraged to maintain extension of the knee to avoid contracture of the hamstrings (posterior thigh muscles).

The patient or a member of the family is taught the care of the stump and the correct application of the bandage. The stump is bathed as necessary with a mild soap and rinsed and dried thoroughly. Lanolin may be applied if the skin is dry and flaky. The patient is taught to inspect the stump twice

Table 24.4 Identification of patients' problems following amputation

Problem	Causative factors	Goals
1. Failure of wound to heal	Infection Poor blood supply Haematoma formation	The wound will heal without any complications
2. Potential for injury	Surgical construction of a residual limb (stump) Altered balance Possible disorientation in the postoperative period Phantom limb phenomenon	1. To achieve a residual limb that will support activity with a prosthesis 2. Physical injury will not occur
3. Discomfort or pain	Surgical intervention Phantom pain phenomenon	1. Patient will be pain free 2. To understand and minimize the experience of phantom sensations
4. Disturbance in body image	Amputation of a body part	1. To express feelings about the loss of a body part 2. To attain an acceptable level of social and physical functioning
5. Nutritional intake lower than body requirements	Surgery and anaesthesia	To maintain nutritional and fluid balance
6. Impaired mobility	Surgery and loss of a body part	1. Complications of immobility will not occur 2. To increase physical activity and ambulation
7. Inadequate knowledge about care of the residual limb and prosthesis, application and use of the prosthesis, and follow-up care	Lack of information, skill and resources	1. To develop self-care skills 2. To develop a plan for follow-up health management

daily, using a mirror, for redness, swelling, irritation and calluses. If any symptoms develop, weight bearing on the stump is avoided and the doctor or clinic consulted. Stump bandaging is resumed if the prosthesis is not worn during this time. Certain activities may be ordered that apply pressure to the stump in preparation for the use of a prosthesis and weight bearing. Contact is first made with something quite soft and, as tolerance is developed, the firmness and resistance of the contact surface and pressure are increased progressively. If the patient complains of muscular spasms and discomfort, massage to the stump may provide relief. Figure 24.13 illustrates points the patient is taught 'not to do' with the stump in order to prevent injury and promote healing.

Prevention of physical injury

The most common cause of falls is that the patient forgets momentarily that he or she has only one leg. The patient may experience the sensation that the limb is still present; this phenomenon is known as *phantom limb*. The majority of amputees experience this phenomenon, which is strongest immediately after surgery. The nerve pathways associated with the amputated limb are still intact and active within the body and the brain, leading to the continued perception of the limb. This can be as real to the patient as if the limb were still present. Awareness that it is a common experience following amputation helps to decrease the patient's anxiety.

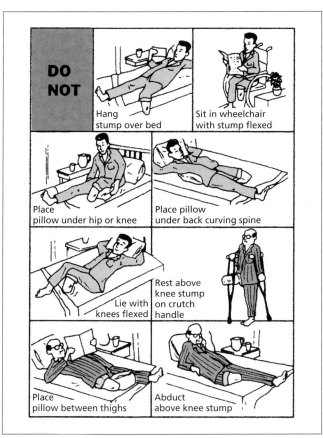

Figure 24.13 Positions to be avoided by lower-extremity amputee during the immediate postoperative period.

Control of pain

An opioid analgesic is usually required by the patient at regular intervals during the first 48 hours after surgery. Persistent **pain** 24–72 hours after operation may indicate haematoma formation. This must be reported to the surgeon immediately, as breakdown of the wound could occur if the haematoma is not evacuated. If pain occurs later in the postoperative recovery period, it may be due to wound infection. If infection is suspected the wound is inspected, a wound swab is taken for microscopy, culture and sensitivity, and the relevant antibiotic is prescribed.

Adjustment to altered body image

Acknowledgement by the nurse of the patient's feelings of depression, anger and frustration, and provision of opportunities for the patient and family members to discuss feelings, help the patient to accept the situation. An understanding of the meaning of the loss is necessary for the health professional to provide constructive support. The nurse and other healthcare workers may set expectations that the patient will increase mobilization, socialization and self-care activities. The patient may feel very differently, however. Support and encouragement are therefore essential. Early mobilization and patient participation in decision-making promote the development of a more positive attitude. A temporary prosthesis is worn as soon as possible so the patient experiences an empty sleeve or empty trouser leg only briefly. The permanent prosthesis is fitted within a few weeks for most patients. As the patient's functional capacity increases, feelings of self-worth and tolerance of the change in body image may begin to emerge. Friends and relatives are encouraged to visit and opportunities for the patient to go home for an evening or weekend are created whenever possible.

Involvement of members of the rehabilitation team prior to surgery and during the postoperative period enables them to provide information about the expectations for functional restoration, to develop plans for rehabilitation and to establish a trusting relationship with the patient and family. Rehabilitation centres usually provide both individual and group sessions to allow patients to share experiences, gain support, and learn new and effective coping strategies.

The patient is encouraged to discuss with the limb-fitter how the artificial limb will look, as well as function. Help is provided in selecting shoes, trousers, skirts, shirts and blouses to promote a favourable and acceptable appearance.

Psychological and social adjustment is generally a longer process than is the re-learning of physical functioning. Those who have been affected by trauma may well have long-term problems with post-traumatic stress disorder.

Maintenance of fluid and nutritional status

Intravenous **fluid** may be necessary during the first 24–48 hours to maintain an adequate intake. Oral fluids are given freely, and the patient progresses to a regular diet as soon as it is tolerated. An explanation is made, if necessary, of the importance of adequate nutrition in maintaining and promoting muscular strength for the exercises that will assist in rehabilitation.

Promotion of mobility

An hourly routine of coughing and deep breathing and frequent change of position are necessary until the patient is allowed up and becomes sufficiently active, to prevent limited ventilation and circulatory stasis.

As soon as the patient is well enough, a daily regimen of exercises is introduced to maintain and promote the muscular strength and joint mobility that are needed for rehabilitation. The tone of the trunk muscles, as well as that of the limb muscles, receives attention because adjustments and compensation are necessary for the amputee to maintain balance. If the leg has been amputated above the knee, the hip extensors and adductors play an important role in re-mobilization, as hip flexion and abduction deformity may occur. The patient should be taught active stump exercises to maintain and improve joint mobility and muscle strength. To prevent flexion contracture of the hip, the patient lies in the prone position for a minimum of 30 minutes two to three times a day. The stump should not be propped up on a pillow for the same reason. If the leg has been amputated below the knee, particular attention is given to quadriceps exercises. Following the amputation of an arm, the shoulder muscles of that limb are exercised to prevent adduction and rounding of the shoulder.

The patient is allowed out of bed as soon as possible. Assistance must be available until he or she can maintain balance and is able to manoeuvre safely. In the case of a lower limb, the patient first learns to stand and gain balance, to transfer safely from bed to chair and from wheelchair to toilet. When fitted with a temporary prosthesis (pylon) the patient mobilizes using a walking aid such as a stick. A walking frame is generally not recommended as there is a risk of the patient falling backwards. Crutches should not be used as they hinder the patient in learning how to weight-bear. To ensure the patient is able to walk safely with walking sticks, he or she is first taught to walk between parallel bars, one hand holding a bar and the other a stick. The patient progresses to walking with the aid of two sticks and then with one stick, held in the opposite hand to the amputation, before the permanent prosthesis is fitted.

When the stump has shrunk sufficiently and is conditioned, measurements are taken and a permanent prosthesis is made.

When learning to use a permanent lower limb prosthesis, the patient uses one or two walking sticks for support. When a satisfactory stable gait has been achieved, the patient is encouraged to discontinue the use of a stick. All of this takes considerable time and perseverance; the amputee will require encouragement and support from family and those working with him or her in rehabilitation.

Inadequate knowledge

After an amputation, the patient and their family are taught to care for the stump and to inspect it several times daily for oedema, redness, drainage or breaks in the skin, and to note any changes in sensation or tenderness. When the prosthesis is fitted, they are taught how to care for it, to assess for proper fit, what to do if the fit alters and when to return to the limb-fitter for reassessment. The physiotherapist helps the patient to develop a plan for continuing the exercise and activity programme at home. The nurse helps the patient and family plan how they may incorporate the recommended healthcare measures and activity programme into the daily routine of the patient. Referrals to a community nurse or resettlement officer are made as indicated. Arrangements are made for follow-up visits to the surgeon's clinic in the outpatient department. Phantom limb pain should be discussed further with the patient as this may persist many years after amputation and be very distressing.

Evaluation

Expected outcomes

1 The skin over the stump is clean, dry and intact.
2 The patient indicates understanding of the phenomena of phantom limb and phantom pain, if present.
3 The patient and family are able to express feelings regarding the loss of a body part and the change in body image.
4 The patient is able to apply the prosthesis and wear it with comfort.
5 The patient follows the planned exercise regimen to maintain and/or increase muscle tone and strength and joint function in all limbs.
6 The patient moves about safely.
7 Suitable body weight to aid mobilization is maintained or achieved.
8 The patient is able to assess the condition of the skin over the stump.
9 The patient knows how to contact the limb-fitting centre should problems occur.
10 The family takes part in the rehabilitation programme and is able to give assistance to the patient if required.

INFLAMMATORY JOINT DISEASE

RHEUMATOID ARTHRITIS

Rheumatoid arthritis (RA) is a long-term systemic disease that occurs worldwide and affects about 1% of the UK population accounting for 46 000 hospital admissions per year (Oliver and Ryan 2004). It first appears in relatively early adult life and a form can develop in childhood (Juvenile Chronic Arthritis, formerly known as Still's disease). The disease also occurs more frequently in women. There is a distinct genetic susceptibility in the disease with a concordance rate of 32% in identical twins and 9% in non-identical twins as compared with the overall population rate of 1% (Black and Hawks 2005). The disease is subsequently provoked by a 'triggering factor' that causes a pathological autoimmune reaction. In effect, the body mistakes the synovial lining of **joints** for a foreign antigen, leading to a chronic and destructive **inflammatory response**. Antibodies called rheumatoid factors are found in the blood of 70–80% of persons with rheumatoid arthritis. These antibodies interact with antigens in various connective tissues, but the reaction is greatest in the synovium of **synovial joints**.

Pathophysiology

Swelling and congestion of the synovial membrane and underlying connective tissue marks the beginning of the disease (synovitis). They become infiltrated by lymphocytes and synovial fluid effusions within the joint space develop during active phases of the disorder. The process is reversible in the early stage, and the joint may be left undamaged and functional. As the inflammation continues, the synovium proliferates and, with the fibrin of the inflammatory exudate, forms a thick spreading membrane of granulation tissue known as a *pannus*. It spreads over the joint surfaces, gradually eroding the cartilage, and may even destroy the denuded bone surfaces. A radiograph may show rarefaction of the ends of the involved **bones**. Instability and irritation of the joint may cause muscle contraction with a resulting flexion or extension deformity or partial dislocation (subluxation) of the joint.

Fibrous scar tissue and adhesions develop between the opposing joint surfaces, leading to fibrous ankylosis of the joint, which becomes fixed and immobile. The exposed, roughened ends of bone tissue may eventually proliferate bone cells into the joint cavity, resulting in calcification and bony ankylosis.

The patient with rheumatoid arthritis may also have diffuse involvement of non-articular connective tissues. Degenerative lesions of the collagen component of the connective tissue may develop in muscles, tendons, blood vessels, pleura, heart or lungs.

Clinical characteristics

The onset is usually insidious: the person experiences a period of general fatigue and non-specific illness. Pain, swelling and morning stiffness of several peripheral joints is the typical beginning of the disease. The small joints of the hands or feet, or the wrists, elbows or knees, are generally the first to be involved. The disease develops symmetrically and, as it progresses, the affected joints become swollen, painful, red and increasingly difficult to move. Their range of motion is reduced. The overlying skin may take on a stretched, smooth, glossy appearance.

Muscle weakness and spasm are common in the early stages and are frequently followed by marked muscular atrophy. Unless early treatment is instituted, progressive joint tissue destruction and deformities develop, leading to permanent disability. Subluxation and flexion contractures occur. Deformities commonly seen include hyperextension of the distal phalanges, flexion contracture or ulnar deviation of the fingers due to metacarpal-phalangeal joint involvement and flexion contraction of the wrists, knees and hips. Subcutaneous nodules (*rheumatoid nodules*) appear principally on extensor surfaces or areas subjected to pressure. These are composed mainly of fibrinoid material (degenerative tissue cells) and granulation tissue.

General constitutional disturbances are manifested; the patient is pale and looks ill; anorexia, loss of weight, fatigue and depression may develop. Low-grade fever, tachycardia, anaemia and a mild leucocytosis may also be present. Later, leucopenia may develop. The widespread effects of the disease on the whole person are summarized in Box 24.4. The erythrocyte sedimentation rate is usually raised and, later in the disease, a blood examination may reveal the presence of the rheumatoid factor.

Classification

The disorder may be classified according to the pathological changes (clinical stages) and the loss of functional capacity (functional classification) (Table 24.5).

Nursing assessment

As rheumatoid arthritis is a systemic disease with a range of signs and symptoms that impact on all aspects of daily life, an extensive nursing history should be obtained that explores the following areas:

- current local and systemic effects on the patient
- self-care abilities
- coping responses to the disease
- knowledge of the disease and its management.

Reliable and valid assessment tools such as the Arthritis Impact Measurement Scale II (Meenan 1992) may be useful as a guide to data collection.

Box 24.4 Major extra-articular features

- Anaemia
- Weight loss, fatigue, fever
- Lymphadenopathy
- Oedema
- Nodules
- Osteoporosis, bursitis and tenosynovitis
- Muscle wasting
- Episcleritis
- Keratoconjunctivitis
- Entrapment neuropathy (e.g. cervical cord compression)
- Nailfold vasculitis
- Peripheral sensory neuropathy
- Splenomegaly
- Cardiac complications (e.g. pericarditis, endocarditis)
- Pleural complications (e.g. effusions, bronchiolitis).

Table 24.5 Classification of rheumatoid arthritis

By clinical stages		By functional classification	
Stage	**Manifestations**	**Class**	**Manifestations**
1 (early)	No evidence of joint destruction or osteoporosis	1	No loss of functional capacity
2 (moderate)	Evidence of some destruction of cartilage and probably of subchondral bone No deformity but full range of motion may be limited Adjacent muscle atrophy present	2	Able to carry out usual activities despite some discomfort and limited joint mobility
3 (severe)	Cartilage and bone destruction quite evident Muscle atrophy and joint deformities such as hyperextension, flexion contracture, ulnar deviation and subluxation present	3	Functional capacity impaired Occupational and self-care activities quite limited
4 (terminal)	Criteria of stage 3 plus fibrous or bony ankylosis present	4	Confined to a wheelchair or bed. Not able to carry out self-care Dependent

Symptoms

The nurse should explore all symptoms the patient is experiencing to obtain some understanding of the extent of the disease. A plan of care can be determined only when the extent of the physical effects the disease has on the patient has been determined together with the psychological consequences. The nurse should determine which joints are involved and obtain a description of the severity, duration, precipitating, aggravating and relieving factors of the common problems: pain, swelling, stiffness and impaired movement. The systemic symptoms of generalized weakness, fatigue, listlessness, anorexia and weight loss should also be explored and enquiry made about the presence of extra-articular symptoms including subcutaneous nodules, sensory loss in one or more of the extremities and dryness of the eyes.

Self-care abilities

Depending on the number and extent of symptoms present, the patient may be able to continue to perform self-care independently or may be completely dependent on others. The ability to walk and use the hands should be assessed along with general mobility. Determine from the patient what activities can be performed and how important each activity is to the patient. Continuing to perform personal hygiene is generally very important to the patient, and giving up household chores may be equally distressing as it represents a loss of independence.

Coping responses

Coping with the pain, stiffness and decreased mobility of rheumatoid arthritis is often overwhelming. Like other chronic illnesses, the symptoms disrupt everyday life, the medical treatment is acknowledged as being only partly effective and the therapeutic regimen further disrupts day-to-day patterns of living. Equally distressing is the uncertainty about when remissions and exacerbations may occur.

The loss of self-care ability coupled with the physical effects of the disease described above can lead to the patient being depressed or very anxious and fearful for the future. The psychological effects of the illness need to be sensitively explored along with the social consequences if the nurse is to be able to plan care for all the patient's needs.

A limited survey by the National Rheumatoid Arthritis Society of 200 patients (note 170 were female) highlighted the psychosocial impact of this disease. Of those surveyed, 88% felt having a job helped them cope with the effects of their RA, yet 85% felt RA had adversely affected their careers. Two-thirds of those surveyed complained of feeling depressed, feeling that pain and chronic tiredness were the biggest factors in their low mood. Note, however, that 85% of the sample were female and depression tends to be reported more by women than men so the nature of the sample may be influencing this finding.

For many women with rheumatoid arthritis, pregnancy brings a relief of all symptoms (Black and Hawks 2005) and there is intense speculation this is linked to the different genetic make-up of the fetus influencing the woman's body in some way. However, following the birth of a baby the symptoms usually return to their previous level.

Knowledge of the disease and its management

In order to maximize independence, the patient must participate in ongoing care and this requires knowledge of the disease process and the treatment regimen. The nurse should determine the patient's knowledge base, interest level, ability to learn and degree of physical comfort in order to promote self-care. Teaching sessions must be based on a thorough assessment of the patient and their level of understanding. Oliver and Ryan (2004) points out that nurse-led review clinics focussing on developing self-care strategies can play a major role in improving the quality of life for those with RA.

Physical assessment

Individual joints or groups of joints and their surrounding tissues are observed, palpated and their range of motion determined. Joints are inspected for swelling, redness, physical deformity, discolouration, scars or discharge. The adjoining muscles are observed for signs of atrophy. Each joint is compared with the corresponding joint for symmetry and degree of change. Painful joints are supported by the examiner's hands, and movements are performed gently and slowly. Illustrations of the human body may be used to record joint assessment and provide an overview of involved joints (Fig. 24.14). A goniometer, which measures angles, may be used to measure degrees of movement of a joint. For example, the normal range of flexion of an elbow is 135–150°, and extension 0–5°; hip abduction varies from 45 to 50°, with hip adduction being approximately 20–30°. Some decrease in mobility of joints occurs with age.

DIAGNOSTIC PROCEDURES

Radiography will usually demonstrate changes within the joint and in adjacent bone (osteopenia or rarefaction of bone). However, as it takes time for these changes to appear, diagnosis is made on clinical presentation and laboratory investigation (below).

Laboratory *blood and serum tests* that may be used in investigation of rheumatoid arthritis and other disorders include the following:

1 Erythrocyte and leucocyte counts

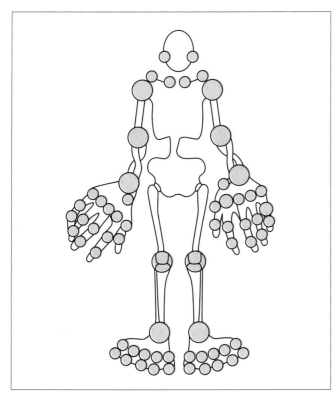

Figure 24.14   Illustration for use in joint assessment.

2 Determination of haemoglobin, erythrocyte sedimentation rate (ESR), serum alkaline phosphatase, calcium and phosphorus concentrations and blood uric acid level
3 Examination for rheumatoid (Rh) factors, antinuclear antibodies (ANAs), lupus erythematosus cells (LE prep), anti-DNA and complement fixation.

The blood cell counts, haemoglobin and ESR are used to determine the presence of anaemia, infection or tissue destruction. The serum phosphatase level is raised in malignant disease, as is the ESR. The phosphorus and calcium concentrations are significant in bone disease, and the blood uric acid level is increased in gout. The presence of rheumatoid factors and autoimmune antibodies in serum occurs in 80% of people with late-stage rheumatoid arthritis. Absence of such factors therefore does not rule out the diagnosis

PATIENT PROBLEMS

Assessment of the patient with rheumatoid arthritis often reveals some or all of the following problems:

● *reduced physical mobility* related to inflammation and deformity of joints, muscle weakness and atrophy, and limitation in range of motion of joints
● *activity intolerance* related to disease process (especially anaemia)
● *pain* related to the disease process and accentuated by movement
● *reduction in self-care activities* related to decrease in activity tolerance
● *depression* related to pain and decreased mobility
● *inadequate nutrition* related to anorexia, pain and decreased mobility
● *lack of knowledge* about rheumatoid arthritis.

GOALS

The goals derive from the identified problems and generally include:

1 To maintain or increase mobility and activity tolerance
2 To obtain relief of pain and discomfort
3 To perform self-care in daily living
4 To achieve an optimal nutritional intake
5 To achieve or maintain a positive mood state.

The overall goal is to achieve a maximum state of wellness within the limitations imposed by a chronic and potentially disabling health problem. Criteria for evaluation of goal attainment should be negotiated with the patient. The nurse uses assessment skills in determining the extent to which each goal is achieved. Criteria may include any of the following:

● demonstrates stable or improved joint mobility
● demonstrates an optimal level of functional mobility
● performs therapeutic measures to minimize further impairment of joint function

● controls pain through appropriate use of treatment measures including medications
● maintains a satisfactory level of independence
● consumes a well-balanced diet
● demonstrates a satisfactory level of psychosocial health.

Nursing intervention

Chapter 5 explores the general problems of long-term illness and many of the issues raised in that chapter are typified in rheumatoid arthritis. Rheumatoid arthritis is a disease for which there is no cure but one in which control is possible by the use of a variety of measures developed and implemented in teamwork between the patient, family, nurse, doctor, physiotherapist, occupational therapist and other healthcare workers. The patient plays a critical role in the management of rheumatoid arthritis and the attainment of the goals of therapy. The disorder has a major social impact in terms of family relationships, ability to work and engage in the normal range of everyday social activity.

As arthritis is a disease characterized by remissions and exacerbations, the patient must be able to adjust management appropriately, including rest, exercise and medications. This requires that the patient learns to make and implement appropriate decisions, and this is possible only if the patient is well informed. Arthritis patient education has been effective in changing knowledge, behaviours, psychosocial status and health status. The most successful programmes use an interactive approach that emphasizes an understanding of the disease and the development of a daily routine of self-management activities. Education that includes coping strategies, problem-solving approaches to common problems, and endurance exercise should supplement the more traditional areas of focus such as joint protection and range-of-motion exercises.

There is an identified need for education and counselling to prepare patients with rheumatoid arthritis for the effect it will have on their family relationships.

Maintain or increase mobility and activity tolerance
Maintenance of joint mobility and the promotion of optimal joint function and activity tolerance are achieved through a combination of planned rest and exercise, and by protecting the joints from unnecessary stress. Planning and implementation of care requires cooperation between the nurse, physiotherapist and occupational therapist, doctor, patient and family.

Rest   Rest is necessary as it helps to control fatigue, inflammation and pain. The patient with limitation of joint function expends excessive energy in movement. Bedrest may be prescribed for a brief period during acute episodes of the disease when many joints are acutely inflamed and when systemic symptoms such as fever, anaemia and severe fatigue are present. Body positioning is important to prevent contractures and deformity during periods of bedrest and during sleep.

The patient should rest and sleep in a position as nearly anatomical as possible, that is with knees and elbows fully extended and with the neck and wrists in a near-neutral position. Pillows may be placed under the full length of the legs to maintain extension of the leg when the patient is supine, but never under a painful knee or elbow as this contributes to the development of contractures.

When an acute episode of the disease has passed, patients are encouraged to continue to have several rest periods daily and to alternate periods of activity with periods of rest. Patients must be convinced that rest is as important a part of their treatment regimen as medications and exercise. Relaxation techniques may also be used by the patient to promote body relaxation and decrease emotional stress.

Joint rest may involve the use of splints to support and protect involved joints. The type of splint that may be applied depends on the purpose to be achieved (Fig. 24.15). Resting splints are used to immobilize inflamed and painful joints and are worn continuously during periods of acute inflammation. They are removed for short intervals for essential activities such as eating and cleansing of the skin. During chronic or inactive phases of joint disease, rest splints are worn only at night. Functional splints are designed to stabilize and support a joint during activity. Corrective or dynamic splints are used to immobilize an involved joint, realign soft tissues, or correct contractures or deformities. Splints are usually made of a lightweight thermoplastic material that is pliable when heated. They are moulded to the affected part and held in place with Velcro straps. The patient's skin is protected from the splint by a layer of cloth material. The protective layer is either placed on the patient (e.g. a tube stocking) or incorporated into the splint. Splints may be used on the fingers, hands, wrists, knees or ankles. Cervical collars may be used to restrict movement of the head and neck, and thus protect the extremely vulnerable joint between the first and second cervical vertebrae.

Patients and family members should learn how to apply the splint and how to prevent any side-effects such as skin breakdown. A demonstration should be given to illustrate the pressure points that are created if the splint is not a proper fit or is not applied correctly. The patient is taught to inspect the skin under the splint for redness and tenderness each time it is removed. Splints may need to be replaced following acute illness, when the oedema has abated, and at regular intervals when used for a long time.

Joints may be afforded protection by means other than splints and patients should be advised as follows (Black and Hawks 2005):

● If an activity is painful, stop
● Take frequent short rests whilst undertaking activities and break them down into smaller manageable sections
● Work out strategies to reduce the loading on joints. For example do not lift when you can slide an object, think about the height objects are stored at
● Preferential use of stronger joints. For example use a shoulder bag not a handbag
● Ensure maximum stability and optimum positioning of joints by concentrating on good posture

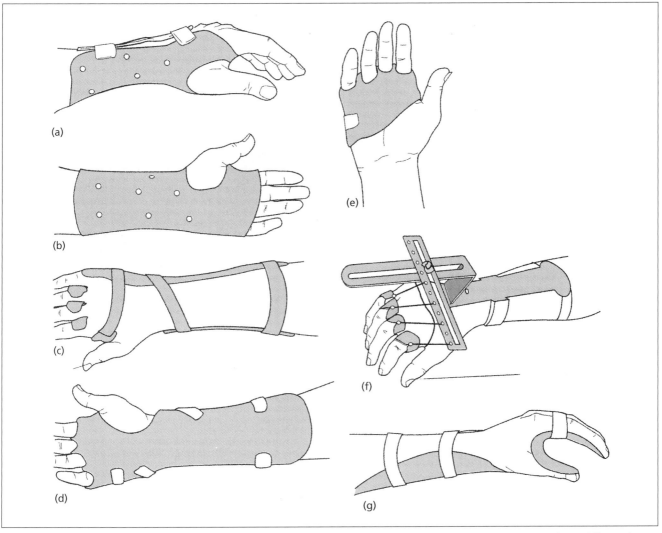

Figure 24.15 Different types of splint. (a)–(e) Resting splints to immobilize joints. (f) Example of a functional splint used to stabilize and support joint during activity. (g) A corrective (dynamic) splint used to immobilize an involved joint, realign soft tissue or correct contractures or deformities.

● Avoid staying in the same position for more than 20 minutes to prevent joint stiffness.

Exercise General exercise and therapeutic exercises contribute to the maintenance and promotion of joint function. An individualized exercise programme is designed by the physiotherapist in consultation with the patient, nurse and medical staff. Patients are told the purpose and importance of exercise in the management of their disease. Although the exercise programme is supervised by a physiotherapist or nurse when it is first begun, it is eventually performed by the patient as independently as possible. Support, including family members, can provide encouragement and assistance to the patient as the exercise programme is incorporated into daily living. Patients are encouraged to report excessive fatigue or increased pain associated with the performance of their exercises so that the programme can be modified.

Any exercise programme includes a *range-of-motion* component. Normally, each joint is capable of a certain range of movement. In a joint disorder, that range of movement may become limited and the muscle fibres shorten. Range-of-movement exercises involve the movement of a limb or part through its maximal potential range of movement to maintain or increase joint function. They may be passive, active or active assisted. Active range of motion involves movements that are performed by the patient unassisted. Active assisted exercises involve movements initiated by the patient that require some assistance in taking the joint through its available range of motion. Passive movements involve the practitioner putting the joint through its range of movement for the patient. These exercises should become as important a part of self-care as brushing teeth or bathing. They are most easily accomplished after initial morning stiffness has subsided or shortly after application of moist heat.

The exercise regimen also includes isometric or isotonic exercises, designed to maintain muscle strength and maintain or promote joint mobility. Isometric (static) exercises involve alternating maximum contraction and relaxation of muscles without movement of the respective part and joint. In isotonic exercise (dynamic), there is active contraction and shortening of muscles to produce movement with a minimal force of contraction. Isotonic exercise should be avoided if the joint is inflamed because pain will be increased and the inflammatory process may increase.

Patients with rheumatoid arthritis exhibit greatly reduced muscle strength, aerobic capacity and physical performance compared with age-matched controls. Patients are encouraged to participate in specially designed long-term fitness and cardiovascular conditioning programmes during periods of remission.

Surgical procedures Various surgical procedures may be used with arthritic patients to facilitate joint function and mobility, to retard disease progress or to correct a deformity. These procedures and the nursing care of the patient are described in the section on osteoarthritis (see p. 863).

Obtain relief of pain and discomfort

The **pain** associated with rheumatoid arthritis is variable in intensity and aggravated by movement. Although the amount of pain does not always correlate with the degree of inflammation present, it generally corresponds to the pattern of joint involvement. Pain is further caused by muscle spasm that develops adjacent to affected joints. Patients should be advised that the therapies for maintenance of joint function are also useful in the relief of pain. Rest, splinting and the continuation of muscle-strengthening exercises all help to prevent and relieve pain. The patient can be helped to identify those activities that aggravate and relieve pain, and take action to improve pain control.

Drug therapy with one or more classes of pharmacological agents has a vital role in the management of rheumatoid arthritis and the associated pain.

Drug therapy *Non-steroidal anti-inflammatory agents* (NSAIDs) provide the first line of therapy in rheumatoid arthritis. Their main purpose is to relieve joint pain and inflammation; however, they all have the same side effects, mainly peptic ulceration. Their anti-inflammatory properties derive from interrupting the synthesis of the prostaglandins. While they all work in the same way, individual responses can vary widely and some experimentation may be needed to find the NSAID that works best for each person. Some prostaglandins are very important for the maintenance of healthy gastric mucosa and as a result, NSAIDs have the unwanted side-effect of damaging the gastric mucosa. Patients with asthma should not use NSAIDs because of the risk of a hypersensitivity reaction leading to bronchospasm. The serious nature of the side-effects caused by NSAIDs has led to much research into a new generation of drugs which would have the beneficial effects of NSAIDs but without

their harmful side-effects. This led to the development of the COX2 inhibitors which had a much more selective effect on prostaglandin synthesis than the traditional NSAIDs. However, this new generation of drugs (such as Vioxx) had to be withdrawn when it became clear they led to a greatly increased risk of cardiovascular problems such as myocardial infarction (British National Formulary 2005).

If the pain and discomfort continue with NSAIDs, low dosage steroids will be introduced to the treatment (5–7.5 mg prednisolone daily) and may even be used as intra-articular injections. Current thinking is now in favour of the early use of steroids as this is when they are most beneficial (Solomon et al 2005). Eventually, however, second-line drugs including gold, methotrexate or penicillamine need to be added to the drug therapy. Collectively, they are known as disease-modifying anti-rheumatic drugs, or DMARDs. They have the capacity to suppress the disease but cannot restore damaged joints. They also take several months to become effective and if one drug is not helping, another should be tried.

Gold compounds are used because of substantial evidence of their efficacy. When a preparation of *gold salts* such as sodium aurothiomalate (Myocrisin) is given, the patient is observed closely for signs of toxic reactions. The initial dose is small to test the patient for adverse reactions. Reactions that may be seen include stomatitis (inflammation of the oral mucous membrane), dermatitis, renal damage and bone marrow depression leading to severe anaemia, leucopenia (agranulocytosis) and thrombocytopenia. Gold therapy usually involves an intramuscular injection (50 mg) given each week for a period of 4–6 months. Most responses occur during the first 16 weeks of treatment. Once a response has been obtained, maintenance therapy should be continued. If no response has occurred after 2 months, it should be discontinued and an alternative drug tried (British National Formulary 2005). Urine analysis and blood cell counts are done weekly, and the patient is checked for possible signs or symptoms of adverse side-effects.

The *antimalarial drugs* such as chloroquine (Avloclor, Nivaquine) and hydroxychloroquine (Plaquenil) may be prescribed over a period of several months for some patients. Toxic effects that may develop include skin eruptions, headache, anorexia, nausea, vomiting, and auditory or visual disturbances. Frequent blood cell counts are done because occasionally bone marrow depression occurs, and frequent eye examinations are required to check for keratopathy, which is reversible or a serious irreversible retinopathy.

Immunosuppressive drugs such as methotrexate or azathioprine have been used to treat the patient with rheumatoid arthritis, using the rationale that the cause is an antigen-antibody reaction. These drugs are prescribed for patients who are unresponsive to any of the drugs mentioned previously in this section. Ciclosporin has become more widespread in its use in recent years.

The suppression of leucocyte and antibody formation makes the patient very susceptible to infection. The rheumatoid arthritic patient is frequently debilitated and already has a lowered resistance. Precautions are necessary to avoid exposure to infection; recognition of early symptoms is reported promptly so that an antibiotic may be prescribed. The patient should be fully informed of the major side-effects that can occur with these drugs. Combination therapy of two or more DMARDs may be used and the patient will need a great deal of support from the nurse in order to manage the side-effects that occur and stay with the drug regimen that has been prescribed.

Cytokine inhibitors (e.g. adalimumab, etanercept) are the most recent development in rheumatoid arthritis treatment. Their action is by inhibition of tumour necrosis factor. They are only used under specialist supervision and are very expensive (adalimumab costs £357 per injection and one injection is required every 2 weeks according to the British National Formulary 2005). Their use should be reserved for very aggressive disease not responding to at least two different DMARDs.

Whatever course of medication the patients are following, they will need a great deal of support and encouragement with working strategies to help them get through their daily routine as things have now become so much harder. Box 24.5 lists general guidelines that help a patient to protect a damaged, inflamed or painful joint from further injury.

Family members must be included in any discussion of self-care, as they must allow the patient to achieve maximum independence. This may be difficult for those who feel that 'doing for' the patient is helpful. Instead, they should encourage the patient to perform activities alone or with help as requested. They need to be aware of the additional time and patience required to allow the patient to achieve various activities that appear simple.

Achieve an optimal nutritional intake

Nutritional problems including anorexia, weight loss and anaemia frequently accompany rheumatoid arthritis. A well-balanced diet, similar to that essential to the health of all persons, is recommended for the arthritic patient. The total calorie intake may require some adjustment with a view to achieving or maintaining the person's normal weight. Obesity increases the strain on joints and may also reduce motivation to exercise.

Breakfast should be easily available and simple to prepare to accommodate the patient's morning stiffness. Eating utensils may be adapted to help the patient. Padded handles on cutlery make them easier to grip; hand supports on cutlery eliminate the need for fine finger movements; special handles on cups and glasses are easier and safer in handling; suction cups stop dishes from sliding; and high edges on dishware prevent food from spilling.

Achieve or maintain a positive mood state

Rheumatoid arthritis may be accompanied by a number of significant losses, both physical (e.g. loss of mobility) and psychosocial (e.g. loss of perceived control, loss of role, loss of relationships). Some patients manage these losses without significant threat to their psychological well-being, whereas others exhibit evidence of decreased psychosocial health, including symptoms of anxiety, depression and a withdrawal from others. Psychosocial health in patients with rheumatoid arthritis is influenced by many factors, including level of perceived support from others and a sense of helplessness toward the disease. The severity of impairment and disability is not a major factor in the mood state of rheumatoid arthritic patients. The nurse has an important role in assisting the patient to achieve and maintain a positive mood state, despite having rheumatoid arthritis. Since emotional and instrumental support from family and friends influences response to illness, the nurse needs to determine with the patient who makes up the patient's social network and who provides the most valuable support. If the patient receives limited support, the nurse can work with the patient to identify alternative sources of support such as self-help groups and home care agencies.

Helping the patient to learn management of the disease is essential. This decreases the feelings of helplessness and hopelessness that the patient may experience and influences the psychological health of the patient. The nurse and other health team members must continue to support the patient and family as they learn about the disease. As this encouragement and support must continue in the community, referral to appropriate community agencies should be made.

Nursing intervention also involves helping the patient to identify feelings about the illness and what it means. By identifying how he or she copes in certain situations, the patient develops insight into his or her behaviour and looks at the consequences of that behaviour and the alternatives open. Is social interaction worth the cost of occasional embarrassment and/or excessive fatigue? Hiding problems and trying to keep up with others drain the patient's energy, but asking for help may reinforce fears of being dependent. Hope may be a positive factor that motivates the patient to comply

---

Box 24.5 Guidelines for joint protection
• Maintain good posture and body alignment at all times
• Change position frequently
• Use the largest muscles and strongest joints available for any task
• Distribute weight of objects over several joints
• Perform activities slowly and smoothly
• Limit repetitive movements
• Minimize use of swollen, painful joints
• Stop activity when pain occurs
• Space activities to provide frequent rest periods
• Use assistive devices in the environment to eliminate unnecessary stress.

with therapy and learn to control symptoms. The patient and family need opportunities to discuss such ideas to help in making decisions about what is best for the patient. Family members and friends also need the opportunity to express their feelings and develop understanding of the patient's illness, limitations and potentials, and how to respond to the daily fluctuations in the patient's behaviour.

Preparation for discharge

Specific actions are required to prepare the patient for discharge from hospital after an acute episode, in addition to the actions taken throughout a patient's hospitalization. The quality of life of the patient with rheumatoid arthritis following discharge depends largely on the severity of the patient's disease and whether or not the pathological process in the joints is arrested. Obviously, if the disease is severe and more and more joints are progressively involved, the patient is less likely to be well enough to return to a former occupation and will require a more active and closely supervised care programme. Many patients are well enough to go to work and adjust their daily life to provide for extra rest as well as continuance of a daily physical exercise regimen. Vocational re-training may be helpful in securing employment.

If the patient is sufficiently handicapped to require physical care, a referral will be made to the community nurse. The community nurse and the occupational therapist can be of assistance in assessing the home situation and making recommendations for adjustments that will simplify the care of the patient and increase mobility and independence.

The patient and family should be acquainted with the societies and organizations that are concerned with rheumatic disease and with publications that may be helpful. Transport is frequently a problem for the person with arthritis. If the patient is required to go regularly for physiotherapy as an outpatient or to a rehabilitation unit, hospital transport may need to be organized.

DEGENERATIVE JOINT DISEASE

OSTEOARTHRITIS

Osteoarthritis is a common chronic joint disorder characterized by degenerative changes in articular cartilage and marginal bony overgrowth. The disorder affects both men and women, but has a higher incidence in women over the age of 55 years. The prevalence of the disease increases with age. At age 65 years, 25% of people have symptoms of osteoarthritis and in 80% of the population, arthritic changes are visible on radiographic examination. There is thought to be a significant genetic pre-disposition towards the disorder (Haslett et al 2002).

Primary osteoarthritis refers to the development of the disease as a result of ageing, whereas secondary osteoarthritis describes a situation where some localizing factor has contributed to the problem. Osteoarthritis occurs when the stresses being placed on a joint become too great for the

joint to carry. This can be due to weakening of the articular cartilage by disease or excess strain being placed on some part of the joint surfaces. This latter factor is implicated in the development of secondary osteoarthritis regardless of age, so that previous joint trauma, intense athletic activity, obesity and strenuous labour are all considered factors in the development of the disease.

Pathophysiology

The pathology of osteoarthritis is associated with biochemical and secondary inflammatory changes that occur in response to ongoing stress on affected joints. The cartilage on the articular ends of the bones becomes thin and worn, and gradually breaks down, leaving the denuded bone exposed. The reaction of the denuded bone (attempting to repair the damage) is manifested in outgrowths of bone from the joint margins, resulting in thickening of the ends of the bones and protruding ridges and spurs (osteophytes), which impair joint movement. Spurs may break off and become loose in the joint, causing further impairment of movement and more pain. There is irritation of the synovium leading to mild synovitis (usually this is the only inflammatory component) and eventually fibrosis of the joint capsule develops.

The weight-bearing joints, such as the hip and knee, and the interphalangeal joints of the fingers are most frequently the site of degenerative joint disease. It may occur in a single joint or may involve several.

Clinical characteristics

The clinical manifestations of the disease include soreness and an aching, poorly localized pain that occurs with use of the involved joint(s) and is relieved by rest. The disorder follows an intermittent course with good periods and bad when symptoms are more pronounced. As the disease progresses, pain occurs even at rest. Joint stiffness is most pronounced in the morning and after periods of activity during the day, and usually lasts for less than 30 minutes. The patient complains of stiffness, soreness and pain in the affected joint(s). Crepitation may be felt or heard on movement. The range of motion becomes increasingly limited because of pain, muscle spasm and the bony outgrowths. Joint enlargement and instability develop, and the joint feels hard and irregular. Bony outgrowths on the dorsal surface of affected interphalangeal joints give the knuckles a knobbly or gnarled appearance. Systemic manifestations do not occur.

Nursing assessment

Pain, stiffness and decreased mobility should be assessed. The PQRST assessment tool can be very useful here (see p. 128):

Provocation or **P**alliation – What brings the pain on and what relieves it?

Quality – What does the pain feel like? (aching, throbbing, burning, etc.)

Region or **R**adiation – Where is the pain? Which joints are affected? Does it radiate or move?

Severity – Ask the patient to rate it on a scale from 0–10. Also ask how the pain affects the patient, does it disrupt sleep? Limit mobility? Make them feel down?

Time – How does the pain vary through the day? How long have you had the pain?

The same approach could be used to assess how much each symptom interferes with the ability to perform self-care and work-related activities and what changes the patient has made in usual daily life. Equally important is an evaluation of the emotional response of the patient to the disease. Some patients feel helpless and hopeless because of the limitations imposed by the disease, whereas others continue to enjoy life despite having osteoarthritis.

The patient's gait, movement and ability to walk are observed. All joints are assessed with particular attention to those that are most troublesome. It is important to gather data in this way, not only to identify problem areas where nursing intervention is required, but also as a baseline against which to measure progress. A pain rating scale of 0–10, for example, allows careful pain control while a progressively reducing stiffness rating allows both patient and nurse to see progress. This can act as a powerful reinforcer for the patient, encouraging maximum participation in a plan of therapy. Assessment should therefore be an ongoing activity rather than a one-off activity performed on presentation.

Patient problems

Assessment of the patient with osteoarthritis often identifies one or all of the following health problems:

- *pain* due to the disease process and accentuated by activity
- *impaired physical mobility* related to limitations in the range of motion of joints
- *reduced self-care* ability due to decreased activity
- *mood alteration* related to discomfort and reduced mobility.

Overall goals for patients with osteoarthritis include achieving optimal physical mobility, relief of pain and discomfort, and attaining realistic levels of independence and hopefulness for the future. Medical and surgical interventions are important components of treatment, as are physiotherapy and occupational therapy. Most patients are treated conservatively but if the pain becomes intractable and the disability severe surgery is indicated.

The nurse has a role in the total care of the patient, including the coordination of the various patient services. The nurse and patient work together to identify patient-centred goals; these may include:

1 a demonstration of optimal physical mobility
2 relief of pain
3 a satisfactory level of independence
4 a satisfactory level of psychosocial health.

Nursing intervention
Achieving optimal physical mobility
Appropriate exercises are prescribed to maintain muscle tone and movement and to promote good alignment and joint stability. Oliver and Ryan (2004) cite evidence showing that regular exercise improves joint stability, functional ability in daily tasks and the person's morale. It also encourages weight loss which is a major factor in lessening the impact of the disease. The patient is encouraged to be posture-conscious and to review regular daily activities and posture. Work should be interspersed with short intervals of rest, and unnecessary walking, climbing stairs, lifting and bending should be eliminated. A firm mattress is recommended to promote good alignment and support for the affected joints.

Relief of pain
Patients with osteoarthritis are encouraged to use the same measures for **pain** relief and joint protection as outlined for the patient with rheumatoid arthritis: splinting; use of assistive devices including a walking stick; good choice of shoes, rest alternating with activity; and the maintenance of an exercise programme.

Medications used in treating the patient with osteoarthritis are prescribed primarily to control pain. They include analgesic agents, initially paracetamol, and the NSAIDs described in the section on rheumatoid arthritis. A systematic review of the evidence by Zhang et al (2004) found NSAIDs offer better pain relief than paracetamol in osteoarthritis but, as expected, cause more gastrointestinal side effects. If the patient does not suffer unduly from gastrointestinal problems, NSAIDs are therefore the first choice over paracetamol. Lin et al (2004) reviewed the evidence comparing the efficacy of topical NSAIDs (which are claimed to avoid gastrointestinal side effects) with oral NSAIDs in the management of osteoarthritis. They found topical NSAIDs were initially less effective than oral versions but between weeks 2 and 4, they were both equally effective. However, they also found the rate of gastrointestinal complications did not differ between topical and oral NSAIDs whilst the topical group reported adverse skin events such as rashes in 7.4% of cases as compared with 1% of the patients on oral NSAIDs. There is therefore little convincing evidence in favour of topical NSAIDs as opposed to oral preparations. No medications are known that halt the disease process of osteoarthritis.

Local corticosteroids injected into the affected joint provide short-term relief. A recent innovation has been the intra-articular injection of hyaluronic acid in patients who have not responded to simple analgesics and other conservative therapies. Hyaluronic acid is a disaccharide that is necessary for the functional integrity of healthy cartilage and extracellular matrix. It is responsible for the viscous and elastic properties of synovial fluid. Sodium hyaluronate and hylan G-F 20 are slow-acting drugs that contain various fractions of hyaluronic acid and which, when injected together at weekly intervals, reduce pain and increase mobility, particularly of the knee joint (British National Formulary 2005). Ultimately joint surgery is indicated for pain and disability that is unrelieved by conservative measures.

As the disease progresses, nursing care in the community is directed towards the promotion of maximum independence through patient education and self-care programmes until such time as surgery is available.

Surgical treatment

When an arthritic or deformed joint causes intractable pain and severe disability, surgical intervention may be undertaken. The main operative procedure involves total replacement arthroplasty. According to Temple (2004) over 30 000 such procedures are carried out each year in the UK. Osteotomy or arthrodesis are the less frequently used alternatives.

Osteotomy is the re-shaping of the bone by cutting or curettement to redistribute the loading on the joint. This operation is used mainly on young patients whose range of motion is still good and whose joint is stable but whose pain requires surgical relief. It is a temporary 'fix' and the person will eventually require a total arthroplasty.

Arthrodesis is the surgical fusion of a joint, which results in loss of joint movement. It is done as a salvage operation if the hip replacement has failed (Girdlestone's arthrodesis) and will provide pain relief at the expense of a fused hip. Arthrodesis is also considered in the treatment of severe osteoarthritis of the cervical spine.

An *arthroplasty* is a reconstructive procedure that may entail replacement of part of a joint, or a whole joint, with a prosthesis. It is done to relieve pain and permit patient mobility.

Total hip arthroplasty

Total hip arthroplasty involves surgical replacement of both articulating surfaces of the joint. If performed on younger patients, there is a risk that the patient will live long enough for the prosthesis to be worn out and the joint then to fail, consequently surgeons are reluctant to perform this surgery on younger people, preferring an osteotomy to buy time and delay the procedure by several years.

The femoral head and neck are removed. The cartilage is removed from the acetabulum and a plastic cup is fitted into the socket. Surgical bone cement may be used to secure the plastic cup to the surface of the acetabulum, or a porous, non-cemented prosthesis may be used. The head and neck of the femur are then replaced with a metal prosthesis consisting of a spherical head and stem (Fig. 24.16). The latter is implanted and may be cemented into the proximal portion of the femoral shaft. The ball part of the prosthesis is fitted into the acetabulum and tested for a range of motions to make sure it does not dislocate on movement.

It is important that the nurse caring for the patient is familiar with the post-surgical position to be maintained and when movement may be resumed in order that the prosthesis does not dislocate accidentally. If surgical cement is not used, the period of immobility is longer. When the wound is closed, a closed drainage system is established to promote drainage of accumulating secretions. Until adduction movements are judged safe by the surgeon, the limb should be kept in abduction.

Preoperative care Pre-admission assessment is increasingly being carried out by nurse practitioners using advanced

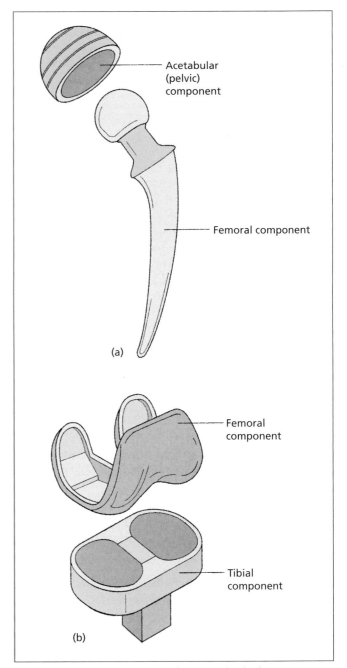

Figure 24.16 (a) Total hip arthroplasty prosthesis. (b) Knee replacement prosthesis.

skills to determine the fitness of the patient for operation. This avoids admitting patients and then cancelling the operation because they are unfit for general anaesthesia. A great deal of patient education and preparation, together with discharge planning, can take place in such a preadmission clinic setting. The patient's psychological assessment should include examining how realistic the person is being about the benefits of surgery in order that unrealistic expectations may be dealt with appropriately. Family and social factors should also be explored.

The patient must also be told what to expect after operation and how to help in the rehabilitation process. The importance of abduction of the hip is explained and techniques to maintain abduction demonstrated. These may include the use of abduction splints, wedge pillows, or two or three pillows between the legs. The limits of hip flexion should be explained (45–60°). An overhead bed frame or pulley can be used to demonstrate how the patient can move about the bed after the operation.

The patient requires instruction in and practice of post-operative exercises. Specific exercises include quadriceps and gluteal contractions, and plantar and dorsiflexion of the toes and ankles are essential to maintain function and aid circulation. Blood is typed and cross-matched and made available for blood replacement during and after the operation, if necessary.

During the preoperative period, an anticoagulant may be prescribed. The anticoagulant is administered to reduce the risk of thrombosis and embolism, and to promote micro-circulation in the operative site.

One further problem that may be encountered is the patient who is reluctant to consent to surgery, despite their pain and immobility. Obviously the patient's autonomy must be respected and if their decision is against surgery, we must respect that, but maintain good communication so that if at some point in the future, the patient changes their mind, they can be rapidly accommodated. There is some interesting work by Clark et al (2004) carried out in Toronto which explores why patients decline surgery. They found patients often succeeded in adapting to the pain and immobility and while the pain might be bad, for some people it was not bad enough to undergo surgery. There was real evidence of the health belief model at work (p. 22) as patients consider the costs, risks and benefits of surgery. Patients also did not always have a realistic picture of the risks (perceiving them as being higher than they were) and the benefits (perceiving them to be less than they were likely to be). This finding led Radwin (2005) to comment on the importance of the nurse in helping patients to make the correct decision at preoperative assessment.

Postoperative care

In the immediate postoperative assessment, the nurse monitors carefully for the complications and sequelae of any operation, including the state of the wound, pain, shock and haemorrhage.

Patient-centred *goals* include the following:

1 The hip is maintained in correct anatomical position
2 The prescribed exercise plan is followed in hospital and plan for exercise after discharge is described
3 The patient is free of pain
4 Infection is prevented in the postoperative period
5 A satisfactory cardiovascular, neurovascular and respiratory function is maintained
6 Anxiety related to surgery is avoided or reduced
7 Mobility is restored to the affected joint.

Preventing dislocation of the hip prosthesis Nursing actions to maintain the prosthesis in position include positioning of the patient in bed, assistance with early ambulation, and instructions for physical mobility at home. The patient returns from surgery supine and will have abductor splints or pillows in place to keep the hip in abduction and maintain neutral rotation. Acute flexion of the hip must be avoided because of the risk of dislocation. Indications of dislocation, including severe hip pain, shortening of the affected extremity, a firm palpable mass in the operative area and rotation of the hip, should be reported immediately. Two nurses are generally required when turning the patient. One nurse supports the limb, maintaining the abducted position, while the second person turns the patient to the unaffected side. Pillows are placed anteriorly and posteriorly to provide support in the side-lying position.

A limited range of movement and slow flexion of the hip are introduced and gradually increased under the supervision of the nurse or physiotherapist. The patient is usually assisted from bed on the first postoperative day but this varies with the individual surgeon. Patients are instructed to avoid flexing the hip joint more than 90° when moving from bed to chair or wheelchair.

Recently, studies have begun to look at whether the various precautions are really necessary to prevent dislocation and one study by Talbot et al (2002) found a dislocation rate of only 0.6%, when no restrictions were imposed. A further study by Peak et al (2005) compared dislocations amongst two groups of patients, one with standard restrictions and the other without. The study looked at 303 hip replacement procedures and found only one dislocation occurred (0.3%) and that was in the group who had the standard restrictions imposed. Those without the restrictions reported statistically significant reductions in return to work times and greater levels of satisfaction and mobility. However, as Forster (2005) commented, this study does not make the case for abandoning restrictions as the numbers of dislocations involved was so low as to render comparisons meaningless due to a high probability of what is known in statistical theory as a Type II error. This means stating there is no difference between two groups when there actually is but the samples sizes are not large enough to reveal the difference. The problem is that the dislocation rates were so low that the samples had to be much larger to provide meaningful statistics. However, there is clearly further research to be undertaken as there are real potential benefits to relaxing these traditional precautions if the evidence reveals no increase in dislocation risk.

Whatever restrictions are in place, eventually the patient is assessed for weight-bearing and, if appropriate, crutches should be used for weight support. Walking is started using crutches or a walking frame. The patient usually remains in hospital for 5–10 days.

Preventing infection Joint infection is disastrous in arthroplasty as it results in destruction of bone and failure of the prosthesis to stabilize and fuse. Strict asepsis is essential in wound care. The appearance of the wound and the colour and amount of any drainage should be assessed for any signs of infection so that they can be detected and reported. Close observations for other signs of infection are also made, including raised temperature and pulse, complaints of pain and pressure in the affected hip, or general malaise.

Preventing thromboembolism Patients undergoing arthroplasty are at high risk for thromboembolism; estimated at between 40 and 70%, owing to a combination of advanced age, immobility and conditions conducive to venous stasis (Temple 2004). Fatal pulmonary embolism is therefore a major risk and low molecular weight heparin therapy and anti-embolic stockings are the standard postoperative precautions most favoured. Careful monitoring is conducted for indications of thromboembolism, such as calf oedema, tenderness or redness.

Reducing pain The patient normally experiences pain following arthroplasty. Pain should be assessed and analgesia provided regularly to control the pain, promote early ambulation and enable the patient to receive adequate rest. Patient-controlled analgesia (PCA) is particularly suitable for this group of patients (see p. 132). Other pain-relieving techniques include ensuring the patient is well informed preoperatively about likely postoperative progress (reducing anxiety) and regular changes in position may also be helpful in maximizing the comfort of the patient. Extreme pain that does not respond to prescribed analgesia should be evaluated carefully and reported to the surgeon as it may indicate a complication such as dislocation of the prosthesis. Critical pathways are particularly helpful for this group of patients as the patient held version keeps the patient on track in assessing their own progress.

Reducing anxiety and maximizing function Patients experience anxiety over many aspects of the operation. Concerns should be assessed and dealt with on an individual basis. Generally, all patients express concern over commencement of activity and ambulation. Having experienced so much pain and instability when walking before the operation, the patient is likely to require repeated reassurance that walking is now possible without discomfort or damage to the new joint. The patient needs much support, both physical and emotional, in the early phase of ambulation. The support is withdrawn very gradually when the patient has sufficient control to be safe and displays confidence.

Another area of potential anxiety concerns the return to sexual activity. Counselling should be offered to all patients, regardless of their age. The patient should refrain from intercourse for about 6 weeks after the operation to avoid extreme hip flexion or adduction that could lead to dislocation of the prosthesis. Healing of the internal capsule takes about 6 weeks, after which sexual intercourse can be resumed.

Preparation for discharge To prepare for going home and becoming as independent as possible, the patient gradually takes over self-care and receives instructions for home-care.

It is likely that the more control exerted by the patient with respect to rehabilitation and recovery, the better the outcome will be. Patients should be taught not to flex the hip by more than 90° and to avoid extremes of other movements of the hip. They should avoid lying on the affected side for at least 2 months. Legs should not be crossed and low, soft chairs should be avoided. A high, firm chair with arms is recommended, along with a raised toilet seat in the bathroom. The importance of continuing the exercises and walking is stressed, while excessive bending, heavy lifting and jogging are discouraged. Support stockings are helpful until no swelling remains in the legs or feet. This information should be reviewed verbally with the patient and written instructions given at discharge.

A referral to the community staff is appropriate to reinforce hospital teaching and to provide support to the patient and family as full activity is resumed. A home visit with the occupational therapist before discharge is helpful. The aim of the visit is to assess the situation and to make suggestions regarding any adaptations that would promote the patient's independence and safety.

Knee replacement

Osteoarthritis of the knee occurs mostly in the over 50s and obesity is a common contributing factor. There may also have been a long standing deformity of the limb causing abnormal loading on the joint. Temporary relief may be obtained by the relatively minor procedure of an arthroscopic washout whilst if there is a pronounced deformity this may be corrected and symptoms relieved by a realignment osteotomy. However, in older patients with advanced disease a replacement arthroplasty will be required (Solomon et al 2005).

Before the operation, the patient is taught and practises quadriceps, hamstring and gluteal setting exercises to maintain optimum strength. These exercises are performed 4-hourly. The patient is also taught to transfer from bed to chair and may practise with a Zimmer frame or crutches before the operation.

Care of the patient following total knee replacement is similar to that after total hip replacement.

Evaluation

Nursing care of the patient with osteoarthritis is effective if the patient is able to achieve a maximum level of self-care while controlling pain and discomfort. For patients undergoing surgical intervention, the nursing care has been effective if complications of surgery are avoided (or detected and treated promptly) and the patient regains a satisfactory level of mobility and independence. Osteoarthritis can be controlled with the ongoing collaboration of the patient, family and the healthcare team.

SEPTIC ARTHRITIS

This condition involves inflammation of the joint due to infection and often effects a knee joint. It tends to occur most often in young adults. Staph aureus is the common cause in adults and the organism enters the joint via a penetrating wound or after the rupture of a bone abscess in osteomyelitis (see p. 869). More rarely, it can occur secondary to high risk behaviours such as i.v. drug use or by the systemic spread of Neisseria gonorrhoeae after a primary infection, whatever the site (genital, oral, or rectal). (See Case Study 24.3 for an example of a case study illustrating many of the problems encountered in this type of patient.) This condition can also occur in children when the causative organism is often Haemophilus influenzae (Solomon et al 2005). Joint aspiration and investigations of the fluid are essential for diagnosis together with radiography of the joint. Intravenous antimicrobials need to be started as soon as possible, the joint needs aspiration and washing out and the limb resting with splintage.

CASE A 26-year-old man called Max limped into a walk-in centre complaining of left knee pain. He looked unkept and thin. When the nurse practitioner (NP) began to take a history, he told her he had had the pain for 4 days and today it is real bad. He also complained that he thought his left knee looked a bit swollen. His right knee felt fine however. When the NP asked if he had any other complaints, he stated he also felt like he was having hot and cold turns and had generally felt poorly that day. He looked feverish (flushed) and sweaty. He had limped into the walk-in centre and confirmed the fact that it was painful to weight-bear on his left knee and walking was becoming more difficult.

As the NP continued with the rest of the history, he revealed that he did not have a regular job and lived with his girlfriend in a small flat. When asked about his previous medical history he admitted to being treated for Chlamydia 3 years ago, but was not on any current medication. He stated he smoked 30/day and often 'gets hammered' on strong lager but was vague about exactly how many units of alcohol he consumed per week. The NP asked him about recreational drug use besides tobacco and alcohol. He admitted to using cannabis and i.v. heroin regularly. He stated he had had no new sexual contacts in the last few months and denied any urethral discomfort or discharge.

Vital signs were checked and revealed a temperature of 38.9°C, P112, BP 130/90 and RR 18. His oxygen saturation was 98% on room air.

The NP carried out a physical examination which revealed no gross abnormalities in the neurological, cardiovascular, respiratory or genitourinary systems, while his abdomen was soft and unremarkable. Head, eyes and ENT (HEENT) examinations were normal. The NP then focused on his legs and compared his left knee with his right knee as a reference. It was swollen, erythematous (red looking), warm, tender to palpation and he could not move it. The NP noted a positive ballottement sign indicating a knee effusion (Walsh 2006). A gentle attempt at passive movement caused severe pain so the NP desisted immediately.

What possibilities do you think the NP was considering as a differential diagnosis?

Pain and inflammation in a single joint in an adult raises the possibility of osteoarthritis, gout trauma or septic arthritis. The fact that this was a young adult and the presentation associated with other signs of sepsis such as fever and malaise, point in the direction of septic arthritis. High risk behaviour such as i.v. drug use and the presence of a recent sexually transmitted infection all again point in the direction of septic arthritis.

The NP decided that a septic arthritis was the most likely cause of the problem and arranged with the local A&E department to have him seen by the orthopedic team. They agreed and took blood for a complete blood count and culture, a urethral swab to check for Chlamydia and Neisseria gonorrhoeae and ordered knee X-rays. Neisseria gonorrhoeae often causes septic arthritis in young adults and is capable of dissemination through the body within a week or two of the primary infection, whatever the site (Filbin et al 2002). They carried out knee aspiration to examine the aspirate which was sent for Gram staining and culture (to try and identify organisms which may be present), cell count, differential crystals and testing for protein and glucose. Crystals would be expected in gout and a leucocyte count of over 50 000 is strongly suggestive of infection (septic arthritis). The ratio of joint fluid to serum glucose levels is often 1:2 or less in septic arthritis.

The aspirate appeared cloudy and the X-ray confirmed the presence of a joint effusion but no sign of bone disease. Laboratory results showed a leucocyte count of 83 000 and the Gram staining suggested the presence of *Staph. Aureus*, which was subsequently confirmed on blood and aspirate cultures. The patient was admitted for irrigation of the knee joint and i.v. antibiotic therapy, rest and elevation of the affected limb. Analgesia presented a difficult problem given his known heroin usage.

There was a need for some urgent interdisciplinary work to address his drug use problem as at that time, he was not known to the drug use team.

OTHER INFLAMMATORY JOINT DISEASES

ANKYLOSING SPONDYLITIS

This is a chronic generalized inflammatory disorder characterized by inflammation and ensuing ankylosis of the sacroiliac joints and spinal articulations. The pathological process is similar to that seen in rheumatoid arthritis, but there is a greater tendency toward calcification. In most instances, the disease remains confined to the joints cited above but occasionally does spread to peripheral joints.

The highest incidence is in the second and third decade of life with a male:female ratio estimated at up to 10:1 (Solomon et al 2005). The disorder has a prevalence of about 1 in 500 amongst Europeans but much lower in other ethnic groups such as Japanese or those of African descent. Underdiagnosis in females is possible, mainly due to the lack of knowledge about female incidence and reluctance to perform pelvic radiography. The asymmetrical inflammatory arthritis of hips and knees, which is the early presenting problem in women years before the onset of any back problem, only adds to the difficulty of 'labelling the problem'. The cause is likely to be an inherited genetic susceptibility which is triggered by some other event.

Clinical characteristics

The onset of this disease is usually insidious; the patient first complains of stiffness in the back in the morning or following a period of inactivity. Progressively, this becomes more noticeable; limitation in the range of spinal flexion develops, chest expansion is reduced, and there is low back pain radiating to the buttocks and thighs along the sciatic nerve pathways. General systemic symptoms may include fatigue and weight loss.

Laboratory examinations indicate an increase in the erythrocyte sedimentation rate, but in most cases, rheumatoid factor is absent. Recently it has been recognized that the histocompatibility antigen HLA-B27 is present in 90% of these patients; this has become a confirming diagnostic of ankylosing spondylitis. Leucocytosis and anaemia may be present and the protein concentration of the cerebrospinal fluid is frequently increased.

Remissions and exacerbations of the acute disease are common. In the most advanced stages, some patients develop some peripheral rheumatoid arthritis. A few develop circulatory complications due to aortitis and aortic valvular insufficiency. Uveitis (inflammation of the iris, ciliary body and choroid of the eye) is also seen in about 25% of the patients.

Progressive involvement of spinal segments may continue over a period of years and eventually leave the patient with practically the whole spine firmly ankylosed, producing what may be referred to as a poker back or poker spine. Rarely, osteospondylitis has an abrupt, acute onset and spreads rapidly through the lumbar, thoracic and cervical segments, leaving the patient with a poker spine in a relatively short period.

Nursing assessment

A patient with this condition may be admitted for review and stabilization. It is important to assess mobility, pain levels and the possible side-effects of long-term non-steroidal anti-inflammatory drug (NSAID) therapy such as gastric disturbance. The patient's social circumstances should be assessed as these may have a profound effect upon mood and self-concept. The condition may be seriously affecting the person's ability to work or may have led to loss of employment. The inability to be involved in favourite recreations or sports, or even to play with children, may contribute to a depressed mood state, while self-concept may be severely damaged.

During the inpatient period, medical staff will be reviewing the patient's condition, drug regimen, etc., and there will also be an intensive physiotherapy review. The nurse should be sensitive to the person's psychological and social problems in

order that the person may achieve maximum benefit from the hospitalization and return home with a positive, but realistic, view of the future based upon an effective mix of physical therapy, psychological support and patient teaching.

Nursing care

In general terms, goals for the patient with ankylosing spondylitis include the relief of pain (usually with NSAIDs), maintenance of good spinal alignment and mobility with preservation of maximum spinal function.

Rest and good posture at all times are extremely important so that ankylosis of the affected joints occurs while they are in the normal neutral position, thus preventing deformity and handicap. The patient is advised of the need for constant attention to good posture when up, with emphasis on contraction of the buttock and lower abdominal muscles and keeping the chest up, shoulders back and head erect. A fracture board and a firm mattress are placed on the bed, and it is suggested that the patient does not use a pillow or, if necessary, only a very small one. The patient is advised to sleep straight and flat on the back or in the prone position to discourage possible flexion of the spine.

A daily physical exercise programme is prescribed with the objective of strengthening the muscles that help to support the spine, maintain good alignment and promote the patient's functional capacity. As ankylosis of the costovertebral joints may occur and reduce the ventilatory capacity, breathing exercises are also included in the suggested exercise regimen.

Heavy lifting and activities that place strain upon the back are restricted. The patient assists in determining the level of tolerance of physical activity; activity that produces pain or exhaustion should be avoided, and additional rest is important.

In some cases, hip arthroplasty may be needed to assist with mobility and pain relief, and to prevent subsequent spinal deformities.

METABOLIC JOINT DISEASE

GOUT

Gout is a disorder of uric acid metabolism, characterized by recurring episodes of acute inflammation, pain and swelling in a joint. Any joint may be affected, but those of the foot are more susceptible; the condition usually develops first in the great toe. Gout occurs more commonly in men and is rarely seen in females, except for post-menopausal women. It is also more common in the European population than those of Afro-Caribbean descent.

The disorder is caused by an excessive concentration of uric acid in the plasma (hyperuricaemia), which may be brought about by an overproduction or faulty disposal by the kidneys. Urate crystals may be precipitated and deposited within joint tissues, setting up irritation and a local inflammatory response. The small masses of crystals, which are called *tophi,* may also form in cartilage, the kidneys or soft tissues in other areas of the body.

Secondary gout may develop in disorders such as blood dyscrasias in which there is a marked breakdown of cellular nucleic acid. Certain medications such as the thiazide diuretics (bendroflumethiazide) or the loop diuretics (furosemide) can precipitate episodes of gout. When the urate crystals are deposited in joints and produce inflammation, the condition may be referred to as *gouty arthritis*.

Clinical characteristics

Acute episodes are characterized by the sudden onset of excruciating pain in the affected joint, usually the base of the big toe, with the hind foot or hand joints the next most frequent. It becomes very tender, red, hot and swollen. Veins in the area stand out because of congestion and distension. The patient may also experience anorexia, headache, fever and constipation. The blood uric acid concentration can be raised (normal 0.18–0.42 mmol/L), although this measurement is not always accurate during an acute attack. Subcutaneous tophi are frequently apparent in the ears or over joints or knuckles. Precipitations of urates may occur in kidney tissue, leading to impaired renal function. In some patients, the excessive concentration of uric acid results in the formation of kidney stones.

The acute attack usually subsides in a few days, and in the early stages of the disease the joint returns to normal. Remissions may gradually become shorter, and the disease may become chronic. More joints become involved, and there are irreversible changes, leading to deformity and loss of function.

Nursing assessment

Patients with gout are usually admitted to hospital only for a severe acute exacerbation. Assessment should include checking the principal vital signs, monitoring pain levels and mobility. As in the case of ankylosing spondylitis, it is important to find out how the condition is affecting the person's everyday life in terms of work, family relationships, recreation, etc. Much unhappiness may result if these areas are adversely affected, which may in turn affect patient compliance with therapy. It may be very beneficial for the patient to use the time in hospital to talk freely and frankly about such worries and anxieties.

The nurse in the community may also encounter a patient with gout if the urate crystal deposits lead to tissue breakdown and the formation of open lesions requiring dressing.

Nursing care

During an attack of gout, the patient may be placed on bedrest and the affected part immobilized. Drug therapy is promptly instituted. Apart from NSAIDs, the other preparation that may be used is colchicine, which is administered orally in a short course to achieve relief. Side-effects include nausea, vomiting, abdominal discomfort and diarrhoea. The drug generally relieves the pain fairly quickly but does not lower the hyperuricaemia.

A fluid intake of 2500–3000 mL is encouraged to promote dilution and renal elimination of the uric acid. This minimum daily intake should be continued during remissions.

The patient is instructed to limit foods high in purines such as organ meats (liver, kidneys), shellfish, sardines and meat extracts, and also to limit the intake of alcoholic beverages. As it is more difficult for uric acid crystals to precipitate as urate crystals in alkaline urine, alkaline-producing foods are encouraged, such as milk, potatoes and citrus fruits.

Prevention of acute episodes may be achieved by drugs that lower serum urate levels. Allopurinol and sulfinpyrazone are very effective as they interfere with the production of uric acid (British National Formulary 2005).

CONNECTIVE TISSUE (COLLAGEN) DISEASE

SYSTEMIC LUPUS ERYTHEMATOSUS (DISSEMINATED LUPUS ERYTHEMATOSUS)

This disorder is a multisystem disease that is characterized by diffuse inflammation and biochemical and structural changes in the collagen fibres of connective tissues in organs and tissues throughout the body. The root of the problem is a severe disturbance of immune regulation.

Systemic lupus erythematosus (SLE) is an autoimmune disorder characterized by antibodies that develop against cells' nuclear components. A sensitivity to the individual's own DNA develops and the antigen-antibody complexes damage the vasculature structure and functions of tissues and organs. Several factors are suspected of having a role in precipitating the onset or an acute exacerbation of the disease; these include exposure to the sun's rays, emotional stress, infection and drugs (e.g. sulfonamide, penicillin, procainamide, isoniazid). The incidence is increasing and many patients are diagnosed with mild forms of lupus. The 15-year survival rate for patients with mild disease is over 90%. Prognosis depends on the age of the patient (it is usually more severe in children; in the elderly it may be mild and respond well to treatment), severity of the disease, the organs affected, and the patient's response to treatment and ability to participate in the treatment plan.

Clinical characteristics

The disease may begin at any age in either sex, but is seen most often in young women between the ages of 20 and 30 years. It also affects Afro-Caribbean women six times more frequently than Caucasians (Haslett et al 2002). The signs and symptoms, especially at the onset, vary greatly from one person to another, depending upon the systems and organs involved. Those most commonly seen include fever, general malaise, excessive fatigue, weakness, anorexia, weight loss and joint pain. An erythematous rash may be evident on the face, neck and/or extremities. The lesions on the face typically spread over the nose and cheeks to form a butterfly pattern. Angioneurotic oedema with burning or itchy sensations, areas of hyperpigmentation, mucosal ulceration and alopecia may develop. (*Angioneurotic oedema* is the temporary appearance of large oedematous areas in the skin or mucous membrane due to a disturbance in the innervation of the vasomotor system.)

In the systemic type of lupus erythematosus, generalized lymphadenopathy occurs. The patient may complain of impaired vision as a result of corneal involvement and retinopathy. Raynaud's phenomenon may be troublesome, especially if the patient is exposed to even slight cold. As the disease progresses, impaired pulmonary, haematological (anaemia), cardiovascular and kidney functions are common. Central nervous system involvement also occurs.

The erythrocyte sedimentation rate is raised and anaemia is a frequent development. The presence of the lupus erythematosus cell factor and other antinuclear antibodies in the serum facilitates diagnosis. The haematocrit falls and thrombocytopenia may be manifested in petechiae and purpura.

Nursing assessment

The patient with SLE is likely to be encountered in hospital either as a result of an acute exacerbation or on admission for joint replacement surgery. However, it should be remembered that the patient may have been admitted for other reasons not directly related to this condition, a consideration that applies to all the types of condition discussed in this chapter. Alternatively, they may present undiagnosed, with early symptoms, in primary care.

If the patient has been admitted with an acute exacerbation of SLE, the nursing assessment must be comprehensive, yet tailored to individual needs, as the disorder can affect the patient in many different ways. Multi-system involvement is possible. The person who has been admitted for joint replacement surgery requires careful assessment to ensure they are fit enough for the anaesthetic and the stress of surgery, in addition to the normal assessment required for a patient undergoing joint replacement surgery.

Nursing care

The care of the patient is mainly supportive and symptomatic; at present, no therapy is considered curative. In remissions, the patient is advised against exposure to sunlight, infection and excessive fatigue which are thought to predispose or precipitate an exacerbation of the disease process. High factor sun block (protection factor 25–50) is recommended (Haslett et al 2002). Cold should be avoided because of the vascular reaction (Raynaud's disease).

Medications that may be prescribed include NSAIDs to control fever and joint involvement, and an antimalarial drug such as hydroxychloroquine (Plaquenil) for skin and joint involvement. If the condition is unresponsive to NSAIDs, an adrenocorticosteroid preparation may be considered. The latter is used for the more severe stage of SLE when there is renal, central nervous system, cardiovascular and haematopoietic involvement. The steroid drug is given in relatively large doses during an acute exacerbation such as oral prednisolone 40–60 mg daily, and then gradually reduced to a maintenance dose or withdrawn completely. If hydroxychloroquine is given, frequent ophthalmological examinations are necessary because the drug may precipitate retinopathy. Intravenous cyclophosphamide may be used when the patient with severe disease is unresponsive to the more conservative drugs. Aspirin may be given if there are thrombotic problems.

Dialysis may be necessary when the disease attacks the kidneys. Infection is treated promptly with antibiotics. Emotional stress should be minimized and fatigue avoided. Plasma exchange and immunosuppressive drug therapy are reserved for advanced cases.

SLE is a serious chronic disease that is unpredictable in nature. The patient experiences remissions and exacerbations. Nursing intervention focuses on assisting the patient to manage the disease and adapt his or her lifestyle to altered functional level. Emphasis is placed on the patient's strengths and the positive aspects of functional ability. The patient is helped to identify factors that precipitate flare-ups or exacerbation of symptoms and to create an environment free of stress. A daily routine is planned to provide adequate rest.

The following points are emphasized in teaching patients and their families about the disease and self-management:

1 Knowledge of the disease process, its management, and signs and symptoms of disease activity.
2 Actions, dosage and possible side-effects of the prescribed drug(s) and adjustment of medication dosage in response to symptom changes.
3 The importance of carrying an identification card if the patient is receiving corticosteroid therapy.
4 Awareness of expected weight gains with corticosteroid therapy and measures to minimize and cope with the weight gain.
5 The necessity for regular medical supervision so that tissue changes can be detected early by laboratory tests and prompt adjustment made in drug therapy to help control tissue damage.
6 The importance of prompt identification of infection and the action to take when infection develops.
7 The importance of regular rest, sleep and good nutrition.
8 Methods of decreasing physical and emotional stress.
9 Knowledge of community resources including self-help groups.
10 Avoidance of overexposure to sunlight and use of high factor sun block.

INFECTIVE BONE DISEASE

OSTEOMYELITIS

When bone tissue becomes infected, the condition is known as osteomyelitis. The pathogenic organisms may be introduced directly through an open fracture or from infected contiguous tissue, but are more commonly carried by the blood to the bone from a distant primary focus such as boils (furuncles), an abscessed tooth or infected tonsils. When the infection is blood-borne, the condition is referred to as *haematogenous osteomyelitis*. The most common bacterial offender is *Staphylococcus aureus*, but the disease may also result from the invasion of streptococci, pneumococci or other strains of staphylococci.

Growing bone is more susceptible to haematogenous osteomyelitis and, as a result, the incidence is highest in children and adolescents. The infection usually develops in long bones at the diaphyseal side of the growth plate. In adults, the pelvis and vertebrae are more often affected. The bone marrow is affected first. Unless it is checked at the onset, the inflammatory process forms a purulent exudate that collects in the minute canals and spaces of the bone tissue. The pressure of the exudate builds up because of the resistant, rigid bone and compresses the blood vessels, causing thrombosis and occlusion. The accumulation under pressure eventually breaks through the cortex of the bone into the subperiosteal space. The periosteum at that site becomes elevated and stripped from the bone, interrupting the blood vessels that lead into the bone. Interference with the blood supply results in an area of dead bone tissue, which is called a *sequestrum*. The periosteum may rupture, and the infection may then extend into the adjacent soft tissues, forming a sinus tract that discharges on to the skin surface. Small sequestra, separated from the living bone tissue, may escape with the exudate through the sinus.

The infection may destroy the growth plate (epiphyseal plate), leading to reduced growth of the limb and deformity, or it may extend into the adjacent joint with ensuing permanent loss of joint function. The periosteum initiates the formation of new bone tissue around the affected area. The new tissue is called the *involucrum* (a covering or sheath, such as contains the sequestrum of a necrosed bone) and may enclose and trap sequestra and infecting organisms. These organisms continue to grow in the confined area and the osteomyelitis becomes chronic, characterized by recurring abscess formation and sequestration. Chronicity is more likely to occur in non-traumatic osteomyelitis.

Patient problems

The actual and potential problems of acute osteomyelitis include the following:

- severe pain in the affected limb (caused by the pressure of accumulating exudate and bone destruction) aggravated by even slight movement
- protection of the limb by avoiding weight bearing, any movement and flexion of the adjoining joints
- tenderness and swelling of the affected part; a draining sinus may develop over the involved area
- restlessness and irritability
- nausea and vomiting
- radiographs begin to show destructive bone changes and periosteal elevation 2 weeks after the disease begins but earlier detection is possible with radio-isotope scans.

Nursing assessment

The patient admitted with this condition after trauma has usually been affected over a lengthy period involving significant loss of mobility and function together with chronic pain. A careful assessment of the patient's social and psychological state is essential if nursing care is to address the patient's main problems, while pain assessment is also of prime importance. A patient who is self-employed may, for example, face bankruptcy as a result of a prolonged period of inactivity and frequent hospitalizations, while the chronic nature of the pain and apparent lack of progress in resolving the condition may severely affect the person's morale. The patient may be aware that in some cases the only way of resolving the condition is amputation.

The initial presentation will usually be in a primary care setting, especially if it involves an adolescent. The person will be unwell, feverish and in pain. The nurse needs to pay particular attention to vital signs as the patient may be very febrile and toxic in the initial stages; pain should also be assessed carefully. An urgent referral to a hospital specialist is required as immediate antimicrobial therapy is needed, but not before a sample of aspirate is obtained, if possible, for culture and sensitivity. The developmental stage of the patient should be assessed together with the family situation as this can have a significant bearing upon care.

Nursing care

Antimicrobial drug therapy and rest in the early stage of osteomyelitis may bring the infection under control with minimal bone damage and before a sinus is formed. Intravenous flucloxacillin and fusidic acid is recommended initially and this regime may be altered in light of the sensitivity of the organism (Solomon et al 2005). The biggest fear is of a MRSA infection and then vancomycin is the drug of choice (p. 146). Efforts made to identify the infecting organism include cultures from blood, nose and throat secretions and discharge from any skin lesions (e.g. boils). In more advanced cases, surgery may be necessary to provide drainage to relieve the pressure within the bone and periosteum and to remove dead bone tissue. Osteomyelitis may occur amongst intravenous heroin users and in these cases, a wide range of infectious organisms may be encountered.

Large doses of antibiotics may be given parenterally over several weeks (usually a minimum of 4 weeks). If the response is favourable and the infective process controlled, antimicrobial therapy is generally continued for several weeks to ensure destruction of the organisms. Effective oral antibiotic therapy has been achieved only recently. Clindamycin is recommended for Gram-positive staphylococcal osteomyelitis, although it has serious toxic effects such as antibiotic-induced colitis (British National Formulary 2005).

The patient is placed at rest, and the affected limb is handled very gently. It is positioned and supported to prevent contractures and deformities. A splint may be used to immobilize the adjacent joint. Careful monitoring of pressure areas and rigorous pressure care are essential. A well balanced high-calorie diet is needed to help cope with the metabolic demands of what is a serious infective process.

If the disease process becomes chronic (as it often does in adults where the original cause is traumatic), surgical drainage or a sequestrectomy is performed and the wound is packed and allowed to heal by granulation from within towards the surface. Antimicrobial therapy may supplement the surgeon's efforts. The dressing is changed often enough to keep the wound clean and to prevent the development of an offensive odour that may become very distressing to the patient and those in his or her environment. Precautions must be taken to observe aseptic technique when dressing or treating the wound to prevent the introduction of secondary infection and the transmission of the patient's infection to others.

When the patient is allowed up, protection must be afforded against falls and injury to the limb. The loss of bone substance may weaken the bone structure, predisposing it to fracture when subjected to even slight injury or pressure. In the case of a lower extremity, weight-bearing may be contraindicated for many weeks while new bone tissue is being formed. The patient may then have to be taught to use crutches and may be discharged from the hospital, but is likely to require guidance and supervision for a considerable period of time. Chronic osteomyelitis is a long haul for the patient and may prove to be extremely difficult to eradicate. The nurse therefore needs to beware of raising patient expectations unrealistically.

OSTEOPOROSIS

Osteoporosis is a disease that results from an imbalance between calcium reabsorption and bone formation. This results in an overall loss of bone mass and increases the risk of fracture, often with little trauma. Women suffer more from this problem than men, as there is accelerated loss of bone mass due to deficiency in oestrogen after the menopause. Osteoporotic fractures will affect one woman in three from the age of 50 onwards, compared with one man in 12 (Prodigy 2005). This disorder is a major cause of fractures amongst elders, especially of the wrist, upper femur and vertebrae, mostly in post-menopausal women.

Primary osteoporosis is age related, genetically influenced, while the female sex is the other major risk factor. Poor diet, anorexia, cigarette smoking, alcohol abuse and lack of exercise especially in early life, have all been implicated as contributory factors. Satisfactory levels of calcium intake and exercise during adolescence play a major part in building up bone mass and hence reducing the risk of primary osteoporosis in later life. Men may also develop osteoporosis due to the decline in levels of androgens which occurs with age, but in men, this occurs later than women and is a more gradual process. Consequently, the problem is more pronounced amongst women than men. Secondary osteoporosis occurs as a result of either another disease process (such as cancer leading to bony metastasis) or drug therapy (e.g. corticosteroid treatment). Immobilization for any reason will promote rapid secondary osteoporosis.

Bone mass is investigated using a dual-energy X-ray densitometer machine which measures X-ray absorption, hence the term DEXA scanning. A scan of the spine takes only 10 minutes, and of the hip region even less. Bone mineral density (BMD) as measured by DEXA scanning is used to define the degree of osteoporosis. Whole-population screening for osteoporosis is not carried out at present, instead it is used to investigate patients who are deemed to be at risk of the condition.

NURSING ASSESSMENT

Osteoporosis is a condition that is likely to be present in many elderly patients, particularly women. The presentation can vary from a 65-year-old woman who sees the nurse practitioner at the health centre complaining of backache, through to the 80-year-old lady admitted to A&E with a facture of the upper femur after a fall. The nurse needs to be aware of the likely existence of this condition in assessing all elderly patients and post-menopausal women, whatever other health problems they may have. A useful screen is the 'get up and go' test. Older people who can get up out of a chair without the assistance of their arms, confidently walk a few steps and then sit down again without using their arms, are at very low risk of having a fall and consequently at a much lower risk of sustaining a fracture (Prodigy 2005).

CLINICAL CHARACTERISTICS

Actual and potential problems may include the following:

- Fractures of any bone but most commonly of the vertebrae between T10 and L2, the femoral neck region and the wrist. Fractures may be impacted (Box 24.2)
- Pain, localized or radiating, and tenderness
- Muscle spasm
- Loss of normal lumbar curve and progressive development of kyphosis (curvature of the spine) due to collapsed vertebrae.

The presence of these problems leads to decreased mobility, which exacerbates the condition, and interferes with normal self-care.

NURSING CARE

As treatment for osteoporosis cannot reverse the condition, it is directed at arresting or slowing the rate of calcium reabsorption, reducing discomfort and maintaining a satisfactory lifestyle. These goals are addressed through medication, diet and exercise. Health promotion has a major role in preventing the condition, especially in younger people.

Medication

In osteoporosis, a calcium intake that is double the recommended daily allowance will reduce the rate of bone loss. A calcium supplement is therefore appropriate and is often given with vitamin D.

Vitamin D is necessary for the use of calcium in building bone mass. It may be prescribed in a range of preparations such as ergocalciferol (calciferol, vitamin D_2). However, to be effective it has to be metabolized in the kidney and consequently is not prescribed if the patient suffers from renal impairment.

Bisphosphonate drugs are used in an attempt to prevent osteoclasts from carrying out their normal function and so slow down the rate of bone resorption and this is now considered the first-line treatment for osteoporosis (Prodigy 2005). Alendronate is the main drug used in this group but it can cause problematical side-effects for some women (especially involving oesophageal reactions). Alendronate contributes to building significant bone mass at key skeletal sites. Studies in the USA have shown a 50% reduction in fractures of the hip, wrist and spine over a 3-year period in elderly women with osteoporosis and previous vertebral fractures after use of alendronate (McClung 1999).

Calcitonin works with parathyroid hormone to regulate bone turnover and may help women who cannot tolerate a bisphosphonate. It can also help to relieve pain after a vertebral fracture.

Hormone replacement therapy (HRT) is no longer considered to be a first-line treatment for osteoporosis because of the potential serious and important side-effects. It works by restoring levels of oestrogen to pre-menopausal levels and therefore slows bone loss and maintains bone levels in most women. There is an increased risk of breast cancer in women taking HRT which increases as the length of time on HRT increases (British National Formulary 2005). If the woman has any family history of breast or uterine cancer, HRT should only be prescribed under specialist supervision. The prodigy guidelines state that HRT should now only be a second-line treatment for osteoporosis which is offered if the benefits look like they will outweigh the risks (Prodigy 2005). The woman should be helped to make an informed decision by providing her with all the latest evidence on the pros and cons of treatment with HRT.

Diet

Diet therapy stresses the importance of the intake of foods high in calcium, supplementary vitamin D and protein, and of fluid intake, and the monitoring of the types of foods chosen to accomplish this.

Exercise

Regular weight-bearing exercise (e.g. dancing, walking, keep fit) places bone under stress, and they respond by becoming stronger. Three 20-minute exercise sessions per week are recommended. The general beneficial effects of exercise are added to the skeletal benefits.

Health promotion

Nurses should be aware that women are more likely to suffer from osteoporosis than men. Nurses have a responsibility to teach health habits related to a lifestyle believed to assist in the prevention of osteoporosis. The target group is pre-menopausal women, and this includes girls still at school so school nurses should also be involved in this work. Convincing a 15 year old to take seriously a risk that will only become apparent in 40 years time is a difficult task. After assessing the patient for the risk factors discussed above, a teaching plan should be developed that covers diet, exercise and any medication the person may be taking, and is directed towards the reduction of any risk factors identified. Dietary advice should cover the importance of a well-balanced diet, high in calcium and low in animal fats. Vitamin D supplements may also be recommended. The fact that excessive intake of alcohol and caffeine can accelerate the onset of osteoporosis as will smoking, should be stressed.

An older person who is given the diagnosis of osteoporosis may be very frightened and anxious. Depression, sleep disturbance, apathy and a loss of self-esteem may ensue (McClung 1999). These feelings have to be brought out into the open and worked through if the nurse is to support the patient and allow him or her to take a positive and healthy approach to the later years of life.

BACK PAIN

Back pain is a common and serious health problem in the developed world. In most cases, there is no significant pathology to be found, the pain is a result of poor posture and/or muscle strain from some heavy physical activity such as lifting or digging (mechanical pain). Such pain is usually transient and will resolve. Back pain may, however, have a degenerative origin located at the articulation of one vertebra with another and involving degeneration of the intervertebral disc. The interaction of the diseased disc with surrounding tissues gives rise to the pain. This may be by pressing on a nerve root when the result is sharp, unilateral pain that radiates down one leg and is associated often with altered sensation (paraesthesia). This is called radicular pain. Degenerative processes may also cause pain by involvement of surrounding ligaments and joint facets. The pain may also indicate a collapsed vertebrae caused by severe osteoporosis or metastatic cancer which has spread from a site such as the breast or prostate (Shelton et al 2004). In this instance, the pain is severe and constant, and unrelieved by simple analgesia. Inflammatory disease of the spine, such as spondylitis, may also cause back ache.

Early treatment in primary care should focus on pain relief with the use of simple analgesia and NSAIDs, maintaining activity and physiotherapy. Chronic disability due to back pain is usually associated with serious psychological and sociological problems, so it is essential to try to maintain a positive approach on the part of the patient. Otherwise, the person becomes increasingly dependent upon others, anxious, and experiences disturbed family relationships associated with these factors, plus sleep disturbance, reduced self-esteem and interpersonal friction.

Current guidelines stress that advice to continue ordinary activity may provide equivalent or even faster symptomatic recovery from acute back pain and lead to less chronic disability and time off work. Bedrest should not be recommended as a treatment for low back pain. Drug therapy with NSAIDs and/or benzodiazepines is effective in relieving the symptoms of an acute attack, but both groups of drugs have side-effects that should be monitored. Physiotherapy is very effective in helping patients with chronic low back pain and all patients benefit from a multidisciplinary approach to treatment.

OSTEOMALACIA

Osteomalacia is an adult disorder comparable with rickets in children and, for this reason, it is occasionally referred to as adult rickets. It is characterized by an insufficient plasma concentration of calcium and inorganic phosphate for normal calcification of bone tissue. It may result from an insufficient amount of calcium reaching the plasma or an excessive urinary excretion of the mineral. The deficiency of calcium may be due to a lack of calcium-containing foods in the diet or insufficient absorption of the mineral from the intestine caused by steatorrhoea or prolonged diarrhoea. Vitamin D is necessary for normal absorption of calcium and its deposition in bone tissue; therefore a diet deficient in vitamin D will lead to osteomalacia. This condition may also occur during pregnancy if the woman does not receive additional calcium to meet the increased demand incurred by the developing fetus. Excessive urinary excretion of calcium is usually the result of acidosis associated with renal failure or of renal tubular damage and malfunction.

Actual and potential *problems* may include:

- softening and weakening of bone
- tenderness and aching
- deformity of the long bones
- loss of weight and muscular strength
- tetany.

The *treatment* consists mainly of the administration of calcium, phosphorus and vitamin D. If the serum calcium concentration is markedly low, calcium (e.g. calcium gluconate 10%) may be given intravenously.

PAGET'S DISEASE (OSTEITIS DEFORMANS)

Paget's disease is a chronic disorder of bone remodelling the cause of which is unknown. Whilst it is relatively common in Northern Europe and North America, occurring in 3% of the over 40 population, Solomon et al (2005) notes that it is virtually unknown in Asia, Africa and the Middle East. Localized areas of bone show abnormally rapid reabsorption due to osteoclasts and subsequent replacement with abnormal new bone that is prone to deformity and fracture. The disease may be limited to one area or occur in several parts of the skeleton. The pelvis and tibia are most commonly affected, followed by the femur, skull and spine.

Bone pain is the most common symptom associated with the skeletal deformity, pathological fractures and symptoms of nerve compression that are attributed to the disease. Rarely, malignant degeneration of the bone may occur leading to sarcoma in about 1% of cases.

NURSING CARE

When the disease is asymptomatic and weight-bearing bones are not involved, no treatment is necessary. Treatment and nursing intervention are supportive and directed toward alleviating presenting symptoms (pain) with the use of NSAIDs. In more advanced cases, calcitonin is frequently used. Bisphosphonates are, however, the drug of choice (see p. 872). The objective of this treatment is to control the metabolic action of the disease, reduce the rate of bone turnover and ease pain. Patients are advised to eat a diet high in calcium and protein, with vitamin C and D supplements. An individualized exercise programme is taught and the person is encouraged to follow it unless symptoms recur.

SARCOMA

The term sarcoma refers to any tumour arising from connective tissue. Bone sarcoma is a self explanatory term indicating a malignant tumour has arisen from bone whilst a soft tissue sarcoma is a malignancy that has arisen from extraskeletal connective tissue. Soft-tissue sarcoma is about three times more common than bone sarcoma (Shelton et al 2004). Additionally, secondary neoplasms may develop in bone tissue having metastasized from malignant disease in another area of the body. This occurs more frequently than primary bone neoplasms.

Most primary bone neoplasms develop in children and adults younger than 40 years. They may be classified by the type of cell from which they originate, whether they are benign or malignant, and whether the tissue response is osteolytic or reactive. The neoplasm may cause a breakdown of the bone structure with loss of calcium from the tissue; this type of reaction is referred to as *osteolytic*. The response of bone tissue to some types of neoplastic cells is the formation of dense bone tissue around the lesion, which may be referred to as a *nidus*. This type of process is called *reactive bone formation*.

The more common primary bone neoplasms are listed in Table 24.6. Little is known about the causes of primary sarcoma but they do account for approximately 1% of all cancers.

CLINICAL CHARACTERISTICS

Neoplasms of bones may be asymptomatic for a period of time and may be discovered only when the person has radiography for some other reason (e.g. sustained injury) or has a pathological fracture. Persistent pain, progressively

Table 24.6 Common primary bone neoplasms

Cell of origin	Neoplasm	Benign or malignant	Comments
Osteocyte	Osteoid osteoma	Benign	Small, reactive lesion. Femur and tibia common sites. Especially painful at night. Treatment involves surgical removal
	Osteochondroma	Benign	Most common benign bone neoplasm; a hamartoma consisting of bony outgrowth with a cartilage cap. Distal end of femur, proximal end of tibia and proximal end of humerus are common sites. Symptoms depend upon impingement on surrounding tissues
	Osteogenic sarcoma (osteosarcoma)	Malignant (rapid spread)	Destroys medullary and cortical bone tissue. Usually develops in end of long bone; almost 50% involve the knee joint. Severe pain and tenderness; area may be hot and swollen. Treatment consists of amputation and chemotherapy, or chemotherapy and endoprosthetic replacement
	Osteoclastoma	Benign – may become malignant	Develops most often in epiphyseal region of femur, tibia or humerus of young adults. Rarefaction of bone occurs. It causes pain, swelling and rarely pathological fracture. Treated by curettage or by resection of the bone and replacement with a bone graft. If malignant, the limb is amputated, or chemotherapy and endoprosthetic replacement
Chondrocyte	Endochondroma	Benign	Growth of tumour cells of the hyaline cartilage may cause a pathological fracture. Treatment is by curettage
	Chondroblastoma	Benign	Develops toward end of adolescence. Common sites are femur, tibia and humerus. Highest incidence in males. Causes pain and swelling in epiphyseal area. Treatment is curettage and bone grafts
	Chondrosarcoma	Malignant (slower spread than osteosarcoma)	Age group most often affected 30–60 years. Common sites are scapula, pelvis, humerus and femur. Treatment involves radical excision, amputation, or chemotherapy and endoprosthetic replacement
Fibrocyte	Non-osteogenic fibroma	Benign	Most common site is end of diaphysis of long bone. If asymptomatic, it may be left untreated. If painful, it is excised
	Fibrosarcoma	Malignant	Rare. Usually in adults. Treated by amputation if in a limb or chemotherapy plus endoprosthetic replacement
Uncertain; reticulocyte suggested	Ewing's tumour or sarcoma	Malignant	May involve ilia, ribs, vertebrae and shafts of long bones. Begins in marrow cavity and gradually erodes the bone tissue. Manifestations include severe pain, swelling, fever and leucocytosis. Treatment is combination of irradiation, chemotherapy and surgery, including endoprosthetic replacement

[a]A hamartoma is a benign tumour formed by an overgrowth of normal mature cells characteristic of the area.

increasing in severity and limitation of activity of the affected part are common characteristics. Local tenderness, swelling and warmth may be present. If the neoplasm is malignant, systemic symptoms such as weight loss and anaemia develop. Diagnosis is made by bone scan as this is more sensitive than radiography, although this may also be performed.

Benign bone neoplasms are treated by excision or curettage. The bone structure may have to be reinforced following the removal of the lesion by filling in the space with bone chips or small grafts. Treatment of primary malignant neoplasms involves a combination of surgery and chemo-therapy. Radical excision is done if the lesion is accessible or, in the case of an extremity, the limb is amputated.

The use of custom-made joints and of bone replacement has preserved the mobility of many patients. Suitable cases may be those where there is no diffuse spread of the tumour into surrounding secondary deposits. Extending prostheses have been developed in the past decade. They can be used in the tibia, femur and humerus of the growing child or adolescent.

Treatment of the patient with skeletal metastases depends principally on the origin of the primary malignant disease. Chemotherapy, hormones and/or irradiation may be used (see Ch. 11). Irradiation may be used to reduce the severity of the pain experienced by the patient. Analgesics are prescribed to keep the patient comfortable; a small dose is used at first, but usually has to be increased as the condition worsens and the patient develops a tolerance for the drug.

NURSING INTERVENTION

Nursing care is directed toward symptom management, psychosocial support and patient and family teaching.

The most common patient problems include pain, nausea and vomiting caused by the treatment of the disease, anxiety and fear. Above all, the patient will have a major knowledge deficit about the condition and be in need of teaching and education if informed decisions about treatment options are to be made.

Pain

Specific points for assessment include the presence, location and degree of **pain**. It is important to determine the exact location of pain in order to learn whether new areas of the skeleton are involved, particularly in metastatic bone cancer.

The *goal* is that the patient will be as free from pain as possible. Alleviation of pain may best be achieved through regular scheduling of optimum doses of opioids with follow-up assessment of the effectiveness of each dose. Time-scheduled medication should prevent patients from experiencing pain. If this is not the result for any individual, the medication regimen should be reassessed with the patient and doctor and necessary changes made.

Potential for nausea and vomiting

The *goal* is that the patient should be free from nausea and should not vomit. The patient should be closely assessed for nausea and vomiting as they have many causes and should not be quickly attributed to any particular one; radiation therapy, additive hormones, opioids and hypercalcaemia may all contribute. Effective intervention to prevent nausea is possible only when the cause has been identified.

Lack of knowledge

Patient and family teaching includes issues related to treatment options and signs and symptoms of further advancing disease, including early indications of spinal cord compression and hypercalcaemia. Family members are taught basic care techniques in order to care for the patient at home. These include positioning, bathing, skin care, assisting the person in ambulation, and safety measures. The nurse also assists the patient and family in understanding the need for a diet high in calories, fibre and fluids. Support from community nursing services is essential.

Anxiety and fear

The *goal* is that the patient may adapt to the disease in a positive way. The psychosocial needs of patients with bone neoplasms and their families are most severe when the neoplasm is malignant, particularly as a malignant neoplasm is usually metastatic. Supportive care in the form of guided questioning, attentive listening, use of touch and information giving is provided. If this proves insufficient, referral for more intensive support should be made.

SUMMARY

Disease and trauma affecting bones and joints may have a short-term limited effect or may result in the patient suffering years of chronic pain with occasional acute episodes. Hospital admission is often during the acute stages of the disease and the nurse must be aware of the patient's normal coping strategies.

In caring for patients with orthopaedic conditions, nurses may develop long-term relationships with them. Individuals with a chronic condition will frequently return to the same ward or unit when they need hospitalization. There is a great scope in this situation for the patient's care to be discussed with the family and multidisciplinary team. For example, the work of the physiotherapist is closely linked to that of the occupational therapist and they both need the cooperation of the family at home for their ideas to be continued in the community. It is the patient's quality of life in the long term that must be of paramount importance. This may require specialist advice for chronic pain counselling, the involvement of social services and support groups for both the patient and/or the relatives in addition to a wide range of therapeutic interventions. The ageing population of the UK means that orthopaedic and trauma services will have increasing demands placed upon them in the future. These demands require new ways of working both in terms of expanded nursing roles, better multidisciplinary teamwork and increasingly coordinated care between hospital and primary care teams.

REFERENCES

Adams N (2004) Knee injuries. Emergency Nurse 11(10): 19–27.

Black J, Hawks H (2005) Medical–surgical nursing. St Louis: Elsevier/Saunders.

Blenkinsopp A, Paxton P (2004) Sprains. Primary Health Care 14(1): 33–34.

British National Formulary (BNF) (2005) British National Formulary. London: British Medical Association/Royal Pharmaceutical Society of Great Britain.

Choong P, Langford A, Dowsey M, Santamaria N (2000) Clinical pathway for fractured neck of femur: a prospective controlled study. Medical Journal of Australia 172: 423–426.

Clark J, Hudak P, Hawker G (2004) The moving target; a qualitative study of elderly patients' decision making regarding total joint replacement surgery. Journal of Bone and Joint Surgery of America 86A: 1366–1374.

Cox J, Newton D (2005) Developing and integrated falls service. Primary Health Care 15(2): 25–28.

Cree M (2000) Mortality and institutionalisation following hip fracture. Journal of the American Geriatric Society 48(3): 283–288.

Filbin M, Tsien C, Caughey A (2002) Clinical cases in emergency medicine. Malden: Blackwell.

Forster F (2005) Relaxing hip precautions increased patient satisfaction and promoted quicker return to normal activities after total hip arthroplasty. Evidence Based Nursing 8(October): 115.

Griffiths P (2005) Review Evidence from individually randomized trials shows that hip protectors do not reduce hip fractures in elderly people. Evidence Based Nursing 8(January): 24.

Haslett C, Chilvers E, Hunter J, Boon N (2002) Davidson's principles and practice of medicine, 19th edn. Edinburgh: Churchill Livingstone.

Hubble C (2005) Ankle fractures. Emergency Nurse 13(4): 32–38.

Hunter D (2005) Diagnosis and management of scaphoid fractures: a literature review. Emergency Nurse 13(7): 22–27.

Lin J, Zhang W, Jones A (2004) Efficacy of non-steroidal anti-inflammatory drugs in the treatment of osteoarthritis: meta-analysis of randomized controlled trials. British Medical Journal 329: 324.

McClung B (1999) Using osteoporosis management to reduce fractures in elderly women. Nurse Practitioner 24(3): 26–47.

Meenan R, Mason J, Anderson J, Guccione A, Kazis L. (1992) The content and properties of a revised and expanded arthritis impact measurement scales health status questionnaire. Arthritis and Rheumatism 35: 1–10.

Minns J, Dodd C, Gardner R, Bamford J, Nabhani F. (2004) Assessing the safety and effectiveness of hip protectors. Nursing Standard 18(39): 33–38.

Oliver S, Ryan S (2004) Effective pain management for patients with arthritis. Nursing Standard 18(50): 43–52.

Parker M, Gillespie L, Gillespie W (2004) Hip protectors for preventing hip fractures in the elderly. Cochrane Database Systematic Review 3: CD001255.

Peak E, Parvizi J, Ciminiello M (2005) The role of patient restrictions in reducing the prevalence of early dislocation following total hip arthroplasty; a randomized prospective study. Journal of Bone and Joint Surgery of America 87-A: 247–253.

Platt B (2004) Supracondylar fracture of the humerus. Emergency Nurse 12(2): 22–29.

Prodigy (2005) Online. Available: www.prodigy.nhs.uk

Radwin L (2005) Arthritis symptoms, Information sources, and a constantly shifting threshold of risk-benefit ratios influenced elderly patients' decisions about total joint replacement. Evidence Based Nursing 8(April): 63.

Shelton B, Ziegfield C, Olsen M (2004) Manual of cancer nursing. Philadelphia: Lippincott.

Solomon L, Warwick D, Nayagam S (2005) Apley's concise system of orthopaedics and fractures, 3rd edn. London: Hodder Arnold.

Stiell IG, Greenberg GH, McKnight RD, Nair RC, McDowell I, Worthington JR. (1992) A study to develop clinical decision rules for the use of radiography in acute ankle injuries. Annals of Emergency Medicine 21: 384–390.

Summers A (2005) Recognizing and treating Colles' type fractures in emergency settings. Emergency Nurse 13(6): 26–33.

Swanson C, Yelland C, Day G (2000) Clinical pathways and fractured neck of femur. Medical Journal of Australia 172: 415–416.

Talbot N, Brown J, Treble N (2002) Early dislocation after total hip arthroplasty: are post operative precautions necessary? Journal of Arthroplasty 17: 1006–1008.

Temple J, Santy J (2005) Pin site care for preventing infections associated with external bone fixators and pins. Cochrane Library 4: CD004551.

Temple J (2004) Total hip replacement. Nursing Standard 19(3): 44–51.

Walsh M (2006) Nurse practitioners; clinical skills and professional issues, 2nd edn. Oxford: Butterworth Heinemann.

Zhang W, Jones A, Doherty M (2004) Does paracetamol reduce the pain of osteoarthritis? A meta-analysis of randomized controlled trials. Annals of Rheumatological Disease 63: 901–907.

25 Caring for the patient with a skin disorder

Mark Collier

INTRODUCTION

Health problems involving the skin range from minor irritants to life-threatening situations. Nurses require a wide range of skills to provide not only the necessary physical care but also much needed psychological support for patients who experience problems with their skin. Many skin problems can be prevented through proactive nursing care and patient education. This chapter aims to provide the novice nurse with the necessary underpinning knowledge to work with patients who either have developed a skin problem or are at risk of developing skin problems. The chapter will not only focus on the physical aspects of care but will also consider the wider implications of living with a skin disorder.

THE SKIN

A typical cross-section of the skin is shown in Figure 25.1a, and the outermost layer, the *epidermis*, is shown in more detail in Figure 25.1b. The epidermis is avascular but is supported by the dermis, a region of the skin that has a rich blood and nerve supply. It is important to remember, especially when assessing patients for signs of damage to the skin such as pressure ulceration, that as an organ, the skin covers a surface area of over 2 square metres.

Cells responsible for the regeneration of skin are produced in the basal (germinating) layer of the epithelium and then gradually move through the other layers to the surface. As they ascend, they progressively undergo degenerative changes. The nuclei disintegrate, the cell substance changes to a water-repellent, waxy, protein-like substance called *keratin*, and the cells become flat. They are continuously reproduced in the basal layer and cast off from the surface. The cells that are shed disintegrate, leaving their keratin on the surface; this keratin helps to protect the skin.

The thickness of the epidermis varies in different areas of the body from a minimum of 0.07 mm to 0.12 mm in depth. It is thickest on the soles of the feet and palms of the hands, and thinnest on the lips and eyelids. This provides maximum 'wear and tear' qualities for areas of maximum stress. Imparting physical strength to the skin and potential wounds, remains, however, the role of the dermis.

The *dermis*, consisting of fibrous and elastic connective tissue, contains many blood and lymphatic vessels, nerves and their end-organs, sebaceous and sweat glands, ducts and hair follicles.

Lying between the epidermal germinating layer and the dermis are the melanocytes, which produce the pigment melanin and deliver it to the epidermal cells. The amount of pigment is determined mainly by the person's genetic inheritance. The activity of the pigment-producing cells may also be influenced by melanocyte-stimulating hormone (MSH), which is released by the anterior pituitary and by exposure to sunlight and friction.

The subcutaneous fatty tissue functions as a heat insulator, a cushion against mechanical pressure and an energy store. The subcutaneous tissue is distributed in varying thicknesses over the entire body surface. The thickness of the skin overall is therefore dependent upon regional anatomy and is also influenced by an individual's sex and age.

The cutaneous sebaceous glands secrete an oily substance (sebum) which reaches the skin surface via the hair follicles. Glands are plentiful in the face and scalp but are absent in the palmar and plantar aspects of the hands and feet. The secretion prevents drying of the hair and skin and helps to keep the skin soft and pliable. Blackheads are discoloured accumulations of sebum in hair follicles and frequently pro-

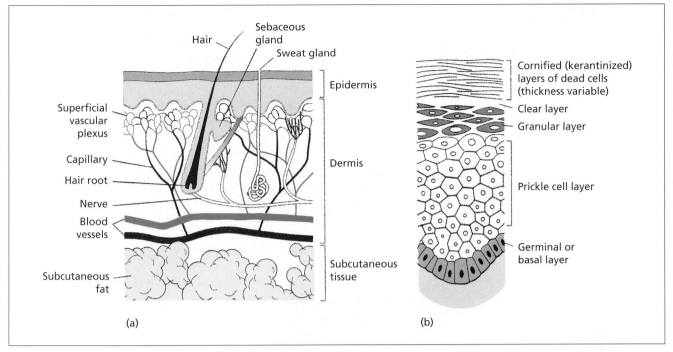

Figure 25.1 (a) Cross-section of the skin. (b) Cell layers of the epidermis.

vide a medium for organisms, causing pimples and this process is linked to the condition called acne. Sebaceous gland activity increases at puberty and decreases in later life due to the influence of gonadal hormones on the output of sebum.

The skin protects the internal structures from injury, acts as a barrier to keep vital fluids and chemicals from leaking out, and prevents invasion of organisms. Its protective functions are enhanced by the water-repellent, waxy nature of the surface cells. Hairs are cylinders of keratinized cells. Distribution of the hair over the body varies with human groups, and with age and sex within each group.

The abundance of sensory receptors and afferent and efferent nerves in the skin influence the sensations of touch, pressure, pain and temperature. These sensations serve as an important protective mechanism for the body and also convey impulses that contribute information about the external environment. For example, through touch we can appreciate shape, composition and texture.

The skin plays an important role in regulating body temperature by varying the calibre of its blood vessels and the activity of the sweat glands. The fluid sweat lying on the surface of the skin cools the body by the process of evaporation. Sweat contains traces of albumin and urea; therefore sweating helps to remove these waste products from the body.

The absorptive function of the skin is limited mainly to the absorption of ultraviolet rays from the sun or special lamps; it then converts sterol substances in the skin to vitamin D. A few drugs, which may be included in ointments or lotions, may be absorbed in small amounts.

The dermis and subcutaneous tissue may act as a storage area for water and fat. For instance, when an excess of water is retained in the body, the accumulation in these tissues becomes evident as oedema. The subcutaneous tissue serves as one of the main fat depots and acts as a pad over muscle and bone, cushioning them from mechanical forces.

The sebaceous glands protect the skin from moisture and prevent desiccation. With advancing years, they become less active, and the skin becomes dry.

Owing to its high proportion of collagen bundles and elastin fibres, the dermis provides mechanical strength and serves to anchor the epidermis to the basal layer of the dermis. The epidermis and its various appendages receive nourishment and support from the dermis. With age, degenerative changes occur in the elastic tissue and collagenous component of fibrous tissue, and the skin becomes wrinkled. Frequently, areas of melanocytes produce more pigment, and 'brown spots' characteristic of ageing skin appear.

From the above introduction, it is apparent that the skin plays an essential role in the maintenance of health. It is also a key component of our self-concept and hence is of fundamental importance in maintaining psychological health. This chapter reviews some of the most common health problems related to the skin that the nurse may encounter.

PROMOTION AND MAINTENANCE OF HEALTHY SKIN

Issues that should be addressed concerning the promotion and maintenance of healthy skin include the following:

Cleansing. Regular cleansing is essential for healthy skin. There are a number of products available to care for the wide variety of skin types – dry, normal, oily, combination. Cleanliness is an integral part of achieving and maintaining healthy skin.

Moisturizing. The skin can become dry due to moisture loss through the use of inappropriate cleansing agents, illness, trauma or exposure to sun, wind, pollution and hot water. Patients should be advised to use emollients to replenish that which has been lost and for the maintenance of healthy, intact skin, which is the body's primary barrier against infection.

Noting changes in the skin's appearance. Nurses should teach the individual to look for any changes in colour, texture or appearance of the skin and changes in moles or other skin lesions. If changes are noted, the person should consult a healthcare professional immediately.

Avoiding exposure to ultraviolet radiation. People are becoming increasingly aware of the dangers associated with exposing the skin to the sun and other sources of ultraviolet radiation (e.g. tanning lamps and beds). The increasing incidence of skin cancer is a cause for alarm, and individuals, health professionals and manufacturers alike are advocating the education of consumers regarding the use of protective practices. These include the use of sunscreens and blocks, decreased time in the sun and the wearing of protective clothing, such as a wide-brimmed hat and a shirt.

In the UK, the incidence of malignant melanoma of the skin has increased by 50% since the mid-1980s and currently there are nearly 6000 new cases diagnosed each year (Savage et al 2004). There is a similar trend across the developed world and there is a proportionately greater increase amongst males and those aged 20–39 years.

Diet. Good nutrition is an essential component in the promotion and maintenance of healthy skin.

GENERAL SKIN CONDITIONS

Patient assessment

In assessing patients suffering from skin diseases it is necessary to assess the whole patient, not just the state of the patient's skin. The extent of the skin disorder should be recorded accurately in order that progress can be monitored and possible allergic substances recorded.

The patient's view of his or her condition should be determined, together with any coping mechanisms used. The patient's self-concept should be explored along with how the illness is affecting everyday life. Other psychosocial factors such as developmental status and family relationships should be explored.

Health history

Skin problems cannot be examined 'in isolation'; information about the patient's total health may reveal very significant diagnostic factors and influence the therapeutic plan. Although skin disorders may present with a striking appearance, it is important to obtain a good history before examining the patient (Walsh 2006). In taking the patient's health history, particular attention is given to eliciting information about:

- any previous skin disorders, their nature, the patient's age, the timing including the season of the year at which they occurred, the treatment used and its effect
- any known allergy or drug reactions
- drugs being taken, and for what reason
- known food(s), fluid(s) or contact substances (e.g. soap, certain material) that worsen the condition
- substances that are brought in contact with the skin throughout daily activities (e.g. cosmetics, chemicals at work)
- dietary habits
- recreational customs (including use of tobacco, alcohol and other drugs) or hobbies
- family history, especially in relation to skin disorders, allergy and systemic disease
- emotional stress resulting from job, interpersonal relations and other situations are identified. Stress and anxiety may influence the severity of skin disorders and the patient's responses to treatment.

The PQRST tool (see p. 128) may be used for symptom analysis in skin disorders:

- **P**rovocation and **P**alliation – what brings on, exacerbates or relieves the problem?
- **Q**uality – the appearance of the skin lesions, itching, soreness, bleeding, discharge, etc.
- **R**egion and **R**adiation – the area affected and whether this has spread
- **S**everity – this should include changes in the severity of skin lesions and how they affect the person's life
- **T**ime – how long the patient has had the problem and whether it varies over time.

PHYSICAL EXAMINATION

The history taking is followed by an examination of the skin. This involves touching, feeling and observing the person's skin. A good light and warm room are essential and the skin must be clean. Care is taken to prevent unnecessary exposure of the patient and to respect dignity by closing curtains or doors and protecting the patient with a gown or sheet.

A general survey of the skin is undertaken noting *colour* (redness, pallor, cyanosis, yellowness or brownness), *vascularity* (any evidence of bruising or bleeding), *moisture* (dryness, sweating, oiliness), *temperature, texture* (roughness and smoothness), *thickness* and *turgor* (the rate at which the skin returns into place when a section is pinched and lifted).

Lesions are inspected, and the nature of the lesion is established and its characteristics recorded according to size, shape, colour and whether it has a dry or wet surface. It is also useful to note if lesions can be located on symmetrical parts of the patient's body or if they appear in one particular unilateral location. It should be noted if an odour is associated with the affected areas. The entire skin surface of the body is examined to determine the general condition of the total skin in addition to the distribution and grouping of the affected areas. The latter is of assistance in diagnosis as certain disorders are known to develop more commonly in certain areas. For example, acne, impetigo and herpes simplex develop most commonly on the face and contact dermatitis on the hand. The oral mucosa is usually included in an examination of the entire skin. The fingernails and toenails are observed and palpated for colour, shape and the presence of lesions. The quantity, texture and distribution of hair is also noted.

DIAGNOSTIC TESTS

The diagnosis of many skin lesions can be made through a process of physical examination and history taking. If the lesions are moist or discharging, a swab of the exudate may be obtained for culture. If the affected areas are dry or scaly, scrapings may be taken for cytological examination, mycology and culture. Other laboratory tests may be undertaken, such as leucocyte and thrombocyte counts, examination for the lupus erythematosus (LE) cell, anti-D test for systemic lupus erythematosus (SLE) and erythrocyte sedimentation rate determination. A biopsy of a lesion may be undertaken if malignancy is suspected or if the lesion is long-standing and obscure in nature. If the condition is dermatitis, patch tests may be performed, ideally during a remission, to identify the allergen or substance to which the person is sensitive. The substances are applied to the skin on the back and observed at intervals over 48 hours. If positive, the reaction is manifested by inflammation and papules or vesicles.

Although the skin lesions prompted the patient to seek medical assistance, the disorder may have internal or systemic components. This may necessitate other investigative procedures, such as urinalysis, radiography, pulmonary function tests or further blood studies.

RISK FACTORS

Health problems involving the skin are related to the presence of one or more risk factors:

1 *Internal factors* – alterations in nutrition, metabolism, circulation, sensation, immune system, mental status, skin turgor, pigmentation, body fat and moisture, thickness and texture of the skin, the presence of infection, and actions of medications.
2 *External or environmental factors* – mechanical forces including pressure and shearing, chemical substances, radiation, temperature extremes, moisture and physical immobilization.
3 *Systemic disorders* such as:
   a) malnutrition
   b) metabolic disorder (e.g. diabetes mellitus, hypothyroidism or hyperthyroidism)
   c) cardiovascular disease
   d) neurological disorders that impair sensation and cause immobility
   e) severe infection and fever
   f) debilitation (such as occurs in cancer and anaemia).

4 *Skin characteristics*:
   a) thickness and texture of the skin vary in different areas of the body and are influenced by the person's genetic code and age
   b) turgor – dehydration and oedema make the skin more fragile and vulnerable to breakdown.
5 *Age* – the older person's skin is drier, less elastic and less turgid, predisposing it to breakdown when subjected to pressure or other mechanical forces or irritants.

MANIFESTATIONS OF SKIN DISORDER

Lesions

Various changes in areas of the skin may occur, and the exact nature of these is important in diagnosis and treatment.

Primary lesions

Characteristic primary lesions in which the skin is usually intact include the following:

● *Erythema* – an area in which the blood vessels become dilated, causing redness, warmth and increased tension of the skin
● *Macule* – a flat non-palpable lesion less than 1 cm in diameter
● *Papule* – a small elevated macule that may or may not be discoloured
● *Vesicle* – an elevated area that contains clear serous fluid
● *Pustule* – similar to a vesicle, elevated and superficial but filled with purulent fluid
● *Nodule* – an elevated firm palpable lesion, more than 0.5 cm in diameter and extending deeper into the dermis than a papule
● *Wheal* – a localized, elevated, irregularly shaped area of cutaneous oedema, which is red at the margins with a blanched centre
● *Bulla* – an elevation larger than 1 cm of superficial skin layers containing serous or purulent fluid
● *Comedo (blackhead)* – a plug of sebum and keratin within a hair follicle
● *Telangiectasia* – a lesion composed of a group of small blood vessels that are abnormally dilated
● *Plaque* – a patch on the skin or mucous membrane.

Secondary lesions

These develop as a result of a break in the skin and destruction of cells. They include:

● *crust (scab)* – a rough, dry area formed by the coagulation and drying of plasma and exudate over a primary lesion
● *scales* – thin, flat, minute plates of dried epidermal cells that have not completely undergone the normal keratinization process before being separated. Desquamation is the term that refers to the separation of scales or patches of cells
● *fissure* – a split or crack in the surface, extending through the epidermal layers and possibly into the dermis. If it extends into the dermis, bleeding occurs. This type of lesion is most likely to occur in a natural skin or surface

crease such as those located over knuckles, at the angles of the mouth, in the groin, between the buttocks and behind the ears

- *erosion (excoriation)* – loss of the epidermis producing a superficial, reddened, weeping lesion as a result of trauma or the prolonged presence of 'toxins' on the skin
- *ulcer* – a denuded area of irregular size and shape extending into the dermis or subcutaneous tissue from, or to, the epidermis due to necrosis of superficial tissue
- *lichenification* – thickening and hardening of skin as a result of continued irritation
- *atrophy* – the skin is thin and wrinkled, resembling tissue paper. Atrophy is seen with ageing
- *corn, callus* – an excessive thickness of the epidermis caused by chronic pressure and/or friction. In the case of a corn, the hyperkeratosis is sharply circumscribed
- *leucoplakia* – a white plaque seen most commonly on the lips or mucous membranes of the oral cavity or tongue. About 10% of patients subsequently develop carcinoma in the lesions
- *scar* – an area of fibrous tissue replacing tissue destroyed by trauma or disease
- *hypertrophic scars* – normally a scar becomes paler and flatter as it matures. Hypertrophic scars become increasingly raised, red and itchy for several months after injury, due to excessive formation of fibrous tissue within the scar. The scar is then classified as hypertrophic. Over the next few years, these scars usually flatten and lose their vascularity, thus becoming paler. The hypertrophy is confined to the site of injury. If these scars are excised, there is some tendency for the hypertrophy to recur. It may be very difficult to determine whether a scar is hypertrophic or keloid (see below)
- *keloids* – histologically, keloids are similar to hypertrophic scars, but keloids behave differently. Fibrous tissue formation is sometimes so excessive that the keloid has the appearance of a tumour, and the initial injury producing the keloid may be so small as to appear insignificant, for example ear piercing or an insect bite. Unlike hypertrophic scars, the keloid extends into surrounding uninjured skin and persists for many years. There is a high tendency for recurrence after excision. The incidence of keloid is highest in the skin of people who are indigenous to central and southern Africa. It appears that tension within a scar encourages hypertrophy and keloid formation; therefore, redistribution of the tension by use of elastic pressure garments usually produces some improvement in scar quality.

Pruritus

Generalized or localized itching is a common complaint in skin disorders. It may be associated with an internal disorder, such as renal failure or obstructive jaundice. Excessive dryness due to overbathing, a dry atmosphere and the ageing process can also cause pruritus. Emotional distress may play an important role in the development and control of this disturbing symptom. The patient is hard-pressed to refrain from scratching, which further irritates the area and is frequently responsible for fissures, abrasions and subsequent secondary infection.

Urticaria

Urticaria is a skin disorder characterized by itching with wheals of varying size, which may develop rapidly and become widespread. The reaction consists of dilatation and increased permeability of the capillaries and arteriolar dilatation.

A severe and possibly life-threatening form of the disorder is known as angioneurotic oedema of the skin and mucous membranes. The lesions frequently disappear in a few hours when the blood vessels return to normal. General malaise and fever may also develop if the urticaria is widespread. The most common cause of angioneurotic oedema is a severe allergic reaction to a drug, food or insect bite.

Pain

The pain associated with skin lesions can cause great discomfort and, depending upon the cause and location, may be described as prickly or burning. Chemical, mechanical or pressure irritation of the cutaneous sensory nerves, actual cellular damage or exposure of the nerve endings due to tissue destruction and erosion may cause it.

Redness

Erythema or redness of the skin indicates vasodilatation and hyperaemia in the area. Erythematous lesions are initially macular but frequently become papular because of the oedema or developing exudate in the affected tissues.

Swelling

A puffy swollen area of the skin is usually due to localized oedema, resulting from increased permeability of the capillaries, or to localized inflammatory reaction.

Systemic disturbances

The skin reflects the individual's general physical and emotional status. Skin lesions are frequently manifestations of a systemic disorder (e.g. measles, systemic lupus erythematosus), or a systemic or emotional disturbance may be secondary to primary skin lesions. A raised temperature is likely to be present if the skin disorder involves infection.

HEALTH PROBLEMS COMMON TO INDIVIDUALS WITH A SKIN DISORDER

Each individual has to cope with varying physiological and psychological problems, depending upon the nature of the disorder. Patients who have lived with their skin condition for a long time are often well informed about the nature of their problem. Others may need more information and the nurse can explain the nature of the disorder to the patient and the rationale behind local skin or wound care, systemic therapy and nutritional support. The patient can then be encouraged to participate in as much of the care as is realistic. Emotional support and health teaching are important nursing functions in assisting the individual to understand and learn to cope with health problems affecting the skin in a positive manner.

GENERAL PRINCIPLES OF CARE FOR PERSONS WITH SKIN DISORDER

The extent of the skin involvement as well as the nature of the condition determines whether or not the patient can continue usual daily activities, is ambulatory and can be treated at home. The patient's reaction to the disease also influences the plan of care and progress. The following are general considerations that will require adaptation and modification according to the individual.

Psychological support

The person is likely to be sensitive about the condition. Many are self-conscious about their appearance, worry constantly and tend to withdraw, believing that a skin disease carries a stigma. The disease may be such that it persists over a long period, interfering with the individual's ability to work or go out socially. Many skin diseases are aggravated by emotional stress. The nurse can help the patient to identify any emotional factors that may contribute to the skin condition and can carefully assess his or her own responses to the person. Where possible, the nurse should make a conscious effort to touch the person's skin, thus reassuring him or her that the appearance and texture of the skin are both accepted. It is important to advise the patient whether or not the disorder is contagious, and there should be no hesitation on the part of the nurse to touch the affected parts when giving care. In accordance with institutional infection control guidelines and the introduction of universal and body substance precautions, gloves may be indicated. The rationale should be explained calmly and in a matter-of-fact way to the patient so as not to add to the psychological distress. An effort is made to convey an appreciation of the patient's feelings, to make the patient aware that he or she is accepted and to provide the necessary support and care which will help to reduce anxiety.

Local care

Cleansing of the skin covering any area of the body should be determined on an individual basis for each patient. In some instances, the application of soap and water may be contraindicated, and an alternative method of cleansing is necessary. For example, cleansing the skin with a bath additive or soap substitute may be necessary. If soap is permitted, it should be mildly alkaline and used very sparingly. A soft flannel is preferable, and the surface is washed lightly and gently to avoid injury and erythema. If there are open, discharging lesions, lint-free sterile gauze or a disposable absorbent cloth may be used. If the skin is dry, it may also be advisable to limit bathing to once or twice a week.

Baths may be used to relieve itching, remove scales or crusts, or apply medications as well as for cleansing purposes. Caution is used against having the water or solution hot: a temperature higher than 35–38°C is likely to be too hot for the sensitive areas. Also, higher temperatures are likely to cause hyperaemia and itching. The patient is usually encouraged to remain in the bath for 10–20 minutes, and an attendant remains with the patient or close by, depending on condition and age. After bathing, the skin should be patted dry gently with a towel avoiding excessive rubbing.

Fingernails should be kept short and clean, and the patient is advised to refrain from scratching due to the threat of skin damage and infection.

Cold applications
Application of cold dressings can cause vasoconstriction and decrease skin sensitivity and itching.

Clothing
Woollens and other irritating clothing should be avoided. Loose-fitting 100% cotton is best. Maintaining a cool environment can enhance the effectiveness of this strategy, when possible.

Topical applications
Many different drug preparations are used in treating skin diseases. Topical applications may be in powder, lotion, oil, cream, paste or ointment form. They may be classified according to their effect:

- *Antipruritic preparations* are applied to relieve itching. Examples are emollients, corticosteroid cream or ointment, and topical antihistamines (although it should be noted these are a common sensitizer causing an allergic or irritant reaction when used topically in some people)
- *Keratolytic agents* soften and remove scales and the horny layer. An example is salicylic acid ointment or paste
- *Antieczematous agents* are applied to relieve itching and remove the vesicular drainage. Examples are corticosteroid cream or ointment. Topical immunomodulators have recently become licensed as a second-line treatment for atopic eczema (e.g. tacrolimus and pimecrolimus) (NICE 2004)
- *Keratolytic preparations* are used for the removal of corns, calluses and warts. An example is a weak salicylic (1–2%) acid ointment
- *Antimicrobial agents* destroy or inhibit the reproduction of bacteria and fungi. Examples are antibiotic ointments such as neomycin and gentamicin or antifungal preparations such as miconazole or clotrimazole. These are also commonly used as combined preparations with other active ingredients such as topical corticosteroids
- *Antiparasitic preparations* destroy or inhibit parasites. Examples are malathion 0.5% aqueous liquid, permethrin 5% dermal cream or phenothrin 0.5% aqueous liquid
- *Emollients* are used to soften the skin. There are many preparations available as lotions, creams, ointments, bath and shower preparations.

Frequently, topical preparations are a combination of two or more agents that can be selected for their specific effect in a particular condition.

Physical agents

Ultraviolet radiation may be prescribed in the treatment of psoriasis. Radiotherapy may used if the lesion is malignant. Cryotherapy (using liquid nitrogen) or cautery may be employed in the removal of warts, leucoplakia and seborrhoeic or senile keratoses (areas of horny thickening of epidermis).

Systemic therapy

If the skin disorder is secondary to a systemic disease, treatment is directed principally toward the primary condition. In addition, some skin conditions require treatment with systemic drugs.

Systemic drugs

The choice of drug depends on the nature of the disorder and the patient's general health and response to the condition. An oral corticosteroid (e.g. prednisolone) may be prescribed in dermatitis, urticaria and pemphigus. If the skin lesions are infected, an oral antibiotic (e.g. flucloxacillin) may be required. An antihistamine such as chlorphenamine may be used in urticaria and for some patients antihistamines are useful in managing pruritus. The older types of antihistamine have a marked sedating effect which the more modern preparations do not. In some situations, a sedating antihistamine may be used specifically because of its sedative effect. For example, concern about the condition and fear of disfigurement and rejection as well as itching may result in a considerable loss of sleep for the patient. A sedative may be necessary to provide rest, which plays an important part in the patient's recovery. In the event of a significant degree of depression, psychiatric services may be appropriate for the patient.

Nutrition

Attention should be paid to the patient's nutritional status (see Ch. 17). Anorexia may be a problem with the dermatological patient because of the skin irritation experienced, as well as the emotional disturbance. Dressings, ointments, lotions or similar applications on the hands may make self-care in feeding difficult. A creative occupational therapist and nurse should be able to assist in choosing appropriate assistive devices if problems with feeding occur. Continuity of such practices in hospital and following discharge are essential if such strategies are to bring about long-term gain.

Patient education

Nurses have a key role in working with the patient and family members of the day-to-day care required and precautionary measures applicable to the prevention of an exacerbation of any skin condition. Verbal and written directions are given about the local applications and taking of medicinal preparations. For example, corticosteroid preparations in the form of an ointment or cream are used topically to suppress inflammation and reduce sensitivity of the tissues. The patient must be cautioned to apply the corticoid preparation sparingly. If compresses or therapeutic baths are to be continued, specific details of the preparation, temperature and application are outlined and demonstrated if necessary.

The need to consider changing employment should be discussed with the patient, and the occupational therapist and social worker may be consulted to discuss retraining facilities if appropriate.

CASE **General skin conditions**

Whilst enjoying a family holiday in Spain, your 16-year-old daughter talks to you 'in confidence' and reports some unusual lumps and bumps that have appeared overnight on her chest and arms – the areas she normally leaves exposed when sunbathing. You are due to come home in a few days time and the nearest health centre to your retreat is over half an hour's drive away. You suddenly remember that in the rush to come away, whilst you and your husband have travel insurance included as part of an incentive package linked to your current banking arrangements, you forgot to arrange holiday insurance cover for your daughter.

Reflective questions

- Describe how you might handle this situation initially and any advice that you would give to your daughter. Highlight the rationale underpinning the advice identified
- On arrival home in the UK, describe any further actions and/or advice that you might give your daughter, again highlighting the rationale for the same.

Dermatological emergencies

Dermatology is a speciality which usually deals with uncomfortable, debilitating and disfiguring conditions but it should be remembered that there are some dermatological conditions which cause the individual to be acutely ill and have a significant risk of mortality. Dermatological conditions which may cause the patient to be acutely ill include:

- Eczema herpeticum, which can occur when a patient with atopic eczema comes into contact with the herpes virus. Patients usually feel generally unwell with an acute infected flare of eczema
- Erythrodermic psoriasis, which is a rare but active form of psoriasis of which one of the causes is withdrawal of potent topical or systemic steroids. The skin has widespread erythema, the patient feels very unwell, hot and shivery and loses heat rapidly. Treatment is copious emollients, weak topical steroids or methotrexate systemically
- Generalized pustular psoriasis, which can also be caused by steroid withdrawal. Patients have small non-follicular blisters which become confluent and the skin may peel off. Treatment is as above
- Autoimmune blistering disorders – pemphigoid and pemphigus which may affect the mucous membranes. Patients feel generally unwell and may experience weakness and weight loss. Treatment is usually high doses of systemic steroids

- Erythema multiforme, Stevens–Johnson syndrome (SJS) and toxic epidermal necrolysis (TEN). These are linked to drug reactions but may also be caused by viral or bacterial infection. The skin is blistered and eroded including mucous membranes, which if severe the patient may require ventilation.

COMMON SKIN DISORDERS

DERMATITIS OR ECZEMA

These two terms are synonymous and refer to an inflammatory disease of the skin that is very common. There are many different types of eczema and they can be classified as exogenous and endogenous. *Irritant contact dermatitis* and *allergic contact dermatitis* are the most common exogenous eczemas. In the former case, previous sensitization by exposure is not necessary, unlike the latter.

Exogenous eczema
Characteristics
- Development of an erythematous area with small papular development 2–4 days after contact, then progression to vesicles
- Vesicles may rupture and discharge contents, followed by crusting and scaling
- Denuded areas may ooze a serous discharge and then be covered by regenerated epidermis.

Risk factors
- Contact with an irritant substance such as strong soaps and some acids/alkalis
- Contact of hypersensitive or allergic skin with an agent such as cosmetics, hair dye, nickel, rubber or cement.

Patient goals
1 The patient will recover from the contact dermatitis with a minimum of scarring and mucosal damage.
2 The patient will maintain or achieve a positive body image and sense of self-esteem.
3 The patient will be able to describe how to avoid future exacerbations and will be able to describe treatment regimens.

Endogenous eczema
Atopic eczema is the most common form of endogenous eczema and is often associated with asthma and a tendency to allergic reactions. This is known collectively as atopy and seems to have a strong genetic component which makes the person susceptible to this group of problems. Other types of endogenous eczema include seborrhoeic, discoid and gravitational eczema. Pompholyx is eczema typically occurring on the palms and soles which involves blistering. The incidence of eczema has increased substantially over recent decades and 1 in 10 UK schoolchildren now have this disorder (Haslett et al 2002).

Characteristics
Diagnosis of atopic eczema is made clinically, based on patient's history, family history and appearance of the skin. The skin is itchy and the most common sites are skin creases such as the antecubital fossa, behind the knees, fronts of ankles and around the neck. Acute lesions may be vesicular and weepy and chronic lesions dry, lichenified and excoriated. Scratching is a major problem and infection of the resulting lesions may occur.

Patient goals
1 The patient will recover from an acute episode of atopic eczema.
2 The patient will manage the condition long-term.
3 The patient will maintain or achieve a positive body image and sense of self-esteem.

Nursing intervention for patients with eczema
- The application of topical emollients
- If extensive, therapeutic baths may be helpful. Explain rationale to the patient
- Education regarding avoidance of irritant or allergens including detergents
- Antibiotic ointment may be applied if there is an infection. Advise the patient regarding use
- Advise the patient to avoid scratching and keep nails short and clean. Mittens may be helpful with children
- The application of topical corticosteroids which can be very helpful for symptom relief but do not treat the underlying disease. They can have serious side-effects such as skin atrophy and the masking of infection. Consequently the minimum strength preparation that is effective should be used, applied thinly only to the affected skin area, no more than twice daily, to prevent side effects (British National Formulary 2006)
- Second-line treatments such as phototherapy or topical immunomodulators may be considered
- Educate patient regarding stress reduction techniques
- Provide the patient and family with psychosocial support
- Arrange for follow-up care.

PSORIASIS

Psoriasis is a condition causing patches or 'plaques' of red scaly skin which may be barely noticeable in some patients and in others it may be all over the body and scalp. The plaques tend to come and go throughout life. Patients may present with nail psoriasis, scalp psoriasis, guttate psoriasis or less commonly, with pustular psoriasis.

Characteristics
- Chronic inflammations of the skin that produce dry scaly lesions, exacerbations and remissions
- Dull, red, papular lesions form
- Silvery white, waxy scales accumulate in layers, with epidermal replacement every 4 days (normal rate is every

28 days); therefore, skin's normal protective layers are not able to form

- Lesions may increase in size, coalesce and form large scaly plaques. Some patients find the lesions do not itch, for others they are intensely itchy
- Small, pinpoint bleeding areas are found when the plaque is removed
- Nail involvement: pitting, discoloration and separation from thick, hard and dry underlying tissue
- Onset may be gradual or sudden
- Duration may be lengthy or short lived.

Risk factors

- Positive family history
- Onset common during adolescence
- Association with rheumatoid arthritis, since raised uric acid level is present in some patients
- May be precipitated by trauma, infections and psychological stress
- Certain medications such as beta blockers, lithium, anti-inflammatory pain killers and chloroquine can trigger flare ups of psoriasis.

Patient goals

1 The patient will recover from the psoriasis with a minimum of scarring.
2 The patient will maintain or achieve a positive body image and sense of self-esteem.
3 The patient will have the information and skills to manage their condition on a daily basis as required.

Nursing intervention

- Teach the individual regarding the rationale and limitations of treatments – to reduce scaling and itchiness, not to cure the condition
- Provide psychosocial support to individual and family, particularly about living with a chronic illness, and assist with the development of adaptive techniques as necessary
- Apply and instruct the patient regarding various treatments – local applications, baths and exposure to ultraviolet rays
- Topical applications may include pastes, ointments or creams, including salicylic acid, coal-tar derivatives, vitamin D derivatives or dithranol. The messy nature of these treatments should not be underestimated
- Caution individual about the use of topical and systemic corticosteroids as discontinuing their use may cause the psoriasis to rebound, in addition to long-term side-effects
- Instruct the patient to soak in prescribed bath for 20–30 minutes and to wipe skin gently with a soft flannel. Daily shampooing may be necessary if the scalp is affected
- If ultraviolet light therapy is used, the phototherapist or nurse will give education and advice regarding the treat-

ment and administer it according to local and national guidelines

- If dithranol paste is used, instruct the patient on the importance of protecting unaffected skin with petroleum jelly, and that it stains everything from skin to baths
- Provide support to the patient as occlusive dressings, plastic bags, vinyl suits and shower caps may be necessary for these time-consuming and aesthetically unappealing treatments
- Explain to the individual and family that topically applied agents such as dithranol will suppress epidermopoiesis, whereas tar therapies retard and inhibit rapid growth of psoriatic tissue
- Encourage the family to accept the individual's condition and not to be fearful that it is contagious or infectious
- Encourage adequate rest, a balanced nutritional diet and prevention of skin irritations and infections
- Arrange for follow-up care.

PARASITIC INFESTATIONS

Pediculosis (lice)

Lice are tiny insects which are passed on by close contact. Head lice are found attached to hairs and pubic lice are found attached to pubic hair and also the hair found on chests, underarms and beards. Lice are not passed on from clothing, bedding or toilet seats as the lice soon die when they are away from a human body.

Characteristics

- Appearance of the empty white egg shells (nits) which look like dandruff or lice on the body, head and/or pubic areas
- In pubic lice, haemorrhagic points may be noted, along with hyperaemia, linear scratches and a slight degree of eczema. In head lice, about one in three people have an allergy to the lice and therefore complain of itch. Many people are completely unaware that they have head lice

Risk factors

- Intimate or close physical contact with an infected person.

Assessment

- *Health history* – ask the patient about their present social situation and contact with infected individuals
- *Physical examination* – visually assess the involved areas in a well-lit room
- *Psychosocial concerns and developmental factors* – assess changes in patient or other interaction due to the contagious nature of the condition. Identify the patient's social situation, i.e. living conditions, health practices and, if previously infected, non-concordance with healthcare treatments
- *Patient and family knowledge* – assess their perceptions of health status, and how they feel about having lice. Assess current understanding of the condition and their willingness to learn.

Patient goals

1 After treatment the patient will have no evidence of pediculosis infestation.
2 The patient will learn preventive healthcare practices to avoid re-infestation.
3 The patient will avoid transmission to other people during the treatment period.

Nursing intervention

Teach the patient and family regarding the cause, nature and prevention of pediculosis.

Pubic lice

● Advise the patient to apply a lotion that kills the lice, such as malathion 0.5% aqueous liquid, permethrin 5% dermal cream or phenothrin 0.5% aqueous liquid. These should be applied from the neck down and in beards and moustaches if necessary. The lotion is left on for 12–24 hours and then the application is repeated in 7 days. During the treatment phase, the patient is instructed not to have close bodily contact with other people. There is no evidence to suggest that cleaning linen and clothing has any impact upon the likelihood of re-infestation
● Close contacts and family should be checked for infestation and treated accordingly.

Head lice

● Advise the patient that treatments can be prescribed or can be bought over the counter from the chemist. Treatments come in the form of lotions or cream rinses and should be applied according to the instructions on the pack. The active ingredients are malathion, permethrin or phenothrin. The lotions are left on for 12 hours (overnight) and then washed off. The creams are left on for 10 minutes and then washed off. The same treatment should be re-applied after 7 days
● 2–3 days after the second application, the hair should be re-checked by detection combing. This involves applying conditioner to the hair and using a fine toothed detection comb to work through the hair, checking the comb for lice after each stroke
● A common cause of re-infestation is the presence of head lice in family members or close contacts. Check family members for infestation and treat as necessary.

Scabies

Scabies is caused by a tiny mite. The female mite burrows into the skin and lays her eggs. The eggs hatch into mites after a few days. The most common site of infestation is the hand, and once infestation has occurred, the condition is passed on to others through close bodily contact, often by holding hands.

Characteristics

● Patients usually complain of a severe itch
● Appearance of greyish-white, slightly elevated, zigzag lines on skin (burrows)

● A rash usually appears soon after the itch has started, it tends to be blotchy red and appears on the inside of the thighs, the loose skin between the fingers, across the abdomen and on the ankles.

Risk factors

Contact with infected people.

Assessment

● *Health history* – enquire about contact with an infected person
● *Physical examination* – inspect the involved site in a well-lit room; common sites include flexor surfaces of the wrist, palms, between the fingers and toes, groin and abdomen. Inspect for secondary lesions such as evidence of bacterial infection
● *Psychosocial concerns and developmental factors* – assess the patient's perception of their health and identify any concerns relating to infection and how they acquired the condition
● *Patient and family knowledge* – assess the patient's understanding of the condition and what effect it might have upon the family and close contacts.

Patient goals

1 After treatment, the patient and their close contacts will have no evidence of scabies infestation.
2 The patient and family will learn preventive healthcare practices to avoid re-infestation and transmission to other people during the treatment period.

Nursing intervention

● Teach the patient and family about the cause, nature and prevention of scabies
● The patient, all household members and sexual partners should be treated even if they have no symptoms as it can take up to 6 weeks for the signs of infection to occur
● Apply a preparation such as permethrin or malathion to cool dry skin over the whole body including soles of the feet, under the nails, scalp, face, neck, ears and penis using cotton wool to apply lotion to sensitive areas. The lotion should be left in place without washing for 8–24 hours depending upon the product used
● Advise the individual and family to wash towels, bedlinen and clothing at 50°C or above. If items cannot be washed, they should be placed in a sealed plastic bag for 72 hours, while the mites die off.

SKIN CANCER

There are various types of skin cancer which can broadly be divided into melanomas and non-melanomas. The non-melanomas include basal cell carcinoma (BCC) and squamous cell carcinoma (SCC). The most common form of skin cancer is BCC and the least common is malignant melanoma. BCC and SCC are most common in people over the age of 60.

Melanoma becomes more common with increasing age but also occurs in younger people.

CHARACTERISTICS

- Changes in moles or other skin lesions that may at first appear innocuous; significant changes include, an increase in size, ulceration, bleeding, serous exudate, asymmetry or itching
- A small nodule that is waxy in appearance with a rolled, translucent border with plaque formation and may ulcerate or bleed from time to time is characteristic of BCC and these are often called 'rodent ulcers'
- Open sores that repeatedly break down and may involve neighbouring structures are characteristic of SCC. If left untreated these can result in total destruction of structures such as the ear or nose and may even metastasize
- Kaposi's sarcoma (KS), a malignancy of lymphatic endothelial cell origin which presents as moderately infiltrated reddish-brown plaques located on the trunk of the body and face, is a complication of HIV infection. KS lesions have particular affinity for the tip of the nose, necessitating body image adjustments for the individual.

RISK FACTORS

- The major cause of skin cancer is prolonged periods of exposure to sunlight and hence ultraviolet radiation. Past episodes of sunburn and excessive exposure to the sun in childhood increase the risks for developing skin cancers
- People who have white skin are more at risk of skin cancer.

ASSESSMENT

- *Health history* – enquire about the patient's age, history of sun exposure, knowledge of changes in moles or skin lesions, occupation, recent changes in general health status, and family history of cancer, in particular skin cancer
- *Physical examination* – visually assess the involved areas in a well-lit room. Common sites include exposed areas, especially of the upper extremities, the face, lower lip, nose, pinna of the ears and forehead. Melanomas can occur anywhere on the body and it is therefore important to examine the patient thoroughly including between the toes, although common sites include the back and legs
- *Psychosocial concerns* – explore the anxiety and fear associated with the word 'cancer' and address the patient and family interactions, concerns and coping abilities
- *Patient and family knowledge* – assess the patient's level of understanding and the implications for family members.

PATIENT GOALS

1 The patient will receive the appropriate treatment for their type of skin cancer.
2 The patient will recover from the skin cancer and will have a minimum of scarring.
3 The patient and family will learn preventive healthcare practices to avoid skin cancer and to detect recurrences.
4 If the cancer has metastasized rapidly and extensively, the goals will include acceptance or adjustment to cancer treatment and/or palliative care measures.

NURSING INTERVENTION

The nurse's role in management of the patient with skin cancer involves education and physical treatments associated with the particular condition.

EDUCATION

Skin cancers can be prevented and many are curable, if diagnosed and treated early. Melanoma remains the most feared form of skin cancer as it can be very aggressive, metastasize rapidly and has a fatal outcome in 20% of cases (Haslett et al 2002). Health promotion programmes and the encouragement of health-seeking behaviours are therefore important for nurses to stress to the public.

Educational points to reinforce with individuals include:

- The avoidance of unnecessary sun exposure, especially between 11.00 a.m. and 3.00 p.m. when the ultraviolet rays are strongest
- The application of sunscreens and/or sunblocks at least to a level of factor 15. In particular, children should be protected from exposure to the sun
- The wearing of protective clothing, i.e. long-sleeved shirts and broad-brimmed hats, but to recognize that sunscreens and blocks are still necessary
- The removal of moles if they are particularly prone to repeated friction and irritation
- An awareness of indicators of potential malignancy, i.e. an increase in size, ulceration, bleeding or serous exudate from a mole or other skin lesion.

TREATMENT

- *Basal cell and squamous cell carcinoma* – discuss with the patient, what the treatment options are and what the individual wishes to do. Options may include surgery, radiation therapy, cryotherapy or chemical destruction of the tumour
- *Malignant melanomas* – prepare the individual educationally and psychologically for surgery to remove the tumour.

Warn the patient that future surgery may be necessary to remove surrounding lymph nodes. An honest appraisal of the likelihood of survival is required and with a great deal of individual and family support.

PRESSURE ULCERS

A pressure ulcer, formerly referred to as a pressure sore, bedsore or decubitus ulcer, is a localized area of tissue damage leading to ulceration of the skin due to the effects of prolonged pressure in combination with a number of other variables. Continual pressure for as little as 20 minutes is sufficient while other contributory factors may be intrinsic or extrinsic in nature. Without immediate intervention the situation deteriorates as the ulcer enlarges, possibly involving deeper structures. The lesion may become infected and lead to the death of the patient in extreme cases. Appropriate preventive measures initiated as soon as a patient's risk status has been established will help to reduce the need for major wound management as any problem associated with the effects of prolonged pressure will be minimized.

The nurse plays a major role in the prevention and management of pressure ulcers and in assisting individuals and families to acquire the necessary knowledge and skill to promote, maintain and restore skin integrity.

RISK FACTORS

The principal factor in pressure ulcer development is excessive tissue pressure that prevents the normal supply of blood to the affected area. The normal mean capillary blood pressure is between 12 and 32 mmHg; therefore, pressure in excess of 30 mmHg for any 'prolonged' period – which may be as little as 10 minutes – will render tissue ischaemic and liable to damage and death (Collier 1999a). By comparison, lying on a hard floor generates surface interface pressures of 240 mmHg on the sacrum. Most healthcare settings now use mattresses with known pressure reducing properties as the standard patient support surface to avoid the problem of high surface interface pressures. The severity of damage therefore depends upon the length of time for which the tissue is exposed to excess pressure which may be due to compression, shear or friction.

Compression is a gravitational force due to the patient's weight and will cause poor lymphatic drainage, local endothelial dysfunction and above all prevent the flow of capillary blood to the area in question. Additionally, bacterial endotoxins may be released in response to hypostasis, increasing the liability of small vessels to thrombose under pressure.

Shearing force on the patient's skin is caused by a mechanical stress acting at an angle to the vertical. This occurs when bone and subcutaneous tissue is trying to move relative to the skin. This will be experienced when the patient's weight is not acting vertically downwards such as when the bed head is raised at an angle and the weight of the upper body acts through the sacrum at an angle which tends to cause the patient to slip down the bed. When a high level of shear is present, the compression force required to produce vascular occlusion is a fraction of that when shear is not present (Grey et al 2006). Friction is the resistance generated when two surfaces attempt to move across each other and in the above example, friction is tending to stop the patient sliding down the bed. Friction may damage skin at the point of contact especially if it is continually repeated, as skin cells will be continually worn away and skin thickness reduced. Knowledge of how these forces are transmitted through a patient's tissues will help to explain why a sinus or cavity may appear due to deep tissue damage, despite the surface skin appearing relatively normal.

Other risk factors for pressure ulcer formation have been identified by NICE (2003):

- Immobility
- Extremes of age – 66% of pressure ulcers occur in patients aged over 70 years as a result of the problems that tend to be associated with old age, but not old age itself
- Sensory impairment
- Acute illness
- Decreased level of consciousness
- Previous history of pressure damage
- Vascular disease
- Severe, chronic or terminal illness
- Poor nutrition and loss of subcutaneous fat
- Excessive moisture; damp skin exacerbates the damage caused by friction and shear as well as being prone to maceration (Grey et al 2006)
- Medical interventions such as drug therapy (steroids) can damage the skin or limit movement (sedatives, analgesics) and increase risk of pressure ulcer development.

In summary, the key to pressure ulcer development is immobility and prolonged unrelieved pressure.

Pressure ulceration in hospitalized elderly patients is linked to a fivefold increase in mortality. Various estimates have been made of the costs of both managing an individual patient with a grade 4 pressure ulcer – £40 000 (Collier 1999b, NICE 2003) and the total cost of pressure ulcers to the NHS – ranging from a minimum of £180m to a maximum of £2bn (Grey et al 2006). Wherever the true figure lies, it is clearly a major item of expense.

Many risk factors are present in elderly patients with fractures of the proximal femur; however, the situation may be compounded by delays and lengthy periods of time spent on trolleys in A&E, X-ray departments and theatres. The development of pressure ulcers is therefore hardly surprising if patients have to lie for lengthy periods on such surfaces without pressure-reducing or relieving equipment (Kenney and Rithalia 1999). Department of Health initiatives such as the Essence of Care Benchmarks (Department of Health 2003) have begun to impact positively on outcomes experienced by all patients, and in particular, the elderly patient who may experience prolonged waiting periods within any A&E department. One effective solution is a fast track pathway through A&E for such a patient.

THE PERSON AT RISK OF DEVELOPING PRESSURE ULCERS

Assessment

Assessment of the person at risk for the development of pressure ulcers includes identification of the contributing factors as listed above. Since the mid-1960s, a great number of tools to assist practitioners assess a patient's risk status have been developed and currently there is evidence of the clinical use of at least 17 throughout Europe (Defloor et al 2001). The forerunner was the *Norton scale* (Box 25.1). The scores derived from this scale can be interpreted to mean those patients with high scores (≥14) are least likely to develop a breakdown of their skin, while those with lower scores (<14) are at greater risk. The maximum score that may be allocated to any individual is 20.

Other scales have since been devised, of which the best known in the UK is the *Waterlow scale* (Fig. 25.2), which adds extra dimensions to the basic Norton scale. When using the Waterlow scale it is important to remember that a low score indicates that the patient is less at risk of developing a pressure ulcer than a patient whose assessment has indicated a high score, the exact reversal of the meaning of scores derived from the Norton tool. The English DoH has emphasized the value of objective risk measurement scales (Department of Health 2001, 2003) in its benchmarking process and this is also reiterated in the NICE guidelines for the prevention of pressure ulcers in primary and secondary care settings (NICE 2003).

Before any risk assessment scale is used in a clinical setting it is important that all practitioners understand the origins of the scale, as well as the applicability, validity, reliability, sensitivity, specificity and usefulness of both the identified risk factors being assessed and the assessment scale being used. Whilst the use of a risk assessment tool can be an important part of an overall pressure ulcer prevention strategy, their limitations must be acknowledged. Furthermore, they should be used by suitably trained practitioners who appreciate the role of the multidisciplinary team in pressure ulcer prevention (Collier 2004).

It should also be remembered that a number of assessment scales are in current clinical use and this can cause some confusion, especially if a patient is transferred from one health setting to another. It is therefore important for all practitioners to remember not only to identify any 'at risk' score on discharge/transfer documentation, but also in brackets to identify the scoring tool that was used to calculate that score.

Figure 25.3 illustrates the areas receiving greatest pressure in different body positions and therefore those areas which are most 'at risk'. Body weight also influences the areas receiving greatest pressure. In the underweight individual, bony prominences are more vulnerable in both the lying and sitting positions. In obese individuals, pressure is redistributed over larger areas. Casts and braces are additional causes of pressure; the skin under these areas should be inspected regularly. Any part of the body in contact with a support surface for a prolonged period of time is susceptible to the effects of pressure. The skin over each potential pressure point should therefore be examined carefully at frequent, regular intervals for redness, swelling, warmth, flaking and signs of erosion.

Patient goals

The goal for the individual at risk for the development of pressure ulcers is to maintain the integrity of the skin.

Nursing intervention

Pressure ulcer prevention

Nursing interventions begin with a thorough assessment and continual reassessment of the patient's skin on a daily basis. Box 25.2 lists the principles for nursing intervention

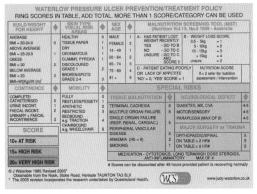

Figure 25.2 Waterlow pressure ulcer prevention/treatment policy. (From Judy-Waterlow.co.uk 2005.)

Box 25.1	The Norton scale for identifying the patient at risk of developing pressure ulcers

A General physical condition		B Mental state		C Activity		D Mobility		E Incontinence	
Good	4	Alert	4	Ambulant	4	Full	4	Not	4
Fair	3	Apathetic	3	Walk with help	3	Slightly limited	3	Occasionally	3
Poor	2	Confused	2	Chair-bound	2	Very limited	2	Usually urinary	2
Very bad	1	Stuporous	1	Bedfast	1	Immobile	1	Double	1

From Norton et al (1962).

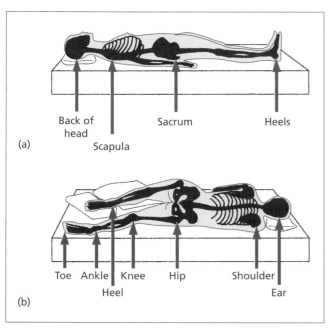

(a)
Back of head — Scapula — Sacrum — Heels

(b)
Toe — Ankle — Heel — Knee — Hip — Shoulder — Ear

Figure 25.3 Risk areas for pressure ulcers. (a) Supine position. (b) Side-lying position.

Box 25.2 Principles of nursing intervention to maintain skin integrity and prevent pressure ulcer development

- Assess individual(s) for risk factors
- Ensure regular changes of position to relieve pressure on 'at-risk' areas 2-hourly, or more frequently if indicated by patient's condition
- Maintain cleanliness and hygiene
- Prevent mechanical, physical and chemical injury
- Ensure adequate nutrition and hydration
- Promote control of incontinence
- Ensure good body alignment and proper positioning
- Utilize devices to redistribute pressure over at-risk anatomical areas
- Inspect the skin at regular intervals during any 24-hour period
- Promote mental alertness and orientation
- Educate the individual, family and caregivers in skin care measures.

---

directed at *maintaining skin integrity* and *preventing pressure ulcer development*. Specific nursing interventions include the following measures:

1 Promote ambulation and range-of-motion activities.
2 Have the patient change position frequently. If the patient is immobile, change his or her position at least every 2–4 hours throughout the day and night, dependent upon the support surface they are resting on and according to an established schedule. If redness is noted and persistent, increase the frequency of the turning schedule or alter the patient support surface to one with better pressure reducing qualities.
3 Provide regular bathing and good perineal care twice daily and immediately after incontinence; keep skin dry but avoid friction and rubbing with towels.
4 Establish a programme to control or manage incontinence.
5 Encourage consistent intake of a nutritionally balanced diet with adequate fluid intake.
6 Use special pressure-redistributing equipment, which will either alternate the area of the body under pressure or redistribute body pressure more evenly over a larger surface area of the body. The former consists of alternating pressure or newer more expensive low air loss, patient support systems. Both of these, however, can be referred to generically as dynamic patient support systems. Low air loss systems are particularly effective. They work by moulding themselves to the contours of the patient's body and redistributing pressure away from the high-risk areas.
7 Keep sheets dry and free of wrinkles and crumbs. Flannelette sheets or pads provide protection from any underlying plastic or rubber covers.
8 Use devices to support specific pressure areas, such as foam pads, gel flotation pads, natural not artificial sheepskins (McGowan et al 2000) and splints or pads over heels and elbows to reduce the effects of *friction* forces on vulnerable areas and thereby prevent epidermal damage.
9 Use a footboard or cradle to prevent pressure on toes.
10 Provide space between the footboard and mattress for heels when the patient is lying supine, or the anterior part of the foot when lying in the prone position.
11 Use pillows and trochanter rolls in positioning the patient to maintain good body alignment and to relieve pressure on known risk areas (see Fig. 25.3).
12 Keep connectors, tubes, pins and clamps from under the patient's body.
13 Avoid shearing forces caused by the patient sliding or slumping down the bed.
14 Those caring for the individual should keep their nails trimmed and remove rings, watches or other jewelry that might scratch or injure the patient during turning or care activities.
15 Teach people to inspect their own skin regularly using a long-handled mirror.
16 Avoid the use of bedpans when possible for persons with sensory loss and paralysis. If the use of a bedpan is unavoidable, a slipper pan should be used.
17 Avoid the use of tight straps on urinary drainage leg-bags.
18 Take steps to prevent at-risk patients from lying for lengthy periods on hospital trolleys or theatre tables

without any pressure-relieving devices placed upon them (NICE 2003).

19 Ensure good nutrition and hydration status.

Evaluation

Strategies to promote skin integrity and to prevent the development of pressure ulcers are effective if the person's skin remains clean, dry and intact. If skin breakdown does occur, reassess the total situation and determine whether the original goal was realistic or whether the person's status or situation has changed.

A quality assurance programme with defined standards for the care of persons at risk of skin breakdown provides a means for nurses to monitor the effectiveness of their practice. For example, it is now recommended that a patient's pressure ulcer risk status be reassessed as a minimum on a weekly basis in an acute care setting and monthly in a primary care setting or whenever there is a significant change in the patient's medical condition (Department of Health 2003). Information obtained from auditing health records can be analyzed by the nurses involved and used to improve care.

THE PERSON WITH A DEVELOPED PRESSURE ULCER

In some cases, even with meticulous attention to preventive measure, pressure ulcers may develop in underlying tissue as a result of internal pressure exerted by the bony prominences on the deep tissues adjacent to the bone. Such deep tissue necrosis may occur without any initial signs of damage to the overlying skin. Subsequently there is an area of swelling and tension and the skin becomes shiny and/or cyanosed. Non-blanching hyperaemia and ultimately a sinus/cavity will develop at a later stage.

The area may appear blanched (for a prolonged time period) and cool at first, followed by redness (non-blanching hyperaemia), warmth and a breakdown of the skin. As the necrotic tissue is sloughed off, an open, moist, inflamed excavation (ulcer) develops which is open to infection and is slow to heal by granulation.

The pressure ulcer area should be examined closely to determine the extent and depth of tissue involvement and must be described accurately. The size of the lesion is monitored either by measuring in centimetres or by tracing its outline on a transparent film at weekly or 2-weekly intervals to assess healing. Several grading systems have been devised to assist with the classification of pressure ulcers. An example of one basic system is given in Box 25.3 and Figure 25.4, but again it must be remembered that a number of classification systems are in current clinical use and this can cause some confusion especially if a patient is transferred from one health setting to another. It is therefore important for all practitioners to identify the grading tool/classification system used on any discharge/transfer documentation.

The pressure lesion should be examined for inflammation, bleeding, sloughing, clinical signs of infection and fibrous scar tissue formation. The area surrounding the lesion is inspected for discolouration, oedema and inflammation which may signify extension of tissue damage.

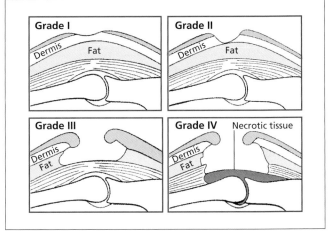

Figure 25.4 Classification of pressure ulcers. (See also Box 25.3.)

Box 25.3 The EPUAP classification of pressure ulcers
Grade I Non-blanchable erythemas of intact skin. Discolouration of the skin, warmth, oedema, induration or hardness may also be used as indicators, particularly on patients with darker skin.
Grade II Partial thickness skin loss involving the epidermis, dermis or both. The ulcer is superficial and presents clinically as an abrasion or blister.
Grade III Full thickness skin loss involving damage to or necrosis of subcutaneous tissue that may extend down to, but not through underlying fascia.
Grade IV Extensive destruction, tissue necrosis, or damage to muscle, bone or supporting structures with or without full thickness skin loss.

The person with a pressure ulcer is at risk of developing further lesions, so vulnerable areas should be inspected at least every 2–4 hours or whenever the patient's position is changed. Nursing care for the individual is designed, whenever possible, to restore skin and tissue integrity and to prevent further skin breakdown.

Nursing intervention

Nursing intervention for a patient with a pressure ulcer has to be individualized, and is based on a detailed assessment of the patient as well as of the pressure ulcer; the general condition is important as well as the grade/classification of the pressure ulcer (Collier 2002). Consistency in carrying out the treatment plan is essential (Black and Hawks 2005).

The measures cited for the preventive care in the preceding pages are still applicable. Further considerations include:

- adequate nutritional intake
- measures to correct existing health problems
- the use of mechanical devices
- care of the lesion
- physical activity
- the control of injurious factors in the environment
- surgical intervention.

Adequate nutritional intake

Nutritional status and dietary intake have been shown to be associated with the presence and healing of pressure ulcers (Black and Hawks 2005). Patients with exuding ulcers have lower serum albumin levels, probably due to the loss of plasma proteins in exudate from pressure ulcers, particularly full-thickness lesions (McLaren and Green 2001). A high-protein, high-vitamin diet is therefore important to combat the tendency toward a negative nitrogen balance and to provide the essentials for healing and continued tissue resistance.

The objectives of nutritional support for the patient may be summarized as follows:

- to maintain optimal body weight
- to optimize the patient's healing potential
- to prevent further tissue breakdown.

Control of existing health problems

Optimal control of health problems such as diabetes mellitus, is essential to promote healing as well as to prevent a break in the skin.

Mechanical devices

The mechanical devices used in the prevention and treatment of pressure ulcers may be divided into three categories:

1 Those designed to support specific pressure areas of the body such as heels, sacrum, buttocks or elbows. These devices include gel flotation pads, natural sheepskins, splints and air-filled wheelchair cushions.
2 Those designed to aid in turning and moving a patient, such as turning frames, rotating beds and hydraulic lifts.
3 Those designed to support the entire body surface by minimizing or equalizing pressure. These can include static pressure-reducing mattresses as well as dynamic alternating pressure mattresses and low air loss beds, which are individually pressurized according to the person's height and weight, and air-fluidized beds.

Turning and positioning of patients is often easier with these beds. The surface moisture level of any pressure ulcer (wound) or the patient's skin can to some extent be controlled, depending upon the type of equipment used and the direction of air flow to the area. These devices supplement the administration of excellent basic skin care and nutritional support.

Wound care for a person with a pressure ulcer

A pressure ulcer is a wound and the principles of wound healing therefore apply to managing and treating an established pressure ulcer (Collier 2003). The essential components of an ideal wound dressing are that it should:

- maintain a high level of humidity at the wound surface
- remove excess exudate and toxic compounds produced in the wound
- allow gaseous exchange
- prevent the wound surface chilling
- form an impenetrable barrier to bacteria
- be free from particles and toxic wound debris
- be able to be changed easily without causing damage to underlying tissue.

The first procedure to be carried out with an established pressure ulcer is the removal of dead and infected material (*debridement*), which may be undertaken 'surgically', as a sharp procedure, chemically or via a process of autolysis. Surgical debridement involves a surgeon cutting/removing dead tissue to expose healthy bleeding tissue within an operating theater with the aid of appropriate anaesthesia, whereas sharp debridement involves a suitably qualified/experienced nurse removing small areas of mobile necrotic tissue with a sterile scissors or a scalpel. For cleansing purposes, normal saline is perfectly adequate.

Autolysis is the natural separation of dead tissue from healthy viable tissue and includes the use of proteolytic enzymes, such as Varidase, which can be applied to the necrotic area. Varidase liquefies dead tissue, thereby de-sloughing the wound and allowing healing to commence. The other types of de-sloughing agents recommended for use are the dextranomer bead or cadexomer iodine preparations, such as Debrisan or Iodosorb respectively. Dextranomer beads absorb wound exudate and bacteria and are very effective in de-sloughing pressure ulcers and other wounds. Iodosorb consists of microbeads of cadexomer iodine (modified starch gel containing iodine 0.9%). Both of these products should be changed once they have become saturated.

Other commonly used agents include hydrogels such as IntraSite and calcium alginate fibre dressings such as Sorbsan both of which are often used to assist the de-sloughing process. Hydrogels are made up mainly of water, and by rehydration of the tissues and the maintenance of a moist wound healing environment assist the process of autolysis.

Box 25.4   Dressings suitable for use on pressure ulcers

Alginates

Alginates are made from seaweed and may be composed of galuronic acid or mannuronic acid, or both, with the proportions of these determining the gel-forming properties of the final fibre. Examples are Sorbsan and AlgiSite M. Alginates with a high proportion of galuronic acid produce firmer fibres, adding strength and shape retention to the dressing material as well as absorption. Alginates have a broad range of clinical uses, but in particular they are useful for absorbing moderate to heavy amounts of exudate and for filling sinuses and cavities (Jones and Milton 2000a, Collier 2003).

Film membranes

Typically, these are transparent sterile elastic thin polyurethane sheets with adhesive properties, which are also vapour permeable, waterproof and extensile. The main differences between products in this category are the moisture vapour transmission rate (MVTR), their ability to act as a carrier and the way in which they are applied. OpSite and Tegaderm are commonly used examples. They are best used on superficial sterile wounds such as operation sites and superficial pressure ulcers; however, they may also be used prophylactically to protect vulnerable areas of the skin that may be at risk of friction forces (Jones and Milton 2000b, Collier 2003).

Foam dressings

These are most suitable for pressure ulcers producing large volumes of exudate. They are made using advanced polymer technology and therefore combine both hydrophilic and hydrophobic properties in varying proportions, depending on the product selected. They are available in both flat sheet and cavity filler forms. Examples are Allevyn, Mepilex, Tielle. They should not be considered for the management of dry necrotic wounds except in conjunction with a suitable debriding agent (Jones and Milton 2000c, Collier 2003).

Hydrogels

Hydrogels come in two basic forms, sheets (Geliperm, Curagel) and gels (AquaForm, IntraSite, Granugel, Nu-Gel). The sheets comprise polysaccharide agarose cross-linked with polyacrylamide. Gels have a high water content, as previously discussed, they are considered to be a very safe primary wound management product and can be used in combination with other secondary dressings to promote and assist the process of autolysis (Jones and Milton 2000d, Collier 2003).

Hydrocolloids

These act on a similar principle to the particulates and alginates in that they interact with wound moisture to form a gel; however, they also have occlusive properties. Granuflex, Comfeel and Tegasorb are common examples where the hydrocolloid layer, consisting of a mixture of pectins, gelatines, sodium carboxymethylcellulose and elastomers, is bonded on to a plastic foam layer with an outer plastic impermeable film. They are designed to absorb low to moderate amounts of fluid. The actual amount of exudate that a hydrocolloid type dressing can absorb will depend upon its MVTR of its backing layer and the amount of hydrocolloid in the dressing product as a whole. These types of dressing may be left in place for up to 5–7 days (Jones and Milton 2000e, Collier 2003).

Particulates

These are occlusive dressings that interact with moisture in the wound to form a paste or gel. Examples are Debrisan and Iodosorb; they are particularly useful for dealing with contaminated and recurrently infected wounds.

Iodine-based materials

The term iodine is used generically to describe all iodine formulations, when in fact there are two distinct preparations, those of PVP-1 (Povidine iodine) – an iodophor composed of elemental iodine and synthetic polymer – and cadexomer iodine – a polysaccharide lattice containing 0.9% elemental iodine that is released on exposure to wound exudate. Both have different physical characteristics that relate to the component parts and the iodine concentration of available iodine that is released when the product is used. As a general rule, PVP-1 products (example – Iodine) are used to prophylactically prevent an increase in bacterial burden on the surface of a wound/pressure ulcer, whereas cadexomer iodine products (example – Iodosorb) have been found to be better for supporting the wound healing process (Jones and Milton 2000f, Collier 2003).

The use of an 'occlusive' or semi-occlusive dressing may also be necessary during the de-sloughing phase and subsequently while healing occurs. There is no place for ordinary gauze as a primary wound management material, as it allows drying of the wound and fibres of gauze may become incorporated in the wound, with the result that dressing removal is very traumatic to the fragile tissues beneath and causes the patient pain at the time of dressings changes. A range of modern interactive wound management products suitable for the management of pressure ulcers is identified in Box 25.4.

Penzer (2002) offers a review of the various modern types of wound management product (dressings) on offer while details may be found in the British National Formulary (2006). The range of new dressing materials can be both bewildering and appear expensive. Nurses must therefore have rational, cost-effective and evidence-based guidelines for their practice, whether for the management of pressure ulcers or any other wounds.

In dealing with chronic wounds such as pressure ulcers, it is important to remember that the presence of bacteria is not uncommon. Wounds may be contaminated but with no sign of multiplication or host reaction; it is only when there is multiplication and a reaction as shown by signs such as localized heat, increased pain, increased exudate and discharge, or cellulitis that it is appropriate to talk about infection. Topical antibiotics and other applications are ineffective in dealing with a wound infection: only systemic antibiotics will be effective. The dressing in this scenario merely helps to clean the wound up, controls the current bacterial burden, prevents further contamination, and facilitates a moist wound healing environment. This in turn facilitates pressure ulcer healing by freeing up the patient's own healing resources. These may be supplemented by antibiotics and other steps to deal with any underlying pathology such as pressure reduction/relief, or the use of compression bandaging to relieve venous congestion as a strategic component of venous leg ulcer management.

Physical activity

Pressure on the area is relieved as much as possible by having the patient change position frequently. If unable to turn unaided, the patient is turned every 2–4 hours throughout the day and night. It is important to remember, however, that 2–4 hourly turning regimens should never be considered absolute and the frequency may need to be varied as the patient's condition either improves or deteriorates, or as a change of patient support surface is indicated. When moving or transferring a patient, precautions are observed to prevent further damage to the skin – especially as a result of unwanted friction forces; the patient is gently lifted clear of the bed or chair, using appropriate aids such as mechanical hoists, to avoid dragging (friction) and exacerbation of any shearing forces already being experienced by the patient.

Patient activity is encouraged; it stimulates metabolism as well as the circulation. A programme of regular exercises adapted to the person's ability to participate actively is established as soon as possible.

Control of environmental factors

A frequent assessment is made of the person's environment for possible sources of pressure and injury to skin. The bedding, wheelchair, bedpan or commode, clothing and appliances such as a prosthesis and drainage tubes or bags are examples of factors in the patient's environment that could be a source of pressure or injury.

Surgical treatment

Minor surgical debridement of a pressure ulcer may be undertaken on the ward by a suitably experienced practitioner such as a Tissue Viability Nurse (TVN), to remove mobile slough and necrotic tissue. Overgranulation of an ulcer in extreme cases may require removal of some of the excess tissue by a surgeon. Some extensive ulcers may require surgical excision and repair by skin flaps in the operating theatre.

Patient and family education

The learning needs of the patient and family are assessed on an ongoing basis and they should be fully involved in the management of the patient's pressure ulcer. They are taught to identify risk factors and to plan and carry out measures to prevent further skin breakdown. If the patient is in the community or returning home before healing is complete, the patient, family and caregivers should be taught the skills necessary to carry out the skin care regimen.

Evaluation

Selection of the treatment and nursing care for the patient with a pressure ulcer should be a cooperative effort by all members caring for the patient and should take into consideration the patient's needs, overall status and resources. For example, if frequent dressing changes cause discomfort for the patient, consideration should be given to a treatment regimen that involves interactive wound-management materials and requires dressing changes less frequently. A variety of interventions are usually required; selection is based on evaluation of the effectiveness of care and assessment of the individual patient, including the amount of pain and discomfort caused by the pressure ulcer.

The evaluation of nursing interventions designed to treat an individual's pressure ulcer(s) includes documented evidence that healing is occurring. The dimensions of the lesions should be decreased, exudate should be reduced or absent, and healthy granulation tissue should be present. When healing is complete, the area will be clean, dry and intact. Other health-related outcomes include the absence of discomfort, and appropriate and realistic improvements in nutritional status, mobility and incontinence.

If documentation indicates that the pressure ulcer is the same or that deterioration has occurred, the patient's status and the identified treatment objectives (goals for care), as well as the suitability of the strategies used, must be re-evaluated. The presence of a pressure ulcer, whether for the short or long term, can have major effects on a patient's quality of life (Franks 2001) and therefore patients must be managed in light of the best available evidence base for any prevention and/or management strategies identified by either a healthcare professional or the patient themselves.

CASE

Pressure ulceration

Mr Morris, an 80-year-old retired coal-miner, is about to be discharged from the acute care setting in which you work, having been treated for a left fractured neck of femur with a hemiarthroplasty that was inserted under spinal anaesthesia. His injury was sustained in the garden at home when he stumbled on uneven ground as he was returning from church one Sunday with his wife.

Mr Morris's wife is herself frail and is registered blind, although she is able to differentiate objects in good light.

Together they are a very independent couple who, although they have a willing supportive family (their oldest daughter lives in the next village), have indicated to you that they want no district nurse visits in the immediate future following Mr Morris's discharge.

Although Mr Morris's mobility is currently improving steadily (he still requires the use of a Zimmer frame), he spends long periods of time in a chair or in his bed, depending on the time of day. His appetite in hospital has been deemed adequate. At the time of his discharge, the skin on Mr Morris's sacral area appeared continually red and the final Waterlow score recorded in the hospital was 18. Previous history included chronic bronchitis and atopic eczema. At home, Mr and Mrs Morris will be sleeping in the divan bed that they were given as a golden wedding present from the family.

Reflective questions

- What factors might increase Mr Morris's risk of developing pressure ulcers, at the time of his discharge from hospital? Highlight any research that could underpin your rationale for the factors identified
- Highlight the relevance of the Waterlow risk assessment score identified here, and identify how this score should be interpreted in a clinical setting
- Identify potential care interventions that could be indicated following the assessment and recording of a Waterlow score of 18, taking account of other information contained within this case scenario.

BURN INJURIES

For most of the population who experience a burn or scald, even in a mild form, there is some understanding of how painful and distressing this type of injury may be. A major burn injury affects not only the skin but every aspect of the patient's life – psychologically, physically and socially. These effects may last a lifetime. Even those with less serious injuries may find their quality of life affected due to pain, wound management and fear of disfigurement. Therefore, it is essential that treatment of a burn patient be delivered by a multidisciplinary team approach, where no single health professional is more important than another. Many burn patients may have other pre-existing health or social problems which complicate their burn injury. The most severe require intensive care nursing, including ventilatory support or haemofiltration due to renal failure, and all need expert nursing care.

CAUSES

Causes of burn injuries include:

- *Scalds* – moist heat such as boiling water, steam or hot liquid at more than 66°C
- *Dry heat* – direct contact with a flame or hot object; may also be associated with a flash or friction injury

- *Friction* – contact with a moving wheel, rope, wire or road surface
- *Radiation* – overexposure to sun or radiant heat sources such as tanning lamps. The ultraviolet radiation involved will cause burns, as may any intense beam of ionizing radiation emitted from a radioactive source
- *Chemical* – acids (sulfuric, nitric, hydrofluoric, hydrochloric), alkalis (caustic soda, oven cleaners) and cement
- *Electrical* – direct passage of current through the body, and lightning injuries.

RELATED FACTORS

A high proportion of burn injuries occur as a result of carelessness, and accidents. The age of the person is an important factor in the type and severity of the burn. Scalds are the most common cause of burn injury in the toddler, for example, and the impact of any given burn injury is more severe in children and the elderly than in other adults.

PREVENTION OF BURN INJURIES

Burn injuries may be prevented by basic safety precautions. Immediate first aid measures will also minimize the complications resulting from a burn injury. Health promotion activities planned for the population at greatest risk such as the elderly, children and their parents, and those with epilepsy, should involve joint collaboration with local fire brigades. Posters in waiting rooms of general practitioners' surgeries or A&E departments are another useful means of getting the message across. Such messages may inform individuals about home safety tips, fire and burn prevention strategies, and give important information on first aid.

CHARACTERISTICS OF BURN INJURIES

The *severity* of a burn injury is determined by five factors:

1 surface area of body burned
2 depth of tissue damage
3 age of patient
4 past medical history
5 part of body burned.

It should be remembered that the severity of the injury is not only related to its depth. Severity will be dependent upon whether the injury is classed as complex or non-complex; the age of the patient; the site, mechanism and nature of the injury; presence of associated inhalation injury; the size of the injury; and the presence of any existing conditions and other associated injuries.

Surface area

The most accurate estimation of the proportion of body surface burned may be based on the Lund and Browder chart (Fig. 25.5). The chart assigns a certain percentage to various parts of the body and includes a table indicating the adjustments necessary for different ages, as the head and

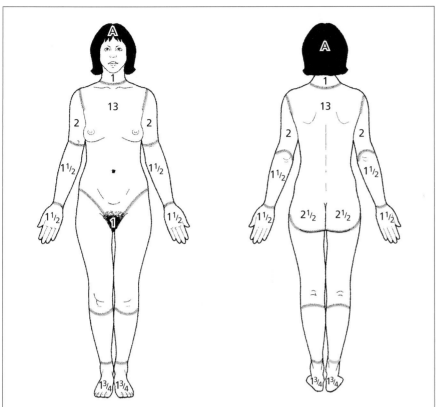

Figure 25.5 The Lund and Browder burn chart.

trunk represent relatively larger proportions of body surface in children. Copies of these charts should be kept available in the emergency department or intensive care unit so that the burned areas can be mapped out when the patient is examined and the percentage estimated.

If the Lund and Browder chart is not available, a quick approximate estimate of the percentage of body surface burned may be made using the Rule of Nines. The Rule of Nines, unlike the Lund and Browder chart, is useful for adult patients only and should not be used for children under the age of 15 years. The body is divided into areas, each of which represents 9% as follows:

● The whole of the upper limb – 9%
● A thigh – 9%
● A leg (below the knee) – 9%
● The anterior chest – 9%
● The posterior chest – 9%
● The abdomen – 9%
● The lower half of the back (lumbar and sacral regions) – 9%
● The head and neck – 9%
● The perineum – 1%.

When neither of the above assessment charts is available, or when the injured area is relatively small, the palmar surface of the patient's hand can be used to approximate the extent of injury, as this is equal to 1% of the patient's total body surface area (TBSA). This assessment technique may also prove to be useful when the burnt areas are scattered over the patient's body.

The TBSA affected by the burn is very closely associated with the incidence of inhalation injury and mortality. According to Walsh and Kent (2001) a major burn requiring immediate i.v. resuscitation is defined as 15% or more TBSA in adults and as 10% or more TBSA in those either under 10 or over 50 years of age (only full- or partial-thickness burns are counted, see below). Burns of less than 10% TBSA in adults and 5% in children may be managed on an outpatient basis, but the patient may require hospitalization for social or medical reasons. Very young children and adults aged over 50 years have higher mortality and morbidity rates associated with burn injury. The mortality rate increases sharply with advancing age.

Depth

The depth of the burn wound is primarily due to the *temperature* of the burning agent and the *duration* of contact or exposure. However, in assessing the wound accurately, many other factors have to be considered including heat source, mechanism of injury, the patient's age, the location of the burn and the wound characteristics. Burn depth is classified as superficial, superficial partial-thickness, deep partial-thickness (deep dermal) or full-thickness (Table 25.1). Superficial burns, such as those that result from sunburn and lead to simple erythema of the skin, are not generally taken into consideration when assessing the area of burns.

Table 25.1 Summary of burn characteristics

Depth	Tissues involved	Usual cause	Characteristics	Pain	Healing
Superficial	Epithelium Epidermis	Sunburn, cooking steam	Dry, no blisters, pink/red, blanches with pressure	Present	Approx. 5 days No obvious scarring
Superficial partial-thickness	Epidermis Minimal dermis	Flash flame, weak chemicals or hot liquid	Moist, pink or red mottled, blisters. Some blanching	Very painful	Approx. 10–21 days. Slight scarring. May appear very red for approx. 6 weeks, then hypopigmented or hyperpigmented depending on amount of remaining intact melanocytes
Deep dermal partial-thickness	Epidermis. Dermis but epidermal-lined. Sweat glands, hair follicles survive	Flame, hot liquids, solids	Few blisters, red with white patches	Sensitive to pressure	6 weeks or more. Hypertrophic scarring. Skin graft early to maximize healing and scar formation and to prevent contractures
Full thickness	As above plus subcutaneous fat and deeper tissues if chemical or electrical injury	Sustained flame, hot liquids or solids, chemicals, electricity	Leathery, cracked, avascular, pale white, brown or charred	Little pain	Cannot self-regenerate, skin grafts needed. Scar will be influenced by genetic predisposition and grafting techniques used

(After Burgess (1991).)

A *full-thickness* burn is characterized by the destruction of the full thickness of the skin and its appendages. Underlying tissues such as the subcutaneous fat, muscles, tendons and bone may also be burned. The skin's re-epithelializing cells are located at the base of the epidermis and line dermal appendages such as the shafts of the hair follicles and sweat glands. Therefore, when the dermis is damaged, spontaneous regeneration and replacement of the skin is not possible. The area may be slowly filled in with granulation tissue and fibrous scar tissue, proliferated from marginal or underlying connective tissue. To avoid the contracture disability that occurs with the fibrous scar tissue, the area may be covered with a skin graft.

PATHOPHYSIOLOGICAL EFFECTS OF BURNS

A burn injury involving 10% TBSA in children and 15% TBSA in adults may significantly alter the body's cardiovascular function leading to a form of hypovolaemic shock known as 'burn shock' (Nowak and Handford 2004). Patients with these types of injury require fluid replacement therapy – known as fluid resuscitation. The result of a significant burn injury is insufficient blood flow through the body to maintain adequate perfusion at the capillary level. This hypovolaemia is a result of both the fluid losses through the burn wound and the movement of intravascular fluid into the interstitial spaces due to the increased permeability and dilatation of the capillaries in the burnt area. The result of this shift of protein-rich fluid out of the vascular compartment leads to the formation of blisters and oedema. There is also a substantial loss of sodium associated with burn oedema. Large volumes of the fluid, which is similar in composition to plasma, may seep into the tissues. Some is carried away via the lymphatics, but they cannot usually cope with the total volume leading to an accumulation of fluid in the tissues. The loss of blood proteins with the fluid and the ensuing reduction in the intravascular colloidal osmotic pressure also promote oedema. As a consequence, oedema also occurs in non-burned tissue, resulting in generalized oedema. Oedema of the lungs from this cause may be life-threatening, even in the absence of any respiratory injury. In a full-thickness burn, the fluid loss is extensive, and in areas of greater vascularization, such as the face, the oedema and swelling may be very severe.

In response to the massive inflammatory reaction postburn, there is an increased release of catecholamines (p. 555). The intravascular volume is reduced, the blood pressure falls, the cardiac output may be decreased by as much as 30–50% (in burns >40%, the decrease occurs within 15–30 minutes of the injury), and the blood flow through the tissues is reduced. Hypovolaemic shock develops rapidly unless there is adequate fluid replacement.

An 8–10% decrease in the number of red blood cells occurs, especially in deep burns, due to trapping and heat injury of the blood cells in the skin capillaries at the time of the injury. Often red cells, including transfused cells, may also be destroyed in the immediate postburn period; blood transfusion may be delayed for at least 48 hours. Normal red blood cell production may also be reduced because of depression of the bone marrow.

Inhalation of smoke and chemical fumes may seriously impair ventilatory function; irritation of the mucosa may cause laryngeal oedema and airway obstruction, or pulmonary oedema and severe respiratory insufficiency.

The urinary output is decreased as a result of the decreased intravascular volume and subsequent hypotension. If the blood supply is markedly reduced in the shock phase, renal tubular damage may also result. A reliable indicator of a good prognosis is the maintenance of urine output at a rate of at least 0.5 mL/kg per hour in adults. This indicates adequate renal perfusion. When there is massive red blood cell destruction, large quantities of haemoglobin are released. These blood pigments may block the renal tubules, causing renal shutdown. Another cause of renal failure in the burn-injured patient is the breakdown of protein from damaged tissue, especially muscle, and the release of these products (e.g. myoglobin) into the renal tubules.

The appearance of brownish-black urine indicates the presence of free haemoglobin and/or myoglobin; this is an ominous sign that requires urgent action to achieve diuresis.

In severe burns gastrointestinal peristalsis is depressed; nausea, vomiting and abdominal distension may occur. Haematemesis or melaena may develop, indicating the presence of stress ulcers.

Electrolyte imbalances develop because of the burn oedema, loss of fluid through the open wound, impaired renal function due to shock, and excessive release of potassium by the damaged tissue cells and erythrocytes. These disturbances are exacerbated by the release of aldosterone from the adrenal cortex in response to the renin-angiotensin pathway (see Ch. ***). This results in sodium and hence water retention by the kidneys (if they are functioning satisfactorily) and potassium excretion. The adrenocortical hyperactivity also accelerates protein catabolism, resulting in a negative nitrogen balance. Immunologically, after a major burn, the patient is compromised, which may have serious consequences, particularly for a patient with an established human immunodeficiency virus (HIV) infection. All burn wounds are colonized with bacteria. Once the bacterial counts become high and infectious organisms enter the lymphatic system, the patient may develop septicaemia. Sepsis is the largest single cause of death in burns patients. Multisystem organ failure, often secondary to sepsis, is a serious and frequently fatal consequence of septicaemia.

The layer of burned tissues may form a dry, charred, coagulated surface, called an *eschar*, or a soft, moist non-coagulated area. Inflammation and oedema develop at the wound margins and below the layers of dead tissue. Many small blood vessels below the devitalized tissue may be thrombosed, promoting further cellular destruction. The de-composition of dead tissue and sloughing produce a favourable culture medium for organisms and the development of serious infection.

ASSESSMENT

Assessment of the person with a burn injury is a collaborative function between the nurse and physician. A significant factor that has helped to reduce the mortality rate associated with major trauma, including burns, has been the introduction and implementation of protocols that are part of the Advanced Trauma Life Support (ATLS) course and other similar courses that are available for healthcare professionals throughout the world. The protocols identify three major stages of patient care. The first, known as the 'primary survey' is intended to find all the immediate life-threatening conditions and to initiate resuscitation accordingly. The second, called the 'secondary survey', is undertaken immediately after the primary survey and its aim is to identify all the patient's injuries, no matter how trivial. Finally, the third stage of patient management is the stage of definitive care, for example, when the patient goes to theatre, intensive care or the burns unit. In the ideal situation, the burnt patient should initially be assessed in an appropriate environment, such as an A&E department or burns unit.

Physical examination

An assessment of the patient should follow as soon as possible after admission to A&E. Although an assessment of the individual's airway, breathing patterns, circulation and cervical spine immobilization will have been performed at the accident scene by paramedics, A&E staff must carry out such an assessment immediately the patient arrives in A&E. The patient should also be assessed for vital signs, pain, shock and concomitant injuries.

The potential for airway obstruction and an ineffective breathing pattern is the primary concern. The airway should be checked for patency, the patient's vital signs and level of consciousness monitored and recorded, and the presence or absence of inhalation injury determined. If the patient is experiencing respiratory distress, the nurse may play an important role in calming the individual and providing support while interventions take place to restore an adequate airway.

Signs and symptoms of smoke inhalation include burns to the head and neck, singed nasal hairs, darkened oral and nasal membranes, carbonaceous sputum, stridor, a history of being burned in an enclosed space, and exposure to flame. Following an assessment of the status of the cervical spine, a laryngoscope and/or fibreoptic bronchoscope may be inserted in the airway to determine the extent of any inhalation injury and subsequent risk of impaired gas exchange. The nurse can provide much needed emotional support to the burned individual during these diagnostic tests.

Circulation to burned and unburned areas should also be assessed and noted. Altered tissue perfusion may occur alongside oedema, as a result of hypovolaemic shock and occlusion of blood vessels due to the constricting effect of eschar in circumferential burns. If the nurse cannot feel the pulses, Doppler ultrasonography should be used to determine their presence or absence.

The previously mentioned severity factors of extent and depth of burn and the part of the body burned are included in the physical assessment and the location of the individual's burns need also to be assessed and noted.

After removal of all constricting items, such as jewelry, belts and remaining clothing, the burn wounds can be inspected more closely. The extent of the burn may be determined by filling in a Lund and Browder form. This exercise should be performed by more than one person (e.g. doctor and nurse) to ensure accuracy. Hypovolaemic shock is likely if the extent of the burn is greater than 15% of the TBSA, making fluid replacement a top priority.

The depth of the burn may be determined using criteria such as those described in Table 25.1. It may take several days of ongoing assessment before an exact determination of depth can be made. Burns can also become deeper either; due to heat retention allowing the burning process to continue, presence of infection, or if the wound is allowed to dry out.

The burned individual's renal and gastrointestinal function needs to be assessed. The nurse can pass a urinary catheter and assess the quantity and quality of the urine produced. Laboratory data such as blood urea and electrolytes, full blood count, and urinalysis (including testing for haemoglobinuria) provide further objective information which will guide treatment. Monitoring bowel sounds, the insertion of a nasogastric tube and the assessment of gastric contents should also be performed.

The burned individual's pain level must be assessed continually and treated effectively with analgesia and perhaps an anxiolytic to relieve anxiety. Initially analgesic therapy should be administered via the intravenous route to ensure the desired outcome.

Once the patient has been transferred or admitted to a burn treatment unit, physical parameters need to be monitored on a consistent basis to note changes in the patient's physical status.

Health history

As soon as it is appropriate, the nursing staff should introduce themselves to the patient or their family or other relatives. This will enable practitioners to collect data about the accident, past medical history, existence of any known allergies and medications the patient may be currently taking as well as to answer any questions that the patient or family may have.

Psychosocial concerns and developmental factors

These include an assessment of the individual's cultural background, usual coping mechanisms and responses to stress, responses to previous hospitalizations or illnesses, and interactions between the patient, family and significant others. Other factors such as financial implications of the

injury, acceptance (adaptation to altered body image), and changes in roles and responsibilities need to be assessed at a later date.

Patient and family knowledge

While the physical examination is taking place, someone from the healthcare team should be providing the family or significant others with information and emotional support. The burned individual should also be made aware of what is, and will be, taking place during the hospitalization and that loved ones are being kept fully informed. To assist with this process, documentary and photographic material may be used over time to demonstrate the progress being made.

HEALTH PROBLEMS COMMON TO THE PERSON WITH A BURN INJURY

Impaired skin and tissue integrity is the major health problem experienced by the individual in relation to the burn injury. The restoration of skin and tissue integrity is a major nursing concern. Much of what has been discussed in the previous sections of this chapter regarding this patient problem will apply to the individual with burns. Nursing care will be discussed in relation to the seven phases of recovery: *rescue, resuscitate, retrieve, resurface, reconstruct, rehabilitate* and *review*. Associated health problems common to persons with burns will be discussed in relation to each highlighted phase.

Rescue, resuscitate and retrieve

Care during these initial phases is directed towards ensuring that the individual receives prompt, knowledgeable and appropriate first aid and initial medical and nursing care to enhance their chances of survival. The following key points require urgent attention:

- The patient should have a patent airway
- The patient's wounds must be protected
- Further injury and contamination of wound(s) should not occur
- The patient's pain should be controlled and relieved
- Prescribed treatment for hypovolaemic shock needs to be implemented immediately
- The patient should be able to talk about concerns and feelings of anxiety
- The patient and family should be able to verbalize awareness of the patient's status and care.

Care during the rescue, resuscitate and retrieve period includes first aid at the site of the injury and the initial medical and nursing care. This initial care is directed toward establishing and maintaining an airway, if necessary, reversing hypovolaemic shock, and cleansing and assessing the severity of the burned areas. These phases may last for 2–7 days.

Nursing intervention

First aid   Initial steps to be taken at the accident scene are listed in Box 25.5.

The overall *aim* of burn first aid is to stop the burning process. With flame burns, the words 'Stop – Drop – Roll –

Box 25.5 First aid at the accident scene for the burned patient

1 Stop the burning process.

2 Maintain airway – resuscitation measures may be necessary.

3 Assess for other injuries.

4 Flush the burn with copious amounts of cold water, except for electrical injuries, facial burns and burns involving certain chemical agents such as metallic sodium, potassium and calcium, as these react violently with aqueous solutions (Fowler 1999).

5 Protect wounds from further trauma.

6 Provide emotional support – have someone remain with patient. Explain that assistance will be available.

7 Transport the patient to where medical care can be obtained.

Cool' apply. Running fans the flames and increases the severity of the injury. Immediate cooling of the burn wound is the next priority. Water is usually accessible. The burned area must be held or immersed under cool running water, or cool moistened towels or compresses can be applied. Burn blisters should be left untouched in the first aid situation as they help protect the wound from contamination. Cooling reduces pain and decreases the effect of heat transmission through the tissues. Ice is avoided because of the sudden vasoconstriction that it produces. Hypothermia is a potential complication which can be decreased by the use of sheets and then blankets over the patient and adjusting the temperature of the cooling agent.

Oils, ointments, lotions and other preparations *should not* be applied, and no attempt should be made to remove clothing that is adherent. The burn area is covered with a moist, sterile or clean material to exclude air and to reduce contamination. Cling film is an excellent first aid dressing. Non-burned areas are covered with warm, dry covers. While awaiting transportation, the patient is kept at rest. A minimal amount of movement and handling is important.

In the case of chemical burns, the area is washed with generous amounts of water for at least 20 minutes or until the pain is lessened. The patient's clothing and consideration should be given to the removal of contact lenses because they may contain some of the chemical substance. Caregivers should also protect themselves from any residual chemical. Neutralizers are no longer indicated as they can produce an undesirable thermal reaction with the acid or alkali.

The patient with severe burns is likely to be conscious unless other injuries interfere with awareness. Simple explanations of what is being done should be provided and repeated frequently. The presence of a nurse can be very supportive and helps to reduce the considerable amount of anxiety and fear experienced by the patient.

Most superficial burns involving *less than* 10% of TBSA may be treated at home or in the review clinic attached to an A&E department, but only after a full and thorough initial assessment has been undertaken. Systemic effects in such cases are usually minimal and are not generally considered sufficiently significant to require hospitalization.

Outpatient management

It is essential that nursing staff ensure the patient will be able to manage at home before discharge from the A&E department is arranged. Attention should be paid to ensuring the wound is securely dressed and the patient has adequate analgesia. The patient should be encouraged to return to the department before their next appointment if they are worried about the state of their injury.

In certain circumstances non-debrided wounds may be managed on an outpatient basis; however, this decision will depend upon discussions between several members of the multidisciplinary team.

TREATMENT OF THE SEVERELY BURNED PATIENT ON ADMISSION

An immediate *assessment* of the patient's general condition is made before attention is directed to the burn wound (Box 25.6). A history as to how the burn was sustained is obtained from the patient or the accompanying person; this may indicate the need to search for other injuries. The burn patient is usually sufficiently alert to provide information; if drowsy, confused or comatose, other disorders or injuries should be suspected (e.g. hypoxia, head injury, cerebral aneurysm or stroke).

POTENTIAL FOR AIRWAY OBSTRUCTION

Damage to the respiratory tract and respiratory insufficiency demands prompt attention. Respiratory impairment is frequently associated with burns of the face or neck, and may be the result of the inhalation of smoke, a gaseous chemical or flames. If an inhalation injury is suspected, 100% oxygen should be given through a non-rebreathing mask. This rule applies even when the patient is known to have chronic airways disease as adjustments can be made easily in the very small number of patients who deteriorate as a result of

---

Box 25.6 Treatment of the severely burned patient on admission

1 Maintain an airway and administer oxygen if necessary.

2 Assess severity of injuries and degree of shock.

3 Initiate fluid replacement – establish an intravenous line.

4 Control pain.

5 Insert a nasogastric tube.

6 Insert an indwelling catheter.

7 Provide emotional support.

8 Provide initial wound care.

9 Initiate protective isolation measures.

10 Administer tetanus prophylaxis.

---

this action. To assess ventilatory function, observe respiratory effects and listen for inspiratory wheezes, check odour of breath (a smoky or chemical odour may be detected which indicates inhalation of smoke or fumes), listen for hoarseness and examine any sputum for blood and carbon particles.

Humidified oxygen is generally administered and suctioning may be helpful to clear the airway of secretions. Intubation may be performed if respiratory embarrassment increases. If there is marked insufficiency, a mechanical ventilator may be used in conjunction with the endotracheal tube. Frequent estimations of the blood gases and expiratory or tidal volume may be done. In addition, a chest radiograph should be taken to establish baseline lung findings and ensure proper placement of invasive tubes and lines.

Respiratory insufficiency may develop later in circumferential or severe chest burns due to the firm, unyielding eschar that forms around the trunk preventing normal chest expansion and hence severely limiting lung ventilation. Several incisions may have to be made in the eschar to relieve the thoracic restriction. This is known as *escharotomy* and may also be performed wherever there is constriction and circumferential burns such as full-thickness limb burns to prevent neurovascular compromise from the tourniquet-like effect of the eschar. After the initial assessment and treatment, the patient is required to breathe deeply and to cough hourly to avoid the risk of chest infection.

When satisfactory ventilation is established, attention is directed toward fluid therapy and assessment of the extent and severity of the burn and any other injuries.

THE MANAGEMENT OF HYPOVOLAEMIC SHOCK

The control of shock resulting from the loss of intravascular volume in a severe burn is dependent upon prompt, adequate fluid replacement. The extent and depth of burn and the patient's age and health status determine the need for fluid therapy. Burns >15% of the total body surface area in adults require intravenous therapy. A reliable intravenous route is established by the insertion of two large intravenous catheters, preferably through unburned tissue. The intravascular fluid shift commences immediately after burning but signs of shock may not appear for a few hours. In the A&E department fluid replacement is based on ATLS guidelines which use crystalloids. Note that colloids should be used with caution in patients with inhalation injury and that the choice of a fluid resuscitation formula is based upon crystalloid or colloid depending upon the attending doctor's and the institution's burn care protocol. In the initial resuscitation stage a plasma substitute such as Haemaccel or Gelofusine may be used to expand the circulation but human albumin solution (4.5%) is needed subsequently to restore plasma volumes. Other fluids that may be used include Ringer's solution to correct electrolyte imbalances (particularly sodium) and fluid loss.

The volume, composition and rate of flow of the intravenous fluids are based on the percentage body surface burned, the weight of the patient, the hourly urinary output, arterial blood pressure, haematocrit and serum electrolyte concentrations, especially potassium and sodium. An adult may require as much as 500–1000 mL/hour intravenously to maintain a minimum acceptable urinary output of 30–60 mL/hour. Close monitoring and frequent adjustment of the intravenous flow rate is essential. If oral fluids are permitted, the amounts ingested are recorded accurately.

Generally, after the first 24–36 hours, fluid extravasation into the tissues lessens and the intravascular volume tends to stabilize gradually. This physiological phenomenon of fluid remobilization signals the end of the emergent period of care. Nursing documentation of intake and output continues to be an essential part of the patient assessment. The intravenous fluid therapy is gradually reduced and may be discontinued when laboratory studies indicate satisfactory concentrations, when the patient is able to take adequate amounts of fluid orally, or their urinary output has increased. As the days go by close observation is needed for signs of circulatory overload, because much of the fluid in the interstitial spaces is reabsorbed into the intravascular compartment as capillary integrity is re-established. Overloading of the circulatory system may be manifested by a urinary output >100 mL per hour within the first 48 hours, pulmonary oedema, a central venous pressure in excess of 13 cm H_2O and a weak pulse. If renal function is satisfactory, the excessive amount can be controlled by diuresis.

An indwelling catheter is passed as soon as the patient requiring fluid resuscitation therapy is admitted so that the hourly urinary output may be noted. This serves as a guide in determining intravenous fluid requirement and also provides information about the patient's general circulatory status and renal function (acute renal failure is possible after burn injury). A bolus of a diuretic (e.g. mannitol 100–200 mL i.v.) may be ordered in the immediate phase of care for electrical burns where there is a high incidence of haemoglobinuria and myoglobinuria. The catheter is removed as soon as the patient's condition is stable and shock is reversed, as the indwelling catheter predisposes to bladder infection and loss of bladder tone.

The patient is observed closely during the early postburn period for signs of shock and continually to monitor their response to treatment. The blood pressure, pulse and level of consciousness are noted every 15–30 minutes and the urinary output and quality is noted continually and should be documented hourly, or as the condition of the patient dictates. A diminishing intravascular volume and subsequent circulatory failure may be reflected by a fall in blood pressure, weak pulse, abnormal drowsiness, disorientation and a urinary output of <30 mL/hour.

Frequent haemoglobin and haematocrit determinations are made; abnormal increases indicate haemoconcentration due to loss of intravascular fluid into the tissues. After 6 or 7 days, a deficiency of erythrocytes and haemoglobin may indicate the need for a blood transfusion. Blood transfusions may be given anyway if escharotomies have been performed. Gastrointestinal motility may cease as a consequence of hypovolaemic shock, a nasogastric tube needs to be inserted to relieve gastric dilatation and the patient is given nothing by mouth until bowel sounds return. H_2 blockers such as ranitidine (to prevent peptic ulceration), antacids, and enteral or parenteral feeds may also be indicated. Serum protein and electrolyte concentrations are also determined frequently; these help in selecting the type of intravenous solutions required.

An accurate record of the fluid intake (oral and intravenous) and output is of paramount importance. The patient is weighed on a regular basis – usually on admission and at the time of every dressing change (naked). A gain is manifested at first because of the increased extracellular fluid and the intravascular infusion. Then a marked weight loss accompanies the diuresis that corresponds with the recovery from shock. Much of the fluid that escaped into the interstitial spaces is reabsorbed into the blood vessels. During this period, the patient is observed for any signs of overhydration. If the intravenous infusion is continued at the previous rate of administration at this time, the vascular system may become overloaded, placing an excessive demand on the heart and causing pulmonary oedema. The reabsorption of the tissue fluid can usually be recognized by a marked increase in the urinary output.

In summary, as well as the nursing responsibilities that have been outlined above, a successful patient outcome is also dependent upon how all the members of the multidisciplinary team care for the severely burnt patient. For example, the anaesthetist and surgeons are responsible for the patient's airway, fluid management, and early excision of tissues and grafting. Rehabilitation starts from the time of admission; the physiotherapist is essential for maintaining passive limb movements and the occupational therapist is required to start making splints (to prevent contractures) as soon as the patient arrives. Both a minister of religion and a counsellor should be available to support the relatives of critically ill patients.

After this initial period of management, the nurse must remain alert for an increase in temperature, rapid pulse, odour and discharge from the burned area, as this may indicate the onset or presence of infection.

The patient's position, especially that of the burned parts of the body, is checked frequently during the day and night for optimal alignment. Flexion contracture may develop very quickly and preclude restoration of function.

PAIN

Pain assessment is a highly individualized and subjective process. Analgesics are administered to decrease pain, and anxiolytics are used to decrease the emotional overtones of the trauma. Many burns units successfully use a pain-control regimen based on continual opiate infusion, delivered by one of the many regulating devices now available. Patient-controlled analgesia (PCA) devices, although encouraged as soon as the patient is able to understand the principles of administration, are usually reserved for use in the later stages of management and postgrafting stage. The intravenous route is always preferred because the circulatory disturbances and oedema previously discussed reduce absorption via alternative routes.

Pain assessment and intervention are ongoing, varying from patient to patient and from day to day in the same patient. The patient's subjective response is the best indicator of the efficacy of a chosen strategy. The nurse's role in pain assessment and management is even more crucial when the patient is ventilated and/or comatose or confused. Particular attention must be paid to providing pain relief while changing dressings, and the use of Entonox gas can be helpful. (For more information on pain management, see Ch. 8.)

ANXIETY

Following a severe burn, the patient and family experience considerable emotional disturbance. As with any severe stress, the reactions and adaptive mechanisms may vary markedly from one person to another, depending mainly on the particular situation and past experiences of each person. Factors that generate fear and anxiety in both the patient and family include the actual threat to life, permanent incapacity and disfigurement, the prolonged period of treatment necessitating dependence as well as separation, and the uncertain future. Feelings of guilt may be lurking near the surface, particularly in the parents of a child who has suffered burn injury. A sensitive approach by the nurse is therefore essential.

The nurse should encourage the patient and family to discuss their concerns and fears. It is important that they are kept informed of all activities and why certain procedures and actions are being carried out. Repetition of information is necessary as the patient and family will be anxious and experiencing varied and rapidly changing phenomena, over which they perceive they have minimal, if any, control. Questions such as 'Will I be scarred for life?' should be given the honest answer, 'Yes – but we cannot predict to what extent or how you will eventually look', and the patient should be encouraged to express fears and anxieties as the nurse explores these issues with sensitivity and empathy.

WOUND CARE

The aim of burn wound care, whatever the size of the burn, is to:

- maintain a clean, moist wound environment
- promote patient comfort
- offer protection from infection or further trauma
- achieve and maintain optimal activity and function.

Before a dressing is applied, burned areas must be gently but thoroughly cleansed with warmed sterile normal saline solution, sterile water or warmed tap water dependent upon local policy. Burned tissue (eschar) may be removed (debrided) carefully, with sterile scissors and forceps, in order to reveal the presence of healthy tissue, and burn blisters may or may not be de-roofed again according to local policy. An example of a dressing guide is shown in Table 25.2. Following a minor burn, the patient should return to the outpatient department or clinic to have the dressing(s) changed every 3–4 days, or more frequently if it is disrupted or if breakthrough drainage occurs. With facial burns, appropriate wound care may need to be performed two or three times a day.

EVALUATION OF THE PERSON FOLLOWING THESE INITIAL PHASES OF MANAGEMENT

The care provided to the person with a severe burn injury during these initial phases is multifaceted and should demonstrate collaboration among first aid workers, paramedics, nurses in A&E and special burns units, doctors, physiotherapists and other health professionals.

The criteria listed in Box 25.7 may be used to evaluate the effectiveness of nursing care during this 'immediate' phase.

RESURFACE AND RECONSTRUCT PHASES

Sepsis is the principal cause of death in patients who die from burn injuries. *Pneumonia* and *cardiovascular, respiratory, gastrointestinal* and *renal system failures* are the other main causes of death. Complications tend to be the rule rather than the exception for individuals with severe burns. Experience of patients with burn injuries indicates the need to take a proactive approach to their care to try to prevent complications.

There are two primary patient *goals* in the intermediate phase for individuals with burns:

1 Healing and closure of the burn wound.
2 Coping with physical and psychosocial complications that cannot be avoided.

Through effective management of the first goal, many of the complications can be avoided or kept to a minimum.

The success of care can be measured using the criteria listed in Box 25.8.

Nursing intervention
Infection risk

It is important to remember that nearly all burns patient's wounds will be colonized (presence of organisms without

---

Box 25.7 Criteria used to evaluate the effectiveness of nursing care during the initial four phases of recovery from burn injury

1 The patient's airway is patent.

2 The patient's breathing pattern is effective.

3 Fluid balance is being maintained.

4 Initial wound assessment has been completed.

5 Initial wound care protocols have been initiated.

6 Pain and discomfort are controlled.

7 The patient and family are able to describe what has happened and the patient's status and progress.

8 The patient and family acknowledge receiving emotional support relevant to the emergency situation.

Table 25.2 Dressing minor burn wounds

Layer of dressing	Rationale
Flamazine cream (silver sulfadiazine)	Antibacterial cream prevents infection of wound
Non-adherent dressing pads (e.g. Melolin, Release) are usually used over skin grafts (ideally not as a primary contact layer) or wound contact material such as Mepitel	Prevents damage to new tissue when dressing removed. Makes dressing changes less painful
Thick gauze pad	Absorbs wound exudates
Tubular bandage for limb(s) (e.g. Tubigrip or TubiFast); may be supplemented by traditional crêpe bandages	Holds dressing securely in place

an associated host reaction); however, the presence of infection (presence of organisms with an associated host reaction) may be reduced by the use of several measures. Avoiding or minimizing infection involves appropriate use of topical antimicrobial agents, primarily silver sulfadiazine (e.g. Flamazine), support for the patient's immune mechanisms, rapid elimination of reservoirs for potential infection and prevention of the transfer of infection.

Fresh frozen plasma may be administered to support the patient's weakened immune system. Strict, aseptic technique is used when inserting invasive lines and when applying sterile dressings. If the patient has dressings in place, standard infection control measures and protective isolation will be undertaken when the patient is first admitted. Infection control measures also focus on the safe handling of all body substances and fluids as potential sources of infection.

Everything in the patient's room is considered a source of contamination to him or her. Hospital personnel serve as potential vectors in the transmission of organisms between patients. The nurse wears a protective isolation gown when rendering physical care to the patient. The importance of handwashing guidelines and strict adherence to them must be stressed.

Septicaemia can develop at any stage until complete wound coverage is achieved. It may have a sudden onset, with rigors and a rapid increase in temperature, or it may develop gradually over 2–3 days. Septicaemia is characterized by high fever that may fluctuate, rapid pulse, drowsiness and disorientation. Paralytic ileus is a common

concomitant. Oozing from the burn wounds or the appearance of purulent exudate or petechiae require wound swabs for microbiology. Blood cultures are necessary for a definitive diagnosis. *Staphylococcus aureus*, haemolytic streptococcus and *Pseudomonas aeruginosa* are common causes of septicaemia.

Nursing interventions for the patient whose wound(s) has shown organisms on culture and is at risk for or has become septic include: careful and continuous monitoring for the early signs of impending sepsis; the administration of antibiotics; assistance with the insertion of invasive lines for more sophisticated diagnostic monitoring; and scrupulous wound and skin care. If a patient does develop a resistant organism, strict isolation procedures must be implemented and enforced at all times. Regardless of the type of isolation employed, however, the most definitive answer to the problem of infection and resultant complications due to burns lies with coverage of the burn wound.

Wound healing and skin grafts

Various forms of local treatment are used to prevent further wound contamination and tissue destruction, to suppress the growth of bacteria in the area, and to promote separation of the devitalized tissue and its replacement with skin. Initially, the burn is cleansed of dirt, foreign substances and detached epithelium, using non-filamented gauze and a mild soapy solution, water or normal saline. Loose, sloughing skin and debris are removed with sterile forceps and the skin may be removed from blisters. The cleansing must be *very gentle* to avoid damage of exposed viable tissue and the area is rinsed with generous amounts of water or saline.

Burn wounds are generally treated using either the open method or the closed method. In the *open method*, (used almost exclusively for the management of facial burns), the wound remains exposed. A thin layer (2–4 mm) of topical antimicrobial ointment may be applied over the wound surface. The exposure results in drying and the formation of a protective coagulum of serum. A cradle is used over the patient to support a sterile sheet and blanket to reduce body heat loss. If infection develops under the coagulum, it is removed and baths and topical antimicrobials used.

With the *closed method*, a dressing may be left intact for 1–7 days. The burned areas may be covered with a topical antimicrobial preparation and non-adherent dressing. The topical applications commonly used include silver sulfadiazine (Flamazine) or povidone-iodine (Betadine). The dressing must be thick enough to absorb fully normal wound exudate (which can be copious), without 'strike through'. In other words, the outside of the dressing must be dry, therefore providing an effective barrier to microorganisms.

The choice and frequency of dressing varies among institutions, and also according to the condition of the burn wound. Flexibility with the wound management approach is very important in burn care (Box 25.9).

If a patient has a circumferential burn on a limb, close observations are made for signs of interference with the circulation or nerve supply, as a result of the constricting effect of the dry, shrinking eschar. If signs of constriction

Box 25.9 Objectives for wound management

- Prevention of conversion to full-thickness burn due to infection or desiccation
- Removal of devitalized tissue
- Preparation of healthy granulation tissue
- Minimization of systemic infection
- Completion of the autograft process
- Limitation of scarring and contracture.

appear, the eschar is surgically divided immediately under aseptic conditions (escharotomy). If the wound is deep enough, fasciotomies may also be performed.

Choice of dressings used will be dependent upon assessment of the burn and a multidisciplinary protocol that should highlight wound management materials to be considered including the rationale for their use. Considerations should include those that promote a moist wound healing environment, optimize the patient's healing potential, alleviate pain, enhance debridement, permit immobilization or mobilization (as desired at the time), preserve function and provide the patient with the least amount of psychological stress.

In a partial-thickness burn, healing (i.e. re-epithelialization) occurs under the coagulum, which gradually separates. When a full-thickness burn is sustained, the non-viable tissue changes in 3–5 days to a hard, tough black layer (eschar). The eschar eventually sloughs off, liquefies and detaches from the viable tissue. There may be considerable drainage before there is complete separation. The wound will not granulate until the eschar has been sloughed off, so treatment in wound care is directed towards the promotion of this process. Alternatively, the wound may be debrided surgically. As the eschar is removed granulation tissue consisting of fibroblasts and capillaries is gradually formed. If the granulation tissue is allowed to mature to fibrous scar tissue, the natural shortening of the collagenous fibres results in contracture of the area and possible deformity or loss of function, depending upon the location. Some marginal growth of epithelium may take place but, unless the burn is very small, this is usually insignificant.

Wounds that are full thickness in nature do not have the capacity for self-healing. These patients have their wounds surgically excised and *skin grafts* placed to provide permanent coverage. The patient's general condition and the size of the burn area determine whether the grafting will require several stages. Priority is given to areas where scarring and contraction produce loss of movement and marked deformity. The grafts may be laid or sutured or stapled, depending on their thickness. They are dressed with a pressure dressing or may be left exposed. If the grafts are around or over a joint surface, a splint or plaster cast may be applied to immobilize the part.

Split-thickness grafts may also be applied to deep partial-thickness burns as they produce a much better scar with improved wear and tear tolerance.

The only graft that is permanent is the *autograft*. As the name implies, the skin is taken from an unburned part of the patient's body (the *donor site*) and placed over the debrided granulation tissue. No tissue rejection is experienced but 100% graft take is not guaranteed with every procedure. If there are not sufficient donor sites available, a temporary skin covering may be used.

Temporary synthetic dressings are available when it is necessary to gain time for the patient awaiting further grafting. Such products include Tegaderm and OpSite.

Donor sites are usually covered with a protective inner dressing at operation. After one to several days following surgery, depending on the unit protocol, the outer dressings are removed and the wound redressed once daily. Great care must be taken with donor sites because they increase the open body surface area and put the patient at greater risk of infection. The donor sites can be re-harvested in about 10 days, once they have healed, providing the patient with the opportunity to have several grafts taken from the same place. Donor sites can be very painful wounds.

Patient teaching related to skin grafts

The nurse who is involved in all stages of wound healing plays a very important role with respect to patient and family teaching and support around this crucial aspect of burn care, as do other members of the multidisciplinary team. When the patient learns that skin grafts are needed, he or she may become apprehensive or have unrealistic expectations regarding graft 'take' and the final appearance. Initially the nurse may re-emphasize what the surgeon tells the patient, with the physiotherapist and occupational therapist also discussing grafts. This support and teaching continue until the wound and scars have fully matured, which may take several years.

Positioning and exercises

The patient is generally turned every 2–3 hours to prevent respiratory congestion and circulatory stasis. If the back is burned, care is facilitated if the patient is nursed on an alternating pressure, low air loss or air-fluidized patient support system, dependent upon the acceptance of the bed to the patient. Because of the oedema, burned extremities are elevated on pillows or other form of support during the initial phase. Frequent attention is paid to body alignment; flexion contractures, outward rotation of thighs and foot-drop must be prevented.

Splints may be applied for immobilization to promote healing and to prevent contracture and deformity. The splint used must fit the contour of the part to which it is applied and be secured well enough to provide stability but not cause pressure or interfere with circulation.

Burned parts that involve joints are moved through their range of motion as soon as possible. Early skin grafting permits the patient to be mobile earlier and prevents contractures. The patient in a bath is encouraged to exercise while soaking. As healing occurs, the activity programme is progressively increased to preserve normal range of motion and function.

Nutrition

In addition to fluid therapy, nutrition plays an important role in the recovery of the burned patient. In the initial shock period in severe burns, intravenous fluids mainly sustain the patient. Intravenous fluids such as dextrose are given as the initial hypovolaemic shock produces depression of gastric motility. Once oral fluid intake can be resumed, it is progressively increased through soft foods, to a full normal diet.

The patient develops a negative nitrogen balance as a result of tissue catabolism which increases susceptibility to infection and debilitation and delays healing. A high-calorie, high-protein and high-vitamin diet is recommended to provide the essentials for tissue repair and the production of antibodies and blood cells.

Supplements of protein concentrates may be added to fluids or given through a fine-bore nasogastric tube. Adequate assistance should be provided so that taking meals does not require too great an effort for the patient. A close check is made of their daily intake and their weight should also be recorded regularly.

Evaluation

After the initial and intermediate periods of care following a severe burn injury, the criteria outlined in Boxes 25.8 and 25.9 may be used to evaluate care. During this intermediate period of care, the nurse assumes both independent and collaborative responsibilities for the assessment and management of the patient's wounds, for the identification of patient and family concerns and anxieties, and for teaching the patient and family about the wound and overall plan of care.

REHABILITATION AND REVIEW PHASES

Rehabilitation of the burned patient is fostered throughout by means of positive communication with the patient and their family, in order to prepare them for the resumption of their lives, and through the earlier stages by conscientious attention to good body alignment, the prevention of infection and contractures, and the maintenance of joint and limb mobility as much as possible. After recovery from the burn, considerable reconstructive surgery may be required before the patient can resume independent and self-supportive functioning. Rehabilitation is a lengthy process for many, and they and their families may require social guidance and financial assistance as well as psychological support throughout. Retraining for a different occupation may be necessary. In some instances, the patient finds it very difficult to resume social contacts and to take his or her place in society because of scarring and gross disfigurement.

Patient goals

1 To achieve maximum function and optimal reconstruction
2 To achieve an acceptable quality of life.

The achievement of these goals may be measured by the criteria outlined in Box 25.10.

Nursing intervention

Skin and tissue integrity

Healed burns must be kept well moisturized because the sebaceous glands are unable to secrete sufficient lubricating oils. Frequent applications of mild, non-perfumed, water-based moisturizers are recommended; oil-based lotions may block pores and do not penetrate into the dermis. When out in the sun, the patient must be reminded to wear sunblock and clothing protection to prevent sunburn and hyperpigmentation.

All wounds heal by the process of contraction. Burn patients must be made aware of the possibility that the splints and other corrective devices they may have been utilizing since the day of admission (in essence, day 1 is when rehabilitation begins) may not bring about a miraculous or 'good as new' result. Further corrective surgery may be needed to release the contracture and insert a skin graft.

Hypertrophic scarring is another result of healing from a burn injury. Some individuals have a greater propensity for scarring than others. The burns team may frequently be unable to give definite answers regarding the need or duration of use of pressure garments or devices for pressure therapy. Counselling should also include information on skin care and cosmetic camouflage. Further surgery may be necessary for these patients, but in the future – for it takes approximately 2 years for the burn scar to mature fully. It is important that, when counselling patients with burns, the

---

> **Box 25.10** Criteria for evaluation of care during rehabilitative and review phases
>
> - Absence of infection
>
> - Intact skin
>
> - Range of movement exercises and functional movement in involved joints
>
> - A plan to continue the prescribed exercise programme
>
> - A diet plan to obtain adequate protein, vitamins, minerals and calories
>
> - Understanding of prescribed skin care routine
>
> - Independence in personal care
>
> - Return to social activities
>
> - Return to employment or plans for job retraining
>
> - Plans for continuing health care.

nurse emphasizes that these timeframes are estimates and that every patient responds to therapy in a unique manner.

Cooperation with positioning and exercises may be a difficult challenge for the burn survivor. Patient education and support from burns team members can be very helpful in meeting these challenges in a positive manner. In addition, the patient is encouraged to undertake more responsibility for self-care. The occupational therapist and nursing staff need to encourage the patient to perform self-care activities, such as personal hygiene, dressing and participating in recreational activities. In order not to lose valuable function, rehabilitation activities must be attended to with much energy by all concerned.

Changes in coping mechanisms

As the burned individual prepares to leave the protective environment of the burns unit, numerous feelings may be experienced. The nursing staff, who have formed a unique and trusting bond with surviving patients and families, should be sensitive to and encourage the need for the patient to verbalize concerns and questions. The burned person may experience feelings of uncertainty, fear and anxiety about what lies ahead. This is linked to decreased confidence due to lengthy dependence on hospital staff, impaired physical mobility and concerns relating to the return to society, potentially with an altered body image and decreased sense of self-esteem. Nervousness about returning home after a prolonged absence and concerns about resumption of previous roles and responsibilities may also be experienced.

It is important to make the person aware that these concerns are very normal for the burn survivor at the same stage of recovery. Knowing that one is not alone can be very comforting. Introduction to previously discharged patients and members of a burns support group, if available, can be a helpful pre-discharge strategy.

Family members generally experience anxiety because they are now assuming the caretaker role once held by burns team members. They may have many questions about their loved one's physical care and emotional readjustment. They may express concerns about how to support the burned individual emotionally as he or she adjusts to being at home, re-enters society and begins to socialize with friends and be seen in the community by strangers and contemplates what the future may bring. Families may have concerns about their own reactions to the burn survivor and should receive support and advice in this regard. Both the patient and family members will experience challenges upon the return home. Coping strategies must either be developed or previous positive strategies reinforced and applied to this particular situation.

A comprehensive discharge teaching programme should begin as soon as possible before discharge. Important topics to discuss include skin care, emotional reactions to returning home, adjusting to alterations in appearance and mobility, coping with discomfort (itchiness and pain), nutrition, rehabilitation needs, family readjustment, and continuity of care (i.e. home care, burns clinic and rehabilitation depart-

ment visits). The information conveyed and the opportunity to talk with nursing staff and other burns team members are both valuable means to support individual and family coping.

Both the individual and the family need to know that nursing staff are anxious to provide support, answer questions, assist in problem solving and conflict resolution, and offer a reassuring pat on the back for the courage and perseverance displayed during a very traumatic time. This supportive and informative presence can do much to assist in the individual's efforts at reaching the optimal level of physical and emotional recovery.

Evaluation

In recent years, a better understanding and delivery of nutritional support, anaesthesia, the provision of enhanced intensive care facilities and skin replacements have all contributed to improved outcomes for patients who suffer from burns injuries, whether major or minor. None-the-less, the importance of evidence-based nursing interventions cannot be stressed enough. Burns nursing is one of the few specialties where practitioners have the opportunity to nurse a patient from the critical stage of their hospital admission, through the continuing care and rehabilitation phases of management up until the patient's discharge home to the care of the primary care team.

As a general rule, all burns patients with complex injuries should be immediately referred to a local Burn Centre or Unit whereas non complex injuries may be dealt with on an outpatient basis by the local A&E department or by the primary care team with the use of appropriate wound management materials. 'In the opinion of the National Burn Care Review Committee and the British Burn Association, there is no justification for injuries requiring hospital admission to be dealt with outside this system' (Pape et al 2001).

Box 25.10 contains the key criteria that may be used to evaluate care in this final phase of treatment.

CASE **Burns**

> On your day off duty, as normal, you go to collect your 6-year-old child from primary school in the local village. On arrival, you are met by the school secretary who is extremely anxious and she asks you to come quickly to her office as apparently there has been an accident involving boiling water from her kettle. As you both move quickly towards the school office, the secretary confirms that the boiling water has been spilled over the chest of an 8-year-old female pupil who was in her office awaiting the anticipated later arrival of her father. He had telephoned the school to report that he was held up in traffic, but expected to be able to collect his daughter at around 4 o'clock.

Reflective questions

- List your initial actions on meeting the injured pupil and highlight your rationale for all items identified on your list
- Describe your anticipated actions when the injured girl's father arrives to collect his daughter.

SUMMARY

This chapter discusses the important role that the skin plays in maintaining overall health and well-being. The skin fulfils a multitude of functions, many of which we are un-aware of until something threatens to alter or impair its integrity. The consequences of an insult to the skin's integrity may be relatively minor, or may be devastating and life threatening. The person with impairment of skin integrity must cope with changes in self-image as well as with minor or major disruptions to physiological functioning.

The nurse plays a key role in the prevention, assessment, planning, administration and evaluation of care strategies to manage potential and actual impairment of skin integrity. Patient and family education is a vital function of the nurse as a primary caregiver and one of those closest to the individual and family.

The care of persons with impaired skin integrity can be challenging and calls upon many facets of the nursing role. The nurse must be knowledgeable about the structure and function of the skin, measures to maintain skin integrity and promote healing and tissue repair, and the impact of changes in body image on the individual and family.

Remember prevention is better than cure – use your opportunities to discuss your patient's skin even if they do not have a skin condition, it is never too late.

REFERENCES

Black J, Hawks J (2005) Medical–surgical nursing. Toronto: Elsevier/Saunders.

BNF (2006) British National Formulary, No. 51. London: BMA and RPSGB.

Collier M (1999a) Fundamental concepts in mattresses and beds. Resource File, Part 1. London: EMAP, p 1–8.

Collier M (1999b) Pressure ulcer prevention and principles for prevention. In: Glover D, Miller M, eds. Wound management: theory and practice. London: EMAP Healthcare Ltd.

Collier M (2002) A ten point assessment plan for wound management. Journal of Community Nursing 16(6): 22–26.

Collier M (2003) Wound care: MIMS for nurses pocket guide. London: Haymarket Medical Imprint.

Collier M (2004) Effective prevention requires accurate risk assessment In: Glover D, Bagshaw S, eds. Pressure ulcer prevention: A guide to product selection. Journal of Wound Care. May(Suppl): 3–7.

Defloor T, Schoonhoven L, Clark M, Halfrens R, Nixon J (2001) Pressure ulcer risk assessment: A draft EPUAP Position Statement. EPUAP Review 3(2): 46–52.

Department of Health (DoH) (2001) The essence of care: patient focused benchmarking for health care practitioners. London: HMSO.

Department of Health (DoH) (2003) Essence of Care. London: DoH.

Fowler A (1999) Burns. In: Glover D, Miller M, eds. Wound management: theory and practice. London: EMAP Healthcare Ltd. p 48–60.

Franks P (2001) Health economics: the cost to nations. In: Morison M, ed. The prevention and treatment of pressure ulcers. Edinburgh: Mosby.

Grey J, Harding K, Enoch S (2006) Pressure ulcers. British Medical Journal 332: 472–475.

Haslett C, Chilvers E, Boon N, Colledge N (2002) Davidson's Principles and Practice of Medicine, 19th edn. Edinburgh: Churchill Livingstone.

Hughes E, Van Onselen J (eds.) (2001) Dermatology nursing: A practical guide. London: Harcourt Publishers Ltd.

Jones V, Milton T (2000a) When and how to use alginates. NT Plus – wound care. Nursing Times 96(Suppl): 2–3.

Jones V, Milton T (2000b) When and how to use adhesive film membranes. NT Plus – wound care. Nursing Times 96(Suppl): 3–4.

Jones V, Milton T (2000c) When and how to use foam dressings. NT Plus – wound care. Nursing Times 96(Suppl): 2–3.

Jones V, Milton T (2000d) When and how to use hydrogels. NT Plus – wound care. Nursing Times 96(Suppl): 3–4.

Jones V, Milton T (2000e) When and how to use hydrocolloid dressings. NT Plus – wound care. Nursing Times 96(Suppl): 5–7.

Jones V, Milton T (2000f) When and how to use iodine dressings. NT Plus – wound care. Nursing Times 96(Suppl): 2–3.

Kenney L, Rithalia S (1999) Technical aspects of support surfaces in mattresses and beds. Resource File, Part 2. London: EMAP, p 1–8.

McGowan S, Montgomery K, Jolley D et al (2000) The role of sheepskins in preventing pressure ulcers in elderly orthopaedic patients. Primary Intention November: 127–134.

McLaren S, Green S (2001) Nutritional factors in the aetiology, development and healing of pressure ulcers. In: Morison M, ed. The prevention and treatment of pressure ulcers. Edinburgh: Mosby. p 195–215.

National Institute for Clinical Excellence (NICE) (2003) The use of pressure relieving devices for pressure ulcer prevention in primary and secondary care. London: NICE.

National Institute for Clinical Excellence (NICE) (2004) Atopic dermatitis (eczema) – pimecrolimus and tacrolimus. Online. Available: http://www.nice.org.uk/ page.aspx?o=217941 [Accessed 31.03.2006].

Norton D, McLaren R, Exton-Smith (1962) An investigation of geriatric nursing problems in hospital. Edinburgh: Churchill Livingstone.

Nowak T, Handford G (2004) Pathophysiology: concepts and applications for health care professionals, 3rd edn. Boston: McGraw Hill.

Pape S, Judkins K, Settle J (2001) Burns: the first five days, 2nd edn. International Edition. Hull: Smith and Nephew.

Penzer R (2002) Nursing care of the skin. Oxford: Butterworth Heinemann.

Savage P, Crosby T, Mason M (2004) Malignant melanoma. Clinical evidence; 12. London: BMJ Books.

Walsh M, Kent A (2001) A&E nursing, 4th edn. Oxford: Heinemann.

Walsh M (2006) Nurse practitioners; clinical skills and professional issues, 2nd edn. Oxford: Butterworth Heinemann.

Waterlow J (2005) Pressure ulcer prevention manual – revised. Online. Available: www.judywaterlow.co.uk

FURTHER READING AND USEFUL WEBSITES

Collier M (2003) Wound care: MIMS for nurses pocket guide. London: Haymarket Medical Imprint.

A comprehensive booklet designed primarily for the practitioner in the primary care setting to support them when dealing with all wound types, including the management of patients with pressure ulcers and minor burns. Sections included: Most common wound types; Normal wound healing and the role of growth factors in the process; Wound assessment and aims for care; How to identify if a wound is infected; Wound management materials and how to use them.

Glover D, Bagshaw S (eds.) (2004) Pressure ulcer prevention: a guide to product selection. Journal of Wound Care May(Suppl.): 3–7.

A useful supplement aimed jointly at the readers of the Journal of Wound Care and Therapy weekly initially, that explores the role of a number of members of the multidisciplinary team – such as Occupational and Physiotherapists – in selecting appropriate equipment to be used primarily for the prevention of pressure ulcers. Specialist patient support surfaces covered include both mattresses and cushions. Sections include: Causes, physiology and assessment of patients at risk of pressure ulceration; Seating – assessment and selection; Choosing the mattress or overlay and Practical, clinical and financial considerations for the selection of the same.

Fowler A (1999) Burns. In: Glover D, Miller M, eds. Wound management: theory and practice. London: EMAP, Ch. 5. p 48–60.

A chapter within an excellent introductory text covering a number of important tissue viability issues. This chapter looks at the assessment and management of patients with burn injuries, both major and minor, and highlights the importance of correct burn assessment, classification and patient management within a holistic care framework.

Hughes E, Van Onselen J (eds.) (2001) Dermatology nursing: a practical guide. London: Harcourt.

A comprehensive overview of this specialist subject area that includes both general principles and information about more specific dermatological conditions.

Morison M (ed.) (2001) The prevention and treatment of pressure ulcers. Edinburgh: Mosby.

An invaluable reference source for all practitioners and other professionals allied to medicine who care for patients at risk of developing pressure ulcers. Written by a team of internationally acknowledged experts, each chapter contains self-assessment questions and activities, and to conclude there is a section containing advanced case studies that allow the reader to reflect on the many complex issues.

NICE (2003) The use of pressure relieving devices for pressure ulcer prevention in primary and secondary care. London: NICE.

The result of extensive work commissioned by NICE, involving the National Collaborating Centre for Nursing and Supportive Care along with a number of key clinical representatives of the multidisciplinary team involved with pressure ulcer prevention, to establish the most clinically and cost effective beds, mattresses and overlays for preventing pressure ulcers. Recommendations for good practice based on the best available evidence of clinical and cost effectiveness are presented for consideration.

Pape S, Judkins K, Settle J (2001) Burns: the first five days, 2nd edn. International Edition. Hull: Smith and Nephew.

An excellent, easily accessible, reference document that covers the management of patients with burns during the initial stages of their management – the first five days. Incorporates and number of very clear and useful flow charts and tables that outline principles for the management of both complex and non-complex burn injuries. Phases of intervention included are at the scene and in the burn unit. Clinical considerations covered include the management of burn shock; principles of resuscitation; the burn wound; inhalation injuries; renal problems; nutrition and principles of care after the first five days.

Royal College of Nursing (2001) Risk assessment and prevention of pressure ulcers. London: RCN.

This technical report and appendices produced by the Royal College of Nursing form the basis of the clinical guideline on pressure ulcer risk assessment and prevention circulated by the National Institute for Clinical Excellence (NICE) in April 2001. There are a number of recommendations highlighted within the document, with the strength of evidence that supports each identified from a continuum. A number of important references are highlighted which cover the vast range of issues related to the prevention of pressure ulcer development.

USEFUL WEBSITES

British Association of Plastic, Reconstructive and Aesthetic Surgeons	www.bapras.co.uk
Burn Survivors Online	www.burnsurvivorsonline.com
National Eczema Society	www.eczema.org
European Pressure Ulcer Advisory Panel	www.epuap.org
Tissue Viability Society	www.tvs.org.uk
Tissue Viability Nurses Association	www.tvna.org
Wound Care Society	www.woundcaresociety.org

26 Caring for the patient with substance misuse or self-harm issues

Mike Walsh

INTRODUCTION

The ever-increasing health, social and economic costs related to drinking alcohol, smoking tobacco and the use of illicit drugs have become a major public health concern. They are important contributing factors in most areas of medical and mental health problems. Indeed, substance misuse remains the largest cause of preventable morbidity and mortality in the UK, and targeted intervention is required to reduce the high costs. Although specialist drug and alcohol services are established to work with substance misusers, it would be both unrealistic and inappropriate to expect them to respond alone to the challenge of prevention and health promotion in this field.

SCALE OF THE PROBLEM

The harm associated with the misuse of alcohol constitutes a major public health problem in both developed and developing countries. The WHO estimates there are 76 million people worldwide with alcohol use disorders. One-quarter of deaths in men aged 15–29 in Europe are due to alcohol (Sargent 2005). To localize the problem further, the Cabinet Office estimates that alcohol abuse costs the UK £1.7 bn/year (Strategy Unit 2004). Finally, in England, we see 27% of men and 17% of women drinking more than the recommended safe maximum weekly amount of alcohol while an extensive survey found that 25% of schoolchildren aged 11–15 had drunk alcohol in the previous week (Department

of Health 2005). According to WHO estimates, there are more than 1 billion smokers in the world – about one-third of the global adult population. Smoking is currently estimated to kill 4.9 million people annually and on current trends this is set to increase to 10 million by the 2020s; 70% of the deaths occurring in developing countries. Smoking is therefore adding considerably to the disease burden of the poorest countries in the world (WHO 2005).

Reliable estimates of the extent and prevalence of illicit drug consumption are difficult to obtain, because users of these substances are unlikely to report on an illegal activity or give truthful responses for fear of reprisals. Despite these difficulties, it is estimated that approximately 15 million people worldwide incur a significant risk to their health as a result of using psychoactive substances. It is further estimated that one-third of these users inject drugs, and many believe this figure to be an underestimate. There are 136 countries in the world who report intravenous drug use as a problem and 93 of them also report the presence of HIV/AIDS (WHO 2005).

Within the UK, the National Treatment Agency for Substance Misuse (NTA) estimates that there were approximately 141 000 problem drug misusers in England alone. This figure represents a 10% increase on the previous year (NTA 2005). The percentage of people who successfully completed treatment or who were retained in treatment at the end of 2002/03 fell from 59% in 2001/02 to 57% in 2002/03. Of the 85 200 who left treatment in 2002/03 the proportion deemed to have successfully completed treatment was only 29%. If one of the wealthiest countries in the world with an advanced healthcare system is struggling to treat half of its problem drug users, this suggests two things:

1 They are a very difficult group to work with due to multiple interacting personal problems and the social context within which they are located.
2 In many other less well-developed parts of the world, drug misuse poses a major threat to the well-being and health of large numbers of people.

When considering the resourcing of drug treatment services it is worth noting that the WHO estimate that for every US$1 spent on drug treatment, US$7 are saved in long-term health and social costs.

SCOPE AND REMIT OF THIS CHAPTER

In this chapter, we will attempt to outline the descriptions, effects and possible interventions associated with a range of commonly misused substances. We will also go on to look at deliberate self-harm and suicide which are often linked to the use of such substances.

DEFINITIONS AND DESCRIPTIONS OF TERMINOLOGY

Substance use. This is used to denote both use and misuse (experimental, recreational, dependent and problematic use). It is a catch-all term that describes the use of substances – drug, alcohol or other – to alter an individual's psychological state.
Problematic use. This is generally accepted to include physical, social, psychological and/or legal problems related to intoxication, excessive consumption or dependence resulting from use of substances.
Drug abuse or misuse. This describes the use of any drug, whether legal or illegal, for a medical or recreational purpose when other alternatives are available, practical or warranted, or when drug use endangers either the user or others with whom he or she may interact. The concept of drug abuse can be viewed as a social construct. The acceptability of using a drug may change in any given society at any given time and will generally be context driven. An example of this could be the growing public acceptance of the use of cannabis as an analgesic in chronic conditions such as cancer, where cannabis is increasingly viewed as an acceptable alternative to prescribed pain relief despite its illegality. However, members of the public still generally view users of cannabis for recreational purposes with suspicion. In this case, the concept of illegality is pushed to the fore, thus denoting cannabis use within the recreational domain as abuse or misuse.

DRUG DEPENDENCE

According to Bennet and Brown (2003) this term refers to:

... a state arising from repeated, periodic or continuous administration of a drug, that results in harm to the individual and sometimes to society. The subject feels a desire, need or compulsion to continue using the drug and feels ill if abruptly deprived of it (abstinence or withdrawal syndrome)

(Bennet and Brown 2003, p.168).

These authors go on to state that dependence is characterized by an initial psychological dependence then physical dependence may develop in some cases. Dependence is also characterized by tolerance.

Psychological dependence. This is more common than physical dependency and may occur with any type of drug. People may use the drug experience as a way of coping with their world, or as a way of maintaining feelings of well-being. The individual will feel that they cannot cope without drugs, although they may not be physically dependent. Individuals can be psychologically dependent on almost anything, such as chocolate or gambling.
Physical dependence. This results from the extended use of drugs such as tranquillizers, heroin and alcohol (i.e. drugs that alter body chemistry). When experiencing physical dependency the individual will require repeated doses of the drug to maintain normal function. Ceasing to use the drug results in symptoms of physical withdrawal.
Tolerance. As an individual takes more of a substance, the body adapts to tolerate increased amounts. More of the drug is needed to sustain the desired effect, i.e. the body has a progressively decreasing responsiveness to the drug.
Cross-tolerance. In this condition, tolerance to one drug results in a lessened response to another drug.
Withdrawal symptoms. These are the symptoms that can result from stopping long-term use of certain drugs, notably opiates such as heroin, benzodiazepines such as diazepam, and also alcohol. Physical effects may include shaking and flu-like symptoms, and will depend on the drug being withdrawn. Examples of the effects of withdrawal from nicotine are irritability, frustration, anger, difficulty concentrating, restlessness, decreased heart rate, and increased appetite or weight gain. Withdrawal from the moderate use of alcohol can cause cravings, irritability and frustration. Withdrawal from high levels of alcohol use may result in *delirium tremens*. This syndrome incorporates tremors with hallucinations, psychomotor agitation, confusion and disorientation, sleep disorders and other associated discomforts, and lasts for several days after alcohol withdrawal.

ADDICTION

This is a non-scientific term which is widely used in general discussion. A simple definition is:

A global pattern in which the person's substance use (and in this case abuse) dominates the person's life

(McDowel and Spitz, 1999 p.4)

Authors such as Bennet and Brown (2003) consider addiction as a situation where dependence has become so severe that compulsive craving dominates the person's everyday life. The term dependence is increasingly preferred as it gets around the rather unhelpful argument of whether a substance is 'addictive' or habit forming. Older definitions of addiction such as that by Donovan and Marlatt (1988) stressed craving as a feature together with withdrawal discomfort when the substance is removed, increasing demands for the substance to achieve the same effect and a tendency to easily go back to the substance after a period of abstinence.

A BIOPSYCHOSOCIAL EXPLANATION FOR SUBSTANCE MISUSE

Many patients that the nurse encounters, whether in primary care or hospital will have significant health problems as a result of drug use, whether they are legal or illegal drugs. In order to practice holistic care we therefore need to understand something of the reasons that underpin this unhealthy behaviour. A number of different theories have been formulated over time to attempt to explain why people abuse drugs and alcohol; these fall broadly into four main categories: moral, biological, psychological and social.

Moral

Moral theories tend to focus on the individual, who is viewed as weak or having a poor character. Interventions associated with moral theories focus the responsibility for change on the individual, and treatment emphasizes deterrence and punishment. An example of a moral intervention would be the incarceration of a drug user for possession of their drug of choice with the hope that they would come to the realization that drug use is bad and leads to negative consequences.

Biological

Biological theories incorporate disease models of substance misuse and genetics. Substance misuse is sometimes also viewed as a primary mental disorder. Treatment is focused around abstinence to halt progression of the disease. Biological approaches tend to remove the focus from the individual's power and responsibility to change, laying the responsibility firmly on medically based interventions. Treatment will vary but may be targeted initially with prescribed medication to break the cycle of drug use, with the overarching principle that once the individual reaches abstinence from their drug of choice medical interventions can be discontinued. An example of a biologically based intervention would be the substitute prescribing of methadone to treat heroin dependence.

Psychological

A readily applied psychological theory of substance misuse is social learning theory. Substance misuse is viewed as a learned behavioural disorder. Interventions associated with psychological explanations focus on the individual's ability to learn more adaptive behaviour as an alternative to substance misuse. This may involve learning new behaviours or substituting known behaviours in place of the substance. An example of this approach might be an individual who drinks to relieve feelings of stress or anxiety, i.e. the function of the drinking is to relax rather than enjoyment of the alcohol per se. The individual may benefit from attending a stress management course focusing on relaxation techniques – the relaxation techniques being an ultimately less damaging coping strategy for stress management than alcohol use.

Social

Social theories view substance misuse as a means for the individual to cope with their environment and social situation. Interventions therefore focus on helping the individual improve their social functioning either by modifying the way they engage with their environment or by changing the environment itself. An example of this approach might be the individual who uses amphetamines on a regular basis when going to the pub. A social approach would focus on why the drug use occurs in that particular environment and look at ways of modifying it. Is it that amphetamine use only happens in the pub; if so, change the meeting place (i.e. modify the environment). Or is it that the dealer frequents that pub, so access to amphetamines is more readily available; thus treatment might be focused towards teaching the individual effective refusal skills (i.e. modifying the way the individual engages with the environment).

Rather than focus on one particular theory as an explanation, clinically it is generally more relevant to combine the different theories according to the individual's expressed need. Thus, substance misuse problems are viewed not merely as a function of the person's self, but as the result of a complex interaction between biological, psychological and social dimensions. The reasons why any individual uses substances will be unique to that individual, and it is important when trying to help the person that a full understanding of the biopsychosocial dimensions is reached before treatment is planned. A number of examples of precipitating and maintaining factors of substance misuse are:

- curiosity
- rites of passage
- pleasure
- experimentation
- relief of underlying distress
- self-adventure
- spiritual meaning or loss of faith
- immediate satisfaction.

ALCOHOL

Alcohol is rapidly absorbed as it is highly lipid soluble and readily diffuses from the stomach and small intestine into the blood stream. Food in the stomach will delay absorption. We metabolize 95% of the alcohol we ingest and excrete the remaining 5% in breath, urine and sweat. The liver is the site of alcohol metabolism, mainly by the enzyme alcohol dehydrogenase. Alcohol has its effect mainly on the central nervous system (being lipid soluble it readily crosses the blood–brain barrier) where it acts as a depressant. Mood changes, excitability or aggressive behaviour are due to the depression of normal inhibitory mechanisms. Eventually in very high doses coma ensues (Bennet and Brown 2003).

Most expert opinion is of the view that alcohol becomes hazardous when consumed by men at a rate of over 21 units per week and women at a rate of over 14 units per week (Haslett et al 2002). Alcohol is also felt to be less harmful if consumed in modest quantities on a regular basis rather than all the units being drunk on one or two nights in the week ('binge drinking').

In order to calculate the patient's alcohol intake as units of alcohol, it is necessary to know the strength the drink that has been consumed as well as the volume. The following will therefore assist:

One unit of alcohol is equal to:

- half a pint of ordinary beer, lager or cider (3.5% ABV)
- one small glass of wine (9% ABV)
- one single pub measure of spirit (40% ABV).

To further assist in patient assessment, note that the number of units in any drink can be calculated by multiplying the volume (in ml) by the %ABV (alcohol by volume) and dividing this by 1000.

The Office of National Statistics Health Survey also outlined that, at any one time, the drinking levels of the adult population of England are approximately as shown in. Of the 8 million or so people exceeding the sensible limits, around 1 700 000 are drinking at 'definitely harmful' levels of more than 50 units per week for men and more than 35 units per week for women. On the basis of the main surveys conducted for the government during the 1990s, at any one time there are probably around 2 million people in the UK experiencing symptoms of alcohol dependence, the male:female ratio being around 3:1 (Institute of Alcohol Studies 1997–2000).

EFFECTS ON HEALTH AND SOCIAL WELL-BEING

Some headline facts compiled by the Institute for Alcohol Studies (2005a) about the impact of alcohol on the British NHS are worth considering:

- 1 in 16 of all hospital admissions are alcohol related
- 35% of A&E attendances and ambulance calls are alcohol related
- between midnight and 5.00 a.m., 70% of A&E attendances are alcohol related while at the busiest periods of the day in A&E, 40% of all patients have a raised blood alcohol level and 13% are intoxicated
- one in five patients presenting in primary care are likely to be excessive drinkers
- problem drinkers consult their GP twice as often as average patients.

In addition, over 60% of cases of chronic pancreatitis are alcohol related, over one-quarter of all assaults and suicides, one-third of all drownings and 40% of fire injuries are alcohol related.

There are three components of drinking behaviour associated with medical and/or social problems: intoxication, regular heavy consumption and alcohol dependence (alcoholism). Examples of such problems are:

1 intoxication:
   a) drunken driving
   b) alcohol poisoning
   c) accidents
   d) violence.
2 regular heavy consumption:
   a) health problems
   b) financial problems
   c) family difficulties
   d) absenteeism from work.
3 alcohol dependence:
   a) psychological problems
   b) health problems
   c) family difficulties
   d) problems of withdrawal.

Alcohol-related problems are often believed to occur predominantly among 'alcoholics' and problem drinkers. Whilst they do experience some of the most severe problems, in terms of the total impact on society as a whole, it appears that most of the problems are contributed or experienced by regular heavy drinkers who are not and may never become 'alcoholics', combined with the results of intoxication experienced by a wide range of drinkers. This paradox occurs because there are so many more of them in the population, collectively contributing the larger share of the total amount of harm, especially in relation to the social problems related to alcohol consumption. Table 26.1 summarizes the medical complications of excess alcohol.

Alcohol is generally found to be a significant factor in:

- hospital admissions
- road traffic deaths
- industrial accidents
- accidental drowning
- homicide
- suicide
- domestic violence
- marital breakdown
- absenteeism from work
- child abuse.

See Case Study 26.1.

CASE Derek is a 38-year-old man who was placed in prison on remand 2 days ago. When he awoke this morning he was shaking, soaked in sweat and vomited shortly afterwards. He was reported as being very agitated and disturbed and had a 'fit' in front of two prison warders whose description matches

Table 26.1 Medical complications of excess alcohol

System or organ	Clinical findings

Nervous system	Acute intoxication
	    Blackouts
	Persistent brain damage
	    Wernicke's encephalopathy
	    Korsakoff's syndrome
	    Cerebellar degeneration
	    Dementia
	Cerebrovascular disease
	    Strokes, especially in the young
	    Subarachnoid haemorrhage
	    Subdural hematoma after head injury
	Withdrawal symptoms
	    Tremor
	    Hallucinations
	    Fits
	Nerve and muscle damage
	    Weakness
	    Paralysis
	    Burning sensation in hands and feet

Liver	Infiltration of liver with fat Alcoholic hepatitis Cirrhosis and eventual liver failure Liver cancer
Gastrointestinal system	Reflux of acid into oesophagus Tearing and occasional rupture of oesophagus Cancer of oesophagus Gastritis Aggravation and impaired healing of peptic ulcers, diarrhoea and impaired absorption of food Chronic inflammation of the pancreas leading in some to diabetes and malabsorption of food
Nutrition	Malnutrition from reduced intake of food, toxic effects of alcohol on intestine, and impaired metabolism, leading to weight loss Obesity, particularly in early stages of heavy drinking
Heart and circulatory system	Abnormal rhythms High blood pressure Chronic heart muscle damage leading to heart failure
Respiratory system	Fractured rib due to trauma Pneumonia from inhalation of vomit Overproduction of cortisol leading to obesity, acne, increased facial hair and high blood pressure Condition mimicking overactivity of the thyroid with loss of weight, anxiety, palpitations, sweating and tremor Severe fall in blood sugar level, sometimes leading to coma Intense facial flushing in many diabetics taking the antidiabetic drug chlorpropamide
Reproductive system	In men, loss of libido, reduced potency, shrinkage in size of testes and penis, reduced or absent sperm formation and so infertility In women, sexual difficulties, menstrual irregularities, and shrinkage of breasts and external genitalia
Occupation and accidents	Impaired work performance Increased risk and severity of accidents

continued

Table 26.1 *Cont'd*

System or organ	Clinical findings
Fetus, child and family	Damage to fetus and fetal alcohol syndrome
	Acute intoxication in young children produces hypothermia, low blood sugar levels, depressed respiration
	Effect on physical development and behaviour of child through heavy drinking by parents
	Interaction of alcohol with medicinal substances
	Increased likelihood of unwanted effects of drugs
	Reduced effectiveness of medicines

Institute of Alcohol Studies Factsheet; Alcohol and Health (2005a).

that of a tonic–clonic seizure. For the next 20 minutes he was confused and drowsy. When the paramedics arrived, they found him very agitated and frightened complaining of spiders and cockroaches running all over him and shouting about rats. They calmed him sufficiently to bring him to the A&E department with a prison escort. The escort confirms he has a lengthy history of alcohol problems and convictions for drunken driving.

On examination: VS. T 38.6, Pulse 128, RR 22, BP 170/105.

He is very distressed and anxious, overweight with evidence of poor dental hygiene. His skin looks well perfused, his face flushed, he is still sweating copiously and his fingers are heavily nicotine stained. Breathing sounds are normal despite rapid RR. A neurological assessment reveals he is over-alert, confused, disoriented in both space and time and he cannot complete the finger to nose test (see p. 667). He has exaggerated reflexes in all limbs.

This combination of fever and delirium with a history of a seizure suggests a serious illness affecting the central nervous system.

Although conditions such as encephalitis, meningitis, hypoglycaemia, sepsis and poisoning are just some of the conditions that can produce many of the features seen here; the history of heavy alcohol intake which was suddenly stopped 48 hours ago, does point towards alcohol withdrawal syndrome or delirium tremens.

Your care should include fixing cot sides, continual observation, cardiac monitor, 100% oxygen via face mask if tolerated, capillary blood glucose test, takes bloods for LFTs, biochemistry, blood cultures and establishing an i.v. line if the paramedics had not already done so. Medical management would involve the use of i.v. benzodiazepines which will suppress the withdrawal symptoms, and probably haloperidol to help deal with the hallucinations. Admission and close observation are essential as seizures and highly disturbing hallucinations are a major risk.

ALCOHOL AND THE FAMILY

In 1997, Alcohol Concern estimated that there are likely to be one million children in Britain living with a parent whose drinking has reached harmful levels (Institute of Alcohol Studies 1997–2000). A paper published by the Institute of Alcohol Studies (IAS) shows that the children of problem-drinking parents have high rates of health, behavioural and emotional problems such as truancy and poor school performance, antisocial behaviour and delinquency, difficulty in forming relationships, and psychiatric problems including depression. They are also at increased risk themselves of abusing alcohol or other drugs in later life (IAS 1997–2000).

ALCOHOL AND WOMEN

In recent decades, it seems that the gap between male and female alcohol consumption has narrowed. The problem is most alarming in young women, as 33% of women between 16 and 24 reported drinking above 14 units per week and if current trends continue they will be drinking three times as heavily as their counterparts in countries such as France and Italy, by 2009. More than one in 10 women aged 16–24 are actually drinking over 35 units per week. There is also a worrying tendency for young women to consume their weekly alcohol in one or two heavy weekend sessions, i.e. 'binge drinking' (IAS 2005b).

Higher than average rates of drinking in British women tends to occur most in the following groups:

● young women aged 16–24
● lone parents with children
● adult women living with one parent
● single women (including separated/divorced)
● students
● residents of urban rather than rural areas.

The IAS (2005b) paper goes on to highlight the fact that approximately 5% of women who drink are 'problem drinkers' meaning they experience problems of psychological or physical dependence. This translates into approximately 747 000 problem female drinkers in the UK (the male equivalent statistic is 1 443 000).

Many of the adverse effects of alcohol consumption are common to women and men, but some are more specific or acute for women:

● Social problems seem to be similar at any level of drinking
● Women suffer some physical problems at lower levels of drinking than men
● Women attain higher blood alcohol concentrations than men, even when allowing for differences in body weight. This is because women have a higher ratio of fat to water in their bodies. Alcohol is highly lipid soluble and with

relatively less water in their bodies, women are less able to dilute any given amount of alcohol down to lower blood concentrations

- Women are more prone to liver damage. They develop cirrhosis and hepatitis quicker than men and at lower levels of daily drinking than men
- Alcohol is a predisposing factor for breast cancer
- Some women report being more affected by alcohol when ovulating or when premenstrual because it takes longer for the alcohol to be metabolized
- Oral contraception delays the absorption of alcohol into the bloodstream, and some women take longer to become intoxicated on this count
- Moderate to heavy drinking may cause infertility, but some evidence suggests much lower levels than previously thought could adversely affect fertility (Jensen 1998)
- Alcohol consumption in pregnancy may result in damage to the fetus. Women who drink heavily during pregnancy also tend to be disadvantaged in other ways such as low income, poor diet, exposure to domestic violence and smoking. There is therefore a complex interplay of factors which are harmful to the fetus, of which alcohol is one
- Women may particularly become the victims of other people's drinking (e.g. domestic violence, sexual assault and rape).

Factors that predispose some women to develop problems in relation to alcohol include (IAS 2005b):

- family background of heavy drinking
- a history of sexual abuse
- low self-esteem
- traumatic life events
- association with eating disorders.

ALCOHOL AND YOUNG PEOPLE

It was not until the 1960s that pubs and drinking became an integral part of the youth scene. By the 1980s, those aged 18–24 years had become the heaviest drinkers in the population, and the group least likely to abstain. This change has been accompanied by a decline in the age of onset of regular drinking.

A survey of 15–16-year-olds found that UK teenagers came at or near the top of the international league for binge drinking, drunkenness and the experience of alcohol problems (IAS 1997–2000):

- 21% of UK teenagers reported individual problems from their own drinking (reduced performance at school)
- 22% reported relationship problems (quarrels or arguments)
- 15% reported sexual problems (unwanted sexual experience or unprotected sex)
- 12% reported delinquency problems (scuffles or fights).

ALCOHOL AND THE ELDERLY

Three types of elderly drinkers may be identified:

1 early onset or 'survivors' – a continuing problem that developed earlier in life
2 late onset or 'reactors' – often in response to traumatic life events
3 intermittent or binge drinkers.

People in categories 2 and 3 are thought to have a high chance of managing their alcohol problem if they have access to counselling and general support.

Ageing tends to be associated with a growing burden of disease, and prolonged heavy drinking is itself a cause of health problems such as liver disease, raised blood pressure and some forms of cancer. Older people are more effected by alcohol for the following reasons:

- Reduction in the ratio of body water to fat meaning there is relatively less water for the alcohol to be diluted
- Decreased hepatic blood flow makes the liver more susceptible to damage
- Liver enzymes become less effective with aging so alcohol is not so efficiently broken down
- Alcohol has a faster effect on the brain (IAS 1999).

As a person ages therefore, the same alcohol intake produces more pronounced effects on the person's behaviour. Alcohol may therefore lead to an increased likelihood of falls, incontinence, cognitive impairment, hypothermia and self-neglect. These sorts of problems may be regarded merely as signs of ageing, by both health professionals and family members. Alcohol misuse can also be obscured by non-specific health problems such as gastrointestinal problems and insomnia, or misdiagnosed as dementia or depression. Health professionals may recognize and diagnose the secondary medical problem, but fail to combat the possible primary cause.

Staff in primary care are generally the first point of contact for elderly people, but some may fail to diagnose alcohol misuse in a population where there are other urgent medical matters, and some believe that it may be better for the individual to continue their established pattern of drinking as altering it could be harmful. Elderly patients may show reluctance at disclosing their alcohol intake, and relatives may wish to hide the evidence of misuse of alcohol and deny existence of the problem. Appropriate screening measures are necessary to identify alcohol or other substance misuse among the elderly – and these measures need to be ongoing. It has been suggested that a full history of alcohol use should be taken at regular intervals, including questions about amounts taken in tea and coffee, which patients may regard as being irrelevant.

Treatment and counselling of older people needs to be based on a thorough assessment and matching of each person's needs to the range of treatment and services available. Emphasis needs to be placed on non-drinking social activities such as day centres and clubs in the context of the person's life circumstances and social support network. It may be necessary to work on redefining a social or family support mechanism. Some specialists argue that there is a need for

TOBACCO

The two main constituents of tobacco smoke are nicotine which produces an immediate effect and various tars which cause long-term effects. Cigarette smoke is acidic (pH 5.3) and this together with the fact that nicotine is largely insoluble in lipids explains why the smoke has to be inhaled into the lungs where it can be absorbed through the large surface area presented by lung tissue and so produce its effects. Nicotine is recognized as a potent drug of dependence, while the psycho-social factors involved in smoking combine to ensure both psychological and physical dependence ensue. The damaging effects of smoke are well-documented and discussed elsewhere in this text. Suffice it to say that the most vivid demonstration of the harm done to the lungs can be gauged from a visit to Gunther van Hagen's Bodyworld Exhibition. Whilst visiting the exhibition as part of a study trip to Vancouver in 2005; the exhibits of plastinated smoker's lungs made a deeply disturbing impact.

In most countries, smoking typically begins in adolescence. Evidence suggests that the longer a person delays the onset of smoking, the less likely they are to take up the habit. Therefore, it is vital that intensive efforts be made to encourage young non-smokers to stay smoke-free.

The process of graduation from first use to addiction may take months or even years. In fact, initial experiences with tobacco are sometimes negative, and social pressure and other factors are required to maintain exposure until the addiction develops. Tolerance to nicotine appears to be acquired over time, and experienced smokers can accept doses of nicotine that would make non-smokers ill.

EFFECTS ON HEALTH AND SOCIAL WELL-BEING

Smoking is estimated to have caused around 3 million deaths a year worldwide in the early 1990s, and the death toll is steadily increasing. Unless current trends are reversed, that figure is expected to rise to 10 million deaths per year by the 2020s or early 2030s, with 70% of those deaths occurring in developing countries. The chief uncertainty is not whether these deaths will occur, but exactly when. Of all the diseases causally associated with smoking, lung cancer is the most well known. However, smoking causes more deaths from diseases other than lung cancer.

The potential for behavioural and pharmacological treatment of the addicted tobacco user and the problems of withdrawal should be recognized. Although 75–85% of smokers (where this has been measured) want to stop and about one-third have made at least three serious attempts, less than half of smokers succeed in stopping permanently before the age of 60 years. Nicotine dependence is clearly a major barrier to successful cessation. Therefore, smoking control policies should contain activities both to strengthen smokers' motivation to quit (health education, public information, price policies, smoke-free policies, behavioural treatment) and to reduce dependence-related difficulties for smokers to quit (behavioural and pharmacological treatment).

An interesting statistic presented by Bennet and Brown (2003) is that only 14% of smokers find it 'very difficult' to stop; it is easier than commonly believed. The problem seems to be that it is also very easy to relapse and many smokers who stop for a short period are unable to remain smoke-free in the long term. Continuing support and motivation therefore are just as important as a focus on getting people to quit in the first place.

To achieve successful cessation of smoking on a very large scale, special 'cessation programmes' are far from enough. All health professionals, including doctors, nurses and pharmacists, should be given both basic and in-service training so that they are capable of providing advice and/or treatment for tobacco dependence.

COMMONLY ABUSED ILLICIT DRUGS

This section of the chapter describes the key characteristics of commonly abused drugs. It is not a definitive guide to all drugs abused, but will give a summary of those that you will commonly come across in nursing practice. It will be structured into three main categories:

1 Stimulants
2 Depressants
3 Hallucinogens.

It is important to bear in mind that drugs will be assigned to the category that describes their main effect. Some drugs cross-over categories depending on, amongst other factors, the quantity they are taken in and the route of ingestion, i.e. the same drug (e.g. cannabis) may have a different subjective effect when smoked (depressant) than when swallowed (hallucinogen).

The groupings of drugs into stimulant, depressant and hallucinogen categories has been used in preference to the categorizations of 'hard' and 'soft' drugs. The terms 'hard' and 'soft' are not based on any description of effect and imply that some drugs are less harmful to all individuals. Drugs produce a spectrum of effects, which will be perceived differently both across and within individuals. In some individuals, 'soft' drugs such as cannabis can have a devastating effect on their ability to function. Conversely, some individuals manage to continue to function and maintain their everyday lives despite reliance on 'hard' drugs such as heroin and methadone.

The terms stimulant, depressant and hallucinogen describe the drugs' primary effects. They also indicate to us the possible effects when individuals simultaneously use drugs from two different categories (e.g. cancelling out the effect of a stimulant by using a depressant on top) or use two different drugs from the same category (e.g. the dangers of mixing two types of depressant – the increased risk of depressing the central nervous system, leading to unconsciousness and cardiac arrest).

DESCRIPTIVE CATEGORIES OF COMMONLY ABUSED DRUGS

Classification

Under the Misuse of Drugs Act 1971, 'controlled drugs' are subdivided into three categories (Class A, B and C). The penalties received by individuals for illegal use of these drugs are defined by their category and the nature of the offence (i.e. possession, intent to supply, or supply):

- *Class A* – e.g. heroin, methadone, cocaine, ecstasy, magic mushrooms (when prepared for consumption). Class A carries the highest penalties
- *Class B* – e.g. amphetamine, methylamphetamine, barbiturate-based tranquillizers. Any Class B drug prepared for injection automatically becomes Class A
- *Class C* – e.g. cannabis, benzodiazepines (diazepam, temazepam, etc.) when not supplied by prescription from a physician; anabolic steroids.

Form and appearance

What forms the drug commonly takes and how it looks.

Street names

It is important to note that street names change across time and across region. The street names described here represent a sample of possibilities but it is worth checking with your local drug service to elicit up-to-date names.

Monetary cost

Costs vary across time and across geographical regions. Knowing the approximate cost of the drug is useful in practice. Patients may often be unable to give you a reliable measure of how much of a drug they are using on a daily or a weekly basis, but they will probably be able to tell you how much they are spending on drugs during that period. By knowing the approximate cost of the drug for your region, you can work out with the patient how much of the drug they are using on a daily or weekly basis. Your local specialist drug service is the best source of up-to-date costs.

Method of use

How the drug is commonly taken. The same drug can be treated and taken in a number of ways. The way the drug is taken affects the strength and often the nature of the effect that the user experiences from it. This is due to the speed and concentration of the drug permeating the blood–brain barrier. For example, smoking cocaine powder with tobacco weakens the effect of the drug, as much of the drug is lost to the air in smoke. In this case, the amount ingested through this method is fairly minimal. Sniffing (snorting) cocaine intranasally means that the majority of the powder goes

into the body and taken into the bloodstream through the capillaries in the nose; thus the effect is quicker and more intense than smoking the drug. However, the process is somewhat slowed by the amount of time the drug takes to be absorbed through the small capillaries in the nose into the bloodstream. Dissolving cocaine powder in water and injecting it directly into the vein ensures maximum take-up of the drug into the body. The drug goes directly into the bloodstream, thus permeating the blood–brain barrier at a higher concentration more quickly, maximizing the drug's effect and causing the user to experience a far faster and more intense 'high'.

Short-term use

The effects of using the drug over the short term. This generally describes the sort of effect the user is aspiring to when using the drug.

Long-term use

Use over a longer period generally decreases the subjective 'positive' effects of the drug, making way for more negative effects. It is during this period with certain drugs that physical dependence may be a problem. In the case of drugs not associated with physical dependence, problems associated with psychological dependence may come to the fore.

STIMULANTS

Amphetamine

Classification

Class B, unless prepared for injection, then Class A.

Forms and appearance

There are three basic types of amphetamine: racemic amphetamines, dextroamphetamines and methylamphetamines. Amphetamine sold on the street today is easily manufactured amphetamine sulfate powder (which may be formed into tablets) rather than amphetamine diverted from legitimate sources. Production is relatively simple. Methylamphetamine is the most potent of the three types.

Street names

Sold under a variety of names: Speed, Billy, Whizz, Sulfate, Buzz, Crystal, Crystal Meth.

Method of use

Amphetamine powder can be sniffed (snorted), swallowed, dissolved in water and injected, or smoked with cannabis and/or tobacco.

Associated equipment

Straws, needles, syringes, metal foil, rolled-up bank notes.

Effects of use

Amphetamines act much like the body's natural adrenaline does in the face of stress, by arousing and activating the user. **Heart rate** and **breathing** speed up, pupils widen and appetite decreases. The user feels more alert, energetic, confident, cheerful and less tired and bored. Higher doses induce feelings of intense exhilaration, rapid flow of ideas and feelings of greatly increased physical and mental capacity. Use of the drug may cause sleeplessness and increased aggression.

For some users, the predominant feeling elicited by using amphetamine may be anxiety, irritability and restlessness, particularly as the body's energy stores become depleted. High doses, especially if repeated over a few days, can cause delirium, panic, hallucinations and feelings of persecution ('amphetamine psychosis'), which should gradually disappear as the drug is eliminated from the body.

The effects of a single dose last about 3–4 hours and leave the user feeling tired; it may take a couple of days for the body to recover fully, even after small doses.

Possible adverse effects

Amphetamine use may lead to lethargy, fatigue, depression, irritability, panic, dry mouth, diarrhoea and increased urination, an increase in blood pressure with increased risk of stroke. Long-term use or a 'run' of use will leave the user feeling depressed, lethargic and ravenously hungry, as amphetamines postpone fatigue, sleep and hunger. The mood-elevating aspects of amphetamine can lead to psychological dependence. Physical dependence is rare, but in frequent users, tolerance may develop to the stimulant effect of amphetamine, so users have a tendency to increase the dose. With increased doses toxic effects may develop, including delusions, hallucinations and feelings of paranoia. Fatal overdose is possible, particularly with inexperienced users.

Szalavitz (2005) cites evidence showing that positron emission tomography of people who had been dependent upon amphetamine and were now abstinent, showed a reduction in dopamine transporter proteins in areas of the brain known to be involved in planning and the experience of positive emotions. They also performed poorly on a range of psycho-motor tests. Amphetamines are now estimated to be the second most popular illicit drug in the world after cannabis yet, despite the known dangers of the drug, we find it is increasingly being prescribed for children as young as 2 years old to treat attention deficit hyperactivity disorder (ADHD). The drug Ritalin for example is methylphenidate, an amphetamine derivative. This has led some researchers to question the long-term safety of such medication in cases of ADHD. There is, however, an alternative point of view which cites evidence showing Ritalin has a dopamine protective effect and suggesting its possible use in Parkinsonism. As Szalavitz (2005) observes, there is a lot more science to be undertaken before we have a complete understanding of Ritalin and similar amphetamine-related medications.

Cocaine

Classification

Class A.

Forms and appearance

Cocaine hydrochloride, white crystalline powder, occasionally in paste form.

Street names

Coke, charlie, snow.

Methods of use

Usually sniffed (snorted) or rubbed on the gums, but may be mixed with water and injected. The paste form may be smoked in a pipe.

Associated equipment

Rolled-up bank notes, shiny surface such as a mirror, straws, pipes, needles and syringes.

Effects of use

As with amphetamine, the drug activates the body's fight or flight mechanism, acting like adrenaline, causing the heart to beat faster and the body to speed up generally. It gives a sense of heightened awareness, euphoria, increased confidence, of being affable and chatty, an energy rush and agitation, and feelings of power.

Possible adverse effects

Users may experience lethargy, fatigue, paranoia, panic, depression, irritability and weight loss (over prolonged periods of use). Cocaine use may also lead to delusions and aggression. Regular use by snorting can damage the nasal passages. Like any injected substance, cocaine use can lead to skin ulcers or collapsed veins at the injection sites. Use may lead to both physical and psychological dependence. Heavy long-term users may experience paranoid psychosis, although this may also occur in some individuals with relatively low levels of use.

Ecstasy (3,4-methylenedioxymethamfetamine; MDMA)

Classification

Class A.

Forms and appearance

Capsules and tablet form in a variety of shapes, colours and sizes. Also available as an off-white powder.

Street names

E, pills, Erics, XTC, love doves, disco biscuits.

Associated equipment

None.

Method of use

Will generally be swallowed, but can also be snorted in powder form or by emptying contents of capsules.

Effects of use

Users experience increased energy, loss of inhibitions, feelings of euphoria and loss of appetite. Less positive aspects may include dry mouth and throat and muscle cramps. Objectively, facial grimacing and increased sweating may be observed. It should be noted that a lot of ecstasy purchased contains very little or no MDMA; rather, it is a combination in variable concentrations of LSD, amphetamine and ketamine. This obviously has implications for the effects experienced by the user, which are highly variable. Thus, a user reporting that they have ingested ecstasy may present with hallucinations more commonly associated with the ingestion of a hallucinogen such as LSD. It is therefore important in assessment to ask the user what they have taken, but also to enquire after the subjective effects. Do not assume that individuals presenting after ingestion of ecstasy will always present with the effects documented above. There is no method of buyers exercising quality control in the drugs market!

Possible adverse effects

The user may experience nausea and vomiting, dehydration, raised blood pressure, over-heating (hyperthermia), convulsions and sudden death, through heart attack or brain haemorrhage. In the aftermath of the drug, the user may feel fatigue and depression.

Crack cocaine

Classification

Class A.

Forms and appearance

Crack is a much stronger form of cocaine consisting of small crystals. It is produced by 'washing up' cocaine hydrochloride with ammonia or baking soda. The crystals are of varying sizes, shapes and colours, ranging from waxy white to pinkish yellow and clear yellow.

Street names

Rock, crack, stone, nuggets, freebase, wash, speedball (mixed with heroin).

Associated equipment

Crack pipe, perforated can, metal foil, Rizla papers, tobacco and cannabis mix (smoked as a 'spliff'; see section on cannabis).

Method of use

Smoked from pipe.

Effects of use

Euphoria and indifference to fatigue.

Possible adverse effects

Depression, fatigue, lethargy, irritability, loss of consciousness, anxiety and severe paranoia. The user may develop a psychosis accompanied by bizarre and often violent behaviour. There is an increased risk of lung damage due to the harsh effects of smoking. Psychological and physical dependence is common. The drug can also cause hypertension, haemorrhagic stroke, cardiac arrhythmias, convulsions and coronary artery spasm of sufficient intensity as to present as acute coronary syndrome (chest pain, myocardial infarction).

Alkyl nitrites

Classification

Not classified under the Act, although amyl nitrite is classified as a pharmacy medicine.

Forms and appearance

Clear, yellow, volatile and flammable liquids (essentially solvents). The two most common are amyl nitrite and butyl nitrite. The main medical use of amyl nitrites is as an antidote to cyanide poisoning.

Street names

Poppers, and by brand name, e.g. TNT, Rush, Rock Hard.

Associated equipment

Small bottle approximately the size of a 'Tippex' bottle.

Method of use

Sniffed in short bursts.

Effects of use

After inhalation, the effects are almost instantaneous. The user experiences a 'rush' as blood vessels dilate, heartbeat quickens and blood rushes to the brain. The person may experience a pounding headache, dizziness, flushed face and neck, and 'light-headedness'. The drug is sold freely in sex shops with the claim that it enhances sexual pleasure, prolonging the sensation of orgasm and preventing premature ejaculation. It may, however, impede erection in some male users.

Possible adverse effects

Irregular heartbeat, rise in blood pressure and strain on the heart. Increased health concerns if injecting, associated with sharing of injecting equipment.

DEPRESSANTS

Cannabis

Classification

Class C.

Forms and appearance

Three main types predominate. Herbal cannabis is a greenish-brown dried plant material. These include Skunk and Sinsemilla. Cannabis resin comes in various colours and shapes in dried and compressed blocks. Cannabis oil is thick and ranges in colour from dark green to brown. It has a distinctive smell like rotting vegetation.

Street names

Hash, draw, puff, blow, dope, herb, weed.

Associated equipment

Rizla papers, home-made pipes, cling-film wraps.

Method of use

Most commonly smoked but can be swallowed raw, added to cooking or made into a drink.

Effects of use

There are many chemicals released by the cannabis leaf of which the most active is tetrahydrocannabinol (THC). That this substance has an effect on the brain, implies that we have neurotransmitter receptor sites sensitive to the molecule in the brain which has led scientists to ask whether we make our own very similar substances which serve as neurotransmitters? The answer is now known and a whole family of substances known as endocannabinoids have been discovered since the mid-1990s (see p. 654). Intensive research is underway as to how they function in order to better understand the brain and also to develop potential new medications. The anecdotal stories about the beneficial uses of cannabis in conditions such as multiple sclerosis therefore have a foundation in fact (Nicoll and Alger 2004).

Cannabis produces relaxation, light intoxication, giggles, increased appetite (the munchies) increased talkativeness and heightened senses. Skunk, which is intensively grown in special circumstances to increase its strength, has a much quicker onset of effects. Users of skunk have reported elation, profound relaxation, alteration of time and perception, and mild hallucinations. As with many drugs, the mood of the person may determine the effects experienced. First-time users of cannabis may feel very little effect from the drug, and may have to learn what effects to look for.

Possible adverse effects

Controversy continues over whether long-term use of cannabis causes lasting damage to physical or mental health. There is still little conclusive evidence either way. However, users may experience inability to concentrate, clumsiness and 'red eye'. Objectively, they may appear drunk. Due to inhalation through smoking either with or without tobacco there may be potential for bronchial problems and cancer. Users may experience short-term memory loss and de-motivation. Withdrawal effects such as anxiety, panic, restlessness and disturbed sleep patterns have also been noted. Research into pharmacological substances related to THC will clearly aim to produce pure compounds without serious side-effects and bypass the need to smoke the substance in order to get it into the body.

Heroin (diamorphine)

Classification

Class A.

Forms and appearance

Heroin is prepared from morphine, a naturally occurring substance derived from the opium poppy. This was first done in 1874 at St Mary's Hospital, London.

Street names

H, skag, smack, junk.

Associated equipment

Needles, syringes and tin foil.

Method of use

Can be injected, smoked ('chasing the dragon'), snorted or taken orally.

Effects of use

Heroin is rapidly converted in the body to morphine and 6-monoacetylmorphine which is a metabolite of morphine and heroin. It is more potent than morphine and 1 mg of heroin is equivalent to 1.5 mg of morphine (Bennet and Brown 2003). The metabolites of heroin act on the bodies own natural opioid receptors designed for the use of our endorphins (mainly μ and κ receptors). The effect is one of comfort, warmth, euphoria, emotional detachment and pain relief. The drug's effect lasts for 3–6 hours.

Possible adverse effects

Heroin, like all opiates, depresses the central nervous system, thus lowering breathing and heart rate. Initially users may experience nausea and vomiting. Users may also suffer from severe constipation. There are a number of well publicized problems associated with intravenous drug use such as the development of abscesses on injecting sites, sharing needles leading to a greatly increased incidence of HIV and hepatitis infection. A total of 1505 intravenous drug users (IDUs) had died from the effects of HIV/AIDS in the UK by late 2004. Annual deaths have dropped from around 170 per year in the mid-1990s to around 60 per year since 2000, presumably due to harm reduction schemes such as needle exchanges. In the UK, people in the age range 40–54 account for the largest single group of HIV infected IDUs (NTA 2005).

In some cities such as Sydney and Vancouver, harm reduction policies have seen the opening of nurse supervised injection centres (Buckis 2005). Such centres are very controversial with opponents claiming they are legitimizing intravenous drug use and a furious debate has been raging in Canada (since late 2005) over whether Toronto should follow Vancouver's lead in opening up such a centre.

There is often claimed to be a high level of physical and psychological dependence associated with the intravenous use of heroin; however, other sources are doubtful of this claim (Bennet and Brown 2003). Opiate use may interfere with a woman's menstrual cycle but will not necessarily stop her from becoming pregnant, which is another major concern. Clearly, the health of the baby is potentially gravely compromised by the multiple risks involved in the mother's drug misuse.

Methadone

Classification

Class A, unless individually prescribed.

Forms and appearance

Clear injectable ampoules, small white tablets, brown, orange or green linctus.

Street names

'Script', juice, red rock, doll, linctus.

Associated equipment
Medicine bottles, needles and syringes.

Method of use
Methadone is a synthetic opiate used as a heroin substitute and prescribed to those engaging in a heroin detoxification or treatment package. It also has a street value and is regularly sold on the drugs market. It is usually swallowed in syrup form but can also be prescribed as tablets. Doctors have, however, been advised by the Department of Health to not prescribe it in tablet form, as tablets are worth more on the illicit market, increasing the likelihood that it will be sold on. Methadone can also be taken in an injectable form.

Effects of use
Methadone has a less intense but longer lasting effect than heroin. Users experience relaxation, bodily warmth and suppression of the withdrawal effects of heroin dependency that lasts for up to 24 hours.

Possible adverse effects
Users may experience bouts of sweating, disruption to the menstrual cycle, constipation, nausea, itching and tiredness, physical and psychological dependence.

Benzodiazepines
Classification
Class C. Supply without prescription is illegal, but it is not illegal to possess benzodiazepines in medicinal form without a prescription, with the exception of temazepam. Benzodiazepines include diazepam (Valium), chlordiazepoxide (Librium), nitrazepam (Mogadon), Nobrium, lorazepam (Ativan), temazepam, flurazepam (Dalmane) and flunitrazepam (Rohypnol).

Forms and appearance
Commonly prescribed tranquillizers and hypnotics, the benzodiazepines are in tablet and capsule form in various colours, shapes and sizes.

Street names
Benzos, jellies, goosies, temazzies, tranx, pills.

Associated equipment
Needles and syringes.

Method of use
Swallowed or melted down or crushed for injection.

Effects of use
Light intoxication, drowsiness, headache, confusion, ataxia. May be used by stimulant users to 'come down' or sleep after a prolonged period of stimulant use. May also be used by injecting opiate users when their drug of choice is unavailable or they cannot afford it. Benzodiazepines may also be used to augment the effect of other depressant drugs such as alcohol or heroin.

Possible adverse effects
Users may experience a 'hangover' effect after use. In high doses aggression, violent mood swings, deep depression, liver damage, lethargy and bizarre sexual behaviour may occur. Physical and psychological dependence is common.

GHB (γ hydroxybutyrate)
Classification
GHB is classed as a medicine, so possession is not an offence, but unauthorized manufacture and distribution could be an offence under the Medicines Act.

Forms and appearance
GHB was developed in the USA as an anaesthetic and is used as a pre-medication to promote sleep before surgery. It has sedative rather than painkilling effects. It is a colourless, odourless liquid that is sold in small bottles or capsule form.

Street names
GBH, liquid E, liquid X.

Associated equipment
GHB bottles.

Method of use
Swallowed.

Effects of use
As GHB is sold in liquid form, it is impossible to tell how concentrated the liquid is: a bottle could contain 3 g of the drug, quite a mild dose, or up to 20 g – a very high dose. At low doses, the drug induces euphoria and loss of inhibitions. At higher doses, however, euphoria gives way to powerful sedative effects along with hallucinations, muscular tremors and facial grimacing. The effects of the drug are experienced between 10 minutes and 1 hour after ingestion, and are reported to last for up to 1 day.

Possible adverse effects
Users may experience nausea, vomiting, disorientation, muscular pain, depression, fatigue, convulsions, coma, respiratory collapse and death.

Ketamine
Classification
Ketamine is not controlled under the Misuse of Drugs Act, so possession is not an offence; however, unauthorized supply is illegal.

Forms and appearance
Tablets, capsules or as a soluble crystalline powder, or in its liquid pharmaceutical form for injecting.

Street names
K, Special K, Vitamin K, kit kat.

Associated equipment
Straws, rolled-up notes, needles and syringes.

Method of use
Swallowed, snorted or injected.

Effects of use
Users experience euphoria in an initial 'rush', intense hallucinations and feelings of depersonalization.

Possible adverse effects

Users may experience fatigue, cramps, severe depression, vomiting, irritability, violent reactions, flashbacks similar to those experienced with LSD, heart failure.

Solvents

Classification

Not controlled under the Act, although it is against the law to sell solvents to known or suspected young solvent misusers.

Forms and appearance

Solvents are commercial products.

Street names

Glue, gas, can, cog.

Method of use

Sprayed directly into the mouth or inhaled from a bag, handkerchief or rag.

Effects of use

The user experiences intense intoxication, loss of balance, and auditory and visual hallucinations. Solvents are manufactured products that generally have a depressant effect on the central nervous system, although in some individuals they may have a stimulant effect. Effects can be heightened by increasing the concentration of the vapour by sniffing from a plastic bag held at the mouth or nose, or in some instances placed over the head, which is extremely dangerous for obvious reasons. It is also equally dangerous to spray the chemicals directly into the mouth.

Possible adverse effects

There is a danger of accidents whilst intoxicated or hallucinating. There is also a danger of loss of short-term memory and cognitive skills, personality changes, kidney damage, liver and bowel disorders, acute brain damage and sudden death. Solvents cause more deaths than any other recreational drugs – apart from alcohol and tobacco.

Barbiturates

Classification

Class B. Barbiturates are known as hypnosedatives. In lower doses they have a calming effect and in higher dose act as sleeping pills.

Forms and appearance

Tablet or capsule form in various sizes and colours.

Street names

Barbs, downers, sleepers.

Associated equipment

Needles and syringes.

Method of use

May be swallowed. Barbiturates do not tend to be popular with younger recreational drug users. They tend to be abused by 'heavy end' dependent drug users. Barbiturates can also be dissolved in water and injected into the vein.

Effects of use

Barbiturates provide temporary relief from fears, tensions and anxiety. The user may appear drunk. Effects are considerably increased when combined with alcohol and other drugs, and can last for up to 16 hours.

Possible adverse effects

Sudden withdrawal from very high doses may be fatal. If there are no complications, withdrawal effects generally subside within a week. Heavy users are susceptible to bronchitis and pneumonia (because the cough reflex is depressed), hypothermia and accidental overdose (as the drugs can cause confusion and tolerance effects). Most of the adverse effects are increased when the drug is injected.

HALLUCINOGENS

LSD (lysergic acid diethylamide)

Classification

Class A.

Forms and appearance

$0.5\,cm^2$ blotters of paper, usually printed with a design from popular culture such as cartoon characters. More rarely, very small tablets and, rarer still, powder form.

Street names

Acid, trips, micros, tabs, dots.

Associated equipment

None.

Method of use

Swallowed or dissolved on the tongue.

Effects of use

LSD is a powerful hallucinogen. Hallucinations may be visual, auditory or tactile. They can range from being very pleasant to extremely unpleasant. This may be influenced by the mood of the user before ingestion. The person's sense of time appears to change, and things take on a new perspective. Effects last between 8 and 12 hours.

Possible adverse effects

Reoccurrence of hallucination many weeks or months after stopping the drug (referred to as 'flashbacks'). Accidents whilst hallucinating; users may believe they have powers above their ability, for example that they can fly. Use may precipitate latent psychiatric disorders.

Magic mushrooms

Classification

The mushrooms are not illegal but their active ingredients psilocin and psilocybin are controlled Class A drugs. It is therefore illegal to boil, crush or make a 'preparation or other product' containing the active ingredients.

Forms and appearance

There are several varieties that are all very different in appearance. Identification may be difficult, and mistakes are easily made.

Street names
Shrooms, mushies.

Associated equipment
None.

Method of use
Swallowed raw, cooked or boiled.

Effects of use
The effects of magic mushrooms are similar to those of a mild LSD experience. Variability in effect due to user's mood: euphoria, high spirits and well-being, bouts of giggling, visual and auditory hallucinations.

Possible adverse effects
Dizziness, nausea, possibility of stimulating latent psychiatric disorders. Accidental ingestion of poisonous mushroom by mistake.

WHAT IF I HAVEN'T A CLUE ABOUT THE DRUG A PATIENT IS TALKING ABOUT?

If, during assessment or care, a patient discloses use of drugs that are not described in this section, there are a number of different sources to contact for information on the effects of the drug. It is easy to feel de-skilled in these circumstances, but accessible information is available in a variety of places. A recommended website is 'TalktoFrank' which both the nurse and patient will find useful as a source of information about everything from current street names to the effects of all the main drugs in use. Your local health promotion unit should also be able to provide information produced by national organizations such as Lifeline or Release. These organizations provide booklets and pamphlets that are readily accessible to both professionals and the general public.

You should also be careful not to fall into the common trap of assuming that because a patient uses certain drugs they have a sound knowledge of the long-term effects of drug use. Drug use is generally focused on short-term gains and clients may often find it difficult to project into the future concerning their use. It is good practice to give the patient as much information about the drugs they are using as possible. The use of pamphlets such as those developed by 'Lifeline' provides an opportunity to give patients objective

Footnote So-called 'psychedelic drugs' such as LSD were originally synthesized as part of serious medical research programmes investigating conditions such as schizophrenia before they became the infamous recreational drugs of the 1960s. It is therefore interesting to note that they are now being re-investigated for possible pharmacological benefits. Horgan (2005) cites basic research work on LSD as a possible treatment for cluster headaches, a rare type of headache so severe it has been known to induce suicide, whilst a project to see if MDMA or ecstasy can help late-stage cancer patients has received US Federal Drug Agency funding.

information without appearing patronizing or pushy. You should also give patients the opportunity to discuss the contents of the leaflet with you wherever possible, to ensure they fully understand the information presented in the leaflet. In these circumstances it is important to be aware of the address of your local drug service, in order to be able to direct the patient there should they require more specialist information or help.

MULTIDISCIPLINARY WORKING AND SERVICE STRUCTURES

With the continued rise of substance misuse in the general population, it is inevitable that nurses will increasingly find they are providing care to individuals with substance misuse problems. Nurses can have a number of pivotal roles when working with individuals with these complex difficulties. This work may occur at the primary care, secondary care or tertiary care level.

A number of the key roles nurses can take are:

- engaging, assessing and appropriately referring on if there is a perceived level of significant harm related to substance use
- screening and early recognition
- harm minimization and prevention
- health promotion and education
- advice and support to the individual
- promotion of risk awareness in relation to substance misuse
- advice and support to the family
- counselling
- ongoing support in the community to individuals on maintenance or withdrawal programmes
- crisis intervention
- shared care
- acting as a key player in policy developments
- use as a consultant and resource for colleagues.

The extent to which each of these roles will be taken on by a nurse is dependent on the context of the service they are working in and their level of experience and interest in working with this client group. However, it should be acknowledged that a number of these roles are core business for any nurse, whatever setting they are working in, namely:

- screening and recognition of substance misuse problems
- promotion of risk awareness to substance-misusing individuals, including basic harm minimization strategies
- ability to engage, assess and refer on to the appropriate agency, according to the individual's expressed need.

The support of an individual with entrenched substance misuse problems often requires a multidisciplinary approach, rather than a response by an individual clinician. A multidisciplinary response takes account of the complexity and difficulties surrounding substance misuse.

For example, an individual with an enduring heroin habit may require support and advice on harm minimization techniques that can be provided by the general nurse. However, he or she may also require a methadone prescription for maintenance or reduction of the use, which will involve a prescribing physician, such as a general practitioner or specialist psychiatrist. The patient could also require the skills of a social worker for a community care assessment, for inpatient detoxification services or housing issues. He or she may have had contact with the criminal justice system, and therefore need to see a probation officer, and might also be seeing a counsellor for mental health-related issues.

As you can see, individuals can quickly develop their own multidisciplinary 'team' around them to meet their complex needs. In some areas, individuals such as this will be referred on to a specialist drug team. In other cases, which may be due to the client's reluctance to engage with the specialist team, or because a specialist team approach is not available in that area, care may be coordinated at a primary or secondary care level. In these cases, communication between each of the workers associated with the individual is imperative. This is where the service model of shared care originates.

SHARED CARE

The government's 2002 updated drug strategy (Department of Health 2002) has stressed the importance of tackling the psycho-social as well as physical damage caused by drug misuse and calls for multi-agency working to be the norm. The joint participation of specialists and GPs (and other agencies where appropriate) in the planned delivery of care for patients with a drug misuse problem is essential. This should be facilitated by enhanced information exchange beyond routine discharge and referral letters. It may involve the day to day management by the GP of the patient's medical needs in relation to his or her drug misuse. Such arrangements would make explicit which clinician was responsible for different aspects of the patient's treatment and care. These may include prescribing substitute drugs in appropriate circumstances.

Policy on guidelines for clinical management of drug misuse and dependence highlights a number of factors, including the need to firm up the process of shared care:

- Shared care aims to deliver a flexible service, based on individual need, utilizing the differing skills of a number of health professionals in the most effective manner
- The general shift towards a better balance of primary and secondary healthcare provision, with the emphasis being placed on a primary care led NHS
- An increasing preference by drug misusers to receive care in a primary care setting in the community wherever possible
- Expansion of the primary healthcare team to include a wide range of specialist mental health staff, including community psychiatric nurses, clinical psychologists, and specialist drug and alcohol workers
- The increasing number of young drug misusers whose natural first point of contact is their family GP.

Shared care should not be limited solely to those drug users who require substitute prescribing, but should aim to include interventions to support and aid drug misusers who wish to give up but do not need substitute prescribing. It should also include specific treatment interventions such as counselling and other therapeutic input, and also interventions carried out between general practice and voluntary drug agencies.

Shared care arrangements already exist in all parts of the UK. However, the success of shared care in any given area will depend heavily on good communication, trust and understanding between all the services involved and the evolution of shared protocols to meet regional needs.

PRIMARY CARE

Over 90% of the population enjoy an occasional drink, one-third of all adults smoke tobacco, minor tranquillizer use is estimated to be in the thousands, and at least 6% of the population are believed to take an illegal drug. About two-thirds of patients consult their general practitioner at least once a year, and more than 90% at least every 5 years. Therefore, nurses working in primary healthcare teams will directly or indirectly come into contact with substance misuse. The importance of screening at this stage lies in the fact that many people accessing primary care may not present with an obvious substance misuse problem. The nurse's knowledge and clinical skills in relation to drugs, solvents and alcohol, and to the risks and consequences of their use, may be the basis for effective interventions with patients, families and communities.

A number of opportunities present for screening in primary care settings:

- prenatal checks
- child and adolescent check-ups
- well-woman clinics
- family planning clinics
- well-men clinics
- new patient registrations
- specialist clinics (e.g. asthma, diabetes)
- routine primary care visits
- attendance at walk-in centres or A&E.

These opportunities are reinforced by factors such as the flexibility of surgery hours, giving more accessibility for consultations, and the reduced stigma of labelling, whereby some people perceive specialist services to be only for 'addicts'. However, the perception of obstacles still impedes some people from seeking help:

- poor previous experiences with health and social care agencies

- treatment of substance misuse being seen as a specialist, rather than primary care, function
- judgemental attitudes towards substance misuse
- being refused treatment and appropriate support
- fear that prescribed medication for other conditions may be stopped
- potential breaches of confidentiality, e.g. to other family members or employers.

ACCIDENT AND EMERGENCY

Nurses working in A&E departments, and minor injuries units, will be well aware of the problems caused by acutely intoxicated people: verbal aggression, physical violence, demanding and uncooperative behaviour. However, the real picture is also one of many people presenting whose alcohol or drug problems go unnoticed.

A&E provides the main interface between primary care and specialist secondary care services. It therefore presents important opportunities for screening, early detection, appropriate assessment and intervention, and referral to the appropriate sources of help and support (Fletcher 2004). For many patients A&E may be the only place they present to health services making this a particularly valuable opportunity for intervention. Consequently, the opportunity to screen, intervene and refer on should not be lost.

When patients are intoxicated, there is an understandable desire to treat the immediate problem such as a laceration and get them out of the department as soon as possible. In some cases, this may require the intervention of security staff or the police. However, in more cooperative patients screening may be possible and one such tool developed for use in Emergency Departments is the Paddington Alcohol Test (Fletcher 2004). This will be reviewed on p. 928 along with other screening tools.

DUAL DIAGNOSIS OR COMORBIDITY (SUBSTANCE MISUSE AND SEVERE MENTAL ILLNESS)

There is a high incidence of cross-over between psychiatric disorders and substance misuse. A number of research studies have found that approximately one-third of heavy drinkers have associated mental health problems, especially depression and anxiety, and one-half of dependent drug users have mental health problems of varying severity (Department of Health 1999). The picture is complicated as the effects of some illicit drugs can mimic psychotic symptoms, both schizophrenia and cocaine can induce paranoia for example. There is also a 'chicken and egg syndrome' here; in some people the mental illness has led to substance abuse, whilst in others the substance abuse came first and this led to mental health problems. It is also possible that both problems developed alongside each other at the same time (McDowell and Spitz 1999). Individuals with these complex needs also tend to be over represented in the prison and homeless populations.

Service structures for this group in the UK are in their infancy. Individuals with these difficulties often rely on a number of services, which require good communication and high levels of coordination. Studies from the USA suggest that integrated services – where the individual receives help for both their mental health problems and their substance misuse difficulties from the same team – show better results than parallel or concurrent service structures (Gournay et al 1997, Manley 1998). Although there are specialist integrated services for those with a 'dual diagnosis' under development in the UK, it is unlikely that specialist teams will serve all such individuals.

The tendency of drug dependent individuals to come into the criminal justice system led to the UK government launching its Drug Intervention Program in 2003, in order that the necessary multi agency working could include the criminal justice system. The aim is to bring drug using offenders into treatment. The system that has been established has made some health professionals wary of the ethos involved (a balance between coercion and motivation), but as Bateman (2005) has demonstrated it is possible to find a way forward with one of the pilot schemes in Wolverhampton being cited as an example of good practice. A single multi-agency team does seem to be making a difference (see Case Study 26.2).

CASE Tom is a 47-year-old man who lives alone in a ground-floor one-bedroom flat. His father and younger sister both live close by and he has regular contact with them when he is sober. They are afraid to visit when Tom is drunk, partly because of his aggressive behaviour and partly because of the other people who congregate at his flat (who are suspected of using alcohol and drugs).

Psychiatric history

Tom is known to local inpatient psychiatric services through 12 hospital admissions over the past 15 years. He has had diagnoses of manic depression and psychotic depressions recorded over this period of time. Most of these admissions record Tom in a depressed and/or agitated state, expressing suicidal ideas. His psychotic symptoms are predominantly in the form of persecutory voices telling him he is worthless, that he is a curse on people he comes into contact with and that he should kill himself. He has made three serious attempts on his own life, including drinking car battery acid, attempted self electrocution and stabbing himself in the stomach with a carving knife. Tom settles quickly on each hospital admission as he reinstates his prescribed medication and ceases to use the alcohol. On occasions, he absconds briefly from the ward, and returns inebriated. He has frequently become lost to contact with community services, through non-attendance at outpatient clinics. Tom's family suggest they are the only people who contact him at home when he is out of hospital.

Substance misuse history

Tom has reported using alcohol from his teenage years and throughout his working life, but it seems to have become a problem for him only since he became unemployed and in contact with psychiatric services. He mainly uses cheap ciders and strong lagers, and when drinking may begin early in the morning when a range of 'friends' visit. Tom smokes about 40 cigarettes a day, denies using any illicit drugs, but does suggest that his visitors use a lot of cannabis.

Assessment

The initiation of an assertive outreach team has enabled some intermittent contact with Tom at his home. He readily engages in discussion when sober. He is accepting of the role prescribed medication plays in keeping away distressing suicidal thoughts, and admits to becoming very forgetful about his tablets when drunk (he is unable to take depot injections because of a previous adverse physical reaction to them during an early hospital admission). Tom says he becomes bored very quickly, which is why he easily reverts to the friends who visit him and engage in substance misuse. People in this social network actively discourage him from taking prescribed medication and encourage him to withdraw amounts from a savings account he built up many years ago.

Care plan interventions

1 Assertive outreach team to engage a working relationship with Tom in the short term through daily, but relatively short, home visits.
2 Establish Tom's use of a dosett box for his oral medication, clearly separating his daily doses (one box holds a week's supply of tablets, refilled weekly by staff of the team).
3 Frequent discussions with Tom about the established pattern of becoming suicidal, to identify and monitor the early warning signs with him.
4 Support family members, by offering education about the psychiatric condition and direct effects of the substance abuse on Tom's suicidal thoughts; also offer them a quick telephone contact when they have concerns about his condition.
5 Actively discuss Tom's interests and talents, and investigate potential options for meaningful activity that may loosen his reliance on current damaging social contacts.
6 Develop a crisis plan for the possible actions if Tom loses contact with the team, or his family express fears of deterioration and/or negative social influences.

ASSESSMENT

A comprehensive, holistic assessment is essential for high-quality care. This requires the nurse to explore areas such as alcohol and substance misuse as a routine part of any patient assessment, whether the patient is a known drug misuser or not. In this context, we can identify assessment as taking place on three levels:

1 triage – for emergency screening
2 screening
3 in-depth assessment.

AIMS OF ASSESSMENT

- Treatment of any emergency or acute problem
- Confirmation that the individual is taking alcohol and/or drugs (history, examination and urine analysis)
- Assessment of the degree of dependence
- Identification of any complications of alcohol or drug misuse, and assessment of risk behaviour
- Identification of other medical, social or mental health problems
- Provision of advice on harm minimization including, if appropriate, access to sterile injecting equipment, testing for hepatitis, HIV and immunization against hepatitis B
- Determination of the individual's expectations of treatment and the degree of motivation to change
- Assessment of the most appropriate level of expertise required to manage the individual (primary care, specialist team, etc.) in order to facilitate a correct referral
- Determination of the need for substitute medication (a specialist team function).

TRIAGE ASSESSMENT

Triage is practised in situations requiring a quick response to emergencies such as A&E departments or telephone help-lines and sometimes other primary care settings. The aim of triage is to establish the degree of emergency for the presenting individual, to determine whether they need immediate intervention or a longer, more specialized, assessment. The aim of triage could be described as a system designed to treat any emergency or acute problem whilst filtering out problems that can be assessed or treated over time.

SCREENING

Screening is an essential part of the assessment process. This part of the assessment should be covered as a matter of course for any individual presenting to health services. It involves a low level of assessment, with generally unobtrusive questioning to establish whether the individual might have problems with substances. A well validated example is the CAGE tool which is used extensively by nurse practitioners and practice nurses to screen for alcohol-related problems in primary care and hospital out patient settings. The tool uses four simple questions:

Cutdown: Ever felt the need to cut down?
Annoyed: Ever felt annoyed by criticism of your drinking?
Guilty: Ever had guilty feelings about your drinking?
Eye-opener: Ever felt the need for a drink to get you started in the morning?

If the person answers yes to any of these questions, this indicates there is a problem. Used in a non-judgemental way this sort of questioning can give people a chance to disclose any 'use' that may have been causing them concern.

The CAGE questionnaire has been refined to make it more appropriate for use with women, given the different effects of alcohol on women compared with men (see p. 915). This has resulted in the TWEAK screen (Table 26.2).

The A&E department offers an excellent screening opportunity and assuming the patient is cooperative, the Paddington Alcohol Test has been found to be a very effective tool to use (Table 26.3).

Screening should always be carried out in a safe, confidential environment, with a non-judgmental attitude and sensitivity towards the individual's personal circumstances. It is also of paramount importance that you are clear about your own attitudes towards these issues, in order that you enable all individuals to obtain equal access to services.

If the results of the screening procedure highlight any issues in need of further consideration, the nurse might take one of the following routes:

1 discussion with or referral to a specialist worker or team
2 brief intervention advice with follow-up
3 in-depth assessment and specialist follow-up.

IN-DEPTH ASSESSMENT

An in-depth assessment of substance misuse should cover at least the following areas:

- reason for presenting to the service
- past substance use
- current substance use (over the past 4 weeks)
- history of injecting and risk of hepatitis and HIV
- medical history
- psychiatric history
- forensic history
- social history (including occupation)
- past contact with treatment services
- other, for example substance misuse in spouse or family members.

The following areas should also be subject to examination:

- assessment of motivation
- assessment of general health
- assessment of mental health
- assessment of social and family situation.

The following special investigations may also be carried out to aid an in-depth assessment:

- haematological – such as testing for **HIV** antibody (before any test of this sort full informed consent should be received from the individual), full blood count, liver function tests, blood alcohol levels
- urine toxicology
- breathalyzer
- physical examination – e.g. gait, track marks, abscesses, injection sites, skin pallor, pupil size, irritability, drowsiness, smell of breath, hair analysis.

Barriers to effective assessment include:

- fear of professional judgement
- fear of being refused treatment
- belief that disclosure of substance use is not appropriate in a particular setting (e.g. A&E)
- poor previous experiences
- fear of 'loss of control'
- difficulty staying in the waiting area due to withdrawal symptoms
- fear of information being placed on medical records
- concern about the family being informed
- concern about police and other agencies being informed
- fear of being labelled 'drug user' or 'alcoholic'
- nurse's experience and confidence
- lack of information about specialist agencies or services
- negative attitudes towards drug and alcohol users
- appropriate skills.

Assessment is not merely for assessment's sake, but should form the basis on which to build a care plan that adequately meets the individual's needs. During the care planning stage,

Table 26.2	The TWEAK screen for alcohol problems in women
Tolerance	How many drinks can you hold? (>6 indicates tolerance)
	or
	How many drinks does it take before you notice a difference in your mood?
	(>3 indicates tolerance)
Worry	Have close friends or relatives worried or complained about your drinking in the last year?
Eye opener	Do you sometimes take a drink in the morning when you first get up?
Amnesia	Has a friend or family member ever told you about things you said or did that you could not remember?
Kut down	Do you sometimes feel the need to '[k]cut down' your drinking?

Scoring: 2 points for a yes to the **T**olerance and **W**orry questions, one point for the others. A total of 2 or more indicates a drinking problem.
Source: Russel 1994.

Table 26.3 The Paddington Alcohol Test

> **'PADDINGTON ALCOHOL TEST'**
> **(PAT)**

N.B. page 3 A&E card

Circle numbers – max. 3 – for specific trigger(s): consider for ALL the **TOP 10** *(include = i):-*

☐ ☐ ☐

1. FALL (L trip)	2. COLLAPSE (i fits)	3. HEAD INJURY (i facial)
4. ASSAULT (i involved)	5. NON-SPECIFIC G.I.	6. "UNWELL"
7. PSYCHIATRIC (i odose)	8. CARDIAC (i palpitations)	9. SELF-NEGLECT
	10. <u>REPEAT Attender</u>	

Other (speficy):-...........................

DATE: ☐ ☐ ☐

PATIENT IDENTIFICATION NUMBER:

After Dealing with patients 'agenda' ie. patient's reason for attendance:-

☐ 1. "Quite a number of people have times when they drink more than usual; what is the most you will drink in any one day?"
(Units, 8 gms alc...for pub measures in brackets, home measures often x3!)

Beer/lager/cider	__Pints (2)	__Cans (1.5)	total Units/day
Strong beer/lager/cider	__Pints (5)	__Cans (4)	= _____
Wine	__Glasses (1.5)	__Bottles (9)	
Fortified wine (sherry, Martini)	__Glasses (1)	__Bottles (12)	
Spirits (gin, whisky, vodka)	__Singles (1)	__Botles (30)	

☐ 2. If this is <u>more than</u> 8 units/day for a man, or 6 units/day for a woman, does this happen

Circle

Once a week or more? = **YES: PAT+ve** (every day: ?)
or
Less frequent ? = **? PAT – neg**

☐ 3. Do you feel your current attendance in A&E is related to alcohol? **YES (PAT+ve)**/NO

If PAT + ve: Would you like to see our Health Worker? **YES/NO**

If Yes: give Alcohol Advice Card with appointment for next Review Clinic + book appt

If NO   1. Still give patient **Alcohol Advice Card** – patient may change mind later and return
      2. Still complete **PAT**; place in notes for reinformcement if patient reattends
      3. Still mark **A&E notes**, p.3: PAT 'POS'. Referred AHW 'NO', to alert staff
      4. Still inform **GP** in **A&E** discharge letter no. 11 letter if alcohol main problem.

If to be **admitted**, note in **AHW** book & state ward if known ....

SIGNATURE   NAME STAMP

PAT 2000

the nurse should help the individual to explore and clarify his or her aims and objectives with regard to substance use. Care planning should always take into account the individual's motivation to change and also the outcomes the individual perceives as desirable. The assessment process should also enable the nurse to identify where the individual's care needs would best be met, for example in the primary care setting or in a specialist service.

TREATMENT INTERVENTIONS

REDUCING ALCOHOL PROBLEMS

There is no single solution to reducing alcohol-related harm. What is required is a comprehensive range of strategies that can address the many causes and dimensions of alcohol problems. These may include:

- controls on price and availability
- minimum age for purchasing alcohol
- legislative measures to curb driving while under the influence of alcohol
- restrictions on the promotion, marketing and advertising of alcohol
- public education and awareness programmes
- primary healthcare and community-based interventions.

In the UK, at a national level, because of the known link between total national consumption and the amount of alcohol-related harm, reducing alcohol problems means reducing the total consumption of alcohol. It is therefore very strange that the UK government, whilst espousing such aims, has extended licensing hours for premises selling alcohol to the extent that the drug is now available 24 hours a day. There is also a need to impact upon patterns of consumption and social attitudes to drinking and drunkenness, e.g. drinking and driving.

At the individual level, people who are already experiencing alcohol problems or who are in danger of doing so need to be encouraged to eliminate the risk by stopping drinking, or to reduce it by cutting down. Depending on the severity of the problems, this could involve getting help from a treatment agency or a process of self-help. People who are alcohol dependent are advised to seek specialist help. Either way, individuals need to make a firm decision to give up or cut down, and then look for ways of maintaining their resolve over time. This is likely to involve:

- recognizing and understanding the harm experienced as a result of drinking
- understanding the functions that alcohol was performing (psychological, social), so as to be able to find alternatives
- identifying high-risk times and situations, so as to be able to learn to cope with them in another way, or avoid them.

AIMS OF TREATMENT FOR DRUG MISUSE

Substance misuse treatment, as befits its complex nature, aims to fulfil a number of individual and social needs. Treatment aims are summarized in Box 26.1.

As previously discussed, no single model can provide us with a full explanation of drug misuse or dependency. It leads to a situation where a pattern of behaviour takes over the whole life of the person with profound biological psychological and social effects. The person tends to lose control over the behaviour despite the harm it is doing to them. Interventions therefore need to be targeted to take account of all of these factors. Every individual will have his or her own unique profile of how each of the factors interrelate, and the aim of a good care plan would be to target each of these factors according to individual need. This further highlights the importance of a thorough and well-structured assessment, as without this a key area maintaining drug and alcohol use may be overlooked.

There are many variations of therapeutic approach that can be used with individuals misusing substances. This section aims to give an overview of some of the common interventions used in clinical practice in the substance misuse field. The interventions are linked to a common model of behaviour change, to highlight how efficacy of intervention may be impeded or increased depending on how ready the individual is, on a psychological level, to maintain that change.

Box 26.1 Treatment aims for substance misuse

- Reduction of the use of illicit or non-prescribed drugs by the individual
- Assist the individual to remain healthy, until, with appropriate care and support, they can achieve a drug-free life
- Deal with the problems related to substance misuse
- Reduce the duration of episodes of substance misuse
- Reduce the dangers associated with substance misuse, particularly the risk of HIV, hepatitis B and C, and other blood-borne infections from injecting and sharing injecting paraphernalia
- Reduce the chance of future relapse to substance misuse
- Reduce the need for criminal activity to finance substance misuse
- Reduce the risk of prescribed drugs being diverted on to the illegal market
- Stabilize the individual, where appropriate, on substitute medication, to alleviate withdrawal symptoms
- Improve overall personal, social and family well-being.

(Adapted from Department of Health 1999).

PROCHASKA AND DICLEMENTE (1982) MODEL OF BEHAVIOUR CHANGE

This model was developed in an attempt to make sense of the processes individuals go through in making changes to their behaviour. It provides a good structure to think about changing drug (including tobacco) and alcohol using behaviours as, not only can the stage the patient is at on a cognitive level be mapped, but the model also give some guidance on the interventions the patient may be able to respond to and make use of at any given time. The model is explained in more detail on p. 23 but the main stages are:

1 Pre-contemplation
2 Contemplation
3 Determination
4 Action
5 Maintenance.

It is important to note that the model is circular in approach rather than linear. This acknowledges that effecting change is difficult and not a direct process. Individuals may journey around the circle any number of times before effecting behaviour change. They may fall out of the stages at any point. When this happens during the active change stage or the maintenance stage it is called relapse. Individuals who experience relapse may then enter back into the circle at any given point. Individuals will also reside in each of the stages for varying lengths of time; for example, they may stay in contemplation for years and then a significant event might occur that focuses them into thinking about how to change.

How does the model of behaviour change fit with intervention?

Substance-using individuals will go round this cycle autonomously, without treatment. Things will happen in their lives that will make them think about their use, and spur decisions to attempt to change their behaviour. Some people will be successful on their own in this; for example, the birth of a child means a couple can no longer attend clubs, so their use of ecstasy is discontinued. But for others, who may be physically or psychologically dependent on the substance, or be in a context where social factors may make it difficult to change, outside help may be required.

The model works as an aid to guide both the clinician and the user toward which interventions would be most useful at a given time. For example, individuals who have been referred to drug services via the criminal justice system may not feel that they have a problem with drug use. They would be in the pre-contemplation stage of the model. They might then benefit from an approach such as motivational interviewing, which would work towards moving them on to look at their drug or alcohol use in a less positive light. They would not generally, however, benefit from an intervention such as relapse prevention at this stage, as they have not yet acknowledged that they have a problem. An intervention such as relapse prevention would be targeted mainly around the maintenance stage.

A SAMPLE OF CLINICAL INTERVENTIONS USED WITH SUBSTANCE MISUSERS

Medical interventions

Medical interventions tend to be focused on the detoxification or maintenance of substance users who are physically dependent on their substances. The major treatment groups for medical interventions are people using heroin, benzodiazepines, cigarettes and alcohol. There is also a limited amount of medical intervention for people with dependency on stimulant drugs.

Why prescribe substitute drugs?

Prescribing is the responsibility of the prescribing practitioner, whether this is the individual's general practitioner or a specialist doctor in a drug treatment facility. Prescribing medication as an alternative to the individual's drug of choice may fulfil a number of different functions, some of which are listed below:

● Offer an opportunity to stabilize drug intake and lifestyle whilst breaking with previous illicit drug use and associated unhealthy behaviours
● Reduce or prevent withdrawal symptoms (Box 26.2)
● Promote the process of change in drug taking (giving the person a 'clean' start)
● Promote the process of change in risk-taking behaviours (e.g. moving to oral methadone from injecting heroin reduces the risk of hepatitis and HIV infection)
● Helping to maintain contact and offer the individual an opportunity to gain support in working towards change.

The prescription of substitute drugs can fulfil two main functions: withdrawal and detoxification. Some individuals

---

Box 26.2 Signs and symptoms of opiate withdrawal

● Sweating
● Lacrimation and rhinorrhea
● Yawning
● Feeling hot and cold
● Anorexia and abdominal cramps
● Nausea, vomiting and diarrhoea
● Tremor
● Insomnia and restlessness
● Generalized aches and pains
● Tachycardia, hypertension
● Gooseflesh
● Dilated pupils
● Increased bowel sounds.

can withdraw from their drug of choice without substitute medication. This might require outside support and changes in the individual's lifestyle and environment. They may be using a drug on which they are not physically dependent, or they may have the support and be prepared to endure the effects of withdrawal in order to become drug free in as short a space of time as possible.

For others, who may have a history of serious withdrawal complications, for example alcohol withdrawal, epileptic fits, or a number of failed attempts at self-detoxification or other problems such as lack of social support, substitute prescribing may be necessary. Substitute prescribing for withdrawal gives the user the opportunity to withdraw from their drug in a controlled manner. This is achieved by titration of the substitute drug (for example methadone as a substitute for heroin) to the user's current level of use of the illicit drug. The level is then reduced in a controlled manner over an agreed period of time. Withdrawal symptoms should therefore be prevented by careful titration of dose and careful management by both the prescribing doctor and the user. Theoretically, detoxification in this way can be slow (possibly over a period of months in the community) or quick (over a period of days or weeks in an inpatient facility).

Withdrawal symptoms are not unified phenomena and differ according to such factors as the pharmacological profile of the individual and the half-life of the drug. The severity of the withdrawal symptoms is not clearly or directly related to the quantity of drugs previously consumed, thus withdrawal cannot be quantified directly. It is therefore probably best to assume that any drug that has been consumed heavily for a significant period of time may give rise to withdrawal effects in the user. This can apply to cocaine, amphetamines and also cannabis, as well as alcohol and the opioid drugs such as heroin and methadone. Box 26.2 gives an example of symptoms and signs of opiate withdrawal.

Detoxification programmes will generally prove to be successful only if the individual is motivated to remain drug-free. Therefore, the individual will generally be in the Action and Maintenance stage of the cycle of change. Controlled drug use is problematic, as tolerance will quickly develop, leading to redevelopment of old patterns of use. There is also a danger of unintentional suicide, particularly with opioid drugs, as the detoxified body will have low tolerance of the old drug of choice, particularly at pretreatment dosage levels. Thus reverting back to the same quantity of drug may result in fatal overdose, owing to the body's low tolerance.

Medical regimens such as detoxification should not be applied in isolation. As we know, substance misuse is a complex biopsychosocial phenomenon, and as such requires a raft of supporting interventions. The newly detoxified individual will need additional support around how to stay drug-free, particularly returning to the very context where drug use was maintained. Concurrent approaches such as relapse prevention and counselling are essential to such a treatment package.

Maintenance prescribing

Substitute prescribing can be used to maintain the individual on a level so that withdrawal does not begin, thus allowing the person to carry out normal tasks of daily living (e.g. manage to keep their job). Methadone maintenance programmes have been shown to be effective in reducing all of the following factors: injecting behaviour, illicit opiate use, criminal activity and costs to society. Maintenance programmes may be used for patients who take longer to work towards abstinence. It is a useful intervention particularly with patients in the Contemplation stage, giving them space and time away from pursuing their addiction to think through the life changes they want to achieve.

Withdrawal profile and substituted drug for opiates

● Untreated heroin withdrawal typically reaches its peak 36–72 hours after the last dose. Symptoms usually subside after 5 days
● Untreated methadone withdrawal typically reaches its peak between 4 and 6 days after the last dose. Symptoms do not usually subside for 10–12 days.

Motivational interviewing

Motivational interviewing is a key therapeutic technique when working with individuals who abuse substances. It is particularly useful as a means of engaging and working with individuals in the primary stages of change, notably pre-contemplation, contemplation and the determination–action stage.

Motivational interviewing adopts the tenet that motivation is not something that an individual *has*, but rather is something that an individual *does*. It recognizes that individuals, in general, are ambivalent to the change process. It is not, therefore, until something happens to tip the balance that individuals work towards change. For example, a person may have spent many years smoking. They may be well aware of the significant health risks involved, but these seem far removed and they enjoy smoking. Therefore, they are fairly ambivalent about changing their behaviour and giving up. They may attempt to give up on 1 January every year, but their motivation to change is not significant enough and they may quickly return to the 'weed'. At this point the positives and negatives of smoking are fairly equally balanced for the individual. When visiting their general practitioner they may discover that they have a tumour of some kind, and have to go for tests to see whether it is cancerous or benign. They may link this to smoking – and suddenly the negatives outweigh the positives. This may move the individual from the pre-contemplation or contemplation stage of the model to the determination and action stages, where they begin actively to formulate plans on how to give up.

Motivational interviewing seeks to tap into this process of behaviour change by working with individuals in stages of pre-contemplation and contemplation to speed up their movement round the cycle. By allowing the individuals space and time to come up with their own list of positive and negative aspects of the behaviour, the process brings to the fore discrepancies and highlights disparities. Its primary aim is to aid individuals to come to their own conclusions about the need to change their substance use; consequently this technique may be as helpful in smoking cessation work as in helping people to give up alcohol and other drugs. There are four main principles of motivational interviewing which are highlighted below.

Express empathy

This involves the nurse reflecting back what they have heard, the use of good 'active' listening skills, paying attention to things such as eye contact, facial expression and body orientation. The therapist attempts to understand the client's 'world', while suspending advice, judgement and questioning.

Develop discrepancy

This involves a process of exploration of the individual's personal goals, prompting him or her to consider the steps that would be needed to achieve the goals. The individual is asked to highlight any possible consequences of substance use. Reflective listening is used selectively to reinforce the individual's recognition that substance abuse interferes with goal attainment.

Avoid arguments

It is better to 'roll with resistance' rather than oppose it. Exploration of resistance is far more useful as arguments tend to strengthen, not weaken, the individual's beliefs and convictions. You should avoid supplying the reasons for behaviour change: individuals should state these themselves. Ambivalence to change should be viewed as 'normal', not pathological.

Support self-efficacy

The therapist should express confidence that change is possible and that the individual has the personal resources to do it. It is important to instill hope, whilst acknowledging past frustrations. It is also useful to explore how the individual has experienced other successes in the past.

Relapse prevention

Relapse prevention is a cognitive behavioural intervention. The basis of the approach is encouraging the individual to use self-management strategies aimed at enhancing maintenance of a change in behaviour, once that change has been achieved. This involves teaching the person a system of self-control requiring behavioural skills training, cognitive interventions and changes in lifestyle.

Dependent behaviours are seen as 'over-learned habits' – certain behaviours that have become a way of coping and that the individual can change. Instead of focusing on avoidance, the therapist as educator seeks to help the client learn different ways of coping with stressful situations.

Relapse prevention work is located in the maintenance stage of the cycle of change model. However, it is useful if a number of skills associated with avoiding relapse are practised during sessions with the individual's keyworker or therapist prior to the maintenance stage. This will give the client a sense of achievement over some of the skills needed to prevent relapse.

McDowell and Spitz (1999) stress the importance of preventing relapse. The person has to be continuously on their guard against even one single use of the substance they have misused (such as a casual drink) as this will easily trigger a return to full blown dependency. Strategies need to be rehearsed that will help avoid this problem and which include family and friends. A common behaviour is to substitute one dependency for another as the new compulsive behaviour helps kick the old habit. Sometimes this can be harmful such as heavy smoking but can be beneficial such as community work or physical exercise. Such beneficial activities should be encouraged. Time management to avoid empty periods when temptation may reappear also helps.

The importance of timed intervention

It is impossible to overstress the importance of the interventions in substance misuse being linked directly to the stage of change of the client, if they are to be effective. In substance misuse, where there is evidence of significant physical dependence, the initial phase of treatment may involve 'detoxification' in an inpatient or community setting (principles of which are described above). These interventions may be physical or psychological, or both.

In substance misuse, where 'detoxification' is not deemed necessary, the initial phase of treatment should involve a clear decision about what the goals are, and what changes need to be made. Motivational interviewing techniques are ideal for working with an individual during this stage. This may involve the individual aiming for abstinence or aiming to cut down on their intake (control).

The initial stage of treatment will comprise assessment and some form of therapeutic technique (e.g. motivational interviewing). With clients who are aiming for abstinence, relapse prevention work is best carried out during the maintenance phase, i.e. once they have stopped using their substances.

For individuals whose goal is control rather than abstinence, relapse prevention techniques can be used soon after they have made the decision to change their behaviour, thereby equipping them with the means to alter both the ways they think about substances and their lifestyle patterns to make it more likely that change will be adhered to.

Relapse prevention may also be an appropriate intervention if an individual has made a 'slip' during a successful period of maintenance. Individuals need regular reviews and support to maintain the change in their behaviour, and any intervention should have a good period of follow-up attached to it.

Self-help groups

Self-help groups have an important role in the maintenance of a drug- or alcohol-free lifestyle once treatment has ended. They may also be used as an adjunct to treatment or as a treatment regimen in their own right. Self-help groups such as Narcotics Anonymous (NA) and Alcoholics Anonymous (AA) aim to help the substance misuser become or remain abstinent. AA and NA are based on a 12-step approach through which a number of objectives are set. The approach aims gradually to build up the individual's refusal skills and sense of self-efficacy by initially getting the individual to pledge to give up their substance(s) of choice for just 1 day. (A shorter time period may be involved if 1 day appears too difficult.) From that, the length of time is extended. The groups provide daily support that the individual can key into, wherever they are. They also provide a buddy system from existing members. As with any treatment approach, it may be highly successful for some individuals but not for others. Good practice would dictate that, for all individuals with drug or alcohol problems, their awareness is raised to the location of any available, relevant self-help groups in their area.

HEALTH PROMOTION AND EDUCATION

Nursing staff should be ideally placed to offer advice on health promotion and education, in any work settings. The aim is to achieve 'prevention' or 'early intervention' through clear information. Ways you might achieve this could be:

- an environment conducive to health promotion (e.g. poster displays)
- contact with local and national health promotion units
- providing information leaflets, with clear explanations
- advice and support, for example on local self-help groups for individuals and/or families or significant others
- advice on legal issues, for instance contact with the Citizens' Advice Bureau
- advice on health hazards of injecting (e.g. abscesses, septicaemia, thrombophlebitis, hepatitis B and C, HIV).

Patients may be advised that the following will help reduce alcohol intake:

- Drinking more slowly and avoid buying rounds when out with groups of people
- Set a budget and stick to it for your expenditure in an evening
- See if a friend will join you in cutting down their alcohol intake
- Try and have 1 or 2 days a week when you do not drink any alcohol
- Think about how much money you could save by not drinking so heavily and what other benefits there may be.

A similar approach may be tried in advising patients about reducing the risk of harm from illegal drug use. Patients may therefore be advised to:

- Avoid sharing any injecting equipment
- Avoid getting hot when using ecstasy
- Try not to use when alone
- Consider socializing with friends who do not use drugs
- Think about alternative activities to drug use

- Seek professional counselling and support
- Go on a first aid course to learn resuscitation skills which will help in the event of a friend collapsing while using drugs.

Finally, smoking cessation advise should suggest setting a definite date at which the person stops and the use of nicotine replacement therapy. They should also be warned that some weight gain is inevitable as nicotine is an appetite suppressant and therefore they need to consider their diet and activity levels also.

Health promotion is also about challenging the many misconceptions that surround substance misuse. In the case of drug taking, the following messages need to be promoted, alongside active measures to reduce the level of drug use:

- Not all young people take drugs
- Not all drug takers are addicts
- Not all drugs kill
- Not all drug takers commit crime
- Illegal drugs are not the unique preserve of people from particular social or ethnic backgrounds
- The majority of people in the UK do not take, nor have they ever taken, an illegal substance
- The majority of those who have are experimenters or casual users
- The majority of illegal drug users do so for 'recreational purposes'
- The minority of illegal drug users become dependent.

SUICIDE

There is no doubt that substance misuse is inextricably linked with the increased incidence of suicide and suicide attempts. A form of substance misuse may all too frequently be the chosen method of suicide. Also, self-medication of a primary psychiatric disorder or a medical condition may lead to increased impulsivity and poor judgement, and thus may enhance the potential for accidental suicide risk. The most recent year for which full UK statistics are available is 2003 and during that year there were 5755 UK adult suicides, the lowest number since 1973 (NSO 2005). Suicide remains much more common in men with a rate of 18.1 per 100 000 compared with 5.8 for women during 2003. Within the male statistics, there was a marked regional variation with Wales having the worst rate averaged over 2000–03; 40% higher than Eastern England, which had the lowest rate. However, Blackpool had the dubious claim of being the town with the highest male suicide rate in the UK at 39.1/100 000. There is one notable variation in the female statistics. Within the UK, women born in India or East Africa have a 40% higher suicide rate than those born in England and Wales (Samaritans 2005). Nurses working with members of these communities should therefore be particularly alert for signs of depression and distress in such women.

Suicides are usually not 'out of the blue' and unexpected. Approximately one-quarter of individuals who have committed suicide have been in contact with mental health services in the year before their death. Of these, there were high rates of alcohol and drug misuse, with 17% misusing both alcohol and drugs.

DEFINITIONS

Self-harm involves self-inflicted injury (e.g. cutting) or harm (poisoning) often as a means of drawing attention to the self or as a means of relieving distress. Only the more extreme cases are suicidal. This broad category of risk includes suicidal behaviours with a planned intent, suicidal behaviours as a call for help, attention through cutting or mutilation, and abusing or addictive behaviours with the intention of inflicting harm or injury. Suicide is therefore the product of total despair with the person unable to see any other course of action open to them.

RISK FACTORS

Risk factors are characteristic of people that are used to attempt to predict the degree of risk for individuals. Effective suicide assessment involves the assessment of these risk factors to attempt to understand the risk to a particular individual, in the context of his or her own environment at this particular moment. They are more effective in predicting risk in the long term than in the immediate future but should not be thought of as automatic causes of suicide. They are predisposing factors whose presence makes suicide more likely.

Many factors are associated with an increased risk of suicide but the main ones are:

- serious mental illness
- previous attempts
- drug/alcohol problems
- male gender
- unemployment and social isolation
- recent contact with caring professions and other helping agencies, suicidal ideation may have been discussed.

The incidence of substance misuse, as a characteristic risk factor in suicide, features prominently in the research and literature. The expression of suicidal ideas was the strongest predictor of suicide; however, some people indicated their risk in less direct ways, for instance through increased alcohol intake.

Alcohol and drug misuse increase the risk of death by suicide dramatically, and are second only to depressive illness as a contributory factor in suicidal behaviour. It has been found, for example, that chronic alcoholics have a 70–80 times greater risk of suicide in the 5 years following discharge from inpatient treatment than the rest of the population. Moreover, post-mortem studies have shown that almost half of the men and one-fifth of the women had taken alcohol a few hours before the actual act of suicide. Alcohol is likely to produce a depression of mood, which in itself is a major factor in suicide. In addition, alcohol tends to reduce inhibition and releases aggressive behaviour in some individuals and thus may prompt precipitate action in those who otherwise would refrain from such behaviour.

The *Safer Services* report (Department of Health 1999), focusing on suicides in the mental health population, found the most common drugs used in overdose were those prescribed to treat mental disorder (psychotropic drugs); people who had committed suicide and who had previously harmed themselves were more likely to have taken an overdose of psychotropic drugs. The most common diagnoses were depression, schizophrenia, personality disorder, and alcohol or drug dependence. Around half also had a second (co-morbid) diagnosis, indicating more complex treatment needs.

Alarmingly, suicide rates for young men have risen to such an extent that this is the leading cause of death in men aged under 35 in the UK. The rate amongst men aged 25–34 in 2002 was 25 per 100 000, compared with an overall UK average of 10 per 100 000. There has been a slight reduction (11%) in these numbers since the worst year which was 1992 (Samaritans 2005). Although it is difficult to identify clear reasons for this, the considerable social and economic changes in society may have contributed. The suicide rate in UK male prison inmates is on average 5 times higher than males of the same age in the general population. In the age range 15–17, suicide rates are 18 times higher (Fazel et al 2005). This disturbing statistic seriously calls into question health care within the prison system and highlights the high levels of mental illness in this difficult environment.

Risk-mitigating factors

Assessment of suicide risk, based on risk factors alone fails to recognize a balance between risk factors and protective factors. People with high scores on risk factors may be mitigated by a counterbalance of protection against each. Similarly, a stable condition may become high risk if the individual's care is reduced.

Assessment

We cannot be effective without acquiring skills at recognizing suicide risk at interview. From the first encounter, we need to engender an alliance based on hope. Caution is advised in the use of the risk factor research because the assessment needs to be individualized, using the research as a secondary check to back up the clinical assessment. Any use of weightings or rating scales should carefully reflect the person's own context – reducing a person to a series of numbers will never accurately reflect their real experience.

When meeting a client there are a number of clues that may indicate the presence of depression or abnormal distress, both of which heighten the risk of suicidal behaviour. Careful observation is required to ensure that such signs are not missed, and a quick ABC test should be applied:

- **A**ppearance – evidence of self neglect in a normally well groomed person should not go unnoticed; conversely, some people will maintain a 'front' by not allowing their appearance to give away important clues to inner feelings.

- **B**ody language – dejection, characterized by loss of spring in step, laboured gait, retarded body movements.
- **C**ontent of speech – negative attitudes towards the future, no point in planning ahead, general lack of concern, no prospect of future improvements.

If there is a suspicion of suicidal thought, you should proceed to sensitively explore this. Jarvis (2004) suggests the following are useful questions to ask:

- Have you ever felt so blue that you thought of hurting yourself?
- Do you feel like hurting yourself now?
- Do you have a plan to hurt yourself?
- What would happen if you were dead?
- How do you think would other people react if you were dead?

Nurses may be very reluctant to enter this kind of conversation with a patient as there is always an element of taboo about death and suicide. However, the patient's life may depend upon recognition of their suicidal intent early enough to offer treatment and prevent an unnecessary death.

High risk factors for suicide are summarized by the mnemonic SAD PERSONS in Box 26.3, while Box 26.4 lists factors associated with a lethal outcome of any attempt.

The assessment of suicide is not easy and some of the problems that may be encountered are:

- deliberate denial of suicide risk by the patient
- variable degrees of risk, linked to ever-changing circumstances
- false improvement
- lack of trust by the patient in services

Box 26.3   Summary of suicide risk factors: SAD PERSONS

Sex – Male

Age – Young

Depression or hopelessness

Previous suicide attempts or psychiatric admissions

Excess alcohol/drug use

Rational thinking deficit

Separated, divorced, bereaved

Organized or serious attempt

No social supports

Stated future intention to commit suicide.

(From Filbin et al 2002)

- staff feeling 'manipulated' by the expression of suicidal intent
- staff or patients avoiding the difficult, and potentially traumatic, issue
- dealing with feelings of anger, resentment and lack of cooperation.

INTERVENTIONS

If the nurse is concerned about a potential suicide risk in a patient, the mental health services and the patient's general practitioner should be involved immediately, whatever the situation. If the nurse finds him- or herself with a crisis situation in which a patient is threatening immediate suicide or actually attempting suicide, the key points to consider are:

- Do I attempt to take control to save the person?
- What can I realistically do in the circumstances?
- Making the patient fully aware of the consequences of his or her actions, stating that there are certain things that are impossible for you to do
- Acknowledge that sometimes, despite the best efforts of staff, patients do kill themselves on hospital wards and in other care environments.

Box 26.4   Assessment of lethality

Plans
- Has the person made any?
- How well formulated are they?
- For how long has the person had them?
- How often does the person think about them?
- How realistic are the plans?

Method
- How lethal is the method chosen?
- Is the method chosen irreversible?
- What does the person know about this method?
- Does the person have access to this method?

Discovery
- How likely is the person to be discovered?
- Has the person made active plans to avoid discovery?

Past history
- Has the person attempted suicide before?
- What were the details and circumstances of the previous attempt?
- Are there current similarities in circumstances?
- Is there a family or significant other history?

(From Gianfrancesco 1999)

The nurse always owes the patient a duty of care and, in the case of a suicidal patient, this includes (Morgan 1998):

- performing professional responsibilities to an accepted standard
- considering all the options with relevant others, where permissible by time and accessibility
- clearly documenting discussions, decisions and interventions
- being explicit about what is possible and what is clearly impossible in the light of:
  - time
  - place
  - available resources
  - expectations.

DELIBERATE SELF-HARM

'Self-injurious behaviour', 'self-destructive behaviour', 'deliberate self-harm', 'self-mutilation', 'self-abuse' are clinical labels used to describe actions by a person towards herself or himself that result in physical harm to the body. Self-injury ranges from mild or superficial effects, to permanent physical damage, to life-threatening dangers. The nurse will encounter patients who have self-harmed in A&E and on overnight short-stay wards, usually after self-poisoning. Recent trends in A&E attendance rates continue upwards but reductions in the size of packets introduced in 1998 do seem to have reduced the number of paracetamol overdoses being seen. Relationship difficulties are the most common reasons for deliberate self-harm attendances and females aged 10–19 are four times more likely than males in the same age group to engage in deliberate self-harm (Hawton et al 2003).

Types of self-harming include:

- cutting
- burning
- scalding
- head banging
- hair pulling
- ligatures around the neck
- scratching
- swallowing objects
- punching
- inserting objects
- overdosing.

Estimates of the prevalence of self-harm vary between 0.4% and more than 10% of the population. Given the prevalence, however, self-harm is still generally misunderstood. Self-injury is often labelled as 'attention seeking' or attempted suicide, and when people who harm themselves come into contact with health and social care agencies they often feel that the treatment they receive exacerbates rather than relieves their distress (Pacitti 1998).

The true figures for people self-injuring are not known. Some people will self-injure in the privacy of their own home and never share their distress. Self-injury is often linked to suicide and the term 'para-suicide' is sometimes used to label the behaviour. Most people who self-injure do not wish to commit suicide. Rather, they want to find some tangible way of relieving their emotional pain and distress. Individuals who harm themselves frequently describe a history of physical or sexual abuse in childhood. Hidden within a shame-bound family system, abusive events are kept secret from outside the family, and are often denied within the family as well. Self-injury can often be an outward, visible signal from the self-injuring person to himself or herself and/or others about the internalized pain of the victimization (MIND 2005).

Myths and fantasies surround deliberate self-harm. These include:

- self-injury is a sign of madness or deep mental disturbance
- people who self-injure are trying to kill themselves
- the severity of the injury represents the severity of the condition
- if it is not an artery, they do not mean it
- people who injure themselves are a danger to others
- self-injury is about attention seeking
- self-injury is used to manipulate others
- self-injury is just a habit to be stopped
- people who self-injure enjoy or do not feel physical pain
- it is masochism.

Self-injury and suicide have an intimate relationship, but they are different. Every individual has their own motivations and mix of self-injuring and suicidal feelings:

- self-injury often represents the prevention of a suicidal period
- self-injury may be one way of averting suicide
- self-injury may be a survival strategy
- self-injury frequently represents the least possible amount of damage and represents extreme self-restraint.

Many people who commit deliberate self-harm repeat the act at some time: 15–25% are re-admitted to hospital within 12 months, the first 3 months being the most risky time. The more social and personal problems that are present, the greater the likelihood of the suicidal behaviour being repeated. Unfortunately, each repetition increases the chances of unintentional suicide and many such people have undoubtedly died unintentionally through misjudgement or bad luck and are recorded under the suicide statistics.

Moreover, there is a subgroup of individuals who chronically repeat their self-harming behaviour and who pose an enormous challenge for the helping agencies. They tend to differ from the repetition group in that they consist of those with much more severe personality problems, criminal records, and abuse of alcohol and drugs. Their lifestyle tends to be rather disorganized with frequent visits to psychiatric hospital, court appearances, prison sentences, etc. They may also have a history of violence to others or property.

ASSESSMENT

Haslett et al (2002) note the following factors are significant in considering the risk of an episode of deliberate self-harm escalating into a future suicide:

- Psychiatric illness such as depression or schizophrenia
- Age over 45
- Male sex
- Living alone
- Unemployed
- Recently bereaved, divorced or separated
- Chronic physical ill health
- Drug or alcohol misuse
- Violent method used in deliberate self-harm such as jumping
- Suicide note was left
- History of previous deliberate self-harm.

INTERVENTION

Staff working in A&E departments may form negative attitudes towards those who self-harm. Perhaps the challenging behaviour we sometimes encounter in those who self-harm is a defence against other people's judgements. Most of these individuals need nothing more than the kind of care that any injured person would expect. While there will be debate over areas of safe practice, cooperation creates trust and allows the individual and the clinician to explore the pain together verbally. Although the behaviour may be seen as an observable manifestation of a person's pain, it is really a consequence of their intervention against that pain, and not a symptom of it. For nurses to be able to help with the problems that underlie self-harm they must first learn to recognize this difference. In the past, nurses were encouraged to ignore or suppress these values when dealing with the distress of individuals who self-harm. This has led to professionals applying unnatural standards in their inter- actions with patients. Basic human qualities in addition to clinical techniques are most effective, particularly when dealing with people who have these sorts of difficulties.

SUMMARY

This chapter has reviewed the effects of alcohol, tobacco and other drug use on health, and offered insights into the assessment and management of these conditions. Nurses working in general hospitals or primary care will spend a great deal of their time caring for people whose health problems stem from the use of drugs, both legal and illegal. The subject is therefore the business of all nurses, not just mental health nurses or nurses working in specialist treatment centres. Whether it be the school nurse, practice nurse, nurse practitioner or A&E nurse, to name but a few, all nurses have a role to play in reducing the harmful effects of drugs in common use today. The principles outlined in this chapter for assessment and for helping people reduce or cease altogether their drug use are valuable whether applied by a practice nurse to smoking cessation clinics in primary care or by specialist nurses in a drug detoxification and treatment centre.

REFERENCES

Bateman M (2005) The Wolverhampton prolific and other priority offenders programme. British Journal of Nursing 14(17): 924–27.

Bennet P, Brown M (2003) Clinical pharmacology. Edinburgh: Churchill Livingstone.

Buckis C (2005) High and dry. Nursing Standard 20(10): 24–25.

Department of Health (DoH) (1999) Safer services: national confidential inquiry into suicide and homicide by people with mental illness. London: The Stationery Office.

Department of Health (DoH) (2002) Updated Government Drug Strategy. Online. Available: www.drugs.gov.uk/drug-strategy

CRITICAL INCIDENT

You are a psychiatric liaison nurse in a busy district general hospital A&E department. On your return from 2 weeks' annual leave, your first consultation is with a 27-year-old woman brought in by her husband with their two children (8 and 4 years old). You already have messages that she has been brought to A&E on four previous occasions during the last fortnight.

She is once again alcohol intoxicated, has re-opened wounds on her forearms, upper arms and abdomen, initially self-inflicted with a cheese-knife. She tells you that she smokes 30 cigarettes a day and occasionally smokes cannabis when her husband is out at work. She has a previous psychiatric history, with two suicide attempts on the ward shortly after admission to the psychiatric unit.

Her Muslim husband and the family's GP are requesting a psychiatric admission. On each recent presentation, she has been kept overnight on the A&E observation ward, and discharged home the following day. She strongly suggests she does not need medication and will only use it to overdose if her home circumstances become too intense.

Reflection

- What is your assessment of the problems presented within the scope of this case scenario?
- What role do you think substance abuse may be contributing to these problems?
- What reasons may this woman have for using the substances mentioned?
- What treatment interventions and support options may be available to use in this situation?

Department of Health (DoH) (2005) Statistics on Alcohol for England 2004. Online. Available: www.dh.gov.uk

Donovan DM, Marlatt GA (1988) Assessment of addictive behaviours. New York: Guilford Press.

Fazel S, Benning R, Danesh J (2005) Suicides in male prisoners in England and Wales 1978–2003. Lancet 366(9493): 1301–1302.

Filbin M, Tsien C, Caughey A (2002) Clinical cases in emergency medicine. Malden: Blackwell.

Fletcher A (2004) Alcohol screening in emergency departments. Emergency Nurse 12(7): 22–27.

Gianfrancesco P (1999) Suicide risk. Presentation at a practitioner workshop for South Islington Crisis Response Team, St Pancreas Hospital, London, 21 April.

Gournay K Sandford T Johnson G (1997) Dual diagnosis of severe mental health problems and substance abuse/dependence: a major priority for mental health nursing. Journal of Mental Health and Psychiatric Nursing 4:1–7.

Haslett C, Chilvers ER, Boon, NA, Colledge NR, Hunter JA (2002) Davidson's principles and Practice of Medicine, 19th edn. Edinburgh: Churchill Livingstone.

Hawton K, Fagg J, Simkin S et al (2003) Deliberate self-harm in Oxford. Report of the Centre for Suicide Research, Oxford University. Oxford: OUP.

Horgan J (2005) The electric kool-aid trial. New Scientist 26 February: 36–39.

Institute of Alcohol Studies (1997–2000). IAS factsheets. London: IAS.

Institute of Alcohol Studies (1999) Factsheet: Alcohol and the elderly. London: IAS.

Institute of Alcohol Studies (2005a) Factsheet: Alcohol and health. London: IAS.

Institute of Alcohol Studies (2005b) Factsheet: Women and alcohol. London: IAS.

Jarvis C (2004) Physical examination and health assessment. Philadelphia: Elsevier.

Jensen TK (1998) Does moderate alcohol consumption affect fertility? British Medical Journal 317: 505–510.

Manley D (1998) Dual diagnosis: approaches to the treatment of people with dual mental health and drug abuse problems. Mental Health Care 1(6): 190–192.

McDowell D, Spitz H (1999) Substance abuse. Philadelphia: Brunner Mazel.

MIND (2005) Factsheet. Deliberate self-harm. Online. Available: www.mind.org

Morgan S (1998) Assessing and managing risk – a practitioner handbook. Brighton: Pavilion.

Nicoll R, Alger B (2004) The brain's own marijuana. Scientific American December: 44–51.

NSO (2005) National Statistics Office. Online. Available: www.statistics.gov.uk/cci/nugget.asp?id=1092

NTA (2005) National Treatment Agency for Substance Misuse. Online. Available: www.nta.nhs.uk

Pacitti R (1998) Damage limitation. Nursing Times 94:27–39.

Prochaska JO, DiClemente CC (1982) Transtheoretical therapy: toward a more integrative model of change. Psychotherapy Theory, Research and Practice 19: 276–288.

Russel M (1994) Screening for pregnancy risk drinking. Alcoholism: Clinical and Experimental Research 18: 1156–1161.

Samaritans (2005) The Samaritans. Online. Available: www.samaritans.org

Sargent S (2005) The aetiology, management and complications of alcoholic hepatitis. British Journal of Nursing 14(10): 556–562.

Strategy Unit (2004) Alcohol harm reduction strategy for England. London: Cabinet Office.

Szalavitz M (2005) Demon healer. New Scientist 23 July: 37–39.

World Health Organization (WHO) (2005) Factsheets. Online. Available: www.who.int/substance_abuse

USEFUL WEBSITES

Department of Health	www.dh.gov.uk
Health Protection Agency	www.hpa.org.uk/hpa/publications
Institute of Alcohol Studies	www.ias.org.uk
MIND	www.mind.org.uk
National Statistics Office	www.statistics.gov.uk
National Treatment Agency for Substance Misuse (NTA)	www.nta.nhs.uk
Oxford Centre for Suicide Research	www.cebmh.warne.ox.ac.uk/crs
The Samaritans	www.samaritans.org
World Health Organization Drug Misuse	www.who.int/substance_abuse
Drug information	www.talktofrank.com

Appendix 1: Resuscitation guidelines

Your actions in the first few seconds after finding a collapsed person, whatever the circumstances, could determine whether the person survives or not. We have therefore presented in this appendix some of the key guidelines, with kind permission, from the UK Resuscitation Council which were revised in 2005. The situations covered are:

- Adult Basic Life Support. What to do if you find a collapsed person anywhere outside a hospital/health centre
- In Hospital Resuscitation. What to do if you find a collapsed person in hospital. Nurses are the most likely group of staff to encounter this situation. You are the first person there with no equipment or crash cart to hand, what do you do next?
- Adult Advanced Life Support. These guidelines explain what will happen when experienced staff take over with the full range of resuscitation equipment.

For further details, discussion of actions and changes that have been made to the old guidelines, please visit the Resuscitation Council website at www.resus.org.uk

ADULT BASIC LIFE SUPPORT

INTRODUCTION

This section contains the guidelines for adult basic life support (BLS). Like the other guidelines, it is based on the document *2005 International Consensus on Cardiopulmonary Resuscitation and Emergency Cardiovascular Care Science with Treatment Recommendations* (CoSTR), which was published in November 2005. Basic life support implies that no equipment is employed other than a protective device.

GUIDELINE CHANGES

There are two main underlying themes in the BLS section of CoSTR: the need to increase the number of chest compressions given to a victim of cardiac arrest, and the importance of simplifying guidelines to aid acquisition and retention of BLS skills, particularly for laypersons.

It is well documented that interruptions in chest compression are common (Van Alem et al 2003) and are associated with a reduced chance of survival for the victim (Eftestol et al 2002). The 'perfect' solution is to deliver continuous

compressions whilst giving ventilations independently. This is possible when the victim has an advanced airway in place, and is discussed in the adult advanced life support (ALS) section. Chest-compression-only CPR is another way to increase the number of compressions given and will, by definition, eliminate pauses. It is effective for a limited period only (about 5 min) (Hallstrom et al 2000). and is not recommended as standard management of out-of-hospital cardiac arrest.

The following changes in the BLS guidelines have been made to reflect the greater importance placed on chest compression, and to attempt to reduce the number and duration of pauses:

1 Make a diagnosis of cardiac arrest if a victim is unresponsive and not breathing normally.
2 Teach rescuers to place their hands in the centre of the chest, rather than to spend more time using the 'rib margin' method.
3 Give each rescue breath over 1 second rather than 2 seconds.
4 Use a ratio of compressions to ventilations of 30:2 for all adult victims of sudden cardiac arrest. Use this same ratio for children when attended by a lay rescuer.
5 For an adult victim, omit the initial 2 rescue breaths and give 30 compressions immediately after cardiac arrest is established.

To aid teaching and learning, the sequence of actions has been simplified. In some cases, simplification has been based on recently published evidence; in others there was no evidence that the previous, more complicated, sequence had any beneficial effect on survival.

There are other changes in the guidelines. In particular, allowance has been made for the rescuer who is unable or unwilling to perform rescue breathing. It is well recorded that reluctance to perform mouth-to-mouth ventilation, in spite of the lack of evidence of risk, inhibits many would-be rescuers from attempting any form of resuscitation. These guidelines encourage chest compression alone in such circumstances.

Guidelines 2000 introduced the concept of checking for 'signs of a circulation'. This change was made because of the evidence that relying on a check of the carotid pulse to diagnose cardiac arrest is unreliable and time-consuming, mainly, but not exclusively, when attempted by non-healthcare professionals (Bahr et al 1997). Subsequent studies have shown

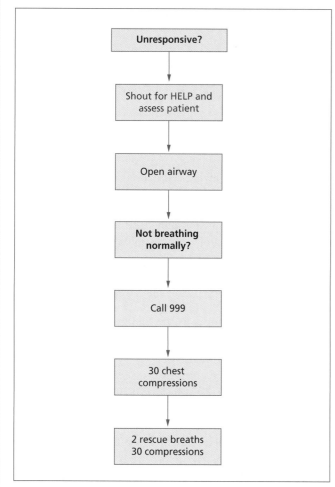

Figure A1.1 Adult Basic Life Support (from the Resuscitation Council, UK, with permission).

that checking for breathing is also prone to error, particularly as agonal gasps are frequently misdiagnosed as normal breathing (Hauff et al 2003). In Guidelines 2005 the absence of breathing, in a non-responsive victim, continues to be the main sign of cardiac arrest. Also highlighted is the need to identify agonal gasps as another, positive, indication to start CPR.

Finally, there is recognition that delivering chest compressions is tiring. It is now recommended that, where more than one rescuer is present, another should take over the compressions (with a minimum of delay) about every 2 minutes to prevent fatigue and maintain the quality of performance.

ADULT BASIC LIFE SUPPORT SEQUENCE

Basic life support (BLS) consists of the following sequence of actions:

1. Make sure the victim, any bystanders, and you are safe.
2. Check the victim for a response.
   - Gently shake his shoulders and ask loudly, 'Are you all right?'

3A If he responds:
- Leave him in the position in which you find him provided there is no further danger
- Try to find out what is wrong with him and get help if needed
- Reassess him regularly.

3B If he does not respond:
- Shout for help
- Turn the victim onto his back and then open the airway using head tilt and chin lift:
  o Place your hand on his forehead and gently tilt his head back
  o With your fingertips under the point of the victim's chin, lift the chin to open the airway.

4. Keeping the airway open, look, listen, and feel for normal breathing:
   - Look for chest movement
   - Listen at the victim's mouth for breath sounds
   - Feel for air on your cheek.
   In the first few minutes after cardiac arrest, a victim may be barely breathing, or taking infrequent, noisy, gasps. Do not confuse this with normal breathing.
   Look, listen, and feel for **no more** than **10 seconds** to determine if the victim is breathing normally. If you have any doubt whether breathing is normal, act as if it is **not** normal.

5A If he *is* breathing normally:
- Turn him into the recovery position (**see below**)
- Send or go for help, or call for an ambulance
- Check for continued breathing.

5B If he is *not* breathing normally:
- Ask someone to call for an ambulance or, if you are on your own, do this yourself; you may need to leave the victim. Start chest compression as follows:
  o Kneel by the side of the victim
  o Place the heel of one hand in the centre of the victim's chest
  o Place the heel of your other hand on top of the first hand
  o Interlock the fingers of your hands and ensure that pressure is not applied over the victim's ribs. Do not apply any pressure over the upper abdomen or the bottom end of the bony sternum (breastbone)
  o Position yourself vertically above the victim's chest and, with your arms straight, press down on the sternum 4–5 cm
  o After each compression, release all the pressure on the chest without losing contact between your hands and the sternum. Repeat at a rate of about 100 times a minute (a little less than 2 compressions a second)
  o Compression and release should take an equal amount of time.

6A Combine chest compression with rescue breaths:
- After 30 compressions open the airway again using head tilt and chin lift

- Pinch the soft part of the victim's nose closed, using the index finger and thumb of your hand on his forehead
- Allow his mouth to open, but maintain chin lift
- Take a normal breath and place your lips around his mouth, making sure that you have a good seal
- Blow steadily into his mouth whilst watching for his chest to rise; take about 1 second to make his chest rise as in normal breathing; this is an effective rescue breath
- Maintaining head tilt and chin lift, take your mouth away from the victim and watch for his chest to fall as air comes out
- Take another normal breath and blow into the victim's mouth once more to give a total of two effective rescue breaths. Then return your hands without delay to the correct position on the sternum and give a further 30 chest compressions
- Continue with chest compressions and rescue breaths in a ratio of 30:2
- Stop to re-check the victim only if he starts breathing normally; otherwise do not interrupt resuscitation.

If your rescue breaths do not make the chest rise as in normal breathing, then before your next attempt:
- Check the victim's mouth and remove any visible obstruction
- Re-check that there is adequate head tilt and chin lift
- Do not attempt more than two breaths each time before returning to chest compressions.

If there is more than one rescuer present, another should take over CPR about every 2 minutes to prevent fatigue. Ensure the minimum of delay during the changeover of rescuers.

6B Chest-compression-only CPR:
- If you are not able, or are unwilling, to give rescue breaths, give chest compressions only
- If chest compressions only are given, these should be continuous at a rate of 100 a minute
- Stop to re-check the victim only if he starts breathing **normally**; otherwise do not interrupt resuscitation.

7 Continue resuscitation until:
- qualified help arrives and takes over
- the victim starts breathing normally, or
- you become exhausted.

IN-HOSPITAL RESUSCITATION

INTRODUCTION

This new section in the guidelines describes the sequence of actions for starting in-hospital resuscitation. Hospital staff are often trained in basic life support (BLS) techniques that are more appropriate for the single lay rescuer in an out-of-hospital environment. These new guidelines are aimed primarily at healthcare professionals who are first to respond to an in-hospital cardiac arrest. Some of the guidelines are also applicable to healthcare professionals in other clinical settings.

The Royal College of Anaesthetists, the Royal College of Physicians of London, the Intensive Care Society and the Resuscitation Council (UK) published a joint statement in 2004, *Cardiopulmonary resuscitation – standards for clinical practice and training* (Gabbott et al 2005). This document provides healthcare institutions with guidance on delivering an effective resuscitation service.

After in-hospital cardiac arrest, the division between BLS and ALS is arbitrary; in practice, the resuscitation process is a continuum and is based on common sense. The public expect that clinical staff should be able to undertake cardiopulmonary resuscitation (CPR). For all in-hospital cardiac arrests, ensure that:

- cardiorespiratory arrest is recognized immediately
- help is summoned using a standard telephone number (e.g. 2222)
- CPR is started immediately using airway adjuncts, for example a pocket mask, and, if indicated, defibrillation attempted as soon as possible (within 3 minutes at the most).

SEQUENCE FOR 'COLLAPSED' PATIENT IN A HOSPITAL

1 Ensure personal safety.
2 Check the patient for a response:
- When a healthcare professional sees a patient collapse, or finds a patient apparently unconscious in a clinical area, he should first shout for help, then assess if the patient is responsive by gently shaking his shoulders and asking loudly, 'Are you all right?'
- If other members of staff are nearby it will be possible to undertake actions simultaneously.

3A If the patient responds:
- Urgent medical assessment is required. Depending on the local protocols this may be by a resuscitation team (e.g. medical emergency team (MET))
- While awaiting this team, assess the patient using the ABCDE approach
- Give the patient oxygen
- Attach monitoring leads
- Obtain venous access.

3B If the patient does not respond:
- Shout for help (if this has not already been done)
- Turn the patient onto his back
- Open the airway using head tilt and chin lift
- Look in the mouth. If a foreign body or debris is visible, attempt to remove it, using suction or forceps as appropriate
- If there is a risk of cervical spine injury, establish a clear upper airway by using jaw thrust or chin lift in combination with manual in-line stabilization (MILS) of the head and neck by an assistant (if sufficient staff are available). If life-threatening airway

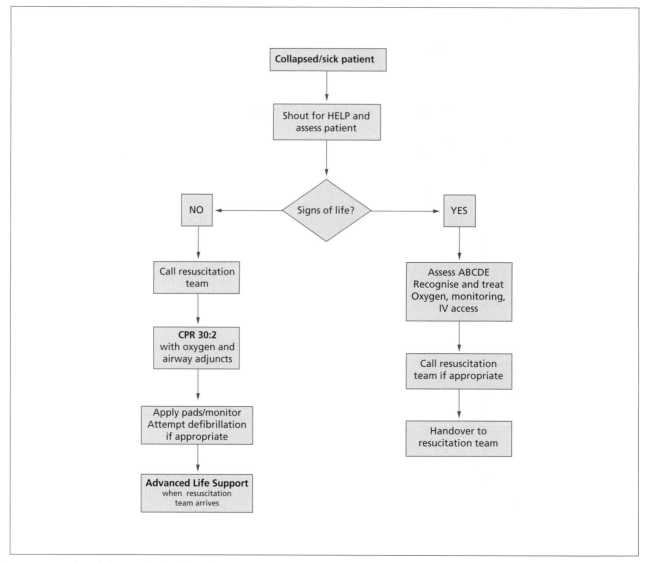

Figure A1.2 In-hospital Resuscitation (from the Resuscitation Council, UK, with permission).

obstruction persists despite effective application of jaw thrust or chin lift, add head tilt a small amount at a time until the airway is open; establishing a patent airway takes priority over concerns about a potential cervical spine injury

- Keeping the airway open, look, listen, and feel for no more than **10 seconds** to determine if the victim is breathing normally:
  o Listen at the victim's mouth for breath sounds
  o Look for chest movement
  o Feel for air on your cheek
- Those experienced in clinical assessment may wish to assess the carotid pulse for not more than 10 seconds. This may be performed simultaneously with checking for breathing or after the breathing check.

The exact sequence will depend on the training of staff and their experience in assessment of breathing and circulation. Agonal breathing (occasional gasps, slow, laboured, or noisy breathing) is common in the early stages of cardiac arrest – it is a sign of cardiac arrest and should not be mistaken for a sign of life.

4A If the patient has a pulse or other signs of life:
- Urgent medical assessment is required. Depending on the local protocols this may take the form of a resuscitation team
- While awaiting this team, assess the patient using the ABCDE approach
- Give the patient oxygen
- Attach monitoring
- Insert an intravenous cannula.

4B If there is no pulse or other signs of life:
- One person should start CPR as others call the resuscitation team and collect the resuscitation equipment and a defibrillator. If only one member of staff is present, this will mean leaving the patient
- Give 30 chest compressions followed by 2 ventilations

- The correct hand position for chest compression is the middle of the lower half of the sternum. The recommended depth of compression is 4–5 cm and the rate is 100 compressions min^{-1}
- Maintain the airway and ventilate the lungs with the most appropriate equipment immediately at hand. A pocket mask, which may be supplemented with an oral airway, is usually readily available. Alternatively, use a laryngeal mask airway (LMA) and self-inflating bag, or bag-mask, according to local policy. Tracheal intubation should be attempted only by those who are trained and experienced in this skill
- Use an inspiratory time of 1 second and give enough volume to produce chest rise as in normal breathing. Add supplemental oxygen as soon as possible
- Once the patient's airway has been secured, continue chest compression uninterrupted (except for defibrillation or pulse checks when indicated) at a rate of 100 min^{-1}, and ventilate the lungs at approximately 10 breaths min^{-1}. Avoid hyperventilation
- If there is no airway and ventilation equipment available, give mouth-to-mouth ventilation. If there are clinical reasons to avoid mouth-to-mouth contact, or you are unwilling or unable to do this, give chest compressions alone until help or airway equipment arrives. A pocket mask should be rapidly available in all clinical areas
- When the defibrillator arrives, apply the electrodes to the patient and analyze the rhythm. The use of adhesive electrode pads or the 'quick-look' paddles technique will enable rapid assessment of heart rhythm compared with attaching ECG electrodes
- If self-adhesive defibrillation pads are available, and there is more than one rescuer, apply the pads without interrupting chest compression. Pause briefly to assess the heart rhythm. If indicated, attempt either manual or automated external defibrillation
- Recommence chest compressions immediately after the defibrillation attempt. Do not pause to assess the pulse or heart rhythm. Minimize interruptions to chest compression
- Continue resuscitation until the resuscitation team arrives or the patient shows signs of life. If using an automated external defibrillator (AED), follow the voice prompts; if using a manual defibrillator, follow the algorithm for ALS (see adult ALS section)
- Once resuscitation is underway, and if there are sufficient people available, prepare intravenous cannulae and drugs likely to be used by the resuscitation team (e.g. adrenaline)
- Identify one person to be responsible for handover to the resuscitation team leader. Locate the patient's records
- Change the person providing chest compression about every 2 minutes to prevent fatigue.

4C If the patient is not breathing but has a pulse (respiratory arrest):

- Ventilate the patient's lungs (as described above) and check for a pulse every 10 breaths (about every minute).

Only those confident in assessing breathing and a pulse will be able to make this diagnosis. If there are any doubts about the presence of a pulse, start chest compression and continue until more experienced help arrives.

5 If the patient has a monitored and witnessed cardiac arrest:

- Confirm cardiac arrest and shout for help
- If a defibrillator is not immediately to hand consider giving a single precordial thump immediately after confirmation of VF/VT cardiac arrest. The precordial thump should be given only by healthcare professionals trained in the technique
- If the initial rhythm is VF/VT and a defibrillator is immediately available, give a shock first
- Start CPR immediately after the shock is delivered as described above
- Continue resuscitation in accordance with the ALS algorithm (see below).

ADULT ADVANCED LIFE SUPPORT

INTRODUCTION

This section on adult advanced life support (ALS) adheres to the same general principles as in Guidelines 2000, but incorporates some important changes. The guidelines in this section apply to healthcare professionals trained in ALS techniques.

GUIDELINE CHANGES

CPR before defibrillation

- In the case of out-of-hospital cardiac arrest attended, but unwitnessed, by healthcare professionals equipped with manual defibrillators, give CPR for 2 minutes (i.e. about 5 cycles at 30:2) before defibrillation
- Do not delay defibrillation if an out-of-hospital arrest is witnessed by a healthcare professional
- Do not delay defibrillation for in-hospital cardiac arrest.

Defibrillation strategy

- Treat ventricular fibrillation/pulseless ventricular tachycardia (VF/VT) with a single shock, followed by immediate resumption of CPR (30 compressions to 2 ventilations). Do not re-assess the rhythm or feel for a pulse. After 2 minutes of CPR, check the rhythm and give another shock (if indicated)
- The recommended initial energy for biphasic defibrillators is 150–200 J. Give second and subsequent shocks at 150–360 J
- The recommended energy when using a monophasic defibrillator is 360 J for both the initial and subsequent shocks.

Fine VF

- If there is doubt about whether the rhythm is asystole or fine VF, do **NOT** attempt defibrillation; instead, continue chest compression and ventilation.

Adrenaline (epinephrine)

VF/VT

- Give adrenaline 1–mg i.v. if VF/VT persists after a second shock
- Repeat the adrenaline every 3–5 minutes thereafter if VF/VT persists.

Pulseless electrical activity/asystole

- Give adrenaline 1 mg i.v. as soon as intravenous access is achieved and repeat every 3–5 minutes.

Anti-arrhythmic drugs

- If VF/VT persists after three shocks, give amiodarone 300 mg by bolus injection. A further dose of 150 mg may be given for recurrent or refractory VF/VT, followed by an infusion of 900 mg over 24 hours
- If amiodarone is not available, lidocaine 1 mg kg⁻¹ may be used as an alternative, but do not give lidocaine if

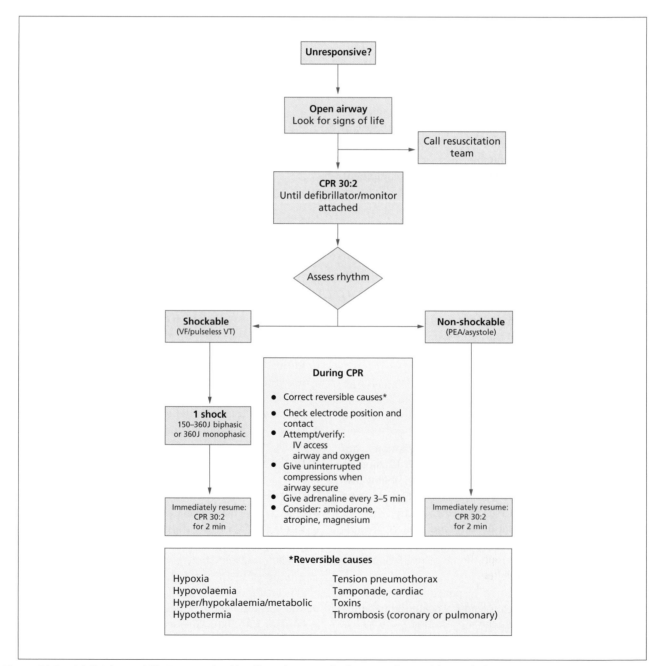

Figure A1.3   Adult Advanced Life Support Algorithm (from the Resuscitation Council, UK, with permission).

amiodarone has already been given. Do not exceed a total dose of 3 mg kg^{-1} during the first hour.

Post-resuscitation care – therapeutic hypothermia

- Unconscious adult patients with spontaneous circulation after out-of-hospital VF cardiac arrest should be cooled to 32–34°C for 12–24 hours
- Mild hypothermia may also benefit unconscious patients with spontaneous circulation after out-of-hospital cardiac arrest due to a non-shockable rhythm, or after cardiac arrest in hospital.

ADVANCE LIFE SUPPORT TREATMENT ALGORITHM

Arrhythmias associated with cardiac arrest are divided into two groups: shockable rhythms (VF/VT) and non-shockable rhythms (asystole and PEA). The principle difference in management is the need for attempted defibrillation in patients with VF/VT. Subsequent actions, including chest compression, airway management and ventilation, venous access, administration of adrenaline, and the identification and correction of reversible factors, are common to both groups. The ALS treatment algorithm provides a standardized approach to the management of adult patients in cardiac arrest.

Shockable rhythms (VF/VT)
Sequence of actions

- Attempt defibrillation (one shock: 150–200 J biphasic or 360 J monophasic)
- Immediately resume chest compressions (30:2) without re-assessing the rhythm or feeling for a pulse
- Continue CPR for 2 minutes, then pause briefly to check the monitor:
  - o If VF/VT persists:
    - Give a further (2nd) shock (150–360 J biphasic or 360 J monophasic)
    - Resume CPR immediately and continue for 2 minutes
    - Pause briefly to check the monitor
    - If VF/VT persists give adrenaline 1 mg i.v. followed immediately by a (3rd) shock (150–360 J biphasic or 360 J monophasic)
    - Resume CPR immediately and continue for 2 minutes
    - Pause briefly to check the monitor
    - If VF/VT persists give amiodarone 300 mg i.v. followed immediately by a (4th) shock (150–360 J biphasic or 360 J monophasic)
    - Resume CPR immediately and continue for 2 minutes
    - Give adrenaline 1 mg i.v. immediately before alternate shocks (i.e. approximately every 3–5 minutes)
    - Give a further shock after each 2-minute period of CPR and after confirming that VF/VT persists.

- o If organized electrical activity is seen during this brief pause in compressions, check for a pulse.
  - If a pulse is present, start post-resuscitation care
  - If no pulse is present, continue CPR and switch to the non-shockable algorithm.
- o If asystole is seen, continue CPR and switch to the non-shockable algorithm.

Precordial thump   Consider giving a single precordial thump when cardiac arrest is confirmed rapidly after a witnessed and monitored sudden collapse, and a defibrillator is not immediately to hand. A precordial thump should be undertaken immediately after confirmation of cardiac arrest but only by healthcare professionals trained in the technique. Using the ulnar edge of a tightly clenched fist, deliver a sharp impact to the lower half of the sternum from a height of about 20 cm, then retract the fist immediately to create an impulse-like stimulus. A precordial thump is most likely to be successful in converting VT to sinus rhythm. Successful treatment of VF by precordial thump is much less likely: in all the reported successful cases the precordial thump was given within the first 10 seconds of VF. There are very rare reports of a precordial thump converting a perfusing to a non-perfusing rhythm.

Explanation for the changes in the treatment of VF/VT
CPR before defibrillation   Although Guidelines 2000 recommended immediate defibrillation for all shockable rhythms, recent evidence indicates that a period of CPR before defibrillation may improve survival after prolonged collapse (>5 minutes) (Wik et al 2003). The duration of collapse is frequently difficult to estimate accurately, so give CPR before attempted defibrillation outside hospital, unless the arrest is witnessed by a healthcare professional or an AED is being used. This advice does NOT apply to lay responders using an AED outside hospital, who should apply the AED as soon as it is available.

In contrast, there is no evidence to support or refute CPR before defibrillation for in-hospital cardiac arrest. For this reason, after in-hospital VF/VT cardiac arrest, give a shock as soon as possible.

REFERENCES

Bahr J, Klingler H, Panzer W, Rode H, Kettler D (1997) Skills of lay people in checking the carotid pulse. Resuscitation 35: 23–26.

Eftestol T, Sunde K, Steen PA (2002) Effects of interrupting precordial compressions on the calculated probability of defibrillation success during out-of-hospital cardiac arrest. Circulation 105: 2270–2273.

Gabbott D, Smith G, Mitchell S et al (2005) Cardiopulmonary resuscitation standards for clinical practice and training in the UK. Resuscitation 64: 13–19.

Hallstrom A, Cobb L, Johnson E, Copass M (2000) Cardiopulmonary resuscitation by chest compression alone or with mouth-to-mouth ventilation. New England Journal of Medicine 342: 1546–1553.

Hauff SR, Rea TD, Culley LL, Kerry F, Becker L, Eisenberg MS (2003) Factors impeding dispatcher-assisted telephone cardiopulmonary resuscitation. Annals of Emergency Medicine 42: 731–737.

Van Alem A, Sanou B, Koster R (2003) Interruption of CPR with the use of the AED in out of hospital cardiac arrest. Annals of Emergency Medicine 42: 449–457.

Wik L, Hansen TB, Fylling F et al (2003) Delaying defibrillation to give basic cardiopulmonary resuscitation to patients with out-of-hospital ventricular fibrillation: A Randomized Trial. Journal of the American Medical Association 289: 1389–1395.

APPENDIX 2
EVIDENCE-BASED PRACTICE

THE TOP 20 THINGS YOU MOST NEED TO KNOW

Previous generations of nurses were taught that nursing should be a research-based profession but within the last decade there has been a pronounced shift towards nursing as an 'evidence-based practice' (EBP). There is more than semantics involved here, as this does represent a real change in emphasis. Increasingly, the literature you read will be peppered by phrases drawn from the lexicon of EBP so we are going to introduce you briefly to the basic idea of EBP and then the top 20 most important terms you need to understand.

There are several definitions of EBP; the following is from Straus et al (2005:1):

The integration of the best research evidence with our clinical expertise and our patient's unique values and circumstances.

Research results are still a key component of EBP but with a change of emphasis and note also that several other things have been added. The research that is most prized is the research that tells us how effective certain treatments or diagnostic and assessment procedures are. This allows us to make choices about what is the most cost-effective and reliable test or screening tool to use and how best to treat the patient. There is therefore a requirement to be numerate and comfortable with statistics. Throwing up your hands and saying 'I was no good at maths at school, where's the qualitative research?' is not an acceptable option, as such an approach will not allow you to decide the best dressing to treat your patient's leg ulcer or assess their risk of pressure ulcers.

Clinical expertise also enters the picture now. This allows practitioners to draw upon their wealth of experience and also intuition as well as the expertise of colleagues. The definition also refers to the *'patient's unique values'*, which is a crucial point. The patient's point of view matters. A strongly supported intervention is useless if the patient does not agree with it and will not accept it. We have to remember each patient is an individual and we must strive to achieve concordance and cooperation, working as partners in care rather than the old model of 'compliance'. Finally, we are reminded about the patient's *circumstances*, which should make us discuss with the patient whether what we propose is feasible in their home circumstances and if they can afford it, along with other factors such as their family circumstances.

As newly qualified nurses you need to understand the evidence base in order to implement its recommendations. The following is only a taster to help you make better sense of the literature that you will be reading during your education. As a lifelong learner, you need to jot down 'Learn more about EBP' on your 'to do after I qualify' list.

EVIDENCE-BASED PRACTICE: THE TOP 20 TERMS

Absolute Risk. The absolute arithmetic difference in incidence rates between an experimental and a control group. If the experimental group has a risk of something harmful (such as a drug side-effect), that is say 5% and the control group has a risk of 7%, then we say the Absolute Risk Reduction of the side-effect with the new drug is 2% (see also 'Relative Risk').

Case Control Study. A study which identifies patients who have the same outcome and another group who do not and then looking to see what makes the first group different from the second. Any factor so identified could well be the cause. This is the design used for example to first identify the possible link between smoking and lung cancer.

Cohort Study. Involves identifying two different groups of people, one of whom has been exposed to a particular substance or event and the other has not. They are then followed-up over time to see if any significant differences emerge which may be attributed to the exposure. Many of the harmful effects of ionizing radiation have been demonstrated in this way.

Confidence Interval (CI). Measures the inevitable uncertainty involved in any measurement. A piece of research may produce an end statistic such as the proportion of patients having a second myocardial infarction within 5 years of the first, this will be followed by CI 95% followed by two more numbers. In other words, the researchers estimate (by various rigorous statistical techniques) that the true value lies between those two final numbers with a 95% probability; their own research result being just the number that applies *to their sample*.

Cross-Over Study Design. Administering two experimental therapies to the same group of patients one after the other to see which produces the best result. Deciding the order in which a patient receives any given therapy can be randomized. There is usually a control group in the study as well.

Gold Standard. The current best measure of an outcome. This is used to assess new diagnostic tests and how sensitive and specific they are and is usually based on a laboratory examination of tissue or an autopsy. For example, the gold standard for detecting breast cancer is examination of a tissue biopsy in the laboratory. Mammography was compared with that standard to assess its sensitivity and specificity.

Incidence. The percentage of a population that develops new cases of a target disorder within a specified time interval – usually 1 year.

Intention to Treat Analysis. This is used in randomized trials and involves analyzing the data according to the group to which patients were allocated regardless of whether they complete the study (drop outs tend to occur). This preserves complete randomization of samples.

Meta-Analysis. A systematic review that uses quantitative methods to synthesize and summarize the results of many research studies of the same problem (see 'Systematic Review').

Number Needed to Harm (NNH). The number of patients who have to be treated to produce one more extra negative event (e.g. drug side-effect). A NNH of 100 means that if 100 patients take a new drug with a known side-effect, one of them will experience the side-effect. The larger the NNH, the safer the treatment.

Number Needed to Treat (NNT). The number of patients who have to be treated to prevent one more extra negative event (e.g. death) or produce one more positive event (e.g. wound healing). A NNT of 10 means that 10 patients have to be treated with the new intervention for one of them to have the desired outcome, so the lower the NNT the more effective the intervention.

Odds. This is measured by dividing the number of people in a group who experience an event by the number who do not. If out of a group of 10 ICU patients, 5 die and 5 do not, the odds of dying are 5/5 = 1.

Odds Ratio (OR). The odds of a patient in an experimental group having an outcome divided by the odds of a patient in the control group having the same outcome. An OR of 1 means that the experimental group are performing exactly the same as the control group and therefore that the new intervention is having no effect, while an OR of 2 tells you the experimental group are doing twice as well (or badly if it is a side-effect being reported on).

Prevalence. The proportion of a population who have a target disorder at any one moment in time. How long they have had the disorder does not matter.

Probability. The likelihood that an event will happen. It is calculated by taking the number of times an event (or case) occurs in a population and dividing it by the total number of possible events (or cases). Toss a coin and there is only one chance it can land on heads out of two possible outcomes (heads or tails) so heads has a 50% probability (or 0.5 if you prefer). If there are 10 AIDS patients and 8 are alive in 2 years time, the probability of any one of them surviving 2 years is 8/10 = 80% or 0.8.

Randomized Controlled Trial (RCT). A study in which subjects are assigned at random to one group receiving a new experimental treatment and another group acting as a control, who do not. The two groups have measurements taken at the start and finish of the study to see if there has been any statistically significant improvement in the experimental group,

Relative Risk. This is similar to 'Absolute Risk' (see above) but with one major difference. We now take the proportion of patients in the experimental group who have the side-effect and *divide* it by the proportion in the control group who have the side-effect to measure the Relative Risk Reduction (or Increase). This has the effect of greatly magnifying an effect and is very controversial, as this is the kind of number that the press report in sensational stories about treatment safety. It scares patients and presents a distorted picture. Always check any story and find the 'Absolute Risk' numbers.

Sensitivity (Se). A measure of a diagnostic test's ability to correctly detect a disorder when it is present. It is expressed as a percentage or a decimal. Most tests have a sensitivity rating and a sensitivity of 95% means that if a person has a disorder, the test is 95% likely to detect it. This also means that there is a 5% chance of failing to detect it. In practice, many tests do not reach even this level of sensitivity.

Specificity (Sp). A measure of a diagnostic test's ability to correctly identify the absence of a disorder in a sample of people who do not have the disorder. Like sensitivity, it is expressed as a percentage or a decimal. A test with a specificity rating of 95% will give a negative result in 95% of patients who genuinely do not have the disorder, however, the test will give a positive result in 5% of people who do not have the disorder. Test results are always interpreted with caution because of these sensitivity and specificity numbers and words such as 'unlikely' and 'probable' are used rather than certainty.

Systematic Review. A rigorous review of all valid research evidence (unpublished and published) using standard explicit methods, to arrive at a critique and summary of the evidence about a specific topic.

REFERENCES

Straus S, Richardson WS, Glasziou P, Haynes RB (2005) Evidence based medicine, 3rd edn. Toronto: Elsevier.

FURTHER READING

DiCenso A, Guyatt G, Ciliska D (2005) Evidence-based nursing: a guide to clinical practice. Philadelphia: Elsevier.

Melnyk B, Fineout-Overholt E (2005) Evidence-based practice in nursing and healthcare. A Guide to Best Practice. Philadelphia: Lippincott Williams and Wilkins.

NOTE: *Evidence-Based Nursing* is a quarterly journal published jointly by the RCN and BMJ publishing companies.

Index

O